CLINICAL VETERINARY ADVISOR

Birds and Exotic Pets

CLINICAL VETERINARY ADVISOR

Birds and Exotic Pets

Editors in Chief

Jörg Mayer, DrMedVet, MSc, DABVP (Exotic Companion Mammal), DECZM (Small Mammal)
Associate Professor of Zoological Medicine
Department of Small Animal Medicine & Surgery
College of Veterinary Medicine
The University of Georgia
Athens, Georgia

Thomas M. Donnelly, BVSc, DipVetPath, DACLAM, DABVP (Exotic Companion Mammal)
The Kenneth S. Warren Institute
Ossining, New York;
Adjunct Associate Professor
Department of Clinical Sciences
Tufts Cummings School of Veterinary Medicine
North Grafton, Massachusetts

With 209 illustrations

ELSEVIER

ELSEVIER
SAUNDERS

3251 Riverport Lane
St. Louis, Missouri 63043

CLINICAL VETERINARY ADVISOR: BIRDS AND EXOTIC PETS ISBN: 978-1-4160-3969-3

978-1-4160-3969-3

Content Strategy Director: Penny Rudolph
Content Manager: Shelly Stringer
Publishing Services Manager: Catherine Jackson
Senior Project Manager: Rachel E. McMullen
Design Direction: Jessica Williams

Printed in the United States of America

Last digit is the print number: 9 8 7 6 5 4

I would like to dedicate this book to my wife and my families in the USA and in Germany. Without their continued support and belief in me, this book and my work would not be possible.
—Jörg Mayer

To the memory of my mentors who are no longer with us— Daria Love, Ernst Friedheim, and Albert Rubin. They encouraged me to pursue both enjoyment and excellence in medicine and research.
And to BHS.
—Thomas M. Donnelly

EDITORS-IN-CHIEF

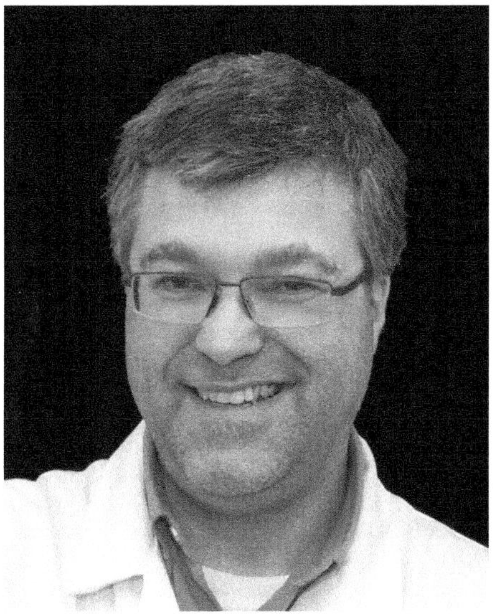

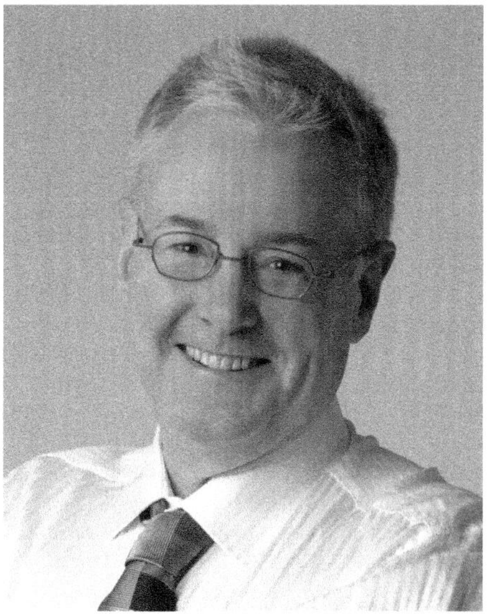

Jörg Mayer, DrMedVet, MSc, DABVP (Exotic Companion Mammal), DECZM (Small Mammal)
Associate Professor of Zoological Medicine
Department of Small Animal Medicine & Surgery
College of Veterinary Medicine
The University of Georgia
Athens, Georgia

Thomas M. Donnelly, BVSc, DipVetPath, DACLAM, DABVP (Exotic Companion Mammal)
The Kenneth S. Warren Institute
Ossining, New York;
Adjunct Associate Professor
Department of Clinical Sciences
Tufts Cummings School of Veterinary Medicine
North Grafton, Massachusetts

EDITORS

Thomas M. Donnelly, BVSc, DipVetPath, DACLAM
Section VI: Zoonoses
The Kenneth S. Warren Institute
Ossining, New York
Adjunct Associate Professor
Department of Clinical Sciences
Tufts Cummings School of Veterinary Medicine
North Grafton, Massachusetts

James G. Fox, DVM, MS, DACLAM, FIDSA, AGAF
Section I: Ferrets
Professor & Director
Division of Comparative Medicine
Massachusetts Institute of Technology
Cambridge, Massachusetts

Christoph Mans, MedVet
Section I: Small Mammals
Clinical Instructor in Zoological Medicine
Special Species Health Service
Department of Medical Sciences
School of Veterinary Medicine
University of Wisconsin-Madison
Madison, Wisconsin

Robert P. Marini, DVM, DACLAM
Section I: Ferrets
Assistant Director
Division of Comparative Medicine
Massachusetts Institute of Technology
Cambridge, Massachusetts

Jörg Mayer, DVM, MS, DABVP (Exotic Companion Mammal), DECZM (Small Mammal)
Section II: Procedures and Techniques
Section III: Differential Diagnosis
Section IV: Laboratory Tests
Section V: Clinical Algorithms
Client Education Sheets
Associate Professor of Zoological Medicine
Department of Small Animal Medicine & Surgery
College of Veterinary Medicine
The University of Georgia
Athens, Georgia

Romain Pizzi, BVSc, MSc, DZooMed (Avian), MACVS (Small Animal Surg), MACVSc (Surg), FRES, FRGS, MRCVS
Section I: Invertebrates
Edinburgh Zoo
Edinburgh, United Kingdom;
Special Lecturer in Zoo & Wildlife Medicine
The University of Nottingham
Sutton Bonnington, United Kingdom
Scottish SPCA National Wildlife Rescue Centre
Fishcross, Clackmannanshire, United Kingdom

Helen E. Roberts, DVM
Section I: Fish
Owner
Aquatic Veterinary Services of Western NY
5 Corners Animal Hospital
Orchard Park, New York

Scott J. Stahl, DVM, DABVP (Avian)
Section I: Reptiles
Owner and Director
Stahl Exotic Animal Veterinary Services
Fairfax, Virginia

Simon R. Starkey BSc (Vet), BVSc, PhD, DABVP (Avian)
Section VI: Zoonoses
Education Veterinarian
PetSmart Inc.
Phoenix, Arizona

Thomas N. Tully, Jr, DVM, MS, DABVP (Avian), DECZM (Avian)
Section I: Birds
Professor Zoological Medicine
Department of Veterinary Clinical Science
School of Veterinary Medicine
Louisiana State University
Baton Rouge, Louisiana

Kevin M. Wright, DVM, DABVP (Reptiles & Amphibians)
Section I: Amphibians
President
Wright Bird and Exotic Pet Hospital
Scottsdale, Arizona

David Vella, BSc, BVSc (Hons), DABVP (Exotic Companion Mammal)
Section I: Rabbits
Owner and Principal Veterinarian
Sydney Exotics and Rabbit Vets
North Shore Veterinary Specialist Centre
Animal Referral Hospital
Sydney, New South Wales, Australia

Beverley Ann Alderton, BVSc (Hons)
Associate Veterinarian
Kincumber Veterinary Hospital
Kincumber, New South Wales, Australia

Jonathan W. Ball, DVM
Emergency Veterinarian
Katonah Bedford Veterinary Center
Bedford Hills, New York

Alberto Rodriguez Barbon, Lic en Vet, CertZooMed DECZM (Avian), MRCVS
Staff Veterinarian
Durrell Wildlife Conservation Trust
Les Augrès Manor, La Profonde Rue
Trinity, Channel Islands

Margaret Batchelder, DVM, DACLAM
Principal Veterinary Scientist
Veterinary Sciences
Bristol-Myers Squibb
Wallingford, Connecticut

Hugues Beaufrère, DrMedVet, DECZM (Avian)
Graduate Assistant, Zoological Medicine
School of Veterinary Medicine
Louisiana State University
Baton Rouge, Louisiana

Michelle Bingley, BSc, BVSc (Hons)
Exotics Associate Veterinarian
Sydney Exotics and Rabbit Vets
North Shore Veterinary Specialist Centre
Sydney, New South Wales, Australia

Michael C. Blanco, DVM, DACLAM
Staff Veterinarian
Department of Comparative Medicine
Mayo Clinic
Rochester, Minnesota

Teresa Bradley Bays, DVM, CertVetAcupuncture, DABVP (Exotic Companion Mammal)
Owner
Belton Animal Clinic and Exotic Care Center
Belton, Missouri

Cynthia J. Brown, DVM, DABVP (Avian)
The Center for Avian and Exotics
New York, New York;
Owner
New England Veterinary Medical Center
Mystic, Connecticut

Anne Burgdorf-Moisuk, DVM
Clinical Veterinarian
San Diego Zoo
San Diego, California

Michael V. Campagna, DVM
Veterinarian
Los Angeles, California

Michelle L. Campbell-Ward, BSc, BVSc (Hons), DZooMed (Mammalian), MRCVS
Veterinarian
Taronga Western Plains Zoo—Wildlife Hospital
Dubbo, New South Wales, Australia

Brendan Carmel, BVSc, MVS (Australasian Wildlife), MANZCVSc (Unusual Pets), GradDipComp
Owner
Warranwood Veterinary Centre
Warranwood, Victoria, Australia
Consultant—Unusual and Exotic Animals
The University of Melbourne
Melbourne, Australia

Cathy T.T. Chan, BVSc (Hons), MANZCVSc (Small Animal Med)
Practice Owner and Director
The Animal Doctors Pte Ltd
Singapore

Jaime Chin, BVSc (Hons), MACVSc (Feline Medicine)
Director
Kowloon Cat Hospital
Hong Kong

John Chitty, BVetMed, CertZooMed, MRCVS
Owner
Anton Vets
Andover, United Kingdom

Deborah Cottrell, DVM
West End Animal Hospital
Newberry, Florida

David A. Crum, DVM
Associate Veterinarian
Stahl Exotic Animal Veterinary Services
Fairfax, Virginia

Julie DeCubellis, DVM
Clinical Instructor
Department of Clinical Sciences
Tufts Cummings School of Veterinary Medicine
North Grafton, Massachusetts

Stephen J. Divers, BVetMed, DZooMed (Reptilian), DECZM (Herp), DACZM, FRCVS
Professor of Zoological Medicine
Department of Small Animal Medicine & Surgery
College of Veterinary Medicine
The University of Georgia
Athens, Georgia

Thomas M. Donnelly, BVSc, DipVetPath, DACLAM, DABVP (Exotic Companion Mammal)
The Kenneth S. Warren Institute
Ossining, New York;
Adjunct Associate Professor
Department of Clinical Sciences
Tufts Cummings School of Veterinary Medicine
North Grafton, Massachusetts

Michael Dutton, DVM, MS, DABVP (Avian/Canine & Feline/Exotic Companion Mammal)
Owner
Weare Animal Hospital;
Owner
Exotic and Bird Clinic of New Hampshire
Weare, New Hampshire;
Medical Director
Veterinary Referral Center of New Hampshire
Concord, New Hampshire

Will Easson, BVMS, MRCVS
Veterinary Emergency Treatment Services
Cardiff, Wales, United Kingdom

David Eshar, DVM, DABVP (Exotic Companion Mammal), DECZM (Small Mammals)
Assistant Professor,
Department of Clinical Sciences
College of Veterinary Medicine
Kansas State University
Manhattan, Kansas

Brian A. Evans, DVM
Owner,
Coastal Animal Hospital
Encinitas, California

Peter G. Fischer, DVM, DABVP (Exotic Companion Mammal)
Director
Pet Care Veterinary Hospital
Virginia Beach, Virginia

James G. Fox, DVM, MS, DACLAM, FIDSA, AGAF
Professor & Director
Division of Comparative Medicine
Massachusetts Institute of Technology
Cambridge, Massachusetts

Amy J. Funk, DVM, DACLAM
Clinical Veterinarian
St. Jude Children's Research Hospital
Memphis, Tennessee

Alexis García, DVM
Research Scientist
Division of Comparative Medicine
Massachusetts Institute of Technology
Cambridge, Massachusetts

Jennifer Graham, DVM, DABVP (Avian/Exotic Companion Mammal), DACZM
Assistant Professor
Department of Clinical Sciences
Tufts Cummings School of Veterinary Medicine
North Grafton, Massachusetts

Caroline Hahn, DVM, MSc, PhD, DECEIM, DECVN, MRCVS
Clinical Research Associate
The Roslin Institute,
Senior Veterinarian
Equine Internal Medicine Service
Royal (Dick) School of Veterinary Studies
University of Edinburgh
Midlothian, Scotland

Katleen Hermans, DVM, PhD, MSc LAS, DECZM (Small Mammal)
Professor of Exotic Mammals and Laboratory Animals
Department of Pathology, Bacteriology and Avian Diseases
Faculty of Veterinary Medicine
Ghent University
Merelbeke, Belgium

Candace Hersey-Benner, DVM
Associate Veterinarian
Roaring Brook Veterinary Hospital
Canton, Connecticut

Gretta Howard, BVSc (Hons), MVS (Small Animal Pract), MANZCVS (Small Animal Med), MRCVS
Senior Associate Veterinarian
Cherrybrook Vet Hospital
Cherrybrook, New South Wales
Australia

Gwendolyn R. Jankowski, DVM
Associate Veterinarian
Denver Zoo
Denver, Colorado

Emma Keeble, BVSc, DZooMed (Mammalian), MRCVS
Exotic Animal Clinician
Exotic Animal and Wildlife Service
Royal (Dick) School of Veterinary Studies
University of Edinburgh
Hospital for Small Animals
Roslin, Midlothian, Scotland

Dominique L. Keller, DVM, PhD
Department of Surgical Sciences
School of Veterinary Medicine
University of Wisconsin-Madison
Madison, Wisconsin

Peter Kerr, BVSc, GradDipSci, PhD
Research Scientist
CSIRO Ecosystem Sciences
Canberra, ACT
Australia

Sharron M. Kirchain, DVM, MBA, DACLAM
Acting Director and Attending Veterinarian
Laboratory Animal Science Center
Boston University Medical Center
Boston, Massachusetts

Megan Kirchgessner, DVM, PhD
Wildlife Veterinarian
Virginia Department of Game and Inland Fisheries
Richmond, Virginia

La'Toya Latney, DVM
Attending Clinician
Exotic Companion Animal Medicine & Surgery Service
School of Veterinary Medicine
University of Pennsylvania
Philadelphia, Pennsylvania

John Henry Lewington, BVetMed, MRCVs
Veterinarian (Retired)
Ferret Advisory Service
Wanneroo
Western Australia, Australia

Brad A. Lock, DVM, DACZM
Assistant Curator of Herpetology
Zoo Atlanta
Atlanta, Georgia

Rebecca L. Malakoff, DVM, DACVIM (Cardiology)
Staff Cardiologist
Cardiology Department
Angell Animal Medical Center
Boston, Massachusetts

Caralee Manley, DVM
Veterinarian
Apple Country Animal Hospital
Stow, Massachusetts

Christoph Mans, MedVet
Clinical Instructor in Zoological Medicine
Special Species Health Service
Department of Medical Sciences
School of Veterinary Medicine
University of Wisconsin-Madison
Madison, Wisconsin

Robert P. Marini, DVM, DACLAM
Assistant Director
Division of Comparative Medicine
Massachusetts Institute of Technology
Cambridge, Massachusetts

Jorge Martínez, DVM, PhD, DECVP
Assistant Professor
Departament de Sanitat i Anatomia Animals
Facultat de Veterinària
Universitat Autònoma de Barcelona
Barcelona, Spain

Jörg Mayer, DrMedVet, MSc, DABVP (Exotic Companion Mammal), DECZM (Small Mammal)
Associate Professor of Zoological Medicine
Department of Small Animal Medicine & Surgery
College of Veterinary Medicine
The University of Georgia
Athens, Georgia

Anna Meredith, MA, VetMB, PhD, CertLAS, DZooMed (Mammalian), MRCVS
Professor of Zoological and Conservation Medicine
Royal (Dick) School of Veterinary Studies
University of Edinburgh
Hospital for Small Animals
Roslin, Midlothian, Scotland

Huynh Minh, DMV, MRCVS
Head of Exotic Department
Centre Hospitalier Vétérinaire Frégis
Arcueil, France

Mark A. Mitchell, DVM, MS, PhD, DECZM (Herpetology)
Professor of Zoological Medicine
Department of Veterinary Clinical Medicine
College of Veterinary Medicine
University of Illinois
Urbana, Illinois

Holly S. Mullen, DVM, DACVS
Chief of Surgery
VCA Emergency Animal Hospital and Referral Center
San Diego, California

Jason Norman, DVM
Veterinarian
Hammond Hills Animal Hospital
North Augusta, South Carolina

Brian S. Palmeiro, VMD, DACVD
Owner
Lehigh Valley Veterinary Dermatology & Fish Hospital
Allentown, Pennsylvania

Jean A. Paré, DVM, DVSc, DACZM
Associate Veterinarian
Zoological Health
Wildlife Conservation Society
Bronx, New York

Mary M. Patterson, MS, DVM, DACLAM
Clinical Veterinarian
Division of Comparative Medicine
Massachusetts Institute of Technology
Cambridge, Massachusetts

David Perpiñán, LV, MSc, DECZM (Herpetology)
Head of the Veterinary Department
Loro Parque & Loro Parque Fundación
Puerto de la Cruz, Tenerife, Spain

Carrie A. Phelps, DVM, CCRT, CertVetAcupuncture
Associate Veterinarian
VCA Delaware Valley Animal Hospital
Fairless Hills, Pennsylvania

Charly Pignon, DVM
Head of the Exotic Service
Alfort University Veterinary Hospital
French National Veterinary School of Alfort
Maisons-Alfort, Paris, France

Anthony A. Pilny, DVM, DABVP (Avian)
Staff Veterinarian
The Center for Avian and Exotic Medicine
New York City, New York

Chantale L. Pinard, DVM, MSc, DACVO
Assistant Professor of Ophthalmology
Department of Clinical Studies
Ontario Veterinary College
University of Guelph
Guelph, Ontario, Canada

Romain Pizzi, BVSc, MSc, DZooMed (Avian), MACVSc (Surg), FRES, FRGS, MRCVS
Edinburgh Zoo
Edinburgh, United Kingdom
Special Lecturer in Zoo & Wildlife Medicine
The University of Nottingham
Sutton Bonnington, United Kingdom

Christal Pollock, DVM, DABVP (Avian)
Veterinary Consultant
Lafeber Company
Cornell, Illinois

Lauren V. Powers, DVM, DABVP (Avian)
Service Chief
Avian and Exotic Pet Service
Carolina Veterinary Specialists
Huntersville, North Carolina

Aidan Raftery, MVB, CertZooMed, CBiol, MIBiol, MRCVS
Clinical Director
Avian and Exotic Animal Clinic
Manchester, United Kingdom

Viviane Silva Raymundo, BVM
Exotics Assistant Veterinarian
Sydney Exotics and Rabbit Vets
Animal Referral Hospital
Sydney, New South Wales, Australia

Drury R. Reavill, DVM, DABVP (Avian), DACVP
Zoo/Exotic Pathology Service
West Sacramento, California

Virgina C.G. Richardson, MA, VetMB, MRCVS
Orchard Veterinary Surgery
Romsey, Hampshire, United Kingdom

Cecilia Robat, DrMedVet, DACVIM (Oncology)
Department of Medical Sciences
School of Veterinary Medicine
University of Wisconsin-Madison
Madison, Wisconsin

Helen E. Roberts, DVM
Owner
Aquatic Veterinary Services of Western NY
5 Corners Animal Hospital
Orchard Park, New York

William Rosenblad, DVM
Clinical Assistant Professor
Tufts Cummings School of Veterinary Medicine
North Grafton, Massachusetts;
Senior Staff
Dentistry/Surgery Department
Angell Animal Medical Center
Boston, Massachusetts

David Sanchez-Migallon Guzman, LV, MS, DECZM (Avian), DACZM
Service Veterinarian,
Avian and Exotic Pet Medicine and Surgery
Department of Medicine and Epidemiology
School of Veterinary Medicine
University of California, Davis
Davis, California

Richard A. Saunders, BSc (Hons), BVSc, MSB, CBiol, DZooMed (Mammalian), MRCVS
Staff Veterinarian
Veterinary Department
Bristol Zoo Gardens
Bristol, Avon, United Kingdom

Shannon N. Shaw, BS, DVM
Staff Veterinarian
San Antonio Zoo
San Antonio, Texas

James L. (Jay) Shelton, Jr, BS, MS, PhD
Associate Professor
Fisheries
Warnell School of Forestry and Natural Resources
The University of Georgia
Athens, Georgia

Alana Shrubsole-Cockwill, BSc, HonsCertSc, DVM, MVSc
Exotics Associate Veterinarian
Sydney Exotics and Rabbit Vets
North Shore Veterinary Specialist Centre
Sydney, New South Wales, Australia

Nico J. Schoemaker, DVM, PhD, DECZM (Small Mammal & Avian), DABVP (Avian)
Faculty Veterinarian and Specialist
Division of Zoological Medicine
Department of Companion Animal Clinical Sciences
Faculty of Veterinary Medicine
Utrecht University
Utrecht, The Netherlands

Jeffrey Smith, BVSc, FACVSc, DACVO
Eye Clinic for Animals
Animal Referral Hospital
Sydney, New South Wales, Australia

Scott J. Stahl, DVM, DABVP (Avian)
Owner and Director
Stahl Exotic Animal Veterinary Services
Fairfax, Virginia

Simon R. Starkey, BSc (Vet), BVSc, PhD, DABVP (Avian)
Education Veterinarian
PetSmart Inc.
Phoenix, Arizona

W. Michael Taylor, DVM, DABVP (Avian)
Avian and Exotics Service Chief
Health Sciences Center
Ontario Veterinary College
University of Guelph
Guelph, Ontario, Canada

Thomas N. Tully, Jr, DVM, MS, DABVP (Avian), DECZM (Avian)
Professor Zoological Medicine
Veterinary Clinical Sciences Department
School of Veterinary Medicine
Louisiana State University
Baton Rouge, Louisiana

Molly Varga, BVetMed, DZooMed (Mammalian), MRCVS
RCVS Specialist Veterinarian in Zoological Medicine
Cheshire Pet
Holmes Chapel, Cheshire, United Kingdom

David Vella, BSc, BVSc (Hons), DABVP (Exotic Companion Mammal)
Owner and Principal Veterinarian
Sydney Exotics and Rabbit Vets
North Shore Veterinary Specialist Centre and
Animal Referral Hospital
Sydney, New South Wales, Australia

Wolf von Bomhard, DrVetMed, DECVP
Specialist in Veterinary Pathology (Fachtierarzt für Pathologie)
Veterinary Specialty Practice for Pathology
Munich, Germany

Narelle Walter, BVSc
Owner and Principal Veterinarian
Melbourne Rabbit Clinic
Melbourne, Victoria, Australia

James F.X. Wellehan, Jr, DVM, MS, DACZM, DACVM
Zoological Medicine Service
College of Veterinary Medicine
University of Florida
Gainesville, Florida

Cameron J.G. Whittaker, BVSc, DipVetClinStud, DACVO
Eye Clinic for Animals
Animal Referral Hospital
Sydney, New South Wales, Australia

Katherine E. Whitwell, BVSc, DECVP, FRCVS, RCVS Specialist in Veterinary Pathology (Equine)
Equine Pathology Consultancy
Newmarket, Suffolk, United Kingdom

Bruce H. Williams, DVM, DACVP
Senior Pathologist
Veterinary Pathology Division
The Joint Pathology Center
Silver Spring, Maryland

Kimberlee B. Wojick, DVM
Associate Veterinarian
Roger Williams Park Zoo
Providence, Rhode Island

Kevin M. Wright, DVM, DABVP (Reptiles & Amphibians)
President
Wright Bird and Exotic Pet Hospital
Scottsdale, Arizona

Nicole R. Wyre, DVM, DABVP (Avian)
Service Head
Exotic Companion Animal Medicine and Surgery
College of Veterinary Medicine
University of Pennsylvania
Philadelphia, Pennsylvania

Trevor T. Zachariah, DVM, MS
Director of Veterinary Services
Brevard Zoo
Melbourne, Florida

Compared with traditional specialties, exotic pet medicine is a vibrant and progressive branch of veterinary medicine that has few ties to a dogmatic past. Yet it has a long tradition based on cumulative knowledge from surprisingly different disciplines in veterinary medicine. From food, fur, and fancy, we have the writings of Oskar Seifried (1937) and Gustave Lesbouyries (1963) on diseases of food rabbits; Helmut Kraft (1959) on diseases of fur chinchillas; and Hans Otto Raebiger (1923) on diseases of fancy guinea pigs. From zoological and laboratory animal medicine, we have ground-breaking authors such as Frederic Frye (1973) on diseases of reptiles; and John Harkness (1977) on diseases of laboratory rabbits and rodents. Such books and numerous pathology and husbandry references over the past 80 years have given our specialty a good foundation in evidence-based medicine.

We have attempted to build on this rich tradition by providing a fresh approach to the management of diseases in the exotic pet. Our emphasis in this book has been on clinical decision making and treatment of individual animals using a template-based format with illustrations. Consequently, the book is organized into six major sections of exotic pet practice: diseases and disorders, procedures and techniques, differential diagnoses, laboratory tests, algorithm-based decision making, and zoonoses.

The first section is Diseases and Disorders. We have presented what information is available as a set of central clinical issues that incorporate clinical findings, etiology, disease manifestations, differential diagnosis, diagnostic tests, prognosis, therapy, and prevention. Selected references allow practitioner self-improvement. Information follows the progression of a case: background information is given first, followed by the reason underlying the veterinary visit (chief complaint) and important or typical elements of the history as it relates to the disorder. After physical examination findings, diagnostic testing is organized into two parts. The initial database contains diagnostic tests that are routinely performed in most general practices. Then we list advanced or confirmatory tests. These cover more specific evaluations that can be done in some general practices or require referral to a university hospital or specialty center. This staged approach reflects the process that we so commonly use with our patients. Treatment is described likewise as initial, acute treatment, and then separately as chronic or long-term treatment for disorders requiring ongoing care. Drug dosages and routes of administration are included directly as we find nothing more frustrating than leafing through a drug formulary for a medication dose and often not finding one for an exotic pet species. The end of each topic in Diseases and Disorders includes a segment for clinical pearls—pieces of valuable information derived from the experience of the author and the editor. These might be given as a counterintuitive point, an easily made mistake to avoid, a concern about the nature of the disease or process, or as other facts that provide medical hints which often escape the written word.

Procedures and Techniques, the second section, illustrates more than 60 diagnostic and therapeutic procedures identifiable in exotic pet practice. The breadth of this material is wide, ranging from the use of E-collars or sexing young exotic small mammals, to reptile, avian, and fish injection techniques, including venipuncture. Specialists who routinely perform these procedures describe the material in a simplified and structured way. Our intent is to allow the reader to feel prepared to perform these procedures if training and skills are adequate, or to realize what is involved in a procedure when referring a patient to another institution to have it performed.

The third section, Differential Diagnosis, regroups tables that list the causes of more than 40 of the most common abnormalities encountered in exotic pet practice. This section is most useful for students and young veterinarians, or for any veterinarian who wishes to review the extent of potential etiologies for a particular disorder.

The fourth section, Laboratory Tests, has been designed to combine the clinical pathologist's expertise with the needs of the general practitioner who sees exotic pets. This section summarizes approximately 40 commonly used laboratory tests. As in other parts of the book, information for each topic is arranged in an intuitive and user-friendly manner. First, we provide basic information (definition, normal range of results for different species of exotic pets). This is followed by causes of abnormal levels, the next test or diagnostic step to consider, and, finally, a listing of artifacts, specimen-handling instructions, and clinical pearls.

Section Five, Clinical Algorithms, approaches the management of some of the more common or challenging disorders in exotic pet practice using the "decision tree" format. Younger veterinarians and those veterinarians looking for information in an unfamiliar part of exotic pet practice may find this section most helpful because it represents a starting point for locating information that is devoid of nuances and caveats. This streamlined approach delivers an initial framework for addressing a particular disorder, from which individual variations can radiate.

Finally, the sixth section, Zoonoses, encompasses 16 of the most important zoonotic diseases seen in exotic pet practice. Veterinarians are often more aware than our medical colleagues of the likelihood of infectious disease transmission from a pet, and our goal is to encourage good liaison between the client's doctor and the exotic pet's doctor. Information is depicted to track the development of a zoonotic case: definition of the disease and infectious agent(s) is first, followed by epidemiology of the zoonosis, including host or carrier exotic pet species, modes of transmission, and clinical presentation of an exotic pet with a zoonotic disease. Often there is no apparent disease in the pet. We then provide a clinical picture of the zoonotic disease in humans. This includes incidence, disease forms, history and primary complaint, physical examination findings, and incubation period. Diagnosis comprises the often wide range of differential diagnoses, as well as diagnostic testing. The initial database includes diagnostic tests that are implemented first in most doctors' offices, followed by advanced or confirmatory tests that require referral to a hospital. Treatment focuses primarily on the affected or carrier pet, but also includes a brief description of medications and therapies used in humans. It includes prevention of zoonosis transmission. Moreover, this segment contains information on whether the disease is notifiable and requires reporting by veterinarians to local or federal official agencies. Next is a brief piece on controversy—for example, should immunosuppressed individuals keep certain exotic pets, or what pets should parents of small children allow to be in the home. The end of each topic in Zoonoses includes a section on client education that offers information for a veterinarian to use when instructing owners on the human health risks of keeping certain exotic pets.

There is a great need in the practice of veterinary medicine to educate clients. It is important that they understand disease processes and to have enough knowledge to monitor their pets' conditions at home. To encourage clients' follow-through on the care we provide to their pets we have created client education sheets. The goal of these sheets is to provide a reference that owners can consult when we have asked them to do something specific to help their companion. Variations and modifications to suit individual patients are inevitable, and these information sheets are written to provide a general summary that practitioners can use as a base for this type of information. We believe these client education sheets will improve client comprehension and understanding.

One of the dominant features of the *Advisor* is the solid link between the print and electronic versions of the book. Since it is only possible to obtain both together (neither website access nor the print book is sold individually), the universal access of the web book and the hands-on gratification of opening the print book are literally bound together. We believe you will enjoy the added value of having the print book in your office or at home, while having the ability to access the book's contents on your PC, laptop, or mobile device.

The companion website includes a digital version of the printed textbook. The online book is fully searchable, which allows quick identification of any topic and its related information in the six different sections. The online book also includes all of the book's images with many in full color. Nearly ninety client education sheets are offered in both English and Spanish to give your clients clear, useful information they can use at home.

Throughout this textbook, information is included on the basis of its clinical importance. Some topics such as dental disease in rabbits are discussed in greater detail than others. To realize our goal, we recruited as contributors some of the best clinicians in their respective fields. In addition, to achieve comprehensive coverage of significant diseases, we actively sought authors from all over the globe. Although the format of the book has been kept as short and precise as possible, we want to ensure that the reader does not regard this book as a "quick reference" on how to manage diseases and problems. Our aim has been to bring together an overview of conditions commonly seen in general practice and to offer a standardized approach on how to evaluate and deal with each clinical scenario.

We hope that in using this book, the reader will be granted the highest rewards and satisfaction of treating exotic pets and their often equally exotic owners. To quote one of the earliest exponents of exotic pet medicine with whom we share a similar belief,

I have therefore ventur'd first to launch forth into this new Science, not being insensible that I shall leave much Room for others to make great Improvements, if any shall hereafter think it worth their while to follow that Track which I have only pointed out to them; and I hope the learned World know how to make Allowances for a first Attempt in the Advancement of any kind of Knowledge.

—John Moore in the Preface to His Columbarium: Or, the Pigeon-House (London, 1735), Page XIII

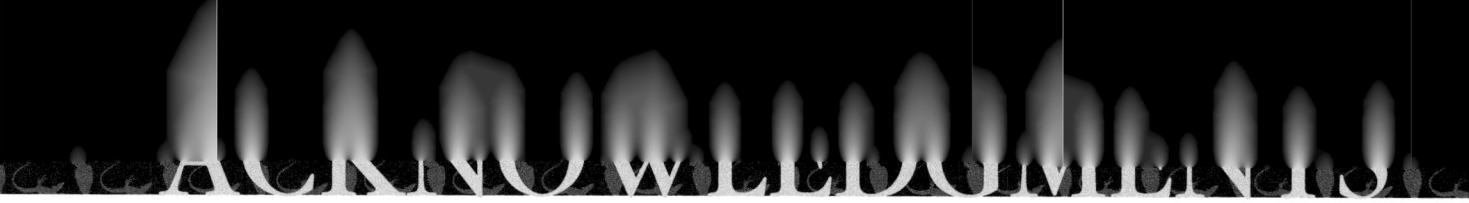

ACKNOWLEDGMENTS

We have tried to keep *Clinical Veterinary Advisor: Birds and Exotic Pets* a reasonable size while ensuring that essential topics are covered. This was easier said than done and required more energy from everyone involved than we ever contemplated when we first undertook to create this book. We are gratefully indebted to many individuals for their verve.

To our loyal section editors, we know how much time and effort you spent to deliver concise, relevant, and up-to-date chapters. Lucille Ball said, "If you want something done, ask a busy person to do it." Lucy was right. Somehow, despite your many professional and personal obligations, you made the time available for writing and exceptional editing. We offer you our unreserved thanks. To our faithful topic authors, many who wrote not one but several topics, we thank you for your contributions and for tolerating our badgering to keep the project on course.

To the wonderful team of Penny, Maureen, Shelly, Whitney, and Rachel at Elsevier, we cannot thank you enough for your patience, encouragement, advice, and professionalism. I fear we pushed you to the limit at times, but you bounced back with enthusiasm and reassurance in your constant communications.

Many colleagues not in avian or exotic pet medicine enhanced the quality of the book by acting as our guinea pigs (no pun intended) for potential readers. To Michael Mulcahy and the veterinarians at Chatswood Veterinary Clinic, North Shore Veterinary Hospital, Tufts Cummings School of Veterinary Medicine, and the University of Georgia College of Veterinary Medicine—thank you all for your belief in our book and for your constructive and frank criticism.

Last, we thank our families and friends for their continuous support and empathy. Although they may have tired of hearing about eventual publication dates, they never showed it.

SECTION I: DISEASES AND DISORDERS

BY SPECIES

INVERTEBRATES

Abscesses/Granulomas, 2
Alopecia, 3
Bacterial Diseases, 4
Dehydration, 5
Dysecdysis, 7
Fungal Infections, Superficial and Systemic, 8
Infectious Diseases of Acroporid Corals, 9
Intoxication, 11
Mites (Acarii), 12
Oral Nematodes (Panagrolaimidae), 13
Trauma, 15
Viral Diseases, 16

FISH

Bacterial Diseases, 17
Dropsy, 20
Ectoparasites, Crustacean, 21
Flukes (Monogenean Parasites), 22
Fungal Diseases, 24
Gastrointestinal Nematode and Cestode Parasites, 27
Gastrointestinal Protozoal Parasites, 28
Head and Lateral Line Erosion (HLLE), 30
Koi Herpes Virus Infection (KHV), 31
Lymphocystis, 32
Protozoal Ectoparasites (Ciliated and Flagellated), 33
Spring Viremia of Carp (SVC), 35
Swim Bladder Disease/Buoyancy Disorders, 36
Trauma and Wound Management, 38
Ulcer Disease in Koi, 40
Viral Diseases, 42
Viral Epidermal Hyperplasia (Carp Pox), 43
Water Quality and Pet Fish Health, 44

AMPHIBIANS

Ammonia Toxicosis, 47
Amoebiasis, 48
Chromomycosis, 49
Cloacal Prolapse, 51
Coccidiosis, 52
Corneal Lipidosis or Xanthomatosis, 53
Flagellate Enterocolitis, 55
Gastrointestinal Foreign Body or Overload, 56
Hypovitaminosis A, 57
Mycobacteriosis, 59
Nematodiasis, 60
Nutritional Secondary Hyperparathyroidism, 62
Saprolegniasis, 64
Septicemia, 65
Trauma and Wound Management, 67
Vomiting, 68
Weight Loss, 70

REPTILES

Abscesses, 71
Adenovirus Infection, 74
Aggression, 75
Bacterial Dermatitis, 77
Calicivirus Infection, 79
CANV/Fungal Disease, 80
Cardiac Disease, 82
Chlamydophilosis, 84
Cloacal Prolapse, 85
Coccidiosis, 87
Cryptosporidiosis, 89
Dermatomycosis, 90
Dermatophilosis (Rain Rot), 92
Diarrhea, 93
Dysecdysis, 95
Ectoparasites, 98
Entamoebiasis, 100
Gout, 101
Hepatic Lipidosis, 103
Herpesvirus Infections, 105
Hyperglycemia, 107
Hypervitaminosis A, 108
Hypovitaminosis A, 110
Inclusion Body Disease of Snakes, 113
Iridovirus Infection, 114
Liver Disease, 115
Mycobacteriosis, 117
Mycoplasma, 118
Nematodiasis, 120
Nutritional Secondary Hyperparathyroidism, 121
Orthopedics and Fracture Repair, 125
Paramyxovirus Infection, 127
Paraphimosis, 128
Pentastomes, 130
Periodontal Disease, 132
Proliferative Spinal Osteoarthropathy, 135
Regurgitation/Vomiting, 136
Renal Disease, 138
Reovirus Infections, 140
Respiratory (Lower) Tract Disease/Pneumonia, 141
Salmonella, 143
Stomatitis, Bacterial, 145

BIRDS

Abscesses, 147
Anemia, 149
Anorexia, 151
Ascites, 153
Aspergillosis, 155
Cardiac Disease, 157
Central Nervous System Signs and Neurologic Conditions, 159
Chlamydophila psittaci, 161
Chronic Egg Laying, 164
Cloacal Prolapse, 165
Conjunctivitis, 167
Constipation (Ileus), 168
Crop Stasis, 170
Dehydration, 171
Diarrhea, 173
Dystocia, 175
Ectoparasitism, 177
Edema, Soft Tissue, 179
Emaciation, 180
Enteritis, 181
Feather Picking, 184
Follicular Stasis, 185

Foreign Bodies, 186
Fractures, 189
Gout, 191
Heavy Metal Toxicity, 192
Hepatic Lipidosis, 194
Hypocalcemia, 197
Hypovitaminosis, 199
Liver Disease, 201
Megabacteriosis, 203
Mycoses, 204
Neurologic Disease, 207
Ocular Lesions, 209
Organophosphate Toxicity, 212
Overgrown Beak and Claws, 213
Papillomas, 215
Pneumonia, 217
Pododermatitis, 219
Polytetrafluoroethylene (Teflon) Toxicity, 221
Proventricular Dilatation Disease, 222
Regurgitation/Vomiting, 225
Renal Disease, 228
Sinusitis, Chronic, 230
Trauma, 232
Tumors, 234
Uropygial Gland Disease Conditions, 237
Viral Diseases, 239

SMALL MAMMALS

RATS
Chromodacryorrhea, 242
Mammary and Pituitary Tumors, 243
Renal Disease, 245
Respiratory Tract Disease, Acute, 248
Respiratory Tract Disease, Chronic, 249
Skin Diseases, 251
GUINEA PIGS
Anorexia, 253
Cheilitis, 254
Dental Disease, 255
Gastric Dilatation and Volvulus, 258
Hyperthyroidism, 260
Hypovitaminosis C, 262
Intestinal Disorders, 263
Neurological Disorders, 266
Ocular Disorders, 268
Ovarian Cysts, 269
Perineal Sac Impaction or Rectal Impaction, 271
Pododermatitis, 273
Pregnancy and Parturient Disorders, 275
Respiratory Tract Disease, 276
Skin Diseases, 278
Streptococcus zooepidemicus (Cervical Lymphadenitis), 280
Urolithiasis, 282
Uterine and Vaginal Disorders, 284
HAMSTERS
Abdominal Distention, 285
Cardiac Disease, 287
Cheek Pouch Disorder, 288
Dental Disease, 290
Intestinal Disorders, 291
Ocular Disorders, 293
Renal Disease, 295
Skin Diseases, 297
GERBILS
Ovarian Disease, 299
CHINCHILLAS
Cardiac Disease, 301
Dental Disease, 302
Fur Disorders, 305
Gastrointestinal Disorders, 308
Ocular Disorders, 311
Penile Disorders, 313
PRAIRIE DOGS
Odontoma, 316
DEGUS
Behavioral Disorders, 318
Dental Disease, 319
Diabetes Mellitus, 322
HEDGEHOGS
Cardiomyopathy, 323
Neoplasia, 324
Skin Diseases—Infectious, 325
Wobbly Hedgehog Syndrome, 327
SUGAR GLIDERS
Behavioral Disorders, 328
Nutritional Disorders, 329

RABBITS
Abscesses, 331
Anorexia, 333
Arthritis, 334
Behavioral Disorders, 337
Buphthalmia and Glaucoma, 338
Cardiovascular Disease, 341
Cataracts, 342
Cherry Eye, 344
Coccidiosis, 346
Conjunctival Disorders, 349
Cutaneous Masses, 351
Dacryocystitis and Epiphora, 352
Dental Disease, 355
Dermatopathies, 360
Dysautonomia (Grass Sickness), 364
Ectoparasites, 366
Electrocution, 368
Encephalitis, 369
Encephalitozoonosis, 371
Endoparasites, 374
Floppy Rabbit Syndrome, 376
Gastric Disorders, 378
Hemorrhagic Disease, 381
Hepatic Disorders, 383
Intestinal Disorders, 385
Lower Respiratory Tract Disorders, 390
Lower Urinary Tract Disorders, 392
Lymphosarcoma, 395
Mammary Gland Disorders, 397
Myxomatosis, 398
Obesity, 401
Otitis, 403
Pasteurellosis, 405
Pododermatitis, 407
Pregnancy Toxemia, 409
Pseudopregnancy, 411
Renal Disorders, 412
Splayleg, 416
Staphylococcosis, 417
Testicular Tumors, 419
Thymoma, 420
Treponematosis, 421
Upper Respiratory Tract Disorders, 423
Uterine Disorders, 424
Uveitis, 426
Vestibular Disease, 428

FERRETS
Adrenal Disease, 430
Aleutian Disease, 433

Campylobacter spp. Infection, 434
Cataracts, 435
Chordoma, 437
Cryptococcosis, 439
Dental Disease, 441
Dirofilariasis, 443
Distemper, 444
Ear Mites, 445
Ectoparasites, 447
Endoparasites, 448
Eosinophilic Gastroenteritis, 450
Epizootic Catarrhal Enteritis, 451
Ferret Systemic Coronaviral Disease (FSCD), 452
Gastrointestinal Foreign Bodies, 454
Heart Disease, AV Block, 456
Heart Disease, Structural, 458
Helicobacter mustelae-Associated Gastritis and Ulcers, 460
Hepatobiliary Disease, 461
Hyperestrogenism-Associated Anemia, 462
Ibuprofen and Acetaminophen Toxicity, 464
Inflammatory Bowel Disease, 465
Influenza, 468
Insulinoma, 469
Lymphoma, 471
Mastitis, 475
Megaesophagus, 477
Myofascitis, 478
Neonatal Disease, 479
Osteoma, 481
Ovarian Neoplasia, 482
Ovarian Remnant Syndrome, 484
Pregnancy Toxemia, 486
Proliferative Bowel Disease, 487
Prostatic Disease, 488
Renal Disorders, 491
Skin Tumors, 495
Splenomegaly, 497
Urolithiasis, 498
Vaccine Reactions, 500

SECTION I: DISEASES AND DISORDERS

ALPHABETICAL LISTING

ABDOMINAL DISTENTION, Hamsters, 285
ABSCESSES,
  Birds, 147
  Rabbits, 331
  Reptiles, 71
ABSCESSES/GRANULOMAS, Invertebrates, 2
ADENOVIRUS INFECTION, Reptiles, 74
ADRENAL DISEASE, Ferrets, 430
AGGRESSION, Reptiles, 75
ALEUTIAN DISEASE, Ferrets, 433
ALOPECIA, Invertebrates, 3
AMMONIA TOXICOSIS, Amphibians, 47
AMOEBIASIS, Amphibians, 48
ANEMIA, Birds, 149
ANOREXIA,
  Birds, 151
  Guinea Pigs, 253
  Rabbits, 333
ARTHRITIS, Rabbits, 334
ASCITES, Birds, 153
ASPERGILLOSIS, Birds, 155
BACTERIAL DERMATITIS, Reptiles, 77
BACTERIAL DISEASES,
  Fish, 17
  Invertebrates, 4
BEHAVIORAL DISORDERS,
  Degus, 318
  Rabbits, 337
  Sugar Gliders, 328
BUPHTHALMIA AND GLAUCOMA, Rabbits, 338
CALICIVIRUS INFECTION, Reptiles, 79
CAMPYLOBACTER SPP. INFECTION, Ferrets, 434
CANV/FUNGAL DISEASE, Reptiles, 80
CARDIAC DISEASE,
  Birds, 157
  Chinchillas, 301
  Hamsters, 287
  Reptiles, 82
CARDIOMYOPATHY, Hedgehogs, 323
CARDIOVASCULAR DISEASE, Rabbits, 341
CATARACTS,
  Ferrets, 435
  Rabbits, 342
CENTRAL NERVOUS SYSTEM SIGNS AND NEUROLOGIC CONDITIONS, Birds, 159
CHEEK POUCH DISORDER, Hamsters, 288
CHEILITIS, Guinea Pigs, 254
CHERRY EYE, Rabbits, 344
CHLAMYDOPHILA PSITTACI, Birds, 161
CHLAMYDOPHILOSIS, Reptiles, 84
CHORDOMA, Ferrets, 437
CHROMODACRYORRHEA, Rats, 242
CHROMOMYCOSIS, Amphibians, 49
CHRONIC EGG LAYING, Birds, 164
CLOACAL PROLAPSE,
  Amphibians, 51
  Birds, 165
  Reptiles, 85
COCCIDIOSIS,
  Amphibians, 52
  Rabbits, 346
  Reptiles, 87
CONJUNCTIVAL DISORDERS, Rabbits, 349
CONJUNCTIVITIS, Birds, 167
CONSTIPATION (ILEUS), Birds, 168
CORNEAL LIPIDOSIS OR XANTHOMATOSIS, Amphibians, 53
CROP STASIS, Birds, 170
CRYPTOCOCCOSIS, Ferrets, 439
CRYPTOSPORIDIOSIS, Reptiles, 89
CUTANEOUS MASSES, Rabbits, 351
DACRYOCYSTITIS AND EPIPHORA, Rabbits, 352
DEHYDRATION,
  Birds, 171
  Invertebrates, 5
DENTAL DISEASE,
  Chinchillas, 302
  Degus, 319
  Ferrets, 441
  Guinea Pigs, 255
  Hamsters, 290
  Rabbits, 355
DERMATOMYCOSIS, Reptiles, 90
DERMATOPATHIES, Rabbits, 360
DERMATOPHILOSIS (RAIN ROT), Reptiles, 92
DIABETES MELLITUS, Degus, 322
DIARRHEA,
  Birds, 173
  Reptiles, 93
DIROFILARIASIS, Ferrets, 443
DISTEMPER, Ferrets, 444
DROPSY, Fish, 20
DYSAUTONOMIA (GRASS SICKNESS), Rabbits, 364

DYSECDYSIS,
Invertebrates, 7
Reptiles, 95
DYSTOCIA, Birds, 175
EAR MITES, Ferrets, 445
ECTOPARASITES,
Ferrets, 447
Rabbits, 366
Reptiles, 98
ECTOPARASITES, CRUSTACEAN, Fish, 21
ECTOPARASITISM, Birds, 177
EDEMA, SOFT TISSUE, Birds, 179
ELECTROCUTION, Rabbits, 368
EMACIATION, Birds, 180
ENCEPHALITIS, Rabbits, 369
ENCEPHALITOZOONOSIS, Rabbits, 371
ENDOPARASITES,
Ferrets, 448
Rabbits, 374
ENTAMOEBIASIS, Reptiles, 100
ENTERITIS, Birds, 181
EOSINOPHILIC GASTROENTERITIS, Ferrets, 450
EPIZOOTIC CATARRHAL ENTERITIS, Ferrets, 451
FEATHER PICKING, Birds, 184
FERRET SYSTEMIC CORONAVIRAL DISEASE (FSCD), Ferrets, 452
FLAGELLATE ENTEROCOLITIS, Amphibians, 55
FLOPPY RABBIT SYNDROME, Rabbits, 376
FLUKES (MONOGENEAN PARASITES), Fish, 22
FOLLICULAR STASIS, Birds, 185
FOREIGN BODIES, Birds, 186
FRACTURES, Birds, 189
FUNGAL DISEASES, Fish, 24
FUNGAL INFECTIONS, SUPERFICIAL AND SYSTEMIC, Invertebrates, 8
FUR DISORDERS, Chinchillas, 305
GASTRIC DILATATION AND VOLVULUS, Guinea Pigs, 258
GASTRIC DISORDERS, Rabbits, 378
GASTROINTESTINAL DISORDERS, Chinchillas, 308
GASTROINTESTINAL FOREIGN BODIES, Ferrets, 454
GASTROINTESTINAL FOREIGN BODY OR OVERLOAD, Amphibians, 56
GASTROINTESTINAL NEMATODE AND CESTODE PARASITES, Fish, 27
GASTROINTESTINAL PROTOZOAL PARASITES, Fish, 28
GOUT,
Birds, 191
Reptiles, 101
HEAD AND LATERAL LINE EROSION (HLLE), Fish, 30
HEART DISEASE, AV BLOCK, Ferrets, 456
HEART DISEASE, STRUCTURAL, Ferrets, 458
HEAVY METAL TOXICITY, Birds, 192
HELICOBACTER MUSTELAE-ASSOCIATED GASTRITIS AND ULCERS, Ferrets, 460
HEMORRHAGIC DISEASE, Rabbits, 381
HEPATIC DISORDERS, Rabbits, 383
HEPATIC LIPIDOSIS,
Birds, 194
Reptiles, 103
HEPATOBILIARY DISEASE, Ferrets, 461
HERPESVIRUS INFECTIONS, Reptiles, 105
HYPERESTROGENISM-ASSOCIATED ANEMIA, Ferrets, 462
HYPERGLYCEMIA, Reptiles, 107
HYPERTHYROIDISM, Guinea Pigs, 260
HYPERVITAMINOSIS A, Reptiles, 108
HYPOCALCEMIA, Birds, 197
HYPOVITAMINOSIS, Birds, 199
HYPOVITAMINOSIS A,
Amphibians, 57
Reptiles, 110
HYPOVITAMINOSIS C, Guinea Pigs, 262
IBUPROFEN AND ACETAMINOPHEN TOXICITY, Ferrets, 464
INCLUSION BODY DISEASE OF SNAKES, Reptiles, 113
INFECTIOUS DISEASES OF ACROPORID CORALS, Invertebrates, 9
INFLAMMATORY BOWEL DISEASE, Ferrets, 465
INFLUENZA, Ferrets, 468
INSULINOMA, Ferrets, 469
INTESTINAL DISORDERS,
Guinea Pigs, 263
Hamsters, 291
Rabbits, 385
INTOXICATION, Invertebrates, 11
IRIDOVIRUS INFECTION, Reptiles, 114
KOI HERPES VIRUS INFECTION (KHV), Fish, 31
LIVER DISEASE,
Birds, 201
Reptiles, 115
LOWER RESPIRATORY TRACT DISORDERS, Rabbits, 390
LOWER URINARY TRACT DISORDERS, Rabbits, 382
LYMPHOCYSTIS, Fish, 32
LYMPHOMA, Ferrets, 471
LYMPHOSARCOMA, Rabbits, 395
MAMMARY AND PITUITARY TUMORS, Rats, 243
MAMMARY GLAND DISORDERS, Rabbits, 397
MASTITIS, Ferrets, 475
MEGABACTERIOSIS, Birds, 203
MEGAESOPHAGUS, Ferrets, 477
MITES (ACARII), Invertebrates, 12
MYCOBACTERIOSIS,
Amphibians, 59
Reptiles, 117
MYCOPLASMA, Reptiles, 118
MYCOSES, Birds, 204
MYOFASCITIS, Ferrets, 478
MYXOMATOSIS, Rabbits, 398
NEMATODIASIS,
Amphibians, 60
Reptiles, 120
NEONATAL DISEASE, Ferrets, 479
NEOPLASIA, Hedgehogs, 324
NEUROLOGIC DISEASE, Birds, 207
NEUROLOGIC DISORDERS, Guinea Pigs, 266
NUTRITIONAL DISORDERS, Sugar Gliders, 329
NUTRITIONAL SECONDARY HYPERPARATHYROIDISM,
Amphibians, 62
Reptiles, 121
OBESITY, Rabbits, 401
OCULAR DISORDERS,
Chinchillas, 311
Guinea Pigs, 268
Hamsters, 293
OCULAR LESIONS, Birds, 209
ODONTOMA, Prairie Dogs, 316
ORGANOPHOSPHATE TOXICITY, Birds, 212
ORTHOPEDICS AND FRACTURE REPAIR, Reptiles, 125
OSTEOMA, Ferrets, 481
OTITIS, Rabbits, 403
OVARIAN CYSTS, Guinea Pigs, 269
OVARIAN DISEASE, Gerbils, 299
OVARIAN NEOPLASIA, Ferrets, 482
OVARIAN REMNANT SYNDROME, Ferrets, 484
OVERGROWN BEAK AND CLAWS, Birds, 213
ORAL NEMATODES (PANAGROLAIMIDAE), Invertebrates, 13
PAPILLOMAS, Birds, 215
PARAMYXOVIRUS INFECTION, Reptiles, 127

PARAPHIMOSIS, Reptiles, 128
PASTEURELLOSIS, Rabbits, 405
PENILE DISORDERS, Chinchillas, 313
PENTASTOMES, Reptiles, 130
PERINEAL SAC IMPACTION OR RECTAL IMPACTION, Guinea Pigs, 271
PERIODONTAL DISEASE, Reptiles, 132
PNEUMONIA, Birds, 217
PODODERMATITIS,
  Birds, 219
  Guinea Pigs, 273
  Rabbits, 407
POLYTETRAFLUOROETHYLENE (TEFLON) TOXICITY, Birds, 221
PREGNANCY AND PARTURIENT DISORDERS, Guinea Pigs, 275
PREGNANCY TOXEMIA,
  Ferrets, 486
  Rabbits, 409
PROLIFERATIVE BOWEL DISEASE, Ferrets, 487
PROLIFERATIVE SPINAL OSTEOARTHROPATHY, Reptiles, 135
PROSTATIC DISEASE, Ferrets, 488
PROTOZOAL ECTOPARASITES (CILIATED AND FLAGELLATED), Fish, 33
PROVENTRICULAR DILATATION DISEASE, Birds, 222
PSEUDOPREGNANCY, Rabbits, 411
REGURGITATION/VOMITING,
  Birds, 225
  Reptiles, 136
RENAL DISEASE,
  Birds, 228
  Hamsters, 295
  Rats, 245
  Reptiles, 138
RENAL DISORDERS,
  Ferrets, 491
  Rabbits, 412
REOVIRUS INFECTIONS, Reptiles, 140
RESPIRATORY (LOWER) TRACT DISEASE/PNEUMONIA, Reptiles, 141
RESPIRATORY TRACT DISEASE, Guinea Pigs, 276
RESPIRATORY TRACT DISEASE, ACUTE, Rats, 248
RESPIRATORY TRACT DISEASE, CHRONIC, Rats, 249
SALMONELLA, Reptiles, 143
SAPROLEGNIASIS, Amphibians, 64
SEPTICEMIA, Amphibians, 64
SINUSITIS, CHRONIC, Birds, 230
SKIN DISEASES,
  Guinea Pigs, 278
  Hamsters, 297
  Hedgehogs, Infectious, 325
  Rats, 251
SKIN TUMORS, Ferrets, 495
SPLAYLEG, Rabbits, 416
SPLENOMEGALY, Ferrets, 497
SPRING VIREMIA OF CARP (SVC), Fish, 35
STAPHYLOCOCCOSIS, Rabbits, 417
STOMATITIS, BACTERIAL, Reptiles, 145
STREPTOCOCCUS ZOOEPIDEMICUS (CERVICAL LYMPHADENITIS), Guinea Pigs, 280
SWIM BLADDER DISEASE/BUOYANCY DISORDERS, Fish, 36
TESTICULAR TUMORS, Rabbits, 419
THYMOMA, Rabbits, 420
TRAUMA,
  Birds, 15
  Invertebrates, 232
TRAUMA AND WOUND MANAGEMENT,
  Amphibians, 67
  Fish, 38
TREPONEMATOSIS, Rabbits, 421
TUMORS, Birds, 234
ULCER DISEASE IN KOI, Fish, 40
UPPER RESPIRATORY TRACT DISORDERS, Rabbits, 423
UROLITHIASIS,
  Ferrets, 498
  Guinea Pigs, 282
UROPYGIAL GLAND DISEASE CONDITIONS, Birds, 237
UTERINE AND VAGINAL DISORDERS, Guinea Pigs, 284
UTERINE DISORDERS, Rabbits, 424
UVEITIS, Rabbits, 426
VACCINE REACTIONS, Ferrets, 500
VESTIBULAR DISEASE, Rabbits, 428
VIRAL DISEASES,
  Birds, 239
  Fish, 42
  Invertebrates, 16
VIRAL EPIDERMAL HYPERPLASIA (CARP POX), Fish, 43
VOMITING, Amphibians, 68
WATER QUALITY AND PET FISH HEALTH, Fish, 44
WEIGHT LOSS, Amphibians, 70
WOBBLY HEDGEHOG SYNDROME, Hedgehogs, 327

SECTION II: PROCEDURES AND TECHNIQUES

BY SPECIES

INVERTEBRATES

Anesthesia, 504
Diagnostic Sampling, 504
Dysecdysis/Ectoparasites, 505
Euthanasia, 506
Exoskeleton Repair, 507
Fluid Administration, 508
Handling and Restraint, 509

FISH

Diagnostic Sampling, 510
Emergency Care, 512
Injections, Intracoelomic (Ice) and Intramuscular (IM), 512
MS 222 Anesthesia, 513
Oral Medication, 514
Surgical Principles, 516
Tank Pond Therapy, 517
Venipuncture, 518

AMPHIBIANS

General Emergency Support, 519
Handling and Restraint, 520

REPTILES

Abscess Removal, 520
Assisting Shedding, 522
Blood Pressure, 523
Cardiopulmonary-Cerebral Resuscitation, 524
Collection of Sampling, 525
Dystocia, 526
Fecal Exam, 529
Glomerular Filtration Rate (GFR) Study, 529
Handling and Restraint, 530
Injections and Medical Administration, 531
Phlebotomy, 533
Tracheal or Lung Wash, 535
Wound Care, 535

BIRDS

Air Sac Tube Placement, 537
Coelomocentesis, 538
Crop Infusion, 538

Duodenostomy, 539
E-collars, 540
Esophagostomy, 540
Fluid Therapy, 541
Handling and Restraint, 543
Nasal Flush, 544
Tracheal or Lung Wash, 545
Venipuncture, 546

SMALL MAMMALS

Anesthesia Monitoring in Rabbits and Rodents, 547
Blood Collection, Volume, and Sites, 549
Blood Transfusion, 551
Bone Marrow Aspiration and Core Biopsy, 552
Bronchoscopy, 553
Castration, 555
Echocardiography, 557
E-Collars, 558
Electrocardiography, 558
Feeding Tube Placement in Rabbits and Rodents, 559
Fluid Therapy in Rabbits and Rodents, 560
Intraosseous Catheters, 561
Intubation Technique in Rabbits and Rodents, 562
Nasolacrimal Cannulation of Rabbits, 563
Ovariohysterectomy, 564
Preventing Hypothermia During Anesthesia, 566
Recognition of Pain in Rabbits and Rodents, 567
Rectal Prolapse and Intussusception Treatment in Hamsters, Mice, and Guinea Pigs, 568
Restraint and Carrying, How to Pick up Rabbits and Rodents, 568
Urethral Catheterization of Ferrets, 570

SECTION II: PROCEDURES AND TECHNIQUES

ALPHABETICAL LISTING

ABSCESS REMOVAL, Reptiles, 520
AIR SAC TUBE PLACEMENT, Birds, 537
ANESTHESIA, Invertebrates, 547
ANESTHESIA MONITORING IN RABBITS AND RODENTS, Small Mammals, 504
ASSISTING SHEDDING, Reptiles, 522
BLOOD COLLECTION, VOLUME, AND SITES, Small Mammals, 549
BLOOD PRESSURE, Reptiles, 523
BLOOD TRANSFUSION, Small Mammals, 551
BONE MARROW ASPIRATION AND CORE BIOPSY, Small Mammals, 552
BRONCHOSCOPY, Small Mammals, 553
CARDIOPULMONARY-CEREBRAL RESUSCITATION, Reptiles, 524
CASTRATION, Small Mammals, 555
COELOMOCENTESIS, Birds, 538
COLLECTION OF SAMPLING, Reptiles, 525
CROP INFUSION, Birds, 538
DIAGNOSTIC SAMPLING,
  Fish, 510
  Invertebrates, 504
DUODENOSTOMY, Birds, 539
DYSECDYSIS/ECTOPARASITES, Invertebrates, 505
DYSTOCIA, Reptiles, 526
E-COLLARS,
  Birds, 540
  Small Mammals, 558
ECHOCARDIOGRAPHY, Small Mammals, 557
ELECTROCARDIOGRAPHY, Small Mammals, 558
EMERGENCY CARE, Fish, 512
ESOPHAGOSTOMY, Birds, 540
EUTHANASIA, Invertebrates, 506
EXOSKELETON REPAIR, Invertebrates, 507
FECAL EXAM, Reptiles, 529
FEEDING TUBE PLACEMENT IN RABBITS AND RODENTS, Small Mammals, 559
FLUID ADMINISTRATION, Invertebrates, 508
FLUID THERAPY,
  Birds, 541
  Rabbits and Rodents, 560
GENERAL EMERGENCY SUPPORT, Amphibians, 519
GLOMERULAR FILTRATION RATE (GFR) STUDY, Reptiles, 529
HANDLING AND RESTRAINT,
  Amphibians, 520
  Birds, 543
  Invertebrates, 509
  Reptiles, 530
INJECTIONS AND MEDICAL ADMINISTRATION, Reptiles, 531
INJECTIONS, INTRACOELOMIC (ICE) AND INTRAMUSCULAR (IM), Fish, 512
INTRAOSSEOUS CATHETERS, Small Mammals, 561
INTUBATION TECHNIQUE IN RABBITS AND RODENTS, Small Mammals, 562
MS 222 ANESTHESIA, Fish, 513
NASAL FLUSH, Birds, 544
NASOLACRIMAL CANNULATION OF RABBITS, Small Mammals, 563
ORAL MEDICATION, Fish, 514
OVARIOHYSTERECTOMY, Small Mammals, 564
PHLEBOTOMY, Reptiles, 533
PREVENTING HYPOTHERMIA DURING ANESTHESIA, Small Mammals, 566
RECOGNITION OF PAIN IN RABBITS AND RODENTS, Small Mammals, 567
RECTAL PROLAPSE AND INTUSSUSCEPTION TREATMENT IN HAMSTERS, MICE, AND GUINEA PIGS, Small Mammals, 568
RESTRAINT AND CARRYING, HOW TO PICK UP RABBITS AND RODENTS, Small Mammals, 568
SURGICAL PRINCIPLES, Fish, 516
TANK POND THERAPY, Fish, 517
TRACHEAL OR LUNG WASH,
  Birds, 545
  Reptiles, 535
URETHRAL CATHETERIZATION OF FERRETS, Small Mammals, 570
VENIPUNCTURE,
  Birds, 546
  Fish, 518
WOUND CARE, Reptiles, 535

SECTION III: DIFFERENTIAL DIAGNOSIS

ACUTE RESPIRATORY DISTRESS SYNDROME, 572
ALOPECIA, 572
ANEMIA, 573
ANOREXIA, 573
ASCITES, 574
AZOTEMIA, 574
BLEEDING DISORDER, 575
BRONCHIAL DISEASE, 575
CENTRAL NERVOUS SYSTEM (CNS) DISORDERS, MULTIFOCAL/DIFFUSE, 575
CENTRAL NERVOUS SYSTEM (CNS) SIGNS, 576
CONJUNCTIVITIS, 577
CONSTIPATION, 577
CONVERSION FACTORS, 578
CORNEAL ULCER, 580
CRANIAL NERVE DEFICITS, 581

DANGEROUS ANTIBIOTICS, 582
DERMATOSIS, 582
DIABETES MELLITUS, 583
DIARRHEA, 583
DISTENDED COELOM, 584
DYSPNEA, 585
DYSTOCIA, 585
EMACIATION, 586
GASTRIC STASIS, 586
HEMATURIA, 587
HEPATIC FAILURE, 587
HYPERCALCEMIA, 588
HYPERKALEMIA, 588
HYPERLIPIDEMIA, 588
INCONTINENCE, URINARY, 588
INFLAMMATORY BOWEL DISEASES, 589
LAMENESS, 589
LIVER FAILURE, 589
NASAL DISCHARGE, 589
NEUROLOGIC SIGNS, 590
POLYPHAGIA, 591
POLYURIA/POLYDIPSIA, 591
REGURGITATION/VOMITING, 592
RENAL FAILURE, 593
SEIZURES, 593
UNDIGESTED FOOD IN DROPPINGS, 595
URATE COLORATION, 595
URIC ACID ELEVATION, 595
WEAKNESS/ATAXIA, 595
WEIGHT LOSS, 596

SECTION IV: LABORATORY TESTS

ADRENAL PANEL (FERRET), 598
ALANINE AMINOTRANSFERASE, 599
ALBUMIN, 600
ALKALINE PHOSPHATASE, 601
AMMONIA, 601
AMYLASE, 602
ASPARTATE AMINOTRANSFERASE, 603
AZUROPHIL COUNT, 604
BASOPHIL COUNT, 604
BILE ACIDS, 606
BILIRUBIN, 608
BLOOD UREA NITROGEN (BUN), 608
BODY SURFACE AREA CONVERSIONS USING THE MEEH COEFFICIENTS, 610
CALCIUM, 610
CHLORIDE, 612
CHOLESTEROL, 613
CREATINE KINASE, 614
CREATININE, 615
EOSINOPHIL COUNT, 616
GAMMAGLUTAMYL TRANSFERASE (GGT), 617
GLOBULINS, 618
GLUCOSE, 619
HEMATOCRIT, 622
LEAD, 623
LIPASE, 624
LYMPHOCYTE COUNT, 625
MONOCYTE COUNT, 628
NEUTROPHIL-HETEROPHIL COUNT, 629
pH, 633
PHOSPHORUS, 636
PLATELET COUNT, 637
POTASSIUM, 640
PROTEIN, TOTAL, 642
RED BLOOD CELL (RBC) COUNT, 643
RETICULOCYTE COUNT, 646
SODIUM, 647
THYROID HORMONES, 648
URIC ACID, 649
ZINC, 650

SECTION V: CLINICAL ALGORITHMS

BY SPECIES

AMPHIBIANS

Sudden Death, 654
Weight, 655

REPTILES

CNS Chelonia, 657
CNS Lizard, 658
CNS Snakes, 659
Constipation, 660
Diarrhea, 661
Parasites, 662
Prolapse, 663
Regurgitation, 664
Swellings, 665
Unspecific Problem/Not Doing Well, 666
Vomiting, 667
Weight Loss, 668

SMALL MAMMALS

Alopecia, 669
Anorexia, 670
CNS Signs, 671
Diarrhea, 672
Dyspnea, 674
Lameness, 677
Lumps and Bumps, 678
Mammary Mass, 680
Ocular Changes, 681
Painful Abdomen, 682
Paresis, 683
Skin/Fur Changes, 684
Vaginal Discharge, 685
Weight Loss, Chronic, 686

RABBITS

Urinary Changes, 687

SECTION V: CLINICAL ALGORITHMS

ALPHABETICAL LISTING

ALOPECIA, Small Mammals, 669
ANOREXIA, Small Mammals, 670
CNS,
  Chelonia, 657
  Lizard, 658
  Snakes, 659
CNS SIGNS, Small Mammals, 671
CONSTIPATION, Reptiles, 660
DIARRHEA,
  Reptiles, 661
  Small Mammals, 672
DYSPNEA, Small Mammals, 674
LAMENESS, Small Mammals, 677
LUMPS AND BUMPS, Small Mammals, 678
MAMMARY MASS, Small Mammals, 680
OCULAR CHANGES, Small Mammals, 681
PAINFUL ABDOMEN, Small Mammals, 682
PARASITES, Reptiles, 662

PARESIS, Small Mammals, 683
PROLAPSE, Reptiles, 663
REGURGITATION, Reptiles, 664
SKIN/FUR CHANGES, Small Mammals, 684
SUDDEN DEATH, Amphibians, 654
SWELLINGS, Reptiles, 665
UNSPECIFIC PROBLEM/NOT DOING WELL, Reptiles, 666
URINARY CHANGES, Rabbits, 687
VAGINAL DISCHARGE, Small Mammals, 685
VOMITING, Reptiles, 667
WEIGHT LOSS, Reptiles, 668
WEIGHT LOSS, CHRONIC, Small Mammals, 686

SECTION VI: ZOONOSES

ACARIASIS, 690
ANIMAL BITES, 694
CHLAMYDIOSIS, 697
CRYPTOSPORIDIOSIS, 699
DERMATOPHYTOSIS, 703
ENCEPHALITOZOONOSIS, 705
HANTAVIRUS, 708
LEPTOSPIROSIS, 711
LYMPHOCYTIC CHORIOMENINGITIS VIRUS, 713
MYCOBACTERIUM MARINUM GRANULOMA, 715
PASTEURELLA MULTOCIDA, 717
PLAGUE, 719
RABIES, 722
RAT BITE FEVER, 724
SALMONELLOSIS, 726
TULAREMIA, 730

CLIENT EDUCATION SHEETS

BY SPECIES

The following Client Education Sheets can be found on the companion website, in both English and Spanish. clinvetadvisorexotics.com

INVERTEBRATES

Husbandry, Tarantula

FISH

Husbandry, Betta
Pet Fish Medicine History Questionnaire
Swim Bladder

AMPHIBIANS

Signs an Amphibian Needs Veterinary Care
Sudden Death

REPTILES

Aural Abscesses in Turtles
Cloacal Prolapse
Dysecdysis, Chelonians
Dysecdysis, General
Dysecdysis, Lizards
Dysecdysis, Snakes
Fracture Management
Husbandry, Bearded Dragons
Husbandry, Iguanas
Husbandry, Red-Eared Sliders
Husbandry, Snakes
Husbandry, Sulcatas
Husbandry, Uromastyx
Inclusion Body Disease, Snakes
Metabolic Bone Disease
Renal Disease
Vitamin A Deficiency

BIRDS

Aspergillosis
Chlamydiosis
Chronic Egg Laying
Cnemidocoptes
Conjunctivitis
Egg Binding
Environmental Enrichment
Feather Picking
Hand Rearing Cockatiels
Husbandry, Chicken
Hypovitaminosis A
Lead Toxicity
Liver Disease, Parrots
Nutrition
Pododermatitis
Proper Housing/Environment
Protecting Your Pet Bird: Common Household Toxins
Proventricular Dilatation Disease
Renal Disease
Vocalization in Companion Parrots
Wing Trim

SMALL MAMMALS

RATS

Mammary Masses
Mycoplasma

GUINEA PIGS

Cystic Ovaries
Husbandry, Guinea Pigs
Pododermatitis
Urinary Calculi

HAMSTERS

Lymphoma
Wet Tail

CHINCHILLAS

Husbandry, Chinchillas

DEGUS

Husbandry, Degus

HEDGEHOGS

Husbandry, Hedgehogs
Wobbly Hedgehog Syndrome (WHS)

RABBITS

Abscesses
Basics
Behavior
Communication
Dental Disease
Hairball
Housing
Introducing a New Rabbit to Your Home
Mastitis
Myiasis
Nutrition
Outdoor Rabbits
Thymoma
Urolithiasis
Uveitis

FERRETS

Adrenal Disease
Aleutian Disease
Analgesic Toxicity
Dental Disease
Diarrhea

Dilated Cardiomyopathy (DCM)
Distemper
Fracture Management
Gastrointestinal Foreign Bodies
Heartworm–*Dirofilaria immitis*
Helicobacter mustelae and Gastric Ulcers
Insulinoma
Irritable Bowel Disease (IBD)
Lymphoma
Post Op
Skin Tumors
Urinary Obstruction

CLIENT EDUCATION SHEETS

ALPHABETICAL LISTING

The following Client Education Sheets can be found on the companion website, in both English and Spanish. clinvetadvisorexotics.com

ABSCESSES, Rabbits
ADRENAL DISEASE, Ferrets
ALEUTIAN DISEASE, Ferrets
ANALGESIC TOXICITY, Ferrets
ASPERGILLOSIS, Birds
AURAL ABSCESSES IN TURTLES, Reptiles
BASICS, Rabbits
BEHAVIOR, Rabbits
CHLAMYDIOSIS, Birds
CHRONIC EGG LAYING, Birds
CLOACAL PROLAPSE, Reptiles
CNEMIDOCOPTES, Birds
COMMUNICATION, Rabbits
CONJUNCTIVITIS, Birds
CYSTIC OVARIES, Guinea Pigs
DENTAL DISEASE
  Ferrets
  Rabbits
DIARRHEA, Ferrets
DILATED CARDIOMYOPATHY (DCM), Ferrets
DISTEMPER, Ferrets
DYSECDYSIS
  Chelonians
  General
  Lizards
  Snakes
EGG BINDING, Birds
ENVIRONMENTAL ENRICHMENT, Birds
FEATHER PICKING, Birds
FRACTURE MANAGEMENT
  Ferrets
  Reptiles
GASTROINTESTINAL FOREIGN BODIES, Ferrets
HAIRBALL, Rabbits
HAND REARING COCKATIELS, Birds
HEARTWORM–*DIROFILARIA IMMITIS*, Ferrets
HELICOBACTER MUSTELAE AND GASTRIC ULCERS, Ferrets
HOUSING, Rabbits
HUSBANDRY
  Bearded Dragons
  Betta
  Chicken
  Chinchillas
  Degus
  Guinea Pigs
  Hedgehogs
  Iguanas
  Red-Eared Sliders
  Snakes
  Sulcatas
  Tarantula
  Uromastyx
HYPOVITAMINOSIS A, Birds
INCLUSION BODY DISEASE, SNAKES, Reptiles
INSULINOMA, Ferrets
INTRODUCING A NEW RABBIT TO YOUR HOME, Rabbits
IRRITABLE BOWEL DISEASE (IBD), Ferrets
LEAD TOXICITY, Birds
LIVER DISEASE, PARROTS, Birds
LYMPHOMA
  Ferrets
  Hamsters
MAMMARY MASSES, Rats
MASTITIS, Rabbits
METABOLIC BONE DISEASE, Reptiles
MYCOPLASMA, Rats
MYIASIS, Rabbits
NUTRITION
  Birds
  Rabbits
OUTDOOR RABBITS
PET FISH MEDICINE HISTORY QUESTIONNAIRE, Fish
PODODERMATITIS
  Birds
  Guinea Pigs, Small Mammals
POST OP, Ferrets
PROPER HOUSING/ENVIRONMENT, Birds
PROTECTING YOUR PET BIRD: COMMON HOUSEHOLD TOXINS, Birds
PROVENTRICULAR DILATATION DISEASE, Birds
RENAL DISEASE
  Birds
  Reptiles
SIGNS AN AMPHIBIAN NEEDS VETERINARY CARE, Amphibians
SKIN TUMORS, Ferrets
SUDDEN DEATH, Amphibians
SWIM BLADDER, Fish
THYMOMA, Rabbits
URINARY CALCULI, Guinea Pigs
URINARY OBSTRUCTION, Ferrets
UROLITHIASIS, Rabbits
UVEITIS, Rabbits
VITAMIN A DEFICIENCY, Reptiles
VOCALIZATION IN COMPANION PARROTS, Birds
WET TAIL, Hamsters
WING TRIM, Birds
WOBBLY HEDGEHOG SYNDROME (WHS), Hedgehogs

SECTION I

Diseases and Disorders

EDITORS

James G. Fox, DVM, MS, DACLAM, FIDSA, AGAF *Ferrets*

Christoph Mans, MedVet *Small Mammals*

Robert P. Marini, DVM, DACLAM *Ferrets*

Romain Pizzi, BVSc, MSc, DZooMed (Avian), MACVSc (Surg), FRES, FRGS, MACVS *Invertebrates*

Helen E. Roberts, DVM *Fish*

Scott J. Stahl, DVM, DABVP (Avian) *Reptiles*

Thomas N. Tully, Jr., DVM, MS, DABVP (Avian), ECZM (Avian) *Birds*

David Vella, BSc, BVSc (Hons) (Exotic Companion Mammals) *Rabbits*

Kevin M. Wright, DVM, DABVP (Reptiles and Amphibians) *Amphibians*

INVERTEBRATES

Abscesses/Granulomas

BASIC INFORMATION

DEFINITION

An abscess/granuloma occurs as a result of a host mounting an inflammatory response to foreign antigens. These antigens can be associated with living organisms, such as bacteria or fungi, or with inanimate objects, such as plant material (e.g., foreign body).

EPIDEMIOLOGY

SPECIES, AGE, SEX Abscesses/granulomas have been documented in both crustaceans and insects, and no apparent age or sex predilections are associated with their formation.

RISK FACTORS

- Abscess/granuloma formation in invertebrates primarily occurs as a result of less-than-optimal captive care conditions.
- Poor hygiene (e.g., poor water quality, dirty environment), inadequate environmental conditions (e.g., low or excessive temperature and humidity), inadequate nutrition, and trauma may predispose invertebrates to abscess formation.

CONTAGION AND ZOONOSIS

- The most common pathogens isolated from invertebrate abscesses/granulomas are opportunistic bacteria.
  - Many of these organisms are Gram-negative (e.g., *Pseudomonas* spp., *Proteus* spp., *Serratia* spp., *Vibrio* spp.), although Gram-positive organisms (e.g., *Clostridium* spp.) can also cause disease.
- Fungal pathogens (e.g., *Mucor* spp., *Paeciliomyces* spp.) have been associated with abscess formation in invertebrates and are most commonly associated with arachnids and crustaceans.
- Most of the pathogens isolated from invertebrates are opportunistic organisms from the host's environment. In collections, it is generally only a single animal that will be found to have disease, although with more virulent organisms, dissemination of the disease into other conspecifics may occur.
- Most of the organisms associated with abscess formation in invertebrates have zoonotic potential.
- Individuals working with these animals should wash their hands and disinfect any equipment used to handle or sample the animals immediately after completing the examination.

CLINICAL PRESENTATION

DISEASE FORMS/SUBTYPES

- Granulomas in gills of crustaceans
- Granulomas in arachnids
- Septicemia in insects

HISTORY, CHIEF COMPLAINT

- Anorexia
- Color change (red or black)
- Lethargy
- Depression
- Death (often acute)

PHYSICAL EXAM FINDINGS

- Focal swelling noted on abdomen or possibly cephalothorax
- Discharge noted from one or more orifices
- Poor body condition
- Dehydration (see Dehydration)
- Inactive: appendages positioned under body segments
- Limited or no response to stimuli
- Gill and/or other tissue necrosis (crustaceans)

ETIOLOGY AND PATHOPHYSIOLOGY

- Most of the abscesses found in invertebrates are associated with opportunistic and ubiquitous bacteria and fungi.
- Invertebrates have a simple immune system that relies mostly on cell-mediated immunity.
- Hemocytes (e.g., archeocytes, plasmacytes, coagulocytes) found in the hemolymph phagocytize pathogens (e.g., bacteria, fungi) and foreign material. Under normal conditions, this material is processed and expelled. Abscesses occur when the response is overwhelming.
- Some invertebrate species may have indigenous bacteria that have an antimicrobial effect on pathogenic bacteria.

DIAGNOSIS

DIFFERENTIAL DIAGNOSIS

- Normal tissue
- Neoplasia

INITIAL DATABASE

- The affected site should be sampled using fine-needle aspiration or biopsy. Samples should be reviewed using a light microscope. Material collected from the sample should be placed on a microscope slide and stained using a general cell stain (e.g., Diff-Quik) and a Gram stain. Based on the findings, a bacterial and/or fungal culture should be submitted.
- A gill biopsy can be collected and processed using the techniques described previously.

ADVANCED OR CONFIRMATORY TESTING

- Bacterial and fungal cultures from invertebrates may need to be processed at room temperature. Placing bacterial cultures at 25°C (75°F) and 37°C (98.7°F) may provide the best results. Fungal cultures can be processed at 25°C (75°F).
- Discuss the samples with the laboratory before the time of submission. If certain pathogens are suspected, specialized media may be needed.
- Histopathologic samples should be submitted to a pathologist with experience processing and interpreting invertebrate tissues.

TREATMENT

THERAPEUTIC GOALS

- Treatment generally has limited success but can be pursued on the basis of culture and sensitivity results. Review the mechanism of action of the drug before starting a therapeutic regimen to ensure that you will not injure the host.
- Therapy should be aimed at improving husbandry and preventing disease in conspecifics.

ACUTE GENERAL TREATMENT

- Supportive care should be focused on improving husbandry conditions.
- Animals that are dehydrated should be provided appropriate fluid therapy.
- Antibacterial and antifungal therapies can be given, but the client should be reminded that all treatments are off-label.

CHRONIC TREATMENT

- Correct environmental deficiencies.
- Minimize stress (e.g., minimize animal densities, provide environmental enrichment/shelter).
- Use routine and appropriate disinfection protocols.

PROGNOSIS AND OUTCOME

The prognosis for these cases is guarded to grave because many invertebrates become septicemic as a result of the infection.

PEARLS & CONSIDERATIONS

COMMENTS

- Clinical medicine of invertebrates is a relatively new facet of the veterinary profession.
- Diagnosis of disease conditions can be frustrating but should be pursued nonetheless.

PREVENTION

- Hygiene and proper husbandry
- Strict quarantine measures for incoming animals

SUGGESTED READINGS

Berzins IK, Smolowitz R: Diagnostic techniques and sample handling. In Lewbart GA, editor: Invertebrate medicine, Ames, IA, 2006, Blackwell Publishing, pp 263–274.
Cooper EL: Comparative immunology, Integr Comp Biol 43:278–280, 2003.
Cooper JE: Insects. In Lewbart GA, editor: Invertebrate medicine, Ames, IA, 2006, Blackwell Publishing, pp 205–219.
Noga EJ, et al: Crustaceans. In Lewbart GA, editor: Invertebrate medicine, Ames, IA, 2006, Blackwell Publishing, pp 179–193.
Pizzi R: Spiders. In Lewbart GA, editor: Invertebrate medicine, Ames, include IA, 2006, Blackwell Publishing, pp 143–168.

AUTHOR: **ANNE BURGDORF-MOISUK**

EDITOR: **ROMAIN PIZZI**

INVERTEBRATES

Alopecia

BASIC INFORMATION

DEFINITION

Deficiency in hair cover caused by failure to grow or loss after growth

SYNONYMS

Hair loss, baldness

EPIDEMIOLOGY

SPECIES, AGE, SEX Tarantulas (Theraphosidae), any age, both genders

RISK FACTORS Common in tarantulas in public display enclosures

ASSOCIATED CONDITIONS AND DISORDERS May be associated with excessive web spinning on enclosure glass and stress-induced anorexia

CLINICAL PRESENTATION

DISEASE FORMS/SUBTYPES Progressive

HISTORY, CHIEF COMPLAINT Hair loss and appearance of a well-demarcated, bald area on the caudodorsal opisthosoma (abdomen) of individual tarantula

PHYSICAL EXAM FINDINGS

- When the body surface is examined under magnification, the hairs are seen to be missing, not broken.
- The underlying cuticle is normal.

ETIOLOGY AND PATHOPHYSIOLOGY

- This condition is most commonly seen in terrestrial New World species such as the commonly kept Chilean rose tarantula (*Grammostola rosea*) and Mexican redknee tarantula (*Brachypelma smithi*).
- In these species, defense against predators is obtained by kicking off urticating (irritant) hairs from this specific region of the opisthosoma into the face of predators.
- A slightly worn, or moth-eaten, appearance of the opisthosoma hairs may be evident when an adult tarantula is approaching ecdysis (moulting) and is normal.
- The underlying cuticle will usually be dark in individuals close to ecdysis owing to the underlying new hairs and cuticle.

DIAGNOSIS

DIFFERENTIAL DIAGNOSIS

- Abrasion or hair damage through rough handling or transportation
- Dysecdysis (abnormal shedding of cuticle) (see Dysecdysis)
- Ectoparasite infections (parasitic or saprophytic mites)
- Endoparasite infections (*Acroceridae larvae*)

INITIAL DATABASE

- Full history
- Examination of affected area under magnification

TREATMENT

THERAPEUTIC GOAL

Prevent recurrence after ecdysis by limiting environmental stress

ACUTE GENERAL TREATMENT

No specific treatment

PROGNOSIS AND OUTCOME

This condition is not life threatening or particularly serious, but it can be an indication of environmental stress (people repeatedly banging on the enclosure glass, prodding spider to induce movement, or overly frequent attempts at handling).

PEARLS & CONSIDERATIONS

COMMENTS

- Do not be tempted to perform cuticle or hair scrapes. The opisthosoma cuticle is thin, friable, and easily ruptured, which may result in death of the tarantula from hemolymph loss. The thin-walled heart lies right, beneath the area of typical hair loss.
- Sticky-tape preparations are not recommended. Parasitic and saprophytic mites are easily visible under magnification and are most commonly seen at the base of the legs (see Mites [Acarii]).
- Gloves and safety glasses are advisable when dealing with New World tarantula species; if irritant hairs become embedded in the cornea it can cause serious chronic keratitis.

CLIENT EDUCATION

- Stress reduction will help prevent this from occurring.

- Tarantulas are photophobic and should be provided with dark retreats.
- Excessive handling should be avoided, and individuals should not be poked to encourage them to move.
- Visitors should be discouraged from taping on the glass of the enclosure.
- The problem will not resolve until the next ecdysis.

SUGGESTED READINGS

Foelix RF: Biology of spiders, Cambridge, 1996, Harvard University Press.

Pizzi R: Spiders. In Lewbart G, editor: Invertebrate medicine, Ames, 2006, Blackwell Publishing, pp 143–168.

Schultz SA, Schultz MJ: The Tarantula keepers' guide, Hauppage, 1998, Barron's Educational Series, Inc.

CROSS-REFERENCES TO OTHER SECTIONS

Mites (Acarii)
Dysecdysis

AUTHOR & EDITOR: **ROMAIN PIZZI**

INVERTEBRATES

Bacterial Diseases

BASIC INFORMATION

DEFINITION

Bacteria are prokaryotic, unicellular microorganisms that are ubiquitous in natural environments.

EPIDEMIOLOGY

SPECIES, AGE, SEX Most exotic pet species in which important bacterial diseases are recognized belong to the phylum Arthropoda. This excludes many well-recognized diseases of invertebrate species used in aquaculture and agriculture.

RISK FACTORS Poor hygiene, inadequate husbandry (e.g., malnutrition, improper temperature and humidity), and integumental defects (e.g., trauma).

CONTAGION AND ZOONOSIS Some bacteria that affect invertebrates as opportunistic pathogens (e.g., *Clostridium* spp., *Pseudomonas* spp., *Proteus* spp., *Serratia* spp., *Vibrio* spp.) can also affect humans. Personal protective equipment and personnel safety should always be considered during any disease investigation.

ASSOCIATED CONDITIONS AND DISORDERS See Risk Factors.

CLINICAL PRESENTATION

DISEASE FORMS/SUBTYPES

- Cyanobacteria (*Oscillatoria* and *Beggiatoa* spp.) in horseshoe crabs (*Limulus polyphemus*)
- Septicemia in arachnids (i.e., spiders and scorpions)
- Septicemia in crustaceans
- *Paenibacillus larvae* (American foulbrood, or AFB) in honey bees (*Apis mellifera*)
- *Melissococcus pluton* (European foulbrood, or EFB) in honey bees

HISTORY, CHIEF COMPLAINT

- Anorexia
- Lethargy
- Depression
- Death (often acute)

PHYSICAL EXAM FINDINGS

- Cyanobacteria in horseshoe crabs
  - Swollen or ruptured gill leaflets
  - Gill and/or other tissue necrosis
- Septicemia in arachnids
  - Possible discharge from one or more orifices
  - Dehydration (manifested as impaired mobility and/or opisthosomal shrinking and deformation)
  - Classic "death pose" (appendages curled ventral to body segments)
- Bacterial septicemia in crustaceans
  - Color changes
  - Lack of response to stimuli
  - Poor muscle tone (manifested as drooping tail or appendages)
  - Postural abnormalities (e.g., lateral or dorsal recumbency)
- AFB in honey bees
  - Sealed cap over affected larval honeycomb cells is dark, moist, sunken, and/or perforated.
  - Dead larva dries into a hard "scale" adhered to the side of the cell after 1 month.
  - Outbreaks can destroy whole colonies.
- EFB in honey bees
  - Affected larva becomes flaccid and shifts to one side of the honeycomb cell.
  - Dead larva turns brown when decomposing.
  - Spontaneous recovery of colonies usually occurs after outbreaks.
- Septicemia in insects
  - Color changes
  - Loose feces
  - Dehydration
  - Liquefaction of internal organs

ETIOLOGY AND PATHOPHYSIOLOGY

- Normal external and internal bacterial florae of most invertebrates have not been described, and it is often difficult to determine whether isolated bacteria from diseased animals are the causative agents.
- Most bacterial disease is caused by opportunistic infection.
- *Bacillus* spp. can cause outbreaks in captive arachnid colonies.
- *Bacillus thuringiensis* causes natural outbreaks of morbidity and mortality in insects, and it has been used extensively by humans for biological control.

DIAGNOSIS

DIFFERENTIAL DIAGNOSIS

- Normal behavior (e.g., preecdysis anorexia in arachnids)
- Debilitation due to inadequate or improper husbandry
- Other infectious diseases (e.g., fungal, viral, parasitic)
- Intoxication (e.g., pesticides)

INITIAL DATABASE

- Culture, cytology, and Gram staining of material from lesions or body cavities
- Hemolymph collection for bacterial culture and determination of biochemistry parameters, color, and clarity
- Appearance of affected honeycomb cells is pathognomonic for AFB of honey bees.
- Introduction of the end of a wooden applicator stick into a cell affected by AFB will produce a viscous thread of material when withdrawn.
- Dissection of honey bee larvae affected by EFB will reveal white clumps in the midgut.

ADVANCED OR CONFIRMATORY TESTING

- Specialized culture media may be needed for bacteria that are not typically cultured from vertebrate species (e.g., AFB and EFB of honey bees).
- Incubation temperatures for invertebrate bacterial pathogens may need to be adjusted to account for the hosts' poikilothermic status (e.g., many bacteria will grow at 25°C [77°F]).
- Polymerase chain reaction analysis is available for both AFB and EFB.
- Biopsy or necropsy and histopathology are important for diagnosis and identification of predisposing or concurrent conditions.
- Specialized fixation techniques may be needed for histopathology.

TREATMENT

THERAPEUTIC GOALS

- Treatment of bacterial disease in invertebrate species is often unrewarding.
- Main goals should be containment and prevention of disease.

ACUTE GENERAL TREATMENT

- Depopulation and destruction of entire colonies may be necessary (e.g., AFB of honey bees).
- Culling and/or isolation of affected individuals in colonies
- Supportive care of individuals (e.g., fluid therapy)
- Empirical antimicrobial therapy may be employed, but almost no data on efficacy and safety are available.

PROGNOSIS AND OUTCOME

Most bacterial infections in invertebrate species have a poor to grave prognosis.

PEARLS & CONSIDERATIONS

COMMENTS

- Clinical medicine of invertebrates is a relatively new facet of the veterinary profession.
- Diagnosis of disease conditions can be frustrating but should be pursued nonetheless.
- AFB and EFB of honey bees are on the Reportable Diseases of Invertebrates List of the Office International des Epizooties (OIE).

PREVENTION

- Strict quarantine measures for incoming animals
- See Chronic Treatment.

CLIENT EDUCATION

- Quarantine for all new animal acquisitions
- Annual examinations for invertebrates
- Proper husbandry practices

SUGGESTED READINGS

Berzins IK, Smolowitz R: Diagnostic techniques and sample handling. In Lewbart GA, editor: Invertebrate medicine, Ames, 2006, Blackwell Publishing, pp 263–274.
Cooper JE: Insects. In Lewbart GA, editor: Invertebrate medicine, Ames, 2006, Blackwell Publishing, pp 205–219.
Noga EJ, et al: Crustaceans. In Lewbart GA, editor: Invertebrate medicine, Ames, 2006, Blackwell Publishing, pp 179–193.
Pizzi R: Spiders. In Lewbart GA, editor: Invertebrate medicine, Ames, 2006, Blackwell Publishing, pp 143–168.
Smith SA: Horseshoe crabs. In Lewbart GA, editor: Invertebrate medicine, Ames, 2006, Blackwell Publishing, pp 133–142.
Williams DL: A veterinary approach to the European honey bee (*Apis mellifera*), Vet J 160:61–73, 2000.
Williams DL: Studies in arachnid disease. In Cooper JE, et al, editors: Arachnida: proceedings of a symposium on spiders and their allies, London, 1992, Chiron Publications Ltd, pp 116–125.

AUTHOR: **TREVOR T. ZACHARIAH**

EDITOR: **ROMAIN PIZZI**

INVERTEBRATES

Dehydration

BASIC INFORMATION

DEFINITION

Negative fluid balance where the body loses more fluid than it takes in.

SYNONYMS

Desiccation, estivation

EPIDEMIOLOGY

SPECIES, AGE, SEX

- All species
- Insects, tarantulas, and snails are particularly prone.

RISK FACTORS

- Abrasive substrates such as sand
- Dry enclosures
- Trauma (see Trauma)

CONTAGION AND ZOONOSIS

- Not contagious
- Not a zoonotic disease

GEOGRAPHY AND SEASONALITY

More common in warm dry months, but also in winter owing to reduced activity

CLINICAL PRESENTATION

HISTORY, CHIEF COMPLAINT

- Anorexia
- Inactivity

PHYSICAL EXAM FINDINGS

- Tarantulas typically will have difficulty ambulating or will be unable to move, with their legs held flexed beneath the body. This is a result of having only limb flexor muscles. Limb extension is totally dependent on adequate hemolymph pressure.
- Snails will become inactive and will retract deep into their shell. They may secrete a dried-out mucoid plug to prevent further dehydration.

ETIOLOGY AND PATHOPHYSIOLOGY

- Most arthropods have a water-proof layer in the cuticle to prevent evaporative fluid loss.
- Abrasive substrates may damage this layer but with no macroscopically visible signs.
- Trauma such as dropping an animal and cracking the cuticle and hemolymph leakage can rapidly result in dehydration.
- Estivation is a normal response in snails, with individuals retracting deep into their shells and secreting a plug to prevent further fluid loss.
- Severe or prolonged dehydration will result in death.

DIAGNOSIS

DIFFERENTIAL DIAGNOSIS

- Intoxication (see Intoxication)
- Bacterial infection (see Bacterial Diseases)
- Fungal infection (see Fungal Infections, Superficial and Systemic)
- Panagrolaimidae nematode infection of tarantulas (see Panagrolaimidae Oral Nematodes in Tarantulas)

INITIAL DATABASE

- Incoordination due to causes such as intoxication; should be differentiated from an inability to ambulate due to dehydration
- Response to provision of water or fluid administration
- Examination for any underlying trauma and ongoing hemolymph hemorrhage

ADVANCED OR CONFIRMATORY TESTING

It can be difficult to assess whether snails deeply retracted into their shells are alive but severely dehydrated, or whether they are simply dead. Placement of a Doppler ultrasound probe with copious gel on the retracted foot will allow one to hear the slow but clearly audible heartbeat in live snails.

TREATMENT

THERAPEUTIC GOALS

- Return normal fluid balance
- Reduce fluid loss

- Increase fluid intake by offering water or high water content food
- Prevent integument damage that may precipitate fluid loss (abrasive substrates)

ACUTE GENERAL TREATMENT

- In less severe cases, provision of fresh green vegetables to herbivorous insects and a very shallow water dish may suffice.
- In very small species, misting surfaces and vegetation in enclosures with a spray is advisable.
- In moderate dehydration cases, arthropods may be placed with their mouthparts in a very shallow container of water.
- Care should be taken to not place the abdomen of insects (spiracles) or the opisthosoma of spiders (booklungs) in the water tray to prevent asphyxiation or drowning.
- In severe cases, lactated Ringer's, Hartmann's solution, or physiologic saline (0.9% NaCl) may be injected into the hemocoel of arthropods.
- In large individuals, this is best administered with a 27-gauge insulin needle through the thin membranes between segments at the bases of the legs (coxa and trochanter).
- In tarantulas, fluid may be injected into the dorsal midline of the opisthosoma, where the heart is situated.
  - This route is not suitable in insects because unlike tarantulas, insects have a tracheolar respiratory system that may be penetrated, and the insect may drown.
- Injection sites should be sealed with cyanoacrylate tissue adhesive or household superglue; otherwise the inelastic membranes often continue to leak fluid and hemolymph afterward.
- Individuals should be kept in a small enclosure on paper towels to monitor for any ongoing hemorrhage of hemolymph.
- In snails, fluid should not be injected.
- Dehydrated snails are best bathed in shallow dishes of lukewarm water twice daily until they exit estivation.

RECOMMENDED MONITORING

Keep affected individuals after treatment in a small enclosure with paper towels used as a substrate to allow detection of any ongoing hemolymph hemorrhage from an unidentified trauma site.

PROGNOSIS AND OUTCOME

Prognosis is dependent on the degree of dehydration (just as in other species), any underlying trauma, and prevention of ongoing hemolymph hemorrhage. Mild to moderate cases have a good prognosis.

PEARLS & CONSIDERATIONS

COMMENTS

- Water dishes should not be so deep that individuals risk drowning; 2-3 mm is a sufficient depth (see figure).
- In very small species, misting surfaces and vegetation in enclosures with a spray is advisable instead of providing a water container in which they may drown.
- Address any underlying husbandry problems predisposing to dehydration or trauma.

PREVENTION

- Provide fresh water or high water content foods.
- Eliminate abrasive substrates that could result in cuticle damage and fluid loss.

SUGGESTED READINGS

Lewbart G, editor: Invertebrate medicine, Ames, 2006, Blackwell Publishing.
Pizzi R: Spiders. In Lewbart G, editor: Invertebrate medicine, Ames, 2006, Blackwell Publishing, pp 143–168.
Williams DL: Invertebrates. In Meredith A, Redrobe S, editors: BSAVA manual of exotic pets, ed 4, Gloucester, 2003, BSAVA, pp 280–287.

CROSS-REFERENCES TO OTHER SECTIONS

Bacterial Diseases
Fungal Infections, Superficial and Systemic
Intoxication
Panagrolaimidae Oral Nematodes in Tarantulas
Trauma

AUTHOR & EDITOR: **ROMAIN PIZZI**

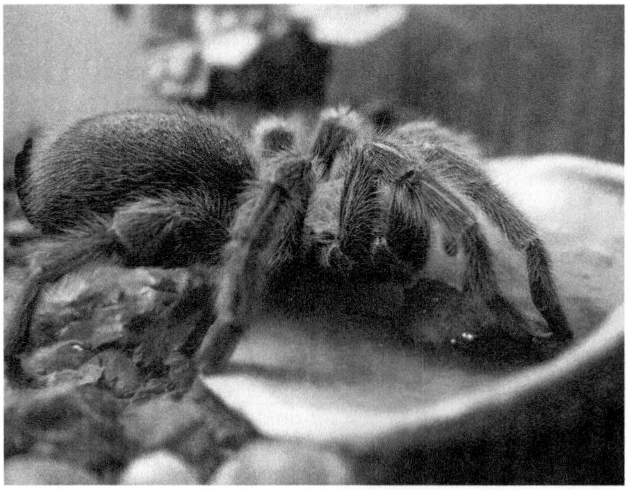

Dehydration A tarantula drinking from a dish; this sign of dehydration is common after shipping or purchase. *(Photo courtesy Jörg Mayer, The University of Georgia, Athens.)*

Dysecdysis

BASIC INFORMATION

DEFINITION

Abnormal shedding, or difficulty in shedding (ecdysis)

SYNONYMS

Abnormal moult, retained moult, retained shed, stuck-in cast, cuticle retention

EPIDEMIOLOGY

SPECIES, AGE, SEX

- All arthropods
- All ages, but groups of juveniles particularly affected in large collections with environmental problems owing to more frequent ecdysis
- Both genders equally affected

GEOGRAPHY AND SEASONALITY

More common in warmer months in arthropods not kept in heated enclosures year round

CLINICAL PRESENTATION

HISTORY, CHIEF COMPLAINT

- Individual stuck in moulted cuticle
- Missing appendages from dysecdysis
- Dismembered arthropod from attempts at assisting ecdysis

PHYSICAL EXAM FINDINGS

- Retained sections of cuticle
- Limbs most commonly affected
- In severe cases, most of the old cuticle may still be retained.
- Abnormal posture
- Unable to move normally
- Distorted legs and anatomy once cuticle has hardened (sclerotized)

ETIOLOGY AND PATHOPHYSIOLOGY

- Shedding of the old cuticle is facilitated by a very thin layer of moisture between old and new cuticles during ecdysis. Dehydration can affect this, so ensure that individuals always have water, and that herbivorous species have fresh food.
- The new underlying cuticle is soft and friable during the process of ecdysis because it needs to expand after ecdysis; the old shed cuticle is dry, rigid, and strong. Intervention should always be left until after the new cuticle has hardened (24-72 hours) to prevent the risk of dismembering the animal. In some species of arthropods, this will be obvious because of a color change and darkening of the cuticle.

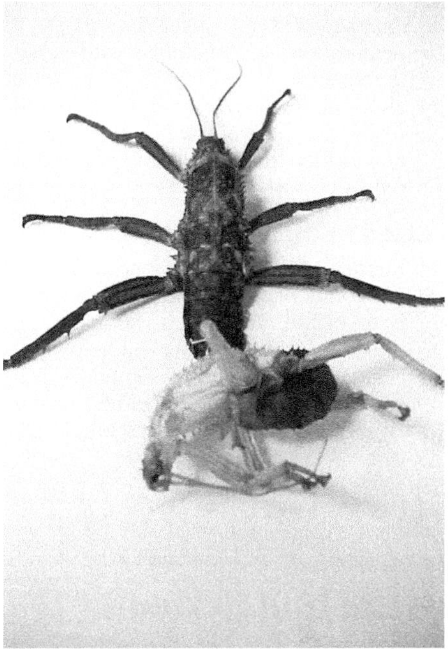

Dysecdysis This stick insect died during shedding; a common cause for dysecdysis is dehydration. *(Photo courtesy Jörg Mayer, The University of Georgia, Athens.)*

DIAGNOSIS

DIFFERENTIAL DIAGNOSIS

- Dehydration (see Dehydration)
- Alopecia (see Alopecia)

INITIAL DATABASE

- Examination under magnification or low-power stereomicroscopy to determine where cuticle is retained, and whether markedly distorted limbs are present that require autotomy or amputation
- Examination of affected individual and enclosures for signs of mites that may also predispose to dysecdysis (see Mites [Acarii])

TREATMENT

THERAPEUTIC GOALS

- Remove retained cuticle ONLY once the new cuticle has hardened (sclerotized) after 48-72 hours
- Perform autotomy or amputation of disfigured limbs if needed
- Provide supportive care of disfigured individuals until next ecdysis
- Prevent recurrence at next ecdysis period

ACUTE GENERAL TREATMENT

- Do NOT try to assist during the actual process of ecdysis. The new cuticle is very soft and friable before it is sclerotized, but the old cuticle is rigid; attempts at removal at this stage will simply result in the arthropod being dismembered.
- If the new underlying cuticle is soft, the only assistance provided should be the application of a lukewarm solution of a household detergent. This will soften the old shed cuticle and will lower the surface tension of the fluid interface between old and new friable cuticles.
- Do NOT try to pull retained cuticle off.
- Application with a fine-tipped artist's brush, or soaking with mild detergent solution even many days after ecdysis, will soften the old retained cuticle but will not affect the new underlying cuticle and will make removal easier and safer.
  - Care should be taken to avoid wetting booklungs and spiracles to prevent drowning.
  - Retained cuticle can be carefully trimmed off with iris scissors.
- Three or more days after dysecdysis, and once the new cuticle has hardened, severely distorted limbs that interfere with locomotion may be amputated or autotomized. Amputation should always be performed through a joint with a thin membrane, rather than attempting to amputate through a rigid section of limb cuticle.
  - The wound must be sealed with several layers of cyanoacrylate tissue adhesive or household "superglue" to prevent hemolymph hemorrhage.
- Autotomy may be performed in tarantulas. This is a conscious process, and individuals should NOT be anesthetized.
  - The femur component of the limb is firmly grasped and is pulled dorsally, while the body is secured on a surface.
  - A natural fracture plane is present in the supporting apodeme of the coxofemoral joint; the joint membrane tears at this point.
  - Although this is a natural process and hemolymph loss may be negligible at the time, the wound should always be sealed with several layers of tissue adhesive to prevent risks of later hemorrhage and death.

CHRONIC TREATMENT

Supportive care of severely affected individuals, or those in which several limbs have needed autotomy or amputation, until the next episode of ecdysis

PROGNOSIS AND OUTCOME

Prognosis is guarded depending on the severity of the retained cuticle. Individuals dismembered through attempts at assistance during ecdysis carry a hopeless prognosis, although attempts can be made to treat as for trauma (see Trauma).

PEARLS & CONSIDERATIONS

COMMENTS

- It is always safest to wait at least 24-48 hours to allow the new cuticle to harden (sclerotize) before trying to trim or remove retained cuticle.
- During ecdysis, application of a lukewarm weak detergent solution with an artist's paintbrush is the only intervention with a chance of success without causing severe damage to the affected animal.
- Application or soaking with mild detergent solution even many days after ecdysis will soften the old retained cuticle but will not affect the new underlying cuticle and will make removal easier and safer.

CLIENT EDUCATION

- Keepers are always convinced that an environment that is insufficiently moist is to blame, and that misting during the approach to ecdysis will help. This is likely an erroneous assumption. The cuticle is water resistant, and misting is unlikely to contribute meaningfully to ecdysis.
- Clients should understand the need to resist the temptation to try to remove the old cuticle during ecdysis.
- In some species of tarantulas, normal ecdysis can take several hours; this does not indicate dysecdysis.

SUGGESTED READINGS

Frye FL: Captive invertebrates: a guide to their biology and husbandry, Malabar, 1992, Krieger.

Lewbart G, editor: Invertebrate medicine, Ames, 2006, Blackwell Publishing.

CROSS-REFERENCES TO OTHER SECTIONS

Alopecia
Dehydration
Mites (Acarii)
Trauma

AUTHOR & EDITOR: **ROMAIN PIZZI**

INVERTEBRATES

Fungal Infections, Superficial and Systemic

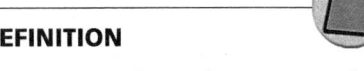

BASIC INFORMATION

DEFINITION

Systemic or surface infections caused by fungi

SYNONYM

Mycoses

EPIDEMIOLOGY

SPECIES, AGE, SEX

- Most common in arthropods, particularly insects and spiders
- Some systemic infections more common in adults

GENETICS AND BREED PREDISPOSITION

- Adult Fregate Island giant tenebrionid beetles (*Polposipus herculeanus*) are particularly sensitive to systemic infection with *Metarhizium anisopliae*, as are many other beetles.
- Silkworm and other caterpillars are susceptible to *Beauveria bassiana* (muscardine).
- *Labyrinthomyxa marina* is the most important fungal pathogen of oysters.

RISK FACTORS

- High-humidity enclosures
- Natural substrates in enclosures
- Infrequently cleaned enclosures and buildup of organic debris
- Previous fungal disease in collection

CONTAGION AND ZOONOSIS

- Entomopathogenic systemic mycoses are very contagious after the appearance of external fruiting bodies, which only occurs after the death of an infected arthropod
- Superficial (opportunistic) mycoses normally not contagious
- Not a zoonosis

ASSOCIATED CONDITIONS AND DISORDERS

- Concomitant mite infestation may indicate poor environmental hygiene.
- Any time of the year
- Heated humid invertebrate enclosures and those with poor ventilation are more likely to be affected.
- May occur as a secondary infection of cuticular wounds

CLINICAL PRESENTATION

DISEASE FORMS/SUBTYPES

- Peracute: Deaths without any external visible fungal growth antemortem (entomopathogenic systemic fungi). Fungal elements are only seen after death (if cadavers are not immediately removed).
- Chronic: Individuals with obvious external fungal growth that otherwise are behaving clinically normally (opportunistic Saprophytes).

HISTORY, CHIEF COMPLAINT

- Reduced appetite and loss of coordination
- Abnormal behavior: Subterranean species rise to the surface, and many species move to high places.
- Many show no clinical signs before death.
- Obvious fungal growth evident on live or dead invertebrates in a collection
- Color changes of the body antemortem or postmortem (also caused by bacterial infection)
- Mummification of adult insects after death. Exceptions are butterfly and moth larvae that may become flaccid with watery contents and may disintegrate if infected with Entomophthorales.
- Small quantities of chalky fungal elements may be evident at the joints, the cloaca, and mouthparts.

PHYSICAL EXAM FINDINGS Most cases where external fungal growth is evident antemortem are due to poor environmental hygiene and to opportunistic Saprophytes.

ETIOLOGY AND PATHOPHYSIOLOGY

- Entomopathogenic fungi will invade via body openings such as the respiratory spiracles or through the oral cavity with ingestion, or they may invade by penetrating the integument, as with chitinolytic fungi such as *Cordyceps* and *Gibellula* species.
- Death is due to nutritional deficiencies, invasion and destruction of tissues, or toxin production.

- Different fungal pathogens may cause peracute death or chronic infection.
  - Some will cause changes in behavior, leading affected individuals to seek out high places to ensure better spore dispersal after death.
- After death, the fungi usually completely invade the hemocoel before producing external fruiting bodies.

DIAGNOSIS

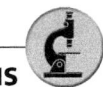

DIFFERENTIAL DIAGNOSIS

- Systemic entomopathogenic fungi
- Opportunistic saprophytic surface fungal growth
- Postmortem fungal invasion (Hyphomycetes)
- Dysecdysis (see Dysecdysis)
- Bacterial infection (see Bacterial Diseases)
- Dried excretory wastes (urates, allantoin, or guanine in spiders)
- Alopecia due to environmental stress in tarantulas (see Alopecia)

INITIAL DATABASE

- Surface cytologic examination (cellotape preparations), light microscopy to confirm fungal elements
- Examination of enclosure substrate and environment for saprophytic fungal growth
- Post mortem to evaluate systemic (hemocoel) fungal invasion

ADVANCED OR CONFIRMATORY TESTING

- Lactophenol cotton blue staining of fungal elements to aid taxonomic identification
- Fungal culture of many entomopathogenic fungi (Entomophthorales) not possible on standard culture media
- Culture of postmortem material may yield only postmortem invaders that grow on standard media (Hyphomycetes).

TREATMENT

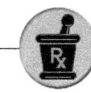

THERAPEUTIC GOALS

- In opportunistic surface infection, eliminate surface fungal growth and remove fungal environmental contamination
- In entomopathogenic fungal disease outbreaks, eliminate infection from the population

ACUTE GENERAL TREATMENT

Topical treatment with povidone-iodine once daily (applied with a cotton tip) or antifungal agents such as clotrimazole

CHRONIC TREATMENT

In entomopathogenic fungal disease outbreaks, quarantine, destocking, fumigation of the rooms while eggs are in a dormant state, or surface antifungal treatment of eggs may be considered dependent on the agent and the host life cycle. Elimination from the premises can be very difficult.

RECOMMENDED MONITORING

- Postmortem examination in collections to evaluate the presence of systemic fungal disease
- The coelom may be replaced with firm chalky, white, pink, or green fungal material, confirmed as fungal in nature by microscopy.

PROGNOSIS AND OUTCOME

- Cases of opportunistic external growth of saprophytic fungi seen antemortem respond well to topical treatment and improved environmental hygiene.
- Outbreaks of entomopathogenic fungal deaths can be very difficult to control in collections. Taxonomic identification is essential to determine the mode of infection (penetration of the integument or via body openings) and to formulate an effective elimination plan.

PEARLS & CONSIDERATIONS

COMMENTS

External fungal growth on pet invertebrates is one of the easiest invertebrate conditions to treat successfully in practice. Entomopathogenic fungal outbreaks in collection are conversely extremely difficult to control.

PREVENTION

- Good enclosure hygiene and timely removal of food remains an organic debris
- Prevention of excessive enclosure humidity and damp substrates

SUGGESTED READINGS

Humber RA: Fungi: identification. In Lacey L, editor: Manual of techniques in insect pathology, London, 1997, Academic Press, pp 153–185.

Lewbart G, editor: Invertebrate medicine, Ames, 2006, Blackwell Publishing.

Tanada Y, Kaya HK: Insect pathology, San Diego, 1993, Academic Press.

Williams DL: Invertebrates. In Meredith A, Redrobe S, editors: BSAVA manual of exotic pets, ed 4, Gloucester, 2003, BSAVA, pp 280–287.

CROSS-REFERENCES TO OTHER SECTIONS

Alopecia
Bacterial Diseases
Dysecdysis

AUTHOR & EDITOR: **ROMAIN PIZZI**

INVERTEBRATES

Infectious Diseases of Acroporid Corals

BASIC INFORMATION

DEFINITION

Bacteria are prokaryotic, unicellular microorganisms that are ubiquitous in natural environments.

EPIDEMIOLOGY

SPECIES, AGE, SEX Corals of the family Acroporidae are found in waters of the Atlantic and Pacific Oceans, where they are found in shallow reef systems. Common species are the staghorn coral (*Acropora cervicornis*) and the elkhorn coral (*A. palmata*).

RISK FACTORS Poor hygiene, inadequate husbandry (e.g., malnutrition, improper temperature and humidity), and traumatic insults

CONTAGION AND ZOONOSIS Some bacteria that affect acroporid corals as opportunistic pathogens (e.g., *Clostridium* spp., *Serratia* spp., *Vibrio* spp.) can also affect humans. Personal protective equipment and personnel safety should always be considered during any disease investigation.

ASSOCIATED CONDITIONS AND DISORDERS See Risk Factors.

CLINICAL PRESENTATION

DISEASE FORMS/SUBTYPES

- Black band disease
- White band disease
- White pox (a.k.a. white patch disease)

- Rapid tissue degeneration (a.k.a. rapid tissue necrosis or shutdown reaction)

HISTORY, CHIEF COMPLAINT

- Color changes
- Death (i.e., living tissue lost and only "skeleton" remains)

PHYSICAL EXAM FINDINGS

- Black band disease
  - Black mat that advances over coral tissue by millimeters per day
  - Leading edge of the mat advances fastest during the day, and the back edge of the mat advances fastest during the night.
- White band disease
  - White band begins at coral base and advances toward branch tips.
  - Two described types
    - Type I: white band of necrosis advances over coral tissue by millimeters per day; tissue sloughs in small masses
    - Type II: similar to type I, but spreading occurs at a faster rate
- White pox
  - Seasonal disease associated with elevated water temperatures
  - Scattered white blotches of tissue loss
  - Rapid expansion of up to 2.5 cm^2 per day
- Rapid tissue degeneration
  - Frequently begins at coral base and advances toward branch tips
  - Increased or decreased production of mucus
  - Prolonged retraction of polyps
  - Tissue sloughing occurs with zooxanthellae intact (no bleaching)

ETIOLOGY AND PATHOPHYSIOLOGY

- Koch's postulates have not been fulfilled for any bacterial disease of acroporid corals.
- Most diseases are likely multifactorial.
- Black band disease
  - The cyanobacterium *Phormidium corallyticum* dominates the microbial community of the band.
  - Other possible pathogens for which evidence has been found include *Beggiatoa* spp., *Desulfovibrio* spp., *Campylobacter* spp., *Arcobacter* spp., *Cytophaga* spp., *Clostridium* spp., *Trichodesmium tenue*.
- White band disease
  - Type I has been associated with Gram-negative bacilli.
  - Type II has been associated with *Vibrio charcharia*.
- White pox
  - *Serratia marcescens* has tentatively been linked to this disease.
- Rapid tissue degeneration
  - *Vibrio vulnificus* has tentatively been linked to this disease.

DIAGNOSIS

DIFFERENTIAL DIAGNOSIS

- Normal behavior (e.g., acroporids may produce mucus capture webs)
- Debilitation due to inadequate or improper husbandry
- Other infectious diseases (e.g., fungal, viral, parasitic)
- Intoxication (e.g., heavy metals, irritants)

INITIAL DATABASE

Culture, cytology, and Gram staining of material from lesions

ADVANCED OR CONFIRMATORY TESTING

- Specialized culture media may be needed for bacteria that are not typically cultured from terrestrial species.
- Incubation temperatures for acroporid bacterial pathogens may have to be adjusted to account for the hosts' poikilothermic status.
- Biopsy or necropsy and histopathology are important for diagnosis and identification of predisposing or concurrent conditions.
- Specialized fixation techniques, including decalcification, may be needed for histopathology.

TREATMENT

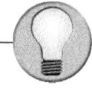

THERAPEUTIC GOALS

- Successful treatment of bacterial disease in acroporid species is highly variable.
- Main goals should be containment and prevention of disease.

ACUTE GENERAL TREATMENT

- Débridement of affected tissues with margins extending into healthy tissue using sharp dissection
- Defects can be filled with a number of different compounds (e.g., plaster of Paris, hydraulic cement, methacrylates, cyanoacrylates, underwater epoxies).
- Empirical antimicrobial therapy may be employed, but almost no data on efficacy and safety are available.

CHRONIC TREATMENT

- Optimization of environmental conditions (especially water quality and light conditions)
- Adequate hygiene

PROGNOSIS AND OUTCOME

Most bacterial infections in acroporid species have a poor to grave prognosis.

PEARLS & CONSIDERATIONS

COMMENTS

- Clinical medicine of invertebrates is a relatively new facet of the veterinary profession.
- Diagnosis of disease conditions can be frustrating but should be pursued nonetheless.

PREVENTION

- Strict quarantine measures for incoming animals
- See Chronic Treatment.

CLIENT EDUCATION

- Quarantine for all new animal acquisitions
- Annual examinations for invertebrates
- Proper husbandry practices

SUGGESTED READINGS

Berzins IK, Smolowitz R: Diagnostic techniques and sample handling. In Lewbart GA, editor: Invertebrate medicine, Ames, 2006, Blackwell Publishing, pp 263–274.

Stoskopf MK: Coelenterates. In Lewbart GA, editor: Invertebrate medicine, Ames, 2006, Blackwell Publishing, pp 19–51.

AUTHOR: **TREVOR T. ZACHARIAH**

EDITOR: **ROMAIN PIZZI**

INVERTEBRATES

Intoxication

BASIC INFORMATION

DEFINITION
Poisoning, the state of being poisoned

SYNONYMS
Poisoning, toxicity, pesticide exposure

EPIDEMIOLOGY
SPECIES, AGE, SEX All invertebrate species, ages, and genders

RISK FACTORS
- Pesticide use in vicinity (adjacent rooms, garden, or in some cases even neighbor's house)
- Enclosures serviced or invertebrates handled by keepers having contact with other animals such as dogs and cats
- Use of topical parasiticides (particularly fipronil) on other animals in vicinity
- Some aerosols, cleaning agents, and aromatic solvents
- Recent painting and building work in building (solvents and sealants)

CONTAGION AND ZOONOSIS
- Not contagious
- Not infectious
- Epidemiology in a group can resemble an infectious disease.
- Not a zoonotic disease

CLINICAL PRESENTATION
DISEASE FORMS/SUBTYPES
- Acute: Most cases of intoxication, particularly with pesticides, will show an acute progression of clinical signs followed by death.
- Chronic: A small number of cases demonstrate chronic and subtle clinical signs such as anorexia and lethargy over several weeks. These cases are difficult to diagnose and are commonly associated with less overtly toxic compounds such as household aerosols and solvents. However, they respond well to timely diagnosis and prevention of further exposure.
- Exposure in a group can sometimes be confused with an infectious disease.

HISTORY, CHIEF COMPLAINT
- History of suspected exposure
- Death
- Abnormal behavior

PHYSICAL EXAM FINDINGS
- Anorexia
- Lethargy
- Paralysis
- Twitching or incoordination
- Poor reproduction (reduced egg hatching)
- The most common sign is simply the finding of dead invertebrates.

ETIOLOGY AND PATHOPHYSIOLOGY
- Fipronil (Frontline) is a common cause of inadvertent captive/pet invertebrate intoxication.
  - It is a widely used agent for the control of ticks and fleas in pet dogs and cats.
  - It is also used for the control of *Ophionyssus* mites in reptiles.
  - Many invertebrate keepers also keep reptiles and may reuse reptile tanks previously treated with fipronil to house invertebrates.
  - The agent appears to be environmentally persistent, and enclosures treated with fipronil for *Ophionyssus* snake mite infestations have consistently killed adult tarantulas placed in the enclosures several months later, despite frequent washing.
- Many unproven cases of intoxication are suspected to be the result of handling of treated dogs and cats by personnel handling invertebrates or servicing invertebrate enclosures.

DIAGNOSIS

DIFFERENTIAL DIAGNOSIS
- Dehydration (see Dehydration)
- Infectious disease

INITIAL DATABASE
- History of exposure or suspected exposure to parasiticide or other chemical compound
- History of pesticide use on other animals in household or collection
- History of fumigation of neighboring house or building
- History of pesticide use in garden in vicinity
- History of crop spraying in area
- History of painting work in building (solvents)
- History of recent invertebrate handling
- History of recent cleaning of invertebrate enclosure

ADVANCED OR CONFIRMATORY TESTING
Toxicologic testing is rarely practical and often is not economically viable.

TREATMENT

THERAPEUTIC GOALS
- Provide supportive care of particularly valuable affected individuals
- Prevent further exposure to toxic compounds

ACUTE GENERAL TREATMENT
- Some cases may respond to supportive care.
- Maintain supportive heating and humidity in enclosures.
- Moribund individuals may be syringed small quantities of water or may be placed with their oral parts in shallow water containers.
- Booklungs and spiracles must not be submerged, or paralyzed individuals will drown.
- Snails may be bathed twice daily in shallow trays of warm water.
- Affected valuable tarantulas have been syringe-fed liquid (aspirated) prey invertebrate species viscera to help with longer-term recovery, although provision of food is of lower priority than administration of fluid.

PROGNOSIS AND OUTCOME
- The prognosis is guarded to poor in most cases.
- After exposure to toxic chemicals, aerosols, and solvents, individuals who show clinical signs before death may respond to supportive care and prevention of further exposure.

PEARLS & CONSIDERATIONS

COMMENTS
- Fipronil (Frontline) is one of the most common causes of inadvertent captive/pet invertebrate intoxication.
- Many unproven cases of intoxication are suspected to be the result of handling of treated dogs and cats by personnel handling invertebrates or servicing invertebrate enclosures.
- Some delicate species such as phasmids may be sensitive to paint and solvent use in the vicinity.

PREVENTION
- Unnecessary handling of pet invertebrates, especially by visitors, who may have dogs or cats, should be discouraged.
- Alternatives to fipronil-based products may be used for the control of fleas in other pets in the household.

- Avoid the use of cleaning products and disinfectants in invertebrate tanks and water dishes.

CLIENT EDUCATION

Clients should discuss their animals with neighbors, so they can be notified well in advance of any household fumigations or pesticide treatments of gardens and can plan accordingly. Some sealants and caulks used in bathrooms and kitchens contain insecticides. These must be avoided if building homemade enclosures for invertebrates.

SUGGESTED READING

Lewbart G, editor: Invertebrate medicine, Ames, 2006, Blackwell Publishing.

CROSS-REFERENCES TO OTHER SECTIONS

Dehydration

AUTHOR & EDITOR: **ROMAIN PIZZI**

INVERTEBRATES

Mites (Acarii)

BASIC INFORMATION

DEFINITION

Small free-living (saprophytic) or parasitic arthropods of the order Acarina, excluding ticks

SYNONYM

Ectoparasites

EPIDEMIOLOGY

SPECIES, AGE, SEX Any species, age, or gender

GENETICS AND BREED PREDISPOSITION Most commonly encountered on Arthropods (Crustacea, Myriapoda, Insecta, and Arachnida) and Molluscs (mainly gastropods).

RISK FACTORS

- Infrequently cleaned enclosures
- High stocking densities
- Mixing of animals from different sources
- Natural substrates in enclosures
- High humidity

CONTAGION AND ZOONOSIS Parasitic species are contagious and appear to be able to affect a wide variety of species. Most species do not appear to be zoonotic, but there is a paucity of specific data.

ASSOCIATED CONDITIONS AND DISORDERS

- Abnormal behavior of host invertebrate species
- Increased activity of some host species
- Anorexia in severe parasitic infections
- Poor growth and reproduction in colony-kept species
- Spread of pathogens and fungal spores between enclosures
- Occlusion of spiracles or booklung surfaces by large numbers of mites

CLINICAL PRESENTATION

HISTORY, CHIEF COMPLAINT Mites seen on individual animals or in enclosures by keeper

PHYSICAL EXAM FINDINGS

- Small, motile white, black, or red mites evident on specimen under magnification or on microscopic examination
- Parasitic mites commonly found in leg joints of arthropods
- Mites found at the mouthparts or on the vent are more likely to be saprophytic.

ETIOLOGY AND PATHOPHYSIOLOGY

- Parasitic mites generally feed on hemolymph, which they access with piercing mouthparts at joints and the thinner part of the cuticle.
- Parasitic mites may have a role in dysecdysis of arthropods (see Dysecdysis).
- Saprophytic mites may be present in very large numbers in larger collections or enclosures, where food residues accumulate or where cleaning is not regularly performed. Saprophytic mites may act as vectors for fungal spores.

DIAGNOSIS

DIFFERENTIAL DIAGNOSIS

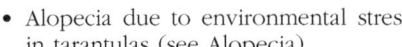

- Alopecia due to environmental stress in tarantulas (see Alopecia)
- Parasitic mites
- Saprophytic mites
- Ants (these can kill captive invertebrates in severe cases)
- Phoridae humpback flies (very small fruit flies that may also act as a vector for Panagrolaimidae nematode infections; see Panagrolaimidae Oral Nematodes in Tarantulas)
- These mechanical methods of mite removal are time consuming. In some cases anesthesia is helpful in performing mite removal with a brush or cotton tip and water based lubricant to trap the mites. Anesthesia will also slow the mites' movements, making them easier to remove.

INITIAL DATABASE

- Examination of the body surface, joints, mouthparts, and vent with magnification for the presence of mites
- Examination of the enclosure or substrate for mites under magnification

ADVANCED OR CONFIRMATORY TESTING

- Microscopy to examine the mouthpart morphology
- Parasitic mites are more likely to have piercing-type mouthparts for feeding on hemolymph.
- Saprophytic mites may have chewing or piercing mouthparts.
- Mite species identification at an agricultural research institution in economically important collections. Specimens should be preserved in 70% to 90% ethanol.

TREATMENT

THERAPEUTIC GOALS

- Eliminate parasitic mites
- Control saprophytic mite population

ACUTE GENERAL TREATMENT

- Removal of substrate and cleaning of enclosures
- Regular cleaning and removal of food residues
- Control of excessive enclosure humidity and substrate moisture
- Place double-sided sticky tape on surfaces surrounding enclosures to limit spread between individual enclosures.
- Parasitic mites may be removed from the joints of valuable individuals with careful use of sticky tape in sturdy arthropods, or in more delicate specimens with a fine-tipped artist's paintbrush and a water-based lubricant such as ultrasound gel or, less preferably, petroleum jelly (this will leave hydrophobic residues).
- Acaricides are generally toxic to the host.
- Ivermectin and an equal quantity of propylene glycol diluted 1:100 with water have been used on cloths to wipe down enclosures walls and have been applied with cotton tips to remove mites directly from limb joints in large tarantulas and arthropods without adverse effects (anecdotal reports only).

CHRONIC TREATMENT

- Commercially available predatory mites such as Hypoaspis miles (Laelapidae) sold to control fungus gnats (Scaridae) and pest thrips (Thripidae) may be used to control parasitic mites in large collections. They appear to not irritate the host invertebrates. Predatory mites will die out once all parasitic and saprophytic mites are gone, and in the event of a new mite outbreak, more predatory mites may be required.
- Isopods (wood lice) have reportedly been used in some collections of tarantulas to minimize food residues that otherwise may encourage mite proliferation.
- Hobbyists routinely microwave substrates, but care must be taken that these are nonflammable.
- Place double-sided sticky tape on surfaces surrounding enclosures to detect mites and limit spread between enclosures.

RECOMMENDED MONITORING

Monitoring of enclosure water dishes and sections of double-sided sticky tape placed around enclosures will help detect whether mites are still present in lower numbers.

PROGNOSIS AND OUTCOME

- Saprophytic mites are of little significance once numbers are reduced with good environmental hygiene.
- Elimination of parasitic mites from individual pet invertebrates is achievable but time-consuming.
- Control can be difficult in large collections, mixed herpetology collections, and old buildings, even with the use of predatory mites.

PEARLS & CONSIDERATIONS

COMMENTS

Quarantine new invertebrate arrivals for at least 1 month in collections, and examine specimens with magnification. Surround quarantine tanks with double-sided sticky tape, and change this regularly. Check water dishes for evidence of drowned mites.

CLIENT EDUCATION

Clients should be made to realize that in individual pet invertebrates, saprophytic mites are common, not zoonotic, and are easily controlled with improved enclosure hygiene.

SUGGESTED READINGS

Breene RG: The ATS arthropod medical manual: diagnosis and treatment, Carlsbad, 1998, American Tarantula Society.

Lewbart G, editor: Invertebrate medicine, Ames, 2006, Blackwell Publishing.

Schultz SA, Schultz MJ: The tarantula keeper's guide, Hauppauge, 1998, Barron's Educational Series.

West RC: Mighty mites. Journal of the British Tarantula Society 10:86–88, 1995.

CROSS-REFERENCES TO OTHER SECTIONS

Alopecia
Dysecdysis
Panagrolaimidae Oral Nematodes in Tarantulas

AUTHOR & EDITOR: **ROMAIN PIZZI**

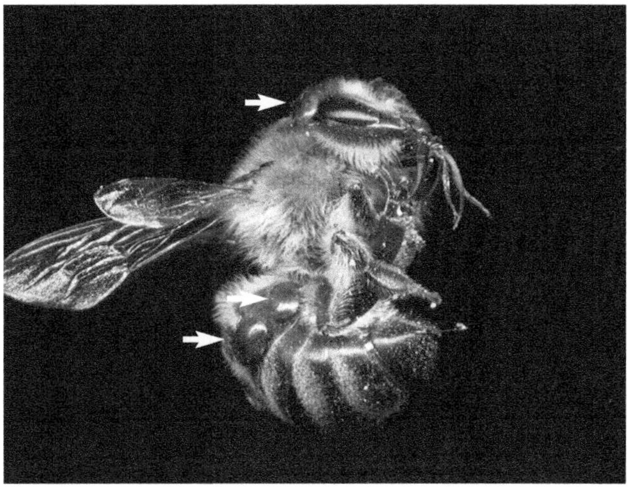

Mites (Acarii) A honey bee with three *Varroa* mites *(arrows on the body)*. Heavy infestation can cause a colony collapse.

INVERTEBRATES

Oral Nematodes (Panagrolaimidae)

BASIC INFORMATION

DEFINITION

Fatal infection of the external mouthparts and oral cavity and pharynx with entomopathogenic Rhabditida nematodes

SYNONYM

Worms

EPIDEMIOLOGY

SPECIES, AGE, SEX Tarantulas (Theraphosidae), spiders

GENETICS AND BREED PREDISPOSITION

- Reported in numerous species from Americas, Africa, and Asia
- Reported in terrestrial and arboreal species

RISK FACTORS Most common after introduction of new tarantulas from other collections

CONTAGION AND ZOONOSIS

- Transmission is so far unclear.
- Infection has been known to spread between isolated enclosures in collections.

- It has been postulated that Phoridae fungus gnats may act as mechanical vectors spreading the infection between individual spiders in separate enclosures.
- Recent work suggests that mealworm beetles *(Tenebrior mollitor)* contaminating cricket cultures could bring the parasite into tarantula collections.
- Unclear whether this is a zoonotic disease
- Closely related nematodes have been reported in difficult to treat deep or anaerobic wounds of humans and mammals.
- Caution is advised given that a bite from an infected tarantula could potentially result in a human infection.

GEOGRAPHY AND SEASONALITY Reported in both the United States and Europe

CLINICAL PRESENTATION

DISEASE FORMS/SUBTYPES Chronic

HISTORY, CHIEF COMPLAINT

- Anorexia
- Lethargy
- Abnormal posture
- Oral discharge

PHYSICAL EXAM FINDINGS

- Viscous white oral discharge between the fangs and on the chelicerae
- Spiders may have a huddled posture or may stand on "tip-toes."
- The nematodes are not usually visible with the naked eye.

ETIOLOGY AND PATHOPHYSIOLOGY

- The mode of transmission and details of the life cycle are currently unknown.
- It has been postulated that Phoridae flies and mealworm beetles may act as mechanical vectors.
- Rhabditida nematode infections are often associated with symbiotic bacterial infections.
- These symbiotic bacteria may cause tissue necrosis, aiding the feeding of the nematodes.

DIAGNOSIS

DIFFERENTIAL DIAGNOSIS

- Bacterial oral infection (see Bacterial Diseases)
- Anorexia before approaching ecdysis (normal moult) (see Dysecdysis)

INITIAL DATABASE

- Light microscopy of the oral discharge, taken by flushing and aspirating the mouth with physiologic saline. Numerous small motile nematodes are easily visible under low-power magnification.
- Bacterial culture is usually unrewarding. Mixed bacterial growth, with overgrowth of *Proteus* on the media, is common.

TREATMENT

THERAPEUTIC GOALS

- Prevent spread of infection in a collection of tarantulas
- Eliminate any zoonotic risk
- Provide humane euthanasia for the affected individual

ACUTE GENERAL TREATMENT

- Numerous treatment trials with varying dosages of benzimidazoles, avermectins, and antibiotics have proved unsuccessful in eliminating infection or prolonging survival.
- Euthanasia is strongly recommended.

RECOMMENDED MONITORING

Remaining spiders and their consumption of prey should be monitored for 3 months following an infection in a collection.

PROGNOSIS AND OUTCOME

- Prognosis is hopeless and affected spiders should be euthanized.
- Numerous treatment attempts with varying dosages of benzimidazoles, avermectins, and antibiotics have proved unsuccessful.

PEARLS & CONSIDERATIONS

COMMENTS

- Microscopy is essential with any oral discharge in a tarantula; the most common error is the presumption that this is a bacterial infection, and that only swabbing of the discharge for culture is necessary.
- What constitutes humane euthanasia in tarantulas is controversial.
  - Keepers will most commonly freeze animals.
  - Alternatives include injection of pentobarbital into the heart in the dorsal midline of the opisthosome, isoflurane anesthesia (5% to 8%) given in an induction chamber, and isoflurane administered on a cotton ball in a sealed plastic container, followed by immersion in 95% ethanol or surgical spirits (for histology) or freezing.
  - Simple immersion in ethanol is not humane, and spiders show long periods of motility after immersion.

PREVENTION

New tarantulas should be quarantined in a separate room from the main collection until confirmed as consuming prey. Avoid feeding mealworms using cricket cultures contaminated with mealworm beetles during an outbreak.

CLIENT EDUCATION

- Owner should be encouraged to quarantine new tarantulas.
- Control of humidity and ventilation discourages movement of Phoridae flies between enclosures.
- Owners should be made aware of the possible zoonotic risk of this infection, euthanasia recommended, and owners discouraged from treatment attempts.

SUGGESTED READINGS

Pizzi R: Disease management in ex-situ invertebrate conservation programs. In Fowler ME, Miller RE, editors: Zoo and wild animal medicine: current therapy 6, St Louis, 2008, Saunders Elsevier, pp 88–96.

Pizzi R: Spiders. In Lewbart G, editor: Invertebrate medicine, Ames, 2006, Blackwell Publishing, pp 143–168.

Pizzi R, Carta L, George S: Oral nematode infection of tarantulas, Vet Rec 152:695, 2003.

CROSS-REFERENCES TO OTHER SECTIONS

Bacterial Diseases
Dysecdysis

AUTHOR & EDITOR: **ROMAIN PIZZI**

Trauma

BASIC INFORMATION

DEFINITION

A wound or injury, damage caused by external force

SYNONYMS

Wound, injury

EPIDEMIOLOGY

SPECIES, AGE, SEX

- Any, but most common in
  - Large terrestrial tarantula species
  - Land snails

RISK FACTORS

- Frequent handling
- Terrestrial species (particularly tarantulas) in high-sided enclosures
- High stocking density or calcium deficiency of land snails
- Interference during ecdysis (moulting) or dysecdysis

CLINICAL PRESENTATION

HISTORY, CHIEF COMPLAINT Reported trauma or visible injury

PHYSICAL EXAM FINDINGS

- Lethargy
- Dehydration (see Dehydration)
- Wounds
- Hemorrhage of hemolymph

ETIOLOGY AND PATHOPHYSIOLOGY

- Owners and vets should not try to "help" invertebrates during ecdysis (moulting). The new cuticle is not sclerotized (hardened) to allow its expansion after ecdysis, and so it is very easily damaged, resulting in a dismembered animal (see Dysecdysis).
- Terrestrial invertebrates may climb high-sided enclosures, especially if inadequate retreats are present.
- A 30-cm fall is sufficient to kill a large terrestrial tarantula because the opisthosome has a thin cuticle that is easily ruptured.
- The hooks on the feet of tarantulas may get caught on mesh tank lids; this can cause damage to the legs of large tarantulas hanging by their feet if caught.

DIAGNOSIS

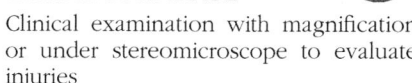

INITIAL DATABASE

Clinical examination with magnification or under stereomicroscope to evaluate injuries

TREATMENT

THERAPEUTIC GOALS

- Provide treatment dehydration for hemolymph hemorrhage (see Dehydration)
- Seal wounds and prevent further hemolymph hemorrhage
- Perform autotomy or amputation of severely damaged limbs

ACUTE GENERAL TREATMENT

- Dehydration due to hemolymph hemorrhage should be treated (see Dehydration).
- Wounds on insects and spiders should be sealed with surgical tissue adhesive, or with household superglue (both consist of cyanoacrylate) if the surgical adhesive is not available.
  - The adhesive should be allowed to dry and numerous layers applied.
  - Superglue gels, liquid skin, and spray-on permeable dressing are not sufficiently strong.
  - Sutures have no holding power in the cuticles of tarantulas, scorpions, and insects, and attempts at suturing wounds only result in increased trauma and larger wounds.
- If amputation of a limb is required in an insect, the limb should be removed by cutting through the thin joint membranes, not the cuticle of a proximal joint. The stump should be sealed with several layers of tissue adhesive.
- If a leg, a pedipalp, or chelicera needs to be removed in a tarantula because of uncontrollable hemolymph hemorrhage or a crushing injury, the limb may be autotomized.
  - The autotomized limb will regrow at the next ecdysis (moult) and will be normal sized within three ecdysis periods.
  - Regrowth will not occur in adult male tarantulas because they are terminal instars with no further ecdysis occurring.
  - Autotomy is a voluntary action; unlike a reptile, the tarantula should not be anesthetized.
- The femur segment of the limb is firmly grasped and is snapped briskly dorsally. The limb always separates between the coxa and the trochanter. Coxal apodeme fractures and joint membranes rupture under tension. Muscles inserting on the joint capsule scleritis contract, closing the joint capsule edges and limiting hemolymph hemorrhage. Several layers of tissue adhesive or superglue should always be applied to the stump to prevent later hemolymph hemorrhage.
- In nontheraphosid spiders, a second autotomy site is present between the patella and tibial segments of the limb.

RECOMMENDED MONITORING

Keep affected individuals on paper towels in a small enclosure after treatment so you can determine whether cyanoacrylate tissue adhesive or superglue has sealed wounds sufficiently, or if hemolymph hemorrhage is ongoing from an unidentified trauma site.

PROGNOSIS AND OUTCOME

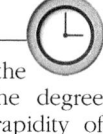

- Prognosis depends on the severity of the trauma, the degree of dehydration, and the rapidity of treatment.
- Severe cases have a poor prognosis.

PEARLS & CONSIDERATIONS

COMMENTS

Tissue adhesive or household superglue (cyanoacrylate) is essential in sealing injuries and preventing hemolymph hemorrhage. Owners with particularly valuable individuals or large collections and those in situations where invertebrates are often handled should keep this on site for first aid.

PREVENTION

- Handle invertebrates over a table to limit the height from which they may be dropped or may jump.
- A 30-cm fall may be sufficient to kill a tarantula.
- Owners and vets should not try to "help" invertebrates during ecdysis (moulting). The new cuticle is not sclerotized (hardened) and is easily torn, resulting in a dismembered animal requiring euthanasia (see Dysecdysis).

CLIENT EDUCATION

Discourage excessive or unnecessary handling of invertebrates.

SUGGESTED READINGS

Lewbart G, editor: Invertebrate medicine, Ames, 2006, Blackwell Publishing.

Pizzi R: Spiders. In Lewbart G, editor: Invertebrate medicine, Ames, 2006, Blackwell Publishing, pp 143–168.

Pizzi R, Ezendam T: So much for sutures, Forum Mag American Tarantula Society 11:122–123, 2002.
Williams DL: Invertebrates. In Meredith A, Redrobe S, editors: BSAVA manual of exotic pets, ed 4, Gloucester, 2003, BSAVA, pp 280–287.

CROSS-REFERENCES TO OTHER SECTIONS

Dehydration
Dysecdysis

AUTHOR & EDITOR: **ROMAIN PIZZI**

INVERTEBRATES

Viral Diseases

BASIC INFORMATION

DEFINITION

Viruses are submicroscopic organisms that contain genetic material surrounded by a protein coat. They require living cells for growth and replication and are thus considered infectious agents.

EPIDEMIOLOGY

SPECIES, AGE, SEX Most exotic pet species in which important viral diseases are recognized belong to the phylum Arthropoda. This excludes many well-recognized diseases of invertebrate species used in aquaculture and agriculture.
RISK FACTORS Exposure to infected conspecifics or a contaminated environment
CONTAGION AND ZOONOSIS Viral diseases of invertebrates are not known to infect or cause disease in humans.

CLINICAL PRESENTATION

DISEASE FORMS/SUBTYPES
- A large number of different viruses have been isolated from invertebrates. Some selected pathogens of species encountered by veterinarians are mentioned here.
- A baculovirus in the nursery web spider (*Pisaura mirabilis*)
- An icosahedral virus in the common yellow scorpion (*Buthus occitanus*)
- Chronic bee paralysis (CBP) in honey bees (*Apis mellifera*)
- Nuclear polyhedrosis viruses (NPVs) in lepidopterans (i.e., butterflies and moths)
- Cytoplasmic polyhedrosis viruses (CPVs) in lepidopterans

HISTORY, CHIEF COMPLAINT
- Anorexia
- Lethargy
- Depression
- Failure to thrive
- Death

PHYSICAL EXAM FINDINGS
- Baculovirus in the nursery web spider
  - None described
- Icosahedral virus in the common yellow scorpion
  - None described
- CBP in honey bees:
  - Two syndromes possible
    - "Bloated abdomen" syndrome: ascites, excessive gastrointestinal fluid excretion (dysentery), death within several days
    - "Black robber" syndrome: black and iridescent-like coloration, alopecia, not recognized by fellow colony bees, attacked and killed by conspecifics
- NPV in lepidopterans
  - Liquefaction of internal organs in larvae
  - Larvae hang head downward until skin ruptures
- CPV in lepidopterans
  - Progressive gastrointestinal failure leading to starvation in larvae
  - Regurgitation in larvae
  - Wing malformations due to dysecdysis in adults

ETIOLOGY AND PATHOPHYSIOLOGY

- Baculovirus in the nursery web spider
  - Attacked the hepatopancreas
- Icosahedral virus in the common yellow scorpion
  - Isolated virus could not be further described.
  - Caused destruction of the hepatopancreas
- CBP in honey bees
  - Single-stranded RNA virus
- NPV and CPV in lepidopterans
  - Baculoviruses
  - NPVs replicate in nuclei of the fat body, hypodermis, and ovarian tissues
  - NPVs are highly host specific
  - CPVs replicate in the cytoplasm of gastrointestinal cells.

DIAGNOSIS

DIFFERENTIAL DIAGNOSIS

- Debilitation due to inadequate or improper husbandry
- Other infectious diseases (e.g., fungal, viral, parasitic)
- Intoxication (e.g., insecticides)

ADVANCED OR CONFIRMATORY TESTING

- Light microscopy of Giemsa-stained hemolymph smears will reveal NPV (nonstaining) and CPV (deeply staining) protein crystals of 0.5-15 μm.
- Electron microscopy
- Virus isolation
- Polymerase chain reaction analysis is available for CBP.
- Biopsy or necropsy and histopathology are important for diagnosis and identification of predisposing or concurrent conditions.
- Specialized fixation techniques may be needed for histopathology.

TREATMENT

THERAPEUTIC GOALS

- Treatment of viral disease in invertebrate species is often unrewarding.
- Main goals should be containment and prevention of disease.

ACUTE GENERAL TREATMENT

- Depopulation and destruction of entire colonies may be necessary.
- Culling and/or isolation of affected individuals in colonies
- Supportive care of individuals (e.g., fluid therapy)

CHRONIC TREATMENT

- Optimization of environmental conditions and husbandry
- Reduction of stressors (e.g., decreased population density, proper grouping of animals)
- Adequate hygiene

PROGNOSIS AND OUTCOME

Most viral infections in invertebrate species have a poor to grave prognosis.

PEARLS & CONSIDERATIONS

COMMENTS

- Clinical medicine of invertebrates is a relatively new facet of the veterinary profession.
- Some invertebrate viruses, such as Iridoviruses, have been isolated from reptiles fed invertebrates.
- Diagnosis of disease conditions can be frustrating but should be pursued nonetheless.

PREVENTION

- Strict quarantine measures for incoming animals

CLIENT EDUCATION

- Quarantine for all new animal acquisitions
- Annual examinations for invertebrates
- Proper husbandry practices

SUGGESTED READINGS

Berzins IK, Smolowitz R: Diagnostic techniques and sample handling. In Lewbart GA, editor: Invertebrate medicine, Ames, 2006, Blackwell Publishing, pp 263–274.

Rivers CF: The control of diseases in insect cultures, Int Zoo Yb 30:131–137, 1991.

Williams DL: A veterinary approach to the European honey bee (*Apis mellifera*), Vet J 160:61–73, 2000.

Williams DL: Studies in arachnid disease. In Cooper JE, et al, editors: Arachnida: proceedings of a symposium on spiders and their allies, London, 1992, Chiron Publications Ltd, pp 116–125.

AUTHOR: **TREVOR T. ZACHARIAH**

EDITOR: **ROMAIN PIZZI**

FISH

Bacterial Diseases

BASIC INFORMATION

DEFINITION

Bacterial disease in fish is often caused by bacteria that are found ubiquitously in the environment and become opportunistic pathogens. Most bacterial infections are caused by Gram-negative organisms, including the genera *Aeromonas, Citrobacter, Edwardsiella, Flavobacterium, Pseudomonas,* and *Vibrio. Aeromonas* is more commonly a pathogen in freshwater fish, whereas *Vibrio* usually affects marine fish. *Streptococcus* is a Gram-positive genus that causes disease in ornamental fish.

SYNONYMS

- Gram-negative yellow-pigmented bacteria (YPB)
  - *Flavobacterium columnare* (freshwater), Columnaris disease, *Flexibacter,* "cotton wool disease," "saddleback"
  - *Flexibacter maritimus* (marine version): "black patch necrosis" or "eroded mouth syndrome"
  - Fin rot: necrosis of fins caused by various bacteria within this group, including *Cytophaga, Flexibacter,* and *Flavobacterium columnare*
- *Aeromonas salmonicida*: furunculosis, ulcer disease
- Motile aeromonad infection (MAI): caused by *Aeromonas hydrophila* complex, *Aeromonas sobria, Aeromonas caviae*; motile *Aeromonas* septicemia (MAS), "red sore"
- Vibriosis: "salt-water furunculosis," *Vibrio* infection, "Hitra" disease
- Enteric septicemia of catfish: *Edwardsiella ictaluri,* ESC
- *Mycobacterium* spp.: Mycobacteriosis is a disease in fish caused by acid-fast bacteria in the genus *Mycobacterium. M. marinum* and *M. fortuitum* are the most common species seen in fish; tuberculosis, "fish TB"
- Streptococcal bacteria: *Streptococcus, Vagococcus, Lactococcus, Enterococcus*

EPIDEMIOLOGY

SPECIES, AGE, SEX All fish of any age, sex, or size can be susceptible to bacterial disease.

GENETICS AND BREED PREDISPOSITION Specific species susceptibilities to certain bacterial infections and individual host immunity variables have been noted.

RISK FACTORS

- Stress is the most common risk factor; poor water quality is the most common stressor that can precipitate an outbreak of bacterial disease in a population of fish.
- Stress can be acute or chronic. Other stressors include shipping, handling, iatrogenic injuries, high temperatures, hypoxia, overcrowding, ectoparasites, poor nutritional status, concurrent viral disease, and predation.

CONTAGION AND ZOONOSIS

- The infectious nature of pathogens depends on bacterial virulence and host immune status/function.
- Mycobacteriosis is a zoonotic disease that can cause nonhealing ulcers (often called "fish tank granuloma") in humans. Humans with the highest risk level are those who are immune suppressed.
- *Edwardsiella tarda,* the causative agent of edwardsiellosis in channel catfish and Japanese eels, can cause enteric disease in humans; it is also implicated in meningitis, liver abscess, and wound infection in humans.
- *Streptococcus iniae,* known to infect certain fish species, has been reported as a cause of infection in humans (increased risk with immune suppression), especially if they suffer cuts or puncture wounds.
- *Vibrio* species are known to cause disease in humans, most often following ingestion of contaminated shellfish. Disease is more serious in individuals with a suppressed immune system.

GEOGRAPHY AND SEASONALITY Although some bacterial diseases are more prevalent at specific times of year, bacterial diseases can occur at any time of year and in most geographic regions. In regions that experience freezing during the winter, the incidence of bacterial infection in fish housed outdoors is very low.

CLINICAL PRESENTATION

DISEASE FORMS/SUBTYPES

- Clinical signs can be peracute, acute, or chronic.
  - Peracute: death without gross evidence of disease (e.g., systemic *Aeromonas salmonicida* infection in salmon fry)
  - Acute onset: short duration of illness
  - Chronic: slowly progressive disease; most common presentation for *Mycobacterium* infections
- Major bacterial pathogens in fish can be divided into the following groups:
  - Ulcer-forming/systemic, Gram-negative: most common groups, including *Aeromonas, Vibrio, Edwardsiella, Pseudomonas, Flavobacterium,* etc.
  - External, Gram-negative: *Flavobacterium columnare, Flexibacter maritimus,* YPB, *Cytophaga* spp., etc.
  - Systemic, Gram-positive, rapidly growing: generally systemic infections; *Streptococcus* and related species
  - Slow-growing, acid-fast bacteria: systemic, chronic, granuloma-forming; most commonly *Mycobacterium*
  - *Rickettsia/Rickettsia*-like organisms and others

HISTORY, CHIEF COMPLAINT

- Clinical signs of bacterial disease include lethargy, anorexia, abnormal

swimming patterns/spinning, hemorrhagic lesions on the skin, abdominal distention/ascites, abnormal position in the water column, exophthalmia ("pop-eye"), external ulcerative lesions, gill necrosis, and mortality.
- With gill involvement, respiratory signs such as increased opercular rate, piping (gasping for air at the water surface), and respiratory distress may be seen.
- Owners may report flashing, often associated with ectoparasites and secondary bacterial infection.
- Mycobacteriosis: Clinical signs are usually nonspecific and can include ulcerative skin lesions, reduced appetite, emaciation, lethargy, exophthalmia ("pop-eye"), swollen abdomen, and fin and tail rot. This disease usually is slowly progressive and causes low to moderate numbers of mortalities.
- Streptococcal infection can cause high mortality and typically presents with abnormal swimming behavior such as spiraling or spinning.

PHYSICAL EXAM FINDINGS
- Presentation varies with pathogen, virulence, associated diseases or conditions, stressors present, and immune status of host.
- Most common clinical findings include the following:
  - Cutaneous ulcerations, petechiation/hemorrhages, necrosis. Chronic skin lesions may be colonized by aquatic molds and algae.
  - Oral lesions (reddened tissue, exposed rostral tissue, ulcerations)
  - Ophthalmic lesions (exophthalmia, keratopathies, hyphema, uveitis, anterior lens luxation)
  - Fin and/or tail ulceration, necrosis
  - Pigmentary changes (lightening or darkening of skin)
  - Gill pathology (ragged edges of primary lamellae, hyperplasia, linear and diffuse necrosis, focal lesions) and associated respiratory signs (piping, increased opercular movements)
  - Coelomic cavity distention (ascitic fluid, organomegaly, swollen gastrointestinal tract), swollen vent
  - Motile aeromonads are the most common pathogen isolated in fish bacterial disease. They can be primary or secondary pathogens and may present as peracute, acute, or chronic disease. Cutaneous ulcers and septicemia are not uncommon.
  - Columnaris disease: perioral, periocular, fin, "saddle" region and tail lesions are common. The synonym "cotton wool" disease describes the fluffy, white cottonlike masses, patches, or plaques seen with *Flavobacterium columnare.*

ETIOLOGY AND PATHOPHYSIOLOGY
- Most secondary pathogens gain entrance through wounds created by trauma, ectoparasites, and/or loss of the protective mucous layer.
- Some bacteria gain access through the intestinal tract.

DIAGNOSIS

DIFFERENTIAL DIAGNOSIS
- *Flavobacterium* may be mistaken for fungal disease because it presents with fluffy, white, raised lesions.
- Viral infections may present with similar clinical signs. Secondary bacterial infections, however, are possible sequelae to some viral infections.
- Parasitic diseases should be ruled out.

INITIAL DATABASE
- Use laboratories that are familiar with aquatic pathogens.
- The diagnostic approach to a fish with bacterial disease should begin with complete history, water chemistry (temperature, salinity, pH, ammonia, nitrites, nitrates, alkalinity, dissolved oxygen), and thorough evaluation of the environment/husbandry.
- Direct observation of the fish in the aquarium or pond
- Complete physical examination
- Skin scrapings
  - Columnaris disease: Diagnosis typically is based on clinical presentation and wet mount examination, revealing characteristic "haystack" protrusions of rod-shaped bacteria.
- Gill snip/scrape
- Culture and sensitivity of ulcers, areas of necrosis (fin rot, mouth rot)
  - Perform culture at room temperature.
  - Request sensitivity patterns for desired medications (enrofloxacin, ceftazidime, etc.).
  - When culturing wounds, tissue cultures obtained aseptically are superior to superficial swabs.
- Cytologic examination of wounds (Diff-Quik and Gram staining)

ADVANCED OR CONFIRMATORY TESTING
- Definitive diagnosis of bacterial disease requires culture and identification of the bacterium.
- Blood culture (nonlethal diagnostic technique)
- Systemic bacterial disease: The organ of choice for bacterial culture/sensitivity is the posterior kidney. Other organs that are cultured include the brain (especially when neurologic signs are present), liver, spleen, and anterior kidney. Moribund fish showing clinical signs should be selected.
- A survival procedure in which the posterior kidney is aspirated and cultured has been described.
- Necropsy/Histopathology
  - Results depend on the bacterial pathogen and organ affected.
  - Mycobacteriosis: Internal organs (kidney, spleen, liver, heart muscle) are usually affected with numerous granulomas. The skin and gills may also be affected. These granulomas may be visible grossly or on wet mount examinations. Once granulomas are seen, an acid-fast stain should be performed. Diagnosis is based on clinical signs, the presence of granulomas, and demonstration of acid-fast bacterial rods in tissues. Culture of these bacteria can be difficult and lengthy.
- Response to therapy

TREATMENT

THERAPEUTIC GOALS
- Control bacterial pathogen
- Eliminate stressors such as poor water quality, overcrowding, whenever possible
- Eliminate secondary parasitic or fungal disease

ACUTE GENERAL TREATMENT
- Correcting environmental abnormalities and removing stressors (poor water quality, other pathogens) are critical steps in decreasing morbidity/mortality.
- Antimicrobials can be administered parenterally, orally, or as a bath.
- Antimicrobial therapy: parenteral
  - Parenteral administration of antibiotics is the most effective method of achieving therapeutic levels. With a large number of fish affected, individual injections may not be practical or financially feasible.
  - Empirical first choice should be effective against Gram-negative bacteria (most common isolates):
    - Examples include enrofloxacin 5-10 mg/kg IM or IC q 3-5 days; ceftazidime 20 mg/kg IM q 3 days
  - Response to therapy is typically seen within 72 hours.
  - Continued therapy should be based on sensitivity data.
- Antimicrobial therapy: orally administered
  - Oral administration of medications is effective only in fish not demonstrating anorexia.
  - Two Food and Drug Administration (FDA)-approved products are available for use in food fish (catfish and salmonids): Terramycin for Fish (oxytetracycline; Pfizer Animal Health, Exton, Pennsylvania) and

Romet-30 (ormetroprim: sulfadimethoxine; Hoffman-LaRoche Inc., Nutley, New Jersey). Both are available over the counter. The withdrawal period for fish fed Terramycin is at least 21 days. The withdrawal period for Romet in catfish is 3 days, and in salmonids 6 weeks.
  - Medication can be added to food. The amount to be added should be calculated by the estimated rate of food consumption by the fish. The range for food consumption is between 1% and 5% of body weight. Fish that are partially anorexic should be dosed at the low end (1%).
  - Antibiotics may be added to the food. This can be accomplished by using a binding agent such as fish or canola oil.
  - Homemade diets or Mazuri aquatic gel diets are convenient for making small batches of food for a single fish or for small groups of fish. Most fish find the commercial gel diets palatable.
  - Extra-label use of antimicrobials on or in animal feeds is prohibited by federal regulations. However, the FDA has published a Compliance Policy Guide (CPG) that details specific conditions under which the agency will not take enforcement action regarding the extra-label use of certain medicated feeds in aquatic animal species ("Extra-label Use of Medicated Feeds for Minor Species, CPG 615-115"). The clinician should be aware of these and any future regulations and guidelines. For more current information, check the FDA website (www.fda.gov/cvm, aquaculture section).
- Bath antibiotics (prolonged immersion therapy) see Sec. II: Tank Pond Therapy
  - Administration of antibiotics in water is commonplace in the aquarium industry. Problems encountered include limited absorption/insufficient dose, damage to the biofilter, and bacterial resistance.
  - Pharmacokinetic data for bath antibiotics are limited. Antibiotics added to water generally are more effective in marine systems. Freshwater fish do not consume much water so are unlikely to receive a therapeutic dose.
  - Bath antibiotics should be limited to cases of external infection (such as Columnaris disease and "fin rot") and to fish that are anorexic. Fish should be switched to oral antibiotics when they resume eating.
  - 75% to 100% water changes should be performed after treatments.
  - The addition of salt at 0.1% to 0.3% in the water of salt-tolerant species may be helpful in reducing osmotic stress and as an aid in healing. Salt can be used with most treatments.
- Topical therapy
  - For external lesions such as superficial or deep ulcerations
  - The authors have used silver sulfadiazine, triple antibiotic ointment, and several other common topical ointments found in veterinary hospitals.
  - Tricide or Tricide Neo (Molecular Therapeutics LLC, Athens, Georgia), available as a powder, can be prepared according to label directions and sprayed topically once daily or used as a dip once daily to aid in healing.
  - Caution should be exercised if topical medications containing corticosteroids are used because they may retard healing.
- *Flavobacterium columnare*
  - Antibiotic bath treatments:
    - Oxytetracycline: 750-3780 mg per 10 gallons for 6-12 hours, repeat daily for 10 days (dose will depend on hardness of water)
  - Potassium permanganate can be administered as a prolonged bath at 2 mg/L.
  - Diquat herbicide (Reward): 2-18 mg/L, 4-hour bath immersions. Repeat daily for 3-4 treatments; large water changes should be performed after bath treatment.
  - Systemic antibiotic therapy may be needed in cases of more severe infection.
- *Streptococcus*
  - Antibiotics that may be effective against *Streptococcus* include erythromycin (1.5 g/lb of food fed for 10-14 days).
  - Other effective antibiotics against *Streptococcus* include amoxicillin/ampicillin and florfenicol.
- Mycobacteriosis:
  - No effective treatment is known for mycobacteriosis in fish. Depopulation of infected fish and disinfection of systems are recommended. Mycobacteria are sensitive to 60% to 85% alcohol. As much as 10,000 ppm chlorine has been reported necessary to kill mycobacteria.
  - Various antibiotics such as rifampicin, erythromycin, streptomycin, kanamycin, doxycycline, and minocycline have been suggested as possible treatments, but a clinical cure is unlikely.

POSSIBLE COMPLICATIONS

Adverse effects can occur in numerous species. A biotest may be performed on a small number of representative fish before widespread usage.

PROGNOSIS AND OUTCOME

- Mycobacteriosis carries a grave prognosis, and no effective treatment is known.
- If environmental/husbandry corrections are made and infections are caught early, the prognosis can be favorable (especially with external/superficial infections).
- With poor environmental conditions and systemic infection, significant mortality may occur.

PEARLS & CONSIDERATIONS

COMMENTS

- Cultures should be interpreted carefully.
- Cultures may grow a secondary pathogen and miss a primary one owing to incorrect specimen handling.
- Inexperienced laboratories may report incorrect names for bacteria cultured.
- Sensitivity patterns often are most important in efficacious treatment of bacterial disease.
- Enteric coliforms can be cultured from cutaneous ulcers found in pet fish. These generally are not associated with fish gastrointestinal flora but more often result from contamination of the environment by other species, including humans.
- It is very common for some ornamental pet fish owners to obtain antimicrobials without a veterinary prescription and at improper doses/duration. Be sure to inquire what treatments have been attempted and what dosages have been used.
- Most bacterial infections can be managed with a single antibiotic, and combining antibiotics is not recommended.
- Many antibiotics commonly used for ornamental fish are sold by different companies; therefore, the percent of active ingredient may vary.

PREVENTION

- Maintain best management practices for feeding, stocking density, water quality, and other environmental concerns.
- Buy fish from a reputable source.
- Vaccinations may be available for some pathogens, such as *Aeromonas salmonicida*. These vaccines have not been found to be as effective as bacterins for other diseases.
- Quarantine new fish (minimum 4 weeks), and promptly evaluate and treat any problems that may arise.
- Avoid "shotgun" or "polypharmacy" treatments without valid indications.

- Antimicrobial resistance can be a problem in certain strains of bacteria. Judicious use and appropriate dosing of antibiotics can help to minimize resistance patterns.

CLIENT EDUCATION

- Finish all medications as prescribed.
- Do not alter the dose or dosing frequency without consulting the veterinarian.
- Monitor water quality with regular testing to minimize stress on recovering fish and as an aid in reducing the incidence of future outbreaks.

SUGGESTED READINGS

Food and Drug Administration (FDA): Judicious use of antimicrobials for aquatic veterinarians, informational booklet, Rockville, Md, 2006, FDA Center for Veterinary Medicine.

Klinger R, et al: Use of blood culture as a nonlethal method for isolating bacteria from fish, J Zoo Wildl Med 34:206–207, 2003.

Noga EJ: Fish disease: diagnosis and treatment, St Louis, 1996, Mosby.

Wildgoose WH: BSAVA manual of ornamental fish, ed 2, Gloucester, 2001, British Small Animal Veterinary Association.

Yanong R: Use of antibiotics in ornamental fish aquaculture, VM-84, Florida Cooperative Extension Service, UF-IFAS, 2006. http://edis.ifas.ufl.edu.

CROSS-REFERENCES TO OTHER SECTIONS

Sec. II: Tank Pond Therapy

AUTHORS: **HELEN E. ROBERTS AND BRIAN S. PALMEIRO**

EDITOR: **HELEN E. ROBERTS**

FISH

Dropsy

BASIC INFORMATION

DEFINITION

Dropsy is an edematous condition of fish in which excessive fluid accumulates in the coelomic cavity and cutaneous tissues.

SYNONYMS

Ascites, "pine-cone" disease, edema

EPIDEMIOLOGY

SPECIES, AGE, SEX Dropsy is seen predominantly in freshwater fish.

RISK FACTORS Poor environmental conditions (crowding, poor water quality) or other stressors (recent shipment/handling, poor nutrition, etc.) may predispose fish to dropsy.

ASSOCIATED CONDITIONS AND DISORDERS Retrobulbar accumulation of fluid may produce unilateral or bilateral exophthalmos.

CLINICAL PRESENTATION

HISTORY, CHIEF COMPLAINT

- The owner will notice abdominal distention and protrusion of the scales.
- Other clinical signs include lethargy and anorexia.

PHYSICAL EXAM FINDINGS

- Symmetric abdominal distention
- Symmetric scale elevation
- Exophthalmos

ETIOLOGY AND PATHOPHYSIOLOGY

- Dropsy can be caused by any condition that causes osmoregulatory dysfunction.
- Tissue damage to the gills, heart, liver, or kidneys may result in organ failure, disruption of normal osmoregulation, and development of edema and/or ascites.
- Systemic bacterial infection (*Aeromonas*, mycobacteriosis, etc.) is one of the most common causes of dropsy in ornamental fish.
- Viral and parasitic infections can cause dropsy.
- Neoplasia causes dropsy in older fish.

DIAGNOSIS

DIFFERENTIAL DIAGNOSIS

- Differential diagnoses include other causes of abdominal distention such as neoplasia, egg binding, granulomas, cysts (e.g., polycystic kidney disease), and obesity. In these cases, abdominal distention is due to mass effect, not to fluid accumulation/edema. Some of these differentials may cause organ dysfunction and may result in dropsy.
- Ectoparasites may cause elevated scales; however, fish with ectoparasites do not typically have bilaterally symmetric scale elevation or abdominal distention.

INITIAL DATABASE

- The diagnostic approach to a fish with dropsy should begin with complete history, water chemistry (temperature, salinity, pH, ammonia, nitrites, nitrates, alkalinity, dissolved oxygen), and thorough evaluation of the environment/husbandry.
- Direct observation of the fish in the aquarium or pond
- Complete physical examination
- Skin scraping and gill biopsy wet mounts should be performed to check for the presence of parasites and/or other abnormalities.
- Fecal examination should be performed to rule out intestinal parasitism.
- Imaging
  - Radiography is useful to rule out other potential causes of abdominal distention such as neoplasia, egg binding, and gas accumulation in the gastrointestinal tract. If ascites is present, radiographs will reveal loss of serosal detail or a "ground glass" appearance.
  - Dental radiographs can be used in smaller patients.
  - Ultrasound examination is very useful to evaluate for the presence of fluid and to rule out other coelomic abnormalities.
- A sterile sample of coelomic fluid should be obtained for cytologic examination, acid-fast stain, and culture/sensitivity.
- Clinical pathology is useful in some cases, but the veterinarian is often limited by patient size and lack of reference intervals.

ADVANCED OR CONFIRMATORY TESTING

- Advanced imaging such as computed tomography (CT) and coelioscopy may be useful in some cases.
- For cases in which systemic bacterial disease is suspected, a bacterial culture/sensitivity should be performed. The organ of choice for bacterial culture/sensitivity is the posterior kidney. Moribund fish showing clinical signs should be selected.
  - A survival procedure in which the posterior kidney is aspirated and cultured has been described.
  - Blood culture (nonlethal diagnostic technique)
- Necropsy/histopathology may be needed to determine the underlying cause of dropsy in some cases.

TREATMENT

THERAPEUTIC GOALS

- Improve environmental conditions/husbandry
- Decrease osmotic stress
- Treat underlying cause

ACUTE GENERAL TREATMENT

- The husbandry should be improved by maintaining excellent water quality, performing frequent water changes, and reducing overcrowding.
- The addition of salt at 0.1% to 0.3% in the water of salt-tolerant species may be helpful in reducing osmotic stress.
- Systemic bacterial infections should be treated with oral or parenteral antibiotics (see Bacterial Diseases).
- Furosemide can be administered at 2-5 mg/kg IM q 12-72 hours.
  - The value of furosemide is questionable in fish because they lack a loop of Henle.

PROGNOSIS AND OUTCOME

The prognosis for dropsy is poor, and affected fish do not typically respond to treatment.

PEARLS & CONSIDERATIONS

COMMENTS

- Systemic bacterial infection is the most common cause of dropsy in young fish, whereas neoplasia is a common cause in older fish.
- If numerous fish are affected, an infectious origin (bacterial, viral, parasitic) is most likely. Diagnostics tests (wet mounts, bacterial culture/susceptibility, and necropsy/histopathology) should be performed to establish the underlying cause and to determine appropriate treatment.

SUGGESTED READINGS

Noga EJ: Fish disease: diagnosis and treatment, St Louis, 1996, Mosby.
Reavill D: Generalized edema of a lionhead goldfish (*Carassius auratus*), Mystic, Conn, 1994, Proceedings International Association of Aquatic Animal Medicine.
Wildgoose WH: BSAVA manual of ornamental fish, ed 2, Gloucester, 2001, British Small Animal Veterinary Association.

CROSS-REFERENCES TO OTHER SECTIONS

Bacterial Diseases

AUTHOR: **BRIAN S. PALMEIRO**

EDITOR: **HELEN E. ROBERTS**

FISH

Ectoparasites, Crustacean

BASIC INFORMATION

DEFINITION

Macroscopic parasites found on the skin, gills, and fins of marine and freshwater fish

SYNONYMS

Copepods, fish louse (*Argulus* spp.), anchor worm (*Lernaea* spp.), gill maggots (*Ergasilus* spp.), isopods (*Gnathia*)

EPIDEMIOLOGY

SPECIES, AGE, SEX Species susceptibility varies. Most affected fish are in outdoor ponds.

RISK FACTORS

- Outdoor housing (ponds, vats, and tanks)
- Failure to quarantine and critically evaluate new fish

CONTAGION AND ZOONOSIS Most of the crustacean parasites have a direct life cycle. There is no zoonotic potential.

GEOGRAPHY AND SEASONALITY No specific season or geographic locations, although parasites may become more problematic during warmer months.

ASSOCIATED CONDITIONS AND DISORDERS Retrobulbar accumulation of fluid may produce unilateral or bilateral exophthalmos.

CLINICAL PRESENTATION

HISTORY, CHIEF COMPLAINT Owner may report "dark spots," "moving color patches or freckles," and/or flashing behavior.

PHYSICAL EXAM FINDINGS

- Parasites are visible to the naked eye.
- Secondary irritation/inflammation or infection may also be present. Cutaneous ulcers may be seen as sequelae to the parasites.

ETIOLOGY AND PATHOPHYSIOLOGY

In most cases of crustacean parasite infestation, damage is done to the epithelium by the mechanical attachment of the parasites as they embed in the fish body wall (Lernaeids) and by parasite feeding behavior.

DIAGNOSIS

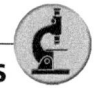

DIFFERENTIAL DIAGNOSIS

Each parasite is unique and should not be mistaken for any other condition.

INITIAL DATABASE

- Visual identification on physical examination
- Low-power (4× objective) microscopic visualization

TREATMENT

THERAPEUTIC GOAL

Control and remove parasites

ACUTE GENERAL TREATMENT

- Organophosphates (OPs) such as trichlorfon (Masoten 80% powder, Neguvon 8% solution, Bayer AG, Barmen, Germany; and several over-the-counter [OTC] products), dichlorvos
  - Prolonged immersion: trichlorfon 0.25 mg/L (0.94 mg/gal) fresh water
    - For *Lernaea:* Treat every 7 days for 1 month.
    - For *Argulus:* One treatment may be sufficient.
  - Bath treatment for Isopods: 2-5 mg/L trichlorfon for 60 minutes
    - Aeration should be provided during treatment.
    - Observe fish for stress and other adverse reactions; remove to clean, aerated water promptly if noted.
  - Fenthion (Spotton, Bayer AG) has been reported as a successful treatment in some ornamental fish species.
  - OPs can be highly toxic to some species of fish (e.g., orfe) and should not be used in species with known sensitivities. Those species should be removed from the environment during treatment and treated with a different medication in a mixed population tank or pond.
  - Resistance has been documented in some parasites.
  - OPs can also be toxic to humans.
- Chitin inhibitors such as diflubenzuron (Dimilin, Union Carbide Company, Brown Brook, New Jersey); PondCare

(Dimilin Aquarium Pharmaceuticals, Chalfont, Pennsylvania; sales restricted in Canada and New Hampshire); and lufenuron (Program, Novartis Animal Health, Basel, Switzerland)
  - Prolonged immersion: difluorobenzuron 0.03-0.06 mg/L (0.11 mg/gal); lufenuron dose anecdotally reported at rate of one crushed 409.8-mg tablet/1000 gal.
  - Chitin inhibitors are toxic to nonparasitic aquatic invertebrates and crustaceans found in freshwater ornamental fish ponds (dragonflies, etc.).
  - Difluorobenzuron and lufenuron are not licensed for use in aquaculture. Dimilin is a restricted-use pesticide.
  - Run off will damage wild crustaceans, and water should not be allowed to drain into natural water bodies.
- Manual removal of parasites
  - Anchor worms and fish lice can be mechanically removed. Wounds must be treated accordingly and monitored for secondary infection. (See Trauma and Wound Management.)
  - Anchor worms can be grasped and gently teased from the body wall at the point of insertion. Lice can be gently removed.
  - Mechanical removal will not eliminate the parasite from the environment, and parasites may be missed on some fish.

DRUG INTERACTIONS

A biotest may be performed on a small sample of fish when organophosphate therapy is considered.

POSSIBLE COMPLICATIONS

- Toxic neurologic effects of OPs
- Death of desired aquatic invertebrates and crustaceans
- Legal issues with unlicensed use of Dimilin

RECOMMENDED MONITORING

Examine all new fish during the quarantine period.

PROGNOSIS AND OUTCOME

Usually favorable

PEARLS & CONSIDERATIONS

COMMENTS

- *Argulus* spp. are sometimes difficult to see on dark fish but are very apparent on light-colored or white fish.
- Some clients may report seeing "sticks" protruding from the body of the fish. These are most likely *Lernaea* spp. (anchor worms).

PREVENTION

- Physical examination and quarantine of new fish
- Disinfection/treatment of new plants, previously used equipment

CLIENT EDUCATION

Examine all new fish closely while in quarantine.

SUGGESTED READINGS

Noga EJ: Fish disease: diagnosis and treatment, St Louis, 1996, Mosby.

Saint-Erne N: Advanced koi care: for veterinarians and professional koi keepers, Glendale, Ariz, 2002, Erne Enterprises.

Wildgoose WH: BSAVA manual of ornamental fish, ed 2, Gloucester, 2001, British Small Animal Veterinary Association.

CROSS-REFERENCES TO OTHER SECTIONS

Trauma and Wound Management

AUTHOR & EDITOR: **HELEN E. ROBERTS**

FISH

Flukes (Monogenean Parasites)

BASIC INFORMATION

DEFINITION

Monogeneans are a group of metazoan parasites that commonly infect the skin and gills of marine and freshwater fish. More than 100 families (approximately 1500 species) of monogeneans may affect fish.

SYNONYMS

Flukes (skin or gill), capsalids (marine species)

EPIDEMIOLOGY

SPECIES, AGE, SEX

- Any fish can be susceptible.
- In one report, monogeneans were commonly found affecting goldfish, *Otocinclus,* Decker Cory catfish, rainbowfish, spotted and figure eight puffers, and Raphael catfish.

RISK FACTORS Poor environmental conditions (crowding, poor water quality) or other stressors (recent shipment/handling, poor nutrition, etc.) may predispose fish to infection.

CLINICAL PRESENTATION

HISTORY, CHIEF COMPLAINT

- Monogeneans typically infest the skin and gills.
- Clinical signs include lethargy, decreased appetite, flashing (rubbing against objects in the pond/aquarium), and excessive production of mucus (from gills or skin).
- When branchial infestations are present, respiratory signs such as increased opercular rate, piping (gasping for air at the water surface), and respiratory distress may be seen.
- Heavy infestation can cause mortality.

PHYSICAL EXAM FINDINGS

- Dermatologic abnormalities include erythema, scale loss, white to gray irregular patches, excessive production of mucus, hemorrhages, erosions, and ulcerations.
- Ophthalmic lesions such as corneal edema can be seen if the parasite affects the corneal epithelium (most commonly seen with *Neobenedenia melleni*).
- Secondary bacterial and fungal infections may be present in areas parasitized by monogeneans.

ETIOLOGY AND PATHOPHYSIOLOGY

- Monogeneans of the genera *Dactylogyrus* and *Gyrodactylus* commonly affect freshwater fish. *Dactylogyrus* predominantly affects the gills, whereas *Gyrodactylus* is more commonly found on the skin.
- Monogeneans affecting marine fish include the capsalids; species such as *Benedenia* and *Neobenedenia* can infest the skin and gills.
- Life cycles: Monogeneans may be oviparous (egg laying) or viviparous (live bearers). Transmission of monogeneans from fish to fish occurs primarily via direct contact. Most monogeneans have direct life cycles. Oviparous monogeneans (Dactylogyridae) release eggs into the water, which hatch into a free-swimming stage (oncomiracidium) that seeks out a fish host. Viviparous monogeneans

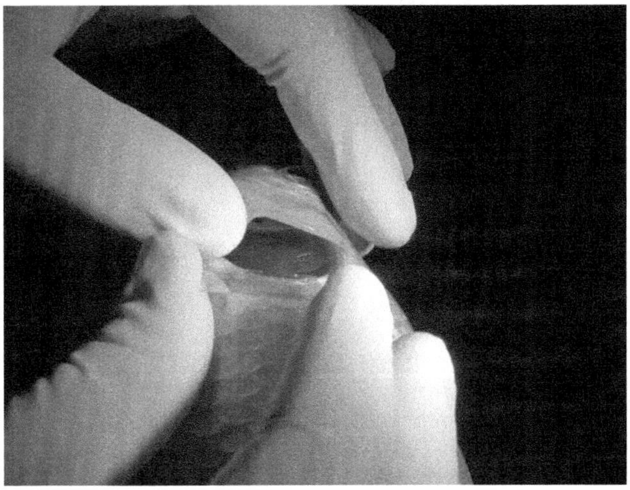

Flukes (Monogenean Parasites) The use of a coverslip to obtain a gill tissue sample for wet mount cytologic examination. *(Courtesy Helen E. Roberts.)*

(Gyrodactylidae) release live larvae that are immediately parasitic.
- Viviparous monogeneans can achieve rapid increases in population with doubling times as short as 24 hours.

DIAGNOSIS

DIFFERENTIAL DIAGNOSIS

Other parasitic infestations, bacterial disease, fungal disease, viral disease, environmental causes of hypoxia (decreased dissolved oxygen, ammonia toxicity, nitrite toxicity, etc.)

INITIAL DATABASE

- The diagnostic approach to a fish with monogeneans should begin with complete history, water chemistry (temperature, salinity, pH, ammonia, nitrites, nitrates, alkalinity, dissolved oxygen), and thorough evaluation of the environment/husbandry.
- Direct observation of the fish in the aquarium or pond
- Complete physical examination
- Definitive diagnosis can be made with wet mounts of the skin or gills.
- Monogeneans are identified on the morphology of the posterior attachment organ (opisthaptor), the mode of reproduction, and the presence/absence of eye spots.
- Monogeneans have a classic jerking, caterpillar-like motion, in which the parasite stretches and recoils.
- Monogeneans affecting freshwater fish can be easily differentiated via light microscopy. *Gyrodactylus* are live bearing and commonly contain intrauterine developing embryos. They do not have eye spots and are found primarily on the skin/fins. *Dactylogyrus* are oviparous and therefore lack developing embryos. They have pigmented light receptors ("eye spots") and are predominantly found on the gills.
- *Neobenedenia* and *Benedenia* are large and are typified by a large, circular opisthaptor on the posterior end and two smaller suckers on the anterior end. *Benedenia* has two pairs of tightly apposed, curved anchors, whereas *Neobenedenia* has three pairs.

ADVANCED OR CONFIRMATORY TESTING

Histopathology is not typically needed for diagnosis. However, sections of monogeneans can be seen on histopathologic examination of the skin and gills.

TREATMENT

THERAPEUTIC GOALS

- Improve environmental conditions
- Control parasites

ACUTE GENERAL TREATMENT

- **Husbandry**
  - Correcting environmental abnormalities and removing stressors (poor water quality) are critical steps in decreasing morbidity/mortality and preventing disease.
  - In oviparous infestations, the water temperature can be increased to hasten the egg incubation rate.
  - Biological control may be helpful in some marine aquaria. "Cleaner fish" such as French angelfish, neon gobies, and Pacific cleaner wrasse may remove parasites from other fish.
- **Medical treatments**
  - Praziquantel is extremely efficacious for both marine and freshwater monogeneans. Dosage: 2 mg/L (ppm). Concentrations up to 10 mg/L have been used successfully and safely in many species of ornamental fish. Praziquantel has few, if any, negative effects on biofiltration.
  - Organophosphates (OPs) such as trichlorfon can be extremely effective for monogeneans. Trichlorfon dosage: 0.25-0.75 mg/L (ppm). As with other products, the fish should be monitored for potential side effects (neurotoxicity may occur with OPs).
  - Formalin (37% formaldehyde) can be administered as a long-term bath at 25 mg/L or as a short-term bath (up to 60 minutes) at 150-250 mg/L. Caution should be taken when treating sick fish with formalin (especially with the short-term bath). Formalin can negatively impact the biofilter and can decrease dissolved oxygen concentrations. The water should be aerated well because each 5 mg/L of formalin added chemically removes 1 mg/L of dissolved oxygen.
  - Potassium permanganate can be administered as a prolonged bath at 2 mg/L.
  - A combination of clostanel (5 mg/mL) and mebendazole (75 mg/mL) (Supaverm, Janssen Animal Health, Beerse, Belgium) has anecdotally been reported to be very effective for treating monogeans in koi (*Cyprinus carpio*). However, this product is uniformly toxic to goldfish, and 100% mortality is expected. The reported dose is 1 mL/400 L. Salt reportedly enhances efficacy.
  - Mebendazole: 1 mg/L
  - Copper treatments applied at 0.2 mg/L can be used to control monogeneans in marine systems. Copper is not safe with certain fish (elasmobranchs) and is toxic to invertebrates. Copper should not be

used in freshwater systems. Copper levels should be monitored daily.
  - Freshwater (for marine fish) and saltwater (for freshwater fish) dips can be performed before fish are introduced into a new system; these dips work best on small monogenean species.
  - A critical step in treating monogeneans is determining whether the monogenean is viviparous or oviparous; the eggs of many monogeneans (*Dactylogyrus*, capsalids) are resistant to treatment. In these cases, several treatments may be required for control. The author treats weekly for 4 treatments, followed by a recheck of wet mount examinations.

DRUG INTERACTIONS

Do not mix formalin and potassium permanganate in the same system.

POSSIBLE COMPLICATIONS

Adverse effects can occur in numerous species. A biotest may be employed on a small number of representative fish before widespread usage.

RECOMMENDED MONITORING

- Wet mount examinations (skin and gills) should be performed routinely to determine response to treatment.
- In large systems/public marine aquaria, ova counts have been used (via 0.1-micron mesh screens on skimmers) to determine infection rates and efficacy of treatment.

PROGNOSIS AND OUTCOME

- If environmental/husbandry corrections are made and infestations are caught early, the prognosis is good.
- With poor environmental conditions and heavy infestations, significant mortality may occur.

PEARLS & CONSIDERATIONS

COMMENTS

The eggs of oviparous monogeneans are very resistant to treatment, and several treatments are usually necessary for control.

PREVENTION

- Provide good husbandry and water quality.
- Reduce crowding.
- Quarantine new fish for a minimum of 4 weeks.

SUGGESTED READINGS

Reed P, Francis-Floyd R, Klinger RE: Monogenean parasites of fish, FA-28, Gainesville, Fla, 2002, Florida Cooperative Extension Service, UF-IFAS. http://edis.ifas.ufl.edu.

Noga EJ: Fish disease: diagnosis and treatment, St Louis, 1996, Mosby.

Wildgoose WH: BSAVA manual of ornamental fish, ed 2, Gloucester, 2001, British Small Animal Veterinary Association.

AUTHOR: **BRIAN S. PALMEIRO**

EDITOR: **HELEN E. ROBERTS**

FISH

Fungal Diseases

BASIC INFORMATION

DEFINITION

Most fungal diseases in pet fish and fish eggs are secondary, opportunistic infections that can be found in fish weakened by stress, epithelial injury, and bacterial, viral, or parasitic disease. Rarely, a fungal pathogen can act as a primary pathogen. Most fungal disease in fish is caused by members of the Saprolegniaceae family (*Saprolegnia* spp., *Achyla* spp., and *Aphanomyces* spp.), *Ichthyophonus*, and *Dermocystidium*.

SYNONYMS

- *Saprolegnia* spp.: "Winter kill," saprolegniasis in channel catfish
- *Branchiomyces* spp.: branchiomycosis, *Branchiomyces demigrans*, gill rot
- *Aphanomyces* spp.: mycotic granulomatosis (MG, Japan), red spot disease (RSD, Australia), epizootic ulcerative syndrome (Asia), ulcerative mycosis (United States), and atypical water mold
- *Ichthyophonus hoferi*: ichthyosporidiosis, ichthyophoniasis

EPIDEMIOLOGY

SPECIES, AGE, SEX

- Any fish (species, age, sex, etc.) can be susceptible. Fungal infection can be found in farmed and wild species; cold water, temperate, and warm water species worldwide.
- Saprolegniasis and *Aphanomyces*: reported in freshwater and brackish species

GENETICS AND BREED PREDISPOSITION

- Tilapia are considered immune to *Aphanomyces* infection; goldfish, *Carassius auratus*, are more susceptible to certain strains.
- Cyprinids, sticklebacks, and eels, seem more susceptible than other species to branchiomycosis.
- *Ichthyophonus hoferi* is observed mainly in marine fish and estuarine fish but has been documented in freshwater species. Infection has been reported in more than 80 species. Goldfish seem to be immune, based on experimentally induced infection.

RISK FACTORS Stress, poor water quality, high organic load in ponds, epithelial injury, water temperature changes, concurrent parasitic, viral, and/or bacterial infections that lead to immune suppression in host animals

CONTAGION AND ZOONOSIS Infection of eggs by *Saprolegnia* spp. is spread from infected infertile and decaying eggs to viable eggs by close or direct contact.

GEOGRAPHY AND SEASONALITY

- In outdoor ponds, an increase in saprolegniasis infection can be seen in the cooler months. *Aphanomyces* outbreaks can occur following water temperature drops.
- The occurrence of branchiomycosis outbreaks increases in ponds with high organic matter, high stocking densities, and high water temperatures 68°F to 77°F (20°C to 25°C).
- *Dermocystidium koi* infections may be observed more frequently when water temperatures are between 63°F and 72°F (17°C and 22°C).

ASSOCIATED CONDITIONS AND DISORDERS Poor water quality; overcrowding; parasitic, viral, and bacterial infections; water temperature changes; excessive use of chemotherapeutics; and any condition that causes epithelial injury or disruption such as rough handling.

CLINICAL PRESENTATION

DISEASE FORMS/SUBTYPES Fungal diseases can occur acutely with high mortality but with chronic duration and frequent recurrences.

ETIOLOGY AND PATHOPHYSIOLOGY

- *Saprolegnia* spp. spores attach to damaged epithelial tissue and mucous layer.
- Hyphal growth of *Branchiomyces* is intravascular, causing infarcts and necrosis of gill tissue.
- *Aphanomyces* spp. spores geminate and can invade the body cavity and internal organs.
- *Ichthyophonus* infections are thought to be transmitted by spore ingestion. The practice of feeding raw fish and raw fish products is thought to spread the disease.

DIAGNOSIS

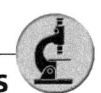

DIFFERENTIAL DIAGNOSIS

- Saprolegniasis: The fluffy, white, cottony appearance may be confused with infection caused by *Flavobacterium columnare.* Wet mount cytology can be used to differentiate.
- *Aphanomyces* infection presenting with cutaneous ulcers may be confused with bacterial ulcers.
- Branchiomycosis: Cytology of affected gill tissue will differentiate from other causes of gill disease, including bacterial gill disease and Cyprinid herpes virus-3 (KHV).
- Skin lesions due to *Dermocystidium* spp. can resemble other diseases known to cause raised nodular skin lesions.

INITIAL DATABASE

- The diagnostic approach to a fish with bacterial disease should begin with complete history, water chemistry (temperature, salinity, pH, ammonia, nitrites, nitrates, alkalinity, dissolved oxygen), and thorough evaluation of the environment/husbandry.
- Direct observation of fish in the aquarium or pond
- Complete physical examination
  - Saprolegniasis:
    - Characteristic superficial, fluffy, white or gray cottonlike growth on skin or eggs
    - Lesions often start at head or on fins of affected fish.
    - Secondary algal growth and debris contamination may be seen on fungal lesions, giving the lesions an overall green, brown, or red fluffy appearance.
    - "Winter kill" is saprolegniasis seen in channel catfish when pond temperatures rapidly drop to below 15°C (59°F). Lesions include endophthalmia, skin feeling rough or "dry" due to loss of protective mucous coating, and proliferative fungal patches on skin.
  - *Aphanomyces*:
    - Deep, ulcerative granulomatous lesions of the skin and muscle tissue
    - Necropsy may reveal ascites and internal granulomatous lesions in multiple organs.
  - Branchiomycosis:
    - Clinical signs are related to pathology of the gill tissue.
    - Fish become weak; demonstrate gasping at surface, piping, and other signs typically related to hypoxia. High mortalities, up to 50%, are not uncommon.
    - The gills appear as hemorrhagic, patchy necrotic lesions, eroded, and pale.
  - *Ichthyophonus hoferi*:
    - Signs vary by anatomical location and severity of the lesions.
    - Skin roughening and darkening (initially along the lateral line), abnormal swimming behavior, lethargy, emaciation, ascites, and skin ulceration can be observed.
    - Scoliosis may be seen occasionally.
    - This disease can mimic mycobacteriosis.
  - *Dermocystidium* spp.
    - *Dermocystidium koi*: smooth, raised skin lesions that range in color from red to white
    - *Dermocystidium salmonis*: raised lesions found in the gills
- Skin scraping/wet mount cytology:
  - Saprolegnia: Long-branched, aseptate hyphae are observed.
  - *Aphanomyces*: presence of nonseptate, fungal hyphae seen in deep cutaneous ulcers
  - Branchiomycosis: Gill tissue cytology reveals light brown, refractile, branching, nonseptate fungal elements and intravascular, intrahyphal, eosinophilic round bodies (apleospores). Lamellar hyperplasia and fusion may also be seen.
  - Ichthyophoniasis: spherical bodies with thick walls seen on wet mount preps of affected organs
  - *Dermocystidium koi*: white filamentous hyphae from wet mount of skin lesion aspirate, spherical spores with a large central refractile vacuole
- Necropsy findings:
  - *Aphanomyces*: deep cutaneous ulcers involving the musculature, internal presence of granulomas and fungal hyphae
  - *Ichthyophonus hoferi*: Internal organs demonstrate white or cream-colored nodules or granulomatous inflammation. Tissues should be reexamined several hours after death as the parasite replicates. Branched germination tubes may be seen in affected tissues.

ADVANCED OR CONFIRMATORY TESTING

- Fungal culture for positive identification
- Histopathologic examination and special staining techniques

TREATMENT

THERAPEUTIC GOALS

- Control secondary or primary fungal pathogen
- Identify and eliminate predisposing stressors such as overcrowding, poor water quality, overfeeding
- Treat any concurrent parasitic and bacterial infections

ACUTE GENERAL TREATMENT

- Saprolegniasis
  - Increase salinity of pond or tank in freshwater systems to 0.1% to 0.3% (1-3 g/L) as an aid with osmoregulatory balance.
  - 35% Perox-Aid (hydrogen peroxide, Western Chemical, Ferndale, Washington) is Food and Drug Administration (FDA) approved to treat freshwater-reared finfish eggs, salmonids, coolwater finfish, and channel catfish for saprolegniasis. A label claim approval is in progress for treatment of saprolegniasis in warmwater fish.
  - Malachite green
    - 1-2 mg/L bath treatment for 30-60 minutes
    - 0.1 mg/L prolonged immersion
  - Formalin (37% formaldehyde) for infection on eggs
    - 1-2 mL/L up to 15-minute bath treatment
    - 0.23 mL/L up to 60-minute bath treatment
  - Daily application of antifungal topical ointment such as Betadine or chlorhexidine can increase survival.
  - Pyceze (bronopol, Novartis UK, Surrey, United Kingdom)
    - Fish and egg treatment
    - Currently not available in the United States
  - Various other treatments attempted with limited success
    - Potassium permanganate
    - Methylene blue
- *Aphanomyces*
  - Malachite green: 0.5 mg/L (0.5 ppm) 1-hour bath treatment
  - Hydrogen peroxide 100-500 ppm 1-hour bath treatment

- Sodium chloride 10-20 ppt (10-20 g/L) 1-hour treatment
- Branchiomycosis
  - Malachite green: prolonged immersion 0.1 mg/L
  - Formalin: 0.15 mL/L followed by repeat treatment of 0.25 mL/L (multiple treatments may be required)
  - Reduce organic loads in ponds.
  - Reduce water temperature to below 20°C (68°F).
- Ichthyophoniasis
  - No effective treatment is known.
- *Dermocystidium* spp.
  - No specific treatment is known.
  - Spontaneous resolution may occur.
  - Surgical excision of granulomas may beneficially influence recovery.
  - Daily application of antifungal topical ointment such as Betadine or chlorhexidine may help.

CHRONIC TREATMENT

- Maintain best management practices, including strict attention to water quality.
- Cull infected fish and remove dead fish promptly.
- Remove and prevent accumulation of decaying organic matter, which can be a food source for many water molds.
- Remove dead eggs promptly (*Saprolegnia* spp.).
- Discourage feeding raw fish and raw fish products (*Branchiomyces*, *Ichthyophonus* spp.).
- If raw fish must be fed, freeze tissue at −20°C (−4°F) or heat to 40°C (104°F) for 3 minutes to kill parasite.
- Dry earthen ponds and expose to ultraviolet light for a long time (*Branchiomyces*, *Ichthyophonus* spp.).
- Disinfect drained ponds with chlorine if possible.
- Spores of *Ichthyophonus* have been shown to survive up to 2 years in seawater at wide temperature ranges and varying pH levels.

DRUG INTERACTIONS

- A biotest should always be done when dealing with a large population of fish because species tolerance to chemotherapeutic agents varies.
- Malachite green stains can be highly toxic to some species (tetras), fry, and some plants.
- Malachite green is more toxic at high water temperatures and low pH.
- Malachite green has been reported as having teratogenic and mutagenic properties.
- Formalin cannot be used to treat eggs within 24 hours of hatching.
- Water stability of Pyceze increases with decreasing hardness and pH.

POSSIBLE COMPLICATIONS

Adverse drug reactions

PROGNOSIS AND OUTCOME

- Saprolegniasis:
  - Prognosis is determined by the locations of lesions and the amount of tissue affected.
  - Lesions restricted to the tail or distal areas of the fins have a better prognosis than those in fish with lesions on the body.
  - Fatalities result from disruption of osmoregulatory control and resultant loss of electrolytes and serum proteins.
  - Gill involvement usually indicates a grave prognosis.
- *Aphanomyces*:
  - Outbreaks can have severe mortality in naïve fish. Subsequent infections within the same populations are usually less severe.
  - Prognosis is dependent on degree of tissue invasion and necrosis.
- Branchiomycosis: poor prognosis if gill pathology is severe
- Ichthyophononiasis: poor prognosis
- *Dermocystidium koi*: good prognosis
- *Dermocystidium salmonis*: poor prognosis if gills severely affected

PEARLS & CONSIDERATIONS

COMMENTS

- Dead fish may develop fungal lesions as decaying tissues provide a good medium for fungal growth. It is important to examine a live fish to diagnose a fungal lesion.
- Use of non–FDA-approved antifungal treatments is prohibited in food fish.
- Reinfection of fungal disease is common unless predisposing factors are identified and eliminated.
- When bath treatments are used, it is considered prudent to observe fish for signs of distress. If distress is noted, fish should be removed immediately and placed in fresh, aerated water.
- *Ichthyophonus hoferi* and *Dermocystidium* demonstrate fungal and protozoan characteristics. Classification as a fungal disease is subject to change.

CLIENT EDUCATION

- Practice best management practices, including safe stocking densities, good nutrition, monitoring of water quality, and prompt removal of infected and dead fish.
- It is impossible to eliminate all water molds from a system.

SUGGESTED READINGS

Noga EJ: Fish disease: diagnosis and treatment, St Louis, 1996, Mosby.
Wildgoose WH: BSAVA manual of ornamental fish, ed 2, Gloucester, 2001, British Small Animal Veterinary Association.
Yanong RPE: Fungal diseases of fish, Vet Clin Exot Anim 6:377–400, 2003.

AUTHOR & EDITOR: **HELEN E. ROBERTS**

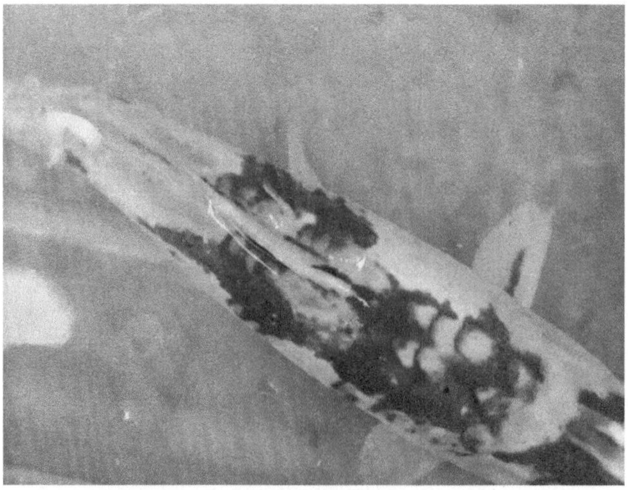

Fungal Diseases Fungal lesion with trapped algae particles on the dorsal aspect of a koi (*Cyprinus carpio*). *(Courtesy Helen E. Roberts.)*

Gastrointestinal Nematode and Cestode Parasites

BASIC INFORMATION

DEFINITION

Gastrointestinal metazoan parasites that affect fish include nematodes and cestodes.

SYNONYMS

- Nematodes: roundworms; common intestinal nematodes include *Capillaria* and *Camallanus*.
- Cestodes: tapeworms; can be divided into *Cestodaria* (infecting mainly Elasmobranchs) and the more common *Eucestoda* (which infect teleosts). One of the most serious intestinal cestodes that affect fish is *Bothriocephalus acheilognathi* (Asian tapeworm).

EPIDEMIOLOGY

SPECIES, AGE, SEX

- Most common in wild caught fish
- Any fish (freshwater and marine) can become infected.
- Juvenile fish are more likely to show clinical signs and have reduced growth rates.

GENETICS AND BREED PREDISPOSITION

- *Capillaria* is common in angelfish/cichlids, *Capillostronyloides* is common in armored catfish, *Camallanus* commonly infects live bearers.
- *Bothriocephalus acheilognathi* (Asian tapeworm) has a wide host range but can cause serious problems in bait minnows, grass carp, and juvenile common carp.

RISK FACTORS Poor husbandry, other ectoparasites and endoparasites may increase morbidity.

CONTAGION AND ZOONOSIS Some larval nematodes can cause larval migrans when ingested by humans (*Anisakis, Pseudoterranova*).

CLINICAL PRESENTATION

DISEASE FORMS/SUBTYPES

- Fish acting as definitive hosts will have adult worms in the gastrointestinal tract.
- When fish act as intermediate hosts, immature stages can be found in almost any part of the body, including the coelomic cavity, various internal organs, skin, or muscle.

HISTORY, CHIEF COMPLAINT

- Many fish infected with cestodes/nematodes show no clinical signs.
- Heavy infestations may cause clinical signs, including lethargy, decreased appetite, weight loss, abnormal feces (white, clear, pale, mucosy, etc.), decreased growth, decreased brood stock production.
- The owner may notice parasites protruding from the vent.
- Nodules may be noted in the skin/muscle from encysted parasites.

PHYSICAL EXAM FINDINGS

- Potential findings include thin/poor body condition, abdominal distention, and abnormal feces.
- The presence of red worms protruding through the anal vent is indicative of *Camallanus* spp.

ETIOLOGY AND PATHOPHYSIOLOGY

- Intestinal cestodes have complex life cycles requiring at least two hosts. Fish may be the second intermediate, paratenic, or definitive host, depending on the species; a copepod is usually the first intermediate host.
- Most intestinal nematodes have complex life cycles involving at least two hosts. Intermediate hosts include copepods, side swimmers, tubifex worms, and insect larvae. Some nematodes such as *Capillaria* spp. have a direct life cycle; these may pose more of a problem in aquaria.
- In nematodes with a direct life cycle, transmission occurs through the water; infective stages are shed in the feces (fecal/oral transmission).
- Migration of immature stages of cestodes/nematodes may cause damage to various tissues.

DIAGNOSIS

DIFFERENTIAL DIAGNOSIS

Other intestinal parasites (protozoans, etc.), other systemic disease (mycobacteriosis, etc.), poor nutrition

INITIAL DATABASE

- The diagnostic approach to a fish with enteric nematode/cestode parasites should begin with complete history, water chemistry (temperature, salinity, pH, ammonia, nitrites, nitrates, alkalinity, dissolved oxygen), and thorough evaluation of the environment/husbandry.
- Direct observation of the fish in the aquarium or pond
- Complete physical examination
- Wet mounts of the skin/gills should be performed to rule out ectoparasites.
- Fecal examination may reveal eggs, proglottids (cestodes), larvae, or adults. Fecal examination should be performed only on fresh feces.
- Necropsy with wet mount examination of intestinal contents/feces and squash preparations of the intestines is most accurate for determining the presence and degree of infection.
- Nematodes are smooth and cylindrical. *Capillaria* eggs have bipolar opercula.
- Cestodes are long, flat, and segmented. They have a scolex (attachment organ) and internal/external segmentation (proglottids).

ADVANCED OR CONFIRMATORY TESTING

- Histopathologic examination is not typically required for diagnosis. However, sections of nematodes/cestodes may be seen on histopathologic examination of the gastrointestinal tract and occasionally other organs.
- Parasite specimens may need to be sent to a reference laboratory for accurate determination of genus/species.

TREATMENT

THERAPEUTIC GOAL

Control parasites

ACUTE GENERAL TREATMENT

- Husbandry
  - Correcting environmental abnormalities while removing stressors (poor water quality) decreases morbidity.
  - Thorough cleaning of the gravel/substrate and filter may help reduce environmental contamination.
  - Eradication/avoidance of known intermediate hosts will prevent perpetuation of the life cycle in parasites with indirect life cycles. Live foods (including side swimmers, insect larvae, tubifex worms, copepods, etc.) that may act as intermediate hosts should be avoided.
  - For nematodes with direct life cycles, infected fish should be isolated and the system cleaned.
  - In situations where fish serve as the intermediate host (e.g., *Eustrongyloides*), the definitive host should be identified (birds, mammals) and contact with these animals eliminated.
- Medical treatments
  - Cestodes
    - Praziquantel
      - Bath treatment: 2 mg/L (ppm). Concentrations up to 10 mg/L

have been used successfully and safely in many species of ornamental fish.
- Oral: 5 mg/kg [0.5%] in feed fed once daily for 3 days; treatment may need to be repeated in 2-3 weeks.

- Nematodes
  - Levamisole
    - Bath treatment: 2 mg/L, weekly treatments for 3 weeks
    - 4 mg/kg [0.4%] in feed (1.8 grams per pound of food) fed once weekly for 3 weeks
  - Fenbendazole
    - Bath treatment: 2 mg/L, weekly treatments for 3 weeks
    - 2.5 mg/kg [0.25%] in feed (1.14 grams per pound of food) fed for 3 days; treatment should be repeated in 3 weeks
- No effective medical treatment for cestodes/nematodes encysted outside the intestinal tract is known. Manual removal can be performed, depending on location.

RECOMMENDED MONITORING

Direct fecal examinations should be performed routinely to determine response to treatment.

PROGNOSIS AND OUTCOME

- Intestinal cestodes/nematodes usually respond well to treatment.
- *Bothriocephalus acheilognathi* (Asian tapeworm) can cause serious problems (and significant mortality) in bait minnows, grass carp, and juvenile common carp.

PEARLS & CONSIDERATIONS

COMMENTS

Free-living nematodes may be found associated with chronic skin lesions, dead fish, and organic debris in an aquarium/pond.

PREVENTION

- Good husbandry and water quality
- Quarantine of new fish for a minimum of 4 weeks
- Eradication/avoidance of known intermediate hosts

SUGGESTED READINGS

Noga EJ: Fish disease: diagnosis and treatment, St Louis, 1996, Mosby.

Wildgoose WH: BSAVA manual of ornamental fish, ed 2, Gloucester, 2001, British Small Animal Veterinary Association.

Yanong RPE: Nematode infections in fish, VM-91, Gainesville, Fla, 2006, Florida Cooperative Extension Service, UF-IFAS. http://edis.ifas.ufl.edu. Accessed Jan. 31, 2007.

AUTHOR: **BRIAN S. PALMEIRO**

EDITOR: **HELEN E. ROBERTS**

FISH

Gastrointestinal Protozoal Parasites

BASIC INFORMATION

DEFINITION

Gastrointestinal protozoal parasites that affect fish include *Hexamita, Spironucleus,* and *Cryptobia,* all of which are flagellated protozoans.

SYNONYMS

- *Hexamita*: three species reported to affect fish: *H. salmonis, H. truttae,* and *H. intestinalis,* commonly called "Hex"
- *Spironucleus: Spironucleus vortens* is reported to be an intestinal parasite in freshwater angelfish.
- *Cryptobia:* Seven species of *Cryptobia* have been associated with the gastrointestinal tract of fish; only *C. iubilans* is reported to be pathogenic and parasitic.

EPIDEMIOLOGY

SPECIES, AGE, SEX

- Most common in freshwater fish
- *Hexamita/Spironucleus* are common in cichlids such as angelfish, discus, oscars, and African cichlids. *Hexamita salmonis* affects salmonids.
- *Cryptobia*: reported in African and Central/South American cichlids; recently reported in juvenile discus

RISK FACTORS

- Poor environmental conditions (crowding, poor water quality) or other stressors (recent shipment/handling, poor nutrition, etc.) may predispose fish to infection.
- Other ectoparasites and endoparasites increase morbidity.

ASSOCIATED CONDITIONS AND DISORDERS

Other intestinal parasites such as *Capillaria* and *Camallanus* may be present.

CLINICAL PRESENTATION

HISTORY, CHIEF COMPLAINT

- Clinical signs include lethargy, decreased appetite, weight loss, abnormal feces (white, pale, mucosy, etc.), erratic swimming, infertility, decreased hatchability of eggs, death of fry, and chronic low-level mortality.
- Angelfish may have buoyancy abnormalities and lay in lateral recumbency at the top of the water column with a distended abdomen.
- *Hexamita/Spironucleus* has been implicated as a potential cause for head and lateral line erosion, but its importance in this syndrome is unclear.
- *Cryptobia* has been implicated as a potential cause for "Malawi bloat," but its importance in this syndrome is unclear.
- Heavy infestations can cause significant mortality.

PHYSICAL EXAM FINDINGS Potential findings include thin/poor body condition, abdominal distention, and abnormal feces.

ETIOLOGY AND PATHOPHYSIOLOGY

- Intestinal protozoans have direct life cycles.
- Transmission likely occurs through the water; infective stages are shed in the feces (fecal/oral transmission).
- Mature trophozoites inhabit the gastrointestinal tract. *Cryptobia* causes granulomatous gastritis but has also been associated with systemic granulomatous disease (kidney, spleen, liver, etc.).

DIAGNOSIS

DIFFERENTIAL DIAGNOSIS

Other intestinal parasites (nematodes, cestodes, etc.), other systemic diseases (mycobacteriosis, etc.), poor nutrition

INITIAL DATABASE

- The diagnostic approach to a fish with protozoal enteric parasites should begin with complete history, water chemistry (temperature, salinity, pH, ammonia, nitrites, nitrates, alkalinity, dissolved oxygen), and thorough evaluation of the environment/husbandry.
- Direct observation of the fish in the aquarium or pond

- Complete physical examination
  - Wet mounts of the skin/gills should be performed to rule out ectoparasites.
  - Direct fecal examination may reveal motile trophozoites. Fecal examination should be performed only on fresh feces.
  - Necropsy examination with wet mount examination of intestinal contents/feces and squash preparations of the intestines is most accurate for determining the presence and degree of infection. Because trophozoites are small, they are best identified at 400× magnification. Grossly, the stomach (*Cryptobia*) or intestines (*Spironucleus/Hexamita*) may be thickened, inflamed, distended, hemorrhagic, and/or edematous.
- *Spironucleus/Hexamita*: Trophozoites are small (12.5-20 μm in length), flagellated, actively motile, with an ellipsoid to pear shape. Trophozoites of *Spironucleus/Hexamita* are often localized in the anterior intestinal lumen and therefore may not be present on fecal examination. They have six anterior and two posterior flagella. Species identification requires electron microscopy.
- *Cryptobia* is most commonly detected by identifying granulomas in squash preparation wet mounts of the stomach. An acid-fast stain should be performed to rule out mycobacteriosis (another common cause of granulomas in ornamental fish). Motile trophozoites are not commonly seen on wet mounts. When present, flagellated trophozoites are elongate (acute infection) to oval/teardrop-shaped (chronic infection) with a characteristic slow undulating movement. The organism has two flagella. Species identification requires electron microscopy.

ADVANCED OR CONFIRMATORY TESTING

- Histopathologic examination is not typically required for diagnosis. However, sections of protozoans may be seen on histopathologic examination of the gastrointestinal tract and occasionally other organs (liver, kidney, spleen, etc.). Histologically, intestinal changes may vary from minimal to severe enteritis. Varying degrees of granulomatous gastritis are seen with *Cryptobia* infestation. Systemic granulomatous disease may also be present (liver, spleen, kidney, etc.) with *Cryptobia* infestation.
- Definitive species identification requires electron microscopy.

TREATMENT

THERAPEUTIC GOALS

- Improve environmental conditions
- Control parasites

ACUTE GENERAL TREATMENT

- Husbandry
  - Correcting environmental abnormalities and removing stressors (poor water quality) is a critical step in decreasing morbidity/mortality and preventing disease.
  - Thorough cleaning of the gravel/substrate and filter may help reduce environmental contamination.
- Medical treatments
  - *Cryptobia*
    - No effective treatment for *Cryptobia* has been reported.
    - *Cryptobia* may be able to survive intracellularly in phagocytic cells, making treatment difficult.
    - Sulfadimethoxine is anecdotally reported to decrease mortality but not eliminate the parasite.
    - Dimetridazole and 2-amino-5-nitrothiazol (additional studies are needed to determine optimal dose and duration) may help to reduce the prevalence of infestation. No significant improvement was illustrated for fish treated with nitrofurazone, primaquine, chloroquine, or metronidazole.
  - *Hexamita/Spironucleus*
    - The treatment of choice for *Hexamita* and *Spironucleus* is metronidazole.
    - Dosage: metronidazole 1.0% (1 gram/100 grams feed) in the feed for 10-14 days; metronidazole can be mixed into a gel diet or top dressed on a commercial diet.
    - Prolonged bath immersion: 5-6 mg/L (250 mg/10 gal [6.6 mg/L] of water); treat every 24-48 hours for 10-14 days. 50% to 75% water changes should be performed between treatments. Metronidazole can damage the biofilter.
    - Infestations respond best to oral treatment. The author reserves bath treatments for anorexic fish.

RECOMMENDED MONITORING

- Direct fecal examinations should be performed routinely to determine response to treatment. However, trophozoites are not always present on direct fecal examination, and necropsy/wet mounts may be necessary to accurately determine treatment response.
- Water quality should be monitored closely because some treatments can damage the biofilter.

PROGNOSIS AND OUTCOME

- *Hexamita/Spironucleus* generally responds well to metronidazole if environmental/husbandry corrections are made and infestations are caught early.
- With poor environmental conditions and heavy infestations, significant mortality may occur.
- No effective treatment for *Cryptobia* is known. Managing concurrent ecto/endoparasites may decrease morbidity/mortality.

PEARLS & CONSIDERATIONS

COMMENTS

- *Protoopalina* is a large, ciliate-like protozoan that is a common, nonpathogenic commensal in discus.
- *Coccidia*, an intracellular protozoan, can potentially cause enteritis in fish.

PREVENTION

- Good husbandry and water quality
- Quarantine of new fish for a minimum of 4 weeks. Some aquariums are quarantining cichlids for 60 days to prevent the introduction of *Cryptobia*.
- Commercial producers should periodically evaluate ornamental cichlids for subclinical infection.

SUGGESTED READINGS

Francis-Floyd R, Reed P: Management of Hexamita in ornamental cichlids, VM-67, Gainesville, Fla, 2002, Florida Cooperative Extension Service, UF-IFAS. http://edis.ifas.ufl.edu.

Francis-Floyd R, Yanong R: Cryptobia iubilans in cichlids, VM-104, Gainesville, Fla, 2002, Florida Cooperative Extension Service, UF-IFAS. http://edis.ifas.ufl.edu. Accessed Jan 24, 2007.

Noga EJ: Fish disease: diagnosis and treatment, St Louis, 1996, Mosby.

Wildgoose WH: BSAVA manual of ornamental fish, ed 2, Gloucester, 2001, British Small Animal Veterinary Association.

Yanong RPE, et al: Cryptobia iubilans infection in juvenile discus, J Am Vet Med Assoc 224:1644–1650, 2006.

AUTHOR: **BRIAN S. PALMEIRO**

EDITOR: **HELEN E. ROBERTS**

FISH

Head and Lateral Line Erosion (HLLE)

BASIC INFORMATION

DEFINITION

Head and lateral line erosion is an important, idiopathic clinical syndrome seen in both marine and freshwater fish.

SYNONYMS

- HLLE
- Freshwater head and lateral line erosion (FHLLE), marine head and lateral line erosion (MHLLE)
- "Hole in the head"

EPIDEMIOLOGY

SPECIES, AGE, SEX

- Can be seen in both freshwater and marine fish
- Freshwater cichlids (discus, oscars, other South American cichlids) are commonly affected.
- Marine fish that are commonly affected include surgeonfishes and tangs (family Acanthuridae) and marine angelfish (family Pomacanthidae).

RISK FACTORS Stressors such as overcrowding, poor water quality, or poor nutrition may predispose fish to HLLE.

ASSOCIATED CONDITIONS AND DISORDERS

Freshwater cichlids may have intestinal infestations with flagellated protozoans (*Hexamita/Spironucleus*).

CLINICAL PRESENTATION

HISTORY, CHIEF COMPLAINT

- This disorder causes chronic progressive dermatologic lesions affecting the head and flanks.
- Affected fish eventually may become anorexic and lethargic.

PHYSICAL EXAM FINDINGS

- Dermatologic examination reveals often symmetric, depigmented erosions and ulcerations that coalesce to produce large crateriform lesions and pits on the head. In some cases, lesions extend down the lateral line/flanks.
- Severely affected fish may become thin and emaciated and may have exophthalmos.
- Secondary bacterial, fungal, and parasitic infections may occur.

ETIOLOGY AND PATHOPHYSIOLOGY

- The exact cause of head and lateral line erosion is unknown.
- Proposed causative agents include hexamitid parasites (such as *Spironucleus vortens*), other infectious agents, activated carbon/carbon dust, heavy metals such as copper, stray electrical voltage, ozone, ultraviolet (UV) radiation products, poor nutrition, nutrient deficiency of vitamins A/C and minerals, and various other stressors.
- A single inciting cause may not be present, and this disease may represent a clinical response to various stressors.

DIAGNOSIS

DIFFERENTIAL DIAGNOSIS

Differential diagnoses include other causes of erosive to ulcerative lesions, including bacterial, parasitic, and fungal disease; however, clinical presentation in previously mentioned species is characteristic.

INITIAL DATABASE

- The diagnostic approach to a fish with head and lateral line erosion should begin with complete history, water chemistry (temperature, salinity, pH, ammonia, nitrites, nitrates, alkalinity, dissolved oxygen), and thorough evaluation of the environment/husbandry.
- Direct observation of fish in the aquarium
- Complete physical examination
  - Skin scraping and gill biopsy wet mounts should be performed to check for the presence of parasites and/or other abnormalities.
  - Fecal examination should be performed to rule out intestinal parasitism.
- Diagnosis typically is based on history and clinical signs.

ADVANCED OR CONFIRMATORY TESTING

Reported histologic findings include acute, multifocal, moderate to severe lymphohistiocytic epidermidis and dermatitis, with multifocal severe keratinocyte ballooning degeneration, necrosis, ulceration, and rare vesicle formation.

TREATMENT

THERAPEUTIC GOALS

- Improve environment, husbandry, and nutrition
- Reduce lesion severity and morbidity
- Control secondary infections

ACUTE GENERAL TREATMENT

- Husbandry
  - Husbandry should be improved by maintaining excellent water quality, performing frequent water changes, and reducing overcrowding.
  - A balanced/varied diet should be provided. Anecdotal reports have described treating HLLE with various vitamin supplements.
  - A grounding device can be installed to remove stray voltage.
  - Activated carbon should be removed from the system.
- Medical treatments
  - Secondary infections (bacterial, fungal, parasitic, etc.) should be treated appropriately.
  - Marine HLLE has been successfully treated with becaplermin 0.01% (Regranex, Ortho-McNeil Pharmaceuticals, Inc., Raritan, New Jersey).
    - This fish is sedated and lesions are débrided with a sterile scalpel blade and gently flushed. Regranex is applied with sterile cotton applicators. Various recommendations have been proposed for contact time. The author typically allows a contact time of 2-3 minutes before placing the fish back into the water.
    - Various protocols have been shown to be effective.
      - Once-weekly application for 8 weeks was successful in sailfin tangs.
      - Successful treatment has been reported in juvenile ocean surgeons with a single application of Regranex, or with one treatment every 3 weeks. However, fish placed in water that was known to induce lesions consistent with HLLE did not improve with Regranex treatment.
      - Regranex has been diluted with 0.9% sodium chloride to a concentration of 50% or 25%, with similar healing rates to fish treated with the full concentration.
    - Use of Regranex in freshwater HLLE has not been reported.
  - When present, *Hexamita/Spironucleus* infestations should be treated with metronidazole.
    - Dosage: metronidazole 1.0% in the feed for 10-14 days (6.6 mL [1 gram/100 grams feed]); metronidazole can be mixed into a gel diet or top dressed on a commercial diet.
    - Prolonged bath immersion: 5-6 mg/L (250 mg/10 gal of water); treat every 24-48 hours for

10-14 days. 50% to 75% water changes should be performed between treatments. Metronidazole can damage the biofilter.
- Infestations respond best to oral treatment. The author reserves bath treatments for anorexic fish.

PROGNOSIS AND OUTCOME

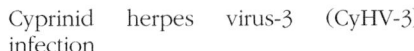

- The mortality rate with head and lateral line erosion is low. Marine HLLE responds well to treatment with Regranex if underlying environmental triggers are removed.
- Affected fish eventually may become anorexic and lethargic, and mortality may result.
- Secondary infection with parasites, bacteria, and fungi can increase morbidity and mortality.

SUGGESTED READINGS

Adams L, Michalkiewicz J: Effect of Regranex gel concentration or post application time on the healing rate of head and lateral line erosions in marine tropical fish. Mystic, Conn, 2005, Proceedings International Association of Aquatic Animal Medicine.

Boerner L, et al: Angiogenic growth factor therapy using recombinant platelet-derived growth factor (Regranex) for lateral line disease in marine fish. Mystic, Conn, 2003, Proceedings International Association of Aquatic Animal Medicine.

Croft L, et al: The effect of dietary vitamin C levels on the development of head and lateral line erosion syndrome in ocean surgeonfish (*Acanthurus bahianus*). Mystic, Conn, 2005, Proceedings International Association of Aquatic Animal Medicine.

Fleming G, et al: Treatment factors influencing the use of recombinant platelet-derived growth factor (Regranex) for head and lateral line erosion syndrome in ocean surgeons (*Acanthurus bahianus*). Mystic, Conn, 2005, Proceedings International Association of Aquatic Animal Medicine.

Francis-Floyd R, et al: Captive nutritional management of Atlantic surgeon fish: effect of dietary vitamin A on development of head and lateral line erosion lesions. Mystic, Conn, 2005, Proceedings International Association of Aquatic Animal Medicine.

Noga EJ: Fish disease: diagnosis and treatment. St Louis, 1996, Mosby.

Paull G, Matthews RA: *Spironucleus vortens*, a possible cause of hole-in-the-head disease in cichlids. Dis Aquat Org 45:197–202, 2001.

Stamper MA, et al: Head and lateral line erosion syndrome in ocean surgeons (*Acanthurus bahianus*): current efforts to determine etiologies. Mystic, Conn, 2005, Proceedings International Association of Aquatic Animal Medicine.

Wildgoose WH: BSAVA manual of ornamental fish. ed 2, Gloucester, 2001, British Small Animal Veterinary Association.

AUTHOR: **BRIAN S. PALMEIRO**

EDITOR: **HELEN E. ROBERTS**

FISH

Koi Herpes Virus Infection (KHV)

BASIC INFORMATION

DEFINITION

Cyprinid herpes virus-3 (CyHV-3) infection

SYNONYM

KHV

EPIDEMIOLOGY

SPECIES, AGE, SEX Common carp and koi, *Cyprinus carpio*, all ages affected, males and females

RISK FACTORS Failure to quarantine

CONTAGION AND ZOONOSIS Highly infectious among susceptible populations at permissive temperatures; not a zoonotic disease

GEOGRAPHY AND SEASONALITY Distribution is worldwide. Clinical signs can be seen 10-14 days following exposure to virus at permissive water temperatures, 15°C to 27°C (59°F to 80°F).

ASSOCIATED CONDITIONS AND DISORDERS

Septicemia, high mortality

CLINICAL PRESENTATION

HISTORY, CHIEF COMPLAINT Mortality, lack of quarantine, permissive water temperatures of 15°C to 27°C (59°F to 80°F)

PHYSICAL EXAM FINDINGS

- No pathognomonic lesions
- Moderate to severe gill necrosis and edema
- Multifocal patches of roughened skin ("sandpaper" texture) with missing scales
- Erratic swimming behavior
- Gasping, piping, congregating in areas of higher oxygen concentration (air stones, surface, waterfalls)
- Enophthalmos, anorexia, and lethargy
- Secondary parasitic and bacterial infections

ETIOLOGY AND PATHOPHYSIOLOGY

- Cyprinid herpes virus-3 (CyHV-3)
- Epitheliotrophic
- Lesions seen on skin, gills, and internal organs such as kidneys and spleen

DIAGNOSIS

DIFFERENTIAL DIAGNOSIS

- Septicemia
- Pathogenic aeromonad infection or other systemic bacterial disease
- Water quality
- Waterborne toxin

INITIAL DATABASE

- High index of suspicion with high mortalities in a population at permissive water temperatures with a history of failure to quarantine. A slower rate of mortalities has been observed in water temperatures at the lower end of KHV permissive range.
- Visualization of typical lesions at necropsy; necrotic and edematous gills, enophthalmos, secondary septicemia, adhesions in the coelomic cavity, and mottled appearance to major organs
- Definitive diagnosis requires testing by a qualified diagnostic laboratory.

ADVANCED OR CONFIRMATORY TESTING

- Polymerase chain reaction (PCR) testing of fresh tissues samples (postmortem)
- PCR of gill swab (antemortem), less reliable owing to sample size
- DNA in situ hybridization of formalin-preserved samples (useful for archived samples or atypical presentations)

TREATMENT

THERAPEUTIC GOALS

- Prevent future outbreaks in new stock
- Provide owner education

ACUTE GENERAL TREATMENT

- No specific treatment
- Anecdotally reported treatment of heating water to 30°C (86°F) may reduce mortalities, but recovered fish may become latent carriers.
- Recurrent outbreaks have been documented with heat treatment.
- Treatment of secondary bacterial and parasitic infections can be attempted, but owners should be warned of the possibility of recrudescence.

- If survivors are present during an outbreak, the owner should be advised to make the pond a closed system with no new fish added.

POSSIBLE COMPLICATIONS

Recrudescence is a possibility in recovered fish, who may become latent carriers.

PROGNOSIS AND OUTCOME

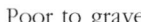

Poor to grave

PEARLS & CONSIDERATIONS

COMMENTS

- Fish can become infected at lower temperatures, but clinical signs may not become apparent until higher water temperatures are reached.
- A positive result on serologic testing indicates only exposure; it is not a prognostic indication of recovery, latency, etc.
- Discussion of this disease is a hot topic on Internet forums and message boards, and much misinformation can be found with regard to infection, diagnosis, and treatment.
- KHV is listed by the OIE (World Organization for Animal Health) as a notifiable disease for member countries. The disease is not reportable to the U.S. Department of Agriculture Animal and Plant Inspection Service (USDA-APHIS). USDA-APHIS will continue to report to OIE that KHV is known to occur in the United States.
- Regulations involving the importation and exportation of ornamental fish have been changing rapidly. The author recommends verifying requirements for import/export prior to arranging shipment.

PREVENTION

- A new attenuated immersion vaccine, Cavoy, was released in the U.S. in 2012 for the prevention of KHV. More information can be found at vaccine informational online site, cavoy.com.
- Provide lengthy quarantine for new koi at KHV permissive temperatures.
- Institute effective biosecurity protocols.
- Disinfect or discard all equipment used in an outbreak situation.
- Ponds should be drained, disinfected, and left to dry before use.
- Refilled ponds should remain empty for a minimum of 7 days before new fish are added.
- Use separate equipment for each system.
- Serologic testing of new fish can indicate previous exposure to virus, assuming that enough time has elapsed for potentially exposed fish to generate antibodies (usually a minimum of 2 weeks).

CLIENT EDUCATION

- Quarantine all incoming fish at permissive water temperatures for KHV for 30-60 days 59°F to 80°F (15°C to 27°C).
- The author quarantines her fish for 1 year in an outdoor quarantine pond.

SUGGESTED READINGS

Petty BD, Fraser WA: Viruses of pet fish. Vet Clin Exot Anim 8:67–84, 2005.

St-Hilaire S, et al: Reactivation of koi herpesvirus infections in common carp Cyprinus carpio, Dis Aquat Org 50:15–23, 2005.

AUTHOR & EDITOR: **HELEN E. ROBERTS**

FISH

Lymphocystis

BASIC INFORMATION

DEFINITION

Infection in susceptible fish with lymphocystivirus (Iridovirus family)

SYNONYMS

Lymphocystis virus disease type 1, lymphocystis virus disease type 2

EPIDEMIOLOGY

SPECIES, AGE, SEX

- Many species of freshwater and marine ornamental fish
- Not seen in catfish, salmonids, or cyprinids (koi, etc.)

RISK FACTORS Stress can cause immune suppression, increase the risk of infection, and precipitate the presence of lesions in exposed fish.

CONTAGION AND ZOONOSIS

- Incubation time can be long but is shorter in higher water temperatures.
- Experimentally, incubation time was 5-12 days at 20°C to 25°C (68°F to 77°F).

CLINICAL PRESENTATION

DISEASEFORMS/SUBTYPES Dermal lesions

HISTORY, CHIEF COMPLAINT Owner reports presence of typical skin lesions on one or more fish.

PHYSICAL EXAM FINDINGS

- Lesions present as raised, white to gray, nodular, verrucous lesions that can occur anywhere on the external surfaces of the body.
- Rarely, lesions can be found on the serosal surfaces of internal organs.
- Not usually fatal
- Can be self-limiting

DIAGNOSIS

INITIAL DATABASE

- History
- Environmental assessment
- Physical examination
- Cytologic examination of lesions (wet mount cytology shows hypertrophy of the epidermal cells)

ADVANCED OR CONFIRMATORY TESTING

- History reveals presence of stressors before appearance of lesions.
- Histopathologic examination is performed.

TREATMENT

THERAPEUTIC GOAL

Reduce adverse effects of infection

ACUTE GENERAL TREATMENT

- No effective treatment is known, although the lesions may become secondarily infected and need antimicrobial therapy.
- Lesions that prevent feeding behavior can be surgically removed.
- Reduce stressors, such as poor water quality, to prevent outbreaks.
- Spontaneous regression of lesions can occur.
- Recovered fish may experience recrudescence.

PEARLS & CONSIDERATIONS

COMMENTS

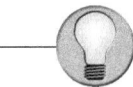

- Lymphocystis is the most common viral disease seen in tropical fish.
- The appearance of an affected fish can affect its retail value and potential fish show value.

- Lesions may leave scars or pigment changes on the skin.
- Latent infections may exist and may become clinical after exposure to stressful conditions.

PREVENTION

- Purchase disease-free fish whenever possible
- Quarantine new fish
- Reduce or prevent stress and presence of stressors in system

CLIENT EDUCATION

As above

SUGGESTED READINGS

Petty BD, Fraser WA: Viruses of pet fish, Vet Clin Exot Anim 8:67–84, 2005.
Wildgoose WH: BSAVA manual of ornamental fish, ed 2, Gloucester, 2001, British Small Animal Veterinary Association.

AUTHOR & EDITOR: **HELEN E. ROBERTS**

FISH

Protozoal Ectoparasites (Ciliated and Flagellated)

BASIC INFORMATION

DEFINITION

Protozoal parasites of fish include Ciliates, Flagellates, Myxozoans, Microsporidians, and *Coccidia*. Ciliated and flagellated protozoal ectoparasites will be discussed in this section. *Ichthyophthirius multifiliis* is the most common disease affecting freshwater tropical fish.

SYNONYMS

- Ciliated ectoparasites
  - *Ichthyophthirius multifiliis*: "Ich," "white-spot disease"; marine equivalent *Cryptocaryon irritans*, "marine ich"
  - *Chilodonella*: marine equivalent *Brookynella*
  - *Tetrahymena*: "guppy killer disease"; marine equivalent *Uronema*
  - *Trichodina*
  - Sessile ciliates: *Epistylis, Ambiphyra (Scyphidia), Apiosoma (Glossatella)*
- Flagellated ectoparasites
  - *Ichthyobodo* (previously *Costia*)
  - Dinoflagellates: *Amyloodinium*, "marine velvet"; freshwater equivalent *Piscinoodinium* (previously *Oodinium*), "freshwater velvet," "gold dust disease," "rust"

EPIDEMIOLOGY

SPECIES, AGE, SEX

- Any fish can be susceptible.
- Scaleless fish such as catfish and loaches may be especially vulnerable to Ich.
- Guppies are predisposed to *Tetrahymena*.

RISK FACTORS

- Poor environmental conditions (crowding, poor water quality) or other stressors (recent shipment/handling, poor nutrition, etc.) may predispose fish to infection.
- Systems with excessive organic debris/detritus are predisposed to some protozoans such as *Trichodina*, *Tetrahymena*, and sessile ciliates.

CLINICAL PRESENTATION

HISTORY, CHIEF COMPLAINT

- Clinical signs include lethargy, decreased appetite, flashing (rubbing against objects in the pond/aquarium), and excessive production of mucus (from gills or skin).
- When branchial infestations are present, respiratory signs such as increased opercular rate, piping (gasping for air at the water surface), and respiratory distress may be seen.
- Heavy infestations can cause significant mortality.
- Ich infestations classically present with white spots on the skin.

PHYSICAL EXAM FINDINGS

- Dermatologic abnormalities include erythema, scale loss, white to gray irregular patches, excessive production of mucus, hemorrhages, discolorations, erosions, and ulcerations. Dinoflagellates may cause an amber or gold dustlike sheen to the skin. With Ich infestations, punctate white nodules (up to 1 mm in size) will be noted on the skin/fins caused by the encysted trophont feeding stage. If infestations are confined to the gills, dermatologic lesions will be absent.
- The gills may become edematous with excessive production of mucus.
- Secondary bacterial and fungal infections may be present in areas parasitized by protozoans.

ETIOLOGY AND PATHOPHYSIOLOGY

- Ciliated/flagellated protozoans have direct life cycles.
  - Life cycle of Ich: The trophont (feeding, encysted stage) enlarges, breaks through the skin, and attaches to substrate forming the encapsulated dividing tomont. These tomonts undergo mitosis, forming hundreds of daughter tomites; tomites develop into free-living theronts (infective stage). Theronts penetrate the skin and gill epithelium and enlarge, forming encysted trophonts. Theronts survive for approximately 48 hours at water temperatures of 75°F to 79°F (24°C). A single trophont can produce more than 1000 theronts.
  - Dinoflagellates have more complex life cycles (similar to Ich), including trophont, tomont, and dinospore stages.
- Parasites damage skin/gill epithelium.

DIAGNOSIS

DIFFERENTIAL DIAGNOSIS

Other parasitic infestations, bacterial disease, fungal disease, viral disease, environmental causes of hypoxia (decreased dissolved oxygen, ammonia toxicity, nitrite toxicity, etc.)

INITIAL DATABASE

- The diagnostic approach to a fish with protozoal ectoparasites should begin with complete history, water chemistry (temperature, salinity, pH, ammonia, nitrites, nitrates, alkalinity, dissolved oxygen), and thorough evaluation of the environment/husbandry.
- Direct observation of the fish in the aquarium or pond
- Complete physical examination
- Definitive diagnosis can be made with wet mounts of the skin or gills. Most protozoal ectoparasites can be identified with 100× magnification.
- Ich: The mature parasite is large (up to 1 mm) and dark brown (cilia distributed over entire cell) and has a horseshoe-shaped macronucleus. The adult parasite has a characteristic tumbling motion, whereas immature stages move quickly and more closely resemble *Tetrahymena*.
- *Tetrahymena/Uronema*: motile teardrop-shaped shaped ciliated parasites
- *Chilodonella/Brookynella*: These ciliates are easily identified microscopically by their heart shape and slow circular motion.

- *Trichodina*: circular, flat ciliates with circular rows of denticles (internal blades) and erratic movement
- Sessile ciliates: cylindrical to conical, apical/oral cilia; *Epistylis* is stalked
- *Ichthyobodo*: very small and best seen at 400× magnification as a comma-shaped organism with a characteristic corkscrew swimming pattern.
- *Amyloodinium/Piscinoodinium*: irregular, variably sized, spherical to pear-shaped trophonts with a dark brown to golden color

ADVANCED OR CONFIRMATORY TESTING

Histopathologic examination is not typically required for diagnosis. However, sections of ciliated/flagellated protozoans can be seen on histopathologic examination of the skin and gills and occasionally deeper tissues.

TREATMENT

THERAPEUTIC GOALS

- Improve environmental conditions
- Control parasites

ACUTE GENERAL TREATMENT

- Husbandry
  - Correcting environmental abnormalities and removing stressors (poor water quality) are critical steps in decreasing morbidity/mortality and preventing disease.
  - The life cycle of Ich is temperature dependent. It lasts 3-6 days at 25°C (77°F), and 10 days at 15°C (59°F). Outbreaks are most common at 15°C to 25°C (59°F to 77°F). Increasing the water temperature speeds the life cycle, allowing for shorter treatment duration.
  - Siphoning the bottom of the aquarium may help control environmental stages of Ich.
- Medical treatments
  - Most ciliated and flagellated protozoal infestations respond to a single chemical treatment. If no improvement is noted, or if signs recur, the fish should be revaluated.
  - Salt effectively controls most protozoal ectoparasites of freshwater fish. Salinity can be maintained at 0.1% to 0.3% (1-3 ppt = 1-3 g/L) as a prolonged immersion. Some species, such as catfish and fish that navigate via the electrical field, can be sensitive to salt.
  - Formalin (37% formaldehyde) can be administered as a long-term bath at 25 mg/L (2 drops/gal; 1 mL/10 U.S. gal). Malachite green/formalin combination products are also effective against protozoal ectoparasites because the two agents are synergistic.
  - Potassium permanganate can be administered as a prolonged bath at 2 mg/L.
  - Prolonged immersion copper is a common method for controlling protozoal ectoparasites in marine fish. Free copper ions levels should be maintained at 0.2 mg/L. Copper is not safe with certain fish (elasmobranchs) and is toxic to invertebrates. Copper is not recommended in freshwater systems. Copper levels should be monitored daily.
  - Freshwater (for marine fish) and saltwater (for freshwater fish) dips are useful for some protozoal ectoparasites but are not recommended for the treatment of Ich because the encysted trophonts are resistant to treatment.
- Ich
  - Only the free-living theront is susceptible to chemical treatment.
  - Detection of even a single Ich trophont warrants treatment.
  - *Cryptocaryon* life cycle is longer (up to 28 days at 75°F to 81°F [24°C to 27°C]) and therefore requires more lengthy treatment.
  - Because only the theront stage is susceptible, multiple treatments are necessary.
  - Formalin (37% formaldehyde) can be administered as a long-term bath at 25 mg/L (2 drops/gal; 1 mL/10 gal). At 77°F to 86°F (25°C to 30°C), affected fish should be treated on alternate days (q 48 h) for three treatments to ensure that all emerging theronts are killed. Fifty percent water changes should be performed before each treatment. In cool water, treatments should be performed every 3-5 days because of the prolonged life cycle.
  - Prolonged immersions of salt (0.1% to 0.3% = 1-3 ppt = 1-3 g/L) can be effective against Ich.
- *Amyloodinium/Piscinoodinium*
  - Only the free-living dinospore is susceptible to treatment.
  - Copper is the most commonly used treatment for marine velvet (*Amyloodinium*).
  - *Piscinoodinium* is less pathogenic and may respond to prolonged salt immersion.
  - *Amyloodinium/Piscinoodinium* can be treated with chloroquine (10 mg/L prolonged bath).
- *Tetrahymena/Uronema*
  - *Tetrahymena/Uronema* can penetrate deep into muscle and internal organs. Cases with muscle/systemic involvement may not respond to treatment. Formalin is the treatment of choice.

DRUG INTERACTIONS

Do not mix formalin and potassium permanganate in the same system.

POSSIBLE COMPLICATIONS

- Adverse side effects can occur in numerous species. A biotest may be performed on a small number of representative fish before widespread usage.
- Formalin can negatively impact the biofilter and decreases dissolved oxygen concentration. The water should be aerated well because each 5 mg/L of formalin added chemically removes 1 mg/L of dissolved oxygen.

RECOMMENDED MONITORING

- Wet mount examinations (skin and gills) should be performed routinely to determine response to treatment.
- Water quality should be monitored closely because some treatments can damage the biofilter.

PROGNOSIS AND OUTCOME

- If environmental/husbandry corrections are made and infestations are caught early, the prognosis can be favorable.
- With poor environmental conditions and heavy infestations, significant mortality may occur.
- Fish with heavy Ich infestations have a guarded prognosis.
- *Tetrahymena/Uronema*: Systemic or deep muscle infections are difficult to treat.

PEARLS & CONSIDERATIONS

PREVENTION

- Provide good husbandry and water quality
- Reduce crowding
- Quarantine new fish for a minimum of 4 weeks

SUGGESTED READINGS

Noga EJ: Fish disease: diagnosis and treatment, St Louis, 1996, Mosby.

Wildgoose WH: BSAVA manual of ornamental fish, ed 2, Gloucester, 2001, British Small Animal Veterinary Association.

AUTHOR: **BRIAN S. PALMEIRO**

EDITOR: **HELEN E. ROBERTS**

Spring Viremia of Carp (SVC)

BASIC INFORMATION

DEFINITION

Reportable viral disease of multiple species caused by spring viremia of carp virus, a rhabdovirus.

SYNONYMS

SVCV, spring viremia

EPIDEMIOLOGY

SPECIES, AGE, SEX

- Koi, goldfish, grass carp, common carp, silver carp, bighead carp, tench, and sheatfish
- Guppies, roach, pumpkinseed, zebra danios pike, and golden shiners have been killed with experimentally induced infection.
- No sex or age specificity

RISK FACTORS Exposure to the virus at permissive water temperatures

CONTAGION AND ZOONOSIS No zoonotic potential

GEOGRAPHY AND SEASONALITY Seen most often in spring but may occur also in fall

CLINICAL PRESENTATION

PHYSICAL EXAM FINDINGS

- No pathognomonic signs
- Exophthalmia, lethargy, pale gills, decreased opercular movements, ascites
- Abnormal swimming (loss of equilibrium), bulging of vent, hemorrhages
- Mortality rates range from 10% to 80%.
- Secondary bacterial and fungal infections may be present.
- Vectors may include *Argulus* spp. (fish louse) and *Pisciola* spp. (leech), fomites, environmental contamination by virus

ETIOLOGY AND PATHOPHYSIOLOGY

- Incubation periods of 7 to 15 days have been reported.
- Clinical disease occurs when water temperature is between 10°C and 18°C (50°F to 64°F).
- Susceptible fish exposed to the virus at water temperatures over (20°C) (68°F) do not usually develop clinical signs.
- Exposure to virus at (16°C to 17°C) (61°F to 62°F) results in 90% death rate in 5 to 17 days (experimentally infected carp).

DIAGNOSIS

DIFFERENTIAL DIAGNOSIS

SVC presents a different, specific clinical picture than most other diseases.

INITIAL DATABASE

- High index of suspicion with clinical signs in multiple species at permissive water temperatures (koi, orfe, and goldfish in an ornamental pond)
- Necropsy findings include hemorrhage in multiple organs, especially the swim bladder, nonspecific inflammation, and edema in coelomic cavity.

ADVANCED OR CONFIRMATORY TESTING

- Samples must be sent to a U.S. Department of Agriculture (USDA)-approved laboratory for testing.
- Any suspicion of SVCV requires the clinician to notify the area veterinarian in charge because of the reportable nature of this disease.

TREATMENT

THERAPEUTIC GOALS

- No treatment for SVC is known.
- Infected populations of fish must be quarantined and destroyed.
- The environment (ponds typically) of the infected fish must be disinfected.
- The virus has been shown to persist at least 42 days in the environment.

PROGNOSIS AND OUTCOME

All fish in the system must be euthanized once the disease has been confirmed.

PEARLS & CONSIDERATIONS

COMMENTS

- Federal regulations instituted in October 2006 require imported SVC-susceptible species to travel with documentation from the competent authority of the exporting country attesting to the fact that the animals being imported have tested negative for SVC according to specific guidelines.
  - An import permit (form VS-135) is required for shipments of SVC-susceptible species entering the United States. There is a fee for the permit.
  - SVC-free status is achieved after 2 years of negative testing (twice-annual testing at appropriate water temperatures).
  - Semiannual testing is required to maintain disease-free status.
  - Importation of SVC-susceptible species requires inspection by a USDA-APHIS VS port veterinarian at port/border of entry with a user fee paid for the inspection.
  - Importers must notify the USDA-APHIS inspector a minimum of 72 hours before arrival.
  - Shipments of SVC-susceptible fish imported into the United States without proper documentation may be held briefly until importers acquire the necessary paperwork. The shipment may be destroyed or returned to the country of origin if the proper documents are not received.
  - All containers used in shipping are made of new material or have been cleaned and disinfected according to protocols listed in the interim rule. If containers are not new, details of cleaning and disinfection (C&D) should be included on the Export Health Certificate or on a separate C&D certificate.
- Currently, no federal program allows a U.S. facility to attain SVC-free status.
- Current and further information can be found by contacting USDA-APHIS VS or http://www.aphis.usda.gov/vs/imports_export/index.shtml.

CLIENT EDUCATION

Quarantine all new fish in a system that allows seasonal temperature fluctuations, including permissive temperatures for koi herpes virus and SVC.

SUGGESTED READINGS

Petty BD, Fraser WA: Viruses of pet fish, Vet Clin Exot Anim 8:67–84, 2005. (U.S. Department of Agriculture, Animal Plant Health Inspection Services). Accessed May 27, 2012

Veterinary Services (USDA APHIS VS): http://www.aphis.usda.gov/import_export/index.shtml and http://www.cfsph.iastate.edu/Factsheets/pdfs/spring_viremia_of_carp.pdf

AUTHOR & EDITOR: **HELEN E. ROBERTS**

FISH

Swim Bladder Disease/Buoyancy Disorders

Client Education Sheet Available on Website

BASIC INFORMATION

DEFINITION

Swim bladder disease is a symptom of various underlying etiologies that results in abnormal buoyancy in the water column. The swim bladder is a gas-filled organ in the dorsal coelomic cavity of fish. Its primary function is maintaining buoyancy, but it is also involved in respiration, sound production, and possibly perception of pressure fluctuations (including sound).

SYNONYMS

Tenpuku (capsized) disease, buoyancy disorder, gyakuten (upside-down) disease

EPIDEMIOLOGY

SPECIES, AGE, SEX

- Can be seen in any species of fish but is especially common in globoid fancy goldfish (Orandas, Ranchus, Lionhead, Moors, Ryukins, fantails, etc.)
- Median age, 3.5 years in one study

CLINICAL PRESENTATION

HISTORY, CHIEF COMPLAINT

- Two clinical presentations of a buoyancy disorder in fish include positive buoyancy ("floaters") and negative buoyancy ("sinkers").
  - "Sinkers" cannot maintain neutral buoyancy and may lay on the bottom of the tank in lateral recumbency.
  - "Floaters" (the more common presentation in fancy goldfish) will float at the surface on one side or upside down.
  - In either presentation, the clinical signs can be transient or permanent.
- Many of these fish remain active and alert with a good appetite.

PHYSICAL EXAM FINDINGS

- Physical examination may reveal abdominal distention.
- Secondary skin changes can occur in both "floaters" and "sinkers" secondary to prolonged contact and desiccation, respectively. Dermatologic findings include erythema, erosions, and ulcerations.

ETIOLOGY AND PATHOPHYSIOLOGY

- Diseases of the swim bladder can result in overinflation or underinflation, causing positive or negative buoyancy, respectively.
- The exact cause of buoyancy disorder is unknown.
- Possibilities include pneumocystis (infectious, idiopathic), swim bladder torsion, anatomic abnormalities of the swim bladder, mechanical obstruction of the pneumatic duct, poor water quality, low water temperature, and neoplasia.
- The condition is especially common in globoid fancy goldfish and may be secondary to conformational changes in the body brought about by selective breeding and genetics.
- Light, floating foods such as flakes and pellets have been incriminated because they are theorized to expand with water in the digestive tract and occlude the pneumatic duct.
- A large number (up to 85%) of fish with buoyancy disorder may have underlying disease.

DIAGNOSIS

DIFFERENTIAL DIAGNOSIS

- Differential diagnoses include other causes of abdominal distention such as ascites, neoplasia, egg binding, granulomas, and cysts (e.g., polycystic kidney disease); gas distention of the intestinal tract; and neurologic disease.
- Gastrointestinal disease (and resultant gas accumulation) is a common cause for buoyancy disorders in non-goldfish species.
- Space-occupying lesions in the coelomic cavity can cause positive or negative buoyancy by altering the normal position of, or compressing, the swim bladder.

INITIAL DATABASE

- The diagnostic approach to a fish with buoyancy disorder should begin with complete history, water chemistry (temperature, salinity, pH, ammonia, nitrites, nitrates, alkalinity, dissolved oxygen), and thorough evaluation of the environment/husbandry.
- Direct observation of the fish in the aquarium or pond
- Complete physical examination
  - Neurologic examination includes checking for the presence of the oculogyration reflex. The upper eye of fish in lateral recumbency should normally be pointed ventrally. Also evaluate the laterally recumbent fish for its ability to right itself in the water column.
  - Skin scraping and gill biopsy wet mounts should be performed to evaluate for the presence of parasites and/or other abnormalities.
  - Fecal examination should be performed to rule out intestinal parasitism.
- Imaging
  - Unfortunately, extreme variability has been noted in the "normal" radiographic appearance of the swim bladder in fancy goldfish. In one study, caudal swim bladder chambers were radiographically present in 29% of diseased goldfish and in 40% of healthy goldfish.
  - Radiography is most useful to rule out other potential causes of abdominal distention and buoyancy disorder such as neoplasia, ascites, egg binding, and gas accumulation in the gastrointestinal tract.
  - Dental radiographs give excellent results in smaller patients.
  - Ultrasound examination may also be useful to look for fluid in the swim bladder and to rule out other coelomic abnormalities.
- If fluid is present in the swim bladder, a sterile sample should be obtained for cytologic examination, acid-fast stain, and culture/sensitivity.
- Clinical pathology is useful in some cases, but the veterinarian is often limited by patient size and lack of reference intervals.

TREATMENT

THERAPEUTIC GOAL

Normalize buoyancy

ACUTE GENERAL TREATMENT

- Husbandry
  - Correcting environmental abnormalities (poor water quality, filtration, etc.) is the first step in treating swim bladder disease.
  - The water temperature should be gradually increased to 24°C to 27°C (75°F to 80°F).
  - Nutrition should be evaluated (see dietary causes earlier), and a diet with a variety of foods including fresh greens/vegetables should be offered.
- Nonpharmacologic and medical treatments
  - If no improvement is noted with husbandry changes, the fish should be fasted for 3 to 5 days. The author then begins a trial with green peas (canned or cooked and lightly crushed) fed once daily for 2 weeks. Green peas have been used successfully to treat buoyancy disorder

in seven fish. Theoretically, the pea forces more buoyant food (such as flake food) through the intestinal tract, unobstructing the pneumatic duct. The high fiber content may also be beneficial.
  - Depending on response to environmental and dietary changes, the author administers metronidazole (concentration 0.5%/5 mg/kg food) in the food for 14 days for possible gastroenteritis. This is equivalent to feeding 50 mg/kg bw when the food is fed at a rate of 1% bodyweight. Oral doses of 25-100 mg/kg bw have been reported. Metronidazole can be mixed into a gel diet or top dressed on a commercial diet. If the fecal examination is positive for flagellated parasites (*Hexamita/Spironucleus*), or if radiographs reveal gas accumulation in the intestines, metronidazole is the first line of treatment.
  - Patients with bacterial swim bladder infection (excluding mycobacteriosis) can respond very well to a 21-day course of parenteral antibiotics. The author's first choice is enrofloxacin 5 to 10 mg/kg IM/ICe q 72-96 h pending culture results.
  - Palliative percutaneous decompressive pneumocystocentesis can be performed in positively buoyant cases. The fish will become negatively buoyant, but the effects are usually transient, and treatment needs to be repeated.
  - Barriers can be placed in the tank to prevent parts of the fish from protruding out of the water.
  - In negatively buoyant cases, buoyancy devices that aid in flotation have been created (with Floy anchor tags and buoyant material/cork fishing float) and are reportedly effective, at least in the short term.
  - If secondary skin changes are significant, treatment with topical medications ± systemic antibiotics may be necessary. Topical medications include silver sulfadiazine, povidone-iodine ointment, and other antibiotic ointments. Noniodized salt can be added to freshwater systems to reduce osmotic stress (salinity 0.1% to 0.3% [1-3 g/L]).
- Surgical treatment
  - Surgical treatment for swim bladder disease has been reported in two fish. In a Ryukin goldfish, surgical clips were used to reduce the volume of the overinflated caudal swim bladder. The fish became negatively buoyant but died 24 days after surgery. Pneumocystectomy was performed in a 5-year-old Midas cichlid, resulting in improved clinical signs.
  - The successful use of intracoelomically placed weights (such as aluminum, quartz, or ball-bearing implants) has anecdotally been reported in positively buoyant cases.

PROGNOSIS AND OUTCOME

Swim bladder disease can be a very frustrating problem. Response to treatment and prognosis are generally poor, especially when underlying disease is present. Cases with fluid accumulation in the swim bladder secondary to bacterial infection (excluding mycobacteriosis) usually respond best to treatment.

PEARLS & CONSIDERATIONS

COMMENTS

- Fish can be categorized by their type of swim bladder into physostomous or physoclistous fish.
  - Physostomous fish (such as goldfish) have a pneumatic duct, which connects the swim bladder to the esophagus, allowing swallowed air to inflate the swim bladder.
  - Physoclistous fish have a prominent countercurrent capillary system (rete mirabile) in the wall of each chamber that regulates the amount of gas in the swim bladder. Many physostomous fish also have vascular rete.

SUGGESTED READING

Lewbart GA: Green peas for buoyancy disorders, Exotic DVM 2:7, 2000.

Lewbart GA, et al: Development of a minimally invasive technique to stabilize buoyancy-challenged goldfish, San Diego, 2005, Proceedings International Association for Aquatic Animal Medicine (IAAAM).

Palmeiro BS: Sink, float or swim: battling tenpuku disease (buoyancy disorder) in goldfish, Schaumburg, Ill, July 2007, Proceedings American Veterinary Medical Association (AVMA).

Tanaka D, et al: Gross, radiological and anatomical findings of goldfish with tenpuku disease, Suisanzoshoku 46:293–299, 1998.

Wildgoose WH: BSAVA manual of ornamental fish, ed 2, Gloucester, 2001, British Small Animal Veterinary Association.

Wildgoose WH: Buoyancy disorders of ornamental fish: a review of cases seen in veterinary practice, Fish Vet J 9:22–37, 2007.

AUTHOR: **BRIAN S. PALMEIRO**

EDITOR: **HELEN E. ROBERTS**

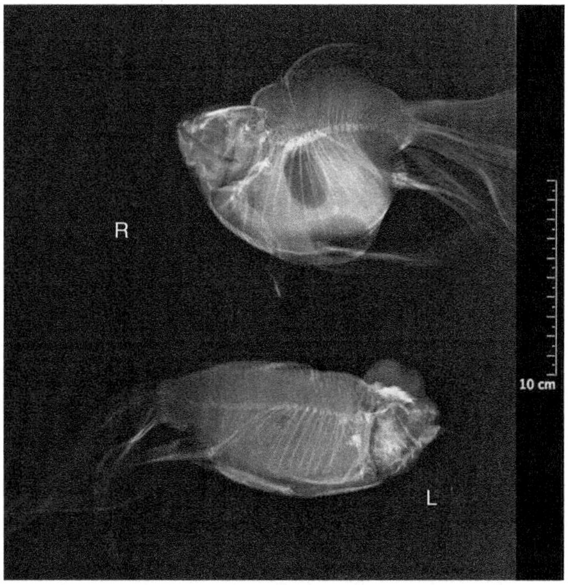

Swim Bladder Disease Two goldfish with severe changes in the swim bladder; in the goldfish, the normal anatomy of the swim bladder is a bilobed bladder, with the caudal part a bit smaller than the cranial part. *(Photo courtesy Jörg Mayer, The University of Georgia, Athens.)*

FISH

Trauma and Wound Management

BASIC INFORMATION

DEFINITION

Trauma is defined as any wound or injury to the body, usually caused by external factors. Wound management is defined as the care required to heal the injury and/or assist with the body's own healing mechanisms.

SYNONYMS

Injury, wounds, cuts, lacerations, bites, fractures

EPIDEMIOLOGY

SPECIES, AGE, SEX
Any fish (species, age, sex, etc.) can be susceptible to injury or trauma.

RISK FACTORS
- Sharp objects in tank or pond
- Careless netting practices
- Predators, including herons, raccoons, mink, and domestic cats
- External parasites may predispose the fish to flashing (scratching against objects or floor of the tank or pond) and the appearance of self-inflicted wounds.
- Fish behavior such as flashing, jumping out of tank/pond, and spawning
- Secondary bacterial infection can progress to internal organ failure and fatal septicemia
- Intraspecies and interspecies aggression
- Overstocking

ASSOCIATED CONDITIONS AND DISORDERS Secondary bacterial/fungal infections, septicemia, cutaneous ulcers

CLINICAL PRESENTATION

HISTORY, CHIEF COMPLAINT Wound or injury on fish as noted by client

PHYSICAL EXAM FINDINGS
- Signs dependent on the body area affected. Usually trauma can be visualized grossly. History may reveal the visit of a predator such as a heron or a raccoon in pond fish or sharp ornamentation in aquaria.
- Wounds may become secondarily infected with bacterial pathogens and fungal organisms. Secondary algal growth may also be present.
- Physical examination is best performed by first observing the fish in its own environment. This makes it easier to evaluate location in the water column, social behavior (isolation vs. schooling in appropriate species), and the presence of abnormal movements such as flashing or rapid opercular movements. Some fish, especially large or aggressive fish, may need to be sedated for a complete physical examination. In most cases, the traumatic injury will be evident on the external body surface or fins. In some circumstances, vertebral/spinal abnormalities may require radiographs to detect fractures and other skeletal injuries.

DIAGNOSIS

DIFFERENTIAL DIAGNOSIS

- Trauma is a condition that has many presentations, but the diagnosis of a traumatically induced injury is usually apparent.
- Cutaneous ulcers may be result from poor water quality/husbandry, external parasitism, or bacterial infection (including mycobacteriosis), or it may be secondary to self-inflicted trauma.
- Nutritional, toxic, chemical, and husbandry-related (e.g., electrical shock) causes should be ruled out with evidence of spinal abnormalities.
- Historical data will usually reveal an inciting cause.

INITIAL DATABASE

- Cultures of infected wounds will usually yield Gram-negative bacteria (e.g., *Aeromonas* spp.) that are secondary or opportunistic pathogens.
- It is important to understand that the routine culture sampling methods used for terrestrial animals may not accurately reveal pathogenic organisms in aquatic animals.
- Handling and transport of samples can affect culture results.
- Preferentially, samples should be submitted to laboratories with experience in aquatic animal diseases.
  - Culture needs to be done at lower temperature than for mammals (usually room temperature is adequate).
- Cytology: Wet mount microscopic evaluation of the lesion can reveal the presence of secondary fungal colonization and algal growth. Inflammatory cells and bacteria may also be seen in cytologic preparations. Skin and gill scrapings should be performed to check for the presence of parasites.

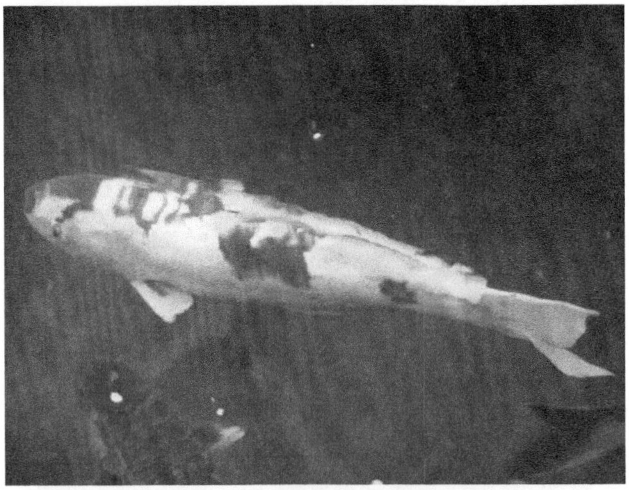

Trauma and Wound Management Wet mount cytology of dorsal lesions in this koi revealed fungal disease and numerous flukes (*Gyrodactylus* spp). Dorsal lesions can also be consistent with sunburn. *(Courtesy Helen E. Roberts.)*

ADVANCED OR CONFIRMATORY TESTING

- Histopathology: Skin biopsies may be helpful for diagnosis and treatment of chronic open wounds or deep wounds. Culture of biopsied specimens may better define bacterial and/or fungal pathogens responsible for the primary infection; superficial cytology may show only contamination by secondary invaders.
- Imaging: Radiographs can be used to rule out skeletal abnormalities but generally are not effective for an accurate assessment of the coelomic cavity. Spinal fractures can occur with stray voltage and iatrogenic causes such as poor handling and netting techniques. Predators such as herons and the "suicidal" jumping behavior of fish can lead to spinal injury. Ultrasonography, computed tomography (CT), and magnetic resonance imaging (MRI) are other modalities that may be used, if available.

TREATMENT

THERAPEUTIC GOALS

- Husbandry
  - Inciting causes such as ectoparasites and poor water quality should be addressed.
  - Remove sharp/harmful objects from the environment.
  - Inexperienced owners should be instructed on netting and fish handling.
  - Pond construction should limit the opportunity for predation by pond design or by protective fencing.
  - Evaluate husbandry practices such as feeding (quantity, food type), water change schedule, additives used by owner, and overall tank or pond hygiene.
  - Life support systems need to be adequate for pond or tank size and bioload.
  - Nutrition should be evaluated (old food discarded).
  - Transfer to a quarantine or a hospital tank usually makes treatment and evaluation of therapeutic response easier if few or one fish is affected. If large numbers of fish are affected, it is best to treat the entire tank or pond.
  - In cases of interspecies or intraspecies aggression, fish that are fighting should be separated.
  - Reduce stocking density if trauma is due to crowding.

ACUTE GENERAL TREATMENT

- Medical treatment
  - Infected wounds should be cultured, and cytologic evaluation/wet mounts should be performed.
  - Empirical treatment with parenteral antibiotics can be started if the wound is deep, infected, or extensive and in cases of suspected septicemia.
  - Most bacterial pathogens in fish are Gram-negative, so the initial choice of an antimicrobial should be one that has a spectrum of activity against Gram-negative bacteria.
  - Careful débridement of the wound to remove necrotic tissue and debris can be done with sterile gauze using sterile saline, dilute chlorhexidine, or povidone-iodine solution.
  - Frequent débridement is not recommended because this disrupts normal reepithelialization.
  - Bandage application to the wound is not feasible in most cases.
  - Liquid "bandages" (Orabase, New Skin) can be used to provide a thin barrier over the healing wound.
- Surgical treatment
  - Primary closure of the wound, once débrided, can be beneficial because it provides an osmotic barrier to the environment; however, this cannot be done in most cases.
  - Monofilament, nonabsorbable or absorbable sutures such as nylon or polydioxanone (PDS) are recommended.
  - Fish do not degrade absorbable sutures as other species do, so all sutures will have to be removed in 10 to 20 days, depending on healing, water temperature, and presence of inflammation or secondary infection.
- Drugs of choice
  - Systemic antibiotics
    - Empirical therapy can be instituted pending culture and sensitivity results
    - Good choices for initial therapy include
      - Enrofloxacin 5 to 10 mg/kg IM, ICe q 72-96 h
      - Ceftazidime 20 mg/kg IM q 72 h
    - Oral medications can be mixed into a gel diet or top dressed on a commercial diet if the patient is eating.
      - Enrofloxacin injectable 2.27% solution can be added at rate of 10 mg/kg pelleted food.
      - Mazuri Aquatic Gel diets (PMI Nutrition International, St Louis, Missouri; www.mazuri.com) are available in powder form and make addition of medications feasible for owners to prepare.
    - Prolonged immersion or bath treatments can be used for treatment of superficial infection; however, parenteral and oral routes of administration are more effective.
  - Topical therapy
    - Topical medications such as silver sulfadiazine, povidone-iodine ointment, and other antibiotic ointments can be applied.
    - Drying the area with gauze will improve the adhesive action of the ointment, although topical therapy should still be considered temporary.
    - The author has successfully used Tricide-Neo (Molecular Therapeutics, LLC, Athens, Georgia) solution as a topical spray on infected wounds on a daily or intermittent basis (treatment interval based on potential stress to the patient).
  - Pain management
    - No analgesic for fish has been approved by the Food and Drug Administration (FDA), although the FDA has approved the anesthetic agent Finquel (MS-222 or tricaine methanesulfonate, Argent Chemical Laboratories, Redmond, Washington), which may provide some analgesia.
    - Butorphanol 0.4 mg/kg IM, carprofen 2.2 mg/kg IM, and ketoprofen 2 mg/kg IM have been used by the author with variable success in some species.

RECOMMENDED MONITORING

- Weekly rechecks or phone calls to the owner to check on healing progress of injuries are recommended.
- Owners living long distances from the clinician can email photos of lesions; however, the photos must be clear and must display the appropriate site of interest.

PROGNOSIS AND OUTCOME

Depending on injury, from good to grave

PEARLS & CONSIDERATIONS

COMMENTS

- It is not uncommon for pet fish hobbyists to gain access to a wide variety of unapproved pharmaceutical agents such as amikacin, enrofloxacin, and others.
- Diplomatic education of the hobbyist should include dosage and dosage intervals of the therapeutics prescribed. Inaccurate dosages and recommended medications are often found on various Internet sites. Discussion should include information on the use of FDA-approved medications in food animal aquatic species.

- Effectiveness and adverse side effects can occur in multiple species. A biotest may be performed to "test" the agent in a system before widespread usage.

CLIENT EDUCATION

- Excellent water quality and stress reduction will help to promote wound healing.
- Noniodized salt should be added to freshwater systems to reduce osmotic stress and aid in healing of wounds. Salt levels of 0.1% to 0.3% (1-3 g/L water) have been found to be helpful.
- Overcrowding, overfeeding, and inadequate life support systems should be corrected.
- New fish should be quarantined to prevent widespread outbreaks of parasitic infestation and introduction of pathogenic bacterial disease and infectious viral disease.
- Routine water changes and water chemistry monitoring will help reduce stress.
- Reevaluation of the environment and the patient is essential. Therapy may be changed pending response to treatment.
- Discontinuation of treatment should be based on advice from the clinician.

SUGGESTED READINGS

Fontenot DK, Neiffer DL: Wound management in teleost fish: biology of the healing process, evaluation and treatment, Vet Clin Exot Anim 7:57–86, 2004.

Wildgoose WH: BSAVA manual of ornamental fish, ed 2, Gloucester, 2001, British Small Animal Veterinary Association.

CROSS-REFERENCES TO OTHER SECTIONS

Husbandry
Physical Examination
Minimum Database

AUTHOR & EDITOR: **HELEN E. ROBERTS**

FISH

Ulcer Disease in Koi

BASIC INFORMATION

DEFINITION

An ulcer is a defect or break in the epidermis that penetrates the basement membrane, exposing the underlying dermis. Ulcers can be superficial and mild or deep, extending into the underlying musculature and, rarely, into the coelomic cavity.

SYNONYMS

Ulcerative dermatitis, ulcerative skin disease, "aeromonas" disease, erythrodermatitis, furunculosis

EPIDEMIOLOGY

SPECIES, AGE, SEX All koi can be affected regardless of age, sex, and type.

RISK FACTORS

- Poor water quality
- Poor husbandry practices
- Poor nutrition
- Environmental hazards (sharp objects)
- Failure to quarantine new fish

CONTAGION AND ZOONOSIS Ectoparasites, poor water quality, some viral diseases, and primary bacterial pathogens will result in higher morbidity, typically with numerous fish affected. Trauma and predation may affect only individual fish.

GEOGRAPHY AND SEASONALITY No specific geographic distribution. In regions of the country that experience seasonal water temperature variations, ulcers may be seen more often in spring and fall owing to decreased immune system function.

ASSOCIATED CONDITIONS AND DISORDERS

- Poor water quality/husbandry can precipitate koi ulcer disease.
- Koi herpes virus (KHV) outbreaks can result in cutaneous ulcers.
- Other associated infections include ectoparasites, secondary bacterial infections, and *Saprolegnia* (oomycetes).
- Systemic bacterial infection

CLINICAL PRESENTATION

DISEASE FORMS/SUBTYPES Acute onset with high morbidity can be seen with virulent primary bacterial pathogens or with koi herpes virus disease outbreaks. Slower onset of clinical signs is usually seen with poor water quality, ectoparasites, etc.

HISTORY, CHIEF COMPLAINT Owner may report a history of flashing, lethargy, failure to thrive, and poor appetite. Ulcers may be seen by owner, but not always. Mortality may be the first observed sign.

PHYSICAL EXAM FINDINGS

- Vary from superficial ulceration of the skin to deep ulcers involving the underlying musculature. Rarely, the coelomic cavity is penetrated by a deep ulcer.
  - Ulcers are commonly surrounded by a peripheral annular region of erythema/hemorrhage with scales that are easily removed.
- Flashing, aimless drifting, lethargy, and abnormal water column positions may be observed by clinicians.
- If secondary septicemia is present, hemorrhagic lesions on the skin (petechiae and ecchymoses), abdominal distention/ascites/dropsy, and exophthalmia ("pop-eye") may be noted.

ETIOLOGY AND PATHOPHYSIOLOGY

- Multiple possible causes
  - The primary pathogen is *Aeromonas salmonicida* (subspecies *achromogenes*) in most cases. *A. salmonicida* was detected via polymerase chain reaction (PCR) in 77% of koi ulcer samples.
  - Lesions are commonly invaded by other species of bacteria (most commonly motile aeromonads) and other microorganisms (including *Saprolegnia*).
  - Ectoparasites may cause cutaneous damage, allowing bacterial invasion.

DIAGNOSIS

DIFFERENTIAL DIAGNOSIS

- An ulcer is fairly unique in presentation but is not pathognomonic for any disease condition.
- Koi herpes virus may cause cutaneous ulcers in koi.
- Ectoparasites
- Other species of bacteria can cause ulcerative skin lesions, including *Mycobacterium* spp.
- Cutaneous neoplasms (squamous cell carcinoma, schwannoma/neurofibroma, various sarcomas, etc.)

INITIAL DATABASE

- Ectoparasite evaluation (skin scrapings, gill biopsies/scrapings, fin biopsy)

- Cytology (wet mount and Gram stain) of ulcer
- Water chemistry testing
- Pond design evaluation, including life support systems
- Environmental hazard analyses (predators, depth of pond, etc.)
- Culture and sensitivity of the lesion
    - It can be very difficult to culture *Aeromonas salmonicida* because cultures can become quickly overgrown by faster growing motile aeromonads and other species.
    - Best culture results are obtained by sampling the peripheral margin of the lesion.

ADVANCED OR CONFIRMATORY TESTING

- Histopathology of affected lesions typically reveals severe ulcerative dermatitis, myositis, and panniculitis.
- With large populations, a representative/moribund fish should be selected for necropsy and culture of caudal kidney tissue.
    - Necropsy is best performed on freshly dead fish.
- KHV PCR testing on gill, spleen, and kidney tissues is recommended in cases where KHV is suspected.
    - If owner is reluctant to sacrifice a fish, a gill swab can be submitted for PCR testing, although this may yield a false negative.
- PCR for *A. salmonicida* can be performed.

TREATMENT

THERAPEUTIC GOAL

Resolve ulcer(s) and treat any associated causes/infections

ACUTE GENERAL TREATMENT

- Maintenance of optimal water quality and husbandry with frequent water changes is necessary for successful management of this disorder.
- Antimicrobial therapy
    - Injectable antibiotics typically give the best results when treating ulcer disease and should be initiated empirically pending culture/sensitivity data. Most pathogens cultured are Gram negative. Choices of the authors include enrofloxacin 5 to 10 mg/kg IM or ICe q 3-5 days (water temperature dependent) or ceftazidime 20 mg/kg IM or ICe q 72 h.
    - A minimum of 3-4 weeks of antimicrobial therapy is needed in many cases.
    - Fish can be given antibiotics orally (mixed in food) if eating.
- Débridement of ulcer under anesthesia (MS 222, 50-100 ppm)
    - Pain management preoperatively may include butorphanol 0.4 mg/kg IM and/or carprofen 2.2 mg/kg.
- Increase salinity
    - Salt should be added to the water to achieve 0.1% to 0.3% (1-3 g/L) to reduce osmotic stress.
- Potential topical therapies
    - Tricide or Tricide Neo (Molecular Therapeutics, LLC, Athens, Georgia) can be sprayed topically or used as a dip once daily to aid in healing.
    - Topical silver sulfadiazine cream
- Increase water temperature
    - Fish kept outdoors in water temperatures below 60°F/15°C should be moved indoors to warmer water. The temperature gradient should not change by more than 1°C per hour if possible. Warmer water promotes the immune response and inhibits bacterial growth. The authors typically recommend water temperatures between 24°C and 27°C (75°F and 80°F). Healing will not usually occur in cold or cool water temperatures.
- Isolation
    - The disease is contagious, and affected fish should be isolated.
- Parasitic infestations should be treated appropriately.
- See Trauma and Wound Management.

CHRONIC TREATMENT

Correct underlying causes, if any are known.

POSSIBLE COMPLICATIONS

- Bacterial septicemia
- Rupture of ulcer into coelomic cavity
- Resistant bacterial strains
- Failure to correct inadequate husbandry practices or poor environment

RECOMMENDED MONITORING

- Monitor for healing (decreasing size) of ulcer.
- Recheck fish in 1-2 weeks, and repeat wet mount cytology if ectoparasites were found.

PROGNOSIS AND OUTCOME

Excellent to grave, depending on the cause

PEARLS & CONSIDERATIONS

COMMENTS

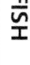

- Correcting underlying water quality/husbandry issues is an integral step in the successful treatment of this disorder.
- It is important to observe the fish in their environment, especially if multiple fish are affected. Ambulatory calls are the best way to accomplish this.

PREVENTION

- Buy healthy fish from reputable dealers.
- Quarantine all new fish and observe for lesions.
- Have quarantined fish examined by aquatic veterinarian if any abnormalities are present.
- Treat/disinfect plants before adding to pond or aquarium to remove potential pathogens.

CLIENT EDUCATION

- Correct husbandry issues.
- Reduce the presence of any other stressors if possible.
- Discuss and set up quarantine protocols.
- Discuss proper dietary management.

SUGGESTED READINGS

Anders BB, et al: Identification of the etiologic agent for ulcerative disease in koi (*Cyprinus carpio*), Proceedings International Virtual Conferences in Veterinary Medicine, 1999.

Goodwin A, Merry G: Are all koi and goldfish ulcers caused by *Aeromonas salmonicida achromogenes*? Proceedings of the Western Fish Disease Workshop American Fisheries Society, June 4-6, 2007, Nanaimo, BC, Canada.

Hunt CJ-G: Ulcerative skin disease in a group of koi carp (*Cyprinus carpio*). Vet Clin Exot Anim 9:723–728, 2006.

Wildgoose WH: BSAVA manual of ornamental fish, ed 2, Gloucester, 2001, British Small Animal Veterinary Association.

CROSS-REFERENCES TO OTHER SECTIONS

Trauma and Wound Management

AUTHORS: **HELEN E. ROBERTS & BRIAN S. PALMEIRO**

EDITOR: **HELEN E. ROBERTS**

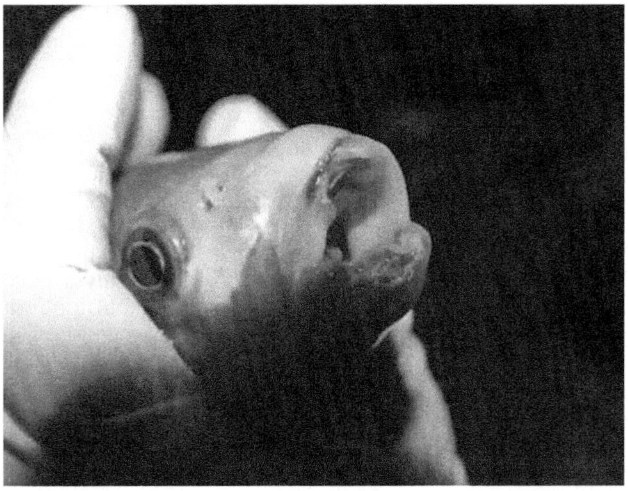

Ulcer Disease in Koi Severe oral erosive and ulcerative bacterial dermatitis ("mouth rot") in a koi (*Cyprinus carpio*) caused by *Aeromonas* spp. Note the exposed underlying cartilage. *(Courtesy Helen E. Roberts.)*

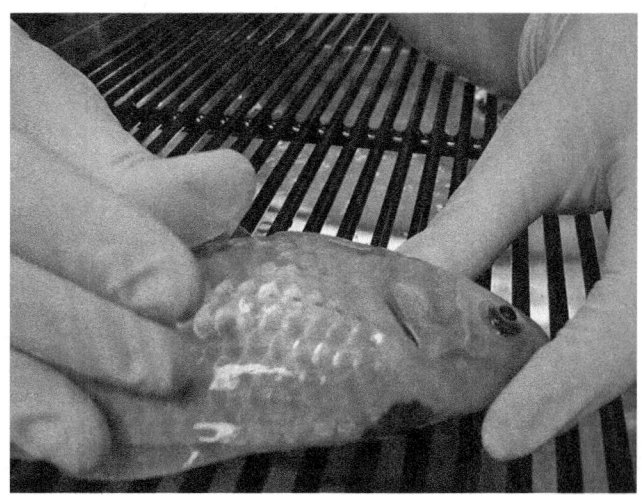

Ulcer Disease in Koi Using a coverslip at a 45-degree angle to obtain a sample of mucus from an anesthetized fish for diagnostic wet mount cytology. *(Courtesy Helen E. Roberts.)*

FISH

Viral Diseases

BASIC INFORMATION

DEFINITION

A few significant viral diseases of pet fish have been identified. Two diseases have recently elicited much discussion in the development of U.S. Department of Agriculture (USDA) import regulations and reporting status. These are koi herpes virus (KHV; Cyprinid herpes virus-3 [CyHV-3]) and spring viremia of carp (SVC).

EPIDEMIOLOGY

SPECIES, AGE, SEX Viral diseases can be found in multiple species of freshwater and marine pet fish. Susceptibility to infection can vary with age in some viral disease situations. Water temperatures are often critical in the appearance of viral disease outbreaks.

GENETICS AND BREED PREDISPOSITION Some viral diseases are host specific; others affect multiples species and age groups.

RISK FACTORS

- Failure to quarantine is the most common risk factor associated with viral disease outbreaks.
- The presence of stressors such as poor water quality, poor husbandry practices, and overcrowding can increase susceptibility to disease.
- Shared equipment between tanks and/or ponds can act as fomites and transmit disease between populations.
- Negligent biosecurity practices in retail, wholesale, and aquacultural settings can increase the likelihood of viral outbreaks and mortalities on a large scale.

CONTAGION AND ZOONOSIS Infectivity varies with viral agent.

GEOGRAPHY AND SEASONALITY Nonspecific. Viral diseases affect fish in cool water and warm water environments.

ASSOCIATED CONDITIONS AND DISORDERS Secondary bacterial infections, fungal infections, and general deterioration of body condition can be associated with some viral diseases.

CLINICAL PRESENTATION

DISEASE FORMS/SUBTYPES

- Most incubation periods and disease outbreaks of viral diseases are water temperature dependent.
- Viral diseases can present acutely, peracutely, or as chronic conditions.

HISTORY, CHIEF COMPLAINT Varies

PHYSICAL EXAM FINDINGS Vary

DIAGNOSIS

DIFFERENTIAL DIAGNOSIS

- Bacterial diseases
- Parasitic diseases
- Environmental disorders such as poor water quality and environmental toxicity, as well as iatrogenic causes of environmental problems

INITIAL DATABASE

- The diagnostic approach to a fish with suspected viral disease should begin with complete history, water chemistry (temperature, salinity, pH, ammonia, nitrites, nitrates, alkalinity, dissolved oxygen), and thorough evaluation of the environment/husbandry.
- Direct observation of the fish in the aquarium or pond
- Complete physical examination

ADVANCED OR CONFIRMATORY TESTING

- Cytologic examination
- Histopathologic examination
- Electron microscopy
- Virus isolation and identification
- Virus specific testing (polymerase chain reaction [PCR], etc.)

TREATMENT

THERAPEUTIC GOALS

- In most cases, no specific treatment is known for an outbreak of viral disease.
- Supportive care may affect the outcome.

ACUTE GENERAL TREATMENT

- Maintain excellent water quality.
- Monitor appetite.

RECOMMENDED MONITORING

- Monitor for resolution of clinical signs.
- Monitor water chemistry parameters.

PROGNOSIS AND OUTCOME

Vary with viral agent from low mortality to widespread fish kills

PEARLS & CONSIDERATIONS

PREVENTION

- Disinfection and quarantine may help prevent spread of the disease.
- Identification of the original source of the infection can aid in preventing further outbreaks.
- Vaccines may be available for specific viral diseases.

CLIENT EDUCATION

- Quarantine for a minimum length of time (30 days to 1 year, depending on species and viral agent) in a fully cycled quarantine tank or pond.
- For koi, owners can ask for KHV serology test results on prospective purchases.
- Use separate equipment for each tank/pond/system, or disinfect equipment between systems.
- Reduce stressors such as poor water quality, overfeeding, overstocking, etc.

SUGGESTED READING

Petty BD, Fraser WA: Viruses of pet fish, Vet Clin Exot Anim 8:67–84, 2005.

AUTHOR & EDITOR: **HELEN E. ROBERTS**

FISH

Viral Epidermal Hyperplasia (Carp Pox)

BASIC INFORMATION

DEFINITION

Infection with Cyprinid herpes virus-1 (CyHV-1) in susceptible species

SYNONYMS

Carp pox, papillosum cyprinid, viral epidermal hyperplasia

EPIDEMIOLOGY

SPECIES, AGE, SEX

- *Cyprinus carpio* (koi) primarily, although infections have been observed in other coldwater species (orfe, rudd) and in some tropical aquarium fish.
- Infection of koi fry younger than 2 months of age can cause systemic disease, and fatalities may occur.

RISK FACTORS Exposure to fish that are shedding the virus. As with other herpes viral infections in fish and other species, herpes infections are lifelong, and latent carriers are plausible.

CONTAGION AND ZOONOSIS

- Incubation period is water temperature dependent, and clinical signs may take up to 2 months to appear.
- Viral replication occurs at an optimum water temperature of 15°C (59°F).

GEOGRAPHY AND SEASONALITY

- Lesions can be seasonal, appearing in water temperatures less than 15°C (59°F).
- Lesions can regress in warmer water (once water temperatures reach 20°C [68°F]).

CLINICAL PRESENTATION

DISEASE FORMS/SUBTYPES

- Systemic infection and mortalities occur in koi fry younger than 2 months.
- In koi over 2 months of age, dermal lesions are the most common manifestation of CyHV-1 infection.

HISTORY, CHIEF COMPLAINT The owner reports the presence of dermal lesions appearing as raised, smooth white to tan patches resembling melted wax.

PHYSICAL EXAM FINDINGS

- Presence of raised, nodular lesions with a waxy appearance that regress in warmer water temperatures raises the index of suspicion for carp pox.
- Some lesions can progress to papillomatous growths.
- Usually seen on head and fins but can appear anywhere

ETIOLOGY AND PATHOPHYSIOLOGY

- Incubation period is water temperature dependent, and clinical signs may take up to 2 months to appear.
- Lesions can be seasonal, appearing in water temperatures less than 15°C (59°F).
- Lesions can regress in warmer water (once water temperatures reach 20°C [68°F]).
- Viral replication occurs at an optimum water temperature of 15°C (59°F).

DIAGNOSIS

DIFFERENTIAL DIAGNOSIS

- The lesions are highly suggestive of infection.
- Other skin lesions may present with a similar appearance, and histopathology will be necessary to determine diagnosis.

INITIAL DATABASE

- A complete history
- Evaluation of the environment, including water testing
- Complete physical examination
- Wet mount cytologic examination for ectoparasites
- Exfoliative cytologic examination of skin lesions

ADVANCED OR CONFIRMATORY TESTING

- Histopathology: hyperplasia of epidermal cells seen in biopsied samples
- Electron microscopy
- Testing for presence of virus can be done on submitted samples.

TREATMENT

ACUTE GENERAL TREATMENT

- No specific treatment is known.
- Lesions usually resolve in warmer weather, only to recur as water cools.

PROGNOSIS AND OUTCOME

- Infection in fish older than 2 months generally is not fatal. Infection results in a fish with cosmetic faults that may not be used in fish shows.
- The presence of infected fish in a population may limit further introductions of new fish.

PEARLS & CONSIDERATIONS

COMMENTS

- The author has seen cases of carp pox that did not regress in warmer temperatures.

- The virus appears to have a low level of infectivity in populations of koi.
- The presence of lesions in adult fish is usually an aesthetic problem, but the virus can be fatal to juvenile fish.

PREVENTION

Quarantine new fish; do not expose naïve fish to populations containing infected fish.

CLIENT EDUCATION

- Quarantine new fish for a period of time that allows water temperature changes (need to have the capacity for increasing and decreasing water temperature).
- Avoid purchasing fish from tanks with infected fish.
- Examine new fish carefully for any external lesions.

SUGGESTED READINGS

Petty BD, Fraser WA: Viruses of pet fish, Vet Clin Exot Anim 8:67–84, 2005.
Szignarowitz B: Update on koi herpes virus, Exotic DVM 7(3):92–95, 2005.
Wildgoose WH: BSAVA manual of ornamental fish, ed 2, Gloucester, 2001, British Small Animal Veterinary Association.

AUTHOR & EDITOR: **HELEN E. ROBERTS**

FISH

Water Quality and Pet Fish Health

BASIC INFORMATION

DEFINITION

- Water quality includes all physical, chemical, and biological characteristics of water that regulate its suitability for maintaining fish.
- Poor water quality is the most common cause of morbidity and mortality in pet fish and the most common stressor that precipitates disease.
- Water quality should be monitored weekly, and records should be maintained to monitor fluctuations.
- Water quality should be performed as part of the minimum database in every fish case.
- Reagents should be replaced yearly.

SYNONYM

Water chemistry

EPIDEMIOLOGY

SPECIES, AGE, SEX

- Any fish may be affected regardless of age, sex, and species.
- Each species has an optimal range for individual water quality parameters.

RISK FACTORS Poor husbandry practices such as overcrowding, overfeeding, and inadequate water flow or filtration predispose to poor water quality.

ASSOCIATED CONDITIONS AND DISORDERS Acute or chronic stress resulting from exposure to poor water quality will often lead to reduced immune system function, predisposing fish to infection by opportunistic pathogens.

CLINICAL PRESENTATION

DISEASE FORMS/SUBTYPES

- Acute exposure to poor water quality can result in sudden and significant mortality.
- Chronic exposure to suboptimal water quality conditions can predispose fish to a variety of infectious diseases that ultimately lead to mortality.

TREATMENT

ACUTE GENERAL TREATMENT

- **Temperature**
  - Fish are poikilothermic.
  - Ideal temperature varies with species. Freshwater tropicals prefer 75°F to 80°F (24°C to 27°C), marine tropicals prefer 78°F to 84°F (25.5°C to 29°C), koi and goldfish prefer 65°F to 77°F (18°C to 25°C).
  - Chronic or rapid hypo/hyperthermia results in stress and immunosuppression.
  - Marine tropical fish are more sensitive to temperature changes than freshwater tropicals.
  - Ideal temperature changes are less than 1°F/day (0.5°C/day).
- **Dissolved oxygen (DO)**
  - Increases in water temperature and salinity decrease oxygen-carrying capacity.
  - DO drops during the night owing to respiration by animals and plants.
  - Expressed in mg/L or ppm
    - Ideal range is greater than 6 mg/L.
- **pH**
  - Measure of the hydrogen ion concentration
  - Logarithmic scale: change of 1 pH unit represents a tenfold difference in concentration.
  - pH of 7.0 is neutral, pH <7.0 is acidic, pH >7.0 is alkaline (basic).
  - Ideal pH varies with species. Most fish live at between 5.5 and 8.5.
    - Freshwater aquaria do best with neutral pH.
    - Marine aquariums: 8 to 8.5
  - More ammonia is present in the toxic form (NH_3) at higher pH.
  - Slow changes in pH are best (0.3-0.5 units/day).
  - Water with low alkalinity is more likely to undergo pH fluctuations.
- **Ammonia**
  - Ammonia is the primary nitrogenous waste product of fish.
    - Nitrifying bacteria oxidize ammonia to nitrites and nitrites to nitrates.
    - New tanks/ponds that lack nitrifying bacteria will have an increase in nitrogenous compounds ("new tank syndrome") that resolves as the biofilter matures.
  - Damages gill tissue, resulting in hyperplasia/hypertrophy and decreased O_2 absorption
  - Two forms
    - Ionized form (NH_4^+/ammonium)
    - Nonionized form (NH_3/ammonia) is much more toxic.
  - Ammonia is more toxic in warm water, at higher pH, and with decreasing salinity.
  - Temperature, pH, and salinity can be used to calculate the actual amount of nonionized ammonia present.
  - Ammonia/chloramine binders can interfere with the Nessler reagent test.
  - High levels of nitrite and nitrate can interfere with the salicylate method.
  - Most test kits report the total ammonia nitrogen in mg/L.
    - The only safe level for ammonia is 0 mg/L; the presence of any ammonia in the water is significant.
- **Nitrite**
  - Ammonia is oxidized to nitrite (NO_2^-) by *Nitrosomonas* and other microbes.
  - Absorbed by the gills and oxidizes hemoglobin (Hb) to methemoglobin (MetHb)
  - Marine fish less sensitive owing to higher levels of chloride in water
  - Less toxic than ammonia but more toxic than nitrate

- Reported in mg/L or ppm
  - Optimal level is 0 mg/L.
- **Nitrate**
  - Nitrite is oxidized to nitrate (NO_3) by *Nitrobacter* and other microbes.
  - Least toxic of nitrogenous compounds, but eggs and fry are more sensitive than adult fish
  - High levels indicative of infrequent water changes
  - High levels stimulate algal blooms and decrease buffering capacity.
  - Reported in mg/L or ppm
    - Maintain below 50 mg/L.
- **Salinity**
  - Measures the concentration of all dissolved salts in water
  - Includes sodium chloride, calcium bicarbonate, calcium carbonate, etc.
  - Most commonly reported as parts per thousand (ppt) or g/L, or as a percentage
    - 1 ppt = 1 g/L = 0.1%
  - Increases can be avoided by performing partial water changes rather than just topping off the pond/tank.
  - Ideal levels vary with species.
  - Marine fish require highest salinity (typically 30-35 ppt).
  - Some plants are extremely sensitive to salt.
  - Maintaining marine fish at suboptimal salinity can result in osmoregulatory stress, impaired growth rates, and reduced disease resistance.
- **Hardness and alkalinity**
  - Hardness represents the concentrations of polyvalent mineral cations in the water, including calcium and magnesium.
    - Expressed as ppm (mg/L) of calcium carbonate. This can be measured with GH test kits.
  - Alkalinity is a measure of the buffering capacity of water (measures the mineral anions). Anions include bicarbonates, carbonates, and hydroxides.
    - Total alkalinity is expressed as ppm (mg/L) calcium carbonate. This sometimes is referred to as KH, or carbonate hardness.
  - Because calcium carbonate is the single largest source of these ions, alkalinity and hardness values as mg/L or ppm usually will be similar.
    - Water softener will result in low GH but will not affect KH.
    - KH can be higher than GH when sodium bicarbonate is added.
  - Hardness, alkalinity, and pH are closely related. Soft water is usually acidic, and hard water usually has a basic pH.
  - Soft water (0-75 ppm), moderately hard water (75-150 ppm), hard water (150-300 ppm), very hard water (>300 ppm)

Water Quality and Pet Fish Health Table

Water Quality Condition	Potential Causes	Historical and Clinical Findings	Corrective Measures
Hypoxia—low dissolved oxygen (DO)	Overcrowding, poor water flow, inadequate aeration, algae die-off, filtration/system failure, increased temperature, chemicals (formalin)	• Acute: high mortality, increased opercular rate, pale gills, piping (gasping at surface), gathering in well-aerated areas • Chronic: lethargy, anorexia, poor growth, opportunistic infections	• Aerate aggressively, monitor ammonia/nitrites, evaluate system and filtration, decrease stocking density. • In emergency, hydrogen peroxide (3%) can be added at a rate of 0.5 mL/L.
Ammonia toxicity	Overcrowding, overfeeding, buildup of organic debris, infrequent water changes, inadequate biological filtration as seen in "new tank syndrome" due to lack of nitrifying bacteria	Mortality, neurologic/behavioral abnormalities, lethargy, anorexia, poor growth, secondary infections, injected fins, gill hyperplasia and hypertrophy	• Reduce or eliminate feeding. • Decrease stocking density. • 25% to 50% water changes • Evaluate and maintain pH (avoid alkaline pH). • Maintain good oxygenation, ammonia binders. • Evaluate biofiltration. • Low doses of salt increase the ionization of ammonia.
Nitrite toxicity, brown blood disease, methemoglobinemia	• See Ammonia Toxicity. • Nitrite oxidizes Hb, MetHb, resulting in hypoxia.	• Respiratory signs: increased opercular rate, piping (gasping at surface), gathering in well-aerated areas, death • Gills and blood may show brown discoloration caused by MetHb.	• Oxygenation • Salt to 0.12%; chloride ions compete with nitrite ions for absorption • See Ammonia Toxicity for other treatments.
Nitrate toxicity	• See Ammonia Toxicity. • Most common cause is infrequent water changes.	Poor growth, lethargy, anorexia, poor growth, opportunistic infections, injected fins	• Water changes: remove organic debris • Aquatic plants may remove nitrates from water.
Temperature	• Rapid temperature fluctuations can result in temperature shock. • Temperature changes can result from equipment malfunction and weather changes.	• Hypothermia: inactive, lying on bottom, lethargy, anorexia, death • Hyperthermia: restlessness, sudden death	• Temperature correction • Fluctuations greater than 1°C/hour may cause temperature shock; however, in life-threatening emergencies, rapid temperature changes may be required.
Chlorine toxicity	Failure to dechlorinate water	Respiratory signs, sudden death	• Dechlorinators such as sodium thiosulfate (3.5 mg/L) • Aeration of water for 24 hours in open-topped container will dissipate chlorine. • Oxygenate water.

Continued

Water Quality and Pet Fish Health Table *(Continued)*

Water Quality Condition	Potential Causes	Historical and Clinical Findings	Corrective Measures
Gas supersaturation, gas bubble disease	Supersaturation of water caused by faulty equipment, sudden elevations in temperature, Venturi effect	• Gas emboli formed in circulation and tissues. Gas bubbles may be seen in eyes, on fins and gills, and under skin. • Behavioral abnormalities, positive buoyancy (small fish), death • Holding a light source close to the fish can help visualization of emboli.	• Elimination of excess gas from water • Repair of faulty equipment
Hydrogen sulfide toxicity	• H_2S is produced under anaerobic conditions at the bottom of ponds/aquaria or in filter beds that are not completely aerated. • Disturbing the bottom can release H_2S into water column.	• Lethargy, anorexia, piping, sudden death • Characteristic rotten egg odor	• Aggressive aeration, water changes: remove decomposing detritus • Maintain aerobic conditions in tank/pond/filter. • Potassium permanganate at 2 mg/L can oxidize/detoxify hydrogen sulfide.
pH	• Rapid pH fluctuations are most problematic. • pH fluctuations are most common in systems with low buffering capacity (alkalinity). • pH can increase during algal blooms and in heavily planted ponds/aquaria. • Buildup of organic debris can decrease pH.	Lethargy, stress, skin lesions, behavioral changes, corneal edema, gill irritation with increased production of mucus, respiratory signs, death	• Many commercial preparations/buffering compounds available for adjusting pH, sodium bicarbonate (improves alkalinity) • Water changes • Limestone or crushed oyster shell can be used to increase alkalinity/pH.

Hb, Hemoglobin; *MetHb,* methemoglobin.

SUGGESTED READINGS

Boyd CE: Water quality: an introduction, Boston, 2000, Kluwer Academic Publishers.
Noga EJ: Fish disease: diagnosis and treatment, St Louis, 1996, Mosby.
Wildgoose WH: BSAVA manual of ornamental fish, ed 2, Gloucester, 2001, British Small Animal Veterinary Association.

AUTHORS: **BRIAN S. PALMEIRO AND JAMES L. (JAY) SHELTON, JR.**
EDITOR: **HELEN E. ROBERTS**

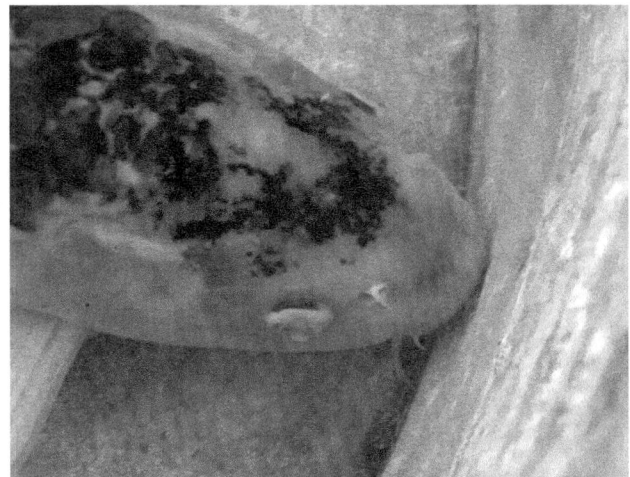

Water Quality and Pet Fish Health Mixed bilateral fungal and bacterial keratitis on a koi *(Cyprinus carpio)*. *(Courtesy Helen E. Roberts.)*

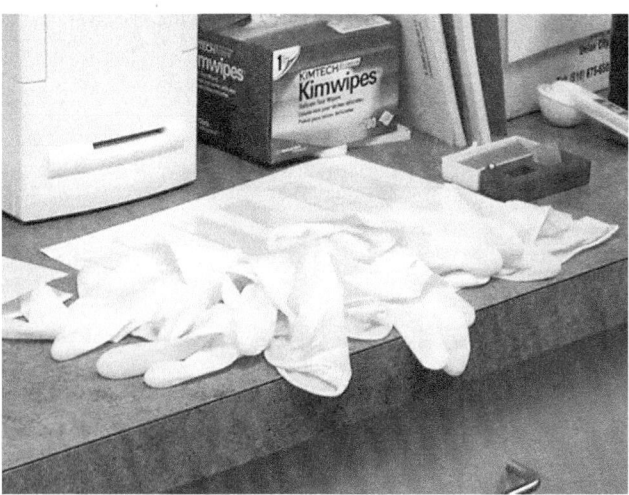

Water Quality and Pet Fish Health Materials (slides, cover slips, and gloves) prepared in advance for wet mount cytology on a fish patient. *(Courtesy Helen E. Roberts.)*

AMPHIBIANS

Ammonia Toxicosis

BASIC INFORMATION

DEFINITION

Amphibian ammonia toxicosis refers to conditions where exogenous sources of ammonia cause elevations of ammonia levels in the blood to the point that various metabolic processes are impaired, often to the point of death.

SYNONYMS

New tank syndrome, ammonia poisoning

EPIDEMIOLOGY

SPECIES, AGE, SEX All. Species that live in streams may be more sensitive to ammonia.

RISK FACTORS

- Water with a pH >7.0 promotes formation of NH_3, which is more toxic than NH_4^+, the form found at lower pH.
- Enclosures with
  - Poor sanitation
  - Unfiltered water (e.g., dump-and-fill water system)
  - Filtered water but lacking adequate biological filtration
  - Recent treatment with antibiotics
- New enclosures that have not had time to develop a biological filtration system
- Enclosures in rooms that have air ducts connecting to rooms holding large numbers of rodents or other mammals
  - Ammonia quickly outgasses from urine excreted by mammals and its decompositional byproducts.
- Recent cleaning of enclosure surfaces with ammonia-containing products such as glass cleaners

CLINICAL PRESENTATION

HISTORY, CHIEF COMPLAINT Owners may observe excess mucus production, a change in or darkening of skin color, a hunched posture or "tip-toe" posture that minimizes contact with substrate, agitation and escape behaviors, or seizures. In many instances, the amphibian is found dead without warning.

PHYSICAL EXAM FINDINGS Affected amphibians typically are producing copious amounts of their protective slime (mucus) layer. The skin may have a grayish cast, and colors are often dull and muted. Muscle fasciculation may be noted. Magnification of toe webs or light-colored skin may reveal dilation of the capillaries. Dyspnea or increased buccal pumping may be noted.

ETIOLOGY AND PATHOPHYSIOLOGY

- Ammonia is found in an un-ionized form, NH_3, at pH above 7.0, and in an ionized form, NH_4^+, at pH less than 7.0. The un-ionized form is more toxic than the ionized form.
- Most amphibians are ammoniotelic and produce large amounts of ammonia as their main nitrogenous waste product. Organic debris containing nitrogen is converted to ammonia through bacterial action. If ammonia is not quickly removed by a flow-through water system, and if it is not converted to less toxic forms of nitrogenous waste such as nitrate via biological filtration, it is rapidly absorbed across the skin and gills of amphibians. With increasing blood levels of ammonia, the liver loses its ability to detoxify the substance, which breaches the blood-brain barrier quickly, resulting in death.
- Ammonia toxicosis may be a rapidly fatal disease.

DIAGNOSIS

DIFFERENTIAL DIAGNOSIS

- Chlorine toxicosis
- Other toxicoses
- Hyperthermia

INITIAL DATABASE

- Obtain temperature, pH, and total ammonia nitrogen (T.A.N.) of water in the enclosure.
  - Temperature must be obtained directly from the tank.
  - Test the T.A.N. content and the pH of the enclosure water.
    - Sample should be taken directly from the tank and immediately tested.
    - If this is not possible, water should completely fill an airtight glass jar and should be analyzed as soon as possible.
    - An ammonia and pH test kit designed for freshwater tropical fish tanks may be used.
    - Most test kits report only T.A.N.
  - T.A.N. >0 ppm is highly suspicious for ammonia toxicosis.

ADVANCED OR CONFIRMATORY TESTING

- The percent of ionized and un-ionized ammonia varies with temperature and pH, so the pH of the water and water temperature must be determined and a T.A.N. table consulted to determine the relative amounts of ionized and un-ionized ammonia present. These tables are available online from many sources and from most texts on aquaculture, tropical fish care, or fish medicine (e.g., Noga, 2000).
  - Multiply the T.A.N. by the un-ionized ammonia (UIA) multiplier in the table. For example, at water temperature of 26°C (78.8°F) and pH of 8.0, the multiplier is 0.0574. If the T.A.N. is 3 ppm, the UIA is 0.17 ppm.
  - T.A.N. levels should be undetectable to rule out ammonia toxicosis.
    - UIA calculations ≥0.02 ppm are of concern.
    - UIA calculations ≥0.05 ppm are adequate for presumptive diagnosis of ammonia toxicosis; levels above 0.1 ppm are confirmatory when coupled with clinical signs.
- A live amphibian with a blood level of ammonia above 0.02 ppm is likely suffering from ammonia toxicosis. Blood must be handled appropriately to prevent outgassing of ammonia before processing.
- Confirmatory testing is not necessary before treatment if clinical signs and history are supportive.

TREATMENT

THERAPEUTIC GOALS

- Remove amphibian from ammonia source and reduce blood levels of ammonia
- Prevent secondary infections resulting from immunocompromise

ACUTE GENERAL TREATMENT

- Remove amphibian from the contaminated water.
  - Move amphibian to a new enclosure with fresh water untainted with ammonia or other chemicals.
  - If this is not practical, rapidly perform a 100% water change with fresh water. Repeat as needed until the T.A.N. is undetectable.
  - If either of these options is not practical
    - Add a commercially available ammonia eliminator (e.g., Am-Quel) to the water in the enclosure
    - Add to the filtration system one or more canister filters containing ammonia-absorbing resin or clay (e.g., clinoptolite, zeolite) to start reducing ammonia levels in the water.

- Supplemental oxygen may be provided by bubbling through the water.

CHRONIC TREATMENT

Four-quadrant antibiotic therapy to prevent secondary bacterial infection (see Septicemia)

PROGNOSIS AND OUTCOME

Guarded to poor. Chronic exposure to UIA concentrations between 0 and 0.02 ppm may result in immunosuppression, weight loss, and poor reproduction. Acute exposure to concentrations between 0.02 and 0.05 ppm has a guarded outcome if treated quickly. Exposure to higher concentrations of UIA and longer exposure times carry a much poorer prognosis. If fasciculation or seizures are noted, the affected amphibian rarely survives.

PEARLS & CONSIDERATIONS

COMMENTS

- Most toxicoses are treated by removal from the suspected source of toxicants and copious flushing with fresh oxygenated water. It is more important to treat the amphibian quickly than it is to have a definitive diagnosis. If you suspect a toxicosis, DON'T DELAY, TREAT WITH FRESH WATER!
- Ammonia-reducing solutions such as Amquel should be immediately available in a clinic that admits amphibians as patients.

PREVENTION

- Appropriate stocking densities
- Daily water changes for dump-and-fill enclosures
- Regular partial water changes for filtered enclosures—a volume of at least 10% per week
- Allow at least 30 days for a new tank to establish a biological filter bed.
- Regular monitoring of water temperature, pH, T.A.N., nitrite, and nitrate to ensure proper working of the biological filter

CLIENT EDUCATION

- Ammonia toxicosis is a life-threatening emergency that requires immediate treatment.
- Appropriate mechanical, chemical, and biological filtration is needed to maintain ammonia-free aquatic and semi-aquatic enclosures. If insufficient time is provided between start-up of a new filter and addition of vertebrates such as amphibians and fish, high concentrations of ammonia will result because the bacteria responsible for the nitrogen cycle have not reached sufficient population levels to handle the incoming load of nitrogenous waste.
- Over-the-counter antibiotics and prescription antibiotics can destroy the capacity of the biological filter until the bacteria have had a chance to recover from the population loss.
- Dump-and-fill water management can quickly lead to high levels of ammonia from amphibian urination and defecation and other sources of organic debris added to the water.
- Some amphibians are exquisitely sensitive to ammonia levels. If ammonia concentrations are strong enough for a human to smell, this is already a potentially lethal level for an amphibian.
- Do not use ammonia-containing compounds around amphibian enclosures.
- In laboratory situations, it is important to keep amphibian rooms separate from mammalian housing. If the ventilation system is shared, the amphibian room needs to be equipped with air filters capable of eliminating ammonia from any air source. When a strong odor of urine is present, ammonia is likely to be sufficient to impact any amphibian. Even if the odor of urine is not detectable, it may be present at a high enough level to impact amphibians.

SUGGESTED READINGS

Diana SF, et al: Clinical toxicology. In Wright KM, Whitaker BR, editors: Amphibian medicine and captive husbandry, Malabar, 2001, Krieger Publications, pp 223–232.

Noga EJ: Ammonia poisoning (new tank syndrome). In Noga EJ, editor: Fish disease: diagnosis and treatment, Ames, IA, 2000, Blackwell Publishing Professional, pp 62–66.

Whitaker BR: Water quality. In Wright KM, Whitaker BR, editors: Amphibian medicine and captive husbandry, Malabar, 2001, Krieger Publications, pp 147–157.

CROSS-REFERENCES TO OTHER SECTIONS

Septicemia

AUTHOR & EDITOR: **KEVIN M. WRIGHT**

AMPHIBIANS

Amoebiasis

BASIC INFORMATION

DEFINITION

Amphibian amoebiasis is infection of any tissue by amoebae of the genera *Acanthamoeba, Copramoeba, Entamoeba, Hartmannella, Mastigamoeba,* and *Vahlkampfia*. Intestinal amoebiasis is most commonly recognized in a clinical setting, although infection of the kidneys, eyes, and central nervous system has been reported.

SYNONYMS

Amoebic enteritis, amoebic nephritis

EPIDEMIOLOGY

SPECIES, AGE, SEX All.

RISK FACTORS

- Stress and debilitation
- Malnutrition
- Starvation
- Concurrent infections such as coccidiosis, nematodiasis, bacterial dermatosepticemia

CONTAGION AND ZOONOSIS

- Directly contagious
- It does not appear to be a zoonotic; given the difficulty of speciating amoebae, caution should be exercised because some of the genera identified to date have species that infect humans.

ASSOCIATED CONDITIONS AND DISORDERS

- Coccidiosis
- Nematodiasis
- Bacterial dermatosepticemia

CLINICAL PRESENTATION

DISEASE FORMS/SUBTYPES Intestinal amoebiasis, renal amoebiasis, and amoebic meningoencephalitis have been reported.

HISTORY, CHIEF COMPLAINT Diarrhea, blood in feces, weight loss, lethargy, hydrocoelom, sudden death. Septic blush (from secondary bacterial infection) may be the presenting complaint.

PHYSICAL EXAM FINDINGS

- Bloody to watery feces
- Amphibians may be dehydrated or may have hydrocoelom or edema.
- Weight loss may be marked.
- Coelom may feel soft or empty on palpation.
- Fat bodies may not be visible via transillumination.

ETIOLOGY AND PATHOPHYSIOLOGY

- Direct life cycle
- Ingestion of trophozoites or cysts
- Lesions may be found in the mucosa of the gastrointestinal tract. Hematogenous spread to the liver, kidneys, and central nervous system may occur. Septicemia may result from intestinal ulcerations.
- Cysts are highly resistant to environmental extremes. Iodine disinfectants typically kill cysts.

DIAGNOSIS

DIFFERENTIAL DIAGNOSIS

- Coccidiosis
- Nematodiasis
- Mycobacteriosis
- Bacterial dermatosepticemia
- Malnutrition
- Starvation

INITIAL DATABASE

- Direct fecal examination or cloacal wash
- Many nonpathogenic amoebae may be found in feces or washes.
- Presumptive intestinal amoebiasis is suggested by the presence of diarrhea, amoebae in the sample, and inflammatory cells and erythrocytes.

ADVANCED OR CONFIRMATORY TESTING

- Identification to genus is difficult and is possible only in special laboratories.
- Histologic examination is required to confirm any form of amoebiasis.

TREATMENT

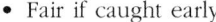

THERAPEUTIC GOALS

- Eliminate amoebae
- Eliminate secondary or contributing infections
- Restore electrolyte and fluid balance
- Restore nutrient intake

ACUTE GENERAL TREATMENT

- Metronidazole: Dosage and treatment depend on the severity of infection and the practicality of dosing the infected amphibian. Injectable forms of metronidazole are most suitable for use as a bath. Because they are acidic, direct topical application is not recommended and would likely result in chemical sloughing of the epidermis.
  - 100 mg PO once
  - 25-50 mg/kg PO SID × 3-5 days
  - 15- to 30-minute bath in 500 mg/L for 5 days
  - 24-hour bath in 50 mg/L
- Four-quadrant antibiotic therapy
  - See Septicemia.
- Bathe in amphibian Ringer's solution.

CHRONIC TREATMENT

- Metronidazole treatments may need to be repeated every 14 days until no evidence of infection remains.
- Place amphibian in a clean environment within 24 hours of each treatment to reduce likelihood of reinfection from amoebic cysts in the environment.
- Provide nutritional support via tube feeding. Enteral solutions designed for cats or ferrets are most appropriate.
  - CatSure or Formula V Enteral Care MHP (PetAg, Hampshire, IL)
  - Carnivore Care (Oxbow Hay Company, Murdock, NE)

PROGNOSIS AND OUTCOME

- Fair if caught early
- Guarded to poor if weight loss is advanced
- Death is common with advanced infection, particularly if the kidneys or central nervous system is involved.

PEARLS & CONSIDERATIONS

COMMENTS

- Amoebiasis is relatively rare but often follows the acquisition of new specimens.
- Quarantine is essential to reduce the risk of outbreaks.

PREVENTION

- Amoeba trophozoites are easily killed with disinfectants such as household bleach or ammonia. Tools and other items that come into contact with amoeba-infected amphibians should be disinfected with povidone-iodine for a minimum contact time of 30 minutes to ensure killing of resistant oocysts. Items must be rinsed thoroughly because povidone-iodine and other disinfectants are toxic to amphibians.
- Prophylactic treatment of incoming amphibians with metronidazole may reduce, but not eliminate, both pathogenic and commensal (nonpathogenic) amoebae.

CLIENT EDUCATION

- Improve husbandry. Ensure that crowding and aggression are not contributing to the problem. Review feeding practices to confirm that malnutrition is not a problem.
- Emphasize the importance of cleaning and disinfecting utensils used in and around amphibian cages.
- Wear disposable gloves and change when moving to a new amphibian cage, or wash hands thoroughly with warm soapy water to reduce the risk of infecting other amphibians.
- Initiate a water quality log.
- Consider adding an ultraviolet (UV) sterilizer to the filtration system to reduce ambient protozoal levels and risk of reinfection.

SUGGESTED READING

Poynton SL, Whitaker BR: Protozoa and metazoa infecting amphibians. In Wright KM, Whitaker BR, editors: Amphibian medicine and captive husbandry, Malabar, 2001, Krieger Publications, pp 193–221.

CROSS-REFERENCES TO OTHER SECTIONS

Septicemia

AUTHORS: **KEVIN M. WRIGHT AND BRAD A. LOCK**

EDITOR: **KEVIN M. WRIGHT**

AMPHIBIANS

Chromomycosis

BASIC INFORMATION

DEFINITION

Amphibian chromomycosis is a systemic granulomatous infection caused by a variety of dark pigmented fungi.

SYNONYM

Chromoblastomycosis

EPIDEMIOLOGY

SPECIES, AGE, SEX All amphibians are most at risk.

RISK FACTORS Debilitated and stressed amphibians are most at risk.

CONTAGION AND ZOONOSIS

- Transmission is by exposure.
- Some of the fungi associated with chromomycosis are zoonotic.

Gloves should be worn to handle amphibians presumptively diagnosed with chromomycosis.

CLINICAL PRESENTATION

DISEASE FORMS/SUBTYPES Chromomycosis often presents as cutaneous nodules or granulomas; however, this is usually a cutaneous manifestation of a systemic disease, and internal granulomas are typically found at necropsy.

HISTORY, CHIEF COMPLAINT Owners typically notice one or more white to gray to tan to black skin nodules. Occasionally, poor coloration, ulcers, anorexia, weight loss, lethargy, or sudden death may occur.

PHYSICAL EXAM FINDINGS "Classic" chromomycosis is seen in an otherwise clinically normal amphibian with nodules of 1 to 3 mm diameter ranging in color from white to brown or black. Hepatic granulomas may be palpated in larger amphibians. Transillumination of the coelomic cavity may reveal granulomas on the liver or other visible internal organs. Ulcers of the toes, ventral skin, and rostrum may be noted in some specimens with no obvious external nodules. Some amphibians may have internal granulomas with no visible cutaneous lesions.

ETIOLOGY AND PATHOPHYSIOLOGY

- The genera of fungi isolated to date include *Cladosporium, Fonseca, Phialophora, Scolecobasidium,* and *Wangiella (Hormiscium).* All of these organisms are ubiquitous in soils and decaying wood and other vegetation.
- Death may occur within 20 days of detection of the first cutaneous lesion.
- Granulomas are typically found in the skin, liver, spleen, kidneys, and other organs, including bone marrow.
- Lesions typically contain a central caseated lesion that may include pigmented fungal hyphae and septate cells. Surrounding layers consist of a mix of monocytes and fibrocytes.
- Experimental transmission by *Fonseca pedrosi* was effective only in debilitated and stressed frogs, strongly suggesting that immunosuppression is a key element leading to chromomycosis.

DIAGNOSIS

DIFFERENTIAL DIAGNOSIS

- Mycobacteriosis
- Cutaneous microsporidiosis
- *Dermocystidium*
- Verminous granulomas

INITIAL DATABASE

- Skin scrape with wet mount may identify pigmented fungal septa or hyphae and may help rule out microsporidiosis and *Dermocystidium.*
- Staining the wet mount with lactophenol blue may help in identification of fungal elements.
- Fixed Gram-stained and acid-fast stained slides may rule out mycobacteriosis.

ADVANCED OR CONFIRMATORY TESTING

- Fungal isolation and identification is difficult. Culture attempts may grow a fungus that fails to sporulate. Without sporulation, identification is impractical.
- Ultrasonography or celioscopy may detect internal granulomas.
- Biopsies are often needed to conclusively identify fungal elements and to rule out other nodular or granulomatous diseases.

TREATMENT

THERAPEUTIC GOALS

- Prevent spread of infection to other specimens
- Prevent spread of infection to human caregivers (No therapeutic treatment has been effective to date.)

ACUTE GENERAL TREATMENT

- Treatments attempted include surgical and cryosurgical débridement and use of antifungals such as itraconazole (10-20 mg/kg PO SID or 10 mg/mL applied as topical solution SID) and amphotericin B (1-2 mg/kg ICe SID). None have proved effective. However, given the variety of species that can cause chromomycosis, a slim possibility exists that therapy may be effective in some cases.
- Euthanasia is recommended owing to the lack of therapeutic treatments to date and the risk of zoonotic disease.
- Gloves should be worn when handling infected amphibians and cage materials.

CHRONIC TREATMENT

Review husbandry to reduce stressors and ensure a high plane of nutrition.

PROGNOSIS AND OUTCOME

- Poor. Euthanasia is recommended.
- Most amphibians die within 20 to 180 days of diagnosis.

PEARLS & CONSIDERATIONS

COMMENTS

Chromomycosis is an indication that husbandry is suboptimal.

PREVENTION

Proper sanitation of the enclosures, appropriate stocking densities, a high-quality diet, and other aspects of good husbandry are key aspects of prevention.

CLIENT EDUCATION

- Review appropriate sanitation practices.
- Initiate a water quality log to monitor temperature, pH, and ammonia levels.
- Review biological filtration as a way to keep ammonia levels in check. Chronic low-level ammonia and spikes of higher concentrations are commonly overlooked stressors. See Ammonia Toxicosis. Consider adding an ultraviolet (UV) sterilizer to the filtration system.
- Ensure that crowding and aggression are not contributing to the problem.
- Review feeding practices to make sure that malnutrition is not a problem. See Hypovitaminosis A.

SUGGESTED READING

Taylor SK: Mycoses. In Wright KM, Whitaker BR, editors: Amphibian medicine and captive husbandry, Malabar, 2001, Krieger Publications, pp 181–191.

CROSS-REFERENCES TO OTHER SECTIONS

Ammonia Toxicosis
Hypovitaminosis A

AUTHORS: **KEVIN M. WRIGHT AND BRAD A. LOCK**

EDITOR: **KEVIN M. WRIGHT**

AMPHIBIANS

Cloacal Prolapse

BASIC INFORMATION

DEFINITION

Cloacal prolapse is the eversion of any tissue out the anus.

SYNONYMS

- Rectal prolapse, oviductal prolapse, bladder prolapse
- "Bubble disease" and "balloon disease" are terms sometimes used by hobbyists because the tissue may swell up and resemble a water balloon.

EPIDEMIOLOGY

SPECIES, AGE, SEX All

RISK FACTORS

- Poor nutrition, especially causing low blood calcium
- Heavy parasite load, especially of gastrointestinal nematodes or pathogenic amoebae
- Intussusception
- GI foreign body
- Septicemia
- Toxicoses

CLINICAL PRESENTATION

HISTORY, CHIEF COMPLAINT Owners may observe pink to red tissue protruding from the cloaca. In aquatic amphibians, this tissue often readily swells in the water and may become edematous and transparent. In terrestrial amphibians, the tissue is more likely to remain pink or red and may start to desiccate if conditions are too dry.

PHYSICAL EXAM FINDINGS Affected amphibians typically have an unidentified tissue prolapsed from the cloaca. Concomitant ventral capillary blush and other signs of infection or distress may be noted.

ETIOLOGY AND PATHOPHYSIOLOGY

- In general, the underlying etiology and pathophysiology remain unknown. It is suspected that patients lose synchronized peristalsis and control of sphincter tone in the event of rectal prolapse. Why the bladder or oviductal tissue may prolapse is unknown.
- Trauma can forcibly evert tissues out the cloaca.
- Some amphibians, such as toads and tree frogs, may naturally evert their stomach. They do this to manually wipe away toxic or nondigestible prey items. Gastric prolapse often happens with anesthesia using eugenol (clove oil) and as a consequence of toxicoses. Its pathophysiology is unknown.
- Once everted, the tissues typically swell with water from the environment. At presentation, osmotically induced swelling is seen along with inflammation. Both must be managed for successful reduction of the tissue.

DIAGNOSIS

DIFFERENTIAL DIAGNOSIS

- Neoplasia
- Granulomatous disease (e.g., mycobacteriosis, fungal infection)
- Parasitism
- Toxicosis
- Hypocalcemia/Nutritional secondary hyperparathyroidism (NSHP)
- Trauma
- GIFB

INITIAL DATABASE

- Water quality test to rule out ammonia toxicosis and other stressors
- Fecal parasite examination using a wet-mounted touch prep of prolapsed tissue.

ADVANCED OR CONFIRMATORY TESTING

- Cloacal endoscopy on amphibians of sufficient size. This will often allow determination of organ prolapse and identification of underlying causes.
- A small red rubber catheter may be introduced into any infoldings of prolapsed tissue in an effort to determine whether it is of GI origin or is composed of some other tissue. GI prolapses often allow the tube to be retrograded far enough forward that it may then be palpated externally as it slides into the normal part of the intestine. Intussusceptions, GI foreign bodies, and other masses may obfuscate these findings.
- Ionized calcium
- Radiographs, with or without contrast material
- Ultrasound

TREATMENT

THERAPEUTIC GOALS

- Reduce the prolapse
- Treat primary underlying cause if determined

ACUTE GENERAL TREATMENT

- Topical and system antiinflammatories to reduce tissue swelling and pain
    - Meloxicam at 0.2 to 0.5 mg/kg IM or ICe; some systemic absorption and direct antiinflammatory effects may be noted if a drop is placed directly on prolapsed tissue.
    - Application of a topical antibiotic cream containing a corticosteroid. It is unknown whether the combination of a nonsteroidal antiinflammatory drug (NSAID) and a corticosteroid puts amphibians at increased risk for gastric ulceration or other side effects expected for mammals. However, in practice, a single application of Animax does not appear to have detectable adverse effects.
- Osmotically reduce tissue swelling.
    - After the antiinflammatories have had a chance to absorb, powdered sugar may be applied to the mucosa.
    - Aquatic amphibians may be held out of the water on damp materials when a prolapse is managed.
    - Placing amphibians into an isotonic electrolyte solution or a slightly hypertonic solution may be helpful to reduce additional swelling of tissues with water.
- Topical and systemic analgesia
    - Risk of adverse effects is associated with applying lidocaine or benzocaine to amphibians. However, dilute solutions may be applied without detectable adverse effects.
    - Opioid narcotics should be considered.
        - Morphine is most effective (38-42 mg/kg SC provides analgesia >4 hr).
        - Buprenorphine may have some effect (38 mg/kg SC provides analgesia >4 hr).
    - Inducing deep anesthesia is often needed to reduce the prolapse without causing debilitating stress to the amphibian.
        - Tricaine methanesulfonate
            - 1 g/L of fresh water buffered to a pH of 7.0 to 7.4
        - Isoflurane gel applied to ventral surface of amphibian
            - 1 mL isoflurane, 1 mL water-soluble gel (e.g., KY gel), 1 mL water
        - Eugenol (clove oil)
            - The formulation found in over-the-counter toothache kits is effective and is readily available.
- Some amphibians may reversibly prolapse their stomachs under eugenol anesthesia, so this is not a first choice for inducing an amphibian with a prolapse.

CHRONIC TREATMENT

- Four-quadrant antibiotic therapy to prevent secondary bacterial infection (see Septicemia)
- Treat underlying cause such as parasitism.

PROGNOSIS AND OUTCOME

Guarded to poor, depending on underlying cause.

PEARLS & CONSIDERATIONS

COMMENTS

Rapid treatment carries the best outcome. Most clients wait too long before bringing amphibians with prolapses for evaluation, and the tissue is devitalized or is seriously injured.

PREVENTION

- Proper nutrition and husbandry
- Appropriate anthelmintic treatments

CROSS-REFERENCE TO OTHER SECTION

Septicemia

AUTHOR & EDITOR: **KEVIN M. WRIGHT**

AMPHIBIANS

Coccidiosis

BASIC INFORMATION

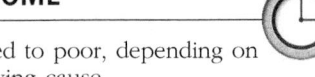

DEFINITION

Amphibian coccidiosis is typically reserved for infections of the gastrointestinal tract or kidneys by apicomplexans of the genera *Eimeria* and *Isospora*. Apicomplexans that infect the blood are typically known as hemogregarines.

SYNONYMS

Eimeria infection, *Isospora* infection

EPIDEMIOLOGY

SPECIES, AGE, SEX Larval and recently metamorphed amphibians are most at risk.

RISK FACTORS Debilitation and stress

CONTAGION AND ZOONOSIS Directly contagious to other amphibians. May quickly build to extremely high levels owing to direct life cycle. Given the biology of other Eimeriidae, it is likely that the different species of amphibian coccidia have a narrow range of host species.

ASSOCIATED CONDITIONS AND DISORDERS

- Diarrhea and weight loss associated with intestinal coccidiosis may be observed with many other diseases.
- Hydrocoelom associated with renal coccidiosis may also be noted with many other diseases.

CLINICAL PRESENTATION

DISEASE FORMS/SUBTYPES

- Intestinal coccidiosis
- Gallbladder coccidiosis
- Renal coccidiosis

HISTORY, CHIEF COMPLAINT

- Weight loss and diarrhea of young, growing amphibians
- Sudden death or higher mortality rates in metamorphs than in previous clutches
- Hydrocoelom
- Occasionally, older amphibians may be affected.

PHYSICAL EXAM FINDINGS

- Loss of muscle mass, a deflated appearance to the coelomic cavity
- Transillumination may reveal reduced or absent coelomic fat bodies.
- Hydrocoelom is rare.

ETIOLOGY AND PATHOPHYSIOLOGY

- These coccidia are intracellular parasites.
- Intestinal coccidiosis may develop, with oocysts sporulating within the gastrointestinal tract of the amphibian followed by subsequent release of sporocysts in the gastrointestinal tract; alternatively, sporulation may occur outside the amphibian, with ingestion of sporulated oocysts being the route of infection. Damage to the intestinal lining causes malabsorption and diarrhea. Secondary infection with bacteria is common.
- Renal coccidiosis disrupts electrolyte and nitrogenous waste and water homeostasis.
- Juvenile amphibians are most at risk. However, stress, debilitation, and other causes of immunosuppression may result in outbreaks among adult amphibians.

DIAGNOSIS

DIFFERENTIAL DIAGNOSIS

- Amoebiasis
- Nematodiasis
- Mycobacteriosis
- Malnutrition

INITIAL DATABASE

- Fecal parasite examination. Oocysts may not be detected because they easily rupture. Collecting a fresh fecal sample may be facilitated by tube feeding an amphibian, then holding it in an empty plastic enclosure lined with a damp paper towel. Check every 15 minutes for feces, and immediately prepare a wet mount of any detected. Refrigeration may cause other protozoa to encyst and may obfuscate the search for coccidian oocysts.
- Wright-Giemsa–stained fixed fecal smears may reveal white blood cells (WBCs) and red blood cells (RBCs), suggesting an inflammatory process in the intestine. Coccidia occasionally may be detected on these slides.

ADVANCED OR CONFIRMATORY TESTING

- Necropsy of clinically ill amphibians with squash preparations of small and large intestinal tissue and histologic examination of the intestine may be needed to detect coccidia.
- *Isospora* have two sporocysts per oocyte; *Eimeria* have four sporocysts per oocyte. Diagnostic laboratories may be able to sporulate oocysts and determine genus.

TREATMENT

THERAPEUTIC GOALS

- Eliminate diarrhea
- Reduce level of coccidial infection
- Eliminate secondary bacterial infection and concomitant intestinal parasites as seen in amoebiasis and nematodiasis
- Eliminate stressors to promote immunocompetence
- Restore nutrient intake

ACUTE GENERAL TREATMENT

- Trimethoprim-sulfa (15 mg/kg PO SID) may have a direct effect on coccidia but more likely simply controls secondary bacterial enteritis. It is unclear whether this has any impact on other forms of coccidiosis. Baycox ???

- Amphibian Ringer's solution (ARS) as a 24-hour bath to restore electrolyte balance. Amphibian Ringer's solution consists of 6.6 g NaCl, 0.15 g KCl, 0.15 g $CaCl_2$, and 0.2 g $NaHCO_3$ dissolved in 1 L distilled water. Alternatively, 5 to 6 g of sodium chloride and 1 g of potassium chloride salt substitute may be added to 1 L of water as temporary therapy until ARS can be prepared.
- Nutritional support via tube feeding. Enteral solutions designed for cats or ferrets are most appropriate.
  - CatSure or Formula V Enteral Care MHP (PetAg, Hampshire, IL)
  - Carnivore Care (Oxbow Hay Company, Murdock, NE)

CHRONIC TREATMENT

- Improve husbandry with particular attention to sanitation.
- Herd health management with prophylactic treatment of at-risk amphibians may be needed until outbreaks of coccidiosis are rare.

POSSIBLE COMPLICATIONS

Concomitant amoebiasis, flagellate infection, or intestinal nematodiasis may be contributing to the problems and may require additional therapeutics (see Amoebiasis, Flagellate Infection, and Nematodiasis).

PROGNOSIS AND OUTCOME

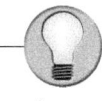

- Guarded to fair. Even with treatment, mortality will occur. Early intervention improves outlook.
- Coccidiostats do not appear to be effective.

PEARLS & CONSIDERATIONS

COMMENTS

Coccidiosis may be very frustrating to manage because no cure is known.

PREVENTION

- High-quality husbandry
- Quarantine to detect carriers before introducing them to a trouble-free collection

CLIENT EDUCATION

- Clinical signs resulting from coccidiosis usually represent failure of husbandry practices, causing stress, debilitation, and immunocompromise. Some amphibians may become stressed from too frequent intrusion into their enclosures. It is difficult to attain balance between providing appropriate sanitation (i.e., removing fresh fecals) and maintaining a low-stress environment.
- Because coccidia are directly infective and current drug therapies are not effective in directly eliminating amphibian coccidia, it is impractical to ever expect to completely eliminate this parasite from an individual amphibian or collection of amphibians.

SUGGESTED READING

Poynton SL, Whitaker BR: Protozoa and metazoa infecting amphibians. In Wright KM, Whitaker BR, editors: Amphibian medicine and captive husbandry, Malabar, 2001, Krieger Publications, pp 193–221.

CROSS-REFERENCES TO OTHER SECTIONS

Amoebiasis
Flagellate Enterocolitis
Nematodiasis

AUTHORS: **KEVIN M. WRIGHT AND BRAD A. LOCK**

EDITOR: **KEVIN M. WRIGHT**

AMPHIBIANS

Corneal Lipidosis or Xanthomatosis

BASIC INFORMATION

DEFINITION

Amphibian corneal lipidosis refers to a specific sign of a lipid storage disorder—the accumulation of cholesterol deposits in the corneal tissues—but it is also used synonymously for the systemic lipid storage disorder called *xanthomatosis*—the deposition of cholesterol-rich deposits in any tissues in the body.

SYNONYMS

Lipid keratopathy, xanthoma, xanthomatosis, hyperlipidosis, hypercholesterolemia, lipid storage disorder

EPIDEMIOLOGY

SPECIES, AGE, SEX Cuban tree frogs *(Osteopilus septentrionalis)* and White's tree frogs *(Litoria caerulea)* are commonly affected, but any adult amphibian may develop this disorder.

RISK FACTORS

- Cholesterol-rich diets, such as crickets that are fed dry dog food or other cholesterol-rich kibbles or mashes
- Overfeeding, particularly of amphibians that consume rodents, goldfish, and other whole-body vertebrate food items
- Maintaining at temperatures below the preferred operating temperature zone (POTZ)

ASSOCIATED CONDITIONS AND DISORDERS

Obesity

CLINICAL PRESENTATION

DISEASE FORMS/SUBTYPES This fat storage disease often may be diagnosed at first as an ophthalmic condition. However, this is only a manifestation of a systemic lipid storage disorder.

HISTORY, CHIEF COMPLAINT A faint haze or a white spot or line is noticed on the cornea of one or both eyes. This may progress to a blob of white material with an irregular surface that gradually infiltrates the entire cornea.

PHYSICAL EXAM FINDINGS

- Early stages present as a white stippling or coalescing lesion on the surface of the cornea.
- Advanced stages may appear three-dimensional, with a white rough surface penetrating the corneal stroma.
- As lipid deposits accumulate and the lesion enlarges, bleeding may occur centrally or along the periphery of the lesion.
- Occasionally, xanthomas may be present in the skin or may be detected on internal organs via transillumination.

ETIOLOGY AND PATHOPHYSIOLOGY

- Most amphibians have evolved by feeding on prey items with inherently low cholesterol levels. It is likely that domestic prey species (e.g., crickets, rodents, mealworms) contain higher amounts of cholesterol than wild prey species and may have a different balance of fatty acids. Amphibians may not be equipped to assimilate and eliminate these unnatural levels of lipids, and cholesterol may accumulate in tissues other than the fat bodies—the normal storage organs for excess fat. Calcium deposits may form within

fat deposits. Inflammation may surround the xanthomas.
- Overfeeding of low-cholesterol items may trigger corneal lipidosis.
- Amphibians that are not able to reach higher temperatures within their POTZ may be prone to corneal lipidosis.
- Amphibians that are not reproducing do not have sufficient turnover of fat stores through egg production or through mate-attracting behaviors, and this may promote corneal lipidosis.
- It is possible that hypovitaminosis A may play a role in this disease through its impact on epithelial cell development, but that theory has not been explored.

DIAGNOSIS

DIFFERENTIAL DIAGNOSIS

- Mycobacteriosis
- Chromomycosis

INITIAL DATABASE

- Plasma cholesterol >400 mg/dL.
- Triglycerides are often similarly elevated.

ADVANCED OR CONFIRMATORY TESTING

Histopathologic examination of lesions will confirm cholesterol clefts (deposits) with or without inflammation.

TREATMENT

THERAPEUTIC GOALS

- Restrict calories
- Prevent intake of excess fat
- Increase use of stored calories
- Control pain and inflammation

ACUTE GENERAL TREATMENT

- Diet should be adjusted to meet the basal metabolic rate so that additional fat is not accumulated. In the case of an adult White's treefrog, four to six adult crickets provide more than enough calories for 1 week.
- Eliminate rodents and goldfish from the diet. Domestic prey insects fed to amphibians should be maintained on low-fat diets such as vegetables and whole grain products and should not be allowed to consume high-cholesterol diets such as kibbled dog food.
- Provide basking spots that meet or exceed the upper level of POTZ, so that the amphibian can reach higher body temperatures, which may help to mobilize lipid deposits.
- Provide exercise opportunities. Some frogs will use "hamster balls" to walk around a room. Swimming is another useful exercise for some amphibians. However, because amphibians do not have a high aerobic scope, exercise periods must be brief to avoid debilitating fatigue.
- Nonsteroidal antiinflammatory drugs (NSAIDs) such as meloxicam (0.05 to 0.1 mg/kg PO q 24-72 h) may reduce inflammation and provide some analgesia.
- Supplementation with vitamin A may be useful (see Hypovitaminosis A).

CHRONIC TREATMENT

- Regular assessment of weight, body condition, and physical signs
- Continue practices initiated during acute phase of treatment.

PROGNOSIS AND OUTCOME

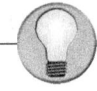

- Guarded to poor. Frogs that have had appropriate nutritional management and have benefited from correction of poor husbandry may live up to 4 years beyond detection of initial corneal opacities. Frogs that have more advanced lesions or internal xanthomas at the time of detection may not live 6 months.
- Amphibians should be euthanized when showing signs of chronic pain that is not responsive to NSAIDs or other forms of analgesia.

PEARLS & CONSIDERATIONS

COMMENTS

- It is often difficult to convince a client that it is time to euthanize an amphibian with corneal lipidosis because the animal will still feed, even with both eyes obscured by fat deposits and ulcerated bleeding lesions present on the surfaces of the eyes. It is important to emphasize that eating is not a measure of pain for most amphibians.
- Assess skin color, posture, and activity as more true measures of how much pain an amphibian is experiencing.
- Critical anthropomorphism, where you ask the owner if he would feel comfortable with the same condition, may help some owners come to terms with their amphibian's quality of life.

PREVENTION

- Provide an appropriate diet with good vitamin supplementation.
- Provide an appropriate thermal environment in the enclosure, so the amphibian can thermoregulate within its POTZ.
- Encourage natural behaviors such as mate calling and reproduction, which require additional energy to turn over stored lipids.

CLIENT EDUCATION

- Amphibians are very efficient at converting food to fat. Most clients overfeed their amphibians, so adherence to a diet that meets but does not exceed a patient's caloric needs is important. Even though it is fun to watch amphibians eat, it is not healthy for them to overeat!
- Cultivate unique invertebrate prey sources, such as grasshoppers, springtails, and firebrats (silverfish), to offer a more varied assortment of fatty acids than is provided by fruit flies, crickets, and mealworms.

SUGGESTED READING

Wright KM: Hypercholesterolemia and corneal lipidosis in amphibians. Vet Clin North Am Exot Anim Pract 6:155–167, 2003.

CROSS-REFERENCES TO OTHER SECTIONS

Hypovitaminosis A

AUTHOR & EDITOR: **KEVIN M. WRIGHT**

Flagellate Enterocolitis

BASIC INFORMATION

DEFINITION

Flagellate enterocolitis refers to the combination of diarrhea with an increased load of flagellate protozoa found on direct fecal parasite examination.

SYNONYMS

Flagellate infection, giardiasis, *Hexamita* infection, trichomoniasis

EPIDEMIOLOGY

SPECIES, AGE, SEX All

RISK FACTORS

- Chronically stressed and debilitated amphibians
- Exposure to new amphibians (e.g., new acquisition from a swap meet that did not undergo quarantine)
- Recent shipping
- Terrestrial anurans are sometimes implicated in outbreaks of flagellate enteritis in salamanders.

CONTAGION AND ZOONOSIS

- Directly contagious to other amphibians via ingestion of contaminated food or water
- Flagellate species that infect amphibians do not appear to be zoonotic.

ASSOCIATED CONDITIONS AND DISORDERS

Concomitant coccidiosis, amoebiasis, nematodiasis, and bacterial gastroenteritis are common.

CLINICAL PRESENTATION

DISEASE FORMS/SUBTYPES

- Flagellates are commensal fauna of the gastrointestinal tract of amphibians.
- Flagellate enterocolitis may occur as a direct invasion of a pathogenic species, or it may be the result of chronic stress that causes a population explosion of commensal flagellates.
- Flagellates typically found in amphibian gut fauna include diplomonads, proteromonads, oxymonads, retortomonads, and trichomonads.

HISTORY, CHIEF COMPLAINT

- Diarrhea
- Weight loss

PHYSICAL EXAM FINDINGS

- Gas-filled intestine
- Poor body condition with loss of intracoleomic fat bodies
- Diarrhea

ETIOLOGY AND PATHOPHYSIOLOGY

- Active and encysted forms of flagellates are directly infective.
- Flagellates are typically found in the large intestine and the cloaca, although occasionally they may be found in the small intestine in low numbers.
- Genera include *Brugerolleia, Chilomastix, Enteromonas, Giardia, Hexamastix, Hexamita, Karotomorpha, Monocercomonas, Monoceromonoides, Octomitus, Proteromonas, Retortomonas, Tetratrichomonas, Trichomitus, Trimitus,* and *Tritrichomonas,* as well as others. It is unknown which species are pathogenic, opportunistic pathogens and which are commensals.
- Diplomonads may be present in the gallbladder.
- Hepatic lesions have been associated with *Tritrichomonas augusta*.
- In otherwise healthy amphibians, repeated fecal examination shows highest concentrations of flagellates immediately after shipping, successively lesser amounts through length of quarantine, and even lower levels once established in long-term housing. Rising levels suggest inappropriate husbandry.
- No specific intestinal lesions have been described from flagellate enterocolitis. All lesions can be ascribed solely to a bacterial infection.
- Severe diarrhea can impair digestion and absorption, resulting in loss of electrolytes.

DIAGNOSIS

DIFFERENTIAL DIAGNOSIS

- Amoebiasis
- Bacterial gastroenteritis
- Coccidiosis

INITIAL DATABASE

- Direct wet mount fecal parasite examination
  - Collecting a fresh fecal sample may be facilitated by tube feeding an amphibian, then holding it an empty plastic enclosure lined with a damp paper towel.
  - Check every 15 minutes for feces, and immediately prepare a wet mount of any detected.
  - Refrigeration may cause flagellates to encyst, making identification problematic.
  - The presence of high levels of flagellate protozoa, typically at least 1 per high power field, along with erythrocytes and leukocytes yields a presumptive diagnosis.
- Wright-Giemsa–stained fixed fecal smears may reveal white blood cells (WBCs) and red blood cells (RBCs), suggesting an inflammatory process in the intestine.

ADVANCED OR CONFIRMATORY TESTING

- Genera may be tentatively identified with special stains.
- Isolation and identification is difficult and is not necessary before treatment is initiated.

TREATMENT

THERAPEUTIC GOALS

- Eliminate diarrhea
- Reduce level of flagellates in intestine
- Eliminate secondary bacterial infection and concomitant intestinal parasites such as amoebiasis, coccidiosis, and nematodiasis (see Amoebiasis, Coccidiosis, and Nematodiasis)
- Eliminate stressors to promote immunocompetence
- Restore nutrient intake
- Restore electrolyte balance

ACUTE GENERAL TREATMENT

- Metronidazole: Dosage depends on the severity of infection and the practicality of dosing the infected amphibian. Injectable forms of metronidazole are most suitable for use as a bath. Because they are acidic, direct topical application is not recommended:
  - 100 mg PO once, repeat in 10-14 days
  - 25 to 50 mg/kg SID × 3-5 days, repeat in 10-21 days
  - 15-30 min bath in 500 mg/L for 5 days
  - 24-hour bath in 50 mg/L, repeat in 7-14 days
- Baths in amphibian Ringer's solution may help restore electrolyte balance.
- If septicemia is suspected,
  - Initiate four-quadrant antibiotic therapy aimed at aerobic and anaerobic organisms (see Septicemia).
- Nutritional support via tube feeding. Enteral solutions designed for cats or ferrets are most appropriate.
  - CatSure or Formula V Enteral Care MHP (PetAg, Hampshire, IL)
  - Carnivore Care (Oxbow Hay Company, Murdock, NE)

CHRONIC TREATMENT

- Improve husbandry with particular attention to sanitation.

- Herd health management with prophylactic treatment of at-risk amphibians may be needed until outbreaks of diarrhea are rare.

PROGNOSIS AND OUTCOME

- Fair with early diagnosis and treatment
- Guarded to poor if weight loss is advanced

PEARLS & CONSIDERATIONS

COMMENTS

- Flagellate enterocolitis often follows the acquisition of new specimens or periods of substandard care.
- Quarantine is essential to reduce the risk of outbreaks.

PREVENTION

- Appropriate water quality and stocking densities are key aspects of prevention.
- Flagellates are easily killed with disinfectants such as household bleach or ammonia. Tools and other items that come into contact with infected amphibians should be disinfected with a minimum contact time of 30 minutes. Items must be rinsed thoroughly because disinfectants are toxic to amphibians.
- Prophylactic treatment of incoming amphibians with metronidazole may reduce, but not eliminate, both pathogenic and commensal (nonpathogenic) flagellates.

CLIENT EDUCATION

- Improve husbandry. Ensure that crowding and aggression are not contributing to the problem. Review feeding practices to make sure that malnutrition is not a problem.
- Emphasize the importance of cleaning and disinfecting utensils used in and around amphibian cages.
- Wear disposable gloves and change when moving to a new amphibian cage, or wash hands thoroughly with warm, soapy water to reduce risk of infecting other amphibians.
- Initiate a water quality log.
- Consider adding an ultraviolet (UV) sterilizer to the filtration system to reduce ambient flagellate levels and risk of reinfection.

SUGGESTED READING

Poynton SL, Whitaker BR: Protozoa and metazoa infecting amphibians. In Wright KM, Whitaker BR, editors: Amphibian medicine and captive husbandry, Malabar, 2001, Krieger Publications, pp 193–221.

CROSS-REFERENCES TO OTHER SECTIONS

Amoebiasis
Coccidiosis
Nematodiasis
Septicemia

AUTHORS: **KEVIN M. WRIGHT AND BRAD A. LOCK**

EDITOR: **KEVIN M. WRIGHT**

AMPHIBIANS

Gastrointestinal Foreign Body or Overload

BASIC INFORMATION

DEFINITION

Gastrointestinal foreign body (GIFB) refers to any item other than food or liquid that is ingested, which results in partial or complete obstruction of the gastrointestinal lumen with an ingested item. Gastrointestinal overload (GIO) refers to distention of the stomach beyond its peak capacity; this may result from ingestion of a large enough volume of food or from subsequent decomposition of food within the stomach, causing gas distention.

SYNONYM

Gastrointestinal impaction

EPIDEMIOLOGY

SPECIES, AGE, SEX

- All
- Horned frogs (*Ceratophrys* spp.) and African bullfrogs (*Pyxicephalus*) are overrepresented for GIO because they are large enough to swallow small rodents, and owners often like to watch them eat such meals. However, large crickets can cause a similar problem for small amphibians.

RISK FACTORS

- GIFB
  - Small pieces of gravel, long-thread sphagnum moss or sheet moss, bark, or other material that may be ingested while feeding
- GIO
  - Feeding items that are longer than the space between an amphibian's eyes, or that weigh more than 5% of the amphibian's body weight
  - Cagemates small enough to be engulfed by another amphibian
  - Temperatures inappropriately cool to maintain the process of digestion and absorption

CLINICAL PRESENTATION

DISEASE FORMS/SUBTYPES

- GIFB
- GIO

HISTORY, CHIEF COMPLAINT

- GIFB
  - Coelomic distention with or without recent defecation
  - Gagging or nonproductive wretching may be noted.
  - Occasionally, a foreign body (FB) may appear, protruding from the cloaca.
  - Careful questioning of the owner may reveal that inappropriate substrates are in the enclosure.
  - With chronic disease, loss of bodily condition may be apparent.
  - Amphibians do not vomit as frequently as mammals with complete obstruction.
- GIO
  - Amphibian has recently eaten a large meal, appears uncomfortable, and has distention of the coelomic cavity.
  - Open-mouth breathing, gagging, and wretching may be noted.
  - Time between feeding and onset of signs is generally short—between 1 and 24 hours.

PHYSICAL EXAM FINDINGS

- The coelomic cavity may feel tense.
- A large mass may be palpable in the cranial half of the coelomic cavity.
- Gaseous bloat may distend the gastrointestinal tract and may be palpable.
- A portion of an FB or meal may be visible in the oropharynx.

ETIOLOGY AND PATHOPHYSIOLOGY

- GIFB

- Distention of the stomach leads to compression of lung fields and associated hypoxia and hypercarbia.
  - It can also decrease cardiac output.
- Loss of electrolytes may occur with vomiting, but this has not been clinically evaluated.
- Depending on where the foreign body lodges, amphibians may continue to eat and develop distention of the lower bowel.

• GIO
  - Distention of the stomach leads to compression of the lung fields and associated hypoxia and hypercarbia.
    - It can also decrease cardiac output.
  - Decomposition of ingesta results in toxicity and overwhelming bacterial populations in the gastrointestinal tract that may lead to septicemia.

DIAGNOSIS

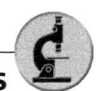

DIFFERENTIAL DIAGNOSIS

- Intussusception
- Gastrointestinal helminthiasis (nematodes, trematodes, or cestodes)

INITIAL DATABASE

Whole-body radiographs

ADVANCED OR CONFIRMATORY TESTING

- Upper GI contrast study with barium. Administer a volume no greater than 0.05 mL barium per 10 g body weight.
- Ultrasonography

TREATMENT

THERAPEUTIC GOALS

- Relieve gas distention and restore respiration and circulation.
- Remove FB or ingesta.
- Control secondary infections.

ACUTE GENERAL TREATMENT

- Supplemental oxygen
- Gastric tube to relieve gas
- Pass rigid endoscope to try to retrieve material.
- Gastric wash may flush out smaller objects like gravel or decomposing ingesta.
- Exploratory celiotomy with gastrotomy or enterotomy
- Four-quadrant antibiotics. See Septicemia.

CHRONIC TREATMENT

- Long-term antibiotics
- Baths in amphibian Ringer's solution may help restore electrolyte balance.
- Nutritional support via tube feeding. Enteral solutions designed for cats or ferrets are most appropriate.
  - CatSure or Formula V Enteral Care MHP (PetAg, Hampshire, IL)
  - Carnivore Care (Oxbow Hay Company, Murdock, NE)

POSSIBLE COMPLICATIONS

- Rupture of the distended gastrointestinal tract is likely with extremely large objects or a large volume of gas.
- Death may occur despite removal of offending material.

PROGNOSIS AND OUTCOME

- Guarded to poor
- Because amphibians have short intestinal tracts, resection of nonviable portions of the intestine may not be possible.
- Immediate recognition of problems and initiation of therapy improve prognosis.

PEARLS & CONSIDERATIONS

COMMENTS

- Intussusceptions are handled in a similar manner as GIFB. Exploratory celiotomy may be curative.
- Inexperienced owners are more likely to overfeed amphibians.

PREVENTION

- Appropriate enclosure design and substrate
- Appropriate feeding practices

CLIENT EDUCATION

- The typical amphibian will be at risk of GIFB/GIO if it is offered prey items that are longer or wider than the distance between the individual amphibian's eyes.
- A decrease in fecal output may be an early sign of disease.

SUGGESTED READING

Wright KM, Whitaker BW: Nutritional disorders. In Wright KM, Whitaker BR, editors: Amphibian medicine and captive husbandry, Malabar, 2001, Krieger Publications, pp 72–87.

CROSS-REFERENCES TO OTHER SECTIONS

Septicemia

AUTHORS: **KEVIN M. WRIGHT AND BRAD A. LOCK**

EDITOR: **KEVIN M. WRIGHT**

AMPHIBIANS

Hypovitaminosis A

BASIC INFORMATION

DEFINITION

Amphibian hypovitaminosis A refers to the condition of squamous metaplasia of mucus-secreting epithelia with concomitant low levels of retinol (vitamin A) in the liver.

SYNONYMS

Short-tongue syndrome, lingual squamous metaplasia, squamous metaplasia

EPIDEMIOLOGY

SPECIES, AGE, SEX Metamorphs and rapidly growing juveniles are most commonly affected, but it may occur at any age. It has been described in anurans and salamanders.

RISK FACTORS

- Diets with absolute low levels of vitamin A
- Diets with a relative imbalance of fat-soluble vitamins A : D:E. Typically, these vitamins should be present at a ratio of 100 IU A:10 IU D:1 IU E. Where vitamin A is <100, risk of developing the disease is increased.
- Aged or inappropriately stored vitamin products (e.g., high heat or humidity)

ASSOCIATED CONDITIONS AND DISORDERS

- Low reproductive success: low fertilization rates, low numbers of eggs produced, early deaths of larvae, and failure of larvae to complete metamorphosis

- Renal insufficiency and hydrocoelom and edema
- Chronic immune suppression with outbreaks of infectious disease lacking a common etiologic agent

CLINICAL PRESENTATION

DISEASE FORMS/SUBTYPES

- Lingual squamous metaplasia, or short-tongue syndrome
- Squamous metaplasia of the bladder, kidney, reproductive organs, and conjunctiva may occur.

HISTORY, CHIEF COMPLAINT

- An anuran may be unable to withdraw prey into its mouth even though the tongue apparently hits the prey.
- Some may present for white raised lesions of the periorbital area.

PHYSICAL EXAM FINDINGS

- Examination of the tongue may suggest squamous metaplasia by decreased mucus production and an opaque appearance to the tongue, but without a normal animal for comparison, this is difficult to ascertain.
- White semicircular swollen areas may be noticed in the lower eyelid, beneath or encompassing one or both eyes (i.e., conjunctival swelling).
- Nonspecific signs such as weight loss and discoloration of the skin may be noted.

ETIOLOGY AND PATHOPHYSIOLOGY

- Lingual squamous metaplasia, or short-tongue syndrome, is seen when the mucus-secreting glands of the tongue become keratinized and are unable to produce the viscous coating that adheres to prey.
- Conjunctival squamous metaplasia may occur and is similar to the vitamin A deficiency noted in aquatic chelonians.
- Squamous metaplasia of the bladder, kidney, reproductive organs, and conjunctiva may occur.

DIAGNOSIS

DIFFERENTIAL DIAGNOSIS

- Presumptive diagnosis of hypovitaminosis A may be based on a history of inability to prehend prey, or of periorbital lesions that are not responsive to antibiotic therapy.
- Nutritional secondary hyperparathyroidism (NSHP)
- Conjunctivitis

INITIAL DATABASE

- Swabs of the tongue may reveal increased numbers of keratinized squamous epithelia.
- Aspirates of periorbital lesions typically lack an inflammatory component and may have large numbers of keratinized squamous epithelia.
- Review vitamin supplementation practices. Certain products that claim to provide vitamin A through beta-carotene are often associated with development of hypovitaminosis A.

ADVANCED OR CONFIRMATORY TESTING

- Submit the entire tongue for histopathologic examination. Squamous metaplasia typically starts at the tip of the tongue rather than at the base. Include samples of bladder, kidney, reproductive organs, and skin.
- Retinol content may be ascertained from frozen liver samples. Levels below 40 μg/g are supportive of hypovitaminosis A. Afflicted Wyoming toads had levels below 10 μg/g.

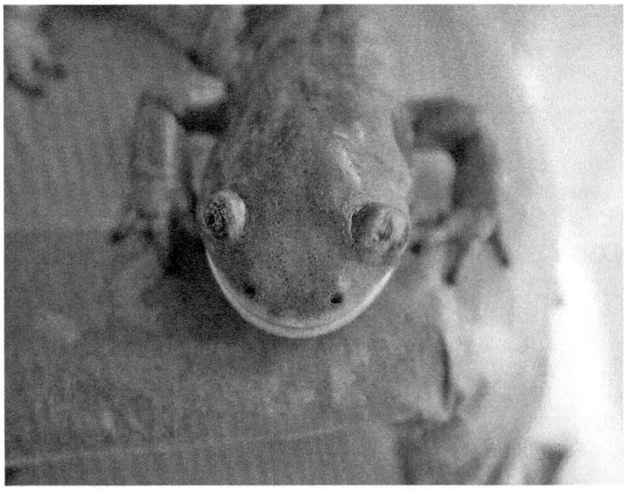

Hypovitaminosis A A salamander with hypovitaminosis A. Note the swollen eyes, a typical lesion for this problem. *(Photo courtesy Jörg Mayer, The University of Georgia, Athens.)*

TREATMENT

THERAPEUTIC GOALS

- Restore circulating and stored vitamin A levels to the point that squamous metaplasia is reversed.
- Treat secondary infections.

ACUTE GENERAL TREATMENT

- Oral supplementation with vitamin A at 1 IU/g daily or 5-50 IU/g weekly
- Topical supplementation is often effective.
- Fat-soluble or water-miscible forms of vitamin A have been used with equal effectiveness.
- As soon as clinical signs resolve, switch to maintenance vitamin supplementation.

CHRONIC TREATMENT

- Dust prey items with a balanced multivitamin supplement at least once weekly, more often with growing or reproductively active adult amphibians.
- Thawed frozen liver from well-nourished rodents (e.g., adult mice or rats) has a high vitamin A content and may be used as a supplement; it typically contains at least 300 μg vitamin A/g liver (equivalent of 1000 IU A/g).

DRUG INTERACTIONS

Excessive levels of vitamin A will inhibit absorption and utilization of vitamins D, E, and K.

POSSIBLE COMPLICATIONS

- Hypervitaminosis A may be induced by oversupplementation with vitamin A.
- Discontinue high dosages of vitamin A if corneal ulcers, hyperkeratotic skin, long bone deformities, or other signs of NSHP are noticed, or if any other unusual signs develop.
- Switch to maintenance vitamin supplementation, and correct NSHP if needed.

PROGNOSIS AND OUTCOME

- Guarded to fair; most amphibians treated will improve within 1 to 2 weeks
- Concomitant infections worsen the prognosis.

PEARLS & CONSIDERATIONS

COMMENTS

- This is an extremely prevalent condition in captive amphibians. Owing to

its prevalence, any ill amphibian should receive vitamin A supplementation as part of initial treatment.
- Some amphibians develop the disease despite being fed items dusted with supplements rich in vitamin A, likely because of inappropriate storage of the product with concomitant degradation of the vitamins. However, species-specific needs for vitamin A may be a factor.

PREVENTION

Proper supplementation with a multivitamin containing vitamin A

CLIENT EDUCATION

- Avoid the use of supplements that list beta-carotene as an ingredient unless a different primary source of vitamin A is clearly stated.
- The ratio of the vitamins is as important as the quantities used.
- Growing and reproductively active amphibians have a higher need for vitamin A than adult nonbreeding amphibians.
- Many other problems, such as sudden death, failure to thrive, and failure to reproduce, may be traced to subclinical hypovitaminosis A.

SUGGESTED READINGS

Kummrow M, et al: What is your diagnosis? Proventriculus and food material in the gizzard, J Avian Med Surg 21:162–166, 2007.
Pessier A, et al: Suspected hypovitaminosis A in captive toads (*Bufo* spp.), Proc AAZV, AAWV, AZA/NAG Joint Conference, p 57.
Wright K: Advances that impact every amphibian patient, Exotic DVM 7:82–86, 2005.

CROSS-REFERENCES TO OTHER SECTIONS

Nutritional Secondary Hyperparathyroidism

AUTHOR & EDITOR: **KEVIN M. WRIGHT**

AMPHIBIANS

Mycobacteriosis

BASIC INFORMATION

DEFINITION

A systemic infection by acid-fast organisms of the genus *Mycobacterium.*

SYNONYMS

- Mycobacterial infection
- Amphibian tuberculosis (This name is a misnomer in that "tubercle" is a description of the lesions mammals form when infected by certain specific species of *Mycobacterium,* notably *M. bovis* and *M. tuberculosis.* Amphibians are not infected by these species.)

EPIDEMIOLOGY

SPECIES, AGE, SEX Any species, age, sex

GENETICS AND BREED DISPOSITION A high incidence has been reported in clawed frogs, *Xenopus* spp., but this is likely the result of these taxa being overrepresented through use in biomedical research.

RISK FACTORS
- Exposure to other known infected amphibians
- Enclosures with rough surfaces such as concrete, degraded fiberglass, and other abrasive substances
- Chronic stress associated with crowding and other poor husbandry practices

CONTAGION AND ZOONOSIS Atypical *Mycobacteria,* such as the taxa that infect amphibians, may infect humans.

ASSOCIATED CONDITIONS AND DISORDERS
- Anorexia
- Weight loss despite good appetite

CLINICAL PRESENTATION

DISEASE FORMS/SUBTYPES
- Granulomatous disseminated infection
- Rarely, infection may be limited to cutaneous nodules, but this usually rapidly progresses to systemic disease spread through the lymphatics.

HISTORY, CHIEF COMPLAINT
- Anorexia
- Weight loss despite good appetite
- Cutaneous nodules that may be gray, tan, or white

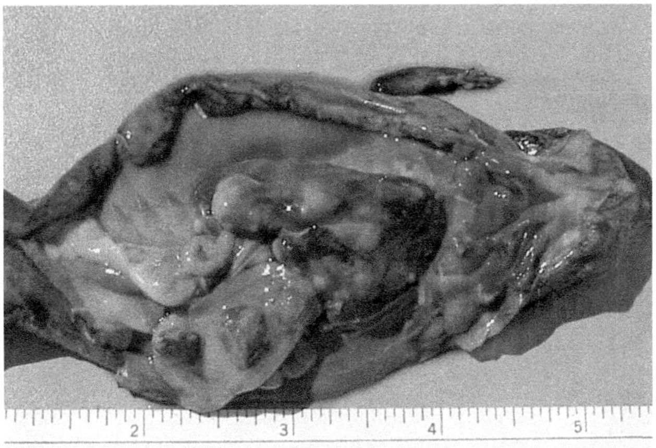

Mycobacteriosis A salamander affected with mycobacteria. Note the granulomatous lesions in the different organs. *(Photo courtesy Jörg Mayer, The University of Georgia, Athens.)*

PHYSICAL EXAM FINDINGS
- Weight loss
- Gray, tan, or white nodules in the skin, with or without ulcerations
- Palpation or transillumination may reveal granulomas of the internal organs.

ETIOLOGY AND PATHOPHYSIOLOGY
- Mycobacteriosis is typically acquired through an open wound or via ingestion of *Mycobacterium* organisms. Lymphatic drainage from the site of initial infection results in disseminated disease.
- Causative species include atypical mycobacteria such as *Mycobacterium avium, M. fortuitum, M. marinum,* and *M. xenopi.*

DIAGNOSIS

DIFFERENTIAL DIAGNOSIS
- Chromomycosis (see Chromomycosis)
- Verminous cysts or verminous granulomas (see Nematodiasis)
- Corneal lipidosis and xanthomatosis (see Corneal Lipidosis and Xanthomatosis)
- Neoplasia (Initially, the histologic lesions caused by mycobacteriosis were erroneously attributed as a transmissible lymphosarcoma; this stimulated decades of work on "infectious cancer.")

INITIAL DATABASE
- Acid-fast stains of any cutaneous lesions, oropharyngeal secretions, and feces
- Transillumination of the coelomic cavity and lungs to detect granulomas

ADVANCED OR CONFIRMATORY TESTING
- Culture of atypical mycobacteria is often unrewarding and requires specialized laboratories for identification to species. Polymerase chain reaction (PCR) tests may become available.
- Histopathologic examination usually confirms acid-fast organisms in lesions.
- Identification to species often is not possible.

TREATMENT

THERAPEUTIC GOALS
- Prevent spread to other amphibians in the collection
- Prevent spread to human caregivers

ACUTE GENERAL TREATMENT
- Euthanasia is strongly recommended owing to lack of effective antimicrobial therapies to date and the risk of zoonotic infection.
- Disposable gloves should be worn by anyone handling the amphibian or materials removed from its cage.

POSSIBLE COMPLICATIONS
- Zoonotic infection often results in ulcerative lesions of the skin.
- *Mycobacterium avium* has been isolated from amphibians and may pose a graver threat to humans in contact with infected amphibians.

PROGNOSIS AND OUTCOME

Most amphibians die within 90 days of diagnosis of mycobacteriosis.

PEARLS & CONSIDERATIONS

COMMENTS
Euthanasia is the best practice to prevent suffering of the amphibian and to reduce the risk of zoonotic infection. Do not let a client talk you into attempting treatment for mycobacteriosis in the home! Because of zoonotic risk, therapy should be attempted only in an appropriate veterinary facility.

PREVENTION
- Quarantine of 180 days or longer may be needed to successfully detect amphibians infected with mycobacteriosis.
- Appropriate disinfection of tools between amphibian cages. Disposable gloves should be worn and exchanged between cages.

CLIENT EDUCATION
- Atypical mycobacteria are part of the normal environment of an amphibian. Infection is typically the result of poor husbandry practices in the home or prior to acquisition of the amphibian.
- Discuss the zoonotic potential of atypical mycobacteriosis, and advise that clients seek the advice of a physician.
- All organic furnishings from the enclosure should be destroyed.
- Appropriate disinfectants should be used to disinfect tools and cage materials that are being retained.
- Cage surfaces should be examined closely to ensure that they are not causing abrasions that would promote infection.

SUGGESTED READINGS

Taylor SK, et al: Bacterial diseases. In Wright KM, Whitaker BR, editors: Amphibian medicine and captive husbandry, Malabar, 2000, Krieger Publications, pp 159–179.
Thoen C, Schliesser T: Mycobacterial infections in cold-blooded animals. In Kubica G, Wayne L, editors: The mycobacteria: a sourcebook, New York, 1984, Dekker-Marcel, pp 1297–1311.

CROSS-REFERENCES TO OTHER SECTIONS

Chromomycosis
Corneal Lipidosis and Xanthomatosis
Nematodiasis

AUTHORS: **KEVIN M. WRIGHT AND BRAD A. LOCK**

EDITOR: **KEVIN M. WRIGHT**

AMPHIBIANS

Nematodiasis

BASIC INFORMATION

DEFINITION
Amphibian nematodiasis is caused by infection with nematodes. Infections may occur in any tissue or within lumens of organs or body cavities. Nematodes infecting the intestine and lungs are of particular importance in captive amphibians.

SYNONYMS
Worms, helminthiasis, lungworms, *Rhabdias* infection, *Strongyloides* infection, hookworms, roundworms, filarid worms

EPIDEMIOLOGY
SPECIES, AGE, SEX All
RISK FACTORS
- Stressed and debilitated amphibians

- Exposure to wild-caught amphibians
- High stocking densities

CONTAGION AND ZOONOSIS

- Nematodes have a variety of life cycles. Important genera in captive amphibians, such as *Rhabdias* and *Strongyloides,* have direct life cycles and can develop superinfection.
- Amphibian nematodes are not known to be zoonotic.

ASSOCIATED CONDITIONS AND DISORDERS Concomitant infections with amoebae, coccidia, and flagellates are common.

CLINICAL PRESENTATION

DISEASE FORMS/SUBTYPES

- Intestinal
- Pulmonary
- Coelomic
- Cutaneous, visceral, and ocular larval migrans
- Verminous granulomas
- Microfilaria and filarids in the circulatory system

HISTORY, CHIEF COMPLAINT

- Weight loss and general unthriftiness are common complaints for all forms of nematodiasis.
- Sudden death is common with intestinal and pulmonary infections, particularly in large groups of amphibians or in groups of recently metamorphed amphibians.
- Diarrhea, bloating, buoyancy issues, and skin lesions may be presenting complaints.

PHYSICAL EXAM FINDINGS

- Dull coloration, loss of muscle mass, reduced coelomic fat bodies
- Transillumination may detect worms and verminous granulomas in the lungs and coelomic cavity
- Intestinal: Diarrhea may be noted. Amphibians may look bloated. Tadpoles may develop buoyancy problems caused by gas in the intestine.
- Pulmonary: Excess oropharyngeal mucus may be noted.
- Coelomic: Typically an incidental finding during transillumination and not something the owner has noticed. In some species, coelomic filarids can reach numbers sufficient to cause organ compromise.
- Cutaneous: White vesicles or crateriform lesions, sloughing of skin, ulcerations. This is a common infection of African clawed frogs, *Xenopus laevis.*
- Visceral and ocular larval migrans: Owner may notice worms in the anterior chamber of the eye. Visceral larval migrans is often undetected by the owner.
- Verminous granulomas: Small nodules in the skin. Transillumination may reveal white spots on dark-colored organs. Occasionally, these may be palpated.
- Microfilaria and filarids in the circulatory system: Occasionally, a lymph sac may be swollen as a result of a worm occluding the lumen of the lymph vessel.

ETIOLOGY AND PATHOPHYSIOLOGY

- *Rhabdias* and *Strongyloides* are important genera in captivity owing to their direct life cycle and the fact that they are self-fertilizing monecious species, thus able to cause superinfections. *Rhabdias* is a lungworm while *Strongyloides* infect the intestine. Direct damage to various organs by migrating larvae and adult worms may result in secondary bacterial infections and debilitation. Low levels of worms may be harbored without clinical signs. Because these genera have free-living generations that can survive in the soil, reinfection can occur from plants and other organic material used in the enclosure. Superinfection results from stress, especially overcrowded enclosures.
- Filarid worms in the coelomic cavity are not associated with inflammation but may occupy a large enough volume of space to compress internal organs. Occasionally, microfilaria and adult filarids may occlude blood and lymph vessels, causing localized fluid accumulations.
- Nematodes may burrow through the epidermis and associated blood supply as larvae and as adult worms (in the case of *Pseudocapillaroides xenopi*). Lesions may develop directly from sloughing of the epidermis or as a result of secondary bacterial infection or vascular occlusion.
- Granulomas develop in response to encysted nematodes that may be in a diapause.
- Hydrocoelom and edema may develop from hypoproteinemia associated with long-term infection.

DIAGNOSIS

DIFFERENTIAL DIAGNOSIS

- Weight loss and a general decline in condition associated with various pulmonary and intestinal worms are similar to these conditions:
  - Chronic stress
  - Coccidiosis
  - Amoebiasis
  - Flagellate infection
  - Mycobacteriosis
  - Malnutrition and starvation
- Cutaneous lesions associated with cutaneous larval migrans and with *Pseudocapillaroides* infection are similar to these conditions:
  - Inappropriately elevated water hardness causing mineralization of the epidermis
  - Trauma
  - Bacterial dermatosepticemia
- Verminous granulomas are similar to these conditions:
  - Mycobacteriosis
  - Chromomycosis
- Hydrocoelom, edema, fluctuant masses
  - Septicemia
  - Mycobacteriosis
  - Renal or hepatic failure
  - Neoplasia

INITIAL DATABASE

- Fecal parasite examination, direct wet mount and float
- Oropharyngeal mucus direct wet mount
- Skin scrapings
  - Direct wet mount
  - Gram-, acid-fast, and Wright-Giemsa–stained slides
- Aspirate of coelomic fluid, edema, or lymph vessel dilations
  - Direct wet mount for detecting microfilaria and filarids
  - Total protein to rule out inflammatory process
- Transillumination to detect internal granulomas

ADVANCED OR CONFIRMATORY TESTING

- Identification of nematodes is difficult. In the case of dioecious species, a male and a female must be submitted. Larval nematodes are difficult to evaluate.
- Ultrasound, double-contrast radiography, and endoscopy may be needed to confirm internal granulomas.

TREATMENT

THERAPEUTIC GOALS

- Reduce numbers of adult nematodes
  - In most cases, it is impossible to eliminate all nematodes.
- Eliminate secondary bacterial infection and concomitant intestinal parasites such as amoebiasis and coccidiosis
- Eliminate stressors to promote immunocompetence
- Restore nutrient intake

ACUTE GENERAL TREATMENT

- Anthelmintic application
  - Ivermectin
  - Fenbendazole
  - Levamisole
  - Milbemycin
- Four-quadrant antibiotic therapy (see Septicemia)
- Baths in amphibian Ringer's solution may help restore electrolyte balance.

- Nutritional support via tube feeding. Enteral solutions designed for cats or ferrets are most appropriate.
  - CatSure or Formula V Enteral Care MHP (PetAg, Hampshire, IL)
  - Carnivore Care (Oxbow Hay Company, Murdock, NE)

CHRONIC TREATMENT

- Improve husbandry with particular attention to sanitation.
- Herd health management with prophylactic treatment of at-risk amphibians may be needed until outbreaks of nematodiasis are rare.

POSSIBLE COMPLICATIONS

Concomitant coccidiosis, flagellate enterocolitis, or amoebiasis may be contributing to the problems and require additional therapeutics (see Amoebiasis, Coccidiosis, Flagellate Enterocolitis).

PROGNOSIS AND OUTCOME

- Guarded
- Many nematodes are resistant to anthelmintic therapy and may be reduced in number but not eliminated.
- Regular monitoring of infected amphibians is needed to develop an effective anthelmintic program.
- Medications should be rotated only when a nematode appears to be thriving despite application of a given anthelmintic.

PEARLS & CONSIDERATIONS

COMMENTS

All incoming amphibians should be considered sources of nematode infection.

PREVENTION

- High-quality husbandry
- Quarantine to detect carriers before they are introduced to a trouble-free collection; prophylactic administration of anthelmintics to all incoming amphibians

CLIENT EDUCATION

- Clinical signs from nematodiasis usually represent failure of husbandry practices, causing stress, debilitation, and immunocompromise. Some amphibians may become stressed from too frequent intrusion into their enclosures. Maintaining balance between appropriate sanitation (i.e., removing fresh fecals) and a low-stress environment is difficult.
- Because some nematodes are directly infective and current drug therapies are not effective in completely eliminating some species, it is impractical to ever expect to completely eliminate this parasite from an individual amphibian or a collection of amphibians.

SUGGESTED READING

Poynton SL, Whitaker BR: Protozoa and metazoa infecting amphibians. In Wright KM, Whitaker BR, editors: Amphibian medicine and captive husbandry, Malabar, 2001, Krieger Publications, pp 193–221.

CROSS-REFERENCES TO OTHER SECTIONS

Amoebiasis
Coccidiosis
Flagellate Enterocolitis
Septicemia

AUTHOR & EDITOR: **KEVIN M. WRIGHT**

AMPHIBIANS

Nutritional Secondary Hyperparathyroidism

BASIC INFORMATION

DEFINITION

A form of metabolic bone disease characterized by hypersecretion of parathormone in response to low blood calcium caused by a diet that does not provide sufficient calcium.

SYNONYMS

Nutritional secondary hyperparathyroidism (NSHP), metabolic bone disease, rubber jaw, brittle bones

EPIDEMIOLOGY

SPECIES, AGE, SEX Any; it is most common in fast-growing postlarval amphibians

RISK FACTORS

- Amphibians adapted for hard alkaline water maintained in soft acidic water
- Fruit flies, crickets, mealworms, king mealworms, or waxworms that have not been supplemented with calcium via gut loading or dusting

ASSOCIATED CONDITIONS AND DISORDERS Pathologic fractures

CLINICAL PRESENTATION

DISEASE FORMS/SUBTYPES

- Hypocalcemia, where the amphibian shows signs of tetany, paralysis, or bloating and has confirmed low levels of ionized calcium
- Normocalcemia, where the amphibian has normal levels of ionized calcium and has signs involving only the mineralized skeleton or calcium storage organs

HISTORY, CHIEF COMPLAINT The amphibian may be anorectic or may have obvious limb or mouth deformities.

PHYSICAL EXAM FINDINGS

- An amphibian that is unable to maintain sufficient levels of circulating calcium may develop bloating, tetany, hydrocoelom, lethargy, and sudden death.
- An amphibian that has normocalcemic NSHP may have a deformed lower jaw, a slightly protruding tongue, slight rounding of the profile of the snout, an inability to elevate itself from the substrate, a curved spine and a kinked tail, and deformed or obviously fractured limb bones.

ETIOLOGY AND PATHOPHYSIOLOGY

- A calcium-to-phosphorus ratio that is significantly different from 1.5:1 or 2:1. Most prey items fed to captive amphibians have an inverse ratio of calcium to phosphorus, typically less than 1:1.
- An absolute lack of calcium despite an appropriate ratio of calcium to phosphorus
- Calcium in the water may be a significant source of this mineral. Amphibians adapted for hard water may develop NSHP if the calcium hardness of their water is too low.
- Lack of vitamin D_3 in the diet may impair calcium absorption and distribution. A ratio of fat-soluble vitamins inappropriately high in vitamin A or vitamin E may impair vitamin D_3 absorption and utilization. Typically, the ratio should be 100 IU D_3 to 10 IU A to 1 IU E. Domestic rodents may have an inappropriate balance of fat-soluble vitamins.
- An inappropriately acidic substrate may interfere with the proton pump

systems needed to maintain normocalcemia and increase the demand for an external source of calcium. This frequently results in gastrointestinal bloating, tetany, seizures, and other signs of hypocalcemia.
- Various other metal ions are present in common calcium supplements such as calcium carbonate and oyster shell flour. These may interfere with calcium uptake if above or below certain levels.
- Oversupplementation with calcium may impair absorption and create NSHP.

DIAGNOSIS

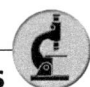

DIFFERENTIAL DIAGNOSIS

- Ammonia toxicosis can cause seizures similar to hypocalcemia.
- Hypervitaminosis A (long bone deformities)
- Septicemia (hydrocoelom, sudden death)
- Trauma (fractures)

INITIAL DATABASE

- Whole-body radiographs to assess radiolucency of bones. Early signs include increased radiolucency of the pelvic bones and lateral spinous processes. With advancing NSHP, additional bones may become radiolucent, and pathologic fractures may occur. Spinal deformities may be present. Endolymphatic sacs may not be mineral dense. Otoliths may be the only significant mineral-dense object visible in very advanced cases.
- A DV digital photo can be used to assess subtle changes in spinal deformities of anurans. Typically, the spine runs in a straight line from between the external nares, between the eyes, and over the center of the urostyle. Deviations are often noticed because the center of the urostyle starts to angle away from the line of the spine.

ADVANCED OR CONFIRMATORY TESTING

Bloodwork should include ionized and total calcium and phosphorus and total protein. An amphibian may have near normal total calcium and still have hypocalcemic signs as the result of low ionized calcium. Inverse plasma levels of calcium-to-phosphorus support a diagnosis of chronic NSHP.

TREATMENT

THERAPEUTIC GOALS

- Correct immediate hypocalcemia
- Correct diet

ACUTE GENERAL TREATMENT

- If tetany, paralysis, or gastrointestinal bloating is noted: 10% calcium gluconate or calcium chloride at 100 mg/kg ICe q 4-6 h until tetany subsides. No sooner than 24 hours after resolution of hypocalcemic signs, consider administration of 1000 IU/kg vitamin D_3 PO or topically. Caution is warranted because this may reinduce a hypocalcemic state.
- Balance the water quality
  - pH and alkalinity/calcium hardness may need to be adjusted. Calcium hardness may need to be above 150 ppm to restore the calcium balance even with diet supplementation.
- Stabilize any fractures.

CHRONIC TREATMENT

- Balance the nutrient intake.
  - Although calcium, phosphorus, and vitamin D_3 are often the sole target of balancing, levels of vitamin A and vitamin E intake should be investigated and balanced if excessively high.
    - Domestic rodents typically have levels of vitamin A that can interfere with vitamin D_3 absorption, so they should be removed from the diet until the disease is corrected.
  - Supplemental calcium may be provided orally by dusting food items with pure calcium carbonate, calcium citrate, or calcium lactate. A liquid calcium source, such as calcium glubionate, may be compounded for direct oral supplementation.
  - Vitamin D_3 may be provided by dusting food items or through oral dosing of 100-400 IU/kg PO weekly.
- Calcium and vitamin D_3 may be absorbed through the skin and may be needed for rapid mineralization of skeletal structures in amphibians with severe deformities.
  - A 2% to 5% solution of calcium gluconate is well tolerated by many species as an 8- to 12-hour daily bath.
  - Vitamin D_3 may be administered in a continuous bath of 3 IU/mL or may be applied topically at 400 IU/kg weekly.
- A minimum of 30 days of supplementation is needed to correct mild to moderate MBD.
- Whole-body radiographs should be taken every 2 to 4 weeks to assess mineralization and conformation of the skeleton.

POSSIBLE COMPLICATIONS

NSHP may be a painful disease in amphibians based on information from human literature. Even though the skeleton may mineralize well following treatment, irreversible deformities in many bones that may affect quality of life are likely.

PROGNOSIS AND OUTCOME

- Fair if major pathologic fractures or deformities are present in the spine, pelvis, long bones, mandible, and hyoid bone.
- Guarded to poor if pathologic fractures involving any of these structures that compromise movement and feeding are present.

PEARLS & CONSIDERATIONS

COMMENTS

This is one of the most common diseases of captive-born and raised amphibians. Although the focus is on dietary correction, a thorough husbandry review is needed to identify any other contributing factors.

PREVENTION

- Supplementation with an appropriate calcium source and a balanced multivitamin supplement
- Proper handling of nutritional supplements
- Proper feeding practices (e.g., dusting, timing of feeding, appropriate prey items)
- Proper environmental conditions (e.g., do not keep hard water–adapted species in acidic conditions)

CLIENT EDUCATION

- Euthanasia may be necessary for amphibians that have significant skeletal lesions or show evidence of chronic pain following remineralization of the skeleton.
- Crickets, fruit flies, mealworms, and waxworms are deficient in calcium and vitamin D_3 and will induce NSHP if fed to young growing amphibians without supplementation.
- All supplements are not created equal. A pure calcium source free of other metals is the best choice for a supplement. Calcium lactate, calcium citrate, and pharmaceutical grade calcium carbonate are excellent sources of pure calcium. Other sources of calcium may contain heavy metals such as lead in quantities that may interfere with normal metabolism.
- Most vitamin sources do not have vitamin D_3 but carry vitamin D_2, which has not been shown to support normal

skeletal mineralization in amphibians. Check with a veterinarian for an appropriate source of vitamin D_3.
- Ultraviolet B may help some amphibians convert vitamin D_2 to vitamin D_3, but this remains unproven.
- Nutritional needs change with age. All things being equal in the captive environment, growing amphibians have a much greater demand for calcium compared with mature amphibians.

SUGGESTED READING

Wright KM: Nutritional disorder. In Wright KM, Whitaker BR, editors: Amphibian medicine and captive husbandry, Malabar, 2001, Krieger Publications, pp 73–87.

AUTHOR & EDITOR: **KEVIN M. WRIGHT**

AMPHIBIANS

Saprolegniasis

BASIC INFORMATION

DEFINITION

Amphibian saprolegniasis is a cutaneous infection by a variety of watermolds (Oomycetes, Diplomastigomycotine; genera include *Achyla, Saprolegnia,* and others).

SYNONYMS

Watermold infection, cotton skin, oomycetosis

EPIDEMIOLOGY

SPECIES, AGE, SEX
- Aquatic amphibians are most at risk.
- Terrestrial amphibians may develop infection if they are in overly wet conditions, but watermolds rarely develop the classic "cotton" appearance that may be seen on completely aquatic amphibians.

RISK FACTORS
- Amphibians maintained at or below 20°C
- Abrasions or other injuries to the epidermis
- Removal of the slime layer from chemical irritants such as an ammonia spike (due to inadequate biological filtration) or contamination of the enclosure with disinfectants, soaps, or detergents
- Malnutrition, particularly hypovitaminosis A
- Crowding

CONTAGION AND ZOONOSIS Transmission is by exposure to the infective forms of watermolds. The contagiousness of different species of watermolds likely varies.

CLINICAL PRESENTATION

DISEASE FORMS/SUBTYPES
- Generalized saprolegniasis can cause severe life-threatening disease by electrolyte disturbance and secondary bacterial septicemia.
- Localized or focal saprolegniasis rarely causes electrolyte imbalance but may offer a route for bacterial septicemia.
- Tadpoles may suffer from infections of the spiracles, resulting in respiratory compromise and death.
- Amphibian eggs are often infected with saprolegniasis, but this usually occurs as a postmortem invasion because healthy eggs appear to be resistant to fungal infection.

HISTORY, CHIEF COMPLAINT
- Owners typically notice a small tuft of white, gray, brown, or green cottony material on the skin of the aquatic amphibian.
- Terrestrial amphibians may have a gray to dull white slime layer. Ulcers may be noted when the fungal mats are removed.
- In some instances, anorexia, weight loss, lethargy, gaping, or sudden death may occur.

PHYSICAL EXAM FINDINGS
- An aquatic amphibian may be covered with one to several small to large fungal mats that are like tangled threads.
- White fungal hyphae suggest an acute infection; gray, brown, or green coloration suggests a more chronic infection that has been dirtied by particles in the water and algae.
- Skin underlying the fungal mats is ulcerated and may erode down to the bone.
- Terrestrial amphibians typically have a white to gray slime layer that bleeds when scraped with a blunt object.
- Systemic signs may include lethargy, weight loss, gaping, vomiting, and anorexia.
- A septic blush consisting of dilated capillaries, petechiae, and ecchymoses may be apparent on pale areas of the body.
- Detecting these early signs of secondary bacterial infection may be enhanced by using a magnification loupe or by photographing with a high-resolution digital camera and enlarging the image.

ETIOLOGY AND PATHOPHYSIOLOGY

- A motile active form, the zoospore, is thought to be the infective form. However, speculation suggests that nonmotile oospores, thick-walled structures designed to resist environmental extremes, may also be directly infective.
- It is unclear whether the host mounts an inflammatory response to the watermold. This may depend on the species of watermold involved.
- Disruption of the mucous layer and epidermis may cause electrolyte and other plasma imbalances and may provide a pathway for invasion by other pathogens. Infection of gills and spiracles may impair gas exchange, electrolyte balance, and elimination of blood ammonia.

DIAGNOSIS

DIFFERENTIAL DIAGNOSIS

- No other disease has clinical signs that closely resemble the cottony tufts of saprolegniasis. However, early stages seen as discoloration of the skin with the presence of ulcers may be mistaken for other diseases.
  - Ectoparasitic ciliated protozoa (e.g., trichodinid ciliates, *Carchesium, Vorticella,* sessile peritrichs)
  - Ectoparasitic flagellated protozoa (e.g., oodinid dinoflagellates such as *Piscinoodinium,* kinetoplastid flagellates such as *Ichthyobodo*)
  - Cutaneous microsporidiosis
  - *Dermocystidium*
  - Traumatic abrasions
  - Granulomatous diseases such as mycobacteriosis and chromomycosis
  - Chemical irritation

INITIAL DATABASE

- Skin scrape with wet mount will identify fungal hyphae and will rule out protozoa.
- Staining the wet mount with lactophenol blue may help identify fungal elements.
- Fixed Gram-stained and acid-fast stained slides will rule out mycobacteriosis and chromomycosis.
- Check water temperature. If it is ≤20°C (68°F), saprolegniasis is a likely diagnosis.

ADVANCED OR CONFIRMATORY TESTING

Fungal isolation is difficult and is not necessary before treatment is initiated.

TREATMENT

ACUTE GENERAL TREATMENT

- Where practical, raise water temperature to above 20°C (68°F). Some species of amphibians may not tolerate warmer temperatures, even when slow acclimation is used.
- Localized lesions
  - Débride and apply a solution of benzalkonium chloride (2 mg/L) to the lesion.
- Generalized lesions
  - Itraconazole at 100 mg/L of 0.6% saline as a bath for 5 to 60 minutes daily for at least 5 days
  - 72-hour bath in benzalkonium chloride (0.25 mg/L)
  - 5- to 30-minute bath in hypertonic salt solution (10-25 g NaCl dissolved in 1 L distilled water)
  - *Note:* Some amphibians, particularly larvae and metamorphs, die when exposed to itraconazole or benzalkonium chloride. Use caution when using these chemicals with an unfamiliar species of amphibian.
- If septicemia is suspected
  - Initiate four-quadrant antibiotic therapy aimed at aerobic and anaerobic organisms (see Septicemia).

CHRONIC TREATMENT

- If the amphibian is developing hydrocoelom or edema, it may need to be maintained in an isotonic or slightly hypertonic electrolyte solution until these signs resolve. Amphibian Ringer's solution may be used as a diluent for benzalkonium chloride or itraconazole for these patients.
- Amphibian Ringer's solution (ARS) consists of 6.6 g NaCl, 0.15 g KCl, 0.15 g $CaCl_2$, and 0.2 g $NaHCO_3$ dissolved in 1 L distilled water. Alternatively, 5 to 6 g of NaCl and 1 g of KCl salt substitute may be added to 1 L of water as temporary therapy until ARS can be prepared.
- Review husbandry, paying particular attention to water filtration and other sanitation practices.
- Maintain water temperature above 20°C (68°F).

POSSIBLE COMPLICATIONS

As previously mentioned, tadpoles and metamorphs may be sensitive to the chemicals used to treat saprolegniasis, even though juveniles and adults may tolerate the treatments.

RECOMMENDED MONITORING

Amphibians should be watched during baths and removed if they are experiencing distress. This may include repeated frantic escape behaviors, hyperemia of pale areas of the skin, excessive production of mucus, and closing the eyes repeatedly. Remove immediately and rinse with fresh water if this happens. Consider reducing the concentration of the solution or the time of exposure for future baths.

PROGNOSIS AND OUTCOME

- Good with early diagnosis and treatment
- Guarded to poor if deep ulcerations and systemic signs of disease are noted

PEARLS & CONSIDERATIONS

COMMENTS

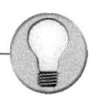

- Saprolegniasis is common when water temperatures are too cool and husbandry is suboptimal.
- Outbreaks are common in laboratories and other situations where hundreds to thousands of specimens are held in large enclosures.

PREVENTION

Appropriate water quality and stocking densities are key aspects of prevention.

CLIENT EDUCATION

- Saprolegniasis typically occurs only when water temperatures are ≤20°C (≤68°F).
- Watermolds are ubiquitous in aquatic environments. High water quality with low amounts of particulate organic matter serves as the first line of defense against outbreaks in an amphibian collection.
- Maintain a water quality log that monitors at least the following factors: temperature, pH, and ammonia levels. Additional tests such as nitrites, nitrates, hardness, and alkalinity may be helpful. Ammonia spikes and temperature drops may lead to outbreaks of saprolegniasis.
- Review biological filtration as a way to keep ammonia levels in check (see Ammonia Toxicosis).
- Consider adding an ultraviolet (UV) sterilizer to the filtration system.
- Ensure that crowding and aggression are not contributing to the problem.
- Review feeding practices to make sure that malnutrition or biological overload of the filtration system is not a problem (see Hypovitaminosis A).

SUGGESTED READINGS

Noga EJ: Watermold infections of freshwater fish: recent advances, Annu Rev Fish Dis 3:291–304, 1993.
Taylor SK: Mycoses. In Wright KM, Whitaker BR, editors: Amphibian medicine and captive husbandry, Malabar, 2001, Krieger Publications, pp 181–191.

CROSS-REFERENCES TO OTHER SECTIONS

Ammonia Toxicosis
Hypovitaminosis A
Septicemia

AUTHORS: **KEVIN M. WRIGHT AND BRAD A. LOCK**

EDITOR: **KEVIN M. WRIGHT**

AMPHIBIANS

Septicemia

BASIC INFORMATION

DEFINITION

Septicemia is an overwhelming systemic infection by one or more bacterial species. Owing to the preponderance of dermatologic lesions in infected amphibians, dermatosepticemia is a more descriptive term.

SYNONYMS

Red leg disease, pink belly disease, dermatosepticemia

EPIDEMIOLOGY

SPECIES, AGE, SEX All are susceptible.

RISK FACTORS

- Poor husbandry with particular emphasis on water quality and inadequate sanitation

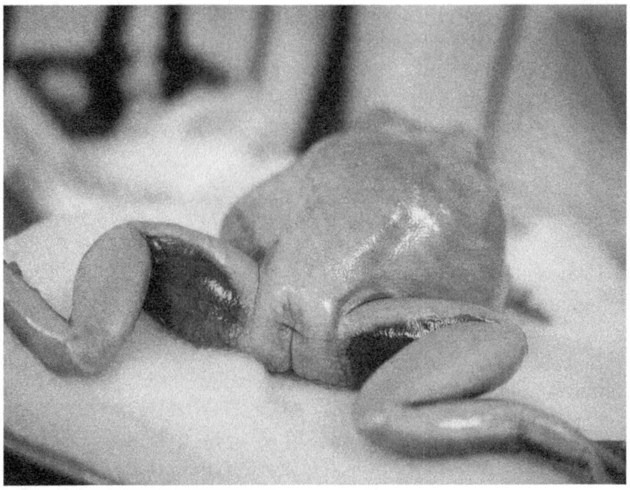

Septicemia Redleg, or dermatosepticemia, is a common clinical sign in amphibians with septicemia. *(Photo courtesy Jörg Mayer, The University of Georgia, Athens.)*

- Recent acquisition through a wholesaler
- Exposure to other infected animals
- Consumption of a diet low in vitamin A

CONTAGION AND ZOONOSIS

- Gram-negative bacteria of many different genera and species
- *Aeromonas* and *Flavobacterium* are common

ASSOCIATED CONDITIONS AND DISORDERS Hypovitaminosis A

CLINICAL PRESENTATION

HISTORY, CHIEF COMPLAINT

- Red to pink skin lesions on pale areas of the body
- Lethargy
- Anorexia
- Prolapse of stomach or cloacal tissue
- Twitching or convulsion
- Sudden death

PHYSICAL EXAM FINDINGS

- Erythema, petechiation, and ecchymosis of the chin, throat, gills, ventral skin, thighs, digital webs, and other pale areas
- Hemorrhagic vesicles
- Hemoptysis
- Hyphema
- Hydrocoelom
- Subcutaneous edema
- Gastric or cloacal prolapse
- Tetany
- Flaccid paralysis

ETIOLOGY AND PATHOPHYSIOLOGY

- Bacteria are able to invade the body (1) through a breach of a physical barrier, such as an abrasion removing the antimicrobial mucous layer on the skin, or (2) through failure of the immune system, often as the result of chronic stress caused by poor husbandry.
- Infection may be noted by the overwhelming presence of a single taxon of bacteria or the synergistic effects of multiple taxa.
- Disruption of electrolyte balance and impairment of cutaneous respiration occur through skin lesions and capillary damage associated with bacterial toxins and septic emboli.
- Hypovitaminosis A is implicated as one of the leading causes of immunosuppression in captive amphibians.

DIAGNOSIS

DIFFERENTIAL DIAGNOSIS

- Iridovirus
- Chlamydophilosis
- Chytridiomycosis
- Chemical irritation
- Mucormycosis
- Mycobacteriosis
- Nematodiasis, cutaneous
- Thermal trauma
- Physical trauma
- Ammonia toxicosis

INITIAL DATABASE

- Aerobic and anaerobic culture and sensitivity of cardiac blood or coelomic fluid from affected and unaffected specimens
- Skin scrapes and wet mounts and stained preps to eliminate fungi, protozoa, and metazoan parasites. On rare occasions, elementary bodies and other signs of chlamydophilosis may be detected with cytologic stains.

ADVANCED OR CONFIRMATORY TESTING

- Biopsy of lesions for histopathologic examination
- Viral isolation may uncover iridovirus or another virus as the underlying cause. Polymerase chain reaction (PCR) may become available.
- PCR tests for *Chlamydophila* may become available.
- At necropsy, longitudinal sections of the tongue may reveal squamous metaplasia supporting the role of hypovitaminosis A in the outbreak.

TREATMENT

THERAPEUTIC GOALS

- Eliminate primary infection
- Treat suspected pathogens such as *Batrachochytrium dendrobatidis* and *Chlamydophila*
- Maintain electrolyte balance
- Support respiration
- Restore positive caloric balance
- Prevent spread of infection to asymptomatic specimens

ACUTE GENERAL TREATMENT

- Itraconazole bath due to ubiquity of chytridiomycosis and rapid fatality without treatment
- Four-quadrant antimicrobials: enrofloxacin and ampicillin; amikacin and ampicillin; amikacin and a third-generation cephalosporin or pencillin; amikacin and oxytetracycline if *Chlamydophila* is suspected; amikacin and metronidazole
- Amphibian Ringer's solution (ARS) as 24-hour bath: ARS consists of 6.6 g NaCl, 0.15 g KCl, 0.15 g $CaCl_2$, and 0.2 g $NaHCO_3$ dissolved in 1 L distilled water. Alternatively, 5 to 6 g of sodium chloride and 1 g of NaCl and KCl substitute may be added to 1 L of water as temporary therapy until ARS can be prepared.
- Supplemental oxygen: Patients may be maintained in clear plastic bags with a small amount of ARS and inflated with

oxygen. The ARS and oxygen are replaced periodically, depending on the size of the patient and the volume of liquid and air in the bag. Typically, this occurs at least every 8 hours.
- Basking spot to permit behavioral fever after an initial 8- to 24-hour period of cooling to slow bacterial growth and allow distribution of antimicrobials

CHRONIC TREATMENT

- Appropriate antimicrobials pending culture and sensitivity (C&S) results. However, if the patient is responding to current treatment, do not switch antibiotics based on C&S findings.
- Correct husbandry: Consider stripping cage and disinfecting and starting over from scratch with new substrate and furnishings.

DRUG INTERACTIONS

Amikacin is usually given 8 to 12 hours apart from other medications to prevent potential interference.

POSSIBLE COMPLICATIONS

- Mortality rates are high once amphibians are showing clinical signs of sepsis.
- Often treatment is aimed at preventing outbreaks in unaffected cagemates.

RECOMMENDED MONITORING

Water and soil samples may be analyzed for the presence of bacterial taxa recovered from ill amphibians.

PROGNOSIS AND OUTCOME

- Poor prognosis for amphibians that present with signs more extensive than mild petechiation
- Guarded to fair prognosis for amphibians that are still eating and have only mild petechiation on presentation

PEARLS & CONSIDERATIONS

COMMENTS

Delaying treatment with itraconazole and antimicrobials will kill more patients than will be killed by either medication's adverse effects.

PREVENTION

- Appropriate quarantine practices
- Proper husbandry and diet with appropriate levels of vitamin A

CLIENT EDUCATION

- Review husbandry specific for the species.
- Review feeding practices and handling of vitamin mixes. A common problem is the use of degraded vitamin products exposed to heat and high humidity or the use of a vitamin product that uses beta-carotene as its source of vitamin A.

SUGGESTED READING

Taylor SK, et al: Bacterial diseases. In Wright KM, Whitaker BR, editors: Amphibian medicine and captive husbandry, Malabar, 2000, Krieger Publications, pp 159–179.

AUTHOR & EDITOR: **KEVIN M. WRIGHT**

AMPHIBIANS

Trauma and Wound Management

BASIC INFORMATION

DEFINITION

Trauma is an injury to the body resulting in damage to one or more organ systems. Wound management is the care required for the injury to heal.

SYNONYMS

Abrasions, bites, fractures, injury, lacerations

EPIDEMIOLOGY

SPECIES, AGE, SEX Any

RISK FACTORS

- Rough surfaces and substrates in the enclosure (e.g., unfinished concrete, pumice and other lava rock, decaying fiberglass)
- Some plants have hairs or crystals that can be irritating to amphibians.
- Cagemate aggression due to inappropriate group composition or enclosure design. Many male amphibians will not tolerate the presence of other males.
- Handling, particular by someone not wearing gloves
- Shipping: Rostral abrasions are particularly common in anurans that have been recently shipped.

ASSOCIATED CONDITIONS AND DISORDERS

- Septicemia
- Saprolegniasis
- Poor water quality

CLINICAL PRESENTATION

HISTORY, CHIEF COMPLAINT Client notices bleeding, skin discoloration, abnormal body posture or movement.

PHYSICAL EXAM FINDINGS Skin damage such as abrasions, lacerations, or burns is often accompanied by internal organ damage. Fractures may be overlooked without a physical examination. Fractures of the hyoid apparatus may be apparent only when an amphibian cannot catch prey by tongue-flicking or has difficulty swallowing its prey.

DIAGNOSIS

DIFFERENTIAL DIAGNOSIS

- Saprolegniasis
- Iridovirus
- Septicemia
- External parasite infection
- Ammonia and other toxicoses
- Nutritional secondary hyperparathyroidism (NSHP)
- Mycobacteriosis

INITIAL DATABASE

- Wet-mounted skin scrapings may help rule out saprolegniasis, ectoparasites, and chromomycosis as causes for skin lesions.
- Cytology of lesions may demonstrate inflammatory cells, suggesting a chronic injury. Acid-fast stains may demonstrate *Mycobacterium*.
- Cultures often are unrewarding and reflect the cutaneous microflora.
- Radiographs are recommended if fractures, particularly of the hyoid bones, are suspected.
- Water quality testing may reveal underlying husbandry problems.

ADVANCED OR CONFIRMATORY TESTING

Histopathologic examination may be needed to completely rule out mycobacteriosis, chromomycosis, and iridovirus.

TREATMENT

THERAPEUTIC GOALS

- Remove inciting causes. Adjust husbandry as needed.
- Promote healing of injuries with appropriate antibiotics, electrolytes, and nutritional support.

ACUTE GENERAL TREATMENT

- Stop bleeding: Corn starch and hemostatic sponges are effective. Sometimes cautery or laser ablation is the best way to stop bleeding from large vessels. Lacerations may be closed with fine absorbable monofilament sutures or tissue glue.
- Topical antibiotics
  - Spraying with "triple sulfa," an over-the-counter product for tropical fish, may help with minor abrasions or ulcers.
  - Baytril Otic Solution, containing enrofloxacin and silver sulfadiazine, is particularly effective in managing abrasions and ulcers. It may cause irritation in some amphibians. Ophthalmic quinolone preparations are also useful as topical treatments.
  - Silver sulfadiazine cream is very effective for many infected wounds.
- Systemic antibiotics
- Stabilize fractures with bandaging; amputation may be required in many cases.
- Flush with fresh water (or amphibian Ringer's solution) frequently if a toxicosis is suspected.
- Meloxicam (0.1 mg/kg PO SID for 3 days) may have some anti-inflammatory and analgesic effects based on clinical experience, but this has not been proven. Morphine and other opioids require very high doses to have much effect and are rarely used to date.

CHRONIC TREATMENT

- Hypovitaminosis A should be suspected whenever wound healing is delayed; supplementation with vitamin A should be initiated.
- Débridement with a dry cotton-tipped applicator is often effective. However, débridement can actually impair healing if performed too frequently. Typically, this is done only on presentation and every 3 to 7 days if needed.
- Rostral abrasions may respond well to hypertonic salt solutions (such as hypertonic ophthalmic drops), topical enrofloxacin, or silver sulfadiazine cream.

POSSIBLE COMPLICATIONS

- Septicemia may result from a breach in the protective slime layer and underlying epithelium.
- Mycobacteriosis and chromomycosis are also possible sequelae.

PROGNOSIS AND OUTCOME

- Fair to good for small lesions that are treated quickly
- Guarded to poor for wounds that are resistant to initial therapy

PEARLS & CONSIDERATIONS

COMMENTS

- Too much handling can create stress, which delays wound healing. A balance needs to be struck so that medical care does not create more issues for the patient.
- Most frogs and toads do quite well with limb amputation. Hind limb amputations are better tolerated than forelimb amputations.
- Many species of salamanders regenerate amputated limbs or tails.

PREVENTION

Proper husbandry is the best prevention. Pay particular attention to group composition and vivarium design.

CLIENT EDUCATION

Correct any defects in husbandry identified through the history.

SUGGESTED READING

Wright KM: Trauma. In Wright KM, Whitaker BR, editors: Amphibian medicine and captive husbandry, Malabar, 2001, Krieger Publications, pp 233–238.

AUTHOR & EDITOR: **KEVIN M. WRIGHT**

AMPHIBIANS

Vomiting

BASIC INFORMATION

DEFINITION

The ejection of partially or wholly digested food or other material from the mouth. This is distinct from regurgitation, where the food is ejected with minimal digestion having occurred.

SYNONYM

Emesis

EPIDEMIOLOGY

SPECIES, AGE, SEX Any

RISK FACTORS

- Infection, especially dermatosepticemia and gastroenteritides caused by parasites and secondary bacterial infection
- Dehydration
- Gastric overload (overconsumption)
- GIFB (gastrointestinal foreign body) or other obstructive lesion
- Toxicosis
- Trauma
- Hyperthermia
- Hypothermia
- Anesthesia, particularly with eugenol

CLINICAL PRESENTATION

DISEASE FORMS/SUBTYPES

- Vomiting due to disease: hemoptysis is a rare occurrence but is a harbinger of death.
- Vomiting due to anesthesia: almost always accompanied by a reversible gastric prolapse; is not considered significant and usually resolves when the anesthetic agent is removed

HISTORY, CHIEF COMPLAINT

- Partially or completely digested food (vomitus) is found in enclosure; rarely only watery mucus or frank blood is present. Occasionally, small nematodes may be seen in the vomitus.
- The owner may see a tan to red organ everted out of the mouth; some bufonids and hylids and other frogs may be able to evert their stomachs and wipe the mucosa with their feet as a way of "vomiting" a toxic insect (such as a firefly) that has been consumed.

PHYSICAL EXAM FINDINGS

- No specific findings
- Hyperemia, petechiation, ecchymosis, or other signs of hemorrhage may suggest a concomitant infection.

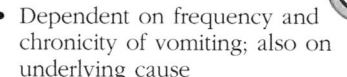

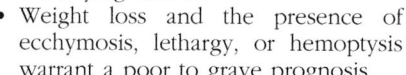

- A hard mass palpable in the coelomic cavity may suggest GIFB, intussusception, abscess, or tumor.

ETIOLOGY AND PATHOPHYSIOLOGY

- The origin of vomiting is triggering of the emetic center of the brain.
- The exact nature of this process in amphibians is poorly known.
  - Emetic compounds in the blood that pass the blood-brain barrier
  - Overstimulation of stretch receptors in the stomach
  - Electrolyte imbalance
  - Dehydration (insufficient bodily fluid stores) may prevent sufficient secretion of gastric juices for digestion or sufficient lubrication for peristalsis.
  - A physical obstruction that prevents peristaltic movement of ingesta through the gastrointestinal tract

DIAGNOSIS

DIFFERENTIAL DIAGNOSIS

- Septicemia
- Nematodiasis
- Amoebiasis
- Coccidiosis
- Gastric overload
- GIFB
- Intussusception
- Tumor
- Abscess/Granuloma
- Ammonia toxicosis
- Chlorine toxicosis
- Pesticide toxicosis
- Other toxicosis
- Trauma
- Hyperthermia
- Hypothermia and subsequent decomposition/fermentation of ingesta within the GI tract
- Anesthesia, particularly from eugenol (clove oil)

INITIAL DATABASE

- Water quality test with particular attention to ammonia, nitrites, chlorine, and copper or other heavy metals
- Husbandry review, with particular attention to other morbidity/mortality within the past 14 days, as well as unusual temperature events, changes in food items or sources of food items, and acquisition of new specimens within the past 30 days
- Vomitus parasite examination + fecal parasite examination
- PCV, TS, albumin, and electrolytes to detect an electrolyte imbalance if present. Normal PCV, TS, albumin, and electrolytes suggest an acute condition; normal PCV, TS, and albumin and low electrolytes suggest a more chronic condition and possible infection (such as chytridiomycosis); elevated PCV, TS, albumin, and electrolytes suggest dehydration.

ADVANCED OR CONFIRMATORY TESTING

- Additional testing to diagnose causes for dehydration can include the following:
  - Blood culture to rule out septicemia
  - Chytrid polymerase chain reaction (PCR) (to explain electrolyte depletion)
  - Radiograph to detect foreign bodies; barium study may be needed to detect obstructive lesions
  - Gastroscopy

TREATMENT

THERAPEUTIC GOALS

- Treat underlying causes (see Amoebiasis, Ammonia Toxicosis, Coccidiosis, Flagellate Enterocolitis, Gastrointestinal Foreign Body or Overload, Nematodiasis, and Septicemia)
- Correct any fluid deficit and provide maintenance fluid requirements

ACUTE GENERAL TREATMENT

- Fluids are best replaced by topical soaking in water or, in the case of electrolyte depletion, a crystalloid such as amphibian Ringer's solution.
- In rare instances, intracoelomic or intravenous fluid therapy may be needed.
- Antiemetics have not been documented for amphibians. In general, vomiting resolves when the underlying problem is resolved.

CHRONIC TREATMENT

- Maintain normohydration.
- Sucralfate may be helpful.

POSSIBLE COMPLICATIONS

Prolonged vomiting may cause electrolyte imbalances resulting in cardiac arrhythmias and death.

RECOMMENDED MONITORING

Electrolyte panel (Na^+, K^+, Cl^-), PCV, and albumin/total protein to assess hydration and electrolyte balance

PROGNOSIS AND OUTCOME

- Dependent on frequency and chronicity of vomiting; also on underlying cause
- Weight loss and the presence of ecchymosis, lethargy, or hemoptysis warrant a poor to grave prognosis.
- If an underlying cause cannot be identified, the prognosis is grave.
- If the inciting factor can be treated, the prognosis is good.

PEARLS & CONSIDERATIONS

COMMENTS

- Vomiting is a sign, not a diagnosis.
- Vomiting is rare and should always be evaluated through a husbandry review and physical examination.
- Do not hesitate to perform gastroscopy or exploratory celiotomy for palpable masses or for signs consistent with an obstructive syndrome.
- Gastric eversion can be seen after certain drugs are given orally.

PREVENTION

Good husbandry with appropriately sized food items

CLIENT EDUCATION

Vomiting should always be reported to your veterinarian.

SUGGESTED READING

Wright KM, Whitaker BR: Amphibian medicine and captive husbandry, Malabar, 2001, Krieger Publications.

CROSS-REFERENCES TO OTHER SECTIONS

Amoebiasis
Ammonia Toxicosis
Coccidiosis
Flagellate Enterocolitis
Gastrointestinal Foreign Body or Overload
Nematodiasis
Septicemia

AUTHOR & EDITOR: **KEVIN M. WRIGHT**

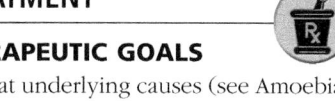

AMPHIBIANS

Weight Loss

BASIC INFORMATION

DEFINITION

Weight loss is clinically relevant when it accounts for a decrease of more than 10% of body mass from ideal body condition, other than when it can be explained by reproductive events or normal volumes of fecal or urine loss for a given individual. Weight loss may result from water loss (dehydration) or from true catabolic states.

SYNONYM

Wasting syndrome

CLINICAL PRESENTATION

HISTORY, CHIEF COMPLAINT Amphibians may have weight loss with or without a decrease in or loss of appetite.

PHYSICAL EXAM FINDINGS Overall loss of musculature. Tailed amphibians show accented pelvic bones and pectoral girdle. Muscles on either side of the spinal column may feel soft and watery. Anurans will have prominent urostyles. The coelomic cavity may appear sunken. The coelomic fat pads are reduced in size and are not easily palpated or detected by transillumination of the body cavity with a cool light source.

ETIOLOGY AND PATHOPHYSIOLOGY

- Weight loss is a sign rather than a diagnosis.
- Weight loss often indicates poor husbandry with associated chronic stress.
- Many different infectious and noninfectious causes of weight loss are known:
  - Weight loss from dehydration is distinct from weight loss caused by loss of body stores of fat, protein, and carbohydrates. However, chronic mild dehydration may decrease even an otherwise healthy amphibian's appetite and may decrease the efficiency of nutrient absorption and assimilation.
  - A commonly overlooked factor is species-specific thermal tolerance. Amphibians that have been exposed to temperatures above their preferred operating temperature zone (POTZ) may have lost the ability to break down and assimilate food even when returned to appropriate temperatures. This may result in thermal damage to certain key enzymes or other proteins involved in digestion.

DIAGNOSIS

DIFFERENTIAL DIAGNOSIS

- Dehydration
  - Often readily diagnosed if physical signs of dehydration (e.g., tacky mucus, dull coloration, water retention posture) are present, and the weight is regained and retained following a 24-hour bath in an appropriate rehydration fluid and correction of husbandry deficiencies
- Geriatric animal
- Prior thermal stress/hyperthermia
  - Difficult to confirm. If the owner has had no lapses in husbandry, this condition may be suspected for any amphibian that has been outside of the current owner's direct care within the past 90 days (e.g., shipping, pet-sitting). Owners may be unaware of temperature fluctuations that occur when they are not around unless they have a maximum-minimum thermometer or another way to detect excessively high temperatures.
- Poor husbandry and associated stress (e.g., water quality, soil pH, humidity, temperature, feeding practices, cagemate aggression)
- Malnutrition (e.g., nutritional secondary hyperparathyroidism, hypovitaminosis A, micronutrient deficiencies, caloric deprivation/starvation, hyperlipidosis/xanthomatosis)
- Endoparasites (e.g., amoebae, coccidia, ciliate overgrowth, flagellates, helminths, hemoparasites)
- Bacterial dermatosepticemia
- Chlamydophilosis
- Mycobacteriosis
- Chromomycosis or other granulomatous fungal infections
- Gastrointestinal foreign body
- Toxicosis (e.g., heavy metal, over-the-counter remedies, ammonia, chlorine, salt, nicotine)
- Ocular disease with vision impairment
- Neurologic disease

INITIAL DATABASE

- Complete husbandry review: Clients should be asked to bring in pictures or videos of the amphibian's enclosure, along with any written records they maintain. These must be thoroughly evaluated for any factors that could be creating stress or unhygienic conditions. The review should also include specific questioning about quarantine practices and the origins of each animal sharing that enclosure.
- Water quality (pH, ammonia, chlorine, copper, water hardness/alkalinity): Although many clients keep water quality records, this sample serves as an independent review of conditions. Clients should bring in a water sample sealed in an airtight container. The water should be chilled on ice to reduce outgassing of ammonia and other volatiles and should not be obtained more than 1 hour before testing.
- Fecal parasite examination, including wet mount, float, fecal acid-fast stain, and fecal cytologic examination
- Oropharyngeal mucus should be examined by wet mount, Wright-Giemsa stain, and acid-fast stain.
- Skin scrape or touch prep of any skin or oral lesions to be examined by wet mount, Wright-Giemsa stain, and acid-fast stain
- Transillumination may reveal parasites, granulomas, and other abnormalities.

ADVANCED OR CONFIRMATORY TESTING

- Gastric wash and cytology and lung wash and cytology may reveal pathogens overlooked by fecal examination or oropharyneal mucus examination.
- Bloodwork particularly focusing on plasma cholesterol, triglycerides, total and ionized calcium, phosphorus, and glucose. CBCs may not be helpful, except where abnormal cell morphologies, abnormal distributions of a particular cell type, or the presence of hemoparasites is present. The buffy coat and plasma from a hematocrit tube and a wet mount of whole blood should be examined by light microscopy to detect hemoparasites.
- Radiographs are helpful in detecting GI foreign bodies, nutritional secondary hyperparathyroidism (NSHP), and a few other conditions.
- Blood, tracheal, and fecal cultures may help identify bacteria that may be pathogens, but interpretation is difficult without specific clinical signs. Viral isolation techniques may be needed too.
- Endoscopy of the GI tract may reveal granulomatous disease or other underlying enteritis. Most amphibians are too small for evaluation other than the stomach or colon.
- Endoscopic biopsy of liver and other organs

TREATMENT

THERAPEUTIC GOALS

- Restore hydration if warranted
- Restore a positive caloric balance with appropriate levels of protein, fat, and carbohydrates

ACUTE GENERAL TREATMENT

- Correct underlying causes.
- Nutritional support via tube feeding. Enteral solutions designed for cats or ferrets are most appropriate.
  - CatSure or Formula V Enteral Care MHP (PetAg, Hampshire, IL)
  - Carnivore Care (Oxbow Hay Company, Murdock, NE)
  - Some amphibians may respond to liquid fry diets designed for rearing carnivorous fish.

POSSIBLE COMPLICATIONS

- Zoonotic infection often results in ulcerative lesions of the skin.
- *Mycobacterium avium* has been isolated from amphibians and may pose a graver threat to humans in contact with infected amphibians.

RECOMMENDED MONITORING

Weigh every 7 to 14 days until the target weight goal is achieved

PROGNOSIS AND OUTCOME

Depends on underlying causes and chronicity of weight loss; usually very good prognosis if weight loss was simply due to poor husbandry practices and weight gain occurs within 14 days of treatment initiation; poor prognosis with any granulomatous disease or hyperlipidosis, or if the patient fails to gain weight within 14 days

PEARLS & CONSIDERATIONS

COMMENTS

Question the owner on exactly how amphibians are being maintained. For example, if an owner puts vitamin-dusted crickets into the cage during the daytime but the amphibian is a species that is only active at night, the crickets will groom off the vitamin before it is consumed. Another example is the owner that does not provide supplemental heat during the winter may be keeping the amphibian too cool for it to feed, even though it did fine during spring and summer months.

PREVENTION

- Proper husbandry practice
- Appropriate treatment of diseases
- Appropriate quarantine practices

SUGGESTED READING

Wright KM, Whitaker BR, editors: Amphibian medicine and captive husbandry, Malabar, 2001, Krieger Publications.

AUTHOR & EDITOR: **KEVIN M. WRIGHT**

REPTILES

Abscesses

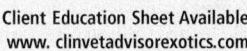

Client Education Sheet Available
www. clinvetadvisorexotics.com

BASIC INFORMATION

DEFINITION

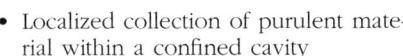

- Localized collection of purulent material within a confined cavity
- Usually associated with bacteria, fungi, parasites, or foreign material trapped within tissue, resulting in inflammation and necrosis
- Reptile abscesses are typically well encapsulated.

SYNONYM

Cellulitis—a more diffuse response to similar trapped infectious or foreign material without the formation of a purulent/caseated center

EPIDEMIOLOGY

SPECIES, AGE, SEX

- Abscesses are common in all reptiles.
- Increased incidence in juvenile reptiles due to:
  - Demands of growth require appropriate husbandry that is often lacking
  - Developing immune system (immune suppression with inappropriate husbandry)
  - Housed in pairs or groups, resulting in increased cagemate aggression/stress
- Male reptiles may develop hemipenal or copulatory organ abscesses.

GENETICS AND BREED PREDISPOSITION

- Lack of proteolytic enzymes in reptilian white blood cells results in solid, caseated purulent material as compared with the liquid pus of mammals.
- Active or highly stressed reptiles that do not acclimate to captive life are predisposed to abscesses.
- Some breed predispositions include:
  - Reticulated pythons (rostral abscesses secondary to trauma of attempting to escape)
  - Asian water dragons and Basilisks (rostral abscesses secondary to trauma from attempting to escape)
  - Old World chameleons (feet/toes, glands at commissure of mouth)

RISK FACTORS

- Poor husbandry/stress (often resulting in immune suppression):
  - Incorrect temperatures
  - Lack of or too much moisture/humidity
  - Incorrect caging (small size, lack of visual barriers/hide areas)
  - Overcrowding
  - Malnutrition (hypovitaminosis A)
- Trauma:
  - Prey items (rodents, insects)
  - Cagemate interactions (bites and scratches)
  - Other house pets
  - Attempting to get out of cage
  - From contact with cage or cage furniture (fiberglass, sharp edges)

CONTAGION AND ZOONOSIS Abscesses may be associated with acid-fast bacteria and salmonella, which may be contagious and zoonotic.

GEOGRAPHY AND SEASONALITY Male reptiles during the breeding season (especially if females are housed nearby) may become restless and injure themselves while attempting to escape their enclosure.

ASSOCIATED CONDITIONS AND DISORDERS Hypovitaminosis A results in squamous metaplasia with secondary bacterial involvement and abscessation.

CLINICAL PRESENTATION

DISEASE FORMS/SUBTYPES

- Aural abscesses
- Hemipenal abscesses
- Scent gland abscesses
- Subspectacular abscesses
- Periodontal disease

HISTORY, CHIEF COMPLAINT
- Cutaneous and subcutaneous abscesses
  - Presented for lump(s), swellings, masses, and/or asymmetry
  - Lameness
  - Nonspecific, including depression, inactivity, and/or anorexia
  - Owners/keepers may (or may not) be aware of trauma/interactions with cagemate or another animal.
- Internal abscesses:
  - Nonspecific, including depression, inactivity, and/or anorexia (e.g., hepatic abscesses)
  - Anorexia with abscesses associated with oral cavity or gastrointestinal tract
  - Specific to internal organs involved, for example:
    - Dyspnea with lung abscesses
    - Diarrhea, melena, hematochezia with gastrointestinal abscessation
    - Ataxia, seizure with abscesses in the brain
- Aural abscesses:
  - Anorexia
  - Swelling on side of head
  - Asymmetry to head (unilateral)
  - Entire head enlarged (bilateral)
  - Head tilt
- Hemipenal abscesses/scent gland abscesses:
  - Swelling associated with cloacal/vent area
  - Fecal and urate accumulation around vent
  - Blood noted from cloacal area
  - Odor from around vent
  - Anorexia
  - Loss of breeding interest
- Subspectacular abscesses:
  - Change in eye(s)
    - Enlarged, swollen, nonsymmetric (if unilateral)
    - No longer clear, cloudy, white, or yellow
    - Owner suspects loss of vision.
  - May be associated with infection in mouth
  - Anorexia

PHYSICAL EXAM FINDINGS
- Cutaneous and subcutaneous abscesses:
  - Enlarged, asymmetric, firm masses evident on examination
  - Injury to the skin over the mass may or may not be evident.
  - Common sites:
    - Head (especially along mandibular and maxillary bones and rostrum)
    - Neck
    - Extremities (legs, feet, digits)
    - Over spine and tail
- Internal abscesses:
  - Nonspecific
  - Abnormal palpation depending on organ involvement and size of abscess
  - Associated with internal organs involved:
    - Dyspnea with lung abscesses
    - Diarrhea, melena, hematochezia with gastrointestinal abscessation
    - Ataxia, seizure, central nervous system (CNS) signs with abscesses in the brain
- Oral cavity:
  - Loss of tissue around oral cavity (especially in rostral area), exposure of oral mucosa and bone
  - Abscessation along gum line may be secondary to periodontal disease in lizards with acrodont dentition (see Periodontal Disease).
  - Commissure of the mouth
    - Asymmetry at corners of mouth, inability to close mouth
    - Associated with gland in Old World chameleons (especially Jackson's)
- Aural abscesses:
  - Common in box and aquatic turtles
  - Swelling under tympanum
  - Asymmetry with unilateral involvement but may be bilateral
- Hemipenal abscesses:
  - Swelling caudal to vent
  - Asymmetric when unilateral but may be bilateral
  - Associated cloacitis with possible odor
  - May be concurrent scent gland involvement
- Scent gland abscesses (snakes):
  - Swelling just cranial, adjacent, and caudal to vent
  - Asymmetric when unilateral (may be bilateral)
  - Associated cloacitis with possible odor
  - May be concurrent hemipenal involvement
- Subspectacular abscesses:
  - Difficult to see eye behind spectacle because of accumulation of purulent debris in subspectacular space
  - Spectacle itself no longer clear; thickened blood vessels may be evident on spectacle
  - Pseudobuphthalmos
  - Oral cavity inspection may reveal stomatitis/lesions in cranial maxillary area (where nasolacrimal ducts empty into oral cavity).

ETIOLOGY AND PATHOPHYSIOLOGY
- Abscesses are cutaneous or subcutaneous but can develop anywhere in the body.
- Lack of proteolytic enzymes in reptilian white blood cells results in solid, caseated purulent material as compared with the liquid pus of mammals.
- Encapsulation of this material typically results in the formation of firm swellings or masses.
- Infection may become locally invasive, moving into soft tissue or bone (osteomyelitis), or may disseminate,

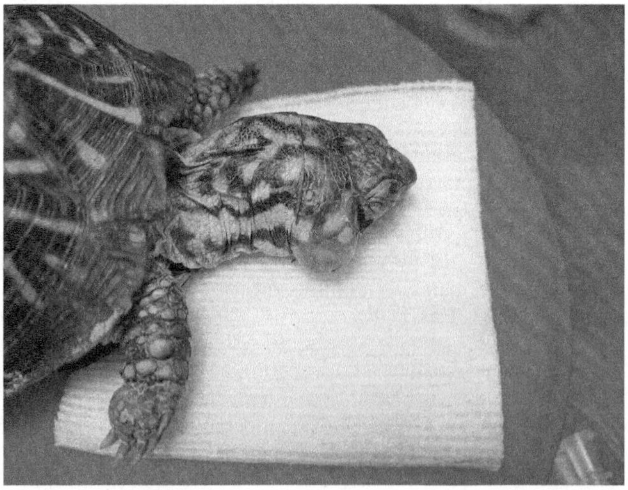

Abscesses Aural abscess in a box turtle. This occurrence is common in this species and may be related to a vitamin deficiency. *(Photo courtesy Jörg Mayer, The University of Georgia, Athens.)*

resulting in sepsis and multiorgan involvement.

- Gram-negative bacteria are the most common primary pathogens:
  - Common Gram-negative organisms include *Pseudomonas, Klebsiella, Proteus, Providencia, Escherichia, Morganella, Salmonella, Aeromonas,* and *Citrobacter.*
- Occasionally, Gram-positive organisms such as *Streptococcus* and *Corynebacteria* are the primary organisms, or can be found concurrently with Gram-negative bacteria.
- Anaerobic bacteria, including *Bacteroides, Fusobacterium,* and *Clostridium,* may be involved, often in conjunction with Gram-negative bacteria.
- Special bacteria such as *Mycobacteria* and *Nocardia* are possible sources.
- Fungi and parasites (protozoa, nematodes, cestodes) are possible sources.
- Foreign material includes plant material, glass, fiberglass, plastic, wood, etc.
- Aural abscesses:
  - Suspicion of organisms migrating from pharyngeal area through the eustachian opening; bacteria as described above are primarily or secondarily involved
  - *Cryptosporidia* spp. (*Iguana iguana*) (see Cryptosporidiosis)
  - Hypovitaminosis A (see Hypovitaminosis A)
  - Exposure to organophosphates
- Hemipenal abscesses:
  - Secondary to trauma from breeding
  - Kept on substrate such as mulch or soil
  - One male being used to breed too many females
  - Low vitamin A
- Scent gland abscesses:
  - In breeding males
  - In male and female snakes can be associated with disuse. From low use, the glands may become "full," and "trapped" glandular material may become inspissated and abscess.
- Subspectacular abscesses:
  - Often caused by:
    - Trauma to the spectacle
    - Migration of organisms from the oral cavity via the nasolacrimal duct is another common cause. Often these cases have active infectious stomatitis. (see Stomatitis, Bacterial)
    - Protozoal organisms
    - Systemic bacterial disease

DIAGNOSIS

DIFFERENTIAL DIAGNOSIS

- Fractures
- Metabolic bone disease (nutritional secondary hyperparathyroidism [NSHP])
- Neoplasia
- Subcutaneous parasites (protozoa, cestodes, nematodes)
- Hematoma/pseudoaneurysm
- Mycobacteria
- Gout/pseudogout
- Sebaceous cysts
- Dermatophilosis (see Dermatophilosis (Rain Rot))
- For subspectacular abscesses:
  - Pseudobuphthalmos (blocked nasolacrimal duct)
  - Pseudobuphthalmos associated with flagellates
  - Retained spectacle

INITIAL DATABASE

- Cytology:
  - Diff-Quik, Gram stains, acid-fast stains, and direct mounts of aspirates or impression smears. Often aspirates are nondiagnostic because material is caseated.
- Culture and sensitivity:
  - Possibly collect both aerobic and anaerobic cultures.
- CBC and chemistry profile:
  - Help determine infectious versus noninfectious disease and related organ involvement with internal abscessation.

ADVANCED OR CONFIRMATORY TESTING

- Biopsy/histopathologic examination:
  - May need special stains such as acid-fast stain, fungal stain, etc.
- Radiographs:
  - Differentiate infectious/inflammatory causes from neoplasia
- Ultrasound:
  - Used to guide collection of diagnostic material with biopsy needle for culture and histopathologic examination
- Endoscopy:
  - Biopsy can then be collected for culture and histopathologic examination.
- Computed tomography (CT)/magnetic resonance imaging (MRI):
  - Useful for internal abscesses, especially for difficult cases such as intracranial, periophthalmic, etc.

TREATMENT

THERAPEUTIC GOALS

- Address husbandry factors that result in stress
- Reduce exposure to trauma from cagemates
- Implement specific dietary changes and supplementation

ACUTE GENERAL TREATMENT

- Initially assess the status of the patient. Warm the patient to the upper end of the reptile's preferred optimal temperature zone (POTZ). For many commonly kept reptiles, this is between 26°C and 32°C (80°F and 90°F). Begin fluid therapy (10-30 mL/kg q 24 h) to rehydrate if clinically indicated.
- When possible, surgical removal of the entire abscess "in toto" is recommended.
- General or local anesthesia is necessary.
- If the abscess cannot be removed (such as the mandible), aggressive surgical débridement of the abscess is needed:
  - Marsupializing the abscess wall to the skin will allow important topical/local treatment.
- Flushing with a variety of solutions such as diluted chlorhexidine solution (1 part chlorhexidine to 30 parts saline) or 50% dextrose solution for 1 or more weeks after surgery is important in management.
- Local treatment should continue before second intention healing is eventually allowed to occur.
- For the surgical description of how to manage abscesses.

CHRONIC TREATMENT

- Most abscesses described in the acute treatment section will require systemic antibiotic therapy. Once the reptile is rehydrated and has an appropriate core body temperature, antibiotic therapy can be initiated.
- For a detailed description of adequate antibiotic treatment.

POSSIBLE COMPLICATIONS

- In cases requiring long-term (longer than 4 to 6 weeks) systemic antibiotics (such as abscesses with associated osteomyelitis), caution should be used with aminoglycoside antibiotics because of possible nephrotoxicity.
- Recurrence may occur in cases where the abscess is not able to be removed "in toto." Premature closure of the surgical site allows re-formation of the abscess. This is especially true with deeper abscesses or abscesses with concurrent bone involvement, internal abscesses or abscesses involving active glandular tissue such as scent gland abscesses, or abscesses involving the glands at the commissure of the mouth in chameleons.

RECOMMENDED MONITORING

- In all cases, a follow-up visit is recommended once the systemic course of antimicrobials is near completion to decide whether longer treatment may be necessary.
- Cases with active flushing and second intention healing should be rechecked before complete closure of the surgery site to ensure that infection has cleared.

- Cases with active osteomyelitis should be rechecked frequently during treatment with follow-up radiographs used to assess progress with any bone change.

PROGNOSIS AND OUTCOME

- With aggressive treatment, isolated abscesses that do not involve bone usually have a favorable prognosis.
- Cases that have a more guarded or a poor prognosis owing to possible sepsis include:
  - Internal abscesses
  - Debilitated patients with multiple abscesses
  - Bone involvement (especially if surgical removal of bone is not possible)

PEARLS & CONSIDERATIONS

COMMENTS

- Correcting the underlying predisposing conditions and risk factors is critical for success.
- Inappropriate husbandry and social stress must be eliminated to avoid continued immune suppression.
- Cagemate aggression and/or overcrowding must be avoided, or recurrence will continue regardless of the clinical treatment provided.

PREVENTION

- With hemipenal abscesses and scent gland abscesses in breeding snakes:
  - Avoid trying to breed one male with too many females.
  - Keep the substrate clean during active breeding.

SUGGESTED READING

Jacobson ER: Bacterial diseases. In Jacobson ER, editor: Infectious diseases and pathology of reptiles, Boca Raton, FL, 2007, CRC Press, pp 461–526.

Lawton MPC: Reptilian ophthalmology. In Mader DR, editor: Reptile medicine and surgery, St Louis, 2006, Elsevier, pp 323–342.

Mader D: Abscesses. In Mader DR, editor: Reptile medicine and surgery, St Louis, 2006, Elsevier, pp 715–719.

Murray MJ: Aural abscesses. In Mader DR, editor: Reptile medicine and surgery, St Louis, 2006, Elsevier, pp 742–746.

Pare JA, et al: Microbiology: fungal and bacterial diseases of reptiles. In Mader DR, editor: Reptile medicine and surgery, St Louis, 2006, Elsevier, pp 217–238.

Stewart JS: Anaerobic bacterial infections in reptiles, J Zoo Wildl Med 21:180, 1990.

Swaim SF, Lee AH: Topical wound medications: a review, J Am Vet Med Assoc 190:1588, 1987.

CROSS-REFERENCES TO OTHER SECTIONS

Periodontal Disease
Stomatitis, Bacterial
Dermatophilosis (Rain Rot)
Cryptosporidiosis
Hypovitaminosis A
Paraphimosis

AUTHOR & EDITOR: **SCOTT J. STAHL**

REPTILES

Adenovirus Infection

BASIC INFORMATION

DEFINITION

Reptilian adenoviruses are DNA, nonenveloped viruses ranging in size from 70-90 nm in diameter. There are numerous adenoviral species identified in reptiles representing at least three different genera.

EPIDEMIOLOGY

SPECIES, AGE, SEX

- Many reptile species can be infected with adenoviruses.
- No sex predilections are known.

GENETICS AND BREED PREDISPOSITION

- Adenoviral disease appears to be most common in bearded dragons, chameleons, kingsnakes, and blue-tongued skinks.
- Reptile adenoviruses characterized to date are fairly species specific, although leopard geckos and fat-tailed geckos have been found to be infected with the same adenovirus.
- Young, geriatric, and immune suppressed animals appear to be at greatest risk for disease.

RISK FACTORS

- Risk factors for adenoviral disease are not well understood.
- Stressed animals appear to be more likely to develop clinical disease.

CONTAGION AND ZOONOSIS

- Adenoviruses are very stable in the environment, and disinfection is difficult.
- Disinfectants effective against other unenveloped viruses, such as parvoviruses, may be expected to be effective against adenoviruses.
- No zoonotic risk is known for any reptile adenovirus.

GEOGRAPHY AND SEASONALITY Agamid adenovirus 1 appears to be widespread and highly prevalent in bearded dragon populations, and highly prevalent in bearded dragon populations in the United States.

ASSOCIATED CONDITIONS AND DISORDERS

- Enteritis and hepatitis are the most common presentations of adenoviral disease.
- Nephritis, bone marrow suppression, and meningitis have also been seen.
- Many adenovirus infections are subclinical.

CLINICAL PRESENTATION

HISTORY, CHIEF COMPLAINT

- Many adenovirus infections are subclinical.
- Enteritis and hepatitis are the most common clinical presentations of adenoviral disease.
- Nephritis, bone marrow suppression, and meningitis have also been seen.
- Common complaints on presentation for adenoviral disease include young that fail to thrive, high death rates in young animals, anorexia, and weight loss.

PHYSICAL EXAM FINDINGS Physical exam findings are generally nonspecific

ETIOLOGY AND PATHOPHYSIOLOGY

- Agamid adenovirus 1, Chameleonid adenovirus 1, Eublepharid adenovirus 1, Gekkonid adenovirus 1, Helodermatid adenovirus 1, Scincid adenovirus 1, Snake adenovirus 1, and Snake adenovirus 2 are all members of the genus *Atadenovirus.*
- Sulawesi tortoise adenovirus 1 is a member of the genus *Siadenovirus,*

and resulted in the most severe viral pathology seen in tortoises to date.

- Several viruses of turtles and tortoises represent a new genus.
- Crocodilian adenoviruses have not been characterized.

DIAGNOSIS

DIFFERENTIAL DIAGNOSIS

- Clinical signs are often fairly nonspecific; many differentials need to be considered.
- If intranuclear inclusions are seen histologically, herpesviral infection is an important differential diagnosis.

INITIAL DATABASE

A thorough husbandry history, physical examination, complete blood count, plasma chemistry, and radiography provide a basic database for animals presenting with nonspecific signs.

ADVANCED OR CONFIRMATORY TESTING

- Nested polymerase chain reaction (PCR) with product sequence analysis is available for all reptile adenoviruses from the University of Florida.
- A real-time PCR specific for Agamid adenovirus 1 is available from Veterinary Molecular Diagnostics in Ohio.
- Cloacal washes are generally the sample of choice.
- Most adenovirus patients are not viremic, so blood is a poor choice for a diagnostic sample.
- Fecal electron microscopy is an option, although this is generally less sensitive and will not identify the species of adenovirus.
- The finding of ballooning intranuclear inclusions on histopathology is suggestive but is not pathognomonic.

TREATMENT

ACUTE GENERAL TREATMENT

- Providing supportive care and addressing husbandry deficiencies are the most important aspects of treating adenoviral disease.
- Cidofovir has been found to be effective in treating adenoviral disease in mammals, but no safety, efficacy, or pharmacokinetic data are available on cidofovir as used in any reptile species.
- Acyclovir is ineffective against adenoviruses.

CHRONIC TREATMENT

Many reptiles remain persistently infected, and continued shedding by recovered animals is a concern.

CROSS-REFERENCES TO OTHER SECTIONS

Coccidiosis
Cryptosporidia
Diarrhea
Entamoebiasis
IBD
Liver Disease
Mycobacteria
Nematodiasis
Renal Disease
Salmonella

PEARLS & CONSIDERATIONS

PREVENTION

The owner should be properly educated about quarantine procedures.

AUTHOR: **JAMES F.X. WELLEHAN, JR.**

EDITOR: **SCOTT J. STAHL**

REPTILES

Aggression

BASIC INFORMATION

DEFINITION

Aggression is defined as any agonistic behavior between cagemates (intraspecies aggression) or between the reptile pet and the handler (interspecies aggression).

EPIDEMIOLOGY

SPECIES, AGE, SEX

- A full review of aggressive behavior in reptiles is beyond the scope of this article.
- Most commonly seen in juveniles kept in high densities and in reproductive age animals and highly territorial species (iguanas, chameleons)
- Less commonly reported in snake species

GENETICS AND BREED PREDISPOSITION Offensive aggression, defensive aggression, and juvenile aggression will be touched on using the green iguana as the main example owing to the common nature of behavioral problems encountered with this species.

RISK FACTORS

- Single large male iguanas in household
- Animals kept in high-density situations, especially juveniles
- Reproductive animals kept in same enclosure
- Multiple males in enclosures
- Competition for resources:
  - Hide areas
  - Basking areas
  - Feed stations
  - Size of enclosure too small for number or gender of animals

ASSOCIATED CONDITIONS AND DISORDERS

- Stress and immune suppression secondary to aggression:
  - Anorexia
  - Failure to thrive
  - Bacterial/fungal septicemias
  - Reductive reproductive output
  - Dysecdysis

CLINICAL PRESENTATION

HISTORY, CHIEF COMPLAINT

- Overt aggression over territory, reproductive aggression, offensive aggression, defensive aggression, and competition for food or basking resources, density aggression
- Observing intraspecies aggressive behavior (fighting, chasing, mounting, biting) or interspecies aggressive behavior (tail whipping, mounting and biting a human in a household)
- If multiple individuals are kept in an enclosure, consider immune suppression/stress (competition for resources, constant attempts at breeding, dominance aggression) leading to secondary septicemias.
- One animal dominating the food station or basking site, preferred hide area, humid hide is common.

PHYSICAL EXAM FINDINGS

- Bite wounds, broken tail tips, lacerations, old scars
- Aggression toward a human may be reported.
- Juvenile animals will often present with a missing tail or toes:
  - Often kept in high densities
- Variable growth in one population

ETIOLOGY AND PATHOPHYSIOLOGY

- Improper husbandry practices:
  - Improper density:
    - High density of animals:
      - This is common in tortoises and herbivorous lizards.
    - Cagemate trauma: missing toes, tail tips, bite wound lesions on body
    - Common in juvenile lizard species (bearded dragons) and juvenile water turtles:
      - Juvenile animals are attracted to movement of cagemates and bite toes and tail tips, thinking these are food items.
  - Gender:
    - Males of many species cannot be kept together as adults:
      - Exhibit territorial and reproductive combat behavior
      - Can lead to direct trauma or competitive immune suppression and secondary disease
  - Territorial behavior:
    - Many species are highly territorial: chameleons, male green iguanas, and some tortoise and turtle species:
      - In small enclosures, this will often lead to a constant battle for territory.
      - This leads to a stress-induced increase in levels of circulating corticosterone.
      - Increased concentrations of corticosterone have been implicated in immune suppression and reduced reproduction.
- Reproductive behavior (offensive aggression):
  - Associated with breeding season or establishment of dominance hierarchies
  - The onset of these usually seasonal reproductive behaviors is variably associated with increased concentrations of circulating androgens (testosterone, dihydrotestosterone).
  - Large male iguanas often see the male human as a threat to territory or as competition for mates (female in household):
    - Ritualized aggression often escalates into physical aggression.
- Defensive behavior:
  - Usually associated with a threat or a perceived threat such as another iguana or a human displacing the animal from a basking site, perch, or food
  - Grabbing the iguana for handling:
    - Most attacks on these animals in the wild occur from above, and this method of handling may be perceived as an attack.
    - Going into the cage and grabbing the animal may be seen as an invasion of the "territory."

DIAGNOSIS

DIFFERENTIAL DIAGNOSIS

- Infectious disease
- Enclosure problems:
  - Lacerations may be secondary to unprotected nails or screws in the enclosure and not from bite trauma.
- Poor husbandry practices:
  - Failure to thrive
  - Anorexia
- Nutritional secondary hyperparathyroidism (NSHP):
  - Hypomotility
- Anorexia

INITIAL DATABASE

- A good thorough history and physical examination
  - History of a seasonal rise in aggressive behavior:
    - Often associated with the male human in the household
    - Characteristic behaviors seen include territorial threat displays (stiff gait with puffed up body turned to the side).
    - Tail whipping and head bobbing leading to biting and aggression associated with contact (handling) of pet
- Commonly seen increase in femoral pore secretions during the breeding season
- History of attacks on female human in household (seen as potential mates) often associated with red clothing or time of menses
  - Often attacks to face and neck because this is the area where iguanas commonly grab female iguanas for breeding
- Missing toes and tail tips, bite wounds will lead to questions to owner about enclosure size, density of enclosures (juveniles will bite at anything that moves for food), and species and gender of animals, which could lead to aggression.
- Questions about competition for limited resources: hide areas, feeding stations, basking sites

TREATMENT

THERAPEUTIC GOALS

- Reduce or eliminate the conditions that may be leading to aggressive behavior
  - Provide client education to help with modification of human behavior
  - Modify husbandry practices to minimize cagemate aggression

ACUTE GENERAL TREATMENT

- Density of enclosure:
  - Increase cage size, reduce density of animals
  - Keep only like size juveniles together.
  - Don't keep male species of territorial animals together.
  - Separate animals that are causing problems.
  - As a general rule, most reptile species should be kept singly, except during breeding attempts.
  - Increase the numbers of basking spots, hide areas, and feed stations:
    - The numbers of these resources should be the same as the number of animals, or enough so that one animal cannot dominate the resource.
- Reproductive (offensive) aggression:
  - Keep a record of aggressive behavior. If attacks are associated with clothing color or are associated with menses/ovulation, then modify clothing choice and remain clear of the animal during those times.
  - See whether pattern of attacks exists (e.g., attacks always when male human is present, when two iguanas are near each other), and then modify that pattern or situation.
  - Provide surrogate for mating behaviors:
    - Stuffed toy or towel has worked well in some situations.
    - Changing the room or enclosure the iguana is in
      - This will often reduce territorial defensive behaviors for a time.
    - Adopting an aggressive posture may help.
      - This may exacerbate the behavior in some instances.
  - Castration: before the breeding season has reduced aggression in a fair percentage of individuals
    - This does not help if the castration is performed during the breeding season.
    - Castration before sexual maturity should be considered.
  - Antiandrogens—tamoxifen and leuprolide—have not been adequately studied and clinically do not seem to be very effective.
  - Reducing illumination of the enclosure to 10 hours a day may help in some situations.
- Defensive aggression:
  - Grab from below or under the animal in a slow gentle manner; attacks on animals are from above and are violent and rapid.
  - Change location of cage.
- Calm gentle movements and handling

CHRONIC TREATMENT

- Continue to monitor that the above treatments are working; each breeding season, repeat the steps that work.

POSSIBLE COMPLICATIONS

- No single treatment will work for all situations; the clinician must modify and use a number of treatments or modifications to find those that will work in each case.

PROGNOSIS AND OUTCOME

- For enclosure problems, the prognosis is good for the long term, but for each individual, outcome will depend on how ill they have become from immune suppression.
- For offensive aggression—guarded to fair—some animals will have to be separated from humans each breeding season; many become very aggressive and are euthanized.

PEARLS & CONSIDERATIONS

COMMENTS

Reproductive and defensive aggression behaviors can be difficult to change and can be very frustrating to deal with.

PREVENTION

- For large iguanas: very early castration seems to have promise
- Research husbandry needs of species being kept

CLIENT EDUCATION

- Client education early on will help to prevent many aggressive behaviors.
- Help the client understand the reproductive and defensive behaviors of large pet lizards.
- No free-roaming animals; they will see the house as "their" territory
- Help the client understand how husbandry, density, and competition can affect behavior and aggression.
- Early castration should be considered.

SUGGESTED READINGS

Hernandez-Divers SJ: Clinical aspects of reptile behavior, Vet Clin North Am 4:599–612, 2001.

Lock BA: Behavioral and morphologic adaptations. In Mader DR, editor: Reptile medicine and surgery, St Louis, 2006, Elsevier, pp 163–179.

AUTHOR: **BRAD A. LOCK**

EDITOR: **SCOTT J. STAHL**

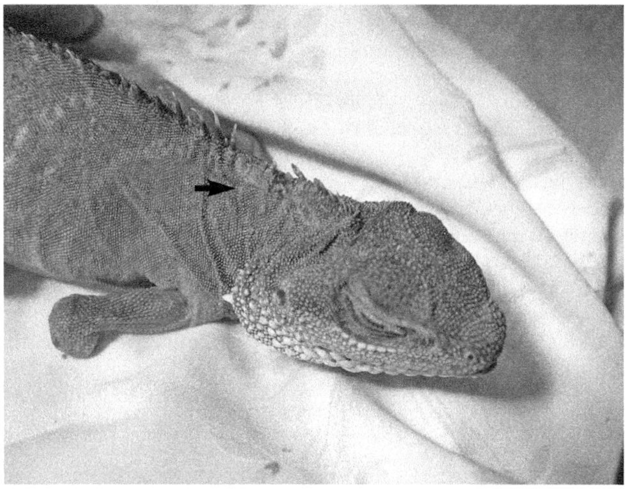

Aggression A female water dragon with typical bite wounds on the back *(arrow)*; these are inflicted by an overly aggressive male during mating. The pair needs to be separated. *(Photo courtesy Jörg Mayer, The University of Georgia, Athens.)*

REPTILES

Bacterial Dermatitis

BASIC INFORMATION

DEFINITION

Superficial or deeper infection of the epidermis and dermis with bacterial organisms

SYNONYMS

- Bacterial skin infection
- Blister disease is sometimes used to describe a bullous/vesiculous bacterial dermatitis in snakes, but fungal skin infection is now known to potentially cause identical lesions.
- Carapacial or plastral infection of chelonians, bacterial or other, is often called *shell rot* in the lay literature.

EPIDEMIOLOGY

SPECIES, AGE, SEX

- Reptiles of all species and ages, and of both sexes, are susceptible to bacterial dermatitis.
- Young and geriatric animals may be more susceptible.
- Wild-caught specimens often fail to adapt to captivity and may be more susceptible.

GENETICS AND BREED PREDISPOSITION No genetic or breed predisposition has been established, although purely anecdotal accounts suggest that color mutants/morphs may be more susceptible.

RISK FACTORS

- Bacterial dermatitis is rare in free-ranging reptiles.
- Deficient or substandard husbandry probably underlies all cases of bacterial dermatitis in reptiles.

CONTAGION AND ZOONOSIS Bacterial dermatitis, other than dermatophilosis, is not contagious, but animals kept in the same deficient captive environment may develop identical skin lesions.

GEOGRAPHY AND SEASONALITY

- Bacterial dermatitis in captive reptiles occurs worldwide, and no seasonality has been documented.
- In temperate climates, animals have no access to sunshine in autumn/winter/spring and may be more susceptible.

ASSOCIATED CONDITIONS AND DISORDERS

- Primary bacterial dermatitis is rare.
- Secondary bacterial dermatitis is common and is due to stress caused by deficient captive husbandry (overcrowding, inadequate temperature, humidity, lighting, nutrition) or to breach of cutaneous integrity from trauma, thermal injury, intraspecific or interspecific trauma, etc.
- Dysecdysis in snakes often leads to skin infection (see Dysecdysis)
- Bacterial dermatitis in aquatic reptiles is usually secondary to poor water quality.
- Generalized bacterial dermatitis in chelonians and in snakes is sometimes a result of hematogenous bacterial or bacterial toxin showering in a septicemic animal.

CLINICAL PRESENTATION

DISEASE FORMS/SUBTYPES

- Bacterial dermatitis is typically focal, or localized, but rarely may be more extensive or generalized.
- Blister disease is a syndrome in which snakes kept under poor husbandry develop multiple vesicular and bullous skin lesions.
- Obvious husbandry deficiencies, such as excessive humidity, inadequate substrate, poor hygiene, or any combination thereof, underlie blister disease.
- Lesions are indistinguishable from mycotic lesions.
- Septicemic cutaneous ulcerative disease (scud) is a generalized infection of the shell in aquatic chelonians characterized by multiple ulcers and lifting and sloughing of scutes.
- Pond turtles, softshell turtles, and snapping turtles appear more susceptible, but that may just reflect their popularity as pets.
- Water quality is typically deficient. Inadequate filtration and/or insufficient water changes are often the cause. This disease may lead to septicemia.
- Cutaneous lesions secondary to bacteremia may also lead to scud, especially in the later stages.
- Certain species of reptiles may be predisposed to trauma.
- Green water dragons and basilisks are flighty lizards that often damage their rostrum.
- Some snakes rub their rostrum against the enclosure walls to the point of damaging it. Rostral abrasions may easily lead to infection.
- Iguanas, bearded dragons, and other long-tailed lizards often damage the extremity of the tail; this may lead to dry gangrene.

HISTORY, CHIEF COMPLAINT

- Reptiles are presented with cutaneous lesions of varying duration and severity.
- Affected reptiles may be in good or poor body condition, and may be alert or depressed depending on the extent and duration of the disease, underlying causes, and/or concurrent disease.
- Hyperkeratotic lesions occur, if the condition becomes chronic.

PHYSICAL EXAM FINDINGS

- Early lesions consist of pustules and/or vesicles. These will rupture and typically ulcerate, exposing the dermis or deeper tissues.
- Lesions may be single or multiple, and if multiple, the lesions may coalesce.
- Trauma, abrasions, or lacerations may be present, indicating an underlying cause.
- Pruritus is almost never reported in reptiles with bacterial dermatitis.
- In aquatic chelonians, clear or blood-tinged fluid may be present under the laminae of carapacial or plastral scutes.
- This may be demonstrated or ascertained by exerting pressure on the scute.
- Shell bone may be exposed when the laminae rupture or slough, and in extreme cases the whole scute may slough off.

ETIOLOGY AND PATHOPHYSIOLOGY

- Bacteria that cause dermatitis in reptiles are often Gram-negative.
- *Pseudomonas* spp., *Aeromonas* spp., and *Citrobacter freundii* are typical offenders among aquatic reptiles.
- *Salmonella* spp. and numerous others such as *Serratia* and *Proteus* are often incriminated and probably represent opportunistic contaminants that proliferate in damaged or breached epithelium.
- Mixed infections are not uncommon.

DIAGNOSIS

DIFFERENTIAL DIAGNOSIS

- Mycotic skin lesions may mimic bacterial lesions.
- Viruses may cause cutaneous vesicles and blisters in mammalian species, but none have yet been documented as causing such lesions in reptiles.
- Pox and other epitheliotropic viruses in reptiles tend to cause hyperkeratotic or crusty lesions that may be confused with more chronic bacterial skin infection, or may lead to it.
- Thermal and caustic burns may cause lesions similar to those of bacterial dermatitis.
- Hypervitaminosis A in chelonians, typically iatrogenic, can cause diffuse sloughing of the epidermis, which may be confused with bacterial dermatitis.

INITIAL DATABASE

- A good review of the husbandry is in order. Particular attention should be given to temperature, humidity, and hygiene. Lighting will also affect the health of reptiles. Any sharp object in a captive environment may cause lacerations or puncture wounds.
- A complete blood count and a serum chemistry panel are needed.
- Radiographs: Deep cutaneous lesions may be assessed for muscle or bone involvement with proper imaging.
- An aspirate from vesicles and blisters should be obtained for cytology and culture.
- Swabs of ruptured or ulcerated lesions are likely to grow contaminants.
- Blood culture may be useful if the reptile shows signs consistent with bacteremia.

ADVANCED OR CONFIRMATORY TESTING

- Biopsy is the preferred and definitive diagnostic test. Excisional biopsies may also be curative.
- If lesions are too numerous, several representative lesions should be excised/biopsied.
- Always freeze some biopsies pending histopathologic examination.
- If the lesion is too large to be resected, collect the biopsy specimen at the demarcation between the lesion and healthy skin, because this is most likely to distinguish whether organisms are involved in the disease process or are merely invaders of dead tissue.

TREATMENT

THERAPEUTIC GOALS

- Stabilize the patient when septicemia underlies cutaneous lesions.
- Provide a proper environment for healing.
- Achieve good tissue levels of appropriate antibiotics at the site of infection.
- Correct husbandry deficiencies.

ACUTE GENERAL TREATMENT

- Stabilize the patient when septicemia underlies cutaneous lesions.
- Débride wounds to allow a healthy granulation bed to develop.
- In most cases, it is best to provide topical and systemic antibacterial coverage.
- Selection of the antibiotic(s) is based on culture and sensitivity.
- Initial coverage should target Gram-negative bacteria, the most common offenders, and is achieved through the use of broad-spectrum antimicrobials (e.g., enrofloxacin, trimethoprim-sulfa, second- or third-generation cephalosporins).
- Topical antiseptics (e.g., silver sulfadiazine cream) may be used.
- Infected skin, except for large defects, typically heals better without a bandage.
- If bandaging is necessary, use wet-to-dry bandages and change them daily.
- Dry-docking (maintaining an aquatic turtle out of the water) for 1-2 hours daily, or longer as necessary, allows topical treatment to be applied more efficiently; the drying may help treat pathogenic bacterial involvement.
- For a detailed antibiotic treatment regimen.

CHRONIC TREATMENT

- Lesions in reptiles may heal slowly; however, they may also heal surprisingly fast.
- If proper husbandry modifications are made, the need for chronic treatment should be rare.

POSSIBLE COMPLICATIONS

The use of antibiotics may lead to potential untoward effects, such as hypersensitivity, gut flora imbalance, organ toxicity, secondary mycotic infection, and others. Patients should be monitored throughout the course of treatment.

RECOMMENDED MONITORING

Treatment typically should not be discontinued before the patient is brought back to the clinic and progress or resolution of lesions has been assessed.

PROGNOSIS AND OUTCOME

- Prognosis will depend greatly on the severity and extent of lesions, the presence or absence and nature of any underlying disease, and the ability to pinpoint and correct husbandry deficiencies.
- Scarring is a common outcome of dermatitis and should not be confused with active lesions.
- Cutaneous scars in reptiles appear as unpigmented, whitish/grayish, smooth, sometimes with a black rim, contracted or wrinkled areas, where lesions previously existed.

PEARLS & CONSIDERATIONS

COMMENTS

Bacterial dermatitis in captive reptiles reflects husbandry inadequacies and/or underlying disease. As our understanding of the captive care of various reptile species increases, the incidence of bacterial dermatitis is likely to decrease.

PREVENTION

Awareness by owners of proper husbandry requirements for the species in their care will minimize the risk for bacterial dermatitis.

SUGGESTED READINGS

Cooper JE: Dermatology. In Mader DR, editor: Reptile medicine and surgery, ed 2, St Louis, 2006, Saunders Elsevier, pp 196–216.

Jacobson ER: Bacterial diseases of reptiles. In Jacobson ER, editor: Infectious diseases and pathology of reptiles: color atlas and text, New York, 2007, CRC Press, Taylor & Francis, pp 461–526.

Paré JA, Sigler L, Rosenthal KL, Mader DR: Microbiology: fungal diseases of reptiles. In Mader DR, editor: Reptile medicine and surgery, ed 2, St Louis, 2006, Saunders Elsevier, pp 196–216.

CROSS-REFERENCES TO OTHER SECTIONS

Dysecdysis

AUTHOR: **JEAN A. PARÉ**

EDITOR: **SCOTT J. STAHL**

REPTILES

Calicivirus Infection

BASIC INFORMATION

DEFINITION

Reptilian caliciviruses

SYNONYMS

Crotalid calicivirus, San Miguel sea lion virus, vesicular exanthema of swine

EPIDEMIOLOGY

SPECIES, AGE, SEX

- Caliciviruses have extremely broad host ranges.
- Sex and age predispositions are not known.

GENETICS AND BREED PREDISPOSITION

- Caliciviruses have been isolated from Aruba Island rattlesnakes (*Crotalus unicolor*), a rock rattlesnake (*Crotalus lepidus*), and an eyelash viper (*Bothrops schlegeli*), as well as from Bell's horned frogs (*Ceratophrys orata*).
- Calicivirus-like particles have also been seen in bearded dragons.

RISK FACTORS Risk factors are not well understood.

CONTAGION AND ZOONOSIS

- As unenveloped viruses, caliciviruses are very stable in the environment.
- Disinfectants effective against other unenveloped viruses may be expected to be effective against caliciviruses.
- Caliciviruses represent the most significant zoonotic risk of any reptile viruses.
- Reptile calicivirus strains have been found to cause disease in pinnipeds. Reptilian caliciviruses are part of a quasi-species that has been found to infect animals ranging from fish to mammals; they have been associated with vesicular lesions and with hepatitis in humans.

GEOGRAPHY AND SEASONALITY Geography and seasonality of reptile caliciviruses are not well understood.

ASSOCIATED CONDITIONS AND DISORDERS

- Disease associated with caliciviruses in reptiles is not well understood.
- In other species, caliciviruses are associated with hepatitis, stomatitis, and vesicular lesions.

CLINICAL PRESENTATION

DISEASE FORMS/SUBTYPES Disease associated with caliciviruses in reptiles is not well understood.

HISTORY, CHIEF COMPLAINT Disease associated with caliciviruses in reptiles is not well understood.

PHYSICAL EXAM FINDINGS Disease associated with caliciviruses in reptiles is not well understood.

ETIOLOGY AND PATHOPHYSIOLOGY

All reptile caliciviruses characterized to date are in the genus *Vesivirus.*

DIAGNOSIS

DIFFERENTIAL DIAGNOSIS

Disease associated with caliciviruses in reptiles is not well understood.

INITIAL DATABASE

A thorough history, physical examination findings, complete blood count, plasma chemistry, and radiographs form the basic database.

ADVANCED OR CONFIRMATORY TESTING

- Nested polymerase chain reaction (PCR) with product sequence analysis is available for caliciviruses from the University of Florida.
- Swabs or biopsy specimens of vesicular lesions or cloacal washes are the samples of choice.
- Electron microscopy may be useful to help identify calicivirus-like particles and is often less expensive when feces are examined, although sequence data are needed for speciation.

TREATMENT

THERAPEUTIC GOAL

Because caliciviruses often establish persistent infection, the goal of treatment is alleviation of clinical disease, and infected animals may be lifelong carriers.

ACUTE GENERAL TREATMENT

Providing supportive care and addressing husbandry deficiencies are the most important aspects of treating caliciviral disease.

CHRONIC TREATMENT

Animals remain persistently infected, and continued shedding by recovered animals is a concern.

PROGNOSIS AND OUTCOME

More study is needed on caliciviral disease in reptiles before prognostic information can be established. Animals often are persistently infected, and introduction of naïve animals to recovered animals should be avoided.

PEARLS & CONSIDERATIONS

COMMENTS

The large host range and rapid evolution of caliciviruses gives them the potential to rapidly jump host species. In cats, related feline caliciviruses have demonstrated the ability to mutate into variants that cause hemorrhagic disease with high mortality.

PREVENTION

Maintenance of a closed group, testing of populations, testing during quarantine, and stringent biosecurity practices are the most effective means of prevention.

SUGGESTED READINGS

Barlough JE, et al: Isolation of reptilian calicivirus *Crotalus* type 1 from feral pinnipeds, J Wildl Dis 34:451–456, 1998.

Neill JD, et al: Genetic relatedness of the caliciviruses: San Miguel sea lion and vesicular exanthema of swine viruses constitute a single genotype within the Caliciviridae, J Virol 69:4484–4488, 1995.

Smith AW, et al: First isolation of calicivirus from reptiles and amphibians, Am J Vet Res 47:1718–1721, 1986.

Smith AW, et al: In vitro isolation and characterization of a calicivirus causing a vesicular disease of the hands and feet, Clin Infect Dis 26:434–439, 1998.

Smith AW, et al: *Vesivirus* viremia and seroprevalence in humans, J Med Virol 78:693–701, 2006.

AUTHOR: **JAMES F.X. WELLEHAN, JR.**

EDITOR: **SCOTT J. STAHL**

REPTILES

CANV/Fungal Disease

BASIC INFORMATION

DEFINITION

Infection of the skin or systemic infection with a fungus called the *Chrysosporium anamorph* of *Nannizziopsis vriesii (CANV)*

SYNONYM

Yellow fungus disease (YFD)

EPIDEMIOLOGY

SPECIES, AGE, SEX

- CANV mycosis has been described mostly in snakes and lizards.
- Infection seems relatively prevalent in aquatic snake species (*Erpeton tentaculatum, Nerodia* spp., *Acrochordus* spp.) and in certain colubrids (e.g., corn snakes, brown tree snakes) but can probably occur in all ophidians.
- Bearded dragons and chameleons appear overrepresented.
- CANV has been documented in the Iguanidae, the Geckonidae, the Agamidae, the Chameleonidae, and the Teiidae and can probably infect all lizards.
- CANV has caused severe dermatomycosis with associated mortality in farmed saltwater crocodile hatchlings.
- No sex predilection has been noted.
- Anecdotally, young lizards may be more vulnerable to CANV infection, and fatal mycosis in saltwater crocodiles was limited to hatchlings.

RISK FACTORS Not known. One study suggests that breaches in cutaneous integrity increase the likelihood of infection with CANV, at least in veiled chameleons.

CONTAGION AND ZOONOSIS

- This disease is contagious among lizards and crocodiles, and probably among snakes.
- Spread seems to occur horizontally through direct or indirect contact and may occur through airborne conidia shed by infected animals.
- CANV was isolated from a brain abscess in a human immunodeficiency virus (HIV)-positive Nigerian man.
- Zoonotic potential likely would be minimal, given that a vast majority of CANV isolates do not grow at 37°C (98.6°F), with the exception of those from bearded dragons, which do grow, albeit very slowly, at 37°C (98.6°F).

GEOGRAPHY AND SEASONALITY

- CANV infection has been documented in North America, Europe, and Australia, but likely occurs worldwide.

- YFD has been reported only in North America.

ASSOCIATED CONDITIONS AND DISORDERS

- Stress, substandard husbandry, and/or any immune suppressive disorders may predispose reptiles to mycotic infection, but the CANV is a primary pathogen capable of causing lesions in seemingly healthy reptiles.
- In bearded dragons, treatment of coccidiosis with sulfa drugs has been anecdotally linked with later onset of YFD.

CLINICAL PRESENTATION

DISEASE FORMS/SUBTYPES

- CANV mycosis is typically a dermatomycosis, and systemic infection usually results from dissemination of cutaneous disease.
- Systemic involvement has been seen in animals with seemingly localized cutaneous disease.
- CANV sometimes causes mycetomas, well-delineated subcutaneous fungal infections, especially in corn snakes.

HISTORY, CHIEF COMPLAINT

- Reptiles with CANV usually are presented with skin disease, often soon after purchase or capture.
- Reptiles with CANV usually are presented because of skin lesions noticed by the owner.

PHYSICAL EXAM FINDINGS

- In early stages of the disease, abnormalities are restricted to cutaneous lesions.
- These may be vesicular, progressing to ulceration and crusting.
- In bearded dragons, the first lesion is often that of retained shed tags, often yellowish in color.
- The tags may appear "melted" and smoother than normal.
- Hyperkeratosis and epidermal necrosis soon follow.
- Necrotic crusts will slough, exposing raw dermis. Especially when on extremities, granulomatous disease may extend to underlying muscles and bones.
- Systemic dissemination typically occurs late in the disease.
- Subcutaneous masses in squamates and particularly snakes, even masses with a gross appearance reminiscent of lipomas, should be submitted for histopathology to dismiss fungal involvement.
- A sample of that mass should be kept frozen for culture.

ETIOLOGY AND PATHOPHYSIOLOGY

- Infection in another reptile probably occurs when conidia colonize dead stratum corneum at the skin surface.
- Hyphae proliferate and eventually penetrate the deeper epidermal layers, then the dermis.

DIAGNOSIS

DIFFERENTIAL DIAGNOSIS

- CANV infection cannot be differentiated clinically from other fungal infections.
- Dermatomycosis may mimic bacterial dermatitis.
- Blister disease and ventral scute necrosis in snakes may present identically to CANV infection.
- Mycetomas may be mistaken for lipomas.
- Lesions of YFD may mimic papillomatous disease or thermal injuries.

INITIAL DATABASE

- Husbandry should be reviewed.
- Cutaneous lesions in reptiles should be biopsied and cultured for bacteria and fungi.
- Alternatively, additional biopsies should be frozen pending histopathology, and cultured if fungal disease is identified.
- Blood work may help identify muscle involvement or dissemination to the liver or kidneys.
- Radiographs may disclose underlying bone involvement.
- Ultrasound, MRI, or CT scans may identify lesions in organ systems.

ADVANCED OR CONFIRMATORY TESTING

- Diagnosis is achieved through biopsy. Biopsy of cutaneous lesions usually is straightforward. Deeper lesions may be accessed through endoscopy/laparoscopy.
- Histopathologic examination will demonstrate the hyphae in tissues.
  - CANV sometimes adopts yeastlike morphology within granulomata, especially in bearded dragons.
  - Dense tufts of arthroconidia at the skin surface of infected reptiles are highly suggestive of CANV.
- Touch preparation cytology of ulcerated or necrotic cutaneous lesions may yield rectangular arthroconidia, highly suggestive of CANV.
- Culture for CANV is best accomplished in a Petri with cycloheximide-containing fungal agar (Mycosel, Mycobiotic), incubated at 25°C (77°F).

TREATMENT

THERAPEUTIC GOALS

- Isolate animal from other reptiles
- Ensure proper husbandry
- Provide fluids and nutritional support as needed
- Provide thermal support and maintain reptile within the upper half of its preferred optimal temperature zone (POTZ), as this may slow or curtail growth of the fungus
- Aggressively débride cutaneous lesions
- Use topical antiseptic (antifungal and antibacterial) dressing.
- Mycetomas need to be surgically excised, and systemic antifungal therapy should follow.
- Involvement of deeper structures carries a very guarded prognosis.
- Surgical débridement/excision should be attempted

ACUTE GENERAL TREATMENT

- Topical treatment alone is bound to fail. Administer a systemic antifungal.
- Voriconazole, terbinafine, and itraconazole are all good choices. If disease is confined to the skin, use itraconazole or terbinafine (or both) pulse therapy, because both drugs tend to accumulate and persist in the skin. Even plasma levels seem to persist after discontinuation of therapy.
- Itraconazole: A pulse therapy consisting of 5 mg/kg SID, 1 week per month (1 week on, 3 weeks off), may be used until resolution of lesions.
- Terbinafine: A starting dose of 10 mg/kg orally SID is administered as pulses, as described for itraconazole.
- Voriconazole: 5-10 mg/kg orally SID or BID

CHRONIC TREATMENT

Ensure that lesions have totally resolved before discontinuing systemic antifungals (treat up to 1 week after resolution of lesions).

DRUG INTERACTIONS

- Largely unknown; a combination of terbinafine and itraconazole may be synergistic
- Pulse therapy could involve 1 week of itraconazole and 1 week of terbinafine per month.

POSSIBLE COMPLICATIONS

- Antifungal drugs may cause toxicity.
- Dosages are largely unknown or have been determined in one or two reptile species.
- Owners should be instructed to call should the patient become anorectic or lethargic, or show any change in its demeanor.
- Blood chemistries taken at regular intervals during treatment may be compared with pretreatment values to identify early organ insult.
- Fecal and urinary output should be monitored.

RECOMMENDED MONITORING

Assess lesions weekly until resolved. Treat for a minimum of 1 week past resolution of lesions. Serum chemistries can be used to try to detect potential hepatic or renal toxicity.

PROGNOSIS AND OUTCOME

- CANV infection is often fatal.
- Treatment is typically prolonged; therefore, owner compliance may fail.
- Even cutaneous infection may be refractory to treatment or may recur once medication is discontinued.
- Prognosis is best if lesions are caught very early and treatment is initiated without delay.
- If limited to an extremity, amputation may be curative.

PEARLS & CONSIDERATIONS

COMMENTS

- Laboratories still often misidentify CANV, largely because it is not yet listed in all veterinary mycology texts.
- *Trichophyton* spp., *Trichosporon* spp., *Geotrichum candidum, Malbranchea* spp., and *Chrysosporium* spp., among other fungi, can be confused with CANV.
- Suspect isolates should be forwarded to a mycology reference laboratory for proper identification. Isolates should be keyed to species. Insist that the laboratory preserve isolates until causation is established or dismissed.
- Confirmed pathogenic isolates should be deposited in a microfungus for preservation. Most deposited CANV isolates are at the University of Alberta Microfungus Collection and Herbarium in Edmonton, Canada (website: http://www.devonian.ualberta.ca/uamh/).

PREVENTION

- Quarantine
- Meticulous hygiene and husbandry

CLIENT EDUCATION

Proper husbandry and hygiene will minimize infectious diseases or their impact. CANV-infected animals are contagious to other reptiles. It is recommended to use gloves when handling and treating patients with CANV infection. Wash hands after handling reptiles.

SUGGESTED READINGS

Bowman MR, et al: Mycotic dermatitis and stomatitis in bearded dragons (*Pogona vitticeps*) caused by the *Chrysosporium* anamorph of *Nannizziopsis vriesii*, Med Mycol 45:371–376, 2007.

Paré JA, et al: Microbiology: fungal and bacterial diseases of reptiles. In Mader DR, editor: Reptile medicine and surgery, St Louis, 2006, Elsevier, pp 217–238.

Paré JA: Mycotic diseases of reptiles. In Jacobson E, editor: Infectious diseases and pathology of reptiles: a color atlas and text, Boca Raton, FL, 2007, CRC Press, pp 527–570.

AUTHOR: **JEAN A. PARÉ**

EDITOR: **SCOTT J. STAHL**

REPTILES

Cardiac Disease

BASIC INFORMATION

DEFINITION

Reptilian cardiac disease refers to any of a number of events that result in some degree of dysfunction of the heart or cardiovascular system.

SYNONYMS

Heart disease, cardiovascular disease

EPIDEMIOLOGY

SPECIES, AGE, SEX

- All adult green iguanas
- Clinical cardiac disease can be primary (idiopathic, cardiomyopathy, congenital defects, and degenerative disease) or secondary to metabolic or nutritional disorders.
- Additionally, infectious, parasitic, and systemic disease may affect the cardiovascular system with clinical signs referable to the heart.

RISK FACTORS

- Diets high in vitamin D_3 and calcium
- Diets consisting of excessively oily fish and/or obese rodents
- Diets low in vitamin E and selenium
- Hypocalcemia
- Suboptimal husbandry practices

ASSOCIATED CONDITIONS AND DISORDERS

- Obesity
- Overfeeding

CLINICAL PRESENTATION

DISEASE FORMS/SUBTYPES Clinical signs of cardiac disease are varied and nonspecific. The form the disease takes is dependent on the etiopathogenesis.

HISTORY, CHIEF COMPLAINT

- A history of poor diet and overfeeding is common.
- Weakness
- Exercise intolerance
- Anorexia
- Weight loss
- Enlargement in the area of the heart

PHYSICAL EXAM FINDINGS

- Nonspecific and rarely if ever pathognomonic
- Swelling in the area of the heart
- Pleural or peripheral edema
- Ascites
- Cyanosis
- Ecchymosis
- Weakness
- Dyspnea
- Slow or increased heart rate
- Slow (greater than 2 seconds) capillary refill (oral or cloacal mucous membranes) time may suggest cardiovascular or circulatory compromise.
  - Patient temperature will have a profound effect on these measurements.

ETIOLOGY AND PATHOPHYSIOLOGY

- Poor husbandry practices:
  - Especially with those species (iguanas, chelonians) that require ultraviolet (UV) B exposure can lead to low dietary levels of calcium (see Nutritional Secondary Hyperparathyroidism [NSHP])
  - Hypocalcemia affects the peripheral nerves, skeletal muscle, and striated cardiac muscle, resulting in dysfunction.
- Inadequate levels of dietary vitamin E may result in cardiac muscle changes similar to classic "white muscle disease."
- Muscle changes similar to cardiomyopathy have been seen in reptiles.
  - Affected individuals (oily fish, obese rodents) have received high-fat diets.

- Small enclosures and reduced exercise in captive reptiles combined with overfeeding can lead to obesity and heart disease.
- Calcification of the tunica media of the large vessels:
  - This condition has been associated with diets high in vitamin D_3 and calcium.
  - Most commonly seen in green iguanas and savannah monitors
- A number of infectious agents have resulted in cardiac disease in reptiles. Most commonly, this results in an endocarditis.
  - Reported agents include *Vibrio damsela*, *Salmonella arizonae*, *Corynebacterium* spp., *Escherichia coli*, *Chlamydophila* spp., *Mycoplasma alligatoris*, and *Mycobacterium* spp.
- Adult filarid worms can live in the vascular system of reptiles, where they can release microfilaria into the circulation.
  - Transmission occurs through bloodsucking arthropods (mosquitoes and ticks).
  - Ischemic necrosis may occur when microfilaria obstruct peripheral capillaries.
- Digenetic spirochid trematodes can also affect the cardiovascular system of reptiles:
  - Chelonians are the group most commonly affected.
  - The most common genera are *Spirochis*, *Henostoma*, *Unicaecum*, *Vasotrema*, and *Hapalorhynchus*.
    - These parasites need a snail to complete their life cycle, so most infestations are seen in wild-caught animals or individuals kept outside, where they may come into contact with the invertebrate host.
  - Adults are found in the heart and great vessels and are associated with minimal clinical disease.
  - Disease from these trematodes is referable to release of eggs within the vascular compartment.
  - Accumulation of eggs may occlude terminal vessels in a variety of organs, including the gastrointestinal tract, liver, spleen, heart, kidneys, and lungs.
  - Vascular occlusion of the vessels in the plastron or carapace may result in ulcerative lesions of the shell.

DIAGNOSIS

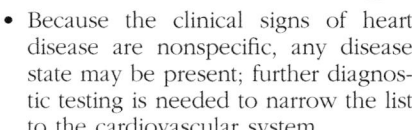

DIFFERENTIAL DIAGNOSIS

- Because the clinical signs of heart disease are nonspecific, any disease state may be present; further diagnostic testing is needed to narrow the list to the cardiovascular system.
- Neoplasia
- Abscess

INITIAL DATABASE

- Physical examination: looking for signs referable to the cardiovascular system (see above)
- CBC/Chemistry: elevated white cell count, morphology changes that may show infection or inflammation
- Radiography: enlarged heart, thrombi, calcification of vessels

ADVANCED OR CONFIRMATORY TESTING

- Echocardiography: Heart shape and size and function, along with blood flow and valve operation, may be evaluated.
- Blood culture with sensitivity profile
- Nonselective angiography: good radiographic images of heart and great vessels (Iohexol 1-2 mL/kg per animal, via IV jugular catheter)
- MRI or CT provides the best images of the chelonian cardiovascular system.

TREATMENT

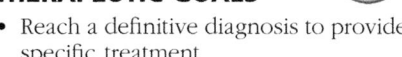

THERAPEUTIC GOALS

- Reach a definitive diagnosis to provide specific treatment
- Treat clinical signs (edema, dyspnea)
- Increase use of stored calories

ACUTE GENERAL TREATMENT

- Initial treatment is based on the cause of the disease present and the state of the patient.
- Optimize husbandry protocols for each individual based on species.
- Provide supportive care (fluids, nutrition) as needed based on physical examination findings and initial diagnostic workup.
- Minimize stress on the patient during treatments: short bouts of interaction followed by longer times in dark quiet holding cage
- Provide calcium in cases of hypocalcemia.
  - Mild signs (low Ca on blood work)
- Oral Ca glubionate: give ≈10 mg/kg orally SID for 1-3 months
  - Severe signs (tremors):
    - Ca lactate/Ca glycerophosphate (Calphosan, Glenwood): give 10 mg/kg SC, Ice q 24 h
    - Ca gluconate: give 100 mg/kg SQ, (into a bolus of fluids or dilated as it is caustic) q 8 h as needed
- Provide vitamin E (12.5 mg/kg) and selenium (0.05 mg/kg) if history suggests deficiencies in the diet.
- Treatment of spirochid infection is difficult and has had limited success.
  - Treatment with praziquantel for a single day at 25 mg/kg (3 doses at hours 0, 3, and 6) can be attempted.
- Filarial nematode infestations have been treated with fenbendazole (10-25 mg/kg PO for 3-5 days, stop for 10-14 days, and then repeat), ivermectin (0.2-0.4 mg/kg PO or IM); do not use in chelonian species and by raising the environmental temperature to 35°C-37°C (95°F-98°F) for 24-48 hours. Note that not all species of reptiles may be able to tolerate this treatment.
- Loop diuretics such as Furosemide (5 mg/kg IV, IM, PO q 12-24 h) should not work in reptiles because the reptilian kidney does not possess a loop of Henle, but clinically they have some positive effects and their use should be considered in cardiac cases that present with ascites and/or edema.

CHRONIC TREATMENT

- Regular assessment of weight, body condition, and physical signs
- Continue practices initiated during acute phase of treatment (optimize husbandry and caloric intake).
- Slow reduction of weight to normal for that species.
- Broad-spectrum antibiotics based on cultures and sensitivities
- Supplementation with calcium: changed from injectable in the acute phase to oral in the chronic phase. Monitor with repeat blood sampling and clinical signs.
- The use of cardiac-specific drugs (cardiac glycosides, vasodilators, and diuretics) has not been adequately evaluated in reptiles; these agents should be used with caution and after discussion with the owner. Understanding these statements enalapril at 5.0 mg/kg PO q 24-48 h can be initiated empirically.

PROGNOSIS AND OUTCOME

- Guarded to poor depending on etiology
- Most cases have been presented in an advanced state of disease.
- Hypocalcemia and hypovitaminosis E causes (if not advanced) have responded well to supplementation.
- Treatments for endocarditis and cardiomyopathy in reptiles have been unrewarding; euthanasia is a viable option that should be discussed with the owner.

PEARLS & CONSIDERATIONS

COMMENTS

- For most cases of cardiac disease in reptiles, treatment will be difficult and unrewarding.

- Frank discussions with the client about treatment options and outcomes are important.
- If treatment attempts are elected, a "team" effort is required, so that all communications as to expectations are clear.

PREVENTION

- Provide appropriate diet with good vitamin supplementation.
- Most captive reptiles are overweight: Strive to not overfeed.
- Provide exercise opportunities.
- Provide appropriate thermal environment with proper ultraviolet (UV) B and UVA light sources for the species.
- Optimize husbandry; this will optimize the immune system.
- Minimize exposure to invertebrates needed to complete the life cycle of some parasitic diseases.

CLIENT EDUCATION

- Reptiles are very efficient at converting food to fat. Most clients overfeed their reptiles, so adherence to a diet that meets but does not exceed a patient's caloric needs is important. Even though it is fun to watch reptiles eat, it is not healthy for them to overeat!
- Educate clients on the differences between direct life cycle and indirect life cycle parasites, and explain how they can minimize their pet's exposure.

SUGGESTED READINGS

Donoghue S: Nutrition. In Mader DR, editor: Reptile medicine and surgery, St Louis, 2006, Elsevier, pp 251–298.

Murry MJ: Cardiology. In Mader DR, editor: Reptile medicine and surgery, St Louis, 2006, Elsevier, pp 181–195.

Schilliger L, et al: Proposed standardization of the two-dimensional echocardiographic examination in snakes, J Herpetol Med Surg 16:76–87, 2006.

Snyder PS, et al: Two-dimensional echocardiographic anatomy of the snake heart (*Python molurus bivittatus*), Vet Radiol Ultrasound 40:66–72, 1999.

CROSS-REFERENCES TO OTHER SECTIONS

Hepatic Lipidosis
Liver Disease
Nutritional Secondary Hyperparathyroidism (NSHP)
Renal Disease

AUTHOR: **BRAD A. LOCK**

EDITOR: **SCOTT J. STAHL**

REPTILES

Chlamydophilosis

BASIC INFORMATION

DEFINITION

Bacterial infection associated with acute or chronic infection in the reptile

SYNONYM

Chlamydiosis. Genera in the Chlamydiae other than *Chlamydophila* that have been found to infect reptiles include *Neochlamydia*, *Parachlamydia*, and *Simkania*.

EPIDEMIOLOGY

SPECIES, AGE, SEX

- Chlamydophilosis is a disease of concern in all vertebrates, including all reptiles.
- Disease due to *Chlamydophila pneumoniae* appears to be especially common in captive emerald tree boas (*Corallus caninus*) in the United States.
- Disease may be seen in all ages. No sex predilections in reptiles are known.

RISK FACTORS

- Immune suppressed animals appear to be at greatest risk for the disease.
- Husbandry deficiencies are a common source of immune suppression.

CONTAGION AND ZOONOSIS

- The elementary body is the life stage of *Chlamydophila* that is most stable in the environment.
- Careful biosecurity practices and disinfection are indicated to prevent spread.
- *Chlamydophila pneumoniae* is a zoonotic pathogen of significant concern.
- Clinical signs in humans often involve the lower respiratory system.
- *Chlamydophila abortus* and other Chlamydiae such as *Simkania* spp. and *Parachlamydia* spp. are also potential zoonotic pathogens.
- Pregnant women are especially at risk. *Chlamydophila felis* and *Neochlamydia* spp. have not yet been clearly established as significant zoonotic pathogens.

GEOGRAPHY AND SEASONALITY

- Chlamydophilosis is cosmopolitan.
- Seasonality has not been reported.

ASSOCIATED CONDITIONS AND DISORDERS

- Chlamydophilosis in reptiles is associated with granulomatous disease.
- Granulomas can be found in all tissues; lung, alimentary tract, liver, heart, and spleen are common sites.

CLINICAL PRESENTATION

DISEASE FORMS/SUBTYPES Chlamydophilosis can vary depending on the species and which tissues are affected.

HISTORY, CHIEF COMPLAINT Common complaints on presentation for chlamydophilosis include nonspecific illness, respiratory disease, regurgitation, and weight loss.

PHYSICAL EXAM FINDINGS Physical exam findings are often nonspecific.

ETIOLOGY AND PATHOPHYSIOLOGY

- A number of species in the phylum Chlamydiae have been identified in reptiles.
- The most common appears to be *Chlamydophila pneumoniae*.
- *Chlamydophila abortus*, *Chlamydophila felis*, *Neochlamydia* spp., *Parachlamydia* spp., and *Simkania* spp. from reptiles have also been identified.
- A *Chlamydophila pecorum*–like organism has been identified in tortoises with nasal discharge, and an unidentified *Chlamydophila* species has been associated with deaths in crocodiles.
- Differences in ecology and zoonotic risk have been noted, and any identified Chlamydiae infection should be speciated.
- Chlamydophilosis in reptiles is associated with granulomatous disease. Granulomas can be found in all tissues; lung, alimentary tract, liver, heart, and spleen are common sites.

DIAGNOSIS

DIFFERENTIAL DIAGNOSIS

Other common causes of granulomatous disease in reptiles include mycobacteriosis, *Dermatophilus* spp., and fungi.

INITIAL DATABASE

- A thorough husbandry history, physical examination findings, complete blood count, plasma chemistry, and radiographs provide a basic database.
- A leukocytosis is often present with chlamydophilosis.
- Inclusions containing elementary bodies and reticulate bodies may be seen in monocytes.

ADVANCED OR CONFIRMATORY TESTING

- Biopsy specimens showing granulomatous disease in reptiles should be examined with a Machiavello stain or by immunohistochemistry.
- In many infections, small numbers of organisms are present, and they may be missed.
- Polymerase chain reaction (PCR) with product sequence analysis is available from the Jacobson Laboratory at the University of Florida College of Veterinary Medicine for identification and speciation of members of the phylum Chlamydiae.

TREATMENT

THERAPEUTIC GOAL

The goal of therapy is eradication of the organism.

CHRONIC TREATMENT

- The organism should be speciated to determine zoonotic potential.
- Any husbandry deficiencies should be addressed and corrected.
  - Zoonotic risks need to be discussed with the owner.
- Tetracyclines and azalides are the best choices for treatment.
- Pharmacokinetic data are available on azithromycin in snakes (ball pythons at 10 mg/kg PO q 48 h), oxytetracycline in American alligators (10 mg/kg IM, IV q 5d), and loggerhead sea turtles (*Caretta caretta*) (at a loading dose of 41 mg/kg IM followed by 21 mg/kg IM q 72 h); these are the current drugs of choice.
- In the absence of further data, treatment should be provided for at least 45-60 days.
- Beta lactams and fluoroquinolones are unlikely to result in successful treatment. Shorter courses appear likely to result in treatment failure.

RECOMMENDED MONITORING

- Biopsy specimens of affected tissues and a CBC should be taken after 6 months to a year to look for recurrence.
- CBCs should be checked every 3 months for several years to look for leukocytosis, which may be a sign of recurrence.

PROGNOSIS AND OUTCOME

- The prognosis for animals with chlamydophilosis varies depending on affected tissues and species.
- Many animals respond well to therapy.

PEARL & CONSIDERATIONS

COMMENTS

- Chlamydophilosis probably is significantly underdiagnosed in reptiles and should be on the differential list of any ill animal.
- Speciation is important; some species cause significant zoonotic concerns, whereas others do not.
- Dual infection with Chlamydiales and *Mycobacterium* spp. has been documented and should be considered in any animal with granulomatous inflammation.
- The shorter, single-drug therapy used for Chlamydiales is likely to result in resistance in any *Mycobacterium* spp. present, and would be of potential zoonotic concern.

PREVENTION

Maintenance of a closed group of known negative status, quarantine, and stringent biosecurity practices are the most effective means of prevention.

CLIENT EDUCATION

Zoonotic risks need to be discussed with the owner.

SUGGESTED READING

Bodetti TJ, et al: Molecular evidence to support the expansion of the host range of *Chamydophila pneumoniae* to include reptiles as well as humans, horses, koalas, and amphibians, Syst Appl Microbiol 25:146–152, 2002.

Homer BL, et al: Chlamydiosis in mariculture-reared green sea turtles (*Chelonia mydas*), Vet Pathol 31:1–7, 1994.

Hotzel H, et al: Evidence of infection in tortoises by *Chlamydia*-like organisms that are genetically distinct from known Chlamydiaceae species, Vet Res Commun 29(Suppl 7):1–80, 2005.

Lock B, et al: An epizootic of chronic regurgitation associated with chlamydophilosis in recently imported emerald tree boas (*Corallus caninus*), J Zoo Wildl Med 34:385–393, 2003.

CROSS-REFERENCES TO OTHER CHAPTERS

Herpesvirus
Mycoplasma
Paramyxovirus
Reovirus
Respiratory (lower) Disease/Phenomenon

AUTHOR: **JAMES F.X. WELLEHAN, JR.**

EDITOR: **SCOTT J. STAHL**

REPTILES

Cloacal Prolapse

Client Education Sheet Available on Website

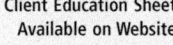

BASIC INFORMATION

DEFINITION

Cloacal prolapse refers to any condition involving protrusion of tissue from the vent (terminal cloacal opening) of the reptile. This tissue can include cloacal mucosa, gastrointestinal tract, reproductive tract, and genitourinary tract.

SYNONYMS

Organ prolapse, tissue prolapse, hemipenile prolapse

EPIDEMIOLOGY

SPECIES, AGE, SEX

- Can be seen in any species, age, or sex
- Common in high-producing, egg-laying female species
- Common in neonate green tree pythons (colonic and cloacal prolapses)

RISK FACTORS

- Poor husbandry and nutrition
- Hypocalcemia
- High reproductive output
- Species: neonate green tree pythons

ASSOCIATED CONDITIONS AND DISORDERS

- Hypocalcemia/Hypovitaminosis D_3
- Dehydration
- Dystocia (see Dystocia)
- Parasitic enteritis
- Bacterial enteritis
- Cystitis
- Intramural or extramural masses
- Nutritional secondary hyperparathyroidism (NSHP)

CLINICAL PRESENTATION

DISEASE FORMS/SUBTYPES

- Tissue mass protruding from the vent opening
- This tissue can have of a variety of origins, including gastrointestinal tract, urinary bladder, phallus (chelonians, crocodilians) or hemipenes (other reptiles), and the oviduct of females.
- In rare cases, the kidney or other organs have been known to prolapse from the vent.

HISTORY, CHIEF COMPLAINT
- Obvious tissue protruding from vent opening
- History of constipation or observation of animal straining to defecate
- History of poor diet and husbandry practices (improper temperatures, inappropriate substrates such as sand)
- For hemipenal or phallus prolapse, a recent history of copulation
- Possible trauma from cagemate or damage to the hemipene from recent probing for sex determination (see Paraphimosis)
- In many cases, no significant history or other clinical signs will be noted.

PHYSICAL EXAM FINDINGS
- Tissue protrusion from the vent opening (see above for possible origin of tissues)
- Often, no other abnormal physical examination findings are obvious.
- Abnormal findings that may be seen include dehydration, poor body condition, and palpable coelomic masses; the animal may present moribund.

ETIOLOGY AND PATHOPHYSIOLOGY
- Cloacal prolapse of tissue or organs is generally secondary to an excessive amount of straining from a variety of causes.
- Inappropriate humidity levels and lack of clean water or improper presentation of water can lead to dehydration, constipation, and straining.
- Husbandry: improper lighting, temperatures, enclosure size (lack of exercise)
- Lack of vitamin D_3 and or calcium in the diet may impair calcium absorption and distribution.
- This condition may lead to hypocalcemia, which will affect contraction of smooth muscle. This can result in constipation and straining.
- NSHP same effect as above (see Nutritional Secondary Hyperparathyroidism [NSHP])
- Infection leading to straining
- Intraluminal or extraluminal masses leading to constipation and straining
- Copulatory organ prolapse most commonly the result of cagemate trauma, forced separation during copulation, or trauma from sex determination (probing). Other reported causes include constipation and neurologic dysfunction.
- Oviductal prolapse: most commonly occurs secondary to dystocia or egg binding
- Urinary bladder prolapse: most often secondary to cystitis, often from cystic calculi
- Colon prolapse: generally the result of tenesmus with constipation, bacterial enteritis, and parasitic enteritis being most commonly implicated

DIAGNOSIS

DIFFERENTIAL DIAGNOSIS
Vent/cloacal trauma (resembles tissue protrusion or prolapse)

INITIAL DATABASE
- Physical examination: observation of prolapsed tissue
- Whole-body radiographs to assess radiolucency of bones and to survey for obvious masses or other abnormalities
- Fecal examination
- CBC/Chemistry profile

ADVANCED OR CONFIRMATORY TESTING
- Ionized calcium concentration: A reptile may have near normal total calcium and may still have hypocalcemic signs due to low ionized calcium (green iguanas; meanionized calcium. 47 ± 0.015 mmol/L).
- Contrast radiographs: to look for evidence of intraluminal and extraluminal masses. MRI and CT scans would also fit into this category and may be more effective in identifying masses.
- Endoscopy to directly visualize masses and provide the ability to take tissue biopsy specimen for culture and histopathologic examination to identify bacterial/fungal enteritis and neoplasia, and to guide antibiotic choice and prognosis

TREATMENT

THERAPEUTIC GOALS
- Determine origin of tissue prolapsed
- Determine cause of prolapse
- Correct immediate hypocalcemia
- Correct diet
- Correct husbandry deficiencies

ACUTE GENERAL TREATMENT
- Prolapses or potential prolapses should be considered and treated as an emergency.
- Instruct client to bring the animal into the clinic as soon as possible.
- Have the client "protect" the tissue by wrapping the cloacal area with a clean, damp facial cloth, diaper, or towel.
- Identify prolapsed tissue before treatment:
  - The urinary bladder generally is very thin walled and translucent; cystitis can cause the bladder wall to be thickened and opaque.
  - A phallus or hemipenile prolapse presents as a solid tissue mass protruding from the vent with no lumen present; a groove or sulcus may be visible on one side.
- Both the colon and the oviduct have lumens that can be identified. The surface of the colon is smooth, and the surface of the oviduct has longitudinal striations present.
- Protruding tissue should be cleaned, lubricated, and gently replaced into the cloaca.
- A moistened cotton-tipped applicator is often helpful for this procedure.
- If the tissue is edematous, glycerin, pure sugar, or concentrated sugar solutions may be helpful in decreasing the size of the enlarged organ.
- A transverse suture is placed on either side of the vent to prevent re-prolapse. Transverse sutures allow for defecation and urination.
- Nonsteroidal antiinflammatory drugs (NSAIDs) to reduce inflammation:
  - Meloxicam: 0.2-0.4 mg/kg, IM, IV q 24 h × 2-3 treatments
  - Ketoprofen: 2 mg/kg SC, IM q 24 h × 2-3 treatments
- Correct hypocalcemia:
  - Ca lactate/Ca glycerophosphate (Calphosan, Glenwood): give 10 mg/kg SC, ICe q 24 h as needed
  - Ca gluconate: give 100 mg/kg IM, ICe q 8 h as needed

CHRONIC TREATMENT
- Leave sutures in for 3-4 weeks after reduction of prolapse. If fecal and urate material can freely pass with the sutures in place, they can be left in longer.
- Discuss and correct any husbandry or dietary problems identified historically.
- Antibiotics based on culture and sensitivity from diagnostic samples taken. Treatment with antibiotics should be provided for 30 days minimum.
- Surgical correction, débridement, amputation of necrotic or friable tissue may be needed:
  - Enlargement of cloacal opening may be required to reduce edematous tissue.
  - Colopexy (externally or via coeleotomy) may be required.
  - Ovariohysterectomy
  - Cystotomy to remove bladder stones
  - Mass removal or foreign body (e.g., sand)

POSSIBLE COMPLICATIONS
If the cause of the prolapse is not identified and corrected, a reoccurrence of the prolapse is likely.

PROGNOSIS AND OUTCOME
- Good to fair if the prolapse is acute, the cause identified, and the problems corrected
- Penile, bladder, and oviduct prolapses are more easily corrected.

- Guarded to poor if the prolapse is more chronic with necrotic, friable tissue present
- Colonic prolapse (especially if chronic) can lead to tissue compromise, subsequent bacterial buildup, possible leakage of colon contents, and septicemia.

PEARLS & CONSIDERATIONS

COMMENTS

- Cloacal prolapse is a common presentation.
- Cloacal prolapse is a clinical sign, not a disease.

PREVENTION

- Supplementation with appropriate calcium source providing a balanced multivitamin supplement
- Proper feeding practices (e.g., dusting, timing of feeding, appropriate prey items)
- Proper husbandry practices (cleaning, density, sex ratios, parasite control, appropriate substrate)

CLIENT EDUCATION

- Crickets, fruit flies, mealworms, and waxworms are deficient in calcium and vitamin D_3 and will induce NSHP if fed to young, growing reptiles without supplementation.
- A pure calcium source free of other metals is the best choice for a supplement. Calcium lactate, calcium citrate, and pharmaceutical grade calcium carbonate are excellent sources of pure calcium.
- Observe captives for cagemate aggression, and remove animals if this occurs (see Aggression).
- Monitor parasite loads through regular fecal examinations.
- Treat a prolapse as an emergency, and contact the veterinarian immediately; do not attempt to reduce by yourself.

SUGGESTED READING

Bennett RA, Mader DR: Cloacal prolapse. In Mader DR, editor: Reptile medicine and surgery, St Louis, 2001, Saunders/Elsevier, pp 751–755.

CROSS-REFERENCES TO OTHER SECTIONS

Aggression
Dystocia (Section II)
Nutritional Secondary Hyperparathyroidism (NSHP)
Paraphimosis

AUTHOR: **BRAD A. LOCK**

EDITOR: **SCOTT J. STAHL**

REPTILES

Coccidiosis

BASIC INFORMATION

DEFINITION

Coccidia are microscopic, spore-forming, single-celled parasites belonging to the Apicomplexan suborder Eimerorina.

SYNONYMS

Acroeimeria, Besnoitia, Caryospora, Choleoeimeria, Eimeria, Goussia, intranuclear coccidiosis, *Isospora, Klossiella, Pythonella, Sarcocystis, Schellackia*

EPIDEMIOLOGY

SPECIES, AGE, SEX

- Coccidiosis is seen in all species of reptiles that have been significantly investigated.
- With intestinal *Coccidia* spp., young animals tend to have the heaviest infestations and show the most significant clinical signs, although older immunologically naïve animals are also at risk.
- No age predilection is apparent for disease seen with extraintestinal coccidia.
- No sex predilection has been noted for any reptile coccidiosis.

RISK FACTORS

- Young animals, animals kept in high population density, and animals kept under conditions of poor hygiene are at greatest risk for clinical coccidiosis.
- For coccidia with indirect life cycles, mixed species collections are at greater risk.

CONTAGION AND ZOONOSIS

- Coccidial oocysts generally are very stable in the environment.
- Fecal-oral transmission is the most common route of infection for coccidia with direct life cycles.
- For coccidia with indirect life cycles, definitive hosts are typically infected by ingesting intermediate hosts, and intermediate hosts are typically infected by fecal-oral transmission from definitive host feces.
- In some *Sarcocystis* spp., the same lizard species may alternate as definitive and intermediate hosts; this is known as a *dihomoxenous life cycle.*
- Zoonotic infection with coccidia of reptiles has not been documented.

GEOGRAPHY AND SEASONALITY The impact of geographic and seasonal factors on coccidiosis in reptiles is not well understood.

ASSOCIATED CONDITIONS AND DISORDERS

- Signs associated with intestinal coccidiosis may include poor growth, weight loss, melena, and diarrhea.
- Signs associated with extraintestinal coccidiosis vary according to the infected tissue, and may include sudden death, rhinitis, anorexia, depression, and reluctance to move.

CLINICAL PRESENTATION

HISTORY, CHIEF COMPLAINT

- History associated with coccidiosis varies according to species of coccidia and host.
- Often, no clinical concerns are present, and coccidia are detected on a routine fecal examination.
- Clinical concerns presented by owners may include poor growth, weight loss, diarrhea, sudden death, rhinitis, anorexia, depression, and reluctance to move.

PHYSICAL EXAM FINDINGS

- Physical examination findings in cases of clinical coccidial infestation vary according to species of coccidia and host.
- Often, no abnormalities are present. Abnormalities may include poor growth, weight loss, and depression.

ETIOLOGY AND PATHOPHYSIOLOGY

- Three families of eimeriorinid coccidia are found in reptiles: Cryptosporidae, which is discussed in a separate section; Eimeriidae, of which the genera *Caryospora, Eimeria,* and *Isospora* have been described in reptiles; and Sarcocystidae, of which the genera *Besnoitia* and *Sarcocystis* have been described in reptiles.
- Most organisms are intracytoplasmic in host cells.
- Tissue cysts consistent with *Besnoitia* have been seen in the kidneys of basilisks (*Basilicus basilicus*); mesentery, intestine, liver, and spleen of ameiva (*Ameiva ameiva*); and heart of wall lizards (*Lacerta dugesii*).
- Known reptile *Caryospora* with indirect life cycles use snakes (viperids

and North American ratsnakes) as definitive hosts, and form tissue cysts in mammals.

- *Caryospora chelonae*, which has a direct life cycle, is a significant pathogen in green turtles (*Chelonia mydas*), causing primarily intestinal lesions, although lesions may also be present in kidney, thyroid, and brain.
- *Choleoeimeria hirbayah* is a significant pathogen of veiled chameleons (*Chamaeleo calyptratus*).
- *Eimeria* spp. are the most commonly described coccidian parasites of reptiles.
  - The number of sporocysts/sporocytes has been used traditionally to classify coccidia as *Eimeria*, but the advent of sequence data has shown that this is not a reliably phylogenetically informative trait.
  - *Eimeria* have direct life cycles and usually are found in the intestinal epithelium.
- Intranuclear coccidiosis: Intranuclear coccidiosis is a significant disease of tortoises, causing high mortality:
  - Organisms are found in cell nuclei of numerous organs, including GI tract, liver, kidney, and spleen.
  - In Sulawesi tortoises, this organism has been associated with erosive rhinitis. The life cycle of this organism is not known.
  - Intranuclear coccidia have been seen in several lizard species, and these lizard coccidia have been called *Isospora* spp. based on sporulation, although no sequence data exist for these organisms.
- *Isospora jaracimrmani* can be a significant pathogen in veiled chameleons (*Chamaeleo calyptratus*), and *I. amphiboluri* can be a significant pathogen in bearded dragons (*Pogona vitticeps*).
- *Klossiella boae* has been reported from the kidneys of a Boa constrictor.
- *Sarcocystis* spp.: *Sarcocystis* spp. have indirect life cycles, forming tissue cysts in intermediate hosts, which then are ingested by carnivorous definitive hosts, where sporogony occurs:
  - Numerous species have been identified in reptiles.
  - Squamates are common definitive hosts, especially snakes.
  - Significant enteric disease has been associated with *Sarcocystis* in a bull snake (*Pituophis melanoleucus sayi*) definitive host.
  - *Sarcocystis* spp. can cause significant disease in mammalian and avian intermediate hosts; this may also prove to be the case in reptile intermediate hosts.
- *Schellackia* spp.: *Schellackia* spp. undergo schizogeny and sporogony in the gut of lizards.
  - Rather than being shed into the lumen of the gut, sporozoites enter the bloodstream and invade erythrocytes or lymphocytes.

DIAGNOSIS

DIFFERENTIAL DIAGNOSIS

- Differential diagnoses for weight loss and diarrhea include poor husbandry and numerous causes of enteritis and metabolic disease.
- Differential diagnoses for depression and systemic disease include malnutrition; bacterial, fungal, viral, and other parasitic diseases; numerous metabolic diseases; and neoplasia.

INITIAL DATABASE

A thorough history, physical examination findings, complete blood count, plasma chemistry, radiographs, and fecal examination form the basic database.

ADVANCED OR CONFIRMATORY TESTING

- Because the clinical significance and approach vary greatly depending on coccidian species, identification of coccidia is essential.
- For enteric forms, fecal flotation may identify the presence of oocysts. Nonenteric forms require samples of infected tissue. *Schellackia* spp. may be seen on blood smears.
- Nested polymerase chain reaction (PCR) with product sequence analysis is available for all coccidia from the University of Florida. Samples containing the organism are the samples of choice.
  - For postmortem samples, collecting two sets of tissues—submitting one in formalin for histopathologic examination to identify infested tissues, and freezing back a second set with no formalin for PCR identification—is advised.
- Images of the different coccidia usually are not reliable for differentiation.
- PCR identification is needed, as stated above.

TREATMENT

THERAPEUTIC GOALS

- The goal of treatment varies according to species of coccidia and host.
- For species that are significantly pathogenic, eradication of coccidia is the goal when feasible.
- When not verifiable ante mortem, as in species found in viscera, the goal may be alleviation of disease.
- For species that are not significantly pathogenic, treatment may not be indicated, especially in nonbreeding situations or where parasites have indirect life cycles.

ACUTE GENERAL TREATMENT

- Treatment varies according to species of coccidia and host.
- For coccidia with direct life cycles, very fastidious hygiene practices are necessary to prevent reinfestation. This is frequently underemphasized, and without this, pharmacologic treatment will fail.
- For debilitated animals, supportive care such as fluid therapy and treatment of secondary infection may be indicated.
- For coccidia with indirect life cycles, access to intermediate hosts needs to be removed.
- Anticoccidials can be used. However, data are lacking on safety, pharmacokinetics, and efficacy of anticoccidials in reptiles; all doses to date are empirical. Some empirical drugs and doses that may be used include the following:
  - Ponazuril (Marquis) 5-20 mg/kg PO q 24 h × 28 d
    - The above dose is based on studies from mammals.
    - An empirical dose of 30 mg/kg (2 doses 48 hours apart) has been used to treat bearded dragons with coccidiosis, and oocysts were not seen following treatment.
  - Toltrazuril (Baycox) 5-20 mg/kg PO q 24 h × 28 d
    - Comment from the editor: Alternatively, 5-20 mg/kg PO q 24 h × 3-5 d has also produced positive results.
  - Nitazoxanide (Navigator) 25 mg/kg PO q 24 h × 5 d, then 50 mg/kg PO q 24 h × 23 d
  - Amprolium hydrochloride 10 mg/kg PO q 24 h × 7-12 d
    - May be less effective, potential thiamine deficiencies
  - Sulfadimethoxine 90 mg/kg PO, then 45 mg/kg PO × 7-10 d
    - May be less effective, potential folic acid deficiencies
  - Trimethoprim/sulfamethoxazole 30 mg/kg PO q 24 h × 2 d, then q 48 h × 26 d
    - May be less effective, potential folic acid deficiencies

RECOMMENDED MONITORING

Enteric coccidia with direct life cycles should have follow-up testing every 6 months until they have gone for 2 years with negative fecal flotation examinations.

PROGNOSIS AND OUTCOME

Prognosis and outcome vary according to species of coccidia and host.

PEARLS & CONSIDERATIONS

COMMENTS

- It is essential to identify coccidia correctly when they are found, because clinical significance and life cycle differ significantly by species.
- It is essential to address husbandry issues. Poor husbandry will result in greater clinical significance of coccidial infection.

PREVENTION

Maintenance of a closed group, testing of populations, strict quarantine, elimination of access to intermediate hosts, and stringent biosecurity practices are the most effective means of prevention.

SUGGESTED READINGS

Godfrey SS, et al: Transmission mode and distribution of parasites among groups of the social lizard *Egernia stokesii*, Parasitol Res 99:223–230, 2006.

Gordon AN, et al: Epizootic mortality of free-living green turtles, *Chelonia mydas*, due to coccidiosis, J Wildl Dis 29:490–494, 1993.

Innis CJ, et al: Antemortem diagnosis and characterization of nasal intranuclear coccidiosis in tortoises, J Vet Diagn Invest 19:660–667, 2007.

Matuschka FR: Reptiles as intermediate and/or final hosts of *Sarcosporidia*, Parasitol Res 73:22–32, 1987.

AUTHOR: **JAMES F.X. WELLEHAN, JR.**

EDITOR: **SCOTT J. STAHL**

REPTILES

Cryptosporidiosis

BASIC INFORMATION

DEFINITION

Cryptosporidiosis or infection by the monogenous (entire life cycle in one host) protozoan Cryptosporidium spp..

SYNONYMS

Cryptosporidium spp., *C. saurophilum*, *C. serpentis*

EPIDEMIOLOGY

SPECIES, AGE, SEX

- Cryptosporidiosis has been documented in squamates and tortoises.
- No age predilection is apparent for disease seen with cryptosporidiosis.
- No sex predilection is known for any reptile cryptosporidiosis.

RISK FACTORS Animals kept under poor husbandry conditions are at greater risk for clinical cryptosporidiosis.

CONTAGION AND ZOONOSIS

- Cryptosporidial sporozoites are very stable in the environment.
- They survive well in bleach and in many other disinfectants.
- Fecal-oral transmission is the route of infection. Zoonotic infection with *Cryptosporidium* of reptiles has not been documented.
- *Cryptosporidium serpentis* has been shown not to infect the only mammal that has been experimentally investigated—the mouse (*Mus musculus*).
- Black rat snakes (*Elaphe obsoleta*) have been found not to be susceptible to several mammal *Cryptosporidium* spp., including *C. parvum*, making carriage of zoonotic species unlikely.

GEOGRAPHY AND SEASONALITY The impact of geographic and seasonal factors on cryptosporidiosis in reptiles is not well understood.

ASSOCIATED CONDITIONS AND DISORDERS Concurrent adenoviral infections appear to work synergistically with *Cryptosporidium* to cause disease.

CLINICAL PRESENTATION

DISEASE FORMS/SUBTYPES Biliary cryptosporidiosis has also been found in snakes with gastric cryptosporidiosis.

HISTORY, CHIEF COMPLAINT

- In some cases, no clinical concerns may be present.
- Clinical concerns presented by owners may include poor growth, weight loss, midbody swelling, regurgitation, diarrhea, sudden death, anorexia, depression, and aural/pharyngeal swellings.

PHYSICAL EXAM FINDINGS

- Vary according to species of *Cryptosporidium* and host
- Often, no abnormalities are present.
- Gastric cryptosporidiosis: poor growth, weight loss, regurgitation, and gastric hypertrophy leading to midbody swelling
- Intestinal cryptosporidiosis: poor growth, weight loss, and diarrhea
- Aural cryptosporidiosis: aural/pharyngeal polyps, which have been documented only in green iguanas

ETIOLOGY AND PATHOPHYSIOLOGY

- Cryptosporidian parasites are epicytoplasmic in host cells rather than intracytoplasmic, unlike most other coccidia, with the exception of *Acroeimeria* spp. All *Cryptosporidium* spp. have direct life cycles.
- *Cryptosporidium serpentis*: typically associated with gastric cryptosporidiosis in snakes and lizards; this was the first species identified in reptiles
- *Cryptosporidium saurophilum*: typically associated with intestinal cryptosporidiosis in snakes and lizards; it is most commonly reported with clinical disease in leopard geckos (*Eublepharis macularius*). It is sometimes incorrectly called *C. saurophilum.*
- Cryptosporidium ducismarci sp. has been associated with intestinal cryptosporidiosis in tortoises.
- An unnamed Cryptosporidium sp. has been associated with gastric cryptosporidiosis in tortoises.
- Unnamed *Cryptosporidium* spp.: A *Cryptosporidium* species has been associated with aural/pharyngeal polyps in green iguanas (*Iguana iguana*).
  - Many other unnamed *Cryptosporidium* spp. have been described in the literature in different reptilian species.

DIAGNOSIS

DIFFERENTIAL DIAGNOSIS

- Differential diagnoses for weight loss and diarrhea include poor husbandry and numerous causes of enteritis and metabolic disease.
- Differential diagnoses for midbody swelling include gastrointestinal obstruction, abscesses, cardiac disease, reproductive disease, and neoplasia.

INITIAL DATABASE

- A thorough history, physical examination findings, complete blood count, plasma chemistry, radiographs, and fecal examination form the basic database.
- For enteric forms, fecal examination may identify the presence of oocysts.
- Nonenteric forms require samples of infected tissue.
- Sporozoites stain acid-fast if they have not been fixed in formalin.

ADVANCED OR CONFIRMATORY TESTING

- *Cryptosporidium* in snakes was detected with greater sensitivity from gastric washes as compared with cloacal swabs. Sensitivity was best when sampled 3 days after feeding.
- Nested polymerase chain reaction (PCR) with product sequence analysis is available from the University of Florida for all *Cryptosporidium* spp. Samples containing the organism are the samples of choice. For postmortem samples, collecting two sets of tissues—submitting one in formalin for histopathologic examination to identify infested tissues, and freezing back a second set with no formalin for PCR identification—is advised.

TREATMENT

THERAPEUTIC GOALS

- The goal of treatment varies according to species of *Cryptosporidium* and specifics of the collection.
- Reliable eradication of the organism has yet to be demonstrated.
- When not outweighed by concerns for the collection, the goal may be alleviation of disease in an individual animal.
- Where animals are very debilitated or where concerns for the collection are significant, euthanasia may be indicated.

ACUTE GENERAL TREATMENT

- Very fastidious hygiene practices are necessary to prevent spread throughout a collection.
- Oocysts are resistant to most disinfectants. Only ammonia (5%) and formal saline solution are effective against oocysts.
- For debilitated animals, supportive care such as fluid therapy and treatment of secondary infection may be indicated.
- Animals without clinical signs often remain healthy with excellent husbandry.
- Some data on the use of hyperimmune anti–*C. parvum* bovine colostrum are available for treatment of cryptosporidiosis in reptiles.
- Anticoccidials can be used. However, data on safety, pharmacokinetics, and efficacy of anticoccidials in reptiles are lacking, and all doses to date are empirical.
- *Cryptosporidium* spp. are not susceptible to many of the older anticoccidials. Some empirical drugs and doses that may be used include the following:
  - Nitazoxanide (Navigator) 25 mg/kg PO q 24 h × 5 d, then 50 mg/kg PO q 24 h × additional 23 d
    - This drug has perhaps the most promise of any currently available anticryptosporidials based on mammalian data. Some data show that azithromycin in combination with nitazoxanide may be useful in mammals.

RECOMMENDED MONITORING

Positive animals should have follow-up testing every 6 months and should be kept separate from naïve animals.

PROGNOSIS AND OUTCOME

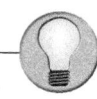

- Prognosis and outcome vary according to species of *Cryptosporidium* and host.
- Animals infected with *C. varanii*, *C. dusismarci*, or *C. serpentis* showing significant clinical signs carry a poor prognosis.

PEARLS & CONSIDERATIONS

COMMENTS

- It is important to identify *Cryptosporidium* spp. correctly when they are found, because clinical significance and host range differ significantly by species.
- It is essential to address husbandry issues. Poor husbandry will result in greater clinical significance of *Cryptosporidium* infection.

PREVENTION

Maintenance of a closed group, testing of populations, strict quarantine, and stringent biosecurity practices are the most effective means of prevention.

SUGGESTED READINGS

Fitzgerald SD, et al: Aural polyp associated with cryptosporidiosis in an iguana (*Iguana iguana*), J Vet Diagn Invest 10:179–180, 1998.

Giacometti A, et al: Activity of nitazoxanide alone and in combination with azithromycin and rifabutin against *Cryptosporidium parvum* in cell culture, J Antimicrob Chemother 45:453–456, 2000.

Graczyk TK, et al: Assessment of the conventional detection of fecal *Cryptosporidium serpentis* oocysts in subclinically infected captive snakes, Vet Res 27:185–192, 1996.

Graczyk TK, et al: Diagnosis of subclinical cryptosporidiosis in captive snakes based on stomach lavage and cloacal sampling, Vet Parasitol 67:143–151, 1996.

Graczyk TK, et al: Hyperimmune bovine colostrum treatment of moribund Leopard geckos (*Eublepharis macularius*) infected with *Cryptosporidium* sp, Vet Res 30:377–382, 1999.

Rossignol JF, et al: Treatment of diarrhea caused by *Cryptosporidium parvum*: a prospective randomized, double-blind, placebo-controlled study of nitazoxanide, J Infect Dis 184:103–106, 2001.

CROSS-REFERENCES TO OTHER SECTIONS

Adenovirus
Coccidiosis
Diarrhea
Mycobacteria
Nematodiasis
Regurgitation
Salmonella

AUTHOR: **JAMES F.X. WELLEHAN, JR.**

EDITOR: **SCOTT J. STAHL**

REPTILES

Dermatomycosis

BASIC INFORMATION

DEFINITION

Fungal infection of the skin and/or adnexae

SYNONYMS

- Fungal skin infection
- Infection with nonpigmented fungi is called *hyalohyphomycosis.*
- Infection with a pigmented fungus is called *phaeohyphomycosis.*
- Infection with a fungus may be called *fusariomycosis, paecilomycosis,* etc., after the causative agent.
- Fungal or any infection of the carapace or plastron in chelonians is sometimes called *shell rot.*
- Yellow fungus disease, or CANV infection in bearded dragon, is addressed separately (see CANV/Fungal Disease).

EPIDEMIOLOGY

SPECIES, AGE, SEX

- All reptiles are considered susceptible.
- Juvenile and senescent individuals may be more at risk.
- No sex predilection is known.
- Some specific fungal infections appear to be restricted to a particular reptile taxon:
  - Necrotizing scute disease in Texas tortoises
  - *Mucor ramosissimus* infection in Marlborough green geckos

RISK FACTORS

- Non-CANV infections in reptiles are typically caused by opportunistic, often ubiquitous fungal agents in immune suppressed individuals.
- Substandard to deficient husbandry practices
- Overcrowding especially in young chelonians
- High humidity, combined with excess organic matter/debris in the enclosure from lack of cleaning, favors conidiation/sporulation.
- Abrupt changes in temperature, especially sudden drops in temperature, may lead to subsequent fungal disease, be it cutaneous or systemic or both.
  - Especially in aquatic turtles; fungal infection is a major concern in recovering cold-stunned sea turtles

CONTAGION AND ZOONOSIS

- Dermatomycosis in reptiles is typically thought to be noncontagious.
- None are known to carry zoonotic potential (excluding CANV).

GEOGRAPHY AND SEASONALITY

- Outbreaks in the wild may have been associated with unusual wet and cold conditions.
- Fungal dermatitis was described in wild wall lizards in Spain during winter.

ASSOCIATED CONDITIONS AND DISORDERS

- Dermatomycosis may be secondary and associated with bacterial or viral disease.
- Traumatic or thermal skin injuries, or any breach of cutaneous integrity, will facilitate fungal infection.

DISEASE FORMS/SUBTYPES

- Necrotizing scute disease in free-living and captive Texas tortoises is a chronic, somewhat insidious shell infection with *Fusarium incarnatum* (formerly *F. semitectum*) resulting in extensive discoloration and blemishes of the carapace. The disease is restricted to the shell.
- Necrotizing mycotic dermatitis is a clinical entity described in snakes.
- Epidermal necrosis affecting primarily (but not only) ventral and ventrolateral scutes may be caused by a variety of fungal isolates.

HISTORY, CHIEF COMPLAINT

- Focal or extensive skin lesions of variable duration
- History of poor response or worsening of skin lesions on antibiotics
- Stressful events and inadequacies or deficiencies in the captive husbandry

PHYSICAL EXAM FINDINGS

- Patients may be alert or depressed.
- They may be in good body condition or may be debilitated.
- They may have concurrent systemic fungal infection that may manifest with digestive, respiratory, or other clinical signs.
- Lesions may be clinically indistinguishable from those of bacterial dermatitis. (see Bacterial Dermatitis)
- Fungal skin lesions are variable. They may be pustular but more commonly appear as short-lived vesicular, bullous lesions that break, ulcerate, and expose underlying dermis. Crusting may occur.
- Fungi invading epidermis may elicit necrosis and hyperkeratosis, especially in the later stages.
- In young crocodilians, fungal lesions may appear as unpigmented thickened, coalescing leathery lesions, which may be confused with scarring. Sometimes, white or grayish felty material may be seen overlying or at the edge of cutaneous lesions.
- In chelonians, especially box turtles, fungal skin infection often affects the toes and feet, causing swelling and necrosis. Shell lesions may consist of blemishes, ulcers, hyperkeratosis, and/or pitting.

ETIOLOGY AND PATHOPHYSIOLOGY

- *Paecilomyces lilacinus* may cause dermatomycosis and systemic mycosis, especially in aquatic reptiles.
- *Fusarium* and *Trichosporon* species have been reliably identified.
- *Mucor* species may also be involved, but these zycomycetous fungi readily invade dead tissues, so they may merely be secondary invaders.
- *Aspergillus* species may cause fungal skin disease, but causality could be difficult to establish because these fungi can easily be cultured from the skin of healthy reptiles.
- Among pigmented fungi, *Exophiala* and *Cladosporium* spp. seem to be most commonly identified.
- Necrotizing scute disease in Texas tortoises is caused by *Fusarium incarnatum* (formerly *F. semitectum*).

DIAGNOSIS

DIFFERENTIAL DIAGNOSIS

- Dermatomycotic lesions may be confused with bacterial lesions or with viral, even neoplastic, lesions.
- Necrotizing mycotic dermatitis in snakes can easily be confused with thermal injuries.

INITIAL DATABASE

- A thorough review of husbandry
- Complete blood count and chemistry profile
- Imaging modalities and endoscopy/laparoscopy to determine whether systemic fungal disease or other concurrent conditions are present.

ADVANCED OR CONFIRMATORY TESTING

- Biopsy of lesions is the preferred diagnostic tool.
  - Special stains (e.g., periodic acid–Schiff [PAS]) may be required.
  - Additional biopsies can be frozen for culture, pending histopathology.
- Fungal isolates from clinical samples should be keyed to species. Have the laboratory preserve the fungal culture.
- Isolates for which causality is established should be forwarded to a national fungus depository, so they are preserved and available for study.

TREATMENT

THERAPEUTIC GOALS

- Ensure proper husbandry
- Provide fluids (10-30 mL/kg q 24 h) and nutritional support, as needed
- Provide thermal support and maintain the reptile within the upper half of the preferred optimum temperature zone (POTZ)
- Achieve adequate levels of an appropriate antifungal in skin tissues

ACUTE GENERAL TREATMENT

- Administer supportive care.
- Administer systemic antifungal. Selection of an antifungal drug should be based ideally on susceptibility patterns of the isolated fungus. In vitro sensitivity testing is routine for yeasts in human mycology laboratories but is not readily available for filamentous fungi (moulds). *Paecilomyces lilacinus* and many *Fusarium* and many *Aspergillus* spp. are resilient organisms with high minimum inhibitory cocentrations (MICs) for commonly used antifungals.
- Voriconazole, terbinafine, and itraconazole are all good choices. If disease is confined to the skin, use itraconazole or terbinafine (or both) pulse therapy because both drugs tend to accumulate and persist in the skin. Even plasma levels seem to persist after discontinuation of therapy.
  - Itraconazole: A pulse therapy consisting of 5 mg/kg SID 1 week per month (1 week on, 3 weeks off) may be used until resolution of lesions.

- Terbinafine: A starting dose of 10 mg/kg orally SID, administered as pulses as described for itraconazole
- Voriconazole: 5 to 10 mg/kg orally SID or BID

- Use topical antiseptic (antifungal and antibacterial) dressing.
  - Silver sulfadiazine cream works well for this purpose.
- Cover for secondary bacterial invaders with systemic antibiotics if needed.
- Ensure that lesions have totally resolved before discontinuing systemic antifungals (treat up to 1 week after resolution of lesions).

CHRONIC TREATMENT

See above.

POSSIBLE COMPLICATIONS

Organ toxicity, mainly liver, may result from the use of antifungals in reptiles.

RECOMMENDED MONITORING

Serum liver enzymes can be monitored throughout treatment and compared with pretreatment levels. Owners should watch for anorexia or any unusual behavior exhibited by the patient.

PROGNOSIS AND OUTCOME

Prognosis depends on the causes, duration, and severity of the disease; the presence of any underlying condition; and the ability to identify and correct deficiencies in husbandry.

PEARLS & CONSIDERATIONS

COMMENTS

- Only with histopathologic examination and with isolation, ideally in pure culture, of a fungus whose hyphae are morphologically consistent with those seen in tissue sections can causality be reasonably demonstrated.
- Diagnosis of dermatomycosis is often made late in the course of the disease, often after empirical antibiotic treatment has failed.

PREVENTION

Attention to proper husbandry should minimize or eliminate the risk for non-CANV dermatomycosis in captive reptiles.

CLIENT EDUCATION

Clients should be encouraged to research captive care of species in their charge.

SUGGESTED READINGS

Paré JA, et al: Cutaneous mycobiota of captive squamate reptiles with notes on the scarcity of *Chrysosporium anamorph* of *Nannizziopsis vriesii*, J Herpetol Med Surg 13:10–15, 2003.

Paré JA, et al: Microbiology: fungal and bacterial diseases of reptiles. In Mader DR, editor: Reptile medicine and surgery, St Louis, 2006, Elsevier, pp 217–238.

Paré JA, et al: Mycotic diseases of reptiles. In Jacobson ER, editor: Infectious diseases and pathology of reptiles: a color atlas and text, Boca Raton, FL, 2007, CRC Press, pp 527–570.

CROSS-REFERENCES TO OTHER SECTIONS

Bacterial Dermatitis
CANV/Fungal Disease

AUTHOR: **JEAN A. PARÉ**

EDITOR: **SCOTT J. STAHL**

REPTILES

Dermatophilosis (Rain Rot)

BASIC INFORMATION

DEFINITION

Infections in reptiles involving *Dermatophilosis* spp. These bacteria have a thick cell wall typical of bacteria of the phylum Acintobacterial.

SYNONYM

In mammals, *Dermatophilus congolensis* infection is called *rain rot.*

EPIDEMIOLOGY

SPECIES, AGE, SEX

- Dermatophilosis is a disease of concern in all reptiles.
- Disease appears to be common in bearded dragons (*Pogona vitticeps*).
- No age or sex predilections are known.

RISK FACTORS

- Immune suppressed animals appear to be at greatest risk for disease.
- Husbandry deficiencies are a common source.

CONTAGION AND ZOONOSIS

- *Dermatophilus* spp. have a thick cell wall typical of the phylum Actinobacteria. Organisms in this genus produce motile cocci called *zoospores.* Therefore, they are very stable in the environment, especially in aquatic or moist environments. Disinfectants that are labeled to have mycobactericidal activity should be selected.
- *Dermatophilus congolensis* has been reported to cause pitted keratolysis and pustular dermatitis in humans. Other *Dermatophilus* spp. have not yet been associated with human disease.

GEOGRAPHY AND SEASONALITY

- Dermatophilosis is more common in warmer climates.
- Seasonality has not been reported.

ASSOCIATED CONDITIONS AND DISORDERS

- Dermatophilosis in reptiles is associated with granulomatous disease.
- Granulomas typically start in the skin and invade deeper tissues.

CLINICAL PRESENTATION

DISEASE FORMS/SUBTYPES Dermatophilosis can vary depending on which tissues are affected.

HISTORY, CHIEF COMPLAINT Common complaints on presentation for dermatophilosis include nonspecific illness, skin disease, and abnormal masses.

PHYSICAL EXAM FINDINGS Physical examination findings often include skin lesions, subcutaneous firmness, or masses.

ETIOLOGY AND PATHOPHYSIOLOGY

- The genus *Dermatophilus* is in the phylum Actinobacteria. The diversity of the genus is poorly understood.
- Before molecular methods were available, *Dermatophilus congolensis* was the only species in the genus.
- Traditional biochemical methods are not very accurate for identification of bacteria in the phylum Actinobacteria, and earlier identifications are somewhat suspect.
- Identification of *D. congolensis* in reptiles using molecular methods has not yet been reported.
- *Dermatophilus chelonae* has been reported to cause disease in chelonians and snakes, and it is likely to be a pathogen in all reptiles.
- Recently, DNA sequencing of the 16S ribosomal RNA genes of *D. chelonae* and *D. congolensis* has suggested that *D. chelonae* may be more closely

related to *Dermacoccus nishinomiyaensis* than to *D. congolensis*; reclassification in the future is not unlikely.
- The name *Dermatophilus crocodyli* has been proposed for a species isolated from crocodiles.
- Dermatophilosis in reptiles is associated with granulomatous disease. Granulomas typically start in the skin and invade deeper tissues.

DIAGNOSIS

DIFFERENTIAL DIAGNOSIS

Other common causes for granulomatous disease in reptiles include *Chlamydophila* spp., *Mycobacterium* spp., and fungi.

INITIAL DATABASE

- A thorough husbandry history, physical examination findings, complete blood count, plasma chemistry, and radiographs form a basic database.
- A leukocytosis is often present with dermatophilosis.
- Biopsy specimens of skin lesions should be taken for histologic examination and potential culture.
- Organisms in this genus have a characteristic branching, filamentous structure and the ability to produce motile cocci called *zoospores*.
- The characteristic "train tracks" seen with *D. congolensis* in mammals are not as obvious in reptile infections.

ADVANCED OR CONFIRMATORY TESTING

- The clinician should communicate in advance with the microbiology laboratory when dermatophilosis is suspected, and the microbiology laboratory should be prepared to look for Actinomycete-like colonies, which may require additional techniques for speciation.
- *D. chelonae* grows faster at 27°C (80.6°F) than at 37°C (98.6°F). 16S polymerase chain reaction (PCR) with product sequence analysis is available for bacterial isolate speciation from Washington State University and the University of Florida.

TREATMENT

THERAPEUTIC GOAL

The goal of therapy is eradication of the organism.

CHRONIC TREATMENT

- Initial therapy should consist of surgical débridement to the greatest extent feasible. Débrided tissue should be examined histologically for margins.
- Significant differences in drug susceptibility have been noted between isolates, and any identified *Dermatophilus* infection should be speciated, and a minimum inhibitory concentration (MIC) profile done.
- Any husbandry deficiencies should be addressed and corrected.
- Successful treatment of dermatophilosis in deep tissues of reptiles has not been documented; one case of treatment of *D. chelonae* in a king cobra (*Ophiophagus hannah*) resulted in relapse a year later.
- It is likely that extensive protocols comparable with mycobacterial treatment protocols may be needed.
- Antibiotic therapy may have to involve multiple drugs given over a course of 6 months to 1 year.
- Single-drug therapy or shorter courses seem likely to result in treatment failure.

RECOMMENDED MONITORING

- Biopsy specimens of affected tissues and a CBC should be taken after 6 months to 1 year to determine whether therapy needs to be continued.
- CBCs should be checked every 3 months for several years to look for leukocytosis, which may be a sign of recurrence.

PROGNOSIS AND OUTCOME

- The prognosis for animals with dermatophilosis varies depending on affected tissues.
- Cutaneous infections are more easily treated than infections involving deeper tissues.

PEARLS & CONSIDERATIONS

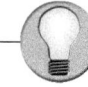

COMMENTS

- Dermatophilosis is probably underdiagnosed in reptiles.
- In a survey of skin diseases of farmed crocodiles in Australia, dermatophilosis was found to be the most common cause.

PREVENTION

Maintenance of a closed group, quarantine, and stringent biosecurity practices are the most effective means of prevention.

CLIENT EDUCATION

Zoonotic risks need to be discussed with the owner if the organism is identified as *D. congolensis*.

SUGGESTED READINGS

Bemis DA, et al: Dermatophilosis in captive tortoises, J Vet Diagn Invest 11:553–557, 1999.

Buenviaje GN, et al: Isolation of *Dermatophilus* sp. from skin lesions in farmed saltwater crocodiles (*Crocodylus porosus*), Aust Vet J 75:365–367, 1997.

Chineme CN, et al: Pathologic changes in lizards (*Agama agama*) experimentally infected with *Dermatophilus congolensis*, J Wildl Dis 16:407–412, 1980.

Masters AM, et al: *Dermatophilus chelonae* sp. nov., isolated from chelonids in Australia, Int J Syst Bacteriol 45:50–56, 1995.

Wellehan JFX, et al: *Dermatophilus chelonae* in a king cobra (*Ophiophagus hannah*), J Zoo Wildl Med 35:553–556, 2004.

CROSS-REFERENCES TO OTHER SECTIONS

Abscesses
Bacterial Dermatitis
CANY
Dermatomycosis
Dysecdysis

AUTHOR: **JAMES F.X. WELLEHAN, JR.**

EDITOR: **SCOTT J. STAHL**

REPTILES

Diarrhea

BASIC INFORMATION

DEFINITION

The production of excessive amounts of soft or liquid feces with increased water content

SYNONYM

Loose stool

EPIDEMIOLOGY

SPECIES, AGE, SEX All species and age categories are potentially susceptible.

GENETICS AND BREED PREDISPOSITION

- Some species of reptiles such as boids have well-formed stools, and some colubrids such as indigo snakes (*Drymarchon* spp.) have significantly more water in their feces.

- An elimination that would be normal for a colubrid would be considered diarrhea in a boid.
- Some reptiles produce excessively voluminous stool for their size.
  - Because of their diet and digestive nature, leopard tortoises (*Geochelone pardalis*) have feces resembling those of a horse.
  - For other tortoise species, a pastelike consistency is normal for the feces.

RISK FACTORS

- Excessive feeding
- Change in diet
- Increased stress (e.g., overcrowding)
- Improper sanitation
- Infection (viral/bacterial)
- Parasites
- Foreign body
- Drug reactions

CONTAGION AND ZOONOSIS Diarrhea itself is a symptom, not a disease, but several infectious agents (e.g., *Entamoeba*) can cause diarrhea.

GEOGRAPHY AND SEASONALITY Typically warm, humid conditions support a wide variety of pathogenic microorganisms that can cause diarrhea.

ASSOCIATED CONDITIONS AND DISORDERS

- Infectious causes of diarrhea are very common.
- Viruses such as parvovirus and adenovirus (see Adenovirus Infection) are known to cause significant disease in colubrids. Chlamydiophylosis is a notable problem that causes diarrhea in lizards.
- *Salmonella* (see Salmonella), *Shigella*, and *Proteus* species cause bacterial gastroenteritis in reptiles, and symptoms of diarrhea are associated.
- Parasites including helminths and protozoans (e.g., *Coccidia* species such as *Cryptosporidium* [see Cryptosporidiosis] and *Eimeria*, and Protozoa such as *Giardia* and *Entamoeba invadens* [see Entamoebiasis]) often cause diarrhea in reptiles. (see Coccidiosis)
- Many of these diseases are spread by fecal-oral and fomite routes.

CLINICAL PRESENTATION

DISEASE FORMS/SUBTYPES

- Reptile diarrhea can be classified as acute or chronic.
  - The acute form is much more common in occurrence than the chronic form.
  - Acute diarrhea is characterized by having a short duration and occurring unexpectedly.
    - In some cases, acute diarrhea may be self-limiting in nature.
  - Chronic diarrhea is more persistent in nature and is not self-limiting.
    - Chronic diarrhea sometimes recurs irregularly.

HISTORY, CHIEF COMPLAINT

- Clients commonly complain of inactivity and poorly formed stool.
- Changes in appetite are commonly noted.
- Observant owners may describe polydipsia.

PHYSICAL EXAM FINDINGS

- An animal with acute diarrhea may present with moderate dehydration and inactivity.
- Reptiles with chronic diarrhea commonly present with moderate to severe dehydration, depression, and cachexia due to insufficient nutrient absorption.
- A display of excessive fecal staining around the cloaca suggests a recent history of diarrhea.

ETIOLOGY AND PATHOPHYSIOLOGY

- Because of this extended transit time of ingesta and the thermoregulatory requirements of reptiles, providing the correct environmental temperature is vital to the health of the animal.
- Extreme temperature may lead to diarrhea because it directly impacts the rate of digestion.
- Reptiles absorb water in their large intestinal tract and cloaca.
- Suspect characteristics of a large bowel problem include hematochezia and increased mucus.
- Changes in diet due to availability or seasonality could potentially cause diarrhea. Animals normally housed outside with access to plant matter and insects that are moved inside to eat a manufactured diet during the winter months could develop diarrhea.

DIAGNOSIS

DIFFERENTIAL DIAGNOSIS

- The reptile stool characteristically consists of three components: feces, urine, and urates.
- Polyuria can sometimes be confused with diarrhea.
- It is important to recognize that an underlying problem must be identified and corrected to discontinue the occurrence of diarrhea.
- Any disease process that causes digestive problems could potentially cause diarrhea.
- In many instances, diarrhea is associated with improper husbandry and mismanagement.

INITIAL DATABASE

- A thorough history, including duration, mode of onset, clinical course, previous treatments, associated signs, appearance of stool, and correlation with any changes for specific agents such as cryptosporidiosis, salmonellosis, etc.
- Fecal analyses:
  - Direct and flotation
  - Acid-fast stains
  - Polymerase chain reaction (PCR) testing
- In cases where no material is immediately available, a cloacocolonic lavage should be performed.
- Survey radiographs, complete blood count, and biochemistry profile are useful.

ADVANCED OR CONFIRMATORY TESTING

- Contrast radiography, coelomic ultrasound, gastrointestinal endoscopy with biopsy for histopathology and microbiology
- For suspected masses, obstructions, and foreign bodies, it may be appropriate to consider advanced imaging.
- Exploratory surgery to evaluate the gastrointestinal tract with subsequent surgical biopsy via enterotomy, etc.

TREATMENT

THERAPEUTIC GOALS

- Stabilize the patient with medical support, and provide species-specific temperature requirements
- Correct any deficits caused by diarrhea, including fluid status, acid-base ratios, and electrolyte imbalances
- Identify the underlying cause of the diarrhea, and correct or treat the specific cause
- Improve husbandry practices, including hygiene, temperature, and diet

ACUTE GENERAL TREATMENT

- Fluid therapy starting with 10-30 mL/kg/24h (intravenous, intraosseous, or intracoelomic) and monitoring of electrolytes; administration of antibacterial or antiparasitic drugs if the presence of pathogenic organisms is detected
- Gastrointestinal motility agents (such as Metoclopramide 0.5-1.0 mg/kg SQ, PO q 24 h or Cisapride 0.5-2.0 mg/kg PO q 24 h) may be useful in some cases.
- Aluminum hydroxide, pectin, and bismuth subsalicylate products can be considered.

CHRONIC TREATMENT

- Correct management issues to species-specific parameters.
- Correct dietary sufficiency or insufficiency.
- Assist feeding with the use of a feeding tube in emaciated patients.

POSSIBLE COMPLICATIONS

- Sepsis

- Starvation
- Dehydration

RECOMMENDED MONITORING

- Monitor weight and food intake.
- Monitor cage temperature.
- Document electrolyte and acid-base levels.
- Log and characterize elimination events.

PROGNOSIS AND OUTCOME

- The prognosis for severe chronic diarrhea is guarded to poor.
- The prognosis for acute diarrhea is good to fair.

PEARLS & CONSIDERATIONS

COMMENTS

- It is often difficult to appreciate diarrhea in aquatic reptiles because of the nature of their environment. It may be necessary to temporarily remove aquatic reptiles from the water to accurately observe and assess a bowel movement.
- It is appropriate to ask the owner to bring a fecal sample in with a sick reptile. This is useful because owners may often confuse regurgitation/vomiting matter (see Regurgitation/Vomiting), or polyuria, with diarrhea.
- Be certain to highlight appropriate sample collection to guard against zoonoses such as salmonellosis.

PREVENTION

- Appropriate management (sanitation, temperature, diet, exercise), along with attempts to simulate natural fasting and hibernation periods, is important in prevention.
- It is important to quarantine, monitor, and perform fecal evaluations on all new animals before introducing them into a healthy population.

CLIENT EDUCATION

Review of ecology and the natural history of the reptile will help the client understand metabolic processes and species-specific requirements.

SUGGESTED READING

Funk RS: Diarrhea. In Mader DR, editor: Reptile medicine and surgery, ed 2, Philadelphia, 2006, WB Saunders, pp 772–773.

CROSS-REFERENCES TO OTHER SECTIONS

Adenovirus Infection
Coccidiosis
Cryptosporidiosis
Entamoebiasis
Regurgitation/Vomiting
Salmonella

AUTHORS: **JASON NORMAN AND STEPHEN J. DIVERS**

EDITOR: **SCOTT J. STAHL**

REPTILES

Dysecdysis

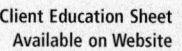

Client Education Sheet Available on Website

BASIC INFORMATION

DEFINITION

- Shedding disorders of reptiles
- The term *dysecdysis* is also used to describe shedding-related problems in other reptiles (besides snakes and geckos) even though they do not actually have a true ecdysis cycle.

SYNONYMS

Shedding disorder, retained shed

EPIDEMIOLOGY

SPECIES, AGE, SEX

- Snakes and certain species of geckos, leopard geckos (*Eublepharis macularius*), fat-tailed geckos (*Hemitheconyx caudicinctus*), etc., with a true ecdysis cycle are more prone to problems with shedding.
- Neonatal and juvenile reptiles:
  - Are growing faster and will shed more often
  - Are under more stress with the demands of growth and thus are more likely:
    - To be malnourished, resulting in problems with the shed cycle
- Female snakes during gestation have hormonally controlled shedding cycles, which can be problematic if underlying health concerns are present.
- Species of reptiles that live in high-humidity environments or microhabitats (burrows in the ground) are more prone to shedding disorders.
- Box turtles (*Terrapin* spp.), green iguanas (*Iguana igauna*), Asian water dragons (*Physignathus cocincinus*), tegus (*Tupinambis* spp.), and rainbow boas (*Epicrates cenchria*)
- Large skinks such as blue tongue skinks (*Tiliqua* spp.) have very small toes for their size; problems with shedding around these toes result in avascular necrosis and sloughing.
- Blue tongue skinks are prone to retaining skin along the oral cavity and the eyelids, resulting in stomatitis and conjunctivitis, respectively.

RISK FACTORS

- Husbandry-related problems:
  - Malnutrition
  - Hypovitaminosis A (see Hypovitaminosis A)
  - Environmental stress
  - Temperature
  - Humidity
  - Hydration
  - Photoperiod
- Intrinsic factors that may increase risk:
  - Age
  - Gender
  - Hormones/Season
  - Thyroid disease
- Infectious (both systemic and specifically associated with the skin):
  - Bacterial
  - Fungal
  - Viral
  - Parasitic
- Previous trauma or damage to skin:
  - Wounds, scars, burns, and surgical incisions will cause shedding problems in these specific sites.

GEOGRAPHY AND SEASONALITY

Reptiles that are housed indoors in the winter may be prone to shedding problems related to lower humidity and temperatures in their captive environments.

ASSOCIATED CONDITIONS AND DISORDERS

- Conjunctivitis
- Abscessation (see Abscesses)
- Stomatitis (see Stomatitis, Bacterial)
- Osteomyelitis secondary to avascular necrosis
- Respiratory disease

CLINICAL PRESENTATION

HISTORY, CHIEF COMPLAINT

- Information on husbandry and diet is the most important diagnostic tool in understanding shedding disorders.
- Patients typically present with a history of suboptimal husbandry and

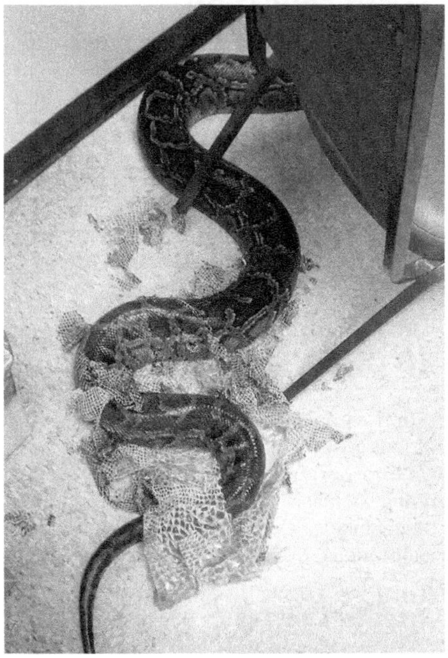

Dysecdysis An incomplete shed of the skin. The old skin should be completely removed to avoid any areas that retain the skin, causing a complication during the next shed. *(Photo courtesy Jörg Mayer, The University of Georgia, Athens.)*

environmental conditions. The owner may or may not be aware of problems with shedding skin.

- Snakes often present with:
  - Incomplete or retained sheds, especially around head and tail
  - Dullness or ulcerations of the skin
  - Change in the color of the skin to pink/red or yellow/brown
  - Respiratory signs: wheezing, open mouth breathing, increased mucus, and blocked nares
  - Abnormalities of the eye(s) such as retained spectacle(s)
- Lizards and chelonians often present with:
  - Incomplete or retained sheds
    - Often involving toes, tail, around oral cavity, eyes/eyelids, and ornamental appendages (e.g., dorsal spines in lizards) and shell scutes of chelonians

PHYSICAL EXAM FINDINGS

- Snakes:
  - The first change noted in the shed cycle is an opaque/blue cloudy change to the eyes.
    - Vision is reduced in snakes during this time, and they may be anxious and agitated.
    - It is best to not handle snakes during this phase because it is easy to damage the skin.
  - Physical examinations should be postponed if snakes are in the middle of the ecdysis cycle.
    - One or more retained spectacles may be present around the eye(s).
    - Retained spectacles often make the eye appear dry and dull, especially when compared with the normal eye, if the condition is unilateral. Magnification is useful.
    - A dimple or crease in a spectacle may be present and should not be mistaken for a retained spectacle(s) (esp. ball python, *Python regius*).
    - The periocular space should be checked for the snake mite and retained skin.
    - The nares may be blocked with dried skin and mucus.
    - Skin lesions often occur when handling a snake just before shedding.
    - Retained shedding skin may trap fluid and debris between old and new layers of skin.
    - Skin may change color to pink, red, yellow, or brown.
    - Retained shedding skin at the end of the tail may cause decreased blood flow, and evidence of necrosis may be seen.
- Lizards/Chelonians:
  - Geckos often will eat the skin as it is shedding off.
  - Physical examinations should be postponed if geckos are in the middle of the ecdysis cycle.
  - Lizards and chelonians are often presented with:
    - Conjunctivitis
    - Retained shedding skin around the oral cavity may trap saliva, mucus, and discharge along the gum line.
      - This may result in an inability to close the mouth properly.
    - Rings of skin retained on digits and the tip of the tail may create distal swelling, ulceration, and necrosis.
    - Retained scutes on the carapace or plastron may trap fluid and debris between old shedding scutes and new scutes.
      - Scutes may appear slightly raised and soft with trapped air bubbles underneath.

ETIOLOGY AND PATHOPHYSIOLOGY

- Dysecdysis is not a disease but is an indicator of an underlying problem in the reptile patient.
- Reptiles routinely lose their keratinized outer layer of skin.
- Chelonians and most lizards continually shed parts (asynchronous shedding) of their body.
- Especially common in species with high humidity requirements, such as tropical or semi-aquatic reptiles.
- Dysecdysis is usually the result of suboptimal environmental conditions.
- Owners handling their reptiles may damage the skin.
- Poor water quality leads to dysecdysis in aquatic and semi-aquatic reptiles.
- Lack of or inappropriate basking/dry-out sites for aquatic and semi-aquatic reptiles may lead to shedding disorders.
- Keeping reptiles at inappropriate temperatures may result in shedding problems.
- Ectoparasites interfere with the normal shedding process, causing retention of skin.
- Retained skin may interrupt and/or restrict blood flow to digits, distal portions of the tail, and ornamental appendages, resulting in swelling, avascular necrosis, osteomyelitis, and sloughing of extremities.
- Retained skin around the nares may occlude airflow through the nostrils, resulting in rhinitis and/or open-mouth breathing.
- Open-mouth breathing may dry the mucous membranes in the oral cavity, leading to stomatitis and possibly lower respiratory tract disease. (see Respiratory (Lower) Tract Disease/ Pneumonia)
- The heads of snakes tend to swell from increased blood flow during the normal ecdysis cycle. This congestion may result in increased noise associated with the respiratory tract; increased saliva may be noted in the oral cavity.
  - This can mimic a true respiratory infection but will resolve once the snake sheds.
- Retained skin around the eyes may lead to epiphora and conjunctivitis in lizards and chelonians.
- Retained skin on the ventrum may trap fluid and contaminants from the substrate surface between old and new layers of skin, resulting in dermatitis or vesicular disease.
- Hyperthyroidism has been associated with excessive shedding cycles.
- Malnutrition and starvation may result in dysecdysis.
- Hypovitaminosis A, which is seen frequently in lizards and chelonians, may lead to dysecdysis in these reptiles.
- When secondary bacterial invasion results in cases of dysecdysis, opportunistic Gram-negative bacteria are usually isolated.
  - Common organisms include *Pseudomonas* spp., *Aeromonas hydrophila*, *Klebsiella* spp., and *Salmonella* spp.
  - Anaerobic bacteria such as *Bacteroides*, *Fusobacterium*, and *Clostridium* are identified with these dysecdysis/dermatitis cases.
- Mycotic organisms, including aspergillosis, candidiasis, phycomycosis,

geotrichosis, fusariosis, and CANV (see CANV/Fungal Disease), have been associated with shedding problems and dermatitis in reptiles.

DIAGNOSIS

DIFFERENTIAL DIAGNOSIS

- Bacterial/fungal dermatitis (see Bacterial Dermatitis)
- Trauma (burns, chemical contact, injury to tail and toes)
- Nutrition-related (e.g., hypovitaminosis A)
- Thyroid disease

INITIAL DATABASE

- A thorough historical review and physical examination findings are usually diagnostic.
- Complete blood count and chemistry profile
- Culture and sensitivity and cytology of obvious infected areas
  - Both aerobic and anaerobic cultures should be submitted when possible.

ADVANCED OR CONFIRMATORY TESTING

- Biopsy and histopathologic examination are the most important diagnostic tools.
- Radiographs in cases involving extremities where avascular necrosis and subsequent osteomyelitis may have occurred
- Consider thyroid testing, although normal clinical biochemical baseline values for thyroid function may not be available.
- Use of ultrasound to evaluate the thyroid gland for changes in size and architecture followed by ultrasound-guided needle aspirate or surgical biopsy may be the more diagnostic approach.
- Scintigraphy will evaluate function of the thyroid.

TREATMENT

THERAPEUTIC GOALS

- Provide support for the presenting patient in the form of heat and hydration as needed
- Gently remove retained skin when possible
- Identify any associated pathogens and direct specific antimicrobial therapy as indicated
- Address and correct specific husbandry such as humidity and nutrition-related issues
- Educate the owner on how to prevent future shedding issues

ACUTE GENERAL TREATMENT

- Retained shedding skin or scutes should be gently removed. Soaking the patient in warm water often softens the retained skin and will facilitate removal.
- Applying topical antimicrobial cream such as silver sulfadiazine cream to damaged skin can help to repair and protect skin.

CHRONIC TREATMENT

- If dysecdysis has resulted in secondary bacterial or fungal dermatitis and/or necrosis topical and parenteral antimicrobials may be indicated. See bacterial dermatitis and dermatomycosis for treatment options.

Owners should be encouraged to provide microhabitats for captive reptiles that allow an area of high humidity within their captive environment to prevent shedding issues (e.g., humidity box).

RECOMMENDED MONITORING

Scars associated with previous injuries, burns, or surgical procedures will require long-term monitoring; many reptiles will need gentle assistance from the owner to shed around these areas.

PROGNOSIS AND OUTCOME

- The prognosis is excellent with gentle and appropriate removal of retained skin and protection of damaged skin until healing occurs.
- Cases involving extremities with associated compromise of blood flow and associated osteomyelitis/necrosis have a more guarded prognosis. However, with amputation and protection from sepsis with the use of systemic antimicrobials, the prognosis is more favorable.

PEARLS & CONSIDERATIONS

COMMENTS

- The skin is an excellent indicator of the general health of a reptile.
- Stressed and chronically ill reptiles will not shed as often as healthy reptiles.
- Identify the species of reptile presenting with dysecdysis to provide proper natural history information to the owner. This is important for understanding the normal shedding cycle and proper captive husbandry for the species.

PREVENTION

- Increase humidity early in the shedding cycle by misting, soaking, or providing a humidity box.
- Whenever possible, do not handle reptiles during the shedding cycle.
- Attempt to provide temperature, humidity, and a lightcycle that mimics the natural history of the captive reptile.
- In species with a true ecdysis cycle such as snakes and geckos, provide rough objects (rocks, branches, etc.) in the reptile enclosure to help initiate the shedding cycle.

CLIENT EDUCATION

- Make sure the client has a good understanding of normal and expected shedding cycles of the reptile patient and how to provide an appropriate environment to encourage proper shedding.
- Counsel clients on how to safely help reptiles with shedding, if dysecdysis occur.

SUGGESTED READINGS

Fitzgerald KT, et al: Dysecdysis. In Mader DR, editor: Reptile medicine and surgery, St Louis, 2006, Elsevier, pp 778–786.

Mader DR: Dysecdysis: abnormal shedding and retained eye caps. In Mader DR, editor: Reptile medicine and surgery, Philadelphia, 1996, WB Saunders.

CROSS-REFERENCES TO OTHER SECTIONS

Abscesses
Assisting Snedding, Sec.II
Bacterial Dermatitis
CANV/Fungal Disease
Hypovitaminosis A
Stomatitis, Bacterial
Respiratory (Lower) Tract Disease/Pneumonia

AUTHOR & EDITOR: **SCOTT J. STAHL**

REPTILES

Ectoparasites

BASIC INFORMATION

DEFINITION

Ectoparasitism refers to an infestation of the reptilian host by one of several groups of Acarids (ticks and mites) of the genera *Ophionyssus, Ixodes, Hyalomma, Haemaphysalis, Amblyomma, Aponomma, Agrasidae*, and *Ornithodoros*.

SYNONYMS

Mite infestation, tick infestation, acariasis, parasites

EPIDEMIOLOGY

SPECIES, AGE, SEX Any.

RISK FACTORS Debilitation and stress, poor husbandry, unsanitary conditions, wild-caught animals, recent imports, unquarantined animals, poor husbandry practices

CONTAGION AND ZOONOSIS

- Feed directly on the reptilian host and can lead directly to health problems in the snake via transmission of blood-borne pathogens
- Zoonotic potential through direct blood feeding on humans:
  - Life cycle cannot be completed on humans, but transmission may occur through bites of a variety of blood-borne pathogens, including but not limited to tularemia (*Francisella tularensis*), Lyme disease (*Borrelia burgdorferi*), *Leptospira pomona*, relapsing fever, bite-associated dermatitis, pruritic papular lesions.
- Possible transmission of vector for heartwater disease *(Ehrlichia ruminatium)* on imported tortoises carrying Amblyomma ticks.

ASSOCIATED CONDITIONS AND DISORDERS

- Anorexia
- Dysecdysis (see Dysecdysis)
- Hyperactivity
- Failure to thrive
- Bacterial septicemias

CLINICAL PRESENTATION

DISEASE FORMS/SUBTYPES Although the disease can manifest in a number of ways, the only form is the presence of ectoparasites—ticks and mites.

HISTORY, CHIEF COMPLAINT

- Finding the parasites on the animal
- Sometimes mites are not easily identified, and the complaint will center on behavior changes or an unthrifty appearance.
- Seeing black dots on the animal or in the water bowl, anorexia, and inability or difficulty in shedding
- Often a history of poor husbandry practices (unsanitary conditions) and recent additions to the collection with no quarantine
- History of behavior changes
  - Staying coiled in water bowls
  - Hyperactivity
  - Rubbing on cage furniture to rid themselves of parasites

PHYSICAL EXAM FINDINGS

- Unthrifty appearance
- Presence of ticks or mites attached to or crawling over the body of the animal
  - Often found in the gular fold, labial pits, conjunctival sac of the eye in snakes, and around the vent
- Often patients are dehydrated and death can result in young animals.
- Associated dermatitis may be extensive; pruritus, dysecdysis, retained eye caps

ETIOLOGY AND PATHOPHYSIOLOGY

- Snake mites (*Ophionyssus natricis*): complicated life cycle
  - Eggs incubate in environment for 28-98 hours
  - Larval stage: nonfeeding, free-living, six-legged (moult 18-47 hours)
  - Protonymph stage: parasitic, four-legged, aggressive feeders (3-14 days)
  - Deutonymph stage: nonfeeding, free-living, four-legged (13-26 hours)
  - Adult stage: parasitic, four-legged, aggressive feeders (10-32 days)
    - Adult females feed two to three times at 1-2 week intervals.
    - 20 eggs are laid after each feeding.
    - Females crawl upward to moist dark areas for oviposition.
  - Life-threatening anemia by direct consumption of host blood is possible when mites are seen in high numbers.
  - Young and small individuals are at greatest risk.
  - Host skin around feeding areas becomes hyperemic, edematous, and infiltrated with heterophils, lymphocytes, and plasma cells.
  - Behavioral changes due to irritation from mite feeding and presence of snakes coiled in water bowls; hyperactivity to rub mites off the body will often lead to anorexia and dysecdysis.
  - Transmission of several pathogens has been documented via hematophagous activity: *Aeromonus hydrophila, Hepatazoon*, and possibly the causative agent of inclusion body disease.
- Trombiculid mites (Chiggers): Trombiculidae
  - Larva: parasitic, six-legged, highly pruritic
  - Nymphs and adults: free living
  - Saliva is injected under the skin of the host and is digested.
  - Mite feeds off this dissolved tissue and lymph: not off blood
  - Clinical signs from irritation
- Ophioptid mites
  - These mites live under the scales and skin of the reptilian host.
  - Cause irritation and subsequent dermatitis—often severe—with raised lesions. Dermatitis resembles bacterial, fungal dermatitis and burn lesions.
- Ticks (various genera; see above)
  - Adults are usually seen on reptilian hosts and are parasitic.
  - Ticks are capable of surviving for months without feeding, so treatment is required.
  - Pathology is through direct blood loss from feeding on host, irritation to the host, and possible disease transmission.
  - Monitor ticks (*Aponomma exornatium* and *A. flavomaculatum*) reside in the nostrils of monitors; heavy infestation has been reported to cause dyspnea and suffocation.

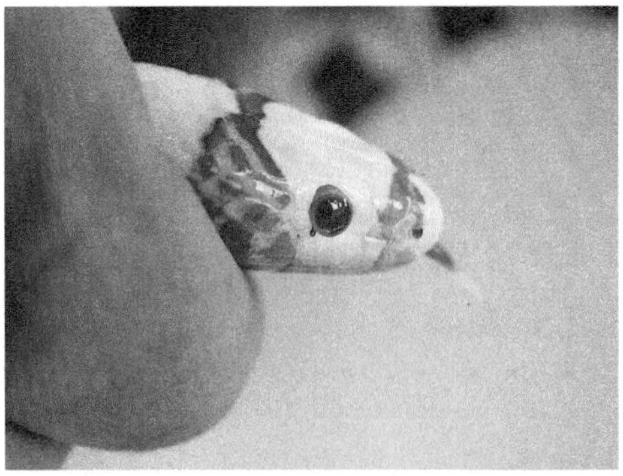

Ectoparasites Note the black adult stage mite just ventral and caudad to the snake eye. This is commonplace for snake mites. The periocular region must be examined closely as this is a common area to find these small mites. *(Photo courtesy Jörg Mayer, The University of Georgia, Athens.)*

DIAGNOSIS

DIFFERENTIAL DIAGNOSIS

- Bacterial, fungal, burn dermatitis (see Bacterial Dermatosis and Dermatomycosis)
- Respiratory disease (monitor ticks)
- Poor husbandry (dysecdysis, unthrifty appearance, extensive time in water bowl)
- Neurologic disease (hyperactivity)

INITIAL DATABASE

- A good physical examination
- Clinical signs of infestation as outlined above

ADVANCED OR CONFIRMATORY TESTING

Ophiotid mites may require a skin scrape or biopsy and microscopic evaluation to identify the mites under scales or skin.

TREATMENT

THERAPEUTIC GOALS

- Eliminate all stages of the life cycle of mites and the adult stages of ticks from the host body, the enclosure, and the surrounding environment
- Identify and treat any secondary bacterial infections diagnosed

ACUTE GENERAL TREATMENT

- Treatment of the animal (snakes and lizards):
  - Ivermectin is applied to the reptile patient (never in turtles or tortoises) as a topical spray; treat three times at 2-week intervals.
    - Spray preparation: 0.5 mL of ivermectin for cattle (10 mg/mL) added to 1 quart of water; applied directly to the animal and the environment using a spray bottle
  - Ivermectin is not water soluble, so the solution must be shaken well before each application; store in an opaque bottle to avoid light degradation.
  - Ivermectin may be used as an injection: 200-400 mcg/kg SC repeated in 10-14 days
- Treatment of the animal (turtles and tortoises):
  - Commercial permethrin spray (Provent-a-Mite) at 0.01% and 0.5%
  - Spray directly on tortoises (from 10 cm distance) and the substrate:
    - Small tortoises: 1-second burst sprayed into each leg opening
    - Large tortoises: two 1-second bursts into each leg opening
  - No signs of toxicity were reported in snakes, lizards, or tortoises at 2 and 10 times the recommended dosage.
- Treatment of enclosure:
  - This is critical. Without treatment of the enclosure, any therapy will fail.
  - Aquarium and smaller commercial fiberglass and plastic enclosures are emptied and thoroughly cleaned with hot (122°F [50°C]), soapy water, with particular attention paid to the upper rim of these cages and lids. Remove and discard all cage furnishings.
  - Large enclosures should be sprayed with the ivermectin solution or a dilute (10%) bleach solution, thoroughly cleaned with soap and water, and allowed to dry completely before the animal is placed back in the enclosure.
  - Use only newspaper as a substrate and minimize cage furnishings (tree branches, rocks, etc.) during treatment. Use Provent-a-Mite spray on newspaper once a month during this time. For the initial, acute treatment, once is enough. Spray from distance of 12-15 inches (30-40 cm) a 1-second burst for each foot of enclosure floor surface. Wait several hours for complete drying and for all vapors to dissipate.
  - For chelonian enclosures: a 0.01% permethrin product (cyfluthrin) is effective for eradication of ticks:
    - Toxic to snakes and lizards in very low concentrations: DO NOT USE.

CHRONIC TREATMENT

- Improved husbandry with particular attention to sanitation
- Quarantine protocols implementation (see prevention section below)
- Careful monitoring of animals for signs of reinfestation
- Once a month, use Provent-a-Mite on enclosure substrate 2-3 months post treatment

POSSIBLE COMPLICATIONS

- Toxicities associated with a number of mite therapies
- Parasiticide toxicities are primarily CNS disorders that vary from reversible to irreversible to even fatal.
- Signs are most common when oil-based products are used, and when animals in poorly ventilated enclosures are treated.

PROGNOSIS AND OUTCOME

- Guarded to good. Depends on owner compliance and health status of the animal before the start of treatment
- Severely affected, debilitated animals must receive supportive treatment before acaricides are used.

PEARLS & CONSIDERATIONS

COMMENTS

In large reptile collections, mites can be extremely difficult and frustrating to manage and eradicate.

PREVENTION

- High-quality husbandry
- Quarantine to detect carriers before they are introduced to a trouble-free collection. This is the most important part of a prevention protocol.

CLIENT EDUCATION

- Importance of quarantine protocols
- Presence of mites usually a failure in proper husbandry: especially sanitation practices
- Treatment of animals and the enclosure is critical for successful treatment.
- More is not better: Safe dosages of many acaricides are unknown, and most toxicities are caused by overdosage.

SUGGESTED READING

Fitzgerald KT, et al: Acariasis. In Mader DR, editor: Reptile medicine and surgery, St Louis, 2006, Saunders/Elsevier, pp 721–738.

CROSS-REFERENCES TO OTHER SECTIONS

Bacterial Dermatitis
Dermatomycosis
Dysecdysis

AUTHOR: **BRAD A. LOCK**

EDITOR: **SCOTT J. STAHL**

REPTILES

Entamoebiasis

BASIC INFORMATION

DEFINITION

Entamoeba invadens is a commensal protozoan living in the gastrointestinal tract of many herbivorous reptiles. However, in snakes and carnivorous lizards/chelonians, this amoeba may cause damage to the intestinal mucosa resulting in hemorrhagic enteritis, colitis, and hepatitis.

SYNONYMS

Protozoal or amoebic enteritis/colitis

EPIDEMIOLOGY

SPECIES, AGE, SEX

- *Entamoeba invadens* is a potential pathogen of all reptiles.
- The organism causes high morbidity and mortality in snakes and lizards.
- Many chelonians and crocodilians may have a commensal relationship with *Entamoeba* spp.
- Epizootics and clinical cases have been reported in a number of reptiles, including:
  - Red-footed tortoises *(Chelonoidis [Geochelone] carbonaria)*
  - Spider tortoises *(Pyxis [Acinixys] planicauda)*
  - Loggerhead musk turtle *(Sternotherus minor minor)*
  - Wood turtles *(Glyptemys insculpta)*
  - Loggerhead sea turtles *(Caretta caretta)*
  - Green sea turtles *(Chelonia mydas)*
  - Monitor lizards, Komodo dragon *(Varanus komodoensis);* water monitor *(V. salvator)* and lace monitor *(V. varus)*.
  - Blue tongue skink *(Tiliqua scincoides)*
  - Green iguana *(Iguana iguana)*
- The author has diagnosed this disease in several collections of crested geckos *(Rhacodactylus cilliatus)*.
- Many species of snakes have been reported, and *E. invadens* is historically one of the most important parasites causing disease in snakes.

RISK FACTORS

- Mixed collections, especially involving aquatic reptiles (turtles and crocodilians)
- Poor quarantine and hygiene practices utilized in the management of a collection of reptiles.
- Insects may carry infected cysts from cage to cage; food items transferred from one cage to another may spread infectious cysts.
- Environmental temperatures at which captive reptiles are maintained may increase the pathogenicity of the organism. In two separate studies in experimentally inoculated snakes, snakes that were maintained at 13°C (55°F), 33°C (91.5°F), and 35°C (95°F) did not develop clinical disease. However, snakes kept at 25°C (77°F) consistently died of clinical disease.

CONTAGION AND ZOONOSIS

- No zoonotic potential is known.
- Chelonians and crocodilians may be subclinical carriers.
- *Entamoeba invadens* is highly contagious and may spread rapidly through a collection.

ASSOCIATED CONDITIONS AND DISORDERS

- Secondary hepatitis with hepatic necrosis and abscessation
- Amoebic encephalitis: *E. invadens* sometimes invade the brain of snakes, resulting in abscess formation, which may lead to seizures and neurologic disease.

CLINICAL PRESENTATION

HISTORY, CHIEF COMPLAINT

- Anorexia
- Dehydration
- Regurgitation
- Constipation
- Diarrhea (see Diarrhea)
- Malodorous and/or bile-stained stools
- Hematochezia
- Weight loss/wasting
- Sudden death
- Seizures (with migration into central nervous system [CNS])

PHYSICAL EXAM FINDINGS

- Poor body condition and muscle tone
- Dehydration
- Emaciation
- Loss of muscle tone
- Palpably thickened colon or colonic mass
- Urate and fecal accumulation and/or staining around vent
- Neurologic signs (with migration into the CNS)

ETIOLOGY AND PATHOPHYSIOLOGY

- *Entamoeba* has a direct life cycle; transmission starts with ingestion of the cyst stage.
- Many turtles and crocodilians are reservoirs for *E. invadens*. These carriers often become a source for potential infection of other reptiles in the collection.
- After the organism damages the gastrointestinal mucosa, secondary bacterial invasion occurs, and a fibrinonecrotic pseudomembrane often forms.
- Protozoal and bacterial dissemination often follows, with invasion of the common bile duct ascending to the gallbladder or with showering of the liver via the portal system.
- Hepatic necrosis and abscessation typically follow, with potential multiple organ involvement followed by bacterial sepsis and death.
- *E. invadens* may migrate into nervous tissue such as the brain, resulting in abscess formation and the inflammatory response, often causing seizures and neurologic signs.

DIAGNOSIS

DIFFERENTIAL DIAGNOSIS

- Other protozoa (small numbers of these protozoa are often considered commensals)
- Other nonpathogenic species of *Entamoeba (E. terrapinae or E testudinis)*
- Flagellates *(Hexamita, Trichomonas, Giardia, Leptomonas)*
- Ciliates *(Balantidium, Nyctotherus)* found primarily in chelonians
- Bacterial enteritis
- Viral enteritis
- Cryptosporidia/coccidiosis (see Cryptosporidiosis, and Coccidiosis)
- Gastrointestinal nematodes (see Nematodiasis)
- Boid inclusion body disease (IBD)
- Foreign body (particulate substrate)
- Associated with poor husbandry (incorrect temperatures and diet)

INITIAL DATABASE

- A thorough history, physical examination, complete blood count, biochemistry, and fecal examination form the initial database.
- Fecal examination (see Fecal Exam, Sec.II)
- Fresh feces may be obtained by gently expressing the colon.

ADVANCED OR CONFIRMATORY TESTING

- Cloacoscopy with warm fluid infusion may be used to evaluate the cloaca and colon and to retrieve biopsies.
- Histopathology and culture and sensitivity
- Necropsy with multiple colonic tissue samples submitted for histopathology

- Periodic acid–Schiff (PAS) stains of tissue sections submitted for histopathologic examination
  - The amoeba may be lost in the fixation and staining processes of histopathologic specimen preparation.
  - In suspect cases, direct smears or impressions of the intestinal tract at the time of the necropsy may be important to confirm a suspected diagnosis.
- *E. invadens* may be cultured, which requires special incubation temperatures of 16°C to 20°C (61°F to 68°F).
- Immunohistochemistry for *E invadens* is available for snakes.

TREATMENT

THERAPEUTIC GOAL

Identify any secondary associated pathogens such as bacteria contributing to the enteritis/colitis, and direct specific antimicrobial therapy as indicated.

ACUTE GENERAL TREATMENT

- The overall status of the patient should be assessed. The patient must be warmed to appropriate temperatures and fluid therapy initiated if indicated.
- The drug of choice is metronidazole 20-50 mg/kg orally.
- The dosage interval varies from every 2-3 days (3-5 doses) for clinically ill reptiles to every 10-14 days (2-3 doses) for reptiles that may have been exposed but are nonclinical.
- Colubrids (e.g., king snakes, milk snakes, indigo) and rattlesnakes may be more sensitive to metronidazole Use the lower dose and frequency.
- For green iguanas and yellow rat snakes, 20 mg/kg orally every 48 hours is recommended.

CHRONIC TREATMENT

Continuing to treat affected reptiles with supportive care, including hydration, assisted alimentation if not feeding, and long-term protective broad-spectrum antimicrobials will be important to increase survival.

POSSIBLE COMPLICATIONS

Metronidazole may be toxic and may cause neurologic disorders such as seizures.

RECOMMENDED MONITORING

- Monitoring fecal output macroscopically for improvement (a more normal appearance) and evidence of continued problems (hematochezia, liquid diarrhea, etc.)
- Follow-up fecal evaluations (as described above) may be useful.
- Monitor patient status such as body weight, hydration status, activity, and interest in feeding.
- Cloacoscopy can be performed to reevaluate the colon and visualize the response to treatment.

PROGNOSIS AND OUTCOME

- Prognosis is poor owing to the rapid progression of this disease.
- Often reptiles are presented acutely dead or in a moribund condition, and treatment is not effective.
- Aggressive specific treatment can be initiated in other clinical reptiles or in those that may have been exposed; the prognosis for these patients will be better.

PEARLS & CONSIDERATIONS

COMMENTS

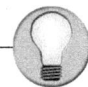

- Avoid inappropriate temperatures for species being maintained.
- Monitor food intake, especially in species that may have a commensal relationship with *Entamoeba* organisms, such as tortoises and turtles.

PREVENTION

- Snakes and lizards should not be kept in enclosures with chelonians and crocodiles, and disinfecting protocols (bleach at a dilution of 1:32 with water is adequate) must be strictly adhered to when working with mixed collections.
- A 60- to 90-day quarantine should be established for all new reptiles entering a collection.
  - During this time, a minimum of three negative fecal results should be obtained.
  - Normal eating and defecating habits should be established before an animal is introduced into a collection.

CLIENT EDUCATION

Educate the owner on biosecurity with emphasis on quarantine protocols and risks associated with mixed collections.

SUGGESTED READINGS

Barrow J, Jr, Stockton JJ: The influences of temperature on the host parasite relationships of several species of snakes infected with *Entamoeba invadens*, J Protozool 7:377–383, 1960.

Jacobson ER: Parasites and parasitic diseases of reptiles. In Jacobson ER, editor: Infectious diseases and pathology of reptiles, Boca Raton, FL, 2007, CRC Press, pp 571–665.

McArthur S, et al: Gastrointestinal system. In Girling SJ, et al, editors: BSAVA manual of reptiles, ed 2, Gloucester, 2004, BSAVA, pp 210–229.

Meerovitch E: Infectivity and pathogenicity of polyxenic and monoxenic *Entamoeba invadens* to snakes kept at normal and high temperatures and the natural history of reptile amoebiasis, J Parasitol 47:791–794, 1961.

Stahl SJ: Crested geckos and other *Rhacodactylus* geckos: common clinical presentations—move over Geico there's a new gecko in town. In Proceedings of the North American Veterinary Conference, Orlando, FL, 2010.

CROSS-REFERENCES TO OTHER SECTIONS

Coccidiosis
Cryptosporidiosis
Diarrhea
Fecal Exam, Sec.II
Mycobacteria
Nematodiasis
Salmonella

AUTHOR & EDITOR: **SCOTT J. STAHL**

REPTILES

Gout

BASIC INFORMATION

DEFINITION

Overproduction of, or failure to excrete, uric acid results in hyperuricemia, which can lead to systemic or localized urate precipitation in tissues.

SYNONYMS

Visceral gout, articular gout

EPIDEMIOLOGY

SPECIES, AGE, SEX Potentially any species, any age, and with no proven gender bias.

RISK FACTORS

- High-protein diets, especially feeding insects or canned dog/cat foods to herbivores
- Dehydration due to low environmental humidity

- Poor or unsuitable water availability (e.g., some reptiles will drink only droplets on foliage)

ASSOCIATED CONDITIONS AND DISORDERS

- Renal failure (see Renal Disease)
- Dehydration
- High-protein diets

CLINICAL PRESENTATION

DISEASE FORMS/SUBTYPES

- Articular gout
- Visceral gout

HISTORY, CHIEF COMPLAINT

- Most cases of gout are the terminal presentation of a chronic disease process (e.g., end-stage renal failure, long-term dehydration, long-term high protein).
- Many owners will miss the slow deterioration and will seek veterinary assistance only when the animal suddenly decompensates.
- Articular gout is commonly cited as a separate condition from visceral gout but is likely to be an earlier presentation that precedes more widespread visceral gout (as is the case in humans).

PHYSICAL EXAM FINDINGS

- A thorough physical examination is always indicated and should include an accurate measurement of weight.
- Reptiles with visceral gout usually will present in a generalized depressed and weakened state.
    - Animals are often cachexic, dehydrated, and moribund.
- Dehydration may be inferred from reductions in skin elasticity and salivary and ocular secretions. White to cream-colored urate tophi may be visible within the mucous membranes.
- Where digital palpation of the kidneys percutaneously or per cloaca is possible, the kidneys may be of abnormal shape and size.
- In cases of articular gout, the joints may appear grossly swollen, and/or nodules or masses may be associated with digit extremities.

ETIOLOGY AND PATHOPHYSIOLOGY

- Reptiles possess paired metanephric kidneys, each containing a few thousand nephrons.
- The main nitrogenous product for most terrestrial reptiles is uric acid (UA).
- UA is actively secreted from the proximal tubule; however, when glomerular filtration rate is severely reduced, UA accumulates in the renal tubule and eventually overcomes active tubular secretion; consequently, blood UA levels rise.
- UA levels above 25 mg/dL (1.47 mmol/L) result in precipitation of UA in soft tissues, causing pronounced inflammation and pain.
- In captive reptiles, hyperuricemia and gout have been associated with excess dietary protein, inadequate water provision, and severe nephropathy.
- The initial predisposition for gout in and around joints is largely unknown.

DIAGNOSIS

DIFFERENTIAL DIAGNOSIS

- Visceral gout and eventual articular gout
- Acute renal failure
- Chronic renal failure
- Constipation
- Renal neoplasia
- Primary water deprivation
- Articular gout (swellings over joints, extremities)
- Abscesses (see Abscesses)
- Cellulitis
- Septic arthritis
- Parasites (cestodes, filarids, etc.)
- Trauma
- Nutritional secondary hyperparathyroidism (NSHP) (see Nutritional Secondary Hyperparathyroidism [NSHP])
- Degenerative arthritis
- Pseudogout (calcium hydroxyapatite)

INITIAL DATABASE

- A thorough history, physical exam, complete blood count, plasma chemistry
- Urinalysis
- Survey radiographs and ultrasonography

ADVANCED OR CONFIRMATORY TESTING

- See Renal Disease
- Renal/joint ultrasonography
- Joint aspirate with cytologic examination and/or soft tissue biopsy for histopathologic examination may be useful.
- Phase contrast microscopy can be used on cytology/direct smears of needles aspirates and joint fluid/material collection at surgery to look for evidence of urate crystals.
- Radiographs of swollen joints and extremities may be useful in differentiating rule-outs:
    - Soft tissue involvement (abscesses, cellulites)
    - Gout (often radiolucent)
    - Pseudogout (more radiodense accumulation of material around joints)
    - Bone involvement (fracture, NSHP, arthritis) (see Orthopedics and Fracture Repair)
- Renal endoscopy and biopsy
- Iohexol excretion study to determine glomerular filtration rate (GFR) (see Glomerular Filtration Rate [GFR] Study Sec.II)

TREATMENT

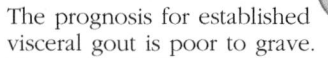

THERAPEUTIC GOALS

- Rehydration to establish urine flow and to normalize any electrolyte abnormalities
- Reduction of plasma UA levels if elevated
- Reduction in dietary protein

ACUTE GENERAL TREATMENT

- Fluid therapy starting at 10-30 mL/kg q 24 h (intravenous, intraosseous, or intracoelomic) and monitoring of hematocrit, electrolytes, and UA
- Diuretics (furosemide, mannitol) if anuric once rehydrated
    - Furosemide 5 mg/kg PO, IM, IV every 12-24 hours
    - Mannitol 0.25-2.0 mg/kg IV slow bolus every 24 hours
- Allopurinol efficacy has been demonstrated in iguanas, and 25 mg/kg daily by mouth reduced UA levels by up to 45%.
- Consider pain management:
    - Morphine:
        - Chelonians: 1.5 mg/kg
        - Lizards: 10 mg/kg
    - Meloxicam: 0.1-0.3 mg/kg PO q 24 h (use with caution if renal disease is present)

CHRONIC TREATMENT

- Rehydration
- Allopurinol
- Dietary correction (reduced protein)
- Improvement in management, especially thermal/humidity/water/quality light provision

POSSIBLE COMPLICATIONS

- Visceral gout causing organ dysfunction/failure
- Articular gout causing arthritis, possible amputation
- Inflammation and pain
- Judicious use of nonsteroidal antiinflammatory drugs (NSAIDs) because these patients may have renal compromise

RECOMMENDED MONITORING

- Monitor UA, electrolytes, total protein, albumin, UA (or urea for aquatic species).
- Weight
- Dietary protein content

PROGNOSIS AND OUTCOME

- The prognosis for established visceral gout is poor to grave.
- The prognosis for acute hyperuricemia is fair if renal function and excretion can be reestablished quickly.

- The prognosis for focal articular gout is fair if the cause has been addressed.

PEARLS & CONSIDERATIONS

COMMENTS

- Reptile kidneys cannot concentrate urine, so urine specific gravity cannot be used as a prognostic indicator.
- Reptile kidneys empty into the cloaca, not directly into the bladder. In those species that have a bladder (all chelonians, some lizards), urine then passes into the bladder, where postrenal modification of urine can occur (electrolyte exchange and water absorption by osmosis).
- Green iguanas fed canned pet food have UA levels almost double those of iguanas fed a vegetarian diet.
- Pseudogout has been noted in veiled chameleons fed a heavily supplemented vitamin D_3- and calcium-based diet in combination with restricted levels of vitamin A.
- Pseudogout deposits usually appear as irregular firm swellings over joints in the limbs and on ribs.
- Fine-needle aspiration and cytologic examination or biopsy can be used to reach a diagnosis.
- Radiology may be useful in screening for metastatic calcification and/or pseudogout.

PREVENTION

- Appropriate water provision
- Appropriate dietary protein
- Appropriate thermal and humidity gradients
- Appropriate lighting and calcium supplementation

CLIENT EDUCATION

Educating clients about the proper diet and husbandry necessary for the specific reptile species presented is critical.

SUGGESTED READINGS

Hernandez-Divers SJ, et al: Effects of allopurinol on plasma uric acid levels in normo- and hyperuricaemic green iguanas (*Iguana iguana*), Vet Rec 162:112–115, 2008.

Hernandez-Divers SJ: Green iguana nephrology: a review of diagnostic techniques, Vet Clin North Am Exot Anim Pract 6:233–250, 2003.

Hernandez-Divers SJ, et al: Renal disease in reptiles: diagnosis and clinical management. In Mader DR, editor: Reptile medicine and surgery, ed 2, St Louis, 2006, Elsevier Publishing, pp 878–892.

Hernandez-Divers SJ, et al: Renal evaluation in the green iguana (*Iguana iguana*): assessment of plasma biochemistry, glomerular filtration rate, and endoscopic biopsy, J Zoo Wildl Med 36:155–168, 2005.

CROSS-REFERENCES TO OTHER SECTIONS

Abscesses
Glomerular Filtration Rate (GFR) Study (Section II)
Nutritional Secondary Hyperparathyroidism (NSHP)
Orthopedics and Fracture Repair
Renal Disease

AUTHOR: **STEPHEN J. DIVERS**

EDITOR: **SCOTT J. STAHL**

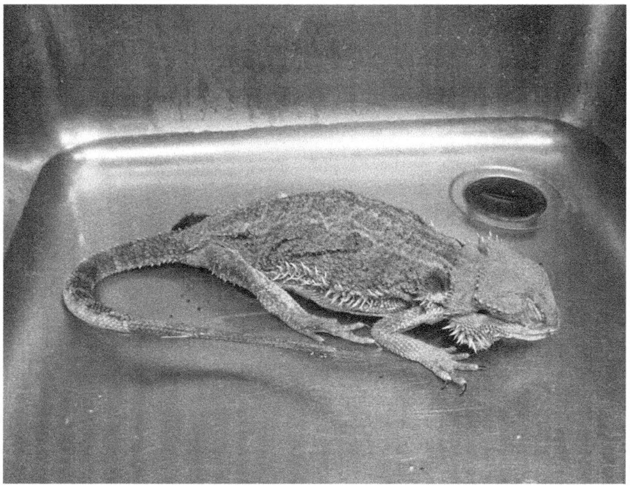

Gout Severely dehydrated bearded dragon. A shallow bath in lukewarm water will stimulate the animal to drink. Never leave an animal unattended because it can easily drown even in shallow water. *(Photo courtesy Jörg Mayer, The University of Georgia, Athens.)*

REPTILES

Hepatic Lipidosis

BASIC INFORMATION

DEFINITION

- Pathologic increase in intrahepatic fat that adversely affects hepatic function
- Hepatic lipidosis must be differentiated from physiologically normal increases in intrahepatic fat associated with hibernation/reproduction.

SYNONYM

Fatty liver disease

EPIDEMIOLOGY

SPECIES, AGE, SEX

- Chelonians, large carnivorous lizards (monitors, tegus), and bearded dragons (*Pogona vitticeps*) well represented clinically
- Excessive feeding in any adult reptile
- Temperate species that would naturally fast (e.g., hibernation) but are maintained year-round appear more prone to hepatic lipidosis if fed ad libitum.
- Unlikely in juveniles
- Females that do not have the opportunity to breed seem particularly at risk.

RISK FACTORS

- Excessive feeding
- Lack of exercise
- Female
- Lack of hibernation or naturally fasting
- Iatrogenic: ivermectin in chelonians

CONTAGION AND ZOONOSIS Infectious causes of hepatic lipidosis are rare.

GEOGRAPHY AND SEASONALITY Temperate species more prone, but can occur in any species that is fed excessively

ASSOCIATED CONDITIONS AND DISORDERS

- Nonbreeding females
- Chronic/acute hepatitis due to toxins, infections, anoxia

CLINICAL PRESENTATION

HISTORY, CHIEF COMPLAINT

- Classified as acute or chronic, inflammatory (hepatitis) or degenerative (hepatosis)
- Usually a gradual reduction in appetite, activity, fecundity, and fertility; retarded weight gain or gradual weight loss; hibernation problems, including post-hibernation anorexia; and changes in fecal character and color
- It may only be during episodes of increased physiologic demand (e.g., hibernation, breeding, concurrent disease) that underlying liver disease becomes clinically apparent.

PHYSICAL EXAM FINDINGS

- When lipidosis is advanced, most affected reptiles are in poor body condition and are flaccid, weak, and cachectic. Regurgitation is considered to be a poor sign, esp. in turtles and lizards.
- Bodyweight (mass) is usually below normal; often the patient is critical.
- In cases of ascites, weight may be artificially maintained or even increased.
- Diarrhea is uncommon.
- Reptiles with acute liver disease usually present in good body condition but with sudden-onset depression and anorexia (see Liver Disease).
- In these cases, diarrhea may be evident, and if the urates are pigmented yellow-green, excretion of biliverdin may indicate severe liver compromise and bile stasis.
- Severely affected animals usually will be depressed, lethargic, and weak; mucous membranes may be pale, hyperemic, or icteric.

ETIOLOGY AND PATHOPHYSIOLOGY

- The functions of the reptile liver are similar to those of mammals and birds, including fat, protein (including globulin), and glycogen metabolism and production of uric acid and clotting factors. These functions may vary markedly as the animal progresses from egg to juvenile to breeding adult, and may be dramatically affected by seasonal changes, especially hibernation and estivation.
- It is important to remember that hepatic lipidosis is a metabolic derangement and is not a single clinical disease.
- In rare situations, toxic insult may cause acute degenerative changes.
  - Ivermectin-induced hepatic lipidosis in chelonians is a well-documented example.

DIAGNOSIS

DIFFERENTIAL DIAGNOSIS

Any disease that causes anorexia or metabolic derangement, including toxins, anoxia, and impaired metabolism of carbohydrate and volatile fatty acids

INITIAL DATABASE

- Blood work
  - Acute inflammation or necrosis of the liver usually will result in a dramatic heterophilia and monocytosis (including azurophilia, in many species).
  - Chronic bacterial hepatitis usually will cause only minor elevations of the total white blood cell count, although shifts in the lymphocyte/monocyte-to-heterophil ratio often occur.
  - Eosinophilia may be seen in cases of parasitic disease.
- Radiographs
  - The radiographic hepatic shadow is often appreciable on horizontal beam radiographs of lizards, less so in snakes, and least of all in chelonian, because of superimposition of the shell.
- Ultrasonography
  - Possible to detect macrohepatic changes

ADVANCED OR CONFIRMATORY TESTING

- Bile acids (3-alpha-hydroxy bile acids) have been investigated only in green iguanas to date. Iguanas fasted for 48 hours have mean resting bile acid values of 7.5 µmol/L, which increase to 33 µmol/L for at least 8 hours after feeding.
- Observations by the author suggest that values greater than 60 µmol/L are often indicative of hepatic dysfunction.
- Endoscopically guided or ultrasound-guided Tru-Cut biopsies of the liver parenchyma
- MRI provides excellent soft tissue detail.

TREATMENT

THERAPEUTIC GOALS

Medical stabilization using fluid therapy is essential, and provision of the species-specific preferred optimum temperature zone (POTZ) can be instrumental in effecting improvement.

ACUTE GENERAL TREATMENT

- Fluids (10-30 mL/kg/d) and nutritional support
- Mild to moderate cases of hepatic lipidosis are usually anorectic on presentation but in good condition; in these cases, oral fluids are adequate.
- Reptiles with severe disease often require intracoelomic, intravenous, or intraosseous infusion. In cases of severe liver pathology, it may be wise to avoid solutions containing lactate.
- Blood samples should be collected before fluid therapy is provided; antibiotic medication should be delayed until after liver biopsy and culture.

CHRONIC TREATMENT

- Hepatic lipidosis is a chronic disease that may take months, if not years, to reverse. Therefore, means of providing long-term fluid and nutritional support should be explored.
- The importance of nutritional support cannot be overemphasized.
- When providing nutritional support, it is important to consider:
  - The patient's energy and nutritional requirements
  - The patient's natural dietary preferences (e.g., herbivorous, omnivorous, carnivorous)
  - Attempting to use natural foods in preference to artificial substitutes
- Carnitine and choline supplementation has been suggested.
  - A daily dose of 250 mg/kg carnitine mixed with the tube-feeding formula appears to be safe in reptiles.
- Methionine, a precursor of choline, may be used:
  - A daily dose of 40-50 mg/kg appears to be safe in reptiles.
- Thyroxine (20 mcg/kg PO q 48 h) and nandrolone (0.5-1 mg/kg IM q 7-28 d) have been advocated.
- Other liver supportive medications that can be empirically used include: Lactulose at 0.5 ml/kg PO q 24 h or Silymarin (milk thistle) at 50-100 mg/kg PO q 24 h. These medications can be mixed together for ease of administration.

POSSIBLE COMPLICATIONS

Be aware that anabolic steroids can cause hepatic disease.

RECOMMENDED MONITORING

- Monitor weight and food intake.
- Liver enzymes and bile acids

- Serial liver ultrasound and endoscopic liver biopsies for repeat histopathology at 3, 6, and 12 months
- Modify management, including diet and exercise.

PROGNOSIS AND OUTCOME

The prognosis for severe chronic hepatic lipidosis is guarded to poor.

PEARLS & CONSIDERATIONS

COMMENTS

- When performing a necropsy on an animal with suspected hepatic lipidosis, care must be taken to ensure that all other body organs are meticulously examined. In particular, note should be taken of other fat deposits, including the size of fat bodies and the presence or absence of adipose tissue under the skin and around the heart.
- In crocodilians, the size of the fat body is carefully assessed as part of postmortem evaluation of the condition—by weighing or by comparing its size with the animal's ventricles. Similar techniques could prove useful in other reptiles.
- In hepatic lipidosis, the color may be pale tan to almost white. The color may also be affected by the natural color of fat in the species, which in turn can be influenced by diet.
- A "fatty liver" is usually swollen, with rounded, nonangular edges, and may weigh more than normal.
- Markedly fatty livers will have a soft, fatty "feel" when held for cutting and are friable—easily torn.
- A diagnosis of hepatic lipidosis cannot usually be confirmed without taking into account:
  - The clinical history and the clinician's assessment of the case (including other laboratory results)
  - The patient's details and circumstances, for example, its species, age, sex, reproductive status, hibernation, estivation, and diet.

PREVENTION

- Appropriate management (temperature, diet, exercise) including simulation of natural fasting/hibernation periods
- Female lizards and chelonians that cannot breed should be considered for elective ovariectomy.

CLIENT EDUCATION

- Clinicians must educate clients about appropriate husbandry, specifically, dietary requirements for the specific reptile species presented.
- Clients should be warned about the risks of overfeeding in all reptiles, but especially in species that are prone to overeating and obesity. Additionally, encouraging clients to offer larger enclosures or the opportunity to exercise these reptiles is important.
- Once the pet (or nonbreeding) reptile has been accurately sexed, discussing the option of elective ovariectomy as a preventive procedure for conditions such as reproductive disease and hepatic lipidosis is important.

SUGGESTED READINGS

Hernandez-Divers SJ, et al: Hepatic lipidosis. In Mader DR, editor: Reptile medicine and surgery, ed 2, Philadelphia, 2006, WB Saunders, pp 806–813.

McBride M, et al: Preliminary evaluation of resting and post-prandial bile acid levels in the green iguana (*Iguana iguana*), J Herpetol Med Surg 16:129–134, 2007.

CROSS-REFERENCES TO OTHER SECTIONS

Liver Disease

AUTHOR: **STEPHEN J. DIVERS**

EDITOR: **SCOTT J. STAHL**

REPTILES

Herpesvirus Infections

BASIC INFORMATION

DEFINITION

Reptilian herpesviruses are DNA, enveloped viruses ranging in size from 120-200 nm in diameter. These viruses replicate in the host nucleus resulting in intranuclear inclusion bodies (INIB).

SYNONYMS

Fibropapillomatosis; Gray patch disease; Lung, eye, and trachea disease (LET); Loggerhead genital-respiratory herpesvirus (LGRV); Loggerhead orocutaneous herpesvirus (LOCV); Tortoise herpesvirus 1; Tortoise herpesvirus 2; herpesvirus 4, Varanid herpesvirus 1; Gerrhosaurid herpesvirus 1; Gerrhosaurid herpesvirus 2; Gerrhosaurid herpesvirus 3; Iguanid herpesvirus 1; Iguanid herpesvirus 2

EPIDEMIOLOGY

SPECIES, AGE, SEX

- It is probable that multiple herpesviruses have co-evolved, along with each reptile host species.
- In their natural hosts, herpesviruses are often associated with mucocutaneous lesions and often cause clinical signs only in stressed or otherwise immune suppressed animals.
- In an aberrant host that is related closely enough that the virus can replicate, disease is more likely to be peracute and fatal.
- Young animals probably are more likely to have significant clinical signs with a herpesvirus that is adapted for their species; aberrant hosts probably do not have an age predisposition.

RISK FACTORS

- Stressed animals appear to be more likely to develop clinical disease.
- Mixed-species enclosures can result in spread of a herpesvirus that is indigenous and relatively benign in one species and may cause peracute fatal disease in another.

CONTAGION AND ZOONOSIS

- As enveloped viruses, herpesviruses are not stable in the environment.
- Direct contact between animals is typically necessary for spread of disease.
- Disinfectants effective against other enveloped viruses (such as sodium hypochlorite 3%) may be expected to be effective against herpesviruses.
- No zoonotic risk for any reptile herpesvirus has been noted, and herpesviruses generally are restricted to species that are at least somewhat related to the normal host species.

GEOGRAPHY AND SEASONALITY

- Herpesviruses are likely to have co-evolved with all reptile species, and may be found wherever reptiles live.
- Clinical disease associated with tortoise herpesvirus 1 is more common in the spring.

ASSOCIATED CONDITIONS AND DISORDERS

- Stomatitis, rhinitis, proliferative skin lesions, and other mucocutaneous lesions are commonly associated with herpesviral disease in native hosts.

- Peracute hepatitis and death are often associated with herpesviral disease in aberrant or immune suppressed hosts.

CLINICAL PRESENTATION

DISEASE FORMS/SUBTYPES

- Many herpesvirus infections are subclinical in native hosts.
- Mucocutaneous lesions are the most common presentations in native hosts.
- Peracute hepatitis and death are often seen in aberrant hosts.

HISTORY, CHIEF COMPLAINT Common complaints on presentation include marked depression, stomatitis, proliferative skin lesions, and high death rates.

PHYSICAL EXAM FINDINGS Physical examination findings often include stomatitis, proliferative skin lesions, and marked depression.

ETIOLOGY AND PATHOPHYSIOLOGY

- It is probable that multiple herpesviruses have co-evolved along with each reptile host.
- All reptile herpesviruses characterized to date are in the subfamily Alphaherpesvirinae.
- Herpesviruses causing proliferative mucocutaneous lesions may progress to neoplasia.
- In the peracute disease seen in aberrant hosts, metabolic derangement may be so severe that the animal may be dead before a significant inflammatory response is present.

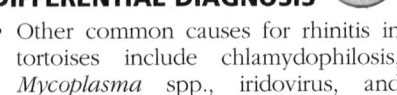

DIAGNOSIS

DIFFERENTIAL DIAGNOSIS

- Other common causes for rhinitis in tortoises include chlamydophilosis, *Mycoplasma* spp., iridovirus, and reovirus.
- Herpesviral disease in tortoises is very similar to disease seen with Ranavirus infection.
- Other differentials for proliferative skin lesions include papillomavirus.

INITIAL DATABASE

A thorough history, physical examination, complete blood count, plasma chemistry, and radiographs form the basic database.

ADVANCED OR CONFIRMATORY TESTING

- Nested polymerase chain reaction (PCR) with product sequence analysis is available from the University of Florida for all herpesviruses.
- Swabs or biopsies of fresh mucocutaneous lesions are the samples of choice.
- For postmortem samples, cranial nerves are also a good sample, and with peracute infection, as seen in aberrant hosts, liver is often a good sample.
- Blood generally is not a good choice for PCR diagnosis of herpesvirus infection in reptiles.
- Histopathologic examination is necessary to establish that any lesions present are consistent with a herpesviral origin; without corresponding lesions, identification of a herpesvirus may be incidental.
- The finding of intranuclear inclusions on histopathology is suggestive but not pathognomonic.
- Although inclusions are common in peracute disease, they may be rare or absent in more chronic lesions, such as fibropapillomatosis in sea turtles.
- If inclusions are present, electron microscopy may be useful to help identify herpesvirus-like particles, although sequence data are needed for speciation.
- In situ hybridization is available from the University of Georgia for identification of the presence of a herpesvirus in tissues, although again, sequence data are needed for speciation.

TREATMENT

THERAPEUTIC GOAL

The goal of treatment is alleviation of clinical disease. Infected animals are lifelong carriers.

ACUTE GENERAL TREATMENT

- Providing supportive care and addressing husbandry deficiencies are the most important aspects.
- Acyclovir has been found to be effective in treating herpesviral disease in mammals, but in vitro studies using tortoise herpesvirus 1 have found it to be effective only at doses that would be expected to be toxic.

CHRONIC TREATMENT

- Animals remain latently infected, and continued shedding by recovered animals is a concern.
- Stress should be minimized to prevent recrudescence.
- Known infected animals should not be brumated.

PROGNOSIS AND OUTCOME

Many animals do well with supportive care. Animals are often latently infected, and introduction of naïve animals to recovered animals should be avoided.

PEARLS & CONSIDERATIONS

COMMENTS

- In mammalian species that have been well studied, it is common to see 80% to 95% infection rates with many herpesviruses in their native hosts. However, the rates for disease are significantly lower. It is likely that herpesviral infections are also common in reptiles.
- Tortoise herpesvirus 1 appears to be very common in Russian tortoises *(Agrionemys [Testudo] horsfieldii)*.

PREVENTION

Maintenance of a closed group, testing of populations, testing during quarantine, and stringent biosecurity practices are the most effective means of prevention.

SUGGESTED READINGS

Wellehan JF, et al: Three novel herpesviruses associated with stomatitis in Sudan plated lizards (*Gerrhosaurus major*) and a black-lined plated lizard *(Gerrhosaurus nigrolineatus)*, J Zoo Wildl Med 35:50–54, 2004.

Wellehan JF, et al: Varanid herpesvirus 1: a novel herpesvirus associated with proliferative stomatitis in green tree monitors *(Varanus prasinus)*, Vet Microbiol 105:83–92, 2005.

Wellehan JFX, et al: A novel herpesvirus associated with hepatic necrosis in a San Esteban Chuckwalla *(Sauromalus varius)*, J Herpetol Med Surg 13:15–19, 2003.

CROSS-REFERENCES TO OTHER SECTIONS

Abscesses
Chlamydophila
Dysecdysis
Hypovitaminosis A
Lower Respiratory (tract) disease/ Pneumonia
Mycoplasma
NSHP
Stomatitis

AUTHOR: **JAMES F.X. WELLEHAN, JR.**

EDITOR: **SCOTT J. STAHL**

Hyperglycemia

BASIC INFORMATION

DEFINITION

- Hyperglycemia is defined as an elevation of blood glucose and is an uncommon clinical abnormality in reptiles.
- Hyperglycemia has not been established as a consistent or specific indicator of pancreatic disease or diabetes mellitus in reptiles.
- Elevations in blood glucose are more often related to other metabolic conditions, systemic diseases, and physiologic variables.
- Persistent hyperglycemia is perhaps a better description for a reptile with elevated blood glucose values until further evaluation can determine possible causes.
- A diagnosis of hyperglycemia in reptiles starts with persistently elevated blood glucose values above 300 mg/dL (16.7 mmol/L).

SYNONYMS

Persistent hyperglycemia, diabetes mellitus (not defined in reptiles)

EPIDEMIOLOGY

RISK FACTORS

- Stress-associated hyperglycemia
- Normal seasonal variation
- Breeding (breeding season influences), esp. in temperate reptiles
- Freshwater turtles show hyperglycemia when diving.
- Post prandial response
- Anorexia/starvation
- Metabolic disease (liver or renal disease)
- Neoplasia

GEOGRAPHY AND SEASONALITY

- A normal seasonal variation in blood glucose levels may occur in many species of reptiles.
- Temperate reptiles generally have higher blood glucose levels during the breeding season.

ASSOCIATED CONDITIONS AND DISORDERS Hyperglycemia has been reported to be associated with metabolic disease (liver and kidney disease) and nonpancreatic neoplasia.

CLINICAL PRESENTATION

HISTORY, CHIEF COMPLAINT

- A complete history is important.
- Information regarding seasonal cycles, including hibernation and reproduction, both past and present, includes important variables that may reflect on blood glucose.

PHYSICAL EXAM FINDINGS

- Physical examination findings are often nonspecific as described above but also may include loss of muscle mass, weakness, loss of righting reflex, stupor, and severe depression. Some reptiles may present overconditioned or obese.
- Polyuria and polydipsia may be present but are not common clinical signs.

ETIOLOGY AND PATHOPHYSIOLOGY

- Damage to the reptile pancreas is expected to elevate blood glucose.
- Variations in blood glucose may be more common in reptiles because of variable metabolic rate, environmental influences and adaptations, and relative insulin resistance.
- Stress-associated hyperglycemia has been reported in a number of reptile species.
- A normal seasonal variation in blood glucose levels may occur in many species of reptiles.
- Tropical reptiles may not show seasonal blood sugar variations.
- Freshwater turtles were found to show marked hyperglycemia when diving.
- Studies indicate that reptiles may exhibit hyperglycemia of several days' duration after a meal. In a laboratory setting, 2 months of starvation at approximately 70°F (21°C) was necessary before blood sugar levels became hypoglycemic.

DIAGNOSIS

DIFFERENTIAL DIAGNOSIS

- Persistent hyperglycemia:
  - Metabolic disease (liver/kidney)
  - Stress
  - Neoplasia
  - Seasonal influences such as breeding/hibernation
  - Postprandial event
  - Starvation

INITIAL DATABASE

- A thorough history, physical examination findings, complete blood count, and full biochemical analysis, including bile acids, fecal examination, radiology, ultrasonography, endoscopy, and surgery, are modalities that can be used.
- Glucosuria:
  - May be noted in reptiles with persistent hyperglycemia
  - Reptile urine typically is not sterile because it is exposed to contents of the proctodeum and copradeum and, in many species, is actually held within the terminal colon before it is released.

ADVANCED OR CONFIRMATORY TESTING

- Blood insulin levels:
  - May prove to be useful to differentiate between diabetes mellitus and other causes of hyperglycemia
- Ketones:
  - Ketoacidosis is a concurrent clinical condition seen commonly with diabetes mellitus in mammals.
- Pancreatic biopsy:
  - Be aware of the location of the islet tissue in the pancreas of the reptile patient.
  - For example, in the savannah monitor (*Varanus exanthematicus*), all of the islet tissue is concentrated in the splenic portion of the pancreas.
- Necropsy and histopathology:
  - Submission of the entire pancreas for histopathologic analysis is imperative.
  - Histopathologic changes have also been found in the kidneys of reptiles with persistent hyperglycemia, including chronic glomerulonephritis, interstitial nephritis, and nephrosclerosis.

TREATMENT

THERAPEUTIC GOALS

- Stabilize patient by providing heat, fluid therapy (10-30 mL/kg q 24 h), and other indicated patient support
- Identify the cause of the persistent hyperglycemia
- Address any possible treatment for underlying metabolic disease of this condition
- Initiate glucose-regulating agents (see below) and monitor blood glucose
- Provide support and follow-up during treatment
- Address husbandry factors that may have contributed, including diet

ACUTE GENERAL TREATMENT

- Supportive care, including hydration, alimentation, liver support (lactulose 0.5 mL/kg PO q 24 h and milk thistle 50-100 mg/kg q 24 h), and other appropriate chemotherapeutics as indicated, should be initiated.

- If all factors indicate that the patient is truly a strong candidate for diabetes mellitus, an uncommon diagnosis in reptiles, and the clinician believes that some glucose-regulating agent must be initiated, a starting point for regular mammalian insulin may be as follows:
  - Lizards and crocodilians: 5-10 IU/kg every 24-48 hours
  - Snakes and chelonians: 1-5 IU/kg every 24-48 hours
- Oral glipizide at 0.25-3 mg was given to a Chinese Water Dragon (*Physignathus cocincinus*) with hyperglycemia with no response.

CHRONIC TREATMENT

- Continued serial sampling of blood glucose and adjustment of dosage regimens may be necessary for weeks to months to establish a response to initial and continued therapy.
- Making recommendations for husbandry changes that may help with long-term management such as increasing fiber in the diet of herbivorous and omnivorous reptiles

POSSIBLE COMPLICATIONS

- Adverse reactions to any glucose-regulating agents based on these empirical recommendations may occur.
- Close monitoring of patients is necessary.

RECOMMENDED MONITORING

Continued serial sampling of blood glucose and adjustment of dosage regimens may be necessary for weeks to months to establish a response to initial and continued therapy. This will likely be followed by lifelong monitoring.

PROGNOSIS AND OUTCOME

- All cases of reptiles with persistent hyperglycemia reported in the literature died.
- Cases of true pancreatic-associated hyperglycemia appear to have a poor prognosis.
- Cases with persistent hyperglycemia related to neoplastic or other secondary metabolic disorders have a guarded to poor prognosis.
- Cases of persistent hyperglycemia that are related to other intrinsic and extrinsic variables in reptiles as described in the differential diagnosis and risk factors above may have a more favorable prognosis depending on the condition of the reptile at presentation.

PEARLS & CONSIDERATIONS

COMMENTS

If a reptile patient presents with persistent hyperglycemia, do not think diabetes mellitus initially. Because true diabetes mellitus is not common, ruling out other causes for the hyperglycemia is prudent.

SUGGESTED READINGS

Frye FL: Spontaneous autoimmune pancreatitis and diabetes mellitus in a western pond turtle, *Clemmys marmorata*, Columbus, Ohio, 1999, Proc Assoc Reptilian Amphibian Veterinarians.

Griswold WG: Hepatocellular carcinoma with associated hyperglycemia in an inland bearded dragon, *Pogona vitticeps*, Orlando, 2001, Proc Assoc Reptilian Amphibian Veterinarians.

Heatley JJ, et al: Persistent hyperglycemia in a Chinese water dragon, *Physignathus cocincinus*, Orlando, 2001, Proc Assoc Reptilian Amphibian Veterinarians.

Lawrence K: Seasonal variation in blood biochemistry of long term captive Mediterranean tortoises (*Testudo graeca* and *T. hermanni*), Res Vet Sci 43:379–383, 1987.

Miller MR: Pancreatic islet histology and carbohydrate metabolism in amphibians and reptiles, Diabetes 9:318–323, 1960.

Penhos JC, et al: Total pancreatectomy in lizards: effects of several hormones, Endocrinology 76:989–993, 1965.

Stahl SJ: Hyperglycemia in reptiles. In Mader DR, editor: Reptile medicine and surgery, St Louis, 2006, Elsevier, pp 822–830.

CROSS-REFERENCES TO OTHER SECTIONS

Hepatic Lipidosis
Liver Disease
Renal Disease

AUTHOR & EDITOR: **SCOTT J. STAHL**

REPTILES

Hypervitaminosis A

BASIC INFORMATION

DEFINITION

Excessive intake or administration of the fat-soluble vitamin A

SYNONYMS

Iatrogenic hypervitaminosis A, vitamin A intoxication

EPIDEMIOLOGY

SPECIES, AGE, SEX

- Vitamin A toxicity
- Tortoises, box turtles, and aquatic turtles
- Seen frequently in chelonians in relation to increased parenteral treatment in this group of reptiles based on assumptions of hypovitaminosis A
- No age or sex differences

RISK FACTORS

- Overzealous treatment with vitamin A, especially parenteral forms of vitamin A
- Inappropriate dietary intake of fat-soluble vitamins

CLINICAL PRESENTATION

HISTORY, CHIEF COMPLAINT

- Vitamin A toxicity
- Parenteral injections of vitamin A given recently (within several weeks or months)
- Skin ulceration, sloughing in chelonians
- Often presented for skin infection or burn
- Depression
- Lethargy
- Anorexia
- Dehydration

PHYSICAL EXAM FINDINGS

- Skin hyperemia, blisters, ulceration, and skin sloughing. In chelonian patients, these skin changes are typically seen in the loose skin around the front legs and neck but can involve any skin area.
- Blisters typically will rupture and expose ulcerated red damaged tissue, which eventually will slough.
- Exposed dermis and muscle
- Secondary bacterial or fungal dermatitis associated with these skin lesions (see Bacterial Dermatosis)
- Depression
- Lethargy
- Dehydration
- Anorexia
- Weight loss

ETIOLOGY AND PATHOPHYSIOLOGY

- The most common cause of vitamin A toxicosis is iatrogenic intoxication involving the use of parenteral vitamin A preparations.
- Protocols for treating sick chelonians have generally included the use of parenteral vitamin A.
- Vitamin A intoxication occurs with dosages about 100 times the recommended intake.
  - Toxic doses for parenteral (water soluble) vitamin A are from 50,000-100,000 IU/kg.
- Intoxication of fat-soluble vitamins A and D from natural foods is uncommon.
- Vitamin A toxicity occurs when excessive levels of retinols overwhelm the liver, not allowing the liver to properly process and store the retinols.
  - It is the excessive levels of retinol not bound to the retinol-binding protein that then become free in tissues that cause damage.
  - Retinol toxicity affects the epidermis, initially causing dry, flaky skin followed by erythematous skin and blisters.
- Death may occur in severe cases secondary to dehydration from fluid loss associated with large areas of skin sloughing and exposing dermis and muscle. Bacterial and fungal invasion may follow, resulting in sepsis.
- Hypervitaminosis A may result in dysecdysis and organ toxicity, especially involving the liver, renal tubules, and pancreas. (see Liver Disease and Renal Disease)

DIAGNOSIS

DIFFERENTIAL DIAGNOSIS

- Skin erythema and ulceration/necrosis:
  - Infectious (bacterial, fungal, viral, parasitic)
- Trauma (thermal, chemical burn, cagemate aggression, etc.)

INITIAL DATABASE

- A thorough history and the physical examination findings
  - Treatment of the patient with parenteral vitamin A within weeks or months is a critical piece of historical information.
- Tissue biopsy of skin lesions performed to look for other primary causes or to evaluate for secondary bacterial or fungal involvement may be useful.
- Culture and sensitivity can be used in cases with suspected secondary microbial invasion, and to assist in choosing the most appropriate antimicrobial therapy.

TREATMENT

THERAPEUTIC GOALS

- Provide support in the form of heat and hydration as needed.
- Address acute life-threatening presentations.
- Treat secondary conditions associated with hypervitaminosis A with aggressive wound management, including systemic antimicrobials and topical treatment.
- Continue treatment over weeks to months until wounds have healed.

ACUTE GENERAL TREATMENT

- Initially, provide supportive care.
- In cases with severe skin sloughing, aggressive fluid therapy (10-30 mL/kg/d) is usually indicated.
- Skin damage should be protected with gentle hydrotherapy and warm-water soaks, followed by 1% silver sulfadiazine cream.
- Systemic antimicrobials may be indicated if secondary infections are associated with sloughing skin.
- Pain management may be initiated for these patients:
  - Morphine:
    - Chelonians: 1.5 mg/kg
    - Lizards: 10 mg/kg
  - Meloxicam (Metacam): 0.2-0.3 mg/kg PO, IM q 24 h
- Often reptile patients with severe skin damage will not eat voluntarily and may require assist feeding, syringe feeding, or tube feeding, or placement of an esophagostomy/pharyngostomy tube until they can eat voluntarily.

CHRONIC TREATMENT

- Long-term wound management and supportive care with analgesia, fluid support, and alimentation will be important for success.
- See Hypovitaminosis A for safe protocols for parenteral treatment of true hypovitaminosis cases and for long-term dietary recommendations for vitamin A and beta carotene.

DRUG INTERACTIONS

In mammals, glucocorticoids have been shown to prolong elevated circulating retinyl and retinol esters and thus are contraindicated in treating cases of hypervitaminosis A.

POSSIBLE COMPLICATIONS

Owner compliance for long-term treatment and follow-up visits may be challenging because healing for these severe skin lesions may take months.

RECOMMENDED MONITORING

Skin lesions may take months to heal, and frequent rechecks will allow the clinician to monitor progress and change treatment protocols as necessary.

PROGNOSIS AND OUTCOME

- The prognosis for skin lesions is fair to good unless large areas of sloughing occur.
- Other variables that will affect the prognosis include the dose and form (water soluble more toxic than fat soluble) of parenteral vitamin A given, the number of doses given, and the general health of the reptile before treatment.
- High and/or multiple doses of parenteral vitamin A can be lethal.

PEARLS & CONSIDERATIONS

COMMENTS

- Oral dosing may be safer than parenteral treatment in avoiding vitamin A intoxication.
- In suspected cases of hypovitaminosis A, the author has had clinical success when using fat-soluble vitamin A preparations orally in lizards and chelonians.

PREVENTION

- Clinicians should avoid the tendency to treat tortoises (and other chelonians) with parenteral vitamin A unless the diet and physical examination reveal true evidence of a deficiency.

CLIENT EDUCATION

- Clients should be educated about the possible side effects of overdosing reptiles with fat-soluble vitamins.
- Clients should be made aware of how easy it is to actually oversupplement companion reptiles with fat-soluble vitamins.

SUGGESTED READINGS

Boyer TH: Hypovitaminosis A and hypervitaminosis A. In Mader DR, editor: Reptile medicine and surgery, St Louis, 2006, Elsevier, pp 831–835.

Donoghue S: Nutrition. In Mader DR, editor: Reptile medicine and surgery, St Louis, 2006, Elsevier, pp 251–298.

Frye FL: Biomedical and surgical aspects of captive reptile husbandry, ed 2, Melbourne, FL, 1991, Krieger Publishing.

CROSS-REFERENCES TO OTHER SECTIONS

Bacterial Dermatitis
Hypovitaminosis A
Liver Disease
Renal Disease

AUTHOR & EDITOR: **SCOTT J. STAHL**

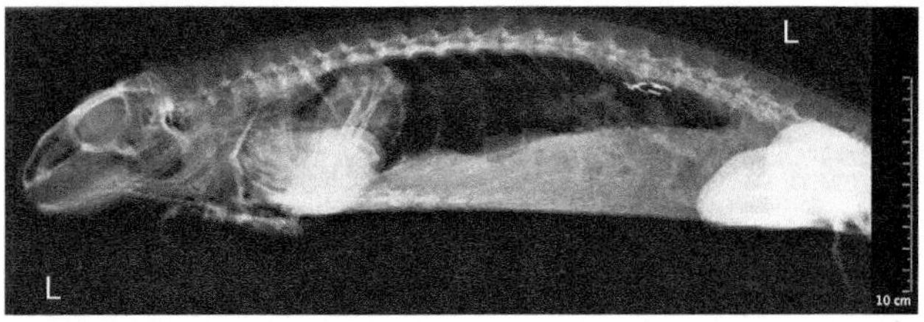

Hypervitaminosis A Severe soft tissue calcification due to hypervitaminosis D. Note the calcified aorta. Usually, these cases are seen in advanced renal failure. *(Photo courtesy Jörg Mayer, The University of Georgia, Athens.)*

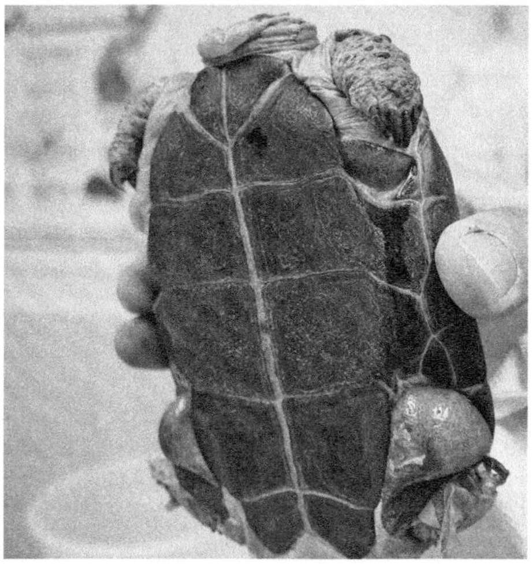

Hypervitaminosis A Iatrogenic hypervitaminosis A due to an injection of vitamin A. Note the skin sloughing. These lesions need to be treated like burn wounds. *(Photo courtesy Jörg Mayer, The University of Georgia, Athens.)*

REPTILES

Hypovitaminosis A

Client Education Sheet Available on Website

BASIC INFORMATION

DEFINITION

Hypovitaminosis A is a clinical condition of reptiles that results from a diet low or lacking in beta carotene (herbivores) and/or preformed vitamin A (carnivores and omnivores).

EPIDEMIOLOGY

SPECIES, AGE, SEX

- Most commonly seen in:
  - Aquatic turtles
  - Box turtles (*Terrapene* spp.)
  - Leopard geckos (*Eublepharis macularius*)
  - Fat-tailed geckos (*Hemitheconyx caudicinctus*)
  - Old World chameleons
  - Anolis lizards
  - Crocodilians
  - Reproductively active female lizards and chelonians
  - Young reptiles
    - Higher demands for vitamin A with growth
- Uncommon in snakes (fed whole prey items such as rodents)

RISK FACTORS Inappropriate diet and husbandry

ASSOCIATED CONDITIONS AND DISORDERS Often linked to aural abscesses in the American box turtle (*Terrapene* spp.)

CLINICAL PRESENTATION

HISTORY, CHIEF COMPLAINT

- Historical information about diet usually involves poor-quality diets low in beta carotene and vitamin A.
- Multivitamin supplements utilized are often lacking preformed vitamin A.
- Anorexia
- Poor growth
- Weight loss
- Lethargy
- Nasal exudates
- Wheezing
- Congestion
- Open-mouth breathing
- Stomatitis, problems with closure of the mouth, discharge
- Lesions on tongue
- Eye problems, swollen eyelids, with or without discharge
- Shedding problems
- Hemipenal swellings
- Dystocia

PHYSICAL EXAM FINDINGS

- Unilateral or bilateral palpebral edema, blepharitis, and conjunctivitis with reduced or loss of vision
- In chronic blepharedema, cases may show bilateral or unilateral white to yellow semi-solid or solid cellular debris filling the conjunctival sac.
- Blindness (post-hibernation blindness in tortoises [*Testudo graeca, T. hermanii*]) from retinal damage
- A clear or purulent nasal discharge may be present, sometimes blocking the nares.
- Increased mucus/discharge is present in the oral cavity, glottis, and trachea.
- Stridor and wheezing are evident from the trachea and the lower respiratory tract.
- Dysecdysis is present and canker material is present in or along the oral cavity.
- Thickened lips, ulcerative cheilitis/stomatitis
- Ulcerations and plaques on tongue
- Inguinal and axillary and gular edema
- Associated with renal disease secondary to vitamin A deficiency
- Swellings, unilateral or bilateral, associated with the hemipenes; retained hemipenal plugs with possible secondary hemipenal abscesses (see Paraphimosis)
- Retained ova

ETIOLOGY AND PATHOPHYSIOLOGY

- Hypovitaminosis A occurs in reptiles fed a diet that is deficient in vitamin A.
- Chelonians seem to be the most susceptible, but it has been seen increasingly in lizards, primarily insectivorous lizards (chameleons and geckos), and crocodilians.
- It is uncommon in captive snakes, which typically are fed a diet of rodents.
- All reptiles need a dietary source of vitamin A. Two forms of vitamin A are available:
  - Animal-based retinol esters (preformed vitamin A):
    - Retinyl acetate
    - Retinyl palmitate
  - Plant-based precursors:
    - Beta carotenes
  - Herbivores are generally efficient in converting beta carotene to vitamin A.

- Carnivores and many turtles and box turtles are less capable of converting beta carotene to vitamin A.
  - Require animal-based retinol esters in the diet
- Nutritional analysis of crickets generally finds them to be low in vitamin A (less than 1 IU /g as fed).
- Vitamin A deficiency is characterized by multifocal squamous metaplasia and hyperkeratosis of epithelium.
- Squamous metaplasia results in changes in ocular and periocular tissues, the respiratory system, the oral cavity, the skin, and all tissues containing epithelium.
- The compromised epithelial barriers of these systems often allow secondary invasion with opportunistic pathogens such as Gram-negative bacteria.
- Respiratory disease, stomatitis/chelitis, dysecdysis, and dermatitis often result from these changes to the epithelium.
- Changes associated with ocular and periocular tissues are one of the most common clinical presentations for hypovitaminosis A. Edema of these structures may affect vision.
- Specifically, inflammation and infection of the periocular anteromedial Harderian gland and the posterolateral lacrimal gland result in dramatic swelling of the eyelids. The eyelids become swollen, trapping cellular debris in the conjunctival sac and allowing secondary microbial invasion.
- Systemic metabolic disease may occur in severe chronic cases of hypovitaminosis A due to epithelial atrophy and necrosis. Cellular debris accumulates and fills spaces between cells, attracting large numbers of granulocytes. Ducts in the pancreas, kidney, and other organs become blocked with desquamated debris.

DIAGNOSIS

DIFFERENTIAL DIAGNOSIS

- Ocular lesions (blepharitis, blepharedema):
  - Infectious, primary or secondary (bacterial, fungal, viral, parasitic)
  - Trauma
  - Foreign bodies
  - Allergy
- Respiratory disease/stomatitis:
  - Infectious, primary or secondary (bacterial, fungal, viral, parasitic)
  - Toxic, trauma, neoplasia
  - Other husbandry related
  - See Respiratory (Lower) Tract Disease/Pneumonia, and Stomatitis, Bacterial.
- Dysecdysis/dermatitis:
  - Infectious, primary or secondary (bacterial, fungal, viral, parasitic)
  - Other husbandry related
  - See Dysecdysis, and Bacterial Dermatitis
- Dystocia:
  - Other nutrition (calcium) or husbandry related
  - Infectious
  - Mechanical
  - See Dystocia.
- Hemipenal abscesses/plugs:
  - Trauma
  - Excessive breeding
  - Other husbandry related
  - See Abscesses.

INITIAL DATABASE

- A thorough historical evaluation of the diet will often reveal vitamin A–deficient intake.
- Careful scrutiny of vitamin/mineral supplements may be necessary to determine which form of vitamin A is being supplemented.

ADVANCED OR CONFIRMATORY TESTING

- For ocular lesions, exfoliative cytologic examination can be performed to look for desquamated keratocytes, granulocytes, and secondary microbial organisms.
- Biopsy of lesions (when possible) and histopathologic examination can be performed in suspicious cases to look for squamous metaplasia and hyperkeratosis.
- Histopathologic examination and special stains are also useful to rule out primary or secondary infectious organisms.
- Culture and sensitivity can then be used to identify secondary bacterial involvement and to determine appropriate antimicrobial treatment choices.
- Vitamin A assays:
  - Liver:
    - Normal liver vitamin A levels in monitor lizards and snakes were found to be greater than 1000 IU/g liver.
    - Values considered to be normal in three Herman's tortoises (*Testudo hermanni*) were 10, 30, and 80 IU/g liver.
    - Guidelines for other animal species are 500 to 1000 IU/g liver.
    - Requires surgery or endoscopy to obtain liver biopsy; thus may not be practical or feasible (small size) in some patients
  - Blood sampling:
    - Vitamin A levels cannot be evaluated with blood sampling, but retinol values can be used as an assessment of vitamin A levels.
    - Turtles have mean plasma retinol values ranging from 0.04-0.6 μm/mL.

TREATMENT

THERAPEUTIC GOALS

- Provide support for the presenting patient in the form of heat and hydration as needed
- Address acute life-threatening presentations
- Provide acute treatment with parenteral or oral preformed vitamin A
- Treat secondary conditions associated with hypovitaminosis A such as secondary bacterial infections (conjunctivitis, respiratory disease, stomatitis, etc.)
- Continue treatment over weeks to months to correct deficiencies of vitamin A
- Correct long-term dietary deficiencies of vitamin A by changing and/or supplementing diet
- Educate the owner on how to prevent deficiencies of vitamin A

ACUTE GENERAL TREATMENT

- Supportive care:
  - The patient should be warmed to appropriate physiologic temperatures, hydration status assessed, and fluid therapy (10-30 mL/kg/d) initiated if necessary.
  - Vitamin A:
    - Water-soluble forms of vitamin A such as Aquasol A (50,000 IU/mL can be used; however, the emulsified/oil-based forms have a greater ability to be stored by the reptile liver and are likely a better choice for acute treatment.
    - Oral dosing may be safer than parenteral treatment in avoiding vitamin A intoxication.
- Initiate vitamin A therapy:
  - Aquatic turtles: 200-300 IU/kg body weight (BW)
  - Box turtles: parenterally 1000-2000 IU/kg BW weekly for 2-6 doses
  - Lizards: orally 2000 IU/30 g BW every 7 days for 2 doses (fat-soluble forms can be used)
  - Subcutaneous injections of fat-soluble vitamin A (500-5000 IU/kg BW for 1 or 2 treatments every 14 days)
  - Clinical improvement may take 2-4 weeks or longer depending on severity.
  - In cases of chronic blepharitis and blepharedema with subsequent cellular debris in the conjunctival sac, warm water and gentle manipulation with a blunt probe will allow removal of this semi-solid or solid material.
  - Saline can then be used to gently flush the conjunctiva. Ophthalmic antimicrobial ointment or drops can be dispensed for the owner to apply

1-2 times daily if secondary bacterial involvement is suspected.
- Patients with respiratory signs, stomatitis, and/or dysecdysis/dermatitis may need to be treated with systemic antimicrobials.
- For patients with dysecdysis, dermatitis and conjunctivitis warm water soaks can be used to soften adhered shedding skin and to gently encourage removal of retained skin and crusts.
- Often reptile patients that are avisual owing to severe ocular involvement will not eat on their own and may require assist feeding, syringe feeding, tube feeding, or placement of an esophagostomy/pharyngostomy tube until they can eat voluntarily.

CHRONIC TREATMENT

- Change the diet to provide more preformed vitamin A (and/or beta carotene for herbivorous reptiles).
- General recommendations for domestic species that can provide a starting point for dietary supplementation are 2.5-15 IU/g diet on a dry matter basis.
- Specific recommendations for dietary levels of preformed vitamin A include:
  - Aquatic turtles: 2-8 IU/g diet DM
  - Box turtles: 3-6 IU/g diet DM
  - Chameleons: dusts containing up to 60 IU/g DM or 5-9 IU/g of cricket DM
- Prevention for herbivorous and omnivorous reptile species includes increasing foods in the diet with high levels of beta carotene, including dark green leafy vegetables and orange and yellow vegetables (sweet potato, carrots, squash, melon, papaya, etc.).
- For insectivores, feed insects an adequate vitamin A diet, such as vegetables or a complete invertebrate or mammalian ration. Dust insects weekly or every other week with a multivitamin that provides adequate levels of preformed vitamin A.
- For more carnivorous reptiles, feed whole food items such as rodents, whole fish, liver, and commercial pelleted diets (depending on formulation and inclusion of preformed vitamin A).
- For omnivorous reptiles such as box turtles and adult aquatic turtles, a combination of the above recommendations is recommended.

DRUG INTERACTIONS

- Caution must be used not to overdose the reptile patient with vitamin A during treatment.
- Dangerous levels may be reached when 100 times the recommended intake is given. This is especially dangerous when parenteral vitamin A is used. (see Hypervitaminosis A)

POSSIBLE COMPLICATIONS

Adequate intakes of other nutrients such as vitamin E, zinc, and protein are important in the metabolism of retinols; therefore these nutrients must also be addressed when a reptile that is suspected to have a vitamin A deficiency is treated.

RECOMMENDED MONITORING

- Follow-up visits for the first 2-3 weeks of treatment are important, especially in cases of severe conjunctivitis, stomatitis, and respiratory disease.
- Continued supportive care may be necessary if vision is impaired because often these patients are not feeding.

PROGNOSIS AND OUTCOME

- Prognosis is good with early diagnosis, aggressive therapy, and appropriate husbandry changes.
- If evidence of metabolic disease such as renal disease (edema) and gout are present, the prognosis is more guarded. (see Renal Disease)

PEARLS & CONSIDERATIONS

PREVENTION

- Ensuring that clients with juvenile reptiles get proper dietary information would prevent many cases.
- Encouraging clients to bring juvenile reptiles in for "new pet" examinations provides a great opportunity to review husbandry and to develop a relationship of trust by which the client will rely on your clinic for future care information.

CLIENT EDUCATION

Educating clients about the proper diet necessary for specific reptile species presented is critical.

SUGGESTED READINGS

Ariel E, et al: Concurrent gout and suspected hypovitaminosis A in crocodile hatchlings, Aust Vet J 75:257–259, 1997.

Boyer TH: Hypovitaminosis A and hypervitaminosis A. In Mader DR, editor: Reptile medicine and surgery, St Louis, 2006, Elsevier, pp 831–835.

Dierenfield ES, et al: Circulating alphatocopherol and retinol concentrations in free ranging and zoo turtles and tortoises, Columbus, OH, 1999, Proc Am Assoc Zoo Vet.

Donoghue S: Nutrition. In Mader DR, editor: Reptile medicine and surgery, St Louis, 2006, Elsevier, pp 251–298.

Elkan E, Zwart P: The ocular disease of young terrapins caused by vitamin A deficiency, Pathol Vet 4:201, 1967.

Finke MD: Complete nutrient composition of commercially raised invertebrates used as a food for insectivores, Zoo Biol 21:269, 2002.

Lawton MPC, Stoakes LC: Post hibernation blindness in tortoises, Orlando, 1989, Third International Colloquium on the Pathology of Reptiles and Amphibians.

Stahl SJ: Captive management, breeding and common medical problems of the veiled chameleon *(Chamaeleo calyptratus)*, Houston, 1997, Proc Assoc Rept Amphib Vet, p 29.

CROSS-REFERENCES TO OTHER SECTIONS

Abscesses
Bacterial Dermatitis
CANV
Dysecdysis
Dystocia
Hypervitaminosis A
Paraphimosis
Renal Disease
Respiratory (Lower) Tract Disease/Pneumonia
Stomatitis, Bacterial

AUTHOR & EDITOR: **SCOTT J. STAHL**

Inclusion Body Disease of Snakes

Client Education Sheet Available on Website

BASIC INFORMATION

DEFINITION

The disease is thought to be due to a retro virus. It is observed in many boid snakes and it is characterized by signs of CNS disease which often leads to mortality. Inclusion bodies in most tissues, especially the brain can be observed at necropsy.

SYNONYM

IBD

EPIDEMIOLOGY

SPECIES, AGE, SEX

- This disease is primarily seen in Henophidia (boas, pythons, and related snake families).
- An identical syndrome has also been identified in palm vipers (*Bothriechis marchi*).
- Age or sex predisposition is not well understood.

RISK FACTORS

- Mixed species collections seem to be at higher risk.
- Collections infested with snake mites (*Ophionyssus natricis*) also seem to be at higher risk, suggesting that these mites may potentially play a role as vectors.

CONTAGION AND ZOONOSIS Because collections with widespread IBD problems often have snake mite problems, these mites may potentially play a role as vectors.

GEOGRAPHY AND SEASONALITY The impact of geographic and seasonal factors on IBD is not well understood.

ASSOCIATED CONDITIONS AND DISORDERS Conditions commonly associated with IBD include immune suppression leading to secondary infection, neurologic abnormalities such as opisthotonos, and round cell tumors.

CLINICAL PRESENTATION

HISTORY, CHIEF COMPLAINT

- The history associated with IBD cases often includes collections with mixed species and poor quarantine.
- *Ophionyssus* spp. mites may be present in the collection.
- Secondary infections due to immune suppression, such as stomatitis, gastritis, or pneumonia, may lead to owner concerns about oral swelling, regurgitation, or dyspnea.
- Neurologic dysfunction may lead to owner concerns of opisthotonos, impaired righting, or decreased mentation.

PHYSICAL EXAM FINDINGS Physical examination findings may include stomatitis, dyspnea, poor body condition, decreased mentation, opisthotonos, and impaired righting.

ETIOLOGY AND PATHOPHYSIOLOGY

- The cause of IBD is unknown.
- Although retroviruses have been suggested as potential causative agents, causality remains to be demonstrated.

DIAGNOSIS

DIFFERENTIAL DIAGNOSIS

- The most common cause of immune suppression in snakes is poor husbandry, often related to improper thermal gradient, humidity, hygiene, or excessive handling.
- Concurrent infection may lead to immune suppression.
- Other common differentials for neurologic dysfunction include trauma, exposure to temperature extremes (heat prostration, etc.), toxic exposure (e.g., ectoparasite treatment with organophosphates), yolk embolism, bacterial or fungal meningoencephalitis, paramyxovirus, reovirus, and adenovirus.

INITIAL DATABASE

- A thorough history, physical examination, complete blood count, plasma chemistry, and radiographs form the basic database.
- Occasionally, inclusions may be seen in peripheral lymphocytes, although this is a very insensitive test.

ADVANCED OR CONFIRMATORY TESTING

- Tissue biopsies may reveal the presence of eosinophilic inclusions, which may be present in large numbers in some cases.
- Liver and esophageal tonsils are good sites for antemortem sample collection.
- Electron microscopic examination of inclusions is needed to ensure that they are consistent with what is seen in this syndrome.
- False-negative biopsy results are possible.

TREATMENT

THERAPEUTIC GOALS

- The goal of treatment is eradication of the disease from a collection.
- Treatment of individual animals is unrewarding.

ACUTE GENERAL TREATMENT

- Confirmed positive animals should be humanely euthanized, and complete necropsies should be performed.
- Mites should be eradicated from the collection.

RECOMMENDED MONITORING

- Biosecurity in the collection should be improved, and no snakes should enter or leave the collection.
- Snakes currently in the collection should be tested by liver and/or esophageal tonsil biopsy and reevaluated after a period of 6 months to a year.
- A negative result on biopsy does not conclusively mean that the snake is free of IBD.

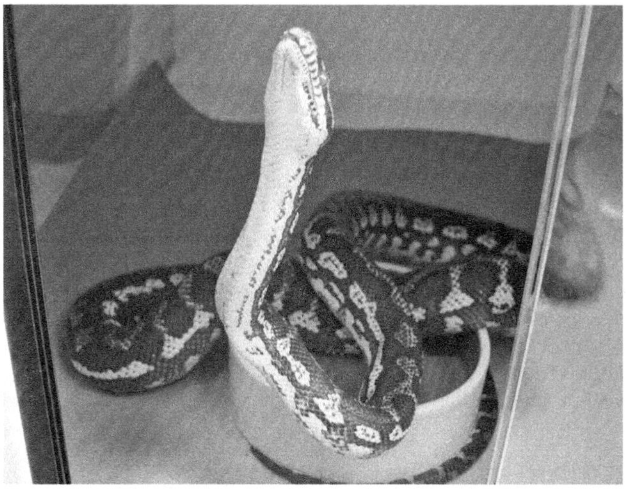

Inclusion Body Disease of Snakes Stargazing is a common clinical sign with inclusion body disease; a liver or kidney biopsy should be scheduled. *(Photo courtesy Jörg Mayer, The University of Georgia, Athens.)*

PROGNOSIS AND OUTCOME

The prognosis for snakes with confirmed IBD is poor.

PEARLS & CONSIDERATIONS

PREVENTION

Maintenance of a closed group, testing of populations, strict quarantine, mite prevention, and stringent biosecurity practices are the most effective means of prevention.

SUGGESTED READINGS

Fleming GJ, et al: Cytoplasmic inclusions in corn snakes, *Elaphe guttata*, resembling inclusion body disease of boid snakes, J Herpetol Med Surg 13:18–22, 2003.

Raymond JT, et al: A disease resembling inclusion body disease of boid snakes in captive palm vipers (*Bothriechis marchi*), J Vet Diagn Invest 13:82–86, 2001.

Schumacher J, et al: Inclusion body disease of boid snakes, J Zoo Wildl Med 25:511–524, 1994.

CROSS-REFERENCES TO OTHER SECTIONS

Adenovirus
Ectoparasites
Paramyxovirus
Reovirus

AUTHOR: **JAMES F.X. WELLEHAN, JR.**

EDITOR: **SCOTT J. STAHL**

REPTILES

Iridovirus Infection

BASIC INFORMATION

DEFINITION

Iridoviruses are icosahedral, enveloped DNA viruses ranging in size from 120-300 nm.

SYNONYMS

Ranavirus, erythrocytic virus, *Toddia*, *Pirhemocyton*

EPIDEMIOLOGY

SPECIES, AGE, SEX

- Many reptile species can be infected with iridoviruses.
- Iridoviral disease appears to be most common in box turtles.
- Evidence indicates that insect iridoviruses in the genus *Iridovirus* can infect lizards, and *Ranavirus* from frogs appears to infect tortoises.
- Young, geriatric, and immune suppressed animals appear to be at greatest risk for disease.
- No sex predilections are known.

RISK FACTORS

- Stressed animals appear to be more likely to develop clinical disease.
- Iridoviral disease also appears to be temperature dependent.

CONTAGION AND ZOONOSIS

- These viruses are very stable in the environment.
- Disinfectants effective against unenveloped viruses may be expected to be effective against iridoviruses.
- No zoonotic risk is known for any reptile iridovirus.

GEOGRAPHY AND SEASONALITY Iridoviral disease appears to be more common in the spring.

CLINICAL PRESENTATION

DISEASE FORMS/SUBTYPES

- Splenitis, bone marrow suppression, and glossitis are the most common presentations of iridoviral disease due to members of the genus *Ranavirus*.
- Anemia with cytoplasmic erythrocytic inclusions is seen with erythrocytic iridoviruses.

HISTORY, CHIEF COMPLAINT Common complaints on presentation for iridoviral disease include marked depression, glossitis, and high death rates.

PHYSICAL EXAM FINDINGS Physical exam findings often include glossitis and marked depression.

ETIOLOGY AND PATHOPHYSIOLOGY

- Two recognized genera of iridoviruses infect reptiles:
  - Members of the genus *Ranavirus* have been found associated with disease in squamates and chelonians.
  - Members of the genus *Iridovirus* have been found in lizards with nonspecific signs.
- Erythrocytic iridoviruses were previously mistakenly identified as protozoal hemoparasites and were formerly named *Toddia* spp. and *Pirhemocyton* spp.

DIAGNOSIS

DIFFERENTIAL DIAGNOSIS

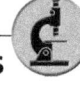

- Herpesviral disease in tortoises is very similar to disease seen with *Ranavirus* infection.
- A large number of differentials are known for nonspecific signs and deaths associated with iridoviruses.

INITIAL DATABASE

A thorough history, physical examination, complete blood count, plasma chemistry, and radiographs form the basic database.

ADVANCED OR CONFIRMATORY TESTING

- Nested polymerase chain reaction (PCR) with product sequence analysis is available from the University of Florida for all iridoviruses.
- Oral swabs are generally the antemortem sample of choice for *Ranavirus* infection.
- Spleen and bone marrow are the best postmortem samples.
- Blood is the sample of choice (any sterile container) for erythrocytic iridoviruses but generally is not a good choice for *Ranavirus* infection.
- Histologic findings of fibrous splenitis are common with *Ranavirus* disease.
- Intracytoplasmic inclusions may be seen, especially in bone marrow, but are not always present.
- Iridoviruses are large viruses that are easily identified on electron microscopy.
- With erythrocytic iridoviruses, cytoplasmic inclusions are often present in significant numbers of mature erythrocytes and may also be seen in leukocytes, endothelial cells, and hepatocytes.

TREATMENT

ACUTE GENERAL TREATMENT

- Supportive care, addressing husbandry deficiencies, and identifying and treating secondary bacterial and fungal infections are the most important aspects of treating iridoviral disease.
- In vitro data suggest that acyclovir is not likely to be useful.
- Increasing the temperature of the warm end of the thermal gradient allows the animal to choose a fever; this appears to help clinically.

CHRONIC TREATMENT

It is not known whether iridoviruses are persistent in reptiles. As large DNA viruses, it is certainly plausible.

PROGNOSIS AND OUTCOME

- The prognosis for animals with *Ranavirus* disease is guarded.
- Animals infected with erythrocytic iridoviruses generally recover well with fluid therapy (10-30 mL/kg q 24 h) supportive care.

PEARLS & CONSIDERATIONS

COMMENTS

- Ranavirus disease is a significant concern in chelonians and should be on the differential list of any acutely debilitated animal.
- Because clinical disease appears to be temperature dependent, raising temperatures can be very clinically useful.

PREVENTION

Maintenance of a closed group, testing of populations, testing during quarantine, and stringent biosecurity practices are the most effective means of prevention.

SUGGESTED READING

De Voe R, et al: Ranavirus-associated morbidity and mortality in a group of captive eastern box turtles (*Terrapene carolina carolina*), J Zoo Wildl Med 35:534–543, 2004.

Hyatt AD, et al: First identification of a ranavirus from green pythons (*Chondropython viridis*). J Wildl Dis 38:239–252, 2002.

Johnson AJ, et al: Experimental transmission and induction of ranaviral disease in Western Ornate box turtles (*Terrapene ornata ornata*) and red-eared sliders (*Trachemys scripta elegans*), Vet Pathol 44:285–297, 2007.

Johnsrude JD, et al: Intraerythrocytic inclusions associated with iridoviral infection in a fer de lance (*Bothrops moojeni*) snake, Vet Pathol 34:235–238, 1997.

Marschang RE, et al: Isolation and characterization of an iridovirus from Hermann's tortoises (*Testudo hermanni*), Arch Virol 144: 1909–1922, 1999.

Marschang RE, et al: Isolation of a ranavirus from a gecko (*Uroplatus fimbriatus*), J Zoo Wildl Med 36:295–300, 2005.

Rojas S, et al: Influence of temperature on *Ranavirus* infection in larval salamanders *Ambystoma tigrinum*, Dis Aquat Organ 63:95–100, 2005.

CROSS-REFERENCES TO OTHER CHAPTERS

Chlamydiophilosis
Herpesvirus
Hypovitaminosis A
Mycoplasma
Reovirus
Respiratory (lower) infection/Pneumonia
Stomatitis

AUTHOR: **JAMES F.X. WELLEHAN, JR.**

EDITOR: **SCOTT J. STAHL**

REPTILES

Liver Disease

BASIC INFORMATION

DEFINITION

Any disease process that adversely affects the liver

SYNONYMS

Hepatic disease, hepatosis, hepatitis

EPIDEMIOLOGY

SPECIES, AGE, SEX None reported

RISK FACTORS

- Malnutrition
- Poor husbandry
- Unhygienic conditions

CONTAGION AND ZOONOSIS Many possible infectious causes, including bacteria, fungi, viruses, and parasites

ASSOCIATED CONDITIONS AND DISORDERS

- Anorexia, depression
- Regurgitation, vomiting
- Biliverdinuria

CLINICAL PRESENTATION

DISEASE FORMS/SUBTYPES

- Bacterial hepatitis
- Viral hepatitis
- Mycotic hepatitis
- Parasitic hepatitis
- Liver neoplasia
- Hepatic lipidosis and hepatoses

HISTORY, CHIEF COMPLAINT

- Owners and keepers should be encouraged to maintain accurate records because this may help in identifying the subtle and often gradual reduction in appetite, activity, fecundity, and fertility; weight gain or gradual weight loss; hibernation problems, including post-hibernation anorexia; and changes in fecal character and color.
- However, it may be only during episodes of increased physiologic demand (e.g., hibernation, breeding, concurrent disease) that the underlying liver disease becomes clinically apparent.
- Unfortunately, many caretakers miss these early signs of disease. As a result, veterinary attention is sought only once the animal has deteriorated to a life-threatening condition.

PHYSICAL EXAM FINDINGS

- In chronic cases, most affected reptiles are in poor body condition and are flaccid, weak, and cachectic.
- The bodyweight (mass) is usually below normal, although in cases of ascites, weight may be artificially maintained or even increased.
- Reptiles with acute liver disease usually present in good body condition but with sudden-onset depression and anorexia.
- If several animals are affected simultaneously, a common cause is most likely, and infection or intoxication should be primarily considered.
- Diarrhea is common in acute cases, and if the urates are pigmented yellow-green, excretion of biliverdin may indicate severe liver compromise and bile stasis.
- Regurgitation is considered to be a poor sign in chelonians and lizards.
- Severely affected animals usually will be depressed, lethargic, and weak; mucous membranes may be pale, hyperemic, or icteric.

ETIOLOGY AND PATHOPHYSIOLOGY

- Many causes for liver disease have been identified, and it is important to remember that "liver disease" is not a diagnosis!
- Can be classified as acute or chronic, inflammatory (hepatitis) or degenerative (hepatosis)
- Acute hepatitis (an inflammatory change) is often associated with infectious agents.
- Bacterial, viral, mycotic, and parasitic hepatitis

- Metabolic changes associated with liver pathology include hepatic lipidosis (see Hepatic Lipidosis) and hepatosis.
- Acute hepatosis (degenerative liver disease) is much less common:
  - Ivermectin-induced hepatic lipidosis in chelonia is well documented.
- Primary neoplasia and metastatic invasion
- In many species, the lobule structure is replaced by cords of hepatocytes, and a variable degree of melanin pigmentation is usually present.

DIAGNOSIS

DIFFERENTIAL DIAGNOSIS

- Any disease that causes anorexia or metabolic derangement
- Septicemia
- Sepsis

INITIAL DATABASE

- A full clinicopathologic investigation is essential to differentiate accurately between acute and chronic liver disease. It is important that pretreatment blood samples are collected before fluid therapy and other supportive measures are initiated.
- Hypoalbuminemia can result in production of an acellular, low-protein, coelomic transudate.
- In cases of chronic hepatopathy, anemia may be evident and can mask serious fluid deficits.
- Acute inflammation or necrosis of the liver usually will result in a dramatic heterophilia and monocytosis (including azurophilia, in many species).
- Chronic bacterial hepatitis (e.g., abscess) usually will cause only minor elevations of the total white blood cell count.
- Eosinophilia may be expected in cases of parasitic disease.
- Hepatocellular damage as noted in mammals may lead to elevations of several enzymes, including AST (aspartate aminotransferase), GGT (gamma-glutamyltransferase), ALP (alkaline phosphatase), ALT (alanine aminotransferase), and LDH (lactate dehydrogenase).
  - Assessment of CPK (creatinine phosphokinase) can be helpful in distinguishing between muscle and nonmuscle sources.
  - In reptiles, tissue distribution of many of these enzymes appears more widespread, and tissue values of GGT may be very low.
  - In cases of chronic hepatopathy with little active damage, enzyme levels may remain normal.
- Hyperglycemia has been associated with some case of hepatic disease (see Hyperglycemia.
- The radiographic hepatic shadow is often appreciable in horizontal beam radiographs of lizards, less so in snakes, and least of all in chelonia, because of the superimposition of the shell.
- Gross hepatomegaly or microhepatica may be discernible in some lizards and snakes.
- Ultrasonography has proved useful for assessment of hepatic size and shape in many reptiles, including chelonia.

ADVANCED OR CONFIRMATORY TESTING

- Bile acids (3-alpha-hydroxy bile acids) have been investigated only in green iguanas to date.
  - Iguanas fasted for 48 hours have mean resting bile acid values of 7.5 μmol/L, which increase to 33 μmol/L for at least 8 hours after feeding.
  - Unpublished observations by the author suggest that values greater than 60 μmol/L are often indicative of hepatic dysfunction.
- Ultrasound-guided Tru-Cut biopsies of the liver parenchyma are possible.
- Endoscopic biopsy is generally safer and might be more precise:
  - Endoscopy requires general anesthesia but permits examination and appreciation of the size, color, shape, and contours of the liver, and allows the collection of multiple tissue biopsy specimens under direct visual control.

TREATMENT

THERAPEUTIC GOALS

- Although specific therapy will depend upon a precise diagnosis, much can be done in general to support a reptile with hepatic dysfunction—whether infectious or noninfectious.
- Medical stabilization using fluid therapy (10-30 mL/kg/d) is essential, and provision of the species-specific preferred optimum temperature zone (within which the reptile can select a preferred body temperature) can be instrumental in effecting improvement.

ACUTE GENERAL TREATMENT

- Fluid and nutritional support: The route of therapy will be directed by the animal's condition at the time of presentation.
- Mild to moderate cases are usually anorectic on presentation; in these cases, oral fluids may be appropriate.
- Reptiles with severe disease will often require intracoelomic, intravenous, or intraosseous infusion. Other medications may be employed at the clinician's discretion, but care should be taken not to invalidate future diagnostic investigations.
- For example, blood samples should be collected before fluid therapy, and antibiotic medication should be delayed until after liver biopsy and culture.

CHRONIC TREATMENT

- In many instances, chronic disease may be present that may take months, if not years, to reverse:
  - Means of providing long-term fluid and nutritional support should be explored.
  - Most lizards and snakes are easily stomach-tubed; however, most chelonia and some squamates are better served by placement of an esophagostomy tube under local and/or light general anesthesia.
- In addition to long-term fluid and nutritional support, the esophagostomy tube can be used to deliver oral medication.
- The importance of fluid and nutritional support cannot be overemphasized.
- When providing nutritional support, it is important to consider:
  - The patient's energy and nutritional requirements:
    - The patient's natural dietary preference (e.g., herbivorous, omnivorous, carnivorous), in an attempt to use natural foods in preference to artificial substitutes
    - General multivitamin supplements have been suggested for animals with liver disease.
    - Methionine and choline may promote hepatic function, especially in cases of hepatic lipidosis (see Hepatic Lipidosis).
    - Other liver supportive medications that can be empirically used include: Lactulose at 0.5 ml/kg PO q24h or Silymarin (milk thistle) at 50-100 mg/kg PO q 24h. These medications can be mixed together for ease of administration.

RECOMMENDED MONITORING

- Monitor weight and food intake.
- Monitor liver enzymes and fasting bile acids.
- Serial liver ultrasound and endoscopic liver biopsies for repeat histopathology
- Modify management, including diet and exercise.

PROGNOSIS AND OUTCOME

The prognosis depends on diagnosis.

PEARLS & CONSIDERATIONS

COMMENTS

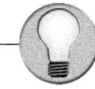

- Biliverdin is the major bile pigment produced by most reptiles because they lack the biliverdin reductase enzyme required to produce bilirubin. However, some snakes do produce bilirubin.
- The gallbladder is located within the liver mass of chelonia and lizards, but in snakes it may appear caudal to, and distinct from, liver.

PREVENTION

Regular health evaluations, including hematology and biochemistry data

CLIENT EDUCATION

Appropriate management (temperature, diet, exercise), including simulation of natural fasting/hibernation periods

SUGGESTED READINGS

Divers SJ: Reptilian liver and gastro-intestinal testing. In Fudge AM, editor: Laboratory medicine: avian and exotic pets, Philadelphia, 2000, WB Saunders, pp 205–209.
Divers SJ, et al: Reptile hepatic lipidosis. Semin Avian Ex Pet Med 9:153–164, 2000.
Hernandez-Divers SJ, et al: Evaluation of an endoscopic liver biopsy technique in green iguanas. J Am Vet Med Assoc 230:1849–1853, 2007.
Hernandez-Divers SJ, et al: Hepatic lipidosis. In Mader DR, editor: Reptile medicine and surgery, ed 2, Philadelphia, 2006, WB Saunders, pp 806–813.
McBride M, et al: Preliminary evaluation of resting and post-prandial bile acid levels in the green iguana (*Iguana iguana*). J Herpetol Med Surg 16:129–134, 2007.

CROSS-REFERENCES TO OTHER SECTIONS

Hepatic Lipidosis
Hyperglycemia

AUTHOR: **STEPHEN J. DIVERS**

EDITOR: **SCOTT J. STAHL**

REPTILES

Mycobacteriosis

BASIC INFORMATION

DEFINITION

Infection with a species of the genus mycobacteria. Mycobacteria are characterized as nonmotile, aerobic or microaerophilic, nonsporulating, slightly curved and slender rod-shaped organisms. In reptiles infections often produce granulomas.

SYNONYM

Mycobacteriosis is sometimes incorrectly referred to by laypeople as *tuberculosis*, a term that is specific for infection with *Mycobacterium tuberculosis*. This should be corrected and clarified.

EPIDEMIOLOGY

SPECIES, AGE, SEX

- Mycobacteriosis is a disease of concern in all vertebrates, including all reptiles.
- Because of the longer time course often seen with mycobacteriosis, diseased animals are more commonly presented as adults.
- No sex predilections are known.

RISK FACTORS

- Immune suppressed animals appear to be at greatest risk for disease.
- Husbandry deficiencies are a common source of immune suppression.

CONTAGION AND ZOONOSIS

- The mycobacterial cell wall is very distinct from that of other bacterial species and protects the organism well.
- Many *Mycobacterium* spp. are very stable in the environment, especially in aquatic or moist environments.
- Disinfectants that are labeled to have mycobactericidal activity should be selected.
- Zoonotic risk varies significantly between different *Mycobacterium* species. Of species reported from natural infections of reptiles, *M. marinum* and *M. ulcerans* present the most significant zoonotic risk.
- Clinical signs of both of these species are nonhealing skin ulcers. Other species, such as *M. agri*, *M. confluentis*, *M. hiberniae*, and *M. phlei*, have not been found to cause disease in immune competent humans.
- All *Mycobacterium* spp. should be considered as presenting risk for immune compromised humans.

GEOGRAPHY AND SEASONALITY

Mycobacteriosis is cosmopolitan. Seasonality has not been reported.

ASSOCIATED CONDITIONS AND DISORDERS

- Mycobacteriosis in reptiles is associated with granulomatous disease.
- Granulomas can be found in all tissues; lung, alimentary tract, heart, and spleen are common sites.

CLINICAL PRESENTATION

DISEASE FORMS/SUBTYPES Mycobacteriosis can vary depending on the *Mycobacterium* sp. present and which tissues are affected.

HISTORY, CHIEF COMPLAINT Common complaints on presentation for mycobacterial disease include nonspecific illness, respiratory disease, and weight loss.

PHYSICAL EXAM FINDINGS Physical examination findings are often nonspecific.

ETIOLOGY AND PATHOPHYSIOLOGY

- A large number of mycobacterial species have been identified in reptile disease, including *M. agri*, *M. avium*, *M. chelonae*, *M. confluentis*, *M. fortuitum*, *M. haemophilum*, *M. hiberniae*, *M. intracellulare*, *M. kansasii*, *M. marinum*, *M. neoaurum*, *M. nonchromogenicum*, *M. phlei*, *M. smegmatis*, and *M. ulcerans*.
- Significant differences in drug susceptibility and zoonotic risk have been noted, and any identified mycobacterial infection should be speciated.
- Mycobacteriosis in reptiles is associated with granulomatous disease.
- Granulomas can be found in all tissues; lung, skin, alimentary tract, heart, and spleen are common sites.

DIAGNOSIS

DIFFERENTIAL DIAGNOSIS

Other common causes for granulomatous disease in reptiles include *Chlamydophila pneumoniae* and fungi.

INITIAL DATABASE

- A thorough husbandry history, physical examination, complete blood count, plasma chemistry, and radiographs form a basic database.
- A leukocytosis is often present with mycobacteriosis.

ADVANCED OR CONFIRMATORY TESTING

- Biopsies showing granulomatous disease in reptiles should always be examined with acid-fast stains.

- Many infections have small numbers of acid-fast organisms present, and they may be missed.
- Polymerase chain reaction (PCR) is more sensitive than histology for detection of the presence of mycobacterial organisms.
- PCR and product sequence ID, culture, and sensitivity profiles for fast-growing mycobacteria are available from the University of Florida.
- Culture and PCR are also available from National Jewish Hospital in Denver, Colorado.

TREATMENT

THERAPEUTIC GOAL

If treated, the goal of therapy is eradication of the organism.

CHRONIC TREATMENT

- Before treatment is initiated, the organism should be speciated to determine zoonotic potential and drug susceptibility.
- Euthanasia should be considered for mycobacterial species of significant zoonotic concern.
- Any husbandry deficiencies should be addressed and corrected.
- Zoonotic risks need to be discussed with the owner, and the clinician needs to determine whether the owner understands the risks and expense and is committed to the long-term therapy necessary. If not, euthanasia should be recommended.
- Antibiotic therapy will need to involve multiple drugs over a course of at least 6 months to a year.
- Single-drug therapy or shorter courses are likely to result in treatment failure and antibiotic resistance.

RECOMMENDED MONITORING

- Biopsy specimens of affected tissues and a CBC should be taken after 6 months to a year to determine whether therapy needs to be continued.
- CBCs should be checked every 3 months for several years to look for leukocytosis, which may be a sign of recurrence.

PROGNOSIS AND OUTCOME

The prognosis for animals with mycobacteriosis varies depending on affected tissues and mycobacterial species.

PEARLS & CONSIDERATIONS

COMMENTS

- Mycobacteriosis is probably significantly underdiagnosed in reptiles and should be on the differential list of any ill animal.
- Speciation is crucial; some species are significant zoonotic concerns, whereas others are not.

PREVENTION

Maintenance of a closed group, quarantine, and stringent biosecurity practices are the most effective means of prevention.

CLIENT EDUCATION

- Zoonotic risks need to be discussed with the owner.
- The clinician needs to determine whether the owner understands the risks and the expense involved with long-term therapy before treatment can be considered.

SUGGESTED READINGS

Clark HF, et al: Effect of environmental temperatures on infection with *Mycobacterium marinum* (Balnei) of mice and a number of poikilothermic species, J Bacteriol 86:1057–1069, 1963.

Marcus LC, et al: Experimental infection of anole lizards (*Anolis carolinensis*) with *Mycobacterium ulcerans* by the subcutaneous route, Am J Trop Med Hyg 124:649–655, 1975.

Soldati G, et al: Detection of mycobacteria and chlamydiae in granulomatous inflammation of reptiles: a retrospective study, Vet Pathol 41:388–397, 2004.

CROSS-REFERENCES TO OTHER SECTIONS

Abscesses
Chlamydophila
Dermatomycosis
Nematodiasis
Respiratory (lower) tract Disease

AUTHOR: **JAMES F.X. WELLEHAN, JR.**

EDITOR: **SCOTT J. STAHL**

REPTILES

Mycoplasma

BASIC INFORMATION

DEFINITION

Mycoplasma refers to a genus of bacteria which lack a cell wall and it is currently considered the smallest known cell at about 0.1 micron (μm) in diameter. Infections in reptiles often cause upper respiratory tract signs.

SYNONYM

Mycoplasma agassizii is one of several causes of upper respiratory tract disease (URTD) in tortoises.

EPIDEMIOLOGY

SPECIES, AGE, SEX

- Infection appears to be much more common than significant disease in most species for most *Mycoplasma* spp.
- *M. agassizii* has been shown to be one cause of significant URTD in California desert tortoises (*Gopherus agassizii*) and Florida gopher tortoises (*Gopherus polyphemus*).
- A different species from California desert tortoises, *M. testudineum*, is also associated with URTD, although a causal relationship has not definitively been shown.
- Another species, *M. testudinis*, isolated from the cloaca of Greek tortoises (*Testudo graeca*), has not been associated with disease and is not currently considered a pathogen.
- A different *Mycoplasma* sp., yet unnamed, has been found in association with URTD in eastern box turtles (*Terrapene carolina*).
- *M. crocodyli* is associated with polyarthritis in Nile crocodiles (*Crocodylus niloticus*).
- *M. alligatoris* has been shown to cause pneumonia, polyserositis, and polyarthritis in American alligators (*Alligator mississippiensis*) and broad-nosed caiman (*Caiman latirostris*), but did not cause disease in Siamese crocodiles (*Crocodylus siamensis*).
- *M. iguanae*, isolated from a green iguana (*Iguana iguana*), did not cause lesions in experimentally infected green iguanas.
- *M. insons* is also likely normal flora in green iguanas.

- An unnamed *Mycoplasma* species has been associated with proliferative tracheitis and pneumonia in a Burmese python (*Python molurus bivittatus*). Mycoplasmal disease may be seen at all ages.
- Seroprevalence of *M. agassizii* in Florida gopher tortoises increases with age.
- No sex predilections are known in reptiles.

RISK FACTORS Mixing of species may result in transfer of *Mycoplasma* spp. from one host to another, with potential resultant disease.

CONTAGION AND ZOONOSIS
- *Mycoplasma* organisms lack a cell wall and therefore are highly susceptible to desiccation.
- They have also evolved dependence on many host cell functions for metabolism and do not survive well in the environment.
- Standard disinfectants should be effective.
- Careful biosecurity practices and disinfection are indicated to prevent spread.
- No zoonotic concerns are known for any of the reptile-associated mycoplasmas.
- Most *Mycoplasma* spp. appear to have evolved closely with their hosts and are somewhat host specific.

GEOGRAPHY AND SEASONALITY
- The geographic ranges of reptilian *Mycoplasma* species are not well studied.
- *M. agassizii* is widespread in North American *G. agassizii* and *G. polyphemus* populations.
- Seasonality has not been reported, but in animals that brumate, clinical disease often presents following brumation.

ASSOCIATED CONDITIONS AND DISORDERS
- In general, mycoplasmal disease in nonreptilian species is often associated with respiratory tract infection and arthritis; this seems to also be the case in reptiles.
- A greater number of *Mycoplasma* spp. among nonreptilian species are not associated with disease, and this seems to be the case in reptiles.
- Mycoplasmosis in *Gopherus* spp. tortoises and box turtles is associated with rhinitis.
- Mycoplasmosis in Nile crocodiles, American alligators, and broad-nosed caiman is associated with polyarthritis/polyserositis.
- Mycoplasmosis in Burmese pythons is associated with tracheitis and pneumonia.

CLINICAL PRESENTATION

DISEASE FORMS/SUBTYPES Common diseases associated with *Mycoplasma* spp. are upper respiratory tract disease, lower respiratory tract disease, and arthritis.

HISTORY, CHIEF COMPLAINT Common complaints on presentation for mycoplasmosis include nonspecific illness, anorexia, nasal discharge, dyspnea, and swollen joints.

PHYSICAL EXAM FINDINGS Physical examination findings often include depression, nasal discharge, dyspnea, and swollen joints.

ETIOLOGY AND PATHOPHYSIOLOGY

Mycoplasmosis in reptiles is usually associated with hyperplasia and inflammation, often lymphoplasmacytic.

DIAGNOSIS

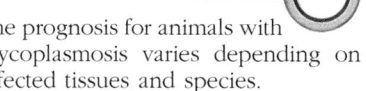

DIFFERENTIAL DIAGNOSIS

- Other common causes for rhinitis in tortoises include chlamydophilosis, herpesvirus, iridovirus, and reovirus.
- Other common causes for polyarthritis in crocodilians include chlamydophilosis and Gram-negative septicemia.
- Other common causes for pneumonia in snakes include chlamydophilosis, paramyxovirus, and reovirus.

INITIAL DATABASE

- A thorough husbandry history, physical examination, complete blood count, plasma chemistry, and radiographs form a basic database.
- A leukocytosis may be present with mycoplasmosis.

ADVANCED OR CONFIRMATORY TESTING

- Because *Mycoplasma* organisms lack a cell wall, they are highly susceptible to desiccation and do not survive standard transport well.
- Because *Mycoplasma* spp. have evolved dependence on many host cell functions for metabolism, special media are required for culture.
- *Mycoplasma* will not grow on standard bacterial media.
- The microbiology lab should be contacted in advance when *Mycoplasma* culture is indicated, and appropriate media obtained.
- Culture success is often improved when swabs are premoistened with *Mycoplasma* media before sample collection.
- Electron microscopy of biopsies may reveal organisms morphologically consistent with *Mycoplasma* spp.
- Serology is available for *M. agassizii* and *M. alligatoris*, and polymerase chain reaction (PCR) with product sequence analysis is available from the Mycoplasma Laboratory at the University of Florida College of Veterinary Medicine for identification and speciation of members of the genus *Mycoplasma*.

TREATMENT

THERAPEUTIC GOALS

- The goal of therapy is treatment of disease.
- Eradication of the organism is a second goal, but *Mycoplasma* spp. are difficult to completely eradicate, and the possibility of having an asymptomatic carrier after treatment is significant.

CHRONIC TREATMENT

- The organism should be speciated to determine disease potential.
- Any husbandry deficiencies should be addressed and corrected.
- Risks of carrier status need to be discussed with the owner.
- Macrolides and tetracyclines are the best choices for treatment.
- In the absence of exact data, treatment should be provided for at least 45-60 days.
- Fluoroquinolones are likely to result in temporary success and relapse.
- Shorter courses appear likely to result in treatment failure.

RECOMMENDED MONITORING

- Patients should be rechecked every 2 months for the first year to look for clinical signs of recurrence.
- Patients that brumate should have regular examinations done both before and after brumation.
- A patient with abnormal examination findings should not be allowed to brumate.

PROGNOSIS AND OUTCOME

- The prognosis for animals with mycoplasmosis varies depending on affected tissues and species.
- Many animals respond well to therapy, but carrier status is common and relapse is possible.

PEARLS & CONSIDERATIONS

COMMENTS

- Mycoplasmosis is well known among reptile owners and veterinarians.
- Although some species can be significant pathogens, it is important to remember that many have not been associated with disease.

- Speciation is important; some species are significant disease concerns, whereas others are not.
- The implications of infection differ between different species. *M. alligatoris* causes disease in American alligators and broad-nosed caiman, but not among Siamese crocodiles (*Crocodylus siamensis*). If a *Mycoplasma* sp. can infect an animal related to the normal host, infection may have significantly different disease implications.
- It is also important to remember that although it is an important differential, *M. agassizii* is only one of a number of differential diagnoses for upper respiratory tract disease in tortoises, and Koch's postulates have been fulfilled only for Florida gopher tortoises and California desert tortoises.
- A *Testudo* sp. with URTD is much more likely to have herpesviral infection; one study found that 10.3% of 155 tortoises with nasal discharge were PCR positive for *Chlamydophila* spp.

PREVENTION

Maintenance of a closed group of known negative status, quarantine, and stringent biosecurity practices are the most effective means of prevention.

CLIENT EDUCATION

The possibility of carrier status after treatment should be discussed with the owner.

SUGGESTED READINGS

Brown DR, et al: *Mycoplasma testudineum* sp. nov. from a desert tortoise (*Gopherus agassizii*) with upper respiratory tract disease, Int J Syst Evol Microbiol 54:1527–1529, 2004.

Brown DR, et al: Mycoplasmosis in green iguanas (*Iguana iguana*), J Zoo Wildl Med 38:348–351, 2007.

Brown MB, et al: *Mycoplasma agassizii* causes upper respiratory tract disease in the desert tortoise, Infect Immun 62:4580–4586, 1994.

Brown MB, et al: Upper respiratory tract disease in the gopher tortoise is caused by *Mycoplasma agassizii*, J Clin Microbiol 37:2262–2269, 1999.

Feldman SH, et al: A novel mycoplasma detected in association with upper respiratory disease syndrome in free-ranging eastern box turtles (*Terrapene carolina carolina*) in Virginia, J Wildl Dis 4:279–289, 2006.

Penner JD, et al: A novel *Mycoplasma* sp. associated with proliferative tracheitis and pneumonia in a Burmese python (*Python molurus bivittatus*), J Comp Pathol 117:283–288, 1997.

CROSS-REFERENCES TO OTHER SECTIONS

Chlamydophila
Dysecdysis
Herpesvirus
Respiratory (lower) disease

AUTHOR: **JAMES F.X. WELLEHAN, JR.**

EDITOR: **SCOTT J. STAHL**

REPTILES

Nematodiasis

BASIC INFORMATION

DEFINITION

Nematodes are found in all orders of reptiles. Nematodes frequently inhabit the intestinal tract of reptiles and their larvae can be seen in the respiratory tract and/or respiratory exudate. Infections often are subclinical but may be associated with secondary bacterial infections.

SYNONYM

Roundworms

EPIDEMIOLOGY

SPECIES, AGE, SEX

- Nematodiasis is seen in all species of reptiles.
- With some nematode species, young animals tend to have the heaviest infestations.
- No sex predilection is associated with nematodiasis.

RISK FACTORS Wild-caught animals, animals kept in enclosures with intermediate hosts, and animals kept under conditions of poor hygiene are at greater risk for clinical nematodiasis.

CONTAGION AND ZOONOSIS

- Contagion varies according to species of nematode and host.
- Fecal-oral contamination, ingestion of intermediate hosts, and arthropod bites are all common routes of infestation.

ASSOCIATED CONDITIONS AND DISORDERS Signs associated with clinical nematode infestation vary according to species of nematode and host, and include poor growth, increased growth, weight loss, subcutaneous swellings, regurgitation, and diarrhea.

CLINICAL PRESENTATION

HISTORY, CHIEF COMPLAINT

- History associated with clinical nematode infestation varies according to species of nematode and host.
- Often, no clinical concerns are present, and nematode ova are detected on a routine fecal examination.
- Other clinical concerns presented by owners include poor growth, weight loss, subcutaneous swellings, regurgitation, and diarrhea.

PHYSICAL EXAM FINDINGS

- Physical exam findings in cases of clinical nematode infestation vary according to species of nematode and host.
- Often, no abnormalities are present.
- Other physical findings include poor growth, increased growth, weight loss, and subcutaneous swellings.

ETIOLOGY AND PATHOPHYSIOLOGY

- Etiology and pathophysiology vary according to species of nematode and host. There are likely thousands of nematode species that use reptiles as hosts.
- Nematodes may be beneficial. *Oxyuroidea* nematodes (pinworms) have been shown to increase growth rates in tadpoles, and it is probable that this is the case in some reptile-host relationships.
- Mechanisms of pathology include direct damage to tissues, host inflammatory response, and diversion of nutrients from the host.

DIAGNOSIS

DIFFERENTIAL DIAGNOSIS

- Differential diagnoses for weight loss, diarrhea, and regurgitation include poor husbandry and numerous causes of enteritis and metabolic disease.
- Differential diagnoses for subcutaneous swellings include bacterial and fungal granulomas, nonnematode parasites, dysplasia, and neoplasia.

INITIAL DATABASE

- A thorough history, physical exam, complete blood count, plasma chemistry, radiographs, and fecal exam form the basic database.
- Microfilaria may be seen on a peripheral blood smear, although this is not a very sensitive test.

ADVANCED OR CONFIRMATORY TESTING

- Because the clinical significance and approach vary greatly depending on nematode species, identification of nematodes is essential, and it is important to develop a relationship with a parasitology lab experienced with reptile parasites.
- Enteric nematodes that are shedding ova usually will be found on fecal flotation examination.
- The presence of microfilaria is more easily identified by examining the buffy coat of an intact spun hematocrit tube under a microscope.
- Subcutaneous nematodes may be removed surgically for identification.
- Gastroscopy is useful for locating gastric nematodes that often do not shed significant numbers of ova, such as *Tanqua* spp.
- Grossly visible nematodes in the coelomic cavity or in other coelomic organs may be found on exploratory coeliotomy.
- Some nematodes may be identified at necropsy on histopathologic exam; complete speciation is often difficult in these cases.

TREATMENT

THERAPEUTIC GOALS

- The goal of treatment varies according to species of nematode and host.
- For species that are pathogenic, eradication of the nematode is the goal when feasible.
- For potentially beneficial species, prevention of significant overgrowth is the goal.

ACUTE GENERAL TREATMENT

- Treatment varies according to species of nematode and host.
- For nematodes with direct life cycles, good hygiene practices are necessary to prevent reinfestation.
- For nematodes with indirect life cycles, access to intermediate hosts needs to be removed.
- For potentially beneficial nematodes, no further treatment beyond good hygiene practices in indicated.
- For filarial nematodes such as *Foleyella* spp. or *Macdonaldius* spp., surgical removal is indicated whenever possible.
    - Chronic microfilarial antigen exposure is a problem, but in cases treated pharmaceutically, the massive inflammatory response to dead worms can be much worse than that to live worms.
- Anthelmintics can be used. However, any drug, including anthelmintics, has potential side effects, and this should be taken into account when anthelmintics are used.
- Some anthelminthic drug doses: Ivermectin 0.2 mg/kg PO or SQ, repeat in 14d. Do not use in turtles or crocodilians. Fenbendazole 25 mg/kg PO, repeat in 14d. Be aware of potential side effects on bone marrow/gut epithelium. Pyrantel pamoate, 5 mg/kg PO, repeat in 14d.
- Ivermectin toxicity is a significant risk in chelonians and crocodilians.
- Benzimidazoles, such as fenbendazole and albendazole, can have a significant negative impact on rapidly dividing cells such as bone marrow and gut epithelium. Deaths have been reported. Heterophil counts may be expected to drop at doses typically used for therapy.
- Many nematode species are not very susceptible to pyrantel.

RECOMMENDED MONITORING

Enteric nematodes with direct life cycles should have follow-up testing every 6 months until the reptile has had negative fecal flotation exams for 2 years.

PROGNOSIS AND OUTCOME

Prognosis and outcome vary according to species of nematode and host.

PEARLS & CONSIDERATIONS

COMMENTS

- It is essential to identify nematodes correctly when they are found.
- Pinworms, which are likely to be beneficial, are often mistaken for hookworms, which are likely to be pathogenic.

PREVENTION

Maintenance of a closed group, testing of populations, strict quarantine, elimination of access to intermediate hosts, and stringent biosecurity practices are the most effective means of prevention.

SUGGESTED READINGS

Garner MM, et al: Pathology of suspected fenbendazole intoxication in three Fea's vipers (*Azemiops feae*). In McKinnell RG, et al, editors: Proceedings of the 6th International Symposium on the Pathology of Reptiles and Amphibians, Minneapolis, 2001, University of Minnesota Printing Service, pp 173–176.

Neiffer DL, et al: Hematologic and plasma biochemical changes associated with fenbendazole administration in Hermann's tortoises (*Testudo hermanni*), J Zoo Wildl Med 36:661–672, 2005.

Pryor GS, et al: Effects of the nematode *Gyrinicola batrachiensis* on development, gut morphology, and fermentation in bullfrog tadpoles (*Rana catesbeiana*): a novel mutualism, J Exp Zoolog A Comp Exp Biol 303:704–712, 2005.

CROSS-REFERENCES TO OTHER SECTIONS

Abscesses
Adenovirus
Coccidiosis
Cryptosporidiosis
Diarrhea
Mycobacteriosis
Regurgitation/Vomiting
Salmonellosis

AUTHOR: **JAMES F.X. WELLEHAN, JR.**

EDITOR: **SCOTT J. STAHL**

REPTILES

Nutritional Secondary Hyperparathyroidism

Client Education Sheet Available on Website

BASIC INFORMATION

DEFINITION

- Nutritional secondary hyperparathyroidism (NSHP) is a clinical condition of reptiles that results from deficiencies of dietary calcium and/or vitamin D_3.
- Most often, it occurs as the result of an imbalance in the calcium-to-phosphorus ratio in the diet and/or inadequate exposure to ultraviolet radiation.
- Persistent hypocalcemia increases the activity of the parathyroid gland (hyperparathyroidism) with a subsequent increase in the production of parathyroid hormone (PTH). Increased PTH results in the resorption of calcium from bones, eventually causing clinical metabolic bone disease. NSHP is the most common form of metabolic bone disease in reptiles.

SYNONYMS

Rubber jaw, nutrition-related metabolic bone disease, fibrous osteodystrophy, rickets, osteomalacia

EPIDEMIOLOGY

SPECIES, AGE, SEX

- Can potentially affect all reptile species but is most common in lizards and aquatic turtles
- NSHP has not been reported in snakes.
- Most commonly seen in neonatal and juvenile reptiles because of the high demand for calcium with bone development and growth
- More common in mature female reptiles as the demand for calcium increases with reproductive activity

RISK FACTORS

- Complexity of husbandry for some species of captive reptiles
- Increased incidence in herbivorous and insectivorous reptile species because their diets are difficult to balance for calcium and mineral
- Diurnal reptiles may be more susceptible because of the increased need for ultraviolet radiation.

GEOGRAPHY AND SEASONALITY In reptiles that breed seasonally, an increased incidence of NSHP may be seen in reproductively active females that are not nutritionally sound.

ASSOCIATED CONDITIONS AND DISORDERS

- Pathologic fractures (see Orthopedics and Fracture Repair)
- Exposure gingivitis/stomatitis
- Neurologic disease
- Gastrointestinal stasis
- Cloacal/intestinal prolapse
- Phallus and hemipenal prolapse
- Dystocia
- Spinal abnormalities (kyphosis, scoliosis, etc.) (see Proliferative Spinal Osteoarthropathy)

CLINICAL PRESENTATION

HISTORY, CHIEF COMPLAINT

- History of inappropriate husbandry, including:
  - Feeding diets low in available calcium or high in phosphorus
  - No supplementation with calcium and vitamin D_3
  - No exposure to unfiltered sunlight or ultraviolet light (UVB in the range of ≈285-320 nm)
  - Improper temperatures
- Chief complaint:
  - Anorexia
  - Lethargy
  - Poor weight gain and stunted growth in juveniles
  - Tremors
  - Paresis/paralysis
  - Bloating
  - Constipation
  - Cloacal/rectal/phallus/hemipenal prolapse
  - Swellings, fractures, and deformities of limbs
  - Spinal deviations (kinking)
  - Abnormal shell growth in chelonians
  - Stomatitis/gingivitis (exposed mucous membranes in oral cavity)
  - Prolapsed or nonfunctioning tongue in Old World chameleons
  - Bleeding (coagulopathies)

PHYSICAL EXAM FINDINGS

- Lizards:
  - Generalized weakness
  - Poor body weight
  - Brachycephalic appearance to head
  - Deformity of mandibular and maxillary bones, soft and pliable
  - Exposure of mucous membranes along mandibular and maxillary surface, often covered with dried yellow/brown secretions/food material (fibrous osteodystrophy of mandibular/maxillary bones)
  - Firm swelling of long bones (fibrous osteodystrophy)
  - Palpable fractures of bones
  - Horizontal rotation of the scapula
  - Kyphosis or scoliosis of spine with/without decreased neurologic function to the rear limbs
  - A large quantity of retained stool or urates may be palpated in the coelom.
  - Palpable gas in the abdomen
  - Bloating and gastrointestinal motility issues are more common in some species of lizard such as juvenile bearded dragons.
  - Hyperreflexia
  - Tremors and fasciculations may be evident, especially during handling
  - Seizure, tetany, and/or flaccid paresis of limbs/tail
  - Poor ability to elevate caudal body and proximal tail off the ground when ambulating
  - Prolapse of cloaca, colon, oviduct, hemipene
  - Gravid female lizards (higher demand for calcium) may present for NSHP with clinical signs, including:
    - Muscle tremors and fasciculations
    - Seizures
    - Dystocia
    - Soft mandibular and maxillary bones
- Chelonians:
  - Generalized weakness
  - Tremors
  - Carapace and plastron may be abnormally soft and pliable, especially in young, growing chelonians.
  - Shape of the shell (especially the carapace) may be abnormal.
  - Often the marginal scutes on the carapace curl upward.
  - The turtle's body may seem too large for its shell.
  - Mandibular and maxillary bones may be soft and pliable (less common than with lizards), and often the anterior maxilla may become elongated.
  - Fractures or swellings of long bones (less common than with lizards)
  - Inability to elevate the caudal plastron off the ground when ambulating
  - With abnormal shell growth of the carapace, conscious proprioceptive deficits or paresis/paralysis of the rear limbs may be noted.
  - Prolapse of cloaca, colon, oviduct, phallus
  - Dystocia

ETIOLOGY AND PATHOPHYSIOLOGY

- NSHP in reptiles results from:

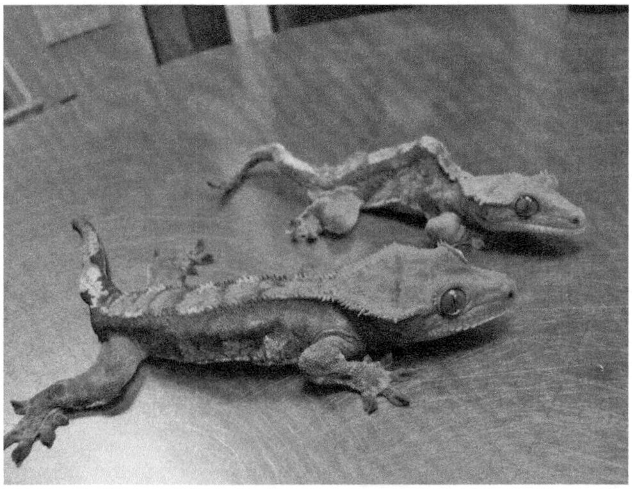

Nutritional Secondary Hyperparathyroidism Typical presentation of reptiles with nutritional secondary hyperparathyroidism (NSHP). Note the severe kyphosis in the crested gecko in the back, and that the animal in front is too weak to lift up its body to walk. *(Photo courtesy Jörg Mayer, The University of Georgia, Athens.)*

  - Dietary imbalance of calcium/phosphorus, typically low dietary calcium with excessive dietary phosphorus
  - Lack of exposure to natural sunlight or full-spectrum lighting or lack of dietary vitamin D_3
  - Calcium deficiencies are common in herbivorous, insectivorous, and omnivorous reptiles.
  - Uncommon in snakes that eat warm-blooded prey.
  - Exacerbated in juvenile reptiles with the same (difficult to balance for calcium) diet but with an increased demand for calcium caused by rapid bone growth and formation
- Subsequent hypocalcemia results in partial depolarization of nerves and muscles (because of an increase in threshold potential), leading to tremors, twitching, and seizures in the reptile patient.
- Eventually, these dietary deficiencies (that result in low calcium uptake) will cause an increase in the production of parathyroid hormone from the parathyroid gland.
- Increased parathyroid hormone results in:
  - An increase in calcium resorption from bone to compensate for the low dietary uptake of calcium
  - Increased renal tubular reabsorption of calcium and increased excretion of phosphorus
  - Increased formation of 1,25-dihydroxycholecalciferol (DHCC), resulting in an increase in absorption of calcium in the intestinal tract
- Paresis and/or paralysis occurs with spinal fractures from weakened vertebral bones or compression of the spinal cord.
- Often innervation to the bowel and bladder is subsequently involved, resulting in elimination problems and constipation.
- Bloating, decreased gastrointestinal motility, and rectal/cloacal prolapse occur because of the effects of decreased calcium on the smooth muscle of the gastrointestinal tract.
- Paresis and paralysis related to spinal changes then result in prolapse of the colon/cloaca or reproductive organs, including the oviduct and hemipenes or phallus (in chelonians).
- NSHP is uncommon in adult reptiles:
  - No longer growing (especially long bones and shell) at the same rate as in a juvenile, so demand for calcium is lessened
  - Exception would be breeding female reptiles that are producing eggs/young, thus still with a demand for calcium.
  - Commonly misdiagnosed as NSHP when other metabolic diseases such as renal secondary hyperparathyroidism are more common in adult reptiles

DIAGNOSIS

DIFFERENTIAL DIAGNOSIS

- For bone changes:
  - Traumatic fractures (normal bone strength)
  - Renal secondary hyperparathyroidism
  - Osteomyelitis
  - Abscesses/cellulitis
  - Gout/pseudogout
  - Hypertrophic osteopathy
  - Osteomalacia
  - Neoplasia
- For neurologic signs:
  - Renal secondary hyperparathyroidism
  - Egg laying in oviparous reptiles
  - Sepsis
  - Toxins/poisons (insecticides, disinfectants)
  - Vitamin E/selenium deficiency
  - Brain/spinal other nervous tissue damage/trauma

INITIAL DATABASE

- Obtain detailed historical information concerning diet and husbandry.
- In many cases, a diagnosis is made with historical dietary and husbandry information and physical exam findings.
- Complete blood cell count:
  - Often normal with NSHP
- Serum/plasma biochemistry panel
  - Reptiles with secondary NSHP usually are normocalcemic; reptiles with renal disease generally are hypocalcemic and hyperphosphatemic (see Renal Disease).
  - Calcium and phosphorus values may provide baseline information needed to initiate calcitonin and monitor the therapeutic plan.
  - Uric acid, sodium, chloride, and total protein will be elevated with severe dehydration.

ADVANCED OR CONFIRMATORY TESTING

- Radiography (lateral and ventrodorsal [VD] or dorsoventral [DV]):
  - Determines the extent and severity of bones involved
  - Often reveals characteristic changes in bones including:
    - Reduced density
    - Loss of definitive cortex and dramatic increase in width and radiolucent appearance of long bones
    - Loss of clear cortical delineation of pelvis and caudal vertebrae
    - Pathologic fractures
- Radiography provides baseline information for use in monitoring the response to therapy.

TREATMENT

THERAPEUTIC GOALS

- Provide support for the presenting patient with supplemental heat and fluid therapy as needed.
- Address acute life-threatening presentations such as controlling seizures and stabilizing broken bones.
- Continue chronic treatment over weeks to months to correct deficiencies of calcium and/or vitamin D_3.
- Correct specific husbandry issues related to NSHP such as diet (calcium and phosphorus intake) and exposure to ultraviolet lighting.

ACUTE GENERAL TREATMENT

- The patient should be warmed to appropriate physiologic temperatures (preferred optimum temperature zone [POTZ]), hydration status assessed, and fluid therapy (10-30 mL/kg q 24 h) initiated if necessary.
- For clinical signs of hypocalcemia, including fasciculations, tetany, and seizures, initiate immediate calcium supplementation with calcium gluconate (100 mg/kg IV or if given SQ give into a bolus of fluid or dilute before injection as it is caustic to tissues). Can be given every 6 h until clinical improvement:
  - Begin oral calcium supplementation with calcium glubionate at 23 mg/kg PO every 12 h.
  - Give 100 IU vitamin D_3/kg IM or SC once weekly for two treatments.
  - If normocalcemic on serum/plasma biochemistry panel, or after treating with oral calcium glubionate for 3-7 days as described above, can give 50 IU/kg synthetic calcitonin intramuscularly weekly for two doses.
- A primary therapeutic goal is to stop bone loss and promote new bone production:
  - Calcitonin decreases circulating calcium and phosphorus.
  - With the use of calcitonin, bone repair may occur as early as 2-3 months as compared with 4-6 months without its use.
- Multiple pathologic fractures in small lizards and chelonians are best treated with strict cage rest:
  - Splinting of one or more limbs may result in stress to the other limbs and increased fractures.
  - All branches and climbing areas should be removed.
- Larger lizards with one fractured limb may have the limb splinted to the body (lateral body wall for front limbs; tail for back limbs) with tape.
- All climbing accessories should be removed from the cage.

- Minimal handling is mandatory during treatment to avoid fracturing weakened bones.
- Reptile patients presented with associated obstipation/constipation may be given warm water soaks and gentle massage and manipulation to express fecal and urate material.
- Warm water enemas may be given using a gentle technique to guide the tube specifically into the colon (not just the cloaca); hydrostatic pressure should be minimized when the enema material is infused.
- During the treatment period (and beyond), optimal temperatures are necessary to allow adequate enzyme activity for gastrointestinal digestion and absorption of oral medications. Temperature gradients must be provided in the environment by focal basking or heat sources.
- If patients are not feeding voluntarily owing to soft mandibular and maxillary bones or other influences of NSHP gentle assist feeding, syringe feeding or tube feeding (chelonians) may be necessary. Start with small volumes, working up to more normal intakes over days to weeks as gastrointestinal motility may be affected by hypocalcemia.

CHRONIC TREATMENT

- Oral calcium glubionate treatment may be continued for a period of 1-3 months or longer.
- Follow-up treatments with parenteral vitamin D_3 and calcitonin
- Correct nutrition and provide appropriate ultraviolet light exposure (natural sunlight or artificial lighting).
- Increase calcium in the diet, and limit phosphorus (calcium-to-phosphorus ratio, 2:1).
- Dietary recommendations are 2-3 mg/kcal of 0.6%-1.5% calcium and 0.5%-0.8% phosphorus on a dry matter basis (DM) for most reptiles.
- Calcium requirements can be higher for turtles and tortoises (1.4% calcium and 0.7% phosphorus DM).
- Excess phosphorus in the diet (bone meal or dicalcium phosphate) will exacerbate secondary hyperparathyroidism.
- Provide endogenous vitamin D_3 through ultraviolet light exposure. Unfiltered sunlight is best, but if this is not feasible, full-spectrum lighting (285-320 nm) should be provided:
  - Positioning of the light is important for fluorescent tubes; they should be within 16-24 inches of the reptile to be useful (may be dangerous if too close to the reptile).
  - Ultraviolet bulbs need to be changed every 6-12 months.
- The level of D_3 as a supplement should range from 500-2000 IU D_3 per kg.
- If a multivitamin is used to supplement oral vitamin D_3, a vitamin A/vitamin D/vitamin E ratio of 100:10:1 is recommended.
- Use of a multivitamin alone typically will not provide enough calcium, and additional calcium must be given.
- Maximum tolerances suggested for many reptile species are 2.5% calcium, 1.6% phosphorus/DM, and 5000 IU/kg vitamin D_3.
- General dietary recommendations for avoiding NSHP include:
  - For carnivores, feed whole animals, including bones and viscera (e.g., rodents, fish). Supplementation with additional calcium or multivitamins is not necessary unless feeding only neonatal prey items (e.g., newborn rodents).
  - For insectivores, feed invertebrate prey items a balanced diet (e.g., complete insect diet, complete mammalian chow). Dust invertebrates with a supplement (e.g., calcium carbonate, limestone) or a calcium/vitamin D_3 combination.
  - Multivitamin supplements do not usually provide sufficient supplemental calcium and must be used in conjunction with a specific calcium source. Dusting is a very unscientific and "haphazard" method of supplementing the diet but has historically been successful. However, overzealous dusting may lead to vitamin toxicity (see Hypervitaminosis A).
  - For herbivores, feed vegetables with a good calcium-to-phosphorus ratio, such as collard greens, endive, parsley, and dandelion greens. For most herbivores, minimize fruit (should be no more than 10%-20% of total diet) in the diet because its high moisture content may dilute out necessary nutrients, and it tends to lack fiber. Salads must be supplemented with a calcium supplement such as calcium carbonate; 1 g (half teaspoon) of calcium carbonate per 100 g of food may be adequate.

DRUG INTERACTIONS

Excessive levels of dietary vitamin D may be toxic, especially if combined with adequate exposure to unfiltered natural sunlight or full-spectrum lighting.

POSSIBLE COMPLICATIONS

Excessive calcium and phosphorus in the diet may interfere with the gastrointestinal absorption of other minerals such as zinc, copper, or iodine to deficiencies of these minerals.

RECOMMENDED MONITORING

- Regular rechecks in the first several weeks of treatment are critical to ensure that the patient is responding to therapy. These recheck visits also allow the clinician to review the husbandry to make sure the recommended changes have been made.
- Radiographic reevaluations can be useful at these follow-up visits to ensure bone healing progress.
- In lizards, malocclusion often occurs in association with fibrous osteodystrophy of the mandibular and maxillary bones. After treatment, the bones may heal, but lifelong malocclusion is a result. Severe underbites and overbites may occur, and management of chronic exposure gingivitis and ptyalism may be necessary. This is a chronic condition that cannot be resolved but can be managed with gentle cleansing and the application of a wax lip balm product to protect exposed tissue.

PROGNOSIS AND OUTCOME

- Prognosis is good with aggressive therapy and appropriate husbandry changes.
- Spinal involvement (scoliosis and kyphosis, changes in the carapace in chelonians) has a more guarded to grave prognosis because neurologic damage may not resolve with treatment.
- If paresis and paralysis are associated with spinal involvement, and elimination complications result in obstipation/constipation, the prognosis is grave. Owners may be trained to help "assist" with elimination, but these patients may be difficult to manage. Often the spinal deformity worsens with growth, and an ascending pyelonephritis may result. Euthanasia may need to be considered in these cases.
- Females with spinal and pelvic changes may present with dystocia due to a narrowed pelvis. Prognosis for survival may be fair but a return to normal morphology poor, and lifelong management may be necessary.
- Prognosis is fair with signs of hypocalcemia such as tremors, ataxia, hyperreflexia, and even cloacal prolapse.
- Prognosis is worse with chronic disease often represented by fibrous osteodystrophy, pathologic fractures, paresis, and paralysis.

PEARLS & CONSIDERATIONS

PREVENTION

- Ensuring that clients with juvenile reptiles get proper husbandry information would prevent many cases.

- Encouraging clients to bring juvenile reptiles in for "new pet" exams provides a great opportunity to review husbandry and develop a relationship of trust, whereby the client will rely on your clinic for future care information.

CLIENT EDUCATION

Educating clients about the proper husbandry necessary for the specific reptile species presented is critical.

SUGGESTED READINGS

Boyer TH: Metabolic bone disease. In Mader DR, editor: Reptile medicine and surgery, Philadelphia, 1996, WB Saunders, pp 385–392.
Donoghue S: Nutrition. In Mader DR, editor: Reptile medicine and surgery, St Louis, 2006, Elsevier, pp 251–298.
Frye FL: Biomedical and surgical aspects of captive reptile husbandry, ed 2, Malabar, FL, 1991, Krieger Publishing.
Mader DR: Metabolic bone disorders. In Mader DR, editor: Reptile medicine and surgery, St Louis, 2006, Elsevier, pp 841–851.

CROSS-REFERENCES TO OTHER SECTIONS

Hypervitaminosis A
Orthopedics and Fracture Repair
Proliferative Spinal Osteoarthropathy
Renal Disease

AUTHOR & EDITOR: **SCOTT J. STAHL**

REPTILES

Orthopedics and Fracture Repair

Client Education Sheet Available on Website

BASIC INFORMATION

DEFINITION

A fracture is a complete or incomplete break in the continuity of bone or cartilage.

EPIDEMIOLOGY

RISK FACTORS

- Inappropriate husbandry and diet
- Free-ranging reptiles are more prone to traumatic injury.
- Juvenile/rapidly growing reptiles

ASSOCIATED CONDITIONS AND DISORDERS

- Poor diet and inappropriate husbandry
- Fibrous osteodystrophy
- Nutritional secondary hyperparathyroidism (NSHP) (see Nutritional Secondary Hyperparathyroidism)
- Renal hyperparathyroidism
- Osetomyelitis
- Osteolytic neoplasia

CLINICAL PRESENTATION

DISEASE FORMS/SUBTYPES

- Closed simple fracture
- Closed comminuted fracture
- Open comminuted fracture
- Open fracture with osteomyelitis
- Shell injuries in chelonians

HISTORY, CHIEF COMPLAINT

- Nonspecific
- Lethargy
- Anorexia
- Swollen limbs
- Inability to use limbs
- Paresis/Paralysis

PHYSICAL EXAM FINDINGS

- Variable depending on location and extent of fracture:
  - Inability to use limb
  - Limping
  - Swollen limb or joint
  - Anorexia and lethargy may result from pain and severe debilitation.
  - Neurologic deficits may be present with damage to spinal cord or associated nerve roots.

ETIOLOGY AND PATHOPHYSIOLOGY

- Most orthopedic injuries in captive reptiles are the result of low-impact injury or nutritional disorders and tend to be closed and simple.
  - In juvenile animals, inappropriate husbandry and diet often lead to NSHP and the development of pathologic fractures.
  - In mature animals, long bone fractures may be associated with metabolic disease, osteomyelitis, or neoplasia of the bone parenchyma.
- Most orthopedic injuries in wild reptiles are the result of high-impact trauma; they are commonly open and highly comminuted with secondary osteomyelitis.

DIAGNOSIS

DIFFERENTIAL DIAGNOSIS

- Infectious
  - Bacterial: Gram-negative, Gram-positive
  - Fungal
- Metabolic
  - Gout/pseudogout
  - Renal disease
- Nutritional
  - Calcium deficiency
  - Calcium/phosphorus imbalance
  - Vitamin D deficiency
- Toxic
  - Lead
  - Zinc
- Neoplastic
- Developmental

INITIAL DATABASE

- Detailed information concerning diet and husbandry
- Radiography (lateral and dorsal ventral [DV] views)
  - Help to determine extent of injury and presence of osteomyelitis
- Complete blood cell count
  - Anemia and heterophilic leukocytosis may be present with osteomyelitis and significant blood loss.
- Serum/Plasma biochemistry panel
  - Creatine kinase may be elevated with significant muscle damage.
  - Reptiles with secondary NSHP usually are normocalcemic; reptiles with renal disease generally are hypocalcemic and hyperphosphatemic.
  - Uric acid, sodium, chloride, and total protein will be elevated with severe dehydration.

ADVANCED OR CONFIRMATORY TESTING

- CT
  - Useful to evaluate structural integrity of associated neurologic, connective, and soft tissues
- Bone biopsy and histopathologic evaluation
- Aerobic and anaerobic culture
  - Fastidious organisms may be difficult to isolate; specialized growth media may be required.
  - Fungal culture should be performed to identify any fungal contamination.
- Impression smears may be collected from the injury site to assess microbial flora.

TREATMENT

THERAPEUTIC GOALS

- Stabilize patient.
- Provide adequate analgesia.
- Establish proper anatomic alignment and rigid stabilization of fracture.

- Address any underlying metabolic disease.
- Correct any underlying dietary or husbandry issues.

ACUTE GENERAL TREATMENT

- Stabilize patient:
  - Stop any hemorrhage if present.
  - Provide supplemental heat consistent with species preferred optimal temperature zone (POTZ).
  - Provide shock therapy if indicated:
    - Fluids: IO or IV boluses of crystalloids (5-10 mL/kg) with colloids (3-5 mL/kg)
- Analgesia
  - Morphine
    - Chelonians: 1.5 mg/kg
    - Lizards: 10 mg/kg
  - Meloxicam (Metacam): 0.1-0.2 mg/kg PO q 24 h
  - Propofol (Rapinovet): provides 20-45 minutes of general anesthesia
    - Lizards: 10 mg/kg IV
    - Snakes: 5 mg/kg IV or ICe
    - Chelonians: 12 mg/kg IV
  - Inhalant anesthesia:
    - Isoflurane can be titrated to needs of patient.
- Select appropriate antibiotic therapy (if indicated):
  - Baytril 22.7 mg/mL: 5-10 mg/kg q 24 h PO, SC, IM, ICe
  - Ceftazidime: 20-40 mg/kg SC, IM, IV q 72 h
  - Amikacin 5 mg/kg IM, then 2.5 mg/kg q 72 h
- Select appropriate fixation method based on patient conformation and location and extent of injury.
  - External coaptation:
    - Useful in cases of simple, noncomplicated fracture
    - Anesthesia is recommended during the application of external coaptation to prevent iatrogenic fractures and to minimize stress and pain.
    - Splint or bandage must restrict the movement of joints both above and below the fracture.
    - Whenever possible, the splint should be placed in a normal "walking" position.
    - Bandages need to be changed regularly (weekly- biweekly) to prevent tendon contracture or additional joint complications.
    - Orthoplast (Johnson & Johnson, New Brunswick, NJ), Hexalite (Hexcel Medical, Dublin, CA), or Thermoplast (VTP; IMEX Veterinary, Inc., Longview, TX) may be used to make custom-fitted splints.
    - Tubular traction splints should be used with care as they may predispose the patient to joint ankylosis.
    - In lizards, the affected limb may be attached to the body for stabilization:
      - Pelvic limb fractures
        - Pelvic limb is secured to the tail.
        - Take care not to cover the vent with the bandage.
      - Thoracic limb fractures
        - Thoracic limb is secured to the body wall.
        - Ensure that the bandage is not too tight to prevent adequate respiration.
    - Chelonians:
      - Used only if fractures are reduced or minimally displaced
      - Affected limb should be flexed into a normal position in the axillary or inguinal fossa.
      - Tape strips or bandaging wrap is used to cover the shell and prevent extension of the affected limb.
      - Radiographs are indicated after bandaging to ensure proper bone alignment.
  - Internal fixation:
    - Useful for fractures that cannot be addressed with external coaptation or for fractious reptiles likely to damage an external fixation apparatus.
    - Preferred method for fracture repair in aquatic species
    - Principles used for surgical approach and application of internal fixators are similar to those used in small mammals.
    - Bone plating is the best choice for femoral and humeral fractures in large reptiles and chelonians, but costs associated with materials and placement may be prohibitive.
  - External fixation:
    - Provides adequate stabilization without interfering with joints and can be used in small reptiles
    - Most often applied parallel to the substrate in a cranial-to-caudal plane rather than a medial-to-lateral plane as in the mammal
    - Pin purchase can be maximized by using pins with the threading applied to the pin and not cut into it.
    - Connecting bars can be made of lightweight materials such as acrylic polymers and Penrose drains filled with polymethylmethacrylate.
  - Chelonian shell fractures:
    - Shell fractures commonly affect surrounding soft tissues and viscera.
    - Provide analgesia before manipulating shell fractures.
    - All shell fractures should be treated as open fractures.
      - If shell fracture is older than 6 hours, treat as a contaminated wound.
      - Systemic antimicrobials should be directed at Gram-positive ground contaminants, Gram-negative pathogens, and anaerobes.
      - All samples for microbiological culture should be collected before initiation of antibiotic therapy.
    - Simple uncontaminated shell fractures:
      - Strict asepsis should be maintained to avoid introducing any opportunistic pathogens.
      - Cerclage wire, metal sutures/plates, and/or plastic zip ties may be used to reduce the fracture.
      - Acrylic polymer can be molded to cover fracture site and provide a protective barrier to the site.
      - Shell repair can take 6-30 months.
    - Contaminated shell fractures:
      - Initiate appropriate systemic antimicrobial therapy.
      - Assess extent of injury and remove devitalized tissues.
        - Irrigate wound with sterile saline.
          - Avoid introduction of large volumes of fluid into the coelomic cavity
        - Wet-to-dry bandages
          - Change every 24 hours.
        - Once wounds have healed, treat as an uncontaminated shell fracture.

CHRONIC TREATMENT

- Daily inspection of pin/fracture site to ensure no premature removal of apparatus or infection
- Exercise restriction for minimum of 8-12 weeks
- Pins or apparatus can be removed based on radiographic evidence of adequate callus formation and complete healing.
- No soaking or limited water exposure until complete fracture healing

DRUG INTERACTIONS

Care should be exercised with the use of aminoglycoside antibiotics and nonsteroidal antiinflammatory drugs (NSAIDs) in severely debilitated or dehydrated patients or in patients with compromised renal function.

POSSIBLE COMPLICATIONS

- Implant loosening
- Pin migration

- Bending of implants
- Osteomyelitis

RECOMMENDED MONITORING

- Surgical sites
- External fixation apparatus
- Radiographs at 4-6 week intervals

PROGNOSIS AND OUTCOME

- In most cases, the prognosis is good if secondary complications are minimal and complete bone healing is achieved.
- Cases of severe or nonresponsive osteomyelitis carry a guarded to poor prognosis, and limb amputation may be indicated.
- Euthanasia should be considered in all cases of severe shell damage in chelonians, especially with exposure or significant contamination of coelomic contents.

PEARLS & CONSIDERATIONS

COMMENTS

- General principles of fracture management and fixation apply to the reptilian patient.
- Bone healing in reptiles is slow. Complete healing may take 6-18 months. Pathologic fractures from NSHP tend to heal faster (4-8 weeks) if the underlying husbandry issues are corrected.
- Some closed fractures may heal without any intervention but may have varying degrees of malunion.

PREVENTION

- Proper nutrition and environmental conditions based on specific species requirements are essential.
- Proper caging

SUGGESTED READINGS

Diethelm G: Reptiles. In Carpenter J, editor: Exotic animal formulary, ed 3, St Louis, 2005, Elsevier, pp 55–131.
Mader D, et al: Surgery. In Mader DR, editor: Reptile medicine and surgery, St Louis, 2006, Elsevier, pp 599–605.
Mitchell MA: Diagnosis and management of reptile orthopedic injuries, Vet Clin North Am Exot Anim Pract 5:97–114, 2002.
Sladky KK, et al: Antinociceptive efficacy and respiratory effects of butorphanol and morphine in three reptile species, Lawrence, KS, 2007, Proc Assoc Reptilian Amphibian Veterinarians, pp 51–52.

CROSS-REFERENCES TO OTHER SECTIONS

Nutritional Secondary Hyperparathyroidism

AUTHOR: **DAVID A. CRUM**

EDITOR: **SCOTT J. STAHL**

REPTILES

Paramyxovirus Infection

BASIC INFORMATION

DEFINITION

Paramyxovirus infections are common in viperid snakes, but have been reported in nonvenomous snakes as well. This highly contagious virus causes predominantly respiratory signs; transmission appears to be from respiratory secretions.

SYNONYM

Genus *Ferlavirus,* consisting of clades A, B, and C in squamates, as well as a tortoise *Ferlavirus,* and a divergent virus known as Sunshine virus.

EPIDEMIOLOGY

SPECIES, AGE, SEX

- Squamates can be infected with Paramyxoviruses. Paramyxoviral disease appears to be most common in viperid snakes.
- Disease has been reported in other snake species, green tree monitors, green iguanas, and Xenosaurus platyceps. A ferlavirus has been identified in a Hermann's tortoise.
- The species specificity of paramyxoviruses is not known, but as small segmented RNA viruses, it is expected that they may be more likely to jump host species than a large DNA virus such as an adenovirus or herpesvirus.
- Young, geriatric, and immune suppressed animals appear to be at greatest risk for disease.
- No sex predilections are known.

RISK FACTORS

- Risk factors for paramyxoviral disease are not well understood.
- Stressed animals appear to be more likely to develop clinical disease.
- Animals with a higher thermal gradient providing the option to have a behavioral fever may be less likely to develop disease.

CONTAGION AND ZOONOSIS

- As enveloped viruses, paramyxoviruses are less stable in the environment. Disinfectants effective against other enveloped viruses may be expected to be effective against adenoviruses.
- No zoonotic risk is known for any reptile paramyxovirus, although ophidian paramyxoviruses have been adapted to primate cell lines in the lab.

ASSOCIATED CONDITIONS AND DISORDERS Pneumonia and encephalitis are the most common presentations of paramyxoviral disease.

CLINICAL PRESENTATION

DISEASE FORMS/SUBTYPES

- Pneumonia and encephalitis are the most common clinical presentations of paramyxoviral disease.
- The immune system of the animal is often overwhelmed, and secondary infections are common.

HISTORY, CHIEF COMPLAINT Common complaints on presentation for paramyxoviral disease include pneumonia, neurologic signs (e.g., loss of righting reflex in snakes), and high death rates.

PHYSICAL EXAM FINDINGS Physical exam findings often include dyspnea and impaired righting reflexes.

ETIOLOGY AND PATHOPHYSIOLOGY

Paramyxoviruses are enveloped RNA viruses that may infect a variety of reptiles.

DIAGNOSIS

DIFFERENTIAL DIAGNOSIS

Reoviral disease in snakes is very similar to paramyxoviral disease.

INITIAL DATABASE

A thorough history, physical exam, complete blood count, plasma chemistry, radiographs, and a pulmonary wash for cytologic examination and PCR form a basic database.

ADVANCED OR CONFIRMATORY TESTING

- Nested PCR with product sequence analysis is available from the University of Florida for all reptile paramyxoviruses.
- Pulmonary washes are generally the antemortem sample of choice.
- Histologic findings of proliferative pneumonia with syncytia are common in both reoviral and paramyxoviral diseases.
- Hemagglutination inhibition is available, but the only assay in North America with experimentally validated cutoffs is for a Group A Ferlavirus. Cross-reactivity for Ferlavirus groups B and C differs.
- Immunohistochemistry and in situ hybridization are available for identification of ophidian paramyxovirus in tissue.

TREATMENT

ACUTE GENERAL TREATMENT

- Providing supportive care, addressing husbandry deficiencies, and identifying and treating secondary bacterial and fungal infections are the most important aspects of treating paramyxoviral disease.
- Increasing the temperature of the warm end of the thermal gradient allows the animal to choose a fever, which appears to help clinically.

CHRONIC TREATMENT

It is not known whether paramyxoviruses are persistent in reptiles. As a small RNA virus, it is considered less likely.

PROGNOSIS AND OUTCOME

The prognosis for animals with paramyxoviral disease is guarded.

PEARLS & CONSIDERATIONS

COMMENTS

- This disease is clinically very similar to reovirus disease.
- Molecular diagnostics need to be done to differentiate the two.
- Although reoviruses have been isolated from tortoises, paramyxoviruses have yet to be isolated from tortoises.

PREVENTION

Maintenance of a closed group, testing of populations, testing during quarantine, and stringent biosecurity practices are the most effective means of prevention.

SUGGESTED READINGS

Bernheim HA, et al: Effects of fever on host defense mechanisms after infection in the lizard *Dipsosaurus dorsalis*, Br J Exp Pathol 59:76–84, 1978.

Clark HF, et al: Fer de Lance virus (FDLV): a probable paramyxovirus isolated from a reptile, J Gen Virol 44:405–418, 1979.

Gravendyck M, et al: Paramyxoviral and reoviral infections of iguanas on Honduran Islands, J Wildl Dis 34:33–38, 1998.

Jacobson ER, et al: Paramyxovirus infection in caiman lizards (*Draecena guianensis*), J Vet Diagn Invest 13:143–151, 2001.

Jacobson ER, et al: Pulmonary lesions in experimental ophidian paramyxovirus pneumonia of Aruba Island rattlesnakes, *Crotalus unicolor*, Vet Pathol 34:450–459, 1997.

Marschang RE, et al: Paramyxovirus and reovirus infections in wild-caught Mexican lizards (*Xenosaurus* and *Abronia* spp.), J Zoo Wildl Med 33:317–321, 2002.

http://www.merckmanuals.com/vet/index.html, access July 10. 2012.

CROSS-REFERENCES TO OTHER SECTIONS

Chlamydophila
Mycobacteria
Mycoplasma
Pentastomes
Respiratory (lower) tract Disease

AUTHOR: **JAMES F.X. WELLEHAN, JR.**

EDITOR: **SCOTT J. STAHL**

REPTILES

Paraphimosis

BASIC INFORMATION

DEFINITION

Inability to retract penis (chelonians) or hemipenis (snakes and lizards)

SYNONYMS

Hemipenal, penis prolapse

EPIDEMIOLOGY

SPECIES, AGE, SEX

- Snakes
  - Seen most frequently in ball pythons and boa constrictors
  - Sexually mature, often actively breeding snakes
- Lizards
  - Common in green iguanas, monitors, chameleons, and leopard geckos
  - Often seen in young, growing herbivorous and insectivorous lizards
  - Nutritional secondary hyperparathyroidism (NSHP) often results in spinal deformities or fractures, which may lead to neurologic damage/deficits.
  - Sexually mature lizards may or may not be actively breeding.
- Chelonians
  - Often seen in aquatic turtles, box turtles, and tortoises
  - Young, growing chelonians
  - NSHP often results in shell (spinal) deformities, which may lead to neurologic damage/deficits.
  - Sexually mature chelonians that may or may not be actively breeding

RISK FACTORS

- Trauma
  - All reptiles
    - Spinal cord damage will result in neurologic deficits that will predispose all reptiles to prolapse.
  - Snakes
    - Especially breeding males that have been courting too many females
    - Increased likelihood if males are breeding on particulate substrates such as mulch or wood shavings
  - Lizards
    - Often seen with underlying nutrition-related issues such as NSHP and hypovitaminosis A
    - As with snakes, may be related to excessive breeding
  - Chelonians
    - Often seen in single pets that are mounting and attempting to breed objects in their environment
    - Also, breeding males that are attempting to court too many females or are relentless in their attempts to breed
    - Associated with NSHP (soft carapace often deformed with associated spinal involvement and neurologic deficits)

GEOGRAPHY AND SEASONALITY

Increased incidence during breeding

season or when perceived seasonal changes result in increased production of sexual hormones.

CLINICAL PRESENTATION

DISEASE FORMS/SUBTYPES

- Abscessation is common in snakes that have been breeding excessively.
- Lizards with underlying vitamin A deficiency may have associated hemipenal plugs (accumulation of seminal material and sloughing skin) that are enlarged and hardened due to the squamous metaplasia.
- Often, inflammation and secondary bacterial involvement are noted in these cases.

HISTORY, CHIEF COMPLAINT

- Penis or hemipenis is exposed or protruding.
- Hemorrhage or discharge associated with exposed and traumatized tissue

PHYSICAL EXAM FINDINGS

- Exposed organ is engorged, discolored, and, in severe cases, necrotic.
- Hemipenis or penis may be only partially prolapsed and may require anesthesia to allow a thorough evaluation of the organ.

ETIOLOGY AND PATHOPHYSIOLOGY

- In cases with associated abscessation, a variety of Gram-negative bacteria can be isolated.
- Test for acid-fast organisms (with biopsy and histopathologic examination) in snakes breeding on mulch.
- With trauma or neurologic damage, the organ may no longer be able to be retracted.
  - The tissue becomes engorged with decreased venous and lymphatic return. This exacerbates the inability for the tissue to be retracted. Ischemia and necrosis often follow.
- Seasonal hypersexuality often leads to paraphimosis as an increase in exteriorizing the penis or hemipenis and its use for breeding, or mounting of physical objects in the environment may result in damage or trauma to the exposed organ.
- In cases with spinal involvement (fracture, scoliosis, kyphosis, etc.), compression of the spinal cord may result in loss of neurologic function distal to a lesion. This reduced neurologic function results in paresis of the muscles that normally retain the penis or hemipenis, leading to prolapse.

DIAGNOSIS

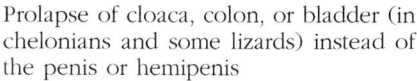

DIFFERENTIAL DIAGNOSIS

Prolapse of cloaca, colon, or bladder (in chelonians and some lizards) instead of the penis or hemipenis

INITIAL DATABASE

Physical exam typically reveals exposed prolapsed penis or hemipenis.

ADVANCED OR CONFIRMATORY TESTING

- Radiographs may be useful to look for spinal involvement that may result in loss of neurologic function distal to a lesion.
- Culture and biopsy/histopathologic examination may be useful in cases with associated infection or abscessation.

TREATMENT

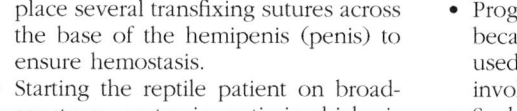

THERAPEUTIC GOALS

- Repair and replace the hemipenis or penis, and keep in place until it can completely heal and stay in place.
- Surgically remove the penis or hemipenis in cases where the organ is considered no longer viable.

ACUTE GENERAL TREATMENT

- Protect and repair the penis or hemipenis, and attempt to replace it as quickly as possible.
- Wound gels and creams (1% silver sulfadiazine cream) can be applied to the organ for protection while waiting for replacement, and with associated abscessation.
- Hypertonic solutions such as sugar or salt solutions can be used along with antiinflammatory drugs to reduce size and swelling.
- Anesthesia is often necessary to successfully replace the penis or hemipenis into the correct anatomic position.

CHRONIC TREATMENT

- After successful replacement, stay sutures may need to be placed across the opening of the hemipene to attempt to keep in place.
  - In chelonians, a purse-string suture may be placed in an attempt to keep the penis in place.
  - The purse-string suture should allow fecal material and urates to pass.
- A necrotic penis or hemipenis may need to be amputated. General anesthesia is recommended. The penis or hemipenis (penis) is clamped with a hemostat near its base; however, the surgeon must leave enough tissue to place several transfixing sutures across the base of the hemipenis (penis) to ensure hemostasis.
- Starting the reptile patient on broad-spectrum systemic antimicrobials is recommended in cases with abscessation and necrosis.
  - Combination therapy such as a quinolone or an aminoglycoside and a third- or fourth-generation cephalosporin or penicillin is often necessary and when possible should be supported by culture and sensitivity.
    - Some examples include:
      - Enrofloxacin (5-10 mg/kg IM, SC, or PO every 24-48 hours) and ceftazidime (20-40 mg/kg IM or SC every 72 hours) or piperacillin (100-200 mg/kg IM or SC every 24-48 hours)
      - Amikacin (5 mg/kg IM or SC initial dose followed by 2.5 mg/kg IM or SC every 72 hours) and ceftazidime (20-40 mg/kg IM or SC every 72 hours) or piperacillin (100-200 mg/kg IM or SC every 24-48 hours)
- Parenteral antibiotic regimens are continued for 3-4 weeks based on severity.

POSSIBLE COMPLICATIONS

- A replaced penis or hemipenis that continues to prolapse over time will likely need to be removed.
- In lizards with hemipenal plugs, gentle removal of the adhered plug material and a "cleaning out" of the hemipenis are necessary. Topical anesthesia or general anesthesia may be necessary to remove this material.
  - Supplementing with vitamin A may be necessary.
- In breeding snakes, hemipenal trauma with subsequent abscessation and cellulitis often involves careful and delicate débridement surgery to remove infected tissue while maintaining as much of the normal architecture as possible (often the owner needs the snake to have the ability to breed in the future).

RECOMMENDED MONITORING

- Watch for reoccurrence of a prolapse.
- Often, hemipenal abscess surgery in breeding snakes may require several surgeries to débride all abscessed tissue.
- Multiple surgeries may be best to maintain as much healthy tissue as possible.

PROGNOSIS AND OUTCOME

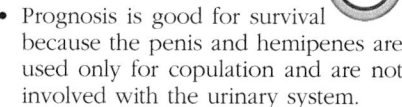

- Prognosis is good for survival because the penis and hemipenes are used only for copulation and are not involved with the urinary system.
- Snakes and lizards have two hemipenes, so losing one will still allow them to potentially breed.
- Chelonians, however, have only one copulatory organ, thus amputation

results in loss of reproductive ability.
- If prolapse is the result of neurologic deficits due to spinal lesions, the overall prognosis is guarded to poor as prolapse of the cloaca and colon may follow.

PEARLS & CONSIDERATIONS

PREVENTION

- Breeding males should not be placed with too many females because overuse of the penis or hemipenis may increase the incidence of trauma, abscessation, and prolapse.
- Keep the environment clean and minimize trauma to the hemipenis from substrates.
- Maintaining adequate levels of vitamin A is important for reducing the incidence of squamous metaplasia and associated hemipenal plug problems in lizards.
- Providing to growing lizards and chelonians a diet with adequate calcium and vitamin D_3 is important to prevent spinal abnormalities that may result from NSHP.

SUGGESTED READINGS

Barten SL: Penile prolapse. In Mader DR, editor: Reptile medicine and surgery, ed 2, St Louis, 2006, Saunders Elsevier, pp 862–864.

DeNardo D: Reproductive biology. In Mader DR, editor: Reptile medicine and surgery, ed 2, St Louis, 2006, Saunders Elsevier, pp 376–390.

Stahl SJ: Veterinary management of snake reproduction, Vet Clin North Am Exotic Anim Pract 5:615–636, 2002.

AUTHOR & EDITOR: **SCOTT J. STAHL**

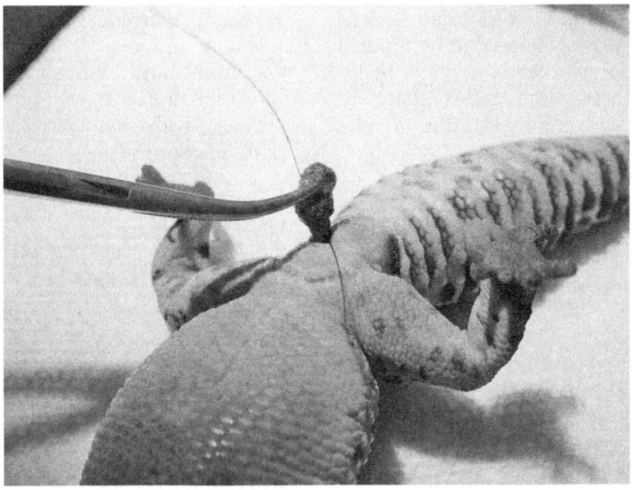

Paraphimosis Prolonged prolapse of the hemipenis required amputation because of extensive tissue trauma; the penis in reptiles can easily be amputated because it is only a copulatory organ and is not needed for urination. *(Photo courtesy Jörg Mayer, The University of Georgia, Athens.)*

REPTILES

Pentastomes

BASIC INFORMATION

DEFINITION

Pentastomes are found in a wide variety of reptiles, with variable pathogenicity. Pentastomid infections are occasionally associated with pneumonic signs.

SYNONYMS

Pentastomiasis, Pentastomida, tongue worms, agema, *Alofia, Armillifer, Cephalobaena, Cubirea, Diesingia, Elenia, Gigliolella, Kiricephalus, Leiperia, Parasambonia, Pelonia, Porocephalus, Raillietiella, Sambonia, Sebekia, Selfia, Subtriquetra, Waddycephalus*

EPIDEMIOLOGY

SPECIES, AGE, SEX

- Pentastomiasis is seen in many diverse species of reptiles.
- No sex predilection is known for pentastomiasis in reptiles.

RISK FACTORS Wild-caught animals, animals kept in enclosures with intermediate hosts, and animals kept under conditions of poor hygiene are at greater risk for clinical pentastomiasis.

CONTAGION AND ZOONOSIS

- Fecal-oral contamination is the typical route of infection for intermediate hosts, and ingestion of intermediate hosts is the typical route of infection for definitive hosts.
- Significant risk of zoonosis is associated with some species of pentastomids.
- Humans are suitable secondary hosts for *Armillifer* spp., which have been associated with a number of human deaths.
- A *Sebekia* spp. has been found to cause parasitic dermatitis in humans.
- *Porocephalus* spp. and have been found to cause fatal disease in dogs.

ASSOCIATED CONDITIONS AND DISORDERS Signs associated with clinical pentastomid infestation vary according to life cycle stage of the pentastomid and include poor growth, subcutaneous swellings, coughing, and dyspnea.

CLINICAL PRESENTATION

HISTORY, CHIEF COMPLAINT

- History associated with clinical nematode infestation usually involves a wild-caught animal or an animal housed in an enclosure with access to intermediate host prey.
- Often, no clinical concerns are present, and pentastomid ova are detected on a routine fecal exam.
- Other clinical concerns presented by owners include poor growth, weight loss, subcutaneous swellings, coughing, and dyspnea.

PHYSICAL EXAM FINDINGS

- Physical exam findings vary according to life cycle stage of the pentastomid.
- Often, no abnormalities are present.
- Abnormalities may include poor growth, weight loss, subcutaneous swellings, coughing, and dyspnea.

ETIOLOGY AND PATHOPHYSIOLOGY

- Most species of pentastomids use reptiles as definitive hosts.
- The adult pentastomid is typically found in the lung, where it lays eggs that are coughed up and passed in the feces.
  - The eggs are ingested by the intermediate host. The intermediate host

is ingested by the definitive host. The nymph then migrates from the gut to the lung.

- Mechanisms of pathology include direct damage to tissues, host inflammatory response, and diversion of nutrients from the host.

DIAGNOSIS

DIFFERENTIAL DIAGNOSIS

- Differential diagnoses for weight loss, coughing, and dyspnea include poor husbandry and numerous causes of pneumonia and metabolic disease.
- Differential diagnoses for subcutaneous swellings include bacterial and fungal granulomas, nonpentastomid parasites, dysplasia, and neoplasia.

INITIAL DATABASE

- A thorough history, physical exam, complete blood count, plasma chemistry, radiographs, and fecal exam form the basic database.
- A pulmonary wash may be useful to screen for pentastomid ova, especially in wild-caught African snakes.

ADVANCED OR CONFIRMATORY TESTING

- Because zoonotic significance and control vary depending on the pentastomid species, identification of pentastomids is essential, and it is important to develop a relationship with a parasitology lab experienced with reptile parasites.
- Pentastomes that are shedding ova may be found by identifying these ova on fecal flotation examination.
- Pentastomes may be removed surgically for identification. Pulmonoscopy is useful for locating pulmonary pentastomes that may not shed significant numbers of ova.
- Grossly visible pentastomes in the coelomic cavity or in other coelomic organs may be found on exploratory coeliotomy.
- Some pentastomes may be identified at necropsy on histopathologic examination.
- Consensus PCR with product sequence analysis is available from the University of Florida for all pentastomids.
  - Samples containing the organism or ova are the samples of choice. Samples should be frozen or stored in ethanol.
  - Samples that have been in formalin for longer than 2 weeks are unsuitable for PCR.

TREATMENT

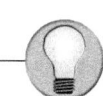

THERAPEUTIC GOALS

- The goal of treatment varies according to the species of pentastomid and the host.
- For *Armillifer*, eradication is the goal.

ACUTE GENERAL TREATMENT

- Treatment varies according to species of pentastomid, site of infestation, life stage, and host.
- For pentastomids with potential direct life cycles, good hygiene practices are necessary to prevent reinfestation.
- Access to intermediate hosts need to be removed.
- Surgical removal is indicated whenever possible. Endoscopic removal of pulmonary adults is often feasible.
- In cases treated pharmaceutically, the massive inflammatory response to dead pentastomids can be much worse than live pentastomids.
- Drugs effective against arthropods can be used, although data on efficacy are lacking.
  - Ivermectin has been used in some case reports.
    - 0.2 mg/ kg SC, repeated in 10 days
  - Ivermectin toxicity is a significant risk in chelonians and crocodilians.
  - Imidacloprid, nitenpyram, selamectin, spinosad, and metaflumizone merit investigation. No safety or efficacy studies have explored use of these drugs in reptiles.
  - Numerous anecdotal stories have described fipronil toxicity in reptiles.

RECOMMENDED MONITORING

Animals should have follow-up testing every 6 months until they have gone for 2 years with negative fecal flotation exams.

PROGNOSIS AND OUTCOME

Prognosis and outcome are variable.

PEARLS & CONSIDERATIONS

COMMENTS

It is essential to identify pentastomids correctly when they are found. *Armillifer* spp. merit greater caution.

PREVENTION

Maintenance of a closed group, testing of populations, strict quarantine, elimination of access to intermediate hosts, avoidance of wild-caught animals, and stringent biosecurity practices are the most effective means of prevention.

SUGGESTED READINGS

Adams L, et al: Fatal pentastomiasis in captive African dwarf crocodile hatchlings (*Osteolaemus tetraspis*), J Zoo Wildl Med 32:500–502, 2001.

Drabick JJ: Pentastomiasis, Rev Infect Dis 9:1087–1094, 2007.

Flach EJ, et al: Pentastomiasis in Bosc's monitor lizards (*Varanus exanthematicus*) caused by an undescribed *Sambonia* species, J Zoo Wildl Med 31:91–95, 2000.

Foster GW, et al: Parasites of Florida softshell turtles (*Apalone ferox*) from southeastern Florida, J Helminthol Soc Washington 65:62–64, 1998.

Junker K, et al: Check-list of the pentastomid parasites crocodilians and freshwater chelonians, Onderstepoort J Vet Res 73:27–36, 2006.

Lavarde V, et al: Lethal infection due to *Armillifer armillatus* (Porocephalida): a snake-related parasitic disease, Clin Infect Dis 29:1346–1347, 1999.

http://www.merckmanuals.com/vet/index.html, access July 10. 2012.

AUTHOR: **JAMES F.X. WELLEHAN, JR.**

EDITOR: **SCOTT J. STAHL**

REPTILES

Periodontal Disease

BASIC INFORMATION

DEFINITION

Bacterial or fungal invasion of the unique periodontal tissue of species of lizards with acrodont dentition

SYNONYMS

Bacterial stomatitis, (see Stomatitis, Bacterial) infectious stomatitis, mouth rot

EPIDEMIOLOGY

SPECIES, AGE, SEX

- Lizards with acrodont dentition are susceptible to periodontal disease.
- Commonly kept species of lizards seen in practice with acrodont dentition include bearded dragons (*Pogona vitticeps*), Asian water dragons (*Physignathus concinnus*), Australian water dragons (*Physignathus lesueurii*), frilled dragons (*Chlamydosaurus kingii*) and all Old World chameleons.
- Acrodont teeth are nonrooted and are ankylosed directly to the mandibular and maxillary bones.
- The fragile nature of the periodontal tissue associated with this type of dentition makes the bones and teeth susceptible to bacterial and fungal invasion.
- No age or sex predilection is known.

RISK FACTORS

- Acrodont dentition:
  - Husbandry factors:
    - Diet: may be related to insects offered. Commonly available cultured insects such as wax worms, mealworms, and crickets are thought to be too soft-bodied compared with natural insects eaten in the wild.
    - Inappropriate heating, lighting, water quality, caging, and/or environmental stress may result in immune compromised lizards that will be more susceptible to opportunistic pathogens with any breakdown of periodontal tissue.
  - Trauma:
    - Trauma to the rostral area, lips, mucous membranes, and/or teeth results in a breakdown in the protective barriers of the oral cavity, allowing organisms to invade.
    - This is common in nervous lizards such as Asian water dragons (*Physignathus concinnus*), which frequently injure the rostral area by jumping into the walls of their enclosure.
  - Wild-caught and/or recently shipped lizards:
    - Lizards that have been shipped and held in holding areas before arrival at suppliers/pet stores have frequently undergone stress and potential trauma to the oral cavity.

CONTAGION AND ZOONOSIS

- Periodontal disease is not considered to be contagious.
- Cases of periodontal disease in which *Salmonella* sp. or *Mycobacterium* have been identified may be zoonotic.

ASSOCIATED CONDITIONS AND DISORDERS Abscesses along lips and perioral tissue associated with active periodontal disease. See Abscesses.

CLINICAL PRESENTATION

HISTORY, CHIEF COMPLAINT

- Lethargy
- Anorexia
- Asymmetry to closure of the mouth
- Swellings or masses on head and perioral area
- Mucus or discharge from mouth or nares
- Swelling and exposure of the mucous membranes of the oral cavity
- Purulent material, discharge, and /or blood evident in oral cavity
- Change in the color of the teeth or of associated bone in the mouth

PHYSICAL EXAM FINDINGS

- Early cases may reveal petechial hemorrhages, increased mucus in the mouth, and asymmetry of mandibular and maxillary bones.
- Inspection of the lateral surfaces of the mandibular and maxillary bones may reveal asymmetric brown/black/green color changes.
- Severe cases often present with deep mandibular and/or maxillary bone involvement, osteomyelitis with associated loss of bone, and pathologic fractures.
- Swellings/abscesses of the soft tissue over the mandibular or maxillary bones may be noted.

ETIOLOGY AND PATHOPHYSIOLOGY

- Acrodont teeth are not replaced when lost and are simply attached/ankylosed to the surface of the mandibular and maxillary bones.
- Occurs when periodontal tissue is damaged or abraded bone is exposed and becomes readily permeable to opportunistic pathogens
- Captive diets of these insectivorous lizards are thought to contribute to this problem because most cultured insects are soft-bodied. It is postulated that the periodontal tissue of these captive lizards does not become "tough" or thickened as it would in wild lizards that are eating a more diverse diet of "rough" insects.
- Severe osteomyelitis with lysis of bone results in weakening of bone and associated fractures.
- Swelling and subsequent abscessation of soft tissues over the involved mandibular and maxillary bones are common as the soft tissue adjacent to periodontal disease becomes involved.
- Gram-negative bacteria are the most common primary pathogens associated with periodontal disease in lizards.
- Commonly isolated Gram-negative organisms include *Pseudomonas, Klebsiella, Proteus, Salmonella, Providencia, Escherichia, Morganella, Aeromonas*, and *Citrobacter.*
- Occasionally, Gram-positive organisms (e.g., *Streptococcus, Corynebacteria*) are the primary organisms, or are found concurrently with Gram-negative bacteria.
- Anaerobic bacteria may also be involved, especially in cases with bone involvement. Often, these anaerobic organisms are found in conjunction with Gram-negative bacteria. Anaerobic organisms frequently isolated include *Bacteroides, Fusobacterium,* and *Clostridium.*
- Fungal organisms (*Aspergillus* sp.) have been identified as pathogens in a case of periodontal disease in a panther chameleon (*Furcifer pardalis*).

DIAGNOSIS

DIFFERENTIAL DIAGNOSIS

- Oral trauma
- Hypovitaminosis A (Old World chameleons) (see Hypovitaminosis A)
- Nutritional secondary hyperparathyroidism (NSHP) (see Nutritional Secondary Hyperparathyroidism)
- Abscesses not involving periodontal tissue
- Neoplasia
- Staining of mandibular and maxillary bones and/or teeth with no associated inflammation/pathology (seen frequently in bearded dragons)

INITIAL DATABASE

- A thorough history, physical exam, complete blood count, plasma chemistry, and fecal exam form the recommended initial database.

- With severe cases, especially those involving bone, elevations of the white blood cell count and/or toxic changes may be noted in heterophils.

ADVANCED OR CONFIRMATORY TESTING

- Culture and sensitivity:
  - A sterile prep should be performed over the site to be sampled, and a sterile scalpel or needle should be used to collect a deep culture sample.
  - Blood cultures may be useful in reptiles with osteomyelitis.
- Cytologic evaluation:
  - Look for bacterial and fungal causes (Diff-Quik, Gram stain, and fresh mounts).
- Biopsy:
  - Pieces of periodontal tissue or damaged/fractured bone and teeth can be submitted for biopsy.
- Radiography:
  - Osteomyelitis in reptiles is characterized radiographically by bone lysis.
  - Radiographs can be used to monitor therapeutic progress.

TREATMENT

THERAPEUTIC GOALS

- Stabilize patient.
- Assess severity of damage to periodontal tissue and bone.
- Attempt to isolate and define specific pathogen(s).
- Perform surgical débridement as necessary using anesthesia and analgesia.
- Provide specific antimicrobials when possible.
- Provide support and follow-up during treatment.
- Discuss and provide long-term preventive care for the oral cavity.
- Address husbandry factors that may have contributed to the periodontal disease/stomatitis.

ACUTE GENERAL TREATMENT

- Initially assess the status of the patient. Warm the patient to the upper end of the reptile's preferred optimal temperature zone (POTZ). For many commonly kept lizards, this is between 80°F and 90°F (between 26°C and 32°C). Begin fluid therapy (10-30 mL/kg/d) to rehydrate if clinically indicated.
- Perform débridement and curettage surgery.
  - Anesthesia may be necessary for these procedures.
- If deep tissue involvement is noted, it may be best to have the patient return once treatment with systemic antimicrobials has been provided for a week. The delineation between healthy and unhealthy tissue will be more evident after this initial systemic treatment, reducing the likelihood of removing any healthy tissue during débridement.
- Necrotic tissue and purulent debris are removed.
- For osteomyelitis, curettage of the bone will be necessary.
  - Unhealthy (soft) or discolored bone should be curetted and removed.
- Multiple surgeries may be necessary.
- Systemic antibiotic therapy:
  - Appropriate initial choices of antibiotics (pending culture and sensitivity results) include amikacin (5 mg/kg IM or SC initial dose followed by 2.5 mg/kg IM or SC every 72 hours), enrofloxacin (5-10 mg/kg IM, SC, or PO every 24-48 hours), and ciprofloxacin (11 mg/kg PO every 48-72 hours).
  - Because anaerobic organisms are commonly associated with osteomyelitis, ceftazidime (20-40 mg/kg IM or SC every 72 hours) is recommended to be combined with one of the above antibiotics.
  - Other antimicrobial choices may be substituted based on the results of sensitivity testing.
  - Systemic antimicrobial regimens are continued for a minimum of 4 weeks in mild cases and potentially for 6-8 weeks in more severe cases involving bone.
  - If fungal organisms are confirmed on culture and cytologic exam/histopathologic exam, systemic itraconazole can be initiated at 5-23.5 mg/kg by mouth every 24-72 hours.
- Topical/local treatment:
  - Dilute chlorhexidine (1 part chlorhexidine to 30 parts saline) can be used to gently clean periodontal lesions.
    - Topical treatment can be stressful and must be done with caution to avoid aspiration.
    - Flushing or cleaning should be done only every 2-3 days, or as necessary.
- Osteomyelitis:
  - Must be reevaluated frequently for continued curettage and débridement until lesions have resolved
  - Topically deep infections involving bone can be treated with 1% silver sulfadiazine cream, or dimethyl sulfoxide (DMSO)/amikacin solution (8 mL of DMSO added to 0.25 mL of amikacin 50 mg/mL) can be used to encourage deep penetration of a topical antibiotic. Depending on culture and sensitivity results, a DMSO/enrofloxacin solution can be used alternatively (add 8 mL of DMSO to 0.5 mL of injectable enrofloxacin 22.7 mg/mL).
  - Topical therapy may need to continue for a minimum of 4 weeks and up to 3-4 months (or longer) depending on severity.
- Pain management:
  - Morphine at 5-10 mg/kg IM or SQ
  - Meloxicam at 0.2-0.3 mg/kg PO, IM q 24 h

CHRONIC TREATMENT

- Oral cleansing gel (e.g., Maxiguard, Oragel) may be used as a long-term/lifetime treatment to clean and protect these damaged tissues.
- After initial therapy for oral disease, developing a strategy for alimentation during treatment for periodontal disease/stomatitis may be necessary. For most lizard patients, gentle assist feeding by hand or with a syringe is acceptable.
- Housing, temperature, humidity, lighting, feeding, water quality, and cagemate interaction are important factors to be evaluated.
- Offering a wide variety of insect prey items, including tough exoskeleton insects such as roaches and beetles, may help to toughen/strengthen periodontal tissue.
- Make specific dietary changes if hypovitaminosis A is suspected to be associated with perioral pathology
- Change housing to decrease rostral damage by providing hide areas and placing visual barriers at the lizard's eye level in the cage.
- Enclosures can be made of solid material instead of glass to reduce visual stress.
- The location of the enclosure can be moved to a low traffic area.
- Meloxicam at 0.2-0.3 mg/kg PO q 24 h can be sent home for use as needed for analgesia during continued treatment.

DRUG INTERACTIONS

Care should be exercised with the use of aminoglycoside antibiotics and nonsteroidal antiinflammatory drugs (NSAIDs) in severely debilitated or dehydrated patients, or in patients with compromised renal function.

RECOMMENDED MONITORING

- Regular oral exams should be performed to inspect the gum line for signs of discoloration, irregularities in the surface, and loss of tissue. If suspicious lesions are present, gentle curettage with dental instrumentation is useful to assess soft tissue and bone.
- In cases with loss of soft tissue or bone, lifelong monitoring by the

owner and the clinician will be necessary because recurrence may occur as the result of changes in the anatomy of the oral cavity.
- Radiographs can be used to monitor therapeutic progress, especially in cases with osteomyelitis.

PROGNOSIS AND OUTCOME

- The prognosis depends on the severity of the periodontal lesions and the state of the reptile at presentation. Aggressive diagnostic measures with early treatment and appropriate adjustments in husbandry will improve the chances for recovery and resolution.
- The prognosis for lizards with periodontal osteomyelitis and loss of bone is guarded to fair depending on severity and progression.
- With chronicity and increased severity of osteomyelitis, the likelihood of hematogenous spread of pathogens to other organs is increased, and the prognosis worsens.
- If *Pseudomonas* sp. are cultured, the prognosis may worsen because these Gram-negative organisms tend to have resistance to many antimicrobials.
- Old World chameleons with severe periodontal disease and associated osteomyelitis have a more guarded prognosis then other lizards because they are easily stressed with treatment.

PEARLS & CONSIDERATIONS

COMMENTS

Clients with lizards that have acrodont dentition should be made aware of the unique oral anatomy of their lizard and how to monitor for early signs of periodontal disease.

PREVENTION

Lifetime dental prophylaxis with an oral cleansing product (e.g., Maxigaurd Oragel, Addison Biological Laboratory, Fayette, MO) will be necessary to reduce progression and minimize the reoccurrence of osteomyelitis.

CLIENT EDUCATION

- It is important to educate owners at the new patient/juvenile checkup and/or at their annual visit about husbandry-related problems that predispose reptiles to periodontal disease, especially for species that are prone to these issues.
- When possible, showing clients how to safely open the mouth of their lizard and evaluate the oral cavity for problems allows them to monitor the health of their lizard.

SUGGESTED READINGS

Heatley JJ, et al: Fungal periodontal osteomyelitis in a Chameleon, *Furcifer pardalis*, J Herpet Med Surg 11:7–12, 2001.
Isaza R, et al: Non-nutritional bone diseases in reptiles. In Kirk RW, editor: Current veterinary therapy, vol 13, Philadelphia, 1995, WB Saunders, pp 1357–1361.
Jacobson ER: Bacterial diseases. In Jacobson ER, editor: Infectious diseases and pathology of reptiles, Boca Raton, FL, 2007, CRC Press, pp 461–526.
McKracken HE: Periodontal disease in lizards. In Fowler ME, et al, editors: Zoo and wild animal medicine, ed 4, Philadelphia, 1999, WB Saunders.
Pare JA, et al: Microbiology: fungal and bacterial diseases of reptiles. In Mader DR, editor: Reptile medicine and surgery, St Louis, 2006, Elsevier, pp 217–238.
Stewart JS: Anaerobic bacterial infections in reptiles, J Zoo Wildl Med 21:180, 1990.
Swaim SF, et al: Topical wound medications: a review, J Am Vet Med Assoc 190:1588, 1987.

CROSS-REFERENCES TO OTHER SECTIONS

Abscesses
Hypovitaminosis A
Nutritional Secondary Hyperparathyroidism
Stomatitis, Bacterial

AUTHOR & EDITOR: **SCOTT J. STAHL**

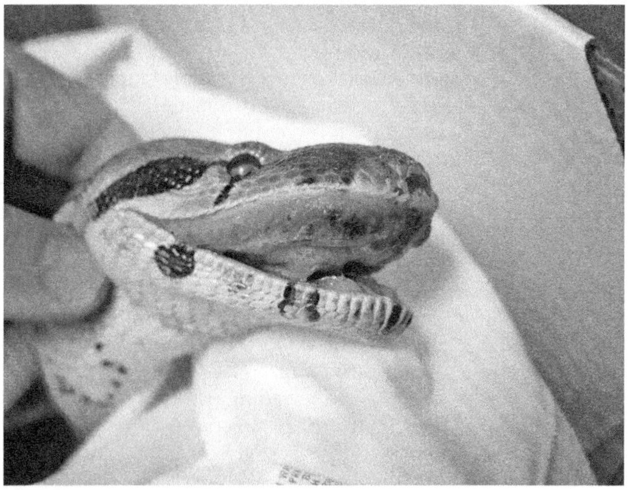

Periodontal Disease Severe stomatitis in a snake, leading to osteomyelitis and swelling of the tissues. Aggressive surgical débridement is needed. *(Photo courtesy Jörg Mayer, The University of Georgia, Athens.)*

REPTILES

Proliferative Spinal Osteoarthropathy

BASIC INFORMATION

DEFINITION

Anomalous displacement or distortion of the spinal column characterized by segmented fusion of affected vertebrae by foci of irregular proliferative bone.

SYNONYMS

Spinal osteopathy, spinal osteoarthropathy, proliferative spinal osteopathy

EPIDEMIOLOGY

SPECIES, AGE, SEX

- All reptilian species, ages, and sexes are possible candidates for this syndrome.
- However, snakes and green iguanas appear to be especially vulnerable.

RISK FACTORS

- Inappropriate husbandry and diet
- Chronic bacterial infections
- Traumatic injury

CONTAGION AND ZOONOSIS *Salmonella* spp. have been associated with some bacterial infections involving the spine, so zoonosis from these bacteria is possible.

ASSOCIATED CONDITIONS AND DISORDERS

- Poor diet and inappropriate husbandry
- Metabolic disease
- Degenerative joint disease
- Osetomyelitis
- Osteolytic neoplasia

CLINICAL PRESENTATION

DISEASE FORMS/SUBTYPES

- Early form
  - Sclerosis of vertebral end plates with or without lysis of the vertebrae
- Advanced form
  - Periarticular bony proliferation involving the dorsolateral articular facets and the costovertebral joints, leading to osseous metaplasia and ankylosis

HISTORY, CHIEF COMPLAINT

- Nonspecific
- Abnormal posture or gait
- Focal swelling on spine
- Irregular spinal conformation
- Lethargy
- Constipation
- Fecal/Urinary incontinence
- Inability to strike, eat, or constrict prey items
- Inability to use limbs
- Paresis/Paralysis

PHYSICAL EXAM FINDINGS

- Variable depending on location and extent of lesion:
  - Decreased mobility
  - Vertebral column stiffness
  - Kyphosis, scoliosis, lordosis
  - Focal swellings along dorsum
  - Pain upon spinal palpation
  - Anorexia and lethargy may result from pain and severe debilitation.
  - Pathologic fractures
  - Neurologic deficits may be present with damage to spinal cord or associated nerve roots:
    - Upper motor neuron signs proximal to lesion
    - Lower motor neuron signs distal to lesion

ETIOLOGY AND PATHOPHYSIOLOGY

- Exact cause is unknown.
- This syndrome may be multifactorial:
  - Inappropriate husbandry
  - Dietary (hypovitaminosis D, hypervitaminosis A)
  - Metabolic disease
  - Bacterial (septicemia)
  - Viral
  - Immune mediated
  - Neoplastic disease
  - Congenital

DIAGNOSIS

DIFFERENTIAL DIAGNOSIS

- Infectious
  - Bacterial: Gram-negative, Gram-positive
  - Fungal
- Metabolic
  - Gout
- Immune mediated
- Nutritional
  - Calcium deficiency
  - Calcium/phosphorus imbalance
  - Vitamin D deficiency
- Neoplastic
  - Osteosarcoma
  - Fibrosarcoma
  - Chondrosarcoma
- Developmental
- Traumatic
- Inappropriate husbandry

INITIAL DATABASE

- Detailed information concerning diet and husbandry
- Radiography (lateral and dorsal ventral [DV] views):
  - Help to determine extent and stage of lesions
- Complete blood cell count:
  - Heterophilic leukocytosis may be present with osteomyelitis.
- Serum/Plasma biochemistry panel
  - Reptiles with secondary nutritional hyperparathyroidism (NSHP) usually are normocalcemic; reptiles with renal disease generally are hypocalcemic and hyperphosphatemic.
  - Uric acid, sodium, chloride, and total protein will be elevated with severe dehydration.

ADVANCED OR CONFIRMATORY TESTING

- CT/MRI:
  - Useful to evaluate structural integrity of associated neurologic, connective, and soft tissues
  - Identify sites of active disease
- Nuclear bone scan:
  - Identifies sites of active disease
- Bone biopsy and histopathologic evaluation
  - Heavy epaxial musculature can make access difficult.
  - Care must be taken not to induce iatrogenic spinal fractures.
- Aerobic and anaerobic culture (bone and blood culture):
  - *Salmonella* spp. and *Streptococcus* spp. have been isolated from both bone and blood culture in snakes with proliferative osteoarthritis and osteoarthropathy of the spine.
  - Lesions may develop 22-36 months after septicemic episode.
  - Fastidious organisms may be difficult to isolate and may require specialized growth media.
  - If bacterial colonies are detected, they are found within the joint spaces, around synovial membranes, along superficial surfaces of cortical bone, or at the interfaces of subchondral bone and articular cartilage.
    - Fine-needle aspiration may be useful for obtaining local culture.
  - Fungal culture should also be performed to identify any fungal contamination.

TREATMENT

THERAPEUTIC GOALS

- Stabilize patient.
- Provide adequate analgesia.
- Address any underlying metabolic disease.
- Determine extent and severity of spinal lesions.
- Select appropriate antimicrobial agent.

- Perform surgical débridement of granulomatous lesions or amputation of affected tail segments.
- Correct any underlying dietary or husbandry issues.

ACUTE GENERAL TREATMENT

- Stabilize patient:
  - Provide supplemental heat consistent with species preferred optimal temperature zone (POTZ).
  - Shock therapy if indicated:
    - Fluids: IO or IV boluses of crystalloids (5-10 mL/kg) with colloids (3-5 mL/kg)
- Analgesia:
  - Morphine:
    - Chelonians: 1.5 mg/kg
    - Lizards: 10 mg/kg
  - Meloxicam (Metacam): 0.1-0.3 mg/kg PO, IM q 24 h
- Select appropriate antibiotic therapy:
  - Baytril (22.7 mg/mL, do not use 100 mg/mL): 5-10 mg/kg q 24-72 h PO, SC, IM, ICe
  - Ceftazidime: 20-40 mg/kg SC, IM, IV q 72 h
  - Amikacin 5 mg/kg IM, then 2.5 mg/kg q 72 h

CHRONIC TREATMENT

- Antimicrobial therapy should be continued for extended periods of time (4-6 weeks or longer):
  - Select antimicrobials that have good bone penetration.
  - Antibiotic-impregnated polymethylmethacrylate beads may be used in conjunction with systemic therapy.
- Surgical intervention:
  - Tail amputation in cases involving coccygeal vertebrae
  - Débridement of granulomatous lesions

DRUG INTERACTIONS

Care should be exercised with the use of aminoglycoside antibiotics and nonsteroidal antiinflammatory drugs (NSAIDs) in severely debilitated or dehydrated patients, or in patients with compromised renal function.

POSSIBLE COMPLICATIONS

Iatrogenic spinal fracture

RECOMMENDED MONITORING

Radiographic evaluation of spinal lesions to assess for improvement or development of new lesions

PROGNOSIS AND OUTCOME

- Because of the advanced state of the lesions at presentation, most cases have a guarded to poor prognosis.
- Euthanasia should be considered in all cases of severe spinal involvement.

PEARLS & CONSIDERATIONS

COMMENTS

- Early detection combined with aggressive long-term antibiotic therapy, surgical débridement, and supportive care may improve the clinical situation but may not result in a true cure of the condition.
- Amputation of as much of the affected tail as surgically possible seemed to result in reduced pain and discomfort in iguanas presenting with coccygeal spinal arthrosis.
- Further investigation into the exact cause and pathogenesis of the syndrome is needed so more effective treatment modalities and preventive strategies can be developed.

PREVENTION

- Proper nutrition and environmental conditions based on specific species requirements are essential.
- Proper caging

SUGGESTED READINGS

Fitzgerald K, et al: Spinal osteopathy. In Mader DR, editor: Reptile medicine and surgery, St Louis, 2006, Elsevier Inc., pp 906–912.

Innis C, et al: Spinal osteoarthropathy in green iguanas (*Iguana iguana*), Lawrence, KS, 2006, Proc Assoc Reptilian Amphibian Veterinarians, pp 40–42.

Isaza R, et al: Proliferative osteoarthritis and osteoarthritis in 15 snakes, J Zoo Wildl Med 31:20–27, 2000.

Ramsay EC, et al: Osteomyelitis associated with *Salmonella enterica* SS *arizonae* in a colony of ridgenose rattlesnakes (*Crotalus willardi*), J Zoo Wildl Med 33:301–310, 2002.

AUTHOR: **DAVID A. CRUM**

EDITOR: **SCOTT J. STAHL**

REPTILES

Regurgitation/Vomiting

BASIC INFORMATION

DEFINITION

- Regurgitation is the passive discharge of undigested food within a few hours of consumption.
- Vomiting is the ejection of food from the stomach or the anterior intestine.
- Vomiting is controlled by the autonomic and somatic nervous systems.

SYNONYM

Emesis

EPIDEMIOLOGY

SPECIES, AGE, SEX

- All species of any age susceptible
- Commonly reported in recently fed snakes in stressful situations (e.g., handled) or kept at a low temperature

RISK FACTORS

- Elevated stress levels due to overstimulation and overcrowding
- Consumption of too large a meal
- Temperature below digestive requirement
- Infection altering physiologic or digestive processes
- Anatomic intestinal obstructions
- Neonatal congenital gastrointestinal defects
- Medication (e.g., tortoises with parenteral enrofloxacin)
- Bufotoxins

CONTAGION AND ZOONOSIS

- Infectious causes are common.
- Cryptosporidiosis in snakes
- Inclusion body disease (IBD) virus in boid snakes (see Inclusion Body Disease in Snakes)
- *Chlamydophyla* in a gaboon viper (*Bitis gabonica*) (see Chlamydophilosis)
- Parasites associated include cryptosporidiosis, amoebiasis, cestodiasis, and ascariasis.

ASSOCIATED CONDITIONS AND DISORDERS Diarrhea (see Diarrhea)

CLINICAL PRESENTATION

HISTORY, CHIEF COMPLAINT

- A complete history and thorough physical exam are needed to narrow down potential causes of regurgitation and vomiting.
- Expelled food found on the cage floor

- It is often difficult for owners to differentiate between regurgitation and vomiting.
- Some clients may provide feeding records that may help clinicians to associate a pattern for the regurgitation/vomiting and to determine the severity of the condition.
- Inactivity and increased basking frequency
- Snakes housed at a temperature that is too cool will expel food that is relatively fresh and undigested.
- Regurgitation and vomiting are uncommon in chelonians and when seen are considered serious symptoms of illness. One exception to this is iatrogenic regurgitation/vomiting associated with parenteral injections of enrofloxacin.
- Animals demonstrating symptoms of regurgitation and vomiting may display prolonged disinterest in feeding.

PHYSICAL EXAM FINDINGS

- Animals suffering from frequent vomiting may present dehydrated with acid-base and electrolyte imbalances.
- Emaciation/cachexia may be evident in an animal that is unable to keep food items down over an extended period of time.
- Animals with advanced symptoms may be dull, inactive, and unresponsive.

ETIOLOGY AND PATHOPHYSIOLOGY

- Improper husbandry is the most common cause of regurgitation and vomiting in reptiles.
- The most common mistakes include keeping the reptile at a lower temperature than required for adequate digestion and postprandial handling, especially in snakes.
- Infectious causes for gastritis and subsequent regurgitation/vomiting are common, including:
  - Gram-negative bacteria
  - *Chlamydophyla*
  - Viral disease such as IBD virus in boid snakes
  - Gastrointestinal parasites, including coccidia (cryptosporidiosis and others), amoebae, cestodes, and nematodes (ascariasis)
  - Toxins such as pesticides, including organophosphates and bufotoxins, may cause vomiting. Iatrogenic vomiting can be caused by drugs such as enrofloxacin, miticides, levamisole, xylazine, and apomorphine.
  - Intestinal obstructions or lesions associated with food consumption, surgery, or disease may induce regurgitation and vomiting.
  - Metabolic disease such as renal or hepatic insufficiency
- These causes disrupt normal esophageal or gastric function and/or motility, resulting in impaired digestion, stasis, putrification, and passive (regurgitation) or active (vomiting) discharge of ingesta.
- Regurgitation typically is associated with an esophageal or pharyngeal problem.
- Gastroesophageal sphincter incompetence is a common gastric issue that causes regurgitation.
  - These events disrupt normal esophageal or gastric functions or motility.
- Both vomiting and regurgitation are symptoms of an underlying problem, not diseases themselves.

DIAGNOSIS

DIFFERENTIAL DIAGNOSIS

- Improper husbandry (temperature, handling)
- Infectious disease (bacterial, *Chlamydophila*, viral [IBD], coccidian, cryptosporidiosis, nematodes, cestodes)
- Toxins
- Iatrogenic from drugs
- Constipation
- Foreign body obstruction
- Neoplasia
- Neonatal gastrointestinal malformations

INITIAL DATABASE

- A thorough history, physical exam, complete blood count, plasma chemistry, fecal parasite analysis, survey radiographs, and ultrasonography
- Acid-fast staining of fecal material or recently regurgitated meal for cryptosporidiosis

ADVANCED OR CONFIRMATORY TESTING

- Gastrointestinal endoscopy with biopsy for histopathologic and microbiological exam
- Contrast radiography
- Surgical biopsy with histopathologic and microbiological exam

TREATMENT

THERAPEUTIC GOALS

- Correction of husbandry practices, including temperature, hygiene, and feeding regiment
- Rehydration (starting at 10:30 mL/kg/24h) to normalize any electrolyte and acid-base abnormalities
- Diagnosis and treatment of specific cause of clinical signs of regurgitation/vomiting
- Removal of obstructions
- Replenishment of dietary deficits

ACUTE GENERAL TREATMENT

- Fluid therapy (starting at 10-30 mL/kg/24h) and monitoring of hematocrit, electrolytes, and uric acid (urea in aquatic species)
- Administration of antibacterial or antiparasitic drugs if these pathogenic organisms are found
- Antibiotics (bacteria):
  - Good initial choices (pending culture and sensitivity) would include combination therapy, such as a quinoline or aminoglycoside, and a third- or fourth-generation cephalosporin or penicillin.
    - For example, enrofloxacin (10 mg/kg IM, SC, PO every 24-48 hours) and ceftazidime (20-40 mg/kg IM or SC every 72 hours) or piperacillin (100-200 mg/kg IM or SC every 24-48 hours)
    - Or amikacin (5 mg/kg IM or SC initial dose followed by 2.5 mg/kg IM or SC every 72 hours) and ceftazidime (20-40 mg/kg IM or SC every 72 hours) or piperacillin (100-200 mg/kg IM or SC every24-48 hours)
    - Systemic antimicrobial regimens are continued for a minimum of 4 weeks. The length of treatment will be based on clinical response and follow-up evaluations.
- Antiparasitics:
  - Nematodes (see Nematodiasis):
    - Fenbendazole at 25 mg/kg PO q 7 days for 3 treatments. Posttreatment fecal examinations should be performed, and treatment repeated as necessary.
  - Cryptosporidiosis:
    - *Cryptosporidium* species are not susceptible to many of the older anticoccidials. Some empirical drugs and doses that may be used include:
      - Nitazoxanide (Navigator) 25 mg/kg PO q 24 h × 5 days, then 50 mg/kg PO q 24 h × additional 23 days. This drug has perhaps the most promise of any currently available anti-cryptosporidial based on mammalian data. Some data show that azithromycin in combination with nitazoxanide may be useful in mammals. See Cryptosporidiosis.
  - Entamoeba/amoeba (see Entamoebiasis):
    - Metronidazole 20-50 mg/kg orally every 2-3 days (3-5 doses) for clinically ill reptiles.
    - Colubrids (e.g., king snakes, milk snakes, indigo) and rattlesnakes may be more sensitive and should use the lower dose. Pharmacokinetic studies in green iguanas and yellow rat snakes

recommended 20 mg/kg orally every 48 hours.
- The effectiveness of specific gastrointestinal supportive medications (used in mammals) for esophagitis and gastritis is unknown in reptiles, and the doses are empirical.
- However, used in conjunction with specific treatments based on diagnostic results, these medications may help to provide comfort from gastrointestinal distress in reptile patients.
- Gastrointestinal supportive medications:
  - Cimetidine 4 mg/kg PO, IM q 8-12 h
  - Sucralfate 500-1000 mg/kg PO q 6-8 h
  - Famotidine 0.25-0.5 mg/kg PO, SC q 24-72 h

CHRONIC TREATMENT

- Assist feeding by feeding tube if necessary to combat severe dietary deficits.
- Improvements in management, especially thermal/humidity/water/quality light provision
- Surgical removal of obstructive masses or foreign bodies

POSSIBLE COMPLICATIONS

- Irreversible metabolic shutdown
- Sepsis
- Starvation

RECOMMENDED MONITORING

- Monitor electrolytes.
- Weight
- Dietary content

PROGNOSIS AND OUTCOME

With appropriate supportive care, dietary management, and chemotherapeutics, the prognosis for acute vomiting is good but guarded if chronic and long-standing.

PEARLS & CONSIDERATIONS

COMMENTS

- Assisted or force feeding without restoring natural physiologic parameters can be detrimental.
- If the underlying cause can be accurately identified, the symptoms of regurgitation and vomiting can be eliminated.
- Snakes with cryptosporidiosis vomit infrequently.
- Reiterate that regurgitation and vomiting are symptoms, not a disease.

PREVENTION

- Appropriate thermal gradients
- Appropriate hygiene
- Appropriate diet

CLIENT EDUCATION

Review of species-specific husbandry requirements, disease risks, hygiene, ecology, and social dynamics. Review of potential zoonoses

SUGGESTED READINGS

Funk RS: Vomiting and regurgitation. In Mader DR, editor: Reptile medicine and surgery, ed 2, Philadelphia, 2006, WB Saunders, pp 939–940.

Mitchell MA, et al: Clinical reptile gastroenterology, Vet Clin North Am Exot Anim Pract 8:277–298, 2005.

Regal PJ: Thermophilic response following feeding of certain reptiles, Copeia 3:588–590, 1966.

CROSS-REFERENCES TO OTHER SECTIONS

Chlamydophilosis
Coccidiosis
Cryptosporidiosis
Diarrhea
Entamoebiasis
Inclusion Body Disease of Snakes
Nematodiasis

AUTHOR: **JASON NORMAN**

EDITOR: **SCOTT J. STAHL**

REPTILES

Renal Disease

Client Education Sheet Available on Website

BASIC INFORMATION

DEFINITION

Infectious and noninfectious causes of reduced function and disease of the urinary system, including renal cysts, interstitial nephritis, glomerulonephritis, pyelonephritis, glomerulosclerosis, nephrosclerosis, glomerulonephrosis, tubulonephrosis, renal edema, amoyloidosis, gout, bacterial nephritis, and neoplasia

EPIDEMIOLOGY

SPECIES, AGE, SEX Potentially any species, any age, and with no proven gender bias

GENETICS AND BREED PREDISPOSITION Commonly reported in green iguanas because of their popularity

RISK FACTORS

- High-protein diets, especially feeding insects or canned dog/cat foods to herbivores
- Dehydration due to low environmental humidity
- Poor or unsuitable water availability (e.g., some reptiles will drink only droplets on foliage)

CONTAGION AND ZOONOSIS

- Infectious causes of renal disease are rare.
- Noninfectious degenerative changes are more common.

ASSOCIATED CONDITIONS AND DISORDERS

- Renomegaly
- Constipation

CLINICAL PRESENTATION

HISTORY, CHIEF COMPLAINT

- A detailed history is most important when investigating any disease.
  - History can often differentiate between true acute renal disease and chronic renal failure.
- Acute renal disease: acute-onset depression, anorexia, and usually cessation of urine and urate output
- Recent exposure to nephrotoxins, including aminoglycoside antibiotics and high doses of vitamin D_3
- Chronic renal disease: reptiles presented with chronic renal disease will often have suffered from long-term mismanagement.
  - High-protein diets rich in purines, in particular, the use of canned dog or cat foods
  - Inadequate humidity or inappropriate water provision (e.g., water bowl instead of daily spraying) can result in chronic dehydration.
- Regular use of oral vitamin D_3 as a substitute for broad-spectrum lighting can cause nephrocalcinosis.
- Reptiles that recover from secondary nutritional hyperparathyroidism may

have sustained chronic renal damage from the cytotoxic effects of excess parathyroid hormone.
- Affected animals tend to have a more protracted history, including deteriorating body condition, capricious appetite, and lethargy that may extend over weeks or months; as a result, most cases present dehydrated and emaciated.
- Rarely will owners report polydipsia or polyuria.

PHYSICAL EXAM FINDINGS
- A thorough physical exam is always indicated and should include an accurate measurement of weight.
- Reptiles with severe renal compromise will present in a depressed and weakened state.
- In cases of acute renal disease, the reptile will often present in good body condition, whereas in chronic renal disease cases, the reptile will likely be underweight.
- Dehydration may be inferred from reductions in skin elasticity and salivary and ocular secretions. Pharyngeal edema is common.
- When digital palpation of the kidneys per cutaneous or per cloaca is possible, the size, shape, and contours of the kidneys should be determined.
- Pronounced renomegaly may cause constipation and cloacal prolapse.

ETIOLOGY AND PATHOPHYSIOLOGY
- Degenerative nephroses represent the most common diseases encountered and usually are characterized by variable degeneration or necrosis of the glomeruli (glomerulonephrosis) and/or tubules (tubulonephrosis).
- In the terminal stages, aberrant calcium metabolism may cause metastatic calcification of the cardiorespiratory and gastrointestinal systems. Calcification of the great vessels and myocardium can lead to congestion of peripheral blood vessels (especially obvious on the sclera of the eye), poor circulation, and ischemic necrosis of the tail. Gastrointestinal effects may include vomiting and passing poorly digested food.
- High-protein diets are considered a predisposing cause of hyperuricemia, gout, and nephrosis in herbivorous reptiles; modern texts now recommend avoiding such foods. Blockage of the renal tubules with secreted urate is another process that impairs renal function and has been associated with chronic dehydration in snakes. Maintenance of high-humidity, rain-forest species in dry captive conditions is suggested as a possible cause of chronic dehydration and nephropathy.

DIAGNOSIS

DIFFERENTIAL DIAGNOSIS
- Acute renal disease
- Chronic renal disease
- Constipation
- Dystocia
- Extrarenal neoplasia
- Secondary nutritional hyperparathyroidism (see Nutritional Secondary Hyperparathyroidism)

INITIAL DATABASE
A thorough history, physical exam, complete blood count, plasma chemistry (especially total calcium, ionized calcium, phosphorus, sodium, potassium, uric acid, urea for aquatic species, total protein, and albumin), urinalysis, survey radiographs, and ultrasonography

ADVANCED OR CONFIRMATORY TESTING
- Renal urography, renal ultrasonography
- Renal endoscopy and biopsy
- Iohexol excretion study to determine glomerular filtration rate (GFR)

TREATMENT

THERAPEUTIC GOALS
- Rehydration to establish urine flow and normalize any electrolyte abnormalities
- Reduction of plasma uric acid (or urea) levels if elevated using allopurinol and dietary reduction in protein

ACUTE GENERAL TREATMENT
- Fluid therapy (intravenous, intraosseous, or intracoelomic) and monitoring of hematocrit, electrolytes, and uric acid (urea in aquatic species)
- Diuretics (furosemide 5 mg/kg PO, IM, IV q 12-24 h) if anuric
- Phosphate binders (aluminum hydroxide 100 mg/kg PO q 12-24 h)
- Calcium therapy if hypocalcemic (calcium glubionate 10 mg/kg PO q 12-24 h)
- Allopurinol (10-20 mg/kg PO q 24 h) to reduce hyperuricemia

CHRONIC TREATMENT
- Allopurinol
- Phosphate binders
- Dietary correction (reduced protein)
- Improvements in management, especially thermal/humidity/water/quality light provision

DRUG INTERACTIONS
Stagger oral phosphate binders and calcium supplements.

POSSIBLE COMPLICATIONS
- Visceral/articular gout (see Gout)
- Soft-tissue mineralization (gastrointestinal tract, great vessels)
- Nonregenerative anemia
- Secondary renal hyperparathyroidism

RECOMMENDED MONITORING
- Monitor electrolytes, total protein, albumin, and uric acid (or urea for aquatic species).
- Weight
- Dietary protein content

PROGNOSIS AND OUTCOME
- The prognosis for chronic renal disease is poor.
- The prognosis for acute renal disease is guarded.

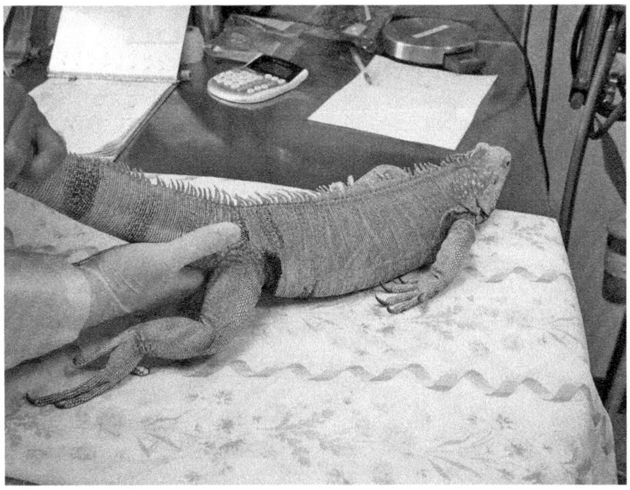

Renal Disease Digital palpation of the cloaca of an iguana with renal disease. The caudal positioning of the kidneys makes it easy to palpate them for enlargement. *(Photo courtesy Jörg Mayer, The University of Georgia, Athens.)*

DISEASES AND DISORDERS

REPTILES

PEARLS & CONSIDERATIONS

COMMENTS

- Reptile kidneys cannot concentrate urine, and so urine specific gravity cannot be used as a prognostic indicator.
- Reptile kidneys empty into the cloaca, not directly into the bladder. In those species that have a bladder (all chelonians, some lizards), urine then passes into the bladder, where postrenal modification of urine can occur (electrolyte exchange and water absorption by osmosis).
- Reptile bladder can act as a water storage organ.
- The reptile renal portal system from the tail and the hind limbs in some species provide blood to the renal tubules, not to the glomeruli.
- Normal glomerular filtration rates for hydrated iguanas are around 15-18 mL/kg/h and can be calculated using an iohexol excretion study:
  - Contact the Diagnostic Center for Population and Animal Health (Michigan State University, East Lansing, MI 48824, USA; Tel 517-353-1683, www.ahdl.msu.edu) to check for any changes to the blood collection and submission requirements for iohexol assay and GFR calculation.
  - Ensure that the reptile is hydrated and fasted for 24 hours.
  - Weigh accurately, and inject 75 mg/kg iohexol intravenously (intravenous catheterization reduces the risks of perivascular injection, which would invalidate the results) at time 0.
- The theoretical ineffectiveness of furosemide in the reptile kidney, lacking a loop of Henle, has not been confirmed experimentally. Indeed, studies in chelonians and lizards have demonstrated that furosemide exerts significant diuretic effects by increasing sodium, chloride, potassium, and water losses from the kidney, colon, cloaca, and bladder.

PREVENTION

- Appropriate thermal and humidity gradients
- Appropriate lighting and calcium supplementation
- Appropriate dietary protein

SUGGESTED READINGS

Hernandez-Divers SJ, et al: Effects of allopurinol on plasma uric acid levels in normo- and hyperuricaemic green iguanas (*Iguana iguana*), Vet Rec 162:112–115, 2008.

Hernandez-Divers SJ, et al: Renal disease in reptiles: diagnosis and clinical management. In Mader DR, editor: Reptile medicine and surgery, ed 2, St Louis, 2006, Elsevier Publishing, pp 878–892.

Hernandez-Divers SJ, et al: Renal evaluation in the green iguana (*Iguana iguana*): assessment of plasma biochemistry, glomerular filtration rate, and endoscopic biopsy, J Zoo Wildl Med 36:155–168, 2005.

CROSS-REFERENCES TO OTHER SECTIONS

Gout

Nutritional Secondary Hyperparathyroidism (NSHP)

AUTHOR: **STEPHEN J. DIVERS**

EDITOR: **SCOTT J. STAHL**

REPTILES

Reovirus Infections

BASIC INFORMATION

DEFINITION

Nonenveloped RNA viruses, 70-85 nm in diameter, spherical icosahedral particles; reoviruses infecting reptiles are found in the genus *Orthoreovirus*.

EPIDEMIOLOGY

SPECIES, AGE, SEX

- Many reptile species can be infected with reoviruses, including snakes, lizards, and tortoises.
- Reoviral disease appears to be most common in snakes.
- The species specificity of reoviruses is not known, but as small segmented RNA viruses, it is expected that they may be more able to jump host species than a large DNA virus, such as an adenovirus or herpesvirus.
- Young, geriatric, and immune suppressed animals appear to be at greatest risk for disease.
- No sex predilections are known.

RISK FACTORS Risk factors for reoviral disease are not well understood. Stressed animals appear to be more likely to develop clinical disease.

CONTAGION AND ZOONOSIS

- Reoviruses are very stable in the environment, and disinfection is difficult.
- Disinfectants effective against other unenveloped viruses, such as parvoviruses, may be expected to be effective against reoviruses.
- No zoonotic risk is known for any reptile reovirus, but a reovirus found to cause encephalitis in baboons is somewhat related to reptile reoviruses.

ASSOCIATED CONDITIONS AND DISORDERS Pneumonia, esophagitis, and encephalitis are the most common presentations of reoviral disease.

CLINICAL PRESENTATION

DISEASE FORMS/SUBTYPES

- Pneumonia and encephalitis are the most common clinical presentations of reoviral disease.
- The immune system of the animal is often overwhelmed, and secondary infections are common.

HISTORY, CHIEF COMPLAINT Common complaints on presentation for reoviral disease include pneumonia, neurologic signs, and high death rates.

PHYSICAL EXAM FINDINGS Physical exam findings often include dyspnea and impaired righting reflexes.

ETIOLOGY AND PATHOPHYSIOLOGY

Reptile reoviruses characterized to date are all in the genus *Orthoreovirus*.

DIAGNOSIS

DIFFERENTIAL DIAGNOSIS

Paramyxoviral disease in snakes is very similar to reoviral disease.

INITIAL DATABASE

A thorough husbandry history, physical exam, complete blood count, plasma chemistry, radiographs, and a pulmonary wash for cytologic exam and PCR form a basic database.

ADVANCED OR CONFIRMATORY TESTING

- Nested PCR with product sequence analysis is available from the University of Florida for all reptile reoviruses. Pulmonary washes are generally the antemortem sample of choice.

- Histologic findings of proliferative pneumonia with syncytia are common in both reoviral and paramyxoviral diseases.

TREATMENT

ACUTE GENERAL TREATMENT

Providing supportive care, addressing husbandry deficiencies, and identifying and treating secondary bacterial and fungal infections are the most important aspects of treating reoviral disease.

CHRONIC TREATMENT

It is not known whether reoviruses are persistent in reptiles. Because they are small RNA viruses, this is considered less likely.

PROGNOSIS AND OUTCOME

The prognosis for animals with reoviral disease is guarded.

PEARLS & CONSIDERATIONS

COMMENTS

- This disease is clinically very similar to paramyxovirus disease.
- Molecular diagnostics need to be done to differentiate the two.
- Although reoviruses have been isolated from tortoises, paramyxoviruses have yet to be isolated from tortoises.

PREVENTION

Maintenance of a closed group, testing of populations, testing during quarantine, and stringent biosecurity practices are the most effective means of prevention.

SUGGESTED READINGS

Ahne W, et al: Isolation of a reovirus from the snake, *Python regius*, Arch Virol 94:135–139, 1987.
Blahak S, et al: Comparison of 6 different reoviruses of various reptiles, Vet Res 26: 470–476, 1995.
Drury SE, et al: Isolation and identification of a reovirus from a lizard, *Uromastyx hardwickii*, in the United Kingdom, Vet Rec 151:637–638, 2002.
Gravendyck M, et al: Paramyxoviral and reoviral infections of iguanas on Honduran Islands, J Wildl Dis 34:33–38, 1998.
Lamirande EW, et al: Isolation and experimental transmission of a reovirus pathogenic in ratsnakes (*Elaphe* species), Virus Res 63: 135–141, 1999.
Vieler E, et al: Characterization of a reovirus isolate from a rattle snake, *Crotalus viridis*, with neurological dysfunction, Arch Virol 138:341–344, 1994.

CROSS-REFERENCES TO OTHER SECTIONS

Adenovirus
Chlamydiophila
Inclusion Body Disease
Mycoplasma
Paramyxovirus
Respiratory (lower) Disease/Pneumonia

AUTHOR: **JAMES F.X. WELLEHAN, JR.**

EDITOR: **SCOTT J. STAHL**

REPTILES

Respiratory (Lower) Tract Disease/Pneumonia

BASIC INFORMATION

DEFINITION

Bacterial invasion of the trachea, bronchi, and lung(s)

EPIDEMIOLOGY

GENETICS AND BREED PREDISPOSITION

- Common in snakes, especially larger species such as boas and pythons
- Commonly affected lizards include monitor lizards, water dragons, and chameleons.
- Not routinely seen in the green iguana
- Aquatic turtles, box turtles, and tortoises are susceptible to both upper and lower respiratory disease.

RISK FACTORS

- Reptile lungs are typically saclike and lack a diaphragm; thus expulsion of respiratory secretions and exudates is functionally difficult.
- Inappropriate temperatures (usually not warm enough) and humidity that is too high or low (e.g., ball pythons) often lead to respiratory disease.
- Poor ventilation, especially with exposure to ammonia gases from urates/uric acid
- Dietary and nutrition-related issues such as hypovitaminosis A, resulting in a compromised respiratory system
- Inappropriate environment may result in damage/trauma to the rostrum with attempts to "push out" and escape.
  - This damage to the oral cavity may predispose the reptile to respiratory disease.
- Stress from shipping and holding conditions
- Captive social stress
- Reproduction-related stress (both males and females)
- Infections or disorders of the oral cavity with subsequent inhalation of mucus and bacteria into the trachea and lungs

CONTAGION AND ZOONOSIS

- Bacterial respiratory infections are not typically contagious from one reptile to another.
- Some special forms of respiratory disease such as *Chlamydia* may have a higher likelihood of being contagious.

ASSOCIATED CONDITIONS AND DISORDERS

- *Chlamydia*
  - Several species of *Chlamydophila* have been associated with lower respiratory tract of boas and pythons.
- *Mycobacterium*
  - *Mycobacterium* spp. can be found to be the primary pathogens in lower respiratory disease.
  - Zoonotic potential
- *Mycoplasma*
  - *Mycoplasma* is the causative agent in the upper respiratory disease found in the California desert tortoise.
  - It may also cause upper respiratory disease in a large number of other tortoise species.
  - It can cause proliferative tracheitis and chronic lower respiratory disease in a Burmese python.
- Salmonellosis
  - Many serotypes of *Salmonella* have been cultured from the respiratory tract of reptiles.
  - Often reptiles are asymptomatic carriers.
  - Treatment is controversial, and some serotypes have zoonotic potential, which may have public health consequences.

CLINICAL PRESENTATION

HISTORY, CHIEF COMPLAINT

- Owner may note a change in the reptile's normal breathing pattern or increased noise with respiration such as wheezing, gurgling, and/or popping sounds.
- Excess mucus in the oral cavity; possible bubbling of fluid from the mouth or nares

- Nasal discharge and/or blockage of the nares often associated with open-mouth breathing
- The head is held in an elevated position with the neck stretched out.
- In lizards and chelonians, an increased amount of discharge from eye(s) or holding an eye(s) closed
- In aquatic chelonians, uneven swimming or an inability to dive
- Inactivity, depression, or anorexia

PHYSICAL EXAM FINDINGS

- Generalized loss of muscle mass and poor body condition
- Conjunctivitis or epiphora
- Fluid or purulent material from nares or blocked nares
- Pale or hyperemic oral cavity, usually with increased "foamy" or "ropey" mucus and saliva
- Obvious fluid or mucopurulent discharge within the choanal area, glottis, and trachea
- Increased respiratory rate or respiratory distress may be noted during or after the examination.
- Obvious wheezing and stridor. It is important to discern whether the noise is originating from the trachea and/or glottis, from the nares, or from both.
    - This can be determined by listening for these sounds with the mouth closed, then with the mouth open (with the mouth open, the nares and upper respiratory system are no longer involved).
- Hyperinflation of the lungs: The reptile may be retaining air in the lungs or air sacs (snakes and some lizards), resulting in a bloated appearance.
- Auscultation with the use of a slightly dampened paper towel or thin cloth between the reptile and the head of the stethoscope may allow detection of abnormal lung sounds such as crackles, wheezes, or pops.

ETIOLOGY AND PATHOPHYSIOLOGY

- Primary pathogens are Gram-negative bacterial organisms:
    - *Pseudomonas* spp. (and others in this same family), *Klebsiella* spp., *Proteus* spp., *Escherichia coli*, *Aeromonas hydrophila*, *Morganella morganii*, *Citrobacter freundii*, *Pasteurella* spp. (primarily in chelonians)
- Anaerobic bacteria are also commonly isolated from cultures.
    - *Clostridium*, *Bacteroides*, *Fusobacterium*, *Propionibacterium*, and *Peptostreptococcus*
- Gram-positive bacteria are occasionally a primary pathogen.
    - *Streptococcus* spp., *Staphylococcus* spp., and *Corynebacterium*
- Increase in mucus and other secretions in the lungs, trachea, glottis, oral cavity, and nares
- Disrupts buoyancy in water turtles, causing uneven swimming or an inability to dive/submerge

DIAGNOSIS

DIFFERENTIAL DIAGNOSIS

- Parasitic disease
- Trematodes (especially in aquatic turtles, indigo snakes, monitor lizards, and any other fish or amphibian eating reptiles)
- Nematodes *(Rhabdias, Strongyloides, Entolomas, Filarids)*
- Pentastomes (monitors, boids such as Boelen's python)
- Protozoa (*Entamoeba invadens, Monocercomonas*)
- Viral disease (paramyxovirus, boid inclusion body disease)
- Fungal (rare)
- Neoplasia (rare)
- Chondromas in the trachea of ball pythons
- Obstruction of nares/nostrils
- Defense "hissing"
- Allergy-related, clear nasal discharge in chelonians
- Aspiration of food material, substrate, or vitamin/mineral powders

INITIAL DATABASE

- Culture and sensitivity
    - Sampling the trachea or glottis rim has been shown to be diagnostic.
    - Swabs of the oral cavity or choanal area are not diagnostic.
    - Anaerobic bacterial culture
- Tracheal or lung wash
- Hematology
- Blood chemistry
- Radiography

ADVANCED OR CONFIRMATORY TESTING

- Endoscopic lung evaluation and biopsy:
    - Directly collect lung samples for histopathologic exam, culture, and DNA PCR testing

TREATMENT

ACUTE GENERAL TREATMENT

- Oxygen and airways:
    - The nares, nostrils, choanae, and glottis should be examined and cleared of any obstruction.
    - It is common for large amounts of mucus and/or purulent material to build up in these areas:
        - This material can be gently removed with cotton-tipped swabs.
        - Suction of material from the glottis may be necessary.
        - Saline or antimicrobial ophthalmic drops can be used to help loosen material in the nostrils.
- Supportive care:
    - The reptile should be warmed to the upper end of the preferred optimal temperature zone (POTZ) for the species.
        - For most reptiles, a range approximately 26°C to 32°C (approximately 80°F to 90°F)
    - Fluid therapy may be warranted.
        - The fluid rate is 10-30 mL/kg/d.
- Antimicrobial therapy:
    - Appropriate initial choices of antibiotics (pending culture and sensitivity results) include:
        - Amikacin (5 mg/kg IM or SC initial dose, followed by 2.5 mg/kg IM or SC every 72 hours) or
        - Enrofloxacin (5-10 mg/kg IM, SC, or PO every 24-48 hours) or
        - Ciprofloxacin (11 mg/kg PO every 48-72 hours)
    - Anaerobic organisms are often involved along with gram negative bacteria so consider combination drug therapy such as:
        - Enrofloxacin (20 mg/kg IM, SC, or PO every 24-48 hours) and ceftazidime (20 mg/kg IM or SC every 72 hours) or
        - Piperacillin (100-200 mg/kg IM or SC every 24-48 hours)
        - Amikacin (5 mg/kg IM or SC initial dose, followed by 2.5 mg/kg IM or SC every 72 hours) and ceftazidime (20 mg/kg IM or SC every 72 hours) or
        - Piperacillin (100-200 mg/kg IM or SC every 24-48 hours)

CHRONIC TREATMENT

- Antibiotic regimens are continued for a minimum of 4 weeks in mild cases, and for 6-10 weeks in severe cases.
- Nebulization in conjunction with systemic antibiotics may be helpful in treating severe respiratory disease.
    - e.g., 1 mL amikacin mixed with 9 mL saline can be nebulized for 30-60 min daily
- This treatment seems more valuable in lizards and chelonians than in snakes.
    - In the author's experience, nebulization in snakes is not a useful adjunct to systemic antibiotic therapy in that it often exacerbates fluid and mucus accumulation in the airways (likely because of the length of the trachea).
- Treatment of *Mycoplasma* (see Mycoplasma):

- Diagnosis of *Mycoplasma* respiratory disease should be based on isolation of the organism by special culture when possible.
- The University of Florida College of Veterinary Medicine (USA) microbiology department can provide services and/or information on sample collection.
- *Mycoplasma* is considered a chronic disease that is usually managed rather than cured.
- A positive diagnosis should result in strict isolation or removal of the affected reptile from a collection to avoid exposure and possible transmission to other reptiles.
- Some treatment regimens for attempting to manage mycoplasma include:
  - Chelonians:
    - Enrofloxacin (5-10 mg/kg IM, SC, PO every 48-72 hours) or as a nasal flush
  - Snakes:
    - Tylosin (5-10 mg/kg IM every 24-48 hours) or
    - Oxytetracycline (5-10 mg/kg IM every 24 hours for 4 weeks or longer). Recurrence is common.

- Treatment of *Chlamydia* (see Chlamydiophila)
  - Chlamydial infection is difficult to eliminate.
  - Snakes:
    - Azithromycin (10 mg/kg PO every 48 hours for 6-8 weeks)
    - Oxytetracycline (5-10 mg/kg IM, SC every 24-48 hours for 6-8 weeks)

PROGNOSIS AND OUTCOME

- The prognosis frequently depends on the state of the animal at presentation.
- In chronic cases, the prognosis is not as favorable.
- If the reptile is wild-caught, the prognosis is poor.
- The prognosis is more favorable with aggressive diagnostic measures and early treatment.
- *Pseudomonas* and respiratory disease related to bacteria in this family often have a high level of resistance.
- Use of culture and sensitivity to select the most effective antibiotic(s) may improve the prognosis in these cases.

PEARLS & CONSIDERATIONS

COMMENTS

- Because many of the causes of respiratory disease are related to husbandry, clients should be educated in proper caging, lighting, heat, humidity, and nutrition to minimize occurrence.
- During routine exams and annual visits, owners should be made aware of early indicators of respiratory disease, so they may present the reptile for treatment before respiratory disease becomes advanced.
- Many lizards and chelonians have salt glands in their nostrils, so evidence of dry white discharge may be seen as normal mineral elimination (e.g., *Iguana iguana*).

SUGGESTED READINGS

Frye FL, et al: The proper method of stethoscopy in reptiles, Vet Med 83:1250–1252, 1988.
Hilf M, et al: A prospective study of upper airway flora in healthy boid snakes and snakes with pneumonia, J Zoo Wildl Med 21:318–325, 1990.
Jacobson ER: Bacterial diseases of reptiles. In Jacobson ER, editor: Infectious diseases and pathology of reptiles, Boca Raton, FL, 2007, CRC Press, pp 461–526.
Murray MJ: Cardiopulmonary anatomy and physiology. In Mader DR, editor: Reptile medicine and surgery, ed 2, St Louis, 2006, Elsevier, pp 124–134.
Murray MJ: Pneumonia and lower respiratory tract disease. In Mader DR, editor: Reptile medicine and surgery, ed 2, St Louis, 2006, Elsevier, pp 865–877.
Stewart JS: Anaerobic bacterial infections in reptiles, J Zoo Widl Med 21:180, 1990.

CROSS-REFERENCES TO OTHER SECTIONS

Chlamydiophila
Herpesvirus
Hypovitaminosis A
Mycobacteria
Mycoplasma
Nematodiasis
Paramyxovirus
Pentastomes

AUTHOR & EDITOR: **SCOTT J. STAHL**

REPTILES

Salmonella

BASIC INFORMATION

DEFINITION

- *Salmonella* organisms are Gram-negative, usually motile, facultative anaerobes from the family Enterobacteriaceae. These bacteria have a cosmopolitan distribution.
- The genus *Salmonella* consists of two species—*S. enterica* and *S. bongori*—and more than 2400 different serotypes.
- All *Salmonella* organisms should be considered pathogenic, although clinical disease in poikilotherms is considered uncommon.

SYNONYM

Salmonellosis

EPIDEMIOLOGY

SPECIES, AGE, SEX

- *Salmonella* has been isolated from chelonians, lizards, snakes, and crocodilians.
- In captivity, animals are most likely exposed soon after hatching, although vertical transmission is also possible.
- All ages should be considered susceptible, as *Salmonella* can colonize both naïve and established intestinal microfloras.
- There does not appear to be a sex predilection for *Salmonella* infection in reptiles.

GENETICS AND BREED PREDISPOSITION

- All species of reptiles should be considered susceptible to infection.
- Turtles, especially red-eared sliders (*Trachemys scripta elegans*), and green iguanas (*Iguana iguana*) are considered important sources of *Salmonella* in humans.
- These animals may have higher carriage rates of this organism because they are captive raised in large numbers.
- However, disease associated with this organism in these species is uncommon.
- Certain species of snakes (e.g., rattlesnakes) may have increased susceptibility to infection.

RISK FACTORS

- Animals housed under high densities are more susceptible to becoming exposed to this organism.

- The likelihood of shedding is higher in animals under stress.
- Herbivorous reptiles offered unwashed and/or contaminated fruits and vegetables, or carnivores offered *Salmonella*-positive prey, are at risk of exposure to *Salmonella.*

CONTAGION AND ZOONOSIS

- Reptile-associated salmonellosis is a major health concern of public health officials.
- In 1975, the U.S. Food and Drug Administration restricted the sale of chelonians <10 cm to limit the incidence of disease in young children.
- More recently, a resurgence of reptile-associated salmonellosis in humans has been associated with the increased popularity of captive reptiles, especially green iguanas.
- The zoonotic potential of this disease is greatest in those cases where reptiles are provided inappropriate husbandry and pet owners do not follow standard hygiene practices.

GEOGRAPHY AND SEASONALITY

- The prevalence of *Salmonella* in farm-raised turtles is greater during the warm summer months. Because it is generally recommended to house pet reptiles indoors under optimized husbandry conditions (e.g., optimized thermal gradient), pet owners should be made aware that environmental conditions for the growth and maintenance of *Salmonella* in the reptile and its environment are also optimized.
- There does not appear to be a geographic distinction for *Salmonella* carriage among reptiles; it has been isolated from animals on all major continents where reptiles reside. The prevalence of *Salmonella* in wild reptiles is generally much lower than in captive animals.

ASSOCIATED CONDITIONS AND DISORDERS

- Reptiles that do develop salmonellosis can show clinical signs consistent with a bacterial septicemia.
- Diarrhea, pneumonia, thromboembolic disease, and osteomyelitis are commonly reported.

CLINICAL PRESENTATION

DISEASE FORMS/SUBTYPES

- Five of the *S. enterica* subspecies are commonly identified in reptiles, including:
  - *Salamae* (subspecies II), *arizonae* (subspecies III), *diarizonae* (subspecies IIIb), *houtenae* (subspecies IV), and *indica* (subspecies V).
  - *S. enterica arizonae* and *S. enterica diarizonae* are most often associated with reptiles.

HISTORY, CHIEF COMPLAINT

- *Salmonella* is most frequently isolated from clinically healthy reptiles and is considered an indigenous component of the microflora.
- Most reptiles presenting to the veterinarian for salmonellosis will have nonspecific systemic signs.
- The history often includes that the animal is lethargic, depressed, or anorectic; has diarrhea; or appears painful (especially when the skeleton is palpated).

PHYSICAL EXAM FINDINGS

- Most reptiles harbor *Salmonella* and show no clinical signs associated with disease (inapparent infection).
- Animals with salmonellosis may present with nonspecific signs such as diarrhea, lethargy, depression, or dyspnea.
- Osteomyelitis is another common finding in reptiles, especially in snakes.

ETIOLOGY AND PATHOPHYSIOLOGY

- *Salmonella* is spread via the fecal-oral route.
- Most captive animals are exposed soon after hatching/birth.
- Reptiles can be exposed to certain serotypes from contaminated food sources.
- *Salmonella* are motile organisms that use their flagella to direct themselves toward enterocytes.
- *Salmonella* organisms appear to rely on invasion genes to penetrate host enterocytes. Invasion genes are believed to mediate an extensive action rearrangement in the host cell, resulting in distortion of the cell membrane and enabling the organism to invade. Disruption of the invasion A gene in a strain of *Salmonella typhimurium* prevents the organism from invading enterocytes. The invasion genes (A-H) are highly conserved among *Salmonella.*
- The chemical composition of the O antigen is also an important consideration in activating complement by the alternate pathway, and may affect the rate of phagocytosis by macrophages.
- Because *Salmonella* can evade host immune functions, the organism can invade most tissues.

DIAGNOSIS

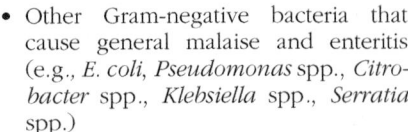

DIFFERENTIAL DIAGNOSIS

- Other Gram-negative bacteria that cause general malaise and enteritis (e.g., *E. coli, Pseudomonas* spp., *Citrobacter* spp., *Klebsiella* spp., *Serratia* spp.)
- Viral diseases that cause general malaise and enteritis
- Parasitic enteritis

INITIAL DATABASE

- Complete blood count:
  - Inflammatory leukograms are common.
  - Heterophilia and monocytosis are common.
  - Animals harboring this organism without clinical disease often have normal white blood cell counts.
- Radiographs:
  - Osteomyelitis may be observed in animals with *Salmonella* bone infection.
- Microbiological culture:
  - This remains the standard for diagnosis of *Salmonella,*
- Only moderate sensitivity and subject to false-negatives
  - Serial cultures can help reduce the likelihood of misclassification.
  - Specificity likely approaches 100%.

ADVANCED OR CONFIRMATORY TESTING

- Enzyme-linked immunosorbent assay:
  - Sensitivity may be higher than for culture.
- Polymerase chain reaction:
  - Higher sensitivity and specificity than culture

TREATMENT

THERAPEUTIC GOALS

- Provide supportive care: Fluid therapy should be provided to reestablish the fluid balance of the patient. Maintenance fluid rates for reptiles are 10-30 mL/kg/day.
- Animals that are anorectc should be provided supplemental calories.
- Administer appropriate antibiotic (based on sensitivity testing preferred).
- Animals that are diagnosed with *Salmonella* but are not showing clinical disease do not need to be treated. The animal should, however, be considered a carrier of the organism, and appropriate hygiene methods should be followed to reduce the likelihood of zoonotic transmission.

ACUTE GENERAL TREATMENT

- Fluid therapy to rehydrate animals with acute or chronic fluid loss from diarrhea
- Antibiotics: enrofloxacin (5-10 mg/kg PO, SQ, IM q 24-72 h) is an excellent first choice while a sensitivity profile is pending.

CHRONIC TREATMENT

Antibiotics may need to be given for 10-14 days to suppress/eliminate the organism. Because *Salmonella* can invade extraintestinal tissues (e.g., gallbladder), treatment may not eliminate all organisms. In these cases, the reptile should be considered a potential latent carrier.

PROGNOSIS AND OUTCOME

- The prognosis for animals that are *Salmonella* culture positive but are not showing clinical signs is good.
- Osteomyelitis carries a guarded prognosis.
- The outcome for most cases associated with enteritis ends positively if the animal is provided supportive care and an appropriate antibiotic.

PEARLS & CONSIDERATIONS

COMMENTS

- *Salmonella* is considered by many public health officials to be a significant zoonotic concern with pet reptiles. Although public health officials often state, "Most, if not all, reptiles have *Salmonella*," this is not necessarily true. *Salmonella* infection of reptiles is primarily a problem associated with captivity. When reptiles are housed in high densities under less than ideal conditions, the potential for exposure to the organism is high.
- In wild, free-ranging reptiles, the prevalence of *Salmonella* is low. This is important to consider when discussing the epidemiology of *Salmonella* in reptiles, because minimizing the densities of animals in captivity and following appropriate hygiene can minimize the likelihood of exposure to both the pet reptile and the human caretaker.
- *Salmonella* organisms are serotyped according to their O (heat-stabile somatic) antigens, Vi (heat-labile capsular) antigens, and H (flagellar) antigens. The Kauffman-White scheme is used to list the antigenic formulae expressed as O antigens and Vi antigens (when present): H antigens phase 1 and H antigens phase 2 (when present).

PREVENTION

- Microbiological culture lacks sensitivity and can lead to the misclassification of infected animals.
- Clients should be informed of the possibility of false-negative results and the importance of collecting sequential samples to confirm *Salmonella* status.
- The use of antimicrobials under appropriate conditions may eliminate *Salmonella*, but no evidence of long-term protection has been found. If the environment of the reptile is not properly sanitized and disinfected, it is possible that reinfection from the animal's own environment will occur. Contaminated food sources, such as fresh produce, could serve as sources of infection.
- Clients should be made aware of the risks of owning reptiles and should be apprised of appropriate husbandry and sanitation procedures.
- Handwashing using soap and warm water is an excellent method of eliminating *Salmonella*. Pet owners should be directed to avoid using bathroom basins or kitchen sinks to clean a reptile or any component of its environment.
- The purchase of a separate washing receptacle, such as a plastic container, is recommended. Dilute bleach solution should be used to clean the environment, as well as food and water bowls. Substrate should be removed and promptly placed into a waste receptacle.

CLIENT EDUCATION

- Always wash your hands after handling a pet reptile or any part of its environment. The wash basin used to wash your hands should not be the primary basin used for handling human food or materials used to cook or serve the food.
- Never use a human wash basin to bathe a reptile or to clean any part of its environment.
- Never bathe a reptile in a water basin used by humans for bathing. Instead, a separate basin should be purchased to be used exclusively for bathing the reptile.
- Infants (<24 months) should not have direct contact with reptiles. Parents should follow strict hygiene practices when handling and cleaning reptiles. Most cases of reptile-associated salmonellosis in infants are associated with indirect reptile contact (e.g., parent served as source of exposure). Parents should always change their clothes and wash after handling/cleaning a reptile/reptile enclosure and prior to handling an infant.
- Toddlers should have only supervised exposure to reptiles. Immediately after handling the reptile, the toddler's hand should be washed and clothes changed.
- Reptiles should not be allowed free roam of a household because they can shed *Salmonella* organisms into the environment.
- Dilute bleach should be used to disinfect a reptile's enclosure and any surface with which a reptile comes into contact.

SUGGESTED READINGS

DuPonte MW, et al: Activation of latent *Salmonella* and *Arizona* organisms by dehydration of red-eared turtles, *Pseudemys scripta-elegans*, Am J Vet Res 39:529–530, 1978.

Grupka LM, et al: *Salmonella* surveillance in a collection of rattlesnakes (*Crotalus* spp.), J Zoo Wild Med 37:306–312, 2006.

Mitchell MA, et al: *Salmonella* in reptiles, Semin Avian Exot Pet Med 10:25–35, 2001.

AUTHOR: **MARK A. MITCHELL**

EDITOR: **SCOTT J. STAHL**

REPTILES

Stomatitis, Bacterial

BASIC INFORMATION

DEFINITION

- Bacterial invasion of the oral cavity, resulting in mucosal inflammation and necrosis
- Deep soft-tissue invasion often will progress to involve mandibular and maxillary bone with subsequent osteomyelitis.

SYNONYMS

Infectious stomatitis, mouth rot, periodontal disease (see Periodontal Disease)

EPIDEMIOLOGY

SPECIES, AGE, SEX

- Bacterial stomatitis is most common in snakes and lizards but is also seen in chelonians.

- Arboreal boid species such as green tree pythons (*Morelia viridis*) and tree boas (*Corallus* sp.) are susceptible to stomatitis.
  - They may strike at movement around their enclosure.
    - Damage the rostrum by hitting the glass or plexiglass, leading to stomatitis.
- Reticulated pythons (*Python reticulatus*), boa constrictors (*Boa constrictor* spp.), and Burmese pythons (*Python molurus bivittatus*) are prone to stomatitis.
  - Often housed in enclosures that do not provide enough space. Continued attempts to escape result in trauma to the oral cavity.
- Mature male snakes during the breeding season may actively try to escape their enclosures to find receptive females. These attempts often cause trauma to the rostrum and perioral area, predisposing them to subsequent bacterial invasion.
- Nervous lizards that run or jump when startled, such as Asian water dragons (*Physignathus concinnus*), are prone to rostral damage from hitting the glass walls of their enclosure. Damage and loss of tissue often result in bacterial stomatitis.

RISK FACTORS

- Lizards with acrodont dentition:
  - Old World chameleons and agamid species such as Asian water dragons (*Physignathus concinnus*) and bearded dragons (*Pogona vitticeps*) have acrodont dentition (nonrooted teeth that are ankylosed to the mandibular and maxillary bones).
  - The fragile nature of periodontal tissue associated with these teeth makes these lizards prone to bacterial and fungal invasion. (see Periodontal Disease)
- Glandular tissue associated with oral cavity:
  - Old World chameleons have glands located in the commissures of the oral cavity that are prone to abscessation and associated stomatitis.
    - Most common in Jackson's chameleons
- Husbandry factors:
  - Malnutrition
  - Inappropriate temperatures
  - Lack of hiding areas, visual barriers, or inappropriate caging
    - Resulting in an intense effort to escape
- Trauma:
  - Trauma to the rostral area, lips, mucous membranes, and/or teeth results in a breakdown in the protective barriers of the oral cavity, allowing organisms to invade.
- Wild-caught and/or recently shipped reptiles:
  - Reptiles that have been shipped and held in holding areas before arriving at pet stores have frequently undergone stress and potential trauma to the oral cavity.

CONTAGION AND ZOONOSIS

- Bacterial stomatitis generally is not considered to be contagious.
- However, a group of reptiles that have been maintained under similar conditions (e.g., stress, poor husbandry, trauma to oral cavity) may have similar lesions and bacterial pathogens.
- Differentials for bacterial stomatitis, such as special organisms like *Mycobacterium* and herpesvirus (see Herpesvirus Infections), may be contagious.
- Cases involving *Salmonella* spp. may be zoonotic.

GEOGRAPHY AND SEASONALITY

- Increased incidence during breeding season may occur as mature reptiles attempt to escape their enclosures to find mates.
- Reptiles that are cooled to hibernate/cycle over winter may have an increased incidence of stomatitis. This is often due to:
  - Hibernating unhealthy or sick reptiles
  - Reptiles being cooled too quickly
  - Hibernating at incorrect temperatures

ASSOCIATED CONDITIONS AND DISORDERS

- Subspectacular abscesses
  - Accumulation of purulent material within the subspectacular space is often associated with bacterial stomatitis. This occurs as a result of the movement of bacteria from the inflamed/infected oral cavity up the nasolacrimal duct and into the subspectacular space.

CLINICAL PRESENTATION

DISEASE FORMS/SUBTYPES Periodontal disease in lizards (see Periodontal Disease)

HISTORY, CHIEF COMPLAINT

- Lethargy
- Anorexia
- Asymmetry to closure of the mouth
- Swellings or masses on head and perioral area
- Mucus or discharge from mouth or nares
- Swelling and exposure of the mucous membranes of the oral cavity
- Purulent material, discharge, and/or blood evident in oral cavity

PHYSICAL EXAM FINDINGS

- Early cases may reveal petechial hemorrhages, increased mucus in the mouth, and asymmetry to closure of the mouth (caseated purulent debris may form a pseudomembrane).
- Severe cases often present with deep abscessation and mandibular and/or maxillary involvement. (see Abscesses)
- Loss of periodontal tissue and teeth often leads to osteomyelitis.
- Concurrent respiratory disease is common (associated with aspiration of purulent debris and discharge).

ETIOLOGY AND PATHOPHYSIOLOGY

- Gram-negative bacteria are the most common primary pathogens:
  - Often, these organisms are part of the normal flora, but they may become opportunistic.
  - Commonly isolated Gram-negative organisms include *Pseudomonas, Klebsiella, Proteus, Salmonella, Providencia, Escherichia, Morganella, Aeromonas,* and *Citrobacter.*
- Occasionally, Gram-positive organisms (e.g., *Streptococcus, Corynebacteria*) are the primary organisms, or are found concurrently with Gram-negative bacteria.
- Often, anaerobic organisms are found in conjunction with Gram-negative bacteria.
  - Anaerobic organisms include *Bacteroides, Fusobacterium,* and *Clostridium.*
- Hypovitaminosis A is often a predisposing factor.

DIAGNOSIS

DIFFERENTIAL DIAGNOSIS

- Oral trauma
- Shedding conditions (associated cephalic edema and congestion in snakes)
- Dysecdysis (see Dysecdysis)
- Hypovitaminosis A (see Hypovitaminosis A)
- Nutritional secondary hyperparathyroidism
- Fungal/protozoal
- *Mycobacterium*
- Viral disease
- Neoplasia

INITIAL DATABASE

- A thorough history, physical exam, complete blood count, plasma chemistry, and fecal exam.
- With severe cases, especially those involving bone, an elevation of the white blood cell count and/or toxic changes may be noted in heterophils.

ADVANCED OR CONFIRMATORY TESTING

- Culture and sensitivity:
  - When possible, anaerobic cultures should be obtained.

- Cytologic evaluation:
  - Look for bacterial, fungal, and protozoan organisms.
- Biopsy:
  - Rule out acid-fast organisms fungal, parasitic, and neoplastic causes.
- Radiography:
  - Assess bone involvement.

TREATMENT

ACUTE GENERAL TREATMENT

See Periodontal Disease for treatment details.

RECOMMENDED MONITORING

In cases with loss of soft tissue or bone, lifelong monitoring by the owner and the clinician will be necessary because recurrence may occur as the result of a change in the anatomy of the oral cavity.

PROGNOSIS AND OUTCOME

- The prognosis depends on the severity of lesions and the state of the reptile at presentation.
- Aggressive diagnostic measures with early treatment and appropriate adjustments in husbandry will improve the chances for recovery and resolution.
- The prognosis is not as favorable if the reptile patient presents with any of the following:
  - Poor body condition (emaciated and/or dehydrated)
  - Deeper lesions likely to result in permanent loss of tissue and chronic exposure of mucous membranes and bone
  - Osteomyelitis
  - If *Pseudomonas* spp. are cultured, this Gram-negative organism tends to have resistance to many antimicrobials.

PEARLS & CONSIDERATIONS

COMMENTS

It is important to educate owners at the new patient/juvenile checkup and/or at their annual visits about husbandry-related problems that predispose reptiles to stomatitis, especially species that are prone to these issues.

PREVENTION

Clients with lizard species that have acrodont dentition should be educated about the unique oral anatomy of their lizard and how to monitor for early signs of periodontal disease.

CLIENT EDUCATION

When possible, showing clients how to safely open the mouth of their reptile and evaluate the oral cavity for problems allows them to monitor the health of their reptile.

SUGGESTED READINGS

McKracken H, et al: Periodontal disease in lizards: a review of numerous cases, Pittsburgh, 1994, Proc Ann Mtg American Association of Zoo Veterinarians Annual Conference, pp 108–115.

Stewart JS: Anaerobic bacterial infections in reptiles, J Zoo Wildl Med 21:180, 1990.

Swaim SF, Lee AH: Topical wound medications: a review, J Am Vet Med Assoc 190:1588, 1987.

CROSS-REFERENCES TO OTHER SECTIONS

Abscesses
Dysecdysis
Herpesvirus Infections
Hypovitaminosis A
Periodontal Disease

AUTHOR & EDITOR: **SCOTT J. STAHL**

BIRDS

Abscesses

Additional Images Available on Website

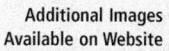

BASIC INFORMATION

DEFINITION

Circumscribed collections of purulent material found in many anatomic locations as a result of heterophilic accumulation

SYNONYMS

Boil, carbuncle, furuncle, pimple, pustule

EPIDEMIOLOGY

SPECIES, AGE, SEX All species, ages, and both sexes

GENETICS AND BREED PREDISPOSITION Waterfowl and raptor species are susceptible to plantar surface abscess, which is referred to as *bumblefoot*.

RISK FACTORS

- Obesity
- Vitamin deficiency (e.g., vitamin A) (see Hypovitaminosis)
- Inadequate nutrition
- Puncture wounds
- Uropygial gland disease (see Uropygial Gland Disease Condition)
- Bacterial infection

ASSOCIATED CONDITIONS AND DISORDERS

- Swelling over the area of the abscess
- Anorexia
- Buphthalmos
- Female reproductive disorders
- Swelling of oral mucosa
- Swelling and asymmetry of nares, infraorbital sinus (see Sinusitis, Chronic)

CLINICAL PRESENTATION

DISEASE FORMS/SUBTYPES

- Plantar surface abscesses—bumblefoot
- Uropygial gland abscesses
- Subcutaneous abscesses
- Oropharyngeal abscesses
- Respiratory tract abscesses
- Periorbital and orbital abscesses
- Reproductive tract abscesses

HISTORY, CHIEF COMPLAINT

- Swelling over affected area
- Depression
- Inappetence
- Difficulty perching or walking
- Female inability to lay eggs
- Protruding globe

PHYSICAL EXAM FINDINGS

- Verification of swelling or presence of mass
- Patient may be "picking" at affected area.

ETIOLOGY AND PATHOPHYSIOLOGY

- In avian species, resolution of heterophilic accumulation as a result of inflammation and/or infection results in formation of a caseous mass (inspissation) rather than liquefaction as found in mammalian species.
- The purulent inflammation associated with abscess formation may be caused by one of four pyogenic bacteria (*Corynebacterium* spp., *Pseudomonas* spp., *Staphylococcus* spp., *Streptococcus* spp.).
- Abscesses are classified as acute or chronic and focal to multiple.
- Variable size range

DIAGNOSIS

DIFFERENTIAL DIAGNOSIS

- Neoplasia
- Granuloma
- Papilloma
- Subcutaneous emphysema
- Seroma

INITIAL DATABASE

- Complete blood count: leukocytosis with concurrent heterophilia may be present. If the abscess is a result of a more chronic infectious process, an associated monocytosis may be present. It is not uncommon to receive normal blood results from avian patients that present with abscess formation due to the physiology of avian abscess formation. The formation of an inspissated abscess allows separation of the affected area from viable tissue.
- Plasma biochemistry panel: creatine kinase (CK) may be elevated

ADVANCED OR CONFIRMATORY TESTING

- Fine-needle aspirate
- Imaging: may help delineate the extent of the abscess, especially oropharyngeal, orbital/periorbital, oviductal, and infraorbital sinus abscesses
  - Radiology
  - Ultrasound
- Culture and sensitivity to try to isolate the causative organism if possible and identify proper treatment

TREATMENT

THERAPEUTIC GOALS

- Stabilize and improve patient's physical condition.
- Confirm diagnosis.
- Treat abscess by removing caseous material.
- Provide supportive therapy to control, anorexia, dehydration, gastroenteritis
- Treat causative bacterial organism, if present.
- Prevent recurrence through client education.

ACUTE GENERAL TREATMENT

- All treatment is to be performed on a stable patient.
  - Nursing care
    - Administer warmed crystalloid fluids SC, IV, IO (50-150 mL/kg/d maintenance plus dehydration deficit factored in if needed) at a rate of 10-25 mL/kg over a 5-minute period or at a continuous rate of 100 mL/kg/q 24 h.
    - Increase environmental temperature to 85°F-90°F (29°C-32°C).
    - Provide a humidified environment by placing warm moist towels in the incubator.
    - Nutritional support is required in most cases.
- Surgical considerations: the patient should be stabilized before any surgical procedure
  - Bumblefoot treatment: see Pododermatitis
  - Oropharyngeal abscesses
    - Location: base of tongue, intermandibular space, choana, pharynx, larynx
    - Highly vascular area
      - Hemostasis is necessary when removing.
      - Intubation is required.
      - Careful dissection
      - After incision, careful cleaning using dilute impregnated cotton-tipped applicators will help reduce the possibility of debris retention within the abscess.
  - Submandibular abscesses
    - Incise the skin covering the masses.
  - Infraorbital sinus abscesses
    - Incise the skin overlying the swelling, which is usually located in the area between the medial canthus of the eye and the nares, to remove the abscess.
  - Reproductive tract abscess
    - Surgical salpingohysterectomy may be required to resolve this condition.
  - Periorbital/orbital abscess formation
    - Enucleation is often the recommended treatment if the abscess cannot be removed and affected area is treated appropriately to prevent recurrence.
  - Uropygial gland abscess
    - Incise over affected lobe(s) of uropygial gland.
    - Culture/sensitivity of affected area
    - Flush with dilute 5% Nolvasan solution.
    - Allow to close by secondary intention.
    - Medications
  - Drugs of choice
    - Antibiotics may be indicated for bacterial infections that are the initiating cause of the abscess formation. Although a broad spectrum antibiotic may be initially prescribed for the patient, ultimately the drug selection should be based on culture and sensitivity of the inciting organism(s).

CHRONIC TREATMENT

Antibiotic treatment as necessary to prevent reinfection or recurrence of abscess formation.

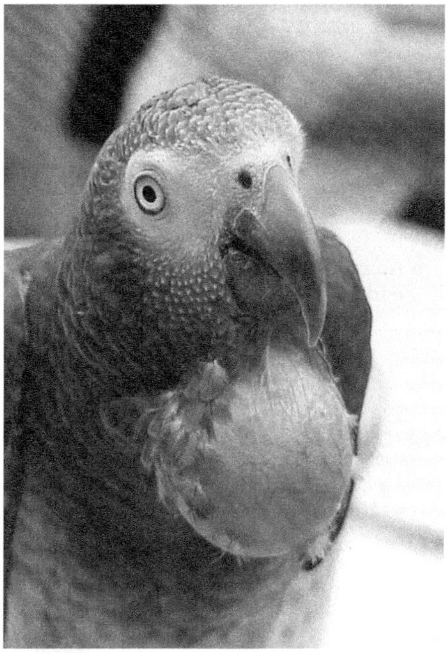

Abscesses Submandibular abscess in an African grey parrot.

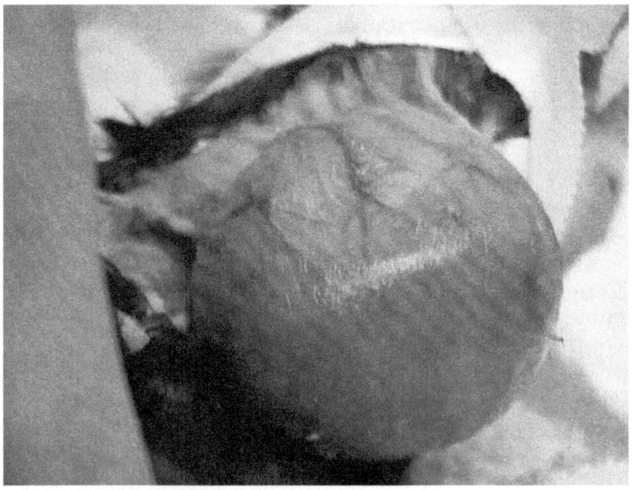

Abscesses Circumscribed abscess in the same African grey parrot. *(Photo courtesy Thomas N. Tully, Jr.)*

RECOMMENDED MONITORING

- Monitor abscess area for recurrence.
- Repeat radiographs if necessary or if the treatment response of internal disease can be assessed through imaging.
- Repeat CBC and plasma chemistry panel to monitor treatment response and recovery.
- Monitor appetite, fecal output, and behavior during treatment.

PROGNOSIS AND OUTCOME

Most abscess cases have a very good prognosis, especially if the abscess can be completely removed and its origins have been identified and appropriately treated.

Depending on the severity of bumblefoot lesions, this disease process can have a good to grave prognosis (see Pododermatitis).

Ocular and reproductive surgery to treat abscess affecting these areas may require removal of tissue, which could affect the bird's ability to see and reproduce. Even with removal of an eye or a female reproductive tract, the patient should have a good quality of life.

PEARLS & CONSIDERATIONS

COMMENTS

- Avian patients commonly present with abscesses.
- Avian abscesses will form into a solid inspissated structure that has to be removed.
- Because of the formation of a thick inspissated mass, CBC may be normal owing to the ability of the abscess to "wall" itself from viable tissue.
- Owners can help prevent oropharyngeal abscesses by providing proper nutrition.

PREVENTION

- Proper nutrition
- Proper husbandry, including toys appropriate for bird in cage
- Proper substrate and perches for waterfowl and raptor species

CLIENT EDUCATION

See Prevention.

SUGGESTED READINGS

Bennett RA, et al: Ophthalmology. In Ritchie BW, et al, editors: Avian medicine: principles and applications, Brentwood, TN, 1994, HBD International Inc., pp 1096–1136.

Coles B: Surgery. In Coles BH, editor: Essentials of avian medicine and surgery, ed 3, Oxford, UK, 2007, Blackwell Publishing Co., pp 142–183.

Williams D: Ophthalmology. In Ritchie BW, et al, editors: Avian medicine: principles and applications, Brentwood, TN, 1994, HBD International Inc., pp 673–694.

CROSS-REFERENCES TO OTHER SECTIONS

Hypovitaminosis
Pododermatitis
Sinusitis, Chronic
Uropygial Gland Disease Conditions

AUTHOR & EDITOR: **THOMAS N. TULLY, JR.**

BIRDS

Anemia

BASIC INFORMATION

DEFINITION

A reduction in the normal erythrocyte or hemoglobin value in a patient's blood sample. A bird's blood sample that has a packed cell volume (PCV) of <35% is often considered the objective delineation of an anemic condition.

EPIDEMIOLOGY

SPECIES, AGE, SEX All species and both sexes. Young birds from 2-6 months of age can have lower PCV values.

GENETICS AND BREED PREDISPOSITION Hemolysis of red blood cells in a blood sample will occur when EDTA is used as an anticoagulant with crows, curasows, hornbills, ostrich, and bush turkeys. This will affect the ability of the clinician to accurately interpret the complete blood count (CBC) results.

RISK FACTORS

- Chronic disease
- Leukemia, lymphosarcoma
- Toxicities
- Iron, folic acid deficiencies
- Hypothyroidism
- Blood loss
- Bacterial septicemias
- Red blood cell parasites
- Viral disease

GEOGRAPHY AND SEASONALITY

- Significant seasonal changes in erythrocyte count have been described in wild birds, associated with moult, reproduction, and food supply.
- Seasonal variation in erythrocyte count has not been described in pet birds.

ASSOCIATED CONDITIONS AND DISORDERS

- Depression
- Anorexia
- Hemorrhage
- Gastroenteritis
- Weakness

CLINICAL PRESENTATION

DISEASE FORMS/SUBTYPES

- Regenerative: blood loss or hemolysis, >10% polychromasia
  - Traumatic injury: response to acute blood loss is faster than in mammals
  - Coagulopathies
    - Primary: conure bleeding syndrome (not common or very well understood)
    - Secondary: intoxication with anticoagulants or toxins released by infectious agents
  - Hematophagous parasite: exposure for long periods to parasites (e.g., red mites, mosquitoes, ticks)
  - Organic disease: ulceration as a result of neoplasia, gastrointestinal ulcers, or organ rupture
  - Hemoparasites: *Plasmodium* spp., *Aegyptianella* spp., trypanosomes, *Hemoproteus* spp., *Leucocytozoon* spp., and *Hemoproteus* spp. usually are not clinically significant but will cause death in severely affected birds
  - Bacterial septicemia
  - Toxicity
    - Chemical products: petroleum products, mustards
    - Diets: rapeseed
    - Copper: in poultry reported to cause hemolytic anemia
  - Immune-mediated disease: rarely noted in avian species
  - Transfusion reaction
- Nonregenerative: incapacity of the body to create new erythrocytes or hemoglobin due to bone marrow suppression, <5% polychromasia
  - Chronic infectious diseases: mycobacteriosis, avian chlamydiosis, aspergillosis, egg peritonitis
  - Viral infections: polyomavirus, circovirus infection can cause pancytopenia in the last stages of the disease
  - Paraneoplastic syndrome

- Hypothyroidism
- Nutritional deficiency: iron, folic acid. This condition has been reported in poultry.
- Toxicity: heavy metals: initially, lead causes a regenerative anemia due to hemolysis, but chronic toxicity leads to bone marrow suppression. Other toxic compounds related to a condition of nonregenerative anemia include zinc and aflatoxins.
- Neoplasia of hematopoietic elements: lymphosarcoma

HISTORY, CHIEF COMPLAINT

- Blood loss
- Trauma
- Bruising
- Depression
- Inappetence
- Blood in stool
- Crop stasis
- Bloody diarrhea
- Polyuria/Polydipsia
- Vomiting
- Broken blood feather

PHYSICAL EXAM FINDINGS

- Subcutaneous hemorrhages
- Blanched mucous membranes
- Hemoglobinuria
- Weakness
- Evidence of trauma or blood loss
- Tachypnea
- Tachycardia

ETIOLOGY AND PATHOPHYSIOLOGY

Blood is vital for the patient to live through oxygenation and removal of physiologic toxins of/from body tissues. The loss of red blood cells will greatly diminish the effectiveness of the remaining blood supply in performing these functions. With regenerative anemias, the body is actively trying to replace the red blood cell deficit; in nonregenerative anemias, the red blood cell–regenerating capacity of the body is not functioning.

DIAGNOSIS

DIFFERENTIAL DIAGNOSIS

- See Disease Forms Subtypes above.
- Anemia associated with improper sampling, transport, or handling of the blood sample

INITIAL DATABASE

- CBC: a low PCV (<35%) is indicative of anemia, although possible hemodilution can be assessed through total protein values
  - PCV and hemoglobin values should be addressed as a general rule. Packed cell volume levels <35% and hemoglobin levels <12 g/L may be suggestive of anemia.
  - Leukocytosis: may be present with infectious and/or inflammatory disease
  - If available, mean corpuscular volume (MCV): defined as erythrocyte size; allows classification of anemic conditions as macro-, micro-, or normocytic. Microcytic anemias are diagnosed in cases of iron deficiency or chronic blood loss. Macrocytic anemias are noted in patients diagnosed with early heavy metal toxicosis or acute blood loss. Normocytic anemias are present in chronic infections. Mean corpuscular value is an important parameter in assessing whether anemia is regenerative or nonregenerative. One should remember that small birds have an MCV that is greater than that of larger avian species.
  - If available, mean corpuscular hemoglobin concentration (MCHC): this parameter enables classification of anemic conditions as hypo-, hyper-, and normochromic. In avian species, hypochromic anemias are noted in cases of chronic blood loss or dietary deficiency, and in patients suffering from heavy metal toxicosis. Normochromic anemias are more common in birds, usually associated with bacterial infection.
  - If available, red cell distribution width % (RDW %): autoanalyzers represent the size of erythrocytes in a bell curve; wider curves mean larger % RDW, suggesting anisocytosis (increase in size variability) that is present with regenerative anemias.
- Plasma biochemistry panel: increases in the levels of intracytoplasmacytic ions may be noted with acute hemolysis
- Fecal parasite examination
- Blood parasite examination

ADVANCED OR CONFIRMATORY TESTING

- Cytology: blood smears made from anemic patients will appear "watery" and thin; blood smears should be examined to differentiate between nonregenerative and regenerative anemias. Variability in the color of erythrocytes (polychromasia) may indicate bone marrow response.
- Viral testing: polyomavirus, circovirus
- Imaging: use of radiographic imaging in cases of avian anemia may be helpful in determining the presence of heavy metal foreign bodies
- Endoscopy: endoscopic examination of the GI tract is indicated when ulceration of the GI mucosa is suspected
- Heavy metal–specific testing (see Heavy Metal Toxicity)
  - A blood smear should be examined for characteristic ballooning of RBC cytoplasm, commonly noted in cases of avian heavy metal toxicosis.
  - Lead tissue concentrations in the liver, kidney, and brain of 3 to 6 ppm wet weight are suggestive of lead toxicosis; greater than 6 ppm is diagnostic. Blood values >0.5 ppm (50 μg/dL, 2.5 μg/dL) are diagnostic.
  - Zinc concentrations in the pancreas of 26.11 μg/g on a dry weight basis were considered normal in cockatiels, and concentrations of 312.4-2418 μg/g were considered toxic. In liver, subclinical birds are less than 40 ppm wet weight, and concentrations greater than 75 ppm were correlated with toxicosis.

TREATMENT

THERAPEUTIC GOALS

- Stop blood loss; stabilize and improve patient's physical condition.
- Determine cause of blood loss.
- Provide supportive therapy to control anemia.
- Determine severity of blood loss and nature of anemia (regenerative/nonregenerative).
- Treat disease condition if possible to prevent recurrence.

ACUTE GENERAL TREATMENT

- All treatment is to be performed on a stable patient.
  - Nursing care
    - Administer warmed crystalloid fluids SC, IV, IO (50-150 mL/kg/d maintenance plus dehydration deficit factored in if needed) at a rate of 10-25 mL/kg over a 5-minute period or at a continuous rate of 100 mL/kg/q 24 h.
    - Increase environmental temperature to 85°C-90°F (29°C-32°C).
    - Provide a humidified environment by placing warm moist towels in the incubator.
    - Nutritional support is required in most cases.
    - Oxygen therapy should be given if respiratory distress is present.
- Hemoglobin-based carriers: these colloidal products carry oxygen to tissues. Oxyglobin, purified polymerized bovine hemoglobin, is being used in birds at a dose of 5-10 mL/kg IV. Oxyglobin has a short half-life and can be very effective in treating acute hemorrhagic presentations, or as initial therapy while a suitable donor for a blood transfusion is located.
- Iron dextran: this agent can be administered at 10 mg/kg IM once and repeated if necessary in 7-10 days to aid in erythropoiesis. Iron dextran must be used with caution in species predisposed to hemochromatosis (e.g., ramphastids, mynah birds) or in patients with possible bacterial infection.

- Blood transfusion: the criteria that may be used to determine whether an avian patient needs a blood transfusion because of an anemic condition include a PCV value of <20% in chronic conditions and <25% in acute presentations, with decreased tissue oxygenation and oxygen-hemoglobin saturation. Only blood transfusions from the same species of bird are recommended. No pretreatment of the recipient is required before the blood transfusion unless the same donor is being used for a repeat transfusion. Pretreatment recommendations consist of a single dose of dexamethasone (2 mg/kg IM) and diphenhydramine (2 mg/kg IM). Clinical signs of a transfusion reaction include increased body temperature, tachycardia, and tachypnea.

CHRONIC TREATMENT

Treat the primary cause of the anemic condition.

DRUG INTERACTIONS

- Use only blood donors from the species of bird needing a blood transfusion.
- Pretreatment of the blood recipient may be required if the same donor is used for multiple transfusions.

POSSIBLE COMPLICATIONS

Iron dextran must be used with caution in species predisposed to hemochromatosis (e.g., ramphastids, mynah birds) and in patients with possible bacterial infection.

RECOMMENDED MONITORING

- Repeat radiographs if monitoring passage of heavy metal particles.
- Repeat CBC and plasma chemistry panel to monitor treatment response and recovery.
- Monitor appetite, fecal output, and behavior during chelation treatment.
- Monitor for clinical signs of a transfusion reaction, including increased body temperature, tachycardia, and tachypnea.

PROGNOSIS AND OUTCOME

Prognosis and outcome are dependent on the cause of the anemic condition, the patient's condition when presented to the hospital, and the ability of the veterinarian to stabilize, diagnose, and properly treat the disease causing the blood loss.

PEARLS & CONSIDERATIONS

COMMENTS

- Blood loss is a serious life-threatening condition that is described in the patient as anemia.
- The veterinarian has little diagnostic help in determining the overall condition of a bird when presented in an anemic state.
- The patient must be stabilized through cessation of blood loss if possible and with supportive care, thereby enabling further investigation into the cause of blood loss if not known.

PREVENTION

- Polyoma vaccination
- Owner awareness of life-threatening nature of blood loss in birds.
- Reduced exposure to animals that may traumatize birds (e.g., dogs, cats, raccoons)
- Parasite control
- Proper nutrition

CLIENT EDUCATION

See Prevention.

SUGGESTED READING

Orosz SE: Diagnostic workup plan. In Olsen GH, et al, editors: Manual of avian medicine, St Louis, 2000, Mosby Inc., pp 1–17.

CROSS-REFERENCES TO OTHER SECTIONS

Heavy Metal Toxicity

AUTHOR: **ALBERTO RODRIGUEZ BARBON**

EDITOR: **THOMAS N. TULLY, JR.**

BIRDS

Anorexia

BASIC INFORMATION

DEFINITION

Lack or loss of appetite for food

SYNONYMS

Inappetence, disinterest in food

EPIDEMIOLOGY

SPECIES, AGE, SEX All species and ages, and both sexes

RISK FACTORS

- Stress factors (e.g., new environment, change in food, environment)
- Disease
- Crop thermal burn
- Polyomavirus infection
- Foreign body ingestion

CONTAGION AND ZOONOSIS *Chlamydophila psittaci* infection

GEOGRAPHY AND SEASONALITY May be more prevalent during the warmer summer months

ASSOCIATED CONDITIONS AND DISORDERS

- Loss of muscle mass—body condition
- Nutritional deficiencies
- Anemia
- Gastroenteritis
- Weakness

CLINICAL PRESENTATION

DISEASE FORMS/SUBTYPES

- Anorexia associated with physical inability to eat
- Anorexia associated with gastrointestinal disease
- Anorexia associated with systemic disease
- Anorexia associated with stress conditions

HISTORY, CHIEF COMPLAINT

- Depression
- Inappetence
- "Going light" (loss of body condition)
- "Sour crop" crop stasis

PHYSICAL EXAM FINDINGS

- Poor body condition
- Weakness

ETIOLOGY AND PATHOPHYSIOLOGY

Any external or disease condition that causes the bird to lack or lose its appetite for food

DIAGNOSIS

DIFFERENTIAL DIAGNOSIS

- Infectious ingluvities
- Infectious gastroenteritis
- Ingested foreign body
- Toxicity
- Neoplasia
- External factors
  - Environment (e.g., high temperature)
  - Abuse by cagemate

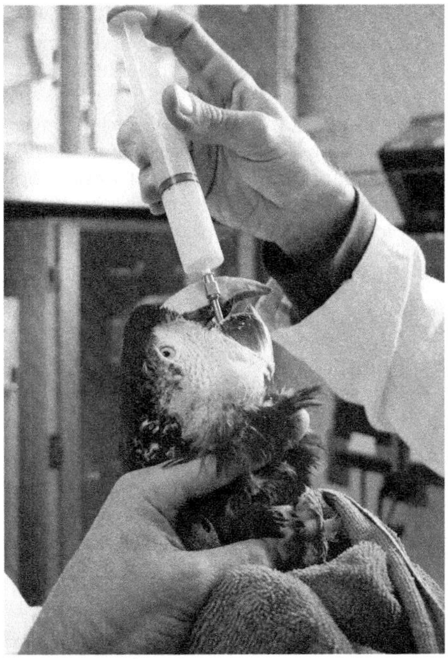

Anorexia If the patient refuses to eat, force-feeding is needed. Specially designed formulas are available. *(Photo courtesy Thomas N. Tully, Jr.)*

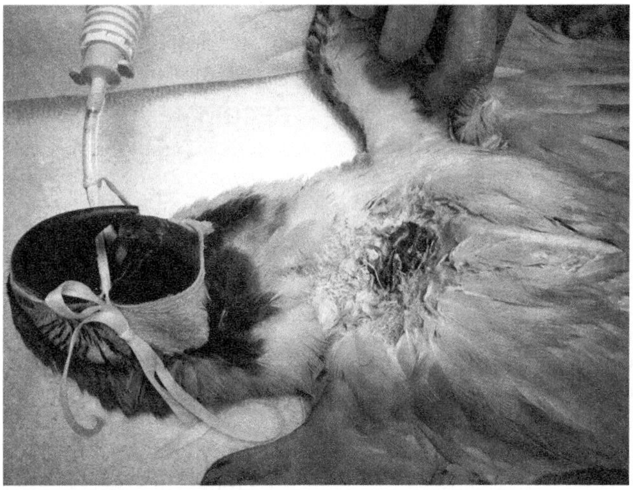

Anorexia Crop thermal burn. *(Photo courtesy Thomas N. Tully, Jr.)*

- Movement of cage
- Change in diet

• Systemic infectious disease
• Systemic illness

INITIAL DATABASE

- Complete blood count (CBC): with infectious diseases, leukocytosis with concurrent heterophilia may be present. Hypochromic regenerative anemia occurs in some cases of lead toxicity.
- Plasma biochemistry panel: lactate dehydrogenase (LDH), creatine kinase (CK), and aspartate aminotransferase (AST) may be elevated. Lipase and amylase may be elevated in zinc toxicity.

ADVANCED OR CONFIRMATORY TESTING

- Imaging: foreign bodies may be noted in the crop and/or the gastrointestinal tract
  - Endoscopic examination of coelomic cavity looking for disease pathology
- Culture and sensitivity of crop, gastrointestinal tract, and/or cloaca
- Heavy metal–specific testing (see Heavy Metal Toxicity)
  - Lead tissue concentrations in the liver, kidney, and brain of 3 to 6 ppm wet weight are suggestive of lead toxicosis; greater than 6 ppm is diagnostic. Blood levels for lead intoxication in birds, 0.25 ppm (significant when associated with clinical signs); >0.5 ppm is considered high.
  - Zinc concentrations in the pancreas of 26.11 µg/g on a dry weight basis were considered normal in cockatiels; concentrations of 312.4-2418 µg/g were considered toxic. In liver, subclinical birds are less than 40 ppm wet weight, and concentrations greater than 75 ppm were correlated with toxicosis. Normal zinc blood levels in parrots is <2.5 ppm. 2.6-3.4 is reported as above normal levels and 3.5-4.4 is high. Any zinc blood levels above 4.5 ppm is considered toxic. Normal zinc levels for waterfowl and poultry are slightly higher than those used for parrots.

TREATMENT

THERAPEUTIC GOALS

- Stabilize and improve patient's physical condition.
- Treat underlying disease conditions if present.
- Improve nutritional status of patient through supplemental nutritional administration.

ACUTE GENERAL TREATMENT

- All treatment is to be performed on a stable patient.
  - Nursing care
    - Administer warmed crystalloid fluids SC, IV, IO (50-150 mL/kg/d maintenance plus dehydration [see Dehydration] deficit factored in if needed) at a rate of 10-25 mL/kg over a 5-minute period or at a continuous rate of 100 mL/kg/q 24 h.
    - Increase environmental temperature to 85°F-90°F (29°C-32°C).
    - Provide a humidified environment by placing warm moist towels in the incubator.
    - Nutritional support is required in most cases.
  - Treat primary and secondary disease conditions.
  - Surgery or endoscopic retrieval may be required to remove foreign body if present.
  - Surgery may be necessary to repair crop burn trauma.
- Medications
  - Drugs of choice
    - Dependent on case presentation and disease diagnosis

CHRONIC TREATMENT

Dependent on case presentation and disease diagnosis

RECOMMENDED MONITORING

- Repeat radiographs to determine whether foreign body has been removed if this was the primary cause of the anorectic condition.
- Repeat CBC and plasma chemistry panel to monitor treatment response and recovery.
- Blood heavy metal levels should be assessed during treatment and after treatment if this was the primary cause of the anorexic condition.
- Monitor appetite, fecal output, and behavior during treatment and recovery period.

PROGNOSIS AND OUTCOME

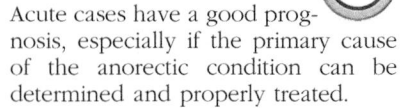

- Acute cases have a good prognosis, especially if the primary cause of the anorectic condition can be determined and properly treated.
- If the patient's body condition is very poor (1/5), the prognosis for recovery is poor to grave.

PEARLS & CONSIDERATIONS

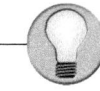

COMMENTS

- Owners should be aware that anorexia may be and often is the first sign of illness in avian species.
- The sooner the bird can start eating on its own, the better chance the patient has of recovering.
- Polyomavirus vaccination is a recommended measure to reduce the incidence of infection in young psittacine birds.
- Many secondary disease conditions develop when birds lose a significant percentage of their muscle mass.
- Birds should be hand-fed by experienced personnel.
- Hand-feeding formula should be fed at a temperature lower than the bird's normal body temperature.

PREVENTION

- Provide excellent nutrition offerings to birds.
- Maintain birds in appropriate environments.
- Provide species-appropriate toys and cage furniture.
- Polyomavirus vaccination

CLIENT EDUCATION

- Owners should be aware of their birds' eating habits.
  - What the birds like to eat
  - How much they normally eat
- Owners should be aware of their birds' fecal/urine output through the use of paper-lined cages.
  - Volume
  - Normal appearance
- If the bird's appetite decreases, or if a decrease in fecal/urine output is noted, a veterinarian should be contacted.

SUGGESTED READINGS

Harcourt-Brown NH: Psittacine birds. In Tully TN, et al, editors: Avian medicine, Oxford, UK, 2000, Butterworth Heinemann, pp 112–144.

Lumeij JT: Gastroenterology. In Ritchie BW, et al, editors: Avian medicine: principles and applications, Brentwood, TN, 1994, HBD International Inc., pp 482–521.

CROSS-REFERENCES TO OTHER SECTIONS

Chlamydophila psittaci
Crop Stasis
Dehydration
Heavy Metal Toxicity
Viral Diseases

AUTHOR & EDITOR: **THOMAS N. TULLY, JR.**

BIRDS

Ascites

BASIC INFORMATION

DEFINITION

The accumulation of serous fluid within one or more of the peritoneal cavities; may be caused by peritoneal and extraperitoneal diseases

SYNONYMS

"Abdominal" fluid, coelomic fluid

EPIDEMIOLOGY

SPECIES, AGE, SEX All species and ages and both sexes

GENETICS AND BREED PREDISPOSITION

- Anseriformes: chronic liver disease, amyloidosis
- Mynahs, toucans, and birds of paradise: iron storage disease
- Budgerigars: coelomic tumors
- Gallinaceous birds and ducklings raised at high altitudes: right ventricular failure

RISK FACTORS

- Bacterial infection leading to endocarditis and myocarditis
- Viral infection: Marek's disease, resulting in heart tumors
- Low environmental temperature and high-sodium diet: right heart failure: chickens, turkeys
- Peritonitis
- Penetrating or nonpenetrating trauma to the abdomen
- Chronic liver disease
- Hypoalbuminemia
- Congestive heart failure
- Exposure to toxins (e.g., chlorinated biphenyls, dioxin, creosol)

CONTAGION AND ZOONOSIS *Mycobacterium* spp. granulomas have been suggested to cause blockage of lymph drainage in some ascites cases. *Mycobacterium* spp. may be zoonotic agents.

ASSOCIATED CONDITIONS AND DISORDERS

- Swelling of the distal coelom
- Anorexia
- Renal: lead damages proximal tubule cells
- Liver disease (see Liver Disease)
- Septicemia
- Weakness
- Heart disease and failure

CLINICAL PRESENTATION

DISEASE FORMS/SUBTYPES

- Ascites associated with liver disease
- Pseudochylous ascites
- Ascites caused by hypoalbuminemia
- Heart disease and failure
- Trauma-induced ascites

HISTORY, CHIEF COMPLAINT

- Dyspnea
- Depression
- Swelling of coelom
- Anorexia
- Difficulty perching
- "Fluffed" feathers

PHYSICAL EXAM FINDINGS

- Dyspnea
- Swelling of the coelom
- Cardiac arrhythmias
- Coelomic fluid

ETIOLOGY AND PATHOPHYSIOLOGY

- Ascites associated with liver disease: caused by increased portal venous hydrostatic pressure and decreased portal venous colloid osmotic pressure
- Cases where an inflammatory exudate is present may be defined as peritonitis.
- Pseudochylous ascites: turbid or milky abdominal fluid is observed; may be associated with abdominal malignancies and infections
- Ascites caused by hypoalbuminemia
- Heart disease and failure: right ventricular failure
- Trauma-induced ascites: urate ascites, bile ascites, pancreatic ascites, and hemoperitoneum due to rupture of the liver, spleen, or kidney

DIAGNOSIS

DIFFERENTIAL DIAGNOSIS

- Neoplasia
- Gravid uterus
- Herniation
- Egg-related peritonitis (see Chronic Egg Laying)
- Obesity
- Granuloma
- Gastrointestinal dilation (see Enteritis)
- Hepatomegaly (see Hepatic Lipidosis)

- Renomegaly
- Splenomegaly

INITIAL DATABASE

- Complete blood count (CBC): heterophilic leukocytosis with peritonitis; monocytosis associated with chronic inflammatory disease (e.g., avian tuberculosis); hypochromic regenerative anemia occurs in some cases of lead toxicity
- Plasma biochemistry panel: lactate dehydrogenase (LDH), creatine kinase (CK), and aspartate aminotransferase (AST) may be elevated. Bile acids may be elevated with hepatic disease. Renal protein may be determined through urinary analysis.
- Triglyceride: plasma triglyceride ratio <1 is suggestive of pseudochylous ascites

ADVANCED OR CONFIRMATORY TESTING

- Imaging: ascites noted radiographically as a diffuse, "ground glass" appearance in the coelomic cavity. Specific organs are often difficult to observe.
  - Cardiohepatic silhouette may appear widened.
  - Air sacs narrowed on ventrodorsal view
  - Individual organs may be enlarged if associated with the presenting condition of ascites.
- Ultrasound is often very useful in evaluating the coelomic cavity of birds that present with ascites.

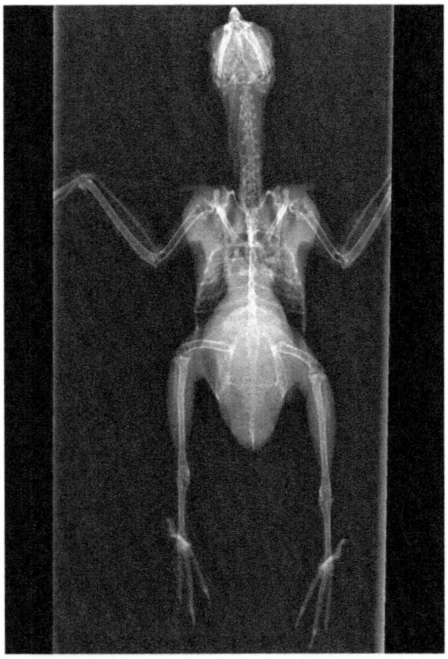

Ascites A radiograph of a mynah bird with ascites. This species is predisposed to hemochromatosis, notice the increase in the liver silhouette. The animal had about 20 ml of fluids in the coelomic cavity. *(Photo courtesy Jörg Mayer, The University of Georgia, Athens.)*

- Abdominocentesis and pathologic examination of fluid sample:
  - When performing abdominocentesis, one must guard against puncture of the air sac system, which would cause aspiration of the coelomic fluid into the respiratory system.
  - Fluid should be obtained with the bird in a ventral recumbent position and removed from the gravity-dependent area caudal to the keel by guiding the needle cranially to the right of center.
    - Transudate clear to pale yellow fluid
      - Low specific gravity (<1.020)
      - Low protein (1 g/dL)
      - Low cellularity
    - Exudate
      - High specific gravity (>1.020)
      - High protein content (3 g/dL)
      - Usually associated with many inflammatory cells
      - Septic conditions may include bacteria.
      - Neoplastic cells may be present with tumors (see Tumors).
      - Urate crystals are indicative of urine in the coelom.
      - Hemorrhagic effusions may be associated with organ trauma.
      - Culture and sensitivity of coelomic fluid if peritonitis present

TREATMENT

THERAPEUTIC GOALS

- Stabilize and improve patient's physical condition.
- Treatment should be focused on primary cause of the condition.
- Removal of fluid is recommended only if life-threatening dyspnea is present.
  - If patient hypoproteinemic: removal of fluid from a hepatically or renally compromised bird may have adverse consequences

ACUTE GENERAL TREATMENT

- All treatment is to be performed on a stable patient.
  - Nursing care:
    - Provide a humidified environment by placing warm moist towels in the incubator.
    - Nutritional support is required in most cases.
- Treatment of primary cause of coelomic fluid accumulation
- Medications
  - Drug of choice
    - Furosemide administered to effect (0.1-2.0 mg/kg PO, SC, IM, IV q 6-24 h)

CHRONIC TREATMENT

Low-sodium diet

POSSIBLE COMPLICATIONS

- Furosemide overdose can lead to dehydration and electrolyte abnormalities.
- Toxicity is characterized by neurologic signs and death.

RECOMMENDED MONITORING

- Repeat radiographs to monitor treatment response.
- Repeat CBC and plasma chemistry panel to monitor treatment response and recovery.
- Monitor appetite, fecal output, and behavior during treatment.

PROGNOSIS AND OUTCOME

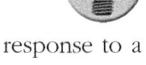

Dependent on primary cause of coelomic fluid accumulation

PEARLS & CONSIDERATIONS

COMMENTS

- Ascites is a physiologic response to a primary cause.
- Identification and treatment of the primary cause of coelomic fluid accumulation will result in cessation of ascites.

PREVENTION

- Prevent birds from ingesting foreign bodies (see Foreign Bodies) through placement of species-appropriate toys in cage.
- Prevent obesity of birds within household.
- Prevent exposure to toxins.
- Furazolidone has been associated with cardiomyopathy in turkeys, chickens, and ducks.

CLIENT EDUCATION

See Prevention.

SUGGESTED READINGS

Lumeij JT: Gastroenterology. In Ritchie BW, et al, editors: Avian medicine: principles and applications, Brentwood, TN, 1994, HBD International Inc., pp 482–521.

Pollock C, et al: Birds. In Carpenter JW, editor: Exotic animal formulary, ed 3, St Louis, 2005, Elsevier/Saunders, pp 135–346.

CROSS-REFERENCES TO OTHER SECTIONS

Chronic Egg Laying
Enteritis
Foreign Bodies
Hepatic Lipidosis
Liver Disease
Tumors

AUTHOR & EDITOR: **THOMAS N. TULLY, JR.**

Aspergillosis

Client Education Sheet and Additional Images Available on Website

BASIC INFORMATION

DEFINITION

Aspergillosis is a noncontagious, opportunistic infection caused by members of the fungal genus *Aspergillus.*

SYNONYM

Mycotic infection, fungal pneumonia (see Pneumonia)

EPIDEMIOLOGY

SPECIES, AGE, SEX All species and ages and both sexes

GENETICS AND BREED PREDISPOSITION Species more at risk for the development of *Aspergillus* spp. infection include African grey parrots *(Psittacus erithacus), Pionus* parrots (*Pionus* spp.), goshawks *(Accipiter gentilis),* rough-legged hawks *(Buteo lagopus),* red-tailed hawks *(Buteo jamaicensis),* golden eagles *(Aquila chrysaetos),* snowy owls *(Nyctea scandiaca),* gyrfalcons *(Falco rusticolus),* swans (*Cygnus* spp.), and penguins (*Spheniscus* spp.).

RISK FACTORS

- Stress
- Adverse environmental conditions (e.g., dusty, dry)
- Inappropriate husbandry
- Nutritional deficiencies (e.g., vitamin A)
- Young or old bird
- Immune suppression
- Long-term corticosteroid and/or antibiotic use
- Recent capture from the wild
- Preexisting disease condition

GEOGRAPHY AND SEASONALITY A combination of humid and dry dusty environmental conditions, especially when hay or grass is present, may predispose exposed birds to this disease.

ASSOCIATED CONDITIONS AND DISORDERS

- Anorexia
- Depression
- Dyspnea
- Weakness
- Nasal granulomas

CLINICAL PRESENTATION

DISEASE FORMS/SUBTYPES

- Air sac plaques diagnosed by endoscopy
- Respiratory granulomas involving nares, trachea, lungs, and/or air sacs

HISTORY, CHIEF COMPLAINT

- Nonspecific
- Depression
- Inappetence
- Breathing difficulty
- Reluctance to fly or perch
- Drooped wings

PHYSICAL EXAM FINDINGS

- Weight loss
- Dyspnea, tachypnea, cyanosis
- Lethargy
- Polyuria/polydipsia
- Vocalization when breathing
- Open beak breathing
- Tail bobbing
- Enlarged nares

ETIOLOGY AND PATHOPHYSIOLOGY

- *Aspergillus* spp. spores are ubiquitous in the environment.
- Birds presenting with an *Aspergillus* spp. infection are usually immune suppressed, which may be induced by a variety of causes.
- Many birds carry spores in their lungs or air sacs for prolonged periods or until immune suppressed, which initiates the onset of clinical disease.

DIAGNOSIS

DIFFERENTIAL DIAGNOSIS

- Mycoplasmosis
- Colibacillosis
- Fowl cholera
- Mycobacteriosis
- Environmental toxicosis
- Avian chlamydiosis

INITIAL DATABASE

- Complete blood count (CBC): aspergillosis generally causes a significant heterophilic leukocytosis (25,000 cells/μL-100,000 cells/μL). A left shift is often present, and white blood cells are usually quite reactive. A nonregenerative anemia is commonly identified, likely in response to the chronic inflammation.
- Plasma biochemistry panel: biochemistry analysis typically reveals elevations in aspartate aminotransferase (AST) and lactate dehydrogenase (LDH). Hypoalbuminemia and hypergammaglobulinemia are characteristic of the disease.
- Fungal culture (see Mycoses): cultures at the base of nasal granulomas and of the affected respiratory tract may help confirm the diagnosis of an aspergillosis infection

ADVANCED OR CONFIRMATORY TESTING

- Imaging
  - Radiology may reveal the distribution and severity of mycotic lesions in the lungs and air sacs but is not a valuable diagnostic tool until late in the course of the disease.
  - Observation of air sac walls, asymmetry, hyperinflation, or consolidation of the air sacs and soft tissue densities in the lungs and air sacs may be observed in birds with aspergillosis infection.
- Serology
  - Serologic tests are often of limited value because of the ubiquitous nature of *Aspergillus* spp. spores in the environment.
  - Indirect ELISA assay measures *Aspergillus* spp. antibody titers, but a positive titer can be attributed to active infection, long-term exposure, or previous infection. A negative titer may be explained by lack of reactivity between the test conjugate and patient immunoglobulins, or by lack of patient humoral response (immune suppression). Paired titers are often more helpful than a single titer.
- Endoscopy
  - Visualization of the trachea, lungs, and air sacs through endoscopic examination is the most useful technique in visualizing granulomas, extracting biopsy samples, and collecting samples for fungal culture.
- Histopathologic examination
  - Granulomatous air sacculitis and pleuritis are commonly diagnosed in cases of aspergillosis infection. More specifically, thickened air sac membranes infiltrated with large numbers of inflammatory cells and germinating conidia are observed.
  - Germinating conidia are also commonly observed in macrophages.
  - Lung lesions typically consist of heterophilic and lymphohistiocytic or granulomatous pleuritis and pneumonia with edema and hemorrhage.

TREATMENT

THERAPEUTIC GOALS

- Stabilize, reduce stress, and improve patient's physical condition.
- Determine extent of disease condition and the cause of immune suppression if not evident, and confirm diagnosis.
- Medical treatment that will result in an expeditious recovery should be initiated.

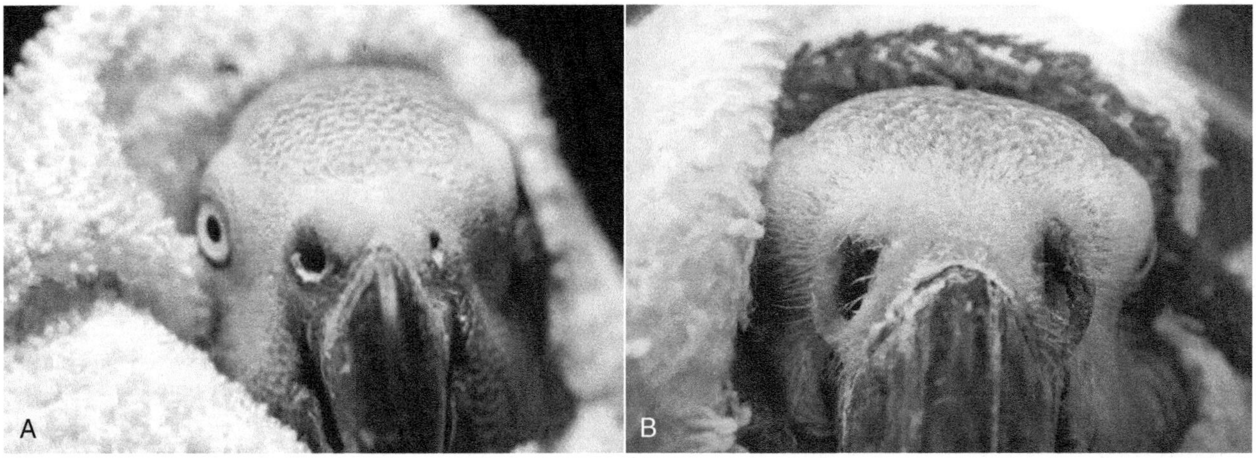

Aspergillosis Enlarged nares of African grey parrot due to growth of a fungal granulomas.

- Obtain complete resolution of infection.

ACUTE GENERAL TREATMENT

- All treatment is to be performed on a stable patient.
  - Nursing care
    - Administer warmed crystalloid fluids SC, IV, IO (50-150 mL/kg/d maintenance plus dehydration deficit factored in if needed) at a rate of 10-25 mL/kg over a 5-minute period or at a continuous rate of 100 mL/kg/q 24 h.
    - Increase environmental temperature to 85°F-90°F (29°C-32°C).
    - Provide a humidified environment by placing warm moist towels in the incubator.
    - Nutritional support is required in most cases.
- Medications
  - Drugs of choice
    - Amphotericin B 1.5 mg/kg IV q 8 h for 3-5 days, in combination with itraconazole (5-10 mg/kg PO q 12 hr for 5 days, then daily; African grey parrots should be treated with 2.5-5 mg/kg q 24 hr), fluconazole (5-15 mg/kg PO q 12 h) or terbinafine (10-15 mg/kg PO q 12-24 h), is recommended. Nebulization therapy 1 mg/mL sterile water or saline × 15 minutes q 12 h. Amphotericin B is usually administered intratracheally at a dose of 1 mg/kg q 8-12 h. Amphotericin B should always be diluted with water before administration.
    - Itraconazole is especially effective when administered with nebulized clotrimazole and/or intravenous or nebulized amphotericin B. The recommended dose of itraconazole is 5-10 mg/kg PO q 12 h for 5 days, then daily for the remainder of treatment. African grey parrots are reportedly more sensitive to the drug; a dose of 2.5-5 mg/kg q 24 h is generally recommended for this species.
    - Fluconazole is reported to be an effective treatment for aspergillosis infection, although less so than itraconazole. It is used primarily for treating mycotic infection of the eye or central nervous system. A dose of 5-15 mg/kg PO q 12 h is generally recommended.
    - Clotrimazole is used as a topical treatment for localized aspergillosis infection that should be treated via nebulization. It is typically administered as a 1% aqueous solution for 30 minutes every 24 hours.
    - Terbinafine hydrochloride has the unique ability to penetrate mycotic granulomas. It is typically administered at a dose of 10-15 mg/kg PO q 12-24 h with itraconazole. It can also be administered via nebulization as a 1 mg/mL aqueous solution for 20 minutes q 8 h.

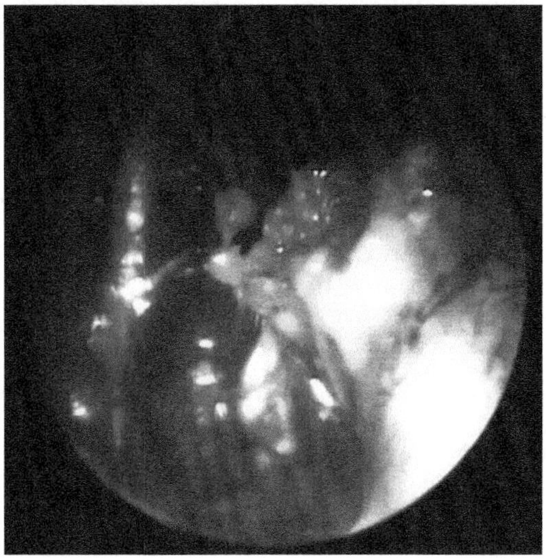

Aspergillosis Fungal plaque in the coelomic cavity of a parrot being examined with a rigid endoscope.

CHRONIC TREATMENT

Surgery and endoscopic treatment: surgery and endoscopic intervention may be considered for extraction or debulking of large, obstructive granulomas

Chronic rhinitis or sinusitis caused by *Aspergillus* spp. infection can be treated via trephination of the frontal sinuses.

DRUG INTERACTIONS

Itraconazole: as an inhibitor of the cytochrome, coadministration with other drugs primarily metabolized by this enzyme system may lead to increased plasma concentrations that could increase or prolong both therapeutic and adverse effects

POSSIBLE COMPLICATIONS

- Amphotericin B is potentially nephrotoxic.
- Fluconazole death observed in budgerigars at dose of 10 mg/kg q 12 h
- Itraconazole will cause anorexia and depression in African grey parrots. If

used with this species, careful monitoring of the patient's condition is required.

RECOMMENDED MONITORING

- Repeat radiographs and endoscopy for treatment response.
- Repeat CBC and plasma chemistry panel to monitor patient's condition during administration of antifungal medication.
- Analgesic/antiinflammatory medication is required in cases of suspected pain and inflammation.
- Monitor appetite, fecal output, and behavior during treatment and until resolution of the disease condition.

PROGNOSIS AND OUTCOME

- Uncomplicated cases have a good prognosis.
- The prognosis degrades depending on immune status of patient, avian species being treated, and chronicity of illness.
- Nasal granuloma presentations may result in permanent deformity of the nasal opening.

PEARLS & CONSIDERATIONS

COMMENTS

- *Aspergillus* spp. infections can be treated.
- Veterinarians must be aware of the side effects associated with drugs commonly used to treat avian aspergillosis cases.
- Often for complete resolution of *Aspergillus* spp. infection in avian patients, therapy can last for months.
- Susceptible species should be monitored or prophylactic antifungal treatment administered if immune suppressed, or if the animal is placed in a stressful environment.

PREVENTION

- Reduce stress.
- Maintain appropriate housing and nutrition for species in question.
- Reduce exposure to *Aspergillus* spp. spores.

CLIENT EDUCATION

Maintain birds in a facility that will reduce stress, exposure to fungal spores, and immune suppression in bird(s).

SUGGESTED READINGS

Jones MP, Orosz SE: The diagnosis of aspergillosis in birds, Semin Avian Exotic Pet Med 9:52–58, 2000.
Orosz SE: Antifungal drug therapy in avian species, Vet Clin North Am Exotic Anim Pract 6:337–350, 2003.
Orosz SE: Overview of aspergillosis pathogenesis and treatment options, Semin Avian Exotic Pet Med 9:59–65, 2000.

CROSS-REFERENCES TO OTHER SECTIONS

Mycoses
Pneumonia

AUTHOR: **MEGAN KIRCHGESSNER**

EDITOR: **THOMAS N. TULLY, JR.**

BIRDS

Cardiac Disease

BASIC INFORMATION

DEFINITION

Cardiac disease may involve the pericardium, myocardium, endocardium, cardiac valves, impulse-forming and conducting systems, and major blood vessels. Pericardial diseases most frequently diagnosed in birds include pericarditis and hydropericardium. Common myocardial diseases include dilatative cardiomyopathy and myocarditis, which can lead to myocardial failure. Endocarditis, valvular insufficiency, and valvular stenosis are disease conditions most often associated with cardiac endothelial tissue.

EPIDEMIOLOGY

SPECIES, AGE, SEX

- All species are susceptible.
- Older birds are more susceptible to cardiac disease (e.g., atherosclerosis).
- Young birds are more often diagnosed with developmental heart abnormalities (e.g., ventricular septal defect).

GENETICS AND BREED PREDISPOSITION

- Psittacine species most commonly affected by atherosclerosis: rose-breasted cockatoos, Amazon parrots, African grey parrots.
- Cockatoos commonly affected by developmental and congenital heart defects

RISK FACTORS

- Poor diet
- Lack of exercise
- Infection
- Toxin
- Idiopathic
- Congenital

ASSOCIATED CONDITIONS AND DISORDERS

- Respiratory distress
- Generalized edema/ascites
- Syncope
- Reduced exercise tolerance

CLINICAL PRESENTATION

DISEASE FORMS/SUBTYPES

- Vegetative endocarditis
- Atherosclerosis
- Congestive heart failure
- Pericarditis
- Pericardial effusion
- Valvular insufficiency/stenosis

HISTORY, CHIEF COMPLAINT

- Usually nonspecific complaint by owner
- Weakness/depression
- Dyspnea

PHYSICAL EXAM FINDINGS

- Respiratory distress (e.g., coughing, wheezing)
- Edema and/or ascites
- Asculted murmur
- Bluish discoloration of periorbital skin
- Anorexia
- Coelomic distention

ETIOLOGY AND PATHOPHYSIOLOGY

- Cardiac disease may lead to congestive heart failure and/or cardiogenic shock.
- Inadequate cardiac function (compensated)
    - Leads to decreased output and increased preload
- Increased atrial and venous pressure due to failing ventricle
- Decreased renal blood flow results in sodium and fluid retention.
- Right heart failure
    - Systemic edema with hepatomegaly, ascites, hydropericardium
- Left heart failure
    - Pulmonary edema

DIAGNOSIS

DIFFERENTIAL DIAGNOSIS

- Dyspnea
    - Respiratory disease
- Coelomic distention
    - Reproductive disease

- Internal ovulation
- Neoplasia
- Systemic infectious disease
- Hepatic disease

INITIAL DATABASE

- Complete blood count
- Plasma chemistry panel (alanine aminotransferase [ALT], aspartate aminotransferase [AST] with mild to moderate elevations)
- Auscultation
- Radiology
  - Useful in assessing position, size, and shape of the heart
  - Measurements of the width of the cardiac silhouette are performed in the ventrodorsal view with perfect superimposition of the keel and spine.
  - In medium-size psittacine patients, the width of the cardiac silhouette should be approximately 51%-61% the width of the thorax.
  - Enlargement of the hepatic silhouette, increased opacity of the lungs, and a fluid-filled coelomic cavity may be observed.

ADVANCED OR CONFIRMATORY TESTING

- Electrocardiography (ECG)
  - Useful in diagnosing cardiac arrhythmias and conductive disorders, and useful in characterizing chamber size
  - Four electrodes (e.g., needle or alligator clip) are attached to the patient: one in the area of each propatagium, and one in the medial aspect of each thigh.
- Echocardiography
  - Allows for identification of abnormalities in heart structure and function
  - With psittacine patients, the recommended window for the machine probe is a ventromedial approach through the midline just behind the sternum, with the bird held in an upright position.
  - Two longitudinal views of the heart are obtained.
  - Measurements have to be taken from two-dimensional (2D) images because a suitable cross-section for M-mode technique cannot be attained.
  - Doppler echocardiography is also possible; general anesthesia is recommended because of the high velocity of flow in the avian heart.
- Angiocardiography
  - Provides additional information, especially in examination of the cardiac vessels
  - Iodinated contrast medium is administered via intravenous catheter at a dose of 2-4 mL/kg of 250 mg/mL at a rate of 1-2 mL of contrast medium/sec.

TREATMENT

THERAPEUTIC GOALS

- Stabilize patient.
- Treat primary disease condition.
- Improve cardiac function.
- Treat secondary heart-induced disease conditions (e.g., ascites, pulmonary edema).

ACUTE GENERAL TREATMENT

- Furosemide 0.15-2 mg/kg PO, IM, IV q 8 h: indicated in pulmonary edema, ascites, and pericardial effusion. Critically dyspneic animals often require high doses (4-8 mg/kg) to be stabilized. Once edema resolves, taper the diuretic to the lowest effective dosage.
- Enalapril 1.25 mg/kg PO q 8-12 h: indicated in heart failure or hypertension
- Digoxin 0.02 to 0.05 mg/kg PO q 12 h: indicated in cardiac failure for acute treatment

CHRONIC TREATMENT

- Pimobendan 3-10 mg/kg q 12-24 h
- Digoxin 0.01 mg/kg PO q 12 h: requires careful monitoring of plasma levels and side effects
- Oxprenolol 2 mg/kg PO q 24 h: has shown a protective effect against the development of atherosclerotic plaques in poultry.

DRUG INTERACTIONS

Combination of high-dose diuretics and angiotensin-converting enzyme (ACE) inhibitors may alter renal perfusion.

POSSIBLE COMPLICATIONS

- Furosemide may predispose the patient to dehydration, prerenal azotemia, and electrolyte disturbances.
- Digoxin should be used with extreme caution in patients with glomerulonephritis and heart failure, idiopathic hypertrophic subaortic stenosis, frequent ventricular premature contractions, ventricular tachycardia, chronic constrictive pericarditis, and/or incomplete atrioventricular (AV) block.

RECOMMENDED MONITORING

- Renal status
- Electrolytes
- Hydration
- Respiratory rate and effort
- Heart rate
- Body weight
- Coelomic distention in patients with congestive heart failure
- ECG—especially in patients with diagnosed cardiac arrhythmias

PROGNOSIS AND OUTCOME

- Guarded for many forms of cardiac disease
- Treatment can stabilize a patient and provide a good quality of life.
- Prognosis depends on severity of the cardiac disease and age of the patient in which it is diagnosed.
- Long-term prognosis for cardiac patients is usually poor because the disease process is often progressive and debilitating to the heart and other major organs.

PEARLS & CONSIDERATIONS

COMMENTS

- Cardiac disease in avian patients is underdiagnosed.
- Basic cardiac evaluation of avian patients will help veterinarians recognize cardiac disease.
- Avian cardiac disease can be diagnosed and treated.

PREVENTION

Nutrition and exercise may help reduce the incidence of cardiac disease in older birds.

SUGGESTED READINGS

Lumeij JT, et al: Cardiovascular system. In Ritchie BW, et al, editors: Avian medicine: principles and applications, Lake Worth, FL, 1994, Wingers Publishing, pp 694–722.

Pees M, et al: Evaluating and treating the cardiovascular system. In Harrison GJ, et al, editors: Clinical avian medicine, vol II, Palm Beach, FL, 2006, Spix Publishing Inc., pp 451–492.

Rosenthal K, et al: Cardiac disease. In Altman RB, et al, editors: Avian medicine and surgery, Philadelphia, 1997, WB Saunders, pp 491–500.

AUTHOR: **DAVID SANCHEZ-MIGALLON GUZMAN**

EDITOR: **THOMAS N. TULLY, JR.**

Central Nervous System Signs and Neurologic Conditions

BASIC INFORMATION

DEFINITION

The central nervous system is the part of the nervous system in birds that consists of the brain and spinal cord, to which sensory impulses are transmitted and from which motor impulses pass out. The central nervous system supervises and coordinates the activity of the entire nervous system. Patients with central nervous system lesions often present with clinical signs affecting proprioception, pain localization, and upper motor neuron abnormalities, but the mental status of the bird is not altered.

SYNONYMS

Convulsions, seizures, ataxia, paresis, paralysis, tremors, circling, head tilt, nystagmus, torticollis

EPIDEMIOLOGY

SPECIES, AGE, SEX All species and ages and both sexes

GENETICS AND BREED PREDISPOSITION African grey parrots are susceptible to an apparent hypocalcemic syndrome. Affected birds often present with a history of seizure activity.

RISK FACTORS
- Hepatic disease
- Renal disease
- Hypoglycemia
- Trauma
- Toxicity (e.g., lead, zinc, chocolate, pesticides, plant ingestion, botulism, organophosphate)
- Iatrogenic drug intoxication (e.g., dimetronidazole, metronidazole)
- Nutritional deficiencies (e.g., calcium, magnesium, selenium, vitamin E, vitamin B complex)
- Neoplasia
- Parasitic infection (e.g., *Baylisascaris procyonis, Sarcocystis* spp., *Chandlerella quiscali*)
- Viral infection (e.g., paramyxovirus, proventricular dilatation disease, polyomavirus, duck viral enteritis, duck viral hepatitis, reovirus, togavirus, flavivirus)
- Bacterial infection (e.g., *Listeria monocytogenes, Chlamydophila psittaci*)
- Fungal infection (e.g., *Dactylaria gallopava, Cladosporius* spp., *Mucomyces* spp.)
- Heart disease

CONTAGION AND ZOONOSIS See *Chalmydophila psittaci.*

ASSOCIATED CONDITIONS AND DISORDERS
- Neurologic disorders (e.g., convulsions, seizures, ataxia, paresis, paralysis, tremors, circling, head tilt, nystagmus, torticollis, anorexia)
- Renal disease
- Anorexia
- Hepatic disease
- Heart disease
- Weakness
- Ophthalmic disorders

CLINICAL PRESENTATION

DISEASE FORMS/SUBTYPES
- Nutritional neuropathies
- Traumatic neuropathies
- Neoplasia
- Metabolic neuropathies
- Idiopathic epilepsy
- Toxic neuropathies
- Infectious neuropathies

HISTORY, CHIEF COMPLAINT
- Neurologic signs (e.g., convulsions, seizures, ataxia, paresis, paralysis, tremors, circling, head tilt, nystagmus, torticollis, anorexia)
- Depression
- Inappetence
- Cachexia

PHYSICAL EXAM FINDINGS
- Neurologic signs (e.g., convulsions, seizures, ataxia, paresis, paralysis, tremors, circling, head tilt, nystagmus, torticollis, anorexia)
- Abrasions and/or feather loss associated with seizure activity
- Muscle atrophy associated with nonfunctioning limb(s)
- Ophthalmic abnormalities

ETIOLOGY AND PATHOPHYSIOLOGY

- Nutritional neuropathies
  - Vitamin E: encephalomalacia
  - Vitamin B_1: polyneuritis and myelin degeneration of peripheral nerves
  - Vitamin B_2: demyelination of peripheral nerves with edema
  - Vitamin B_{12}: multifocal white matter necrosis
- Traumatic neuropathies: when blunt injury causes pathology to brain, or spinal cord adversely affects its function
- Neoplasia: space-occupying lesions that affect function of brain and/or spinal cord
- Metabolic neuropathies
  - Hepatic encephalopathy: high circulating neurotoxins (present in blood because of normal digestive processes and physiologic activity) not properly processed by liver
  - Hypocalcemia: low serum calcium levels prevent normal neurologic function
- Idiopathic epilepsy
- Toxic neuropathies
  - Lead toxicity: demyelination of the vagus nerve, block of presynaptic transmission by competitive inhibition of calcium; also encephalopathy due to diffuse perivascular edema, increases in cerebrospinal fluid, and necrosis of nerve cells
  - Botulism toxicity: toxin interferes with release of acetylcholine at motor endplates
  - Organophosphate toxicity: acetylcholinesterase inhibitors
- Infectious neuropathies: infectious organisms (e.g., bacterium, virus, fungus, parasite) directly or indirectly (through produced toxins) affect neurologic function of avian patient

DIAGNOSIS

DIFFERENTIAL DIAGNOSIS

- Hepatic disease
- Renal disease
- Hypoglycemia
- Trauma
- Toxicity
- Iatrogenic drug intoxication
- Nutritional deficiency
- Neoplasia
- Parasitic infection
- Viral infection
- Bacterial infection
- Fungal infection
- Heart disease

INITIAL DATABASE

- CBC
- Plasma biochemistry panel
- Ophthalmic examination
- Fecal parasite examination
- Neurologic examination
  - Spinal reflex evaluation
    - Hemostat to pinch wing and toe for response
    - Hemostat pinch to the cloacal or vent epithelium
    - Decreased muscle tone usually associated with lower motor neuron disease
    - Increase muscle tone usually associated with upper motor neuron disease
    - Examination of cranial nerves
- Nutritional evaluation

ADVANCED OR CONFIRMATORY TESTING

- Specific neurologic testing
  - Electroencephalography
  - Electromyography
  - Electroretinography
- Imaging
  - Radiography
  - Computed tomography
  - Magnetic resonance imaging
- Organophosphate testing
- Heavy metal–specific testing
  - Lead tissue concentrations in the liver, kidney, and brain of 3 to 6 ppm wet weight are suggestive of lead toxicosis; greater than 6 ppm is diagnostic. Blood levels for lead intoxication in birds, 0.25 ppm (significant when associated with clinical sign), >0.5 ppm is considered high.
  - Zinc concentrations in the pancreas of 26.11 μg/g on a dry weight basis were considered normal in cockatiels; concentrations of 312.4-2418 μg/g were considered toxic. In liver, subclinical birds are less than 40 ppm wet weight, and concentrations greater than 75 ppm were correlated with toxicosis.
- Cerebrospinal fluid evaluation if possible.

TREATMENT

THERAPEUTIC GOALS

- If bird presents with seizure activity, treat to prevent seizure and self-trauma associated with inability to control physical activity.
- Stabilize and improve patient's physical condition.
- Try to establish diagnosis for proper treatment of condition.
- Initiate chelation therapy if heavy metal toxicosis (see Heavy Metal Toxicity) is a differential diagnosis; before treatment, collect samples for diagnostic testing (if patient stable enough); if not stable enough, initiate treatment anyway.
- Provide supportive therapy.
- Remove heavy metal foreign body to reduce exposure.

ACUTE GENERAL TREATMENT

- All treatment is to be performed on a stable patient.
  - Nursing care
    - Administer warmed crystalloid fluids SC, IV, IO (50-150 mL/kg/d maintenance plus dehydration deficit factored in if needed) at a rate of 10-25 mL/kg over a 5-minute period or at a continuous rate of 100 mL/kg/q 24 h.
    - Increase environmental temperature to 85°F-90°F (29°C-32°C).
    - Provide a humidified environment by placing warm moist towels in the incubator.
    - Nutritional support is required in most cases.
- Surgical considerations: the patient should be stabilized and on chelation therapy before any surgery procedure is attempted. Removal of heavy metal objects from the gastrointestinal tract or affected joints should be attempted on the stable patient. Surgical procedures to remove objects from the gastrointestinal tract include the following:
  - Use of a small, very strong magnet, glued to the tip of an enteral feeding tube to remove zinc-coated ferrous items
  - Endoscopic removal of heavy metal particles or gastric lavage can be attempted in stable patients that are of sufficient size.
  - Occasionally, proventriculotomy or enterotomy procedures may be necessary if other attempts to remove the metal particles fail.
- Medications
  - Drugs of choice
    - Clonazepam 0.5 mg/kg PO q 12 h: seizure activity
    - Levetiracetam 100 mg/kg PO q 8 h: seizure activity
    - Zonisamide 20 mg/kg PO q 8 h: seizure activity
    - Gabapentin 20 mg/kg PO q 12 h: seizure activity
    - Phenobarbital sodium—therapeutic levels may not be achieved in African grey parrots through oral administration.

      Normal zinc blood levels in parrots is <2.5 ppm. 2.6-3.4 is reported as above normal levels and 3.5-4.4 is high. Any zinc blood levels above 4.5 ppm is considered toxic. Normal zinc levels for waterfowl and poultry are slightly higher than those used for parrots.
      - 1-5 mg/kg IV bolus: status epilepticus; begin at low end of dosage range and increase for refractory seizure activity
      - 2-7 mg/kg PO q 12 h: seizure activity
      - 50-80 mg/L drinking water: seizure activity
    - Diazepam 0.5 mg/kg IV for controlling seizures. Repeat if necessary. Higher doses may be needed IM.
    - Calcium disodiumversenate (CaEDTA) 35 mg/kg IM or SC q 12 h for 5 days, then off for 3 days, then repeated as needed; chelation
    - Bulk diets and cathartics (e.g., Psyllium [Metamucil, 0.5 tsp/60 ml water or hand feeding formula], mineral oil [5-10 ml/kg] via gavage, peanut butter [peanut butter and mineral oil 2:1 via gavage]) to evacuate particles from the gastrointestinal tract
    - Grit (e.g., ground oyster shell) may be effective in expediting the passage of metallic foreign bodies from the gastrointestinal tracts of birds.
    - Antibiotics may be indicated for bacterial infection
      - Chloramphenicol succinate 50 mg/kg IM, IV q 6-12 h crosses the blood-brain barrier.
      - Enrofloxacin 15 mg/kg PO, SC q 12 h
    - Atropine sulfate 0.01-0.02 mg/kg SC, IM: organophosphate toxicity
    - Dexamethasone sodium phosphate 2-6 mg/kg SC, IM, IV q 6-24 h: higher doses for head trauma, shock
    - Prednisolone 0.5-1.0 mg/kg IM, IV once: shock, trauma
    - Prednisolone sodium succinate
      - 10-20 mg/kg IM, IV q 15 min prn: head trauma
    - Vitamin B_1 complex (dose based on thiamine) 1-3 mg/kg IM q 7 d
    - Vitamin E 0.06 mg/kg IM q 7 d
    - Calcium gluconate 10% 50-100 mg/kg IM once: (slow bolus) hypocalcemia: (dilute 50 mg/mL)
    - Calcium lactate/calcium glycerophosphate 5-10 mg/kg IM q 7 d prn
    - Dextrose 50% 50-100 mg/kg IV slow bolus: hypoglycemia
  - Alternative drugs
    - D-Penicillamine 30-55 mg/kg PO q 12 h for 7-14 days. Highly unpalatable when compounded and administered PO, may elicit a severe adverse reaction from patient: chelation
    - Dimercaptosuccinic acid (DMSA) 25-35 mg/kg PO q 12 h × 5-7 day/wk × 3-5 wk: preferred oral chelation drug

CHRONIC TREATMENT

- Potassium bromide 25 mg/kg PO q 24 h: long-term seizure activity management; may not be effective in treating African grey parrots that present with seizure activity
- CaEDTA for increased blood lead levels that may occur because of adsorption of lead impregnated bone

DRUG INTERACTIONS

Depletion of zinc, iron, and manganese with long-term chelation therapy

POSSIBLE COMPLICATIONS

- D-Penicillamine: do not give if lead is present in the gastrointestinal tract (increases absorption of heavy metal particles)

- D-Penicillamine: extremely unpalatable even when mixed with liquid corn syrup; birds may have severe reaction (e.g., retching, convulsions) when this drug is given orally
- Cathartics may cause diarrhea and are contraindicated in dehydrated and hypovolemic birds.

RECOMMENDED MONITORING

- Monitor treatment of seizure activity and ability of patient to normally function.
- Repeat CBC and plasma chemistry panel to monitor treatment response and recovery.
- Monitor appetite, fecal output, and behavior during treatment period.

PROGNOSIS AND OUTCOME

- Cases that have a treatable disease causing neurologic signs have a good prognosis if the disease process has not caused permanent skeletal or organ damage (e.g., infectious, foreign body that can be removed, nutritional).
- Most neurologic cases have a guarded prognosis for recovery at best.

PEARLS & CONSIDERATIONS

COMMENTS

- Neurologic conditions are often difficult to diagnose.
- If specific treatment can be implemented to treat a diagnosed neurologic disease, the chance for recovery is greatly improved.
- Appropriate nutritional offerings for avian species will prevent many neurologic conditions associated with dietary deficiencies.
- Removal of heavy metal foreign objects in the gastrointestinal system is often required for faster resolution of neurologic signs associated with toxicity.
- Neurologic signs in budgerigars are often associated with pituitary tumors.

PREVENTION

- Provide proper nutrition.
- Prevent trauma.
- Become knowledgeable about sources of heavy metals, and remove from the patient's environment.

CLIENT EDUCATION

- Owners should be aware that African grey parrots are susceptible to hypocalcemic syndrome.
- See Prevention.

SUGGESTED READINGS

Beaufrere H, Pariaut R, Nevarez J, et al: Diagnosis of presumed ischemic stroke and associated seizure management in a Congo African grey parrot, JAVMA 236(5):540–547, 2010.

Bennett RA: Neurology. In Ritchie BW, et al, editors: Avian medicine: principles and applications, Brentwood, TN, 1994, HBD International Inc., pp 723–747.

Pollock CG, et al: Birds. In Carpenter JW, editor: Exotic animal formulary, ed 3, St Louis, 2005, Elsevier/Saunders, pp 135–264.

Tully TN: Neurology and ophthalmology. In Harcourt-Brown N, et al, editors: BSAVA manual of psittacine birds, ed 2, Quedgeley, Gloucester, 2005, British Small Animal Veterinary Association Woodrow House, pp 234–244.

CROSS-REFERENCES TO OTHER SECTIONS

Chlamydophila psittaci
Heavy Metal Toxicity
Hypocalcemia
Hypovitaminosis
Mycoses
Ocular Lesions
Organophosphate Toxicity
Trauma
Viral Diseases

AUTHOR & EDITOR: **THOMAS N. TULLY, JR.**

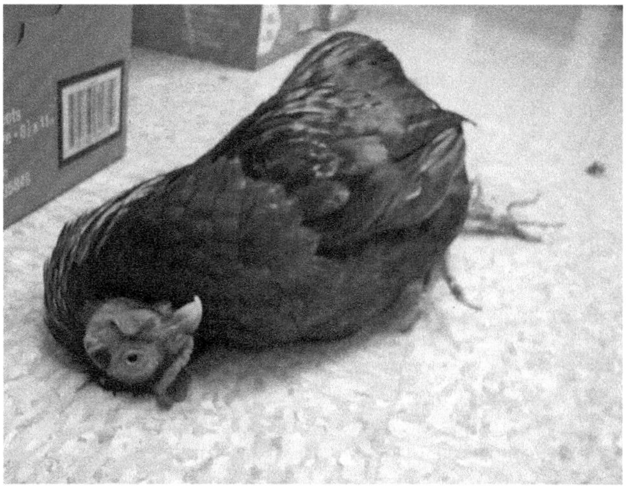

Central Nervous System Signs and Neurologic Conditions Severe CNS signs in this chicken; supportive care and focus on quality of life are the most important aspects in managing these cases. *(Photo courtesy Jörg Mayer, The University of Georgia, Athens.)*

BIRDS

Chlamydophila psittaci

Client Education Sheet Available on Website

BASIC INFORMATION

DEFINITION

Chlamydophila psittaci is an obligate, intracellular, Gram-negative bacterium. Three morphologically distinct forms of the *C. psittaci* organism have been identified: (1) elementary body (infectious form), (2) reticulate body (intracellular metabolically active form), and (3) intermediate form (intermediate form between elementary and reticulate morphs).

SYNONYMS

- Avian chlamydiosis (term used to describe avian illness)
- Psittacosis (term used to describe human illness)
- Ornithosis
- Parrot fever

EPIDEMIOLOGY

SPECIES, AGE, SEX

- All species and ages and both sexes may be infected.
- Older, younger, and immune suppressed individuals will be more susceptible to infection and clinical illness.

GENETICS AND BREED PREDISPOSITION None specific, but in the pet bird population, cockatiels are commonly diagnosed with the disease

RISK FACTORS

- Stress
- Adverse environmental conditions
- Inappropriate husbandry

- High reproductive activity
- Exposure to other birds
- Younger and older birds
- Immune suppressed individuals

CONTAGION AND ZOONOSIS *Chlamydophila psittaci* is arguably the most common zoonotic pathogen associated with pet bird ownership. If improperly diagnosed, a *C. psittaci* infection may be fatal to a human patient. All clients must be informed of the zoonotic potential of *C. psittaci*. *C. psittaci* infection in humans is commonly known as psittacosis (preferred term), *parrot fever*, or *ornithosis*. Similarly to avian infections, human infections induce a wide range of clinical signs that vary from inapparent illness to mild influenza-like symptoms to fulminant pneumonia. Gastrointestinal, hepatic, cardiac, and neurologic conditions have also been described in humans infected with *C. psittaci*. Most humans are infected via inhalation of aerosolized organisms.

ASSOCIATED CONDITIONS AND DISORDERS

- Anorexia
- Depression
- Dyspnea
- Hepatomegaly
- Weakness
- Splenomegaly
- Biliverdinuria
- Conjunctivitis (see Conjunctivitis)
- Diarrhea
- Nasal discharge

CLINICAL PRESENTATION

DISEASE FORMS/SUBTYPES

- Subclinical carrier: the bird is infected but shows no overt signs of clinical illness. Diagnostic testing of the bird may yield negative results owing to the very low levels of organisms in the patient's body and the effective immune status of the bird.
- Clinical disease: the bird is observed with nonspecific disease signs. Diagnostic testing for *C. psittaci* for patients exhibiting clinical disease is often confirmatory.
- Chronic disease: this very rare presentation is often associated with patients presenting with neurologic signs (e.g., ataxia)

HISTORY, CHIEF COMPLAINT

- Nonspecific
- Depression
- Inappetence
- Sneezing
- Dyspnea
- "Greenish" diarrhea
- "Fluffed" feathers

PHYSICAL EXAM FINDINGS

- Depressed patient
- Conjunctivitis
- Inflammation of the choanal slit
- Ocular/nasal discharge
- Dyspnea

ETIOLOGY AND PATHOPHYSIOLOGY

- *Chlamydophila psittaci* is excreted via nasal discharge and feces and usually is spread by inhalation of infected aerosols. Fecal-oral transmission has been documented as well. Although the average amount of time between exposure to *C. psittaci* and onset of clinical disease varies from 3 days to several weeks, a subclinical carrier state has been described. Infected but subclinical birds may be infected by the organism intermittently for extended periods of time. Shedding is usually associated with a stressful event (e.g., relocation, crowding, poor husbandry).
- Birds are primarily infected via aerosolization of the infectious form of the organism (elementary body). The warm moist upper respiratory tract is the principal site of replication. Respiratory epithelial cells become infected in this manner. Subsequently, epithelial cells of the lower respiratory tract become infected, along with macrophages throughout the respiratory system, with ensuing replication. At this time, the *C. psittaci* organism can usually be detected in plasma, monocytes, epithelial cells, and macrophages in various tissues throughout the body.

DIAGNOSIS

DIFFERENTIAL DIAGNOSIS

- Mycoplasmosis
- Bacterial and/or fungal respiratory disease
- Colibacillosis
- Pasteurellosis
- Avian influenza

INITIAL DATABASE

- Complete blood count (CBC): a significant heterophilic leukocytosis (30,000-80,000 cells/μL) is often observed with avian *C. psittaci* infection. Heterophils are usually quite reactive in appearance. Concurrent monocytosis is a common finding.
- Plasma biochemistry panel: evaluation of the plasma biochemistry analysis typically reveals an elevation in creatine kinase (CK) and aspartate aminotransferase (AST), especially if the liver is involved
- Imaging: an enlarged liver and/or spleen may be detected on radiographs

ADVANCED OR CONFIRMATORY TESTING

- Specific testing
  - Isolation: choanal and cloacal swabs are used to isolate and culture the *C. psittaci* organism. The organism is shed in the greatest numbers during early stages of the disease process.
  - Serology and other testing methods: a fourfold increase in antibody titers on paired sera samples (separated by 10-14 days) is generally required to definitively diagnose avian chlamydiosis. Direct immunofluorescence, DNA PCR, ELISA, elementary body agglutination, indirect fluorescent antibody test, complement fixation, and immunochromatography are also viable options for detection of the *C. psittaci* antigen or DNA. It is not recommended to use serology alone to diagnose avian chlamydiosis owing to shortcomings in both sensitivity and specificity.
  - Direct visualization by staining: the *C. psittaci* organism can be visualized in smears and paraffin-embedded tissue sections via Gimenez, modified Gimenez, and Giemsa staining techniques. Immunohistologic staining is another method used for detection of avian chlamydiosis.
- Gross necropsy/histopathologic examination: necropsies performed on infected birds often reveal hepatosplenomegaly. Less frequently, the heart may be enlarged and covered with thick fibrin plaques or encrusted with a yellow, flaky exudate. The air sacs may be covered with a fibrin exudate. Virulent strains frequently induce lung congestion and production of fibrinous exudate in the pleural cavity. The fibrinous exudate likely reflects vascular damage and the severe inflammatory response caused by continued multiplication of *C. psittaci* organisms. Histopathologic examination frequently detects fibrinous air sacculitis, pericarditis, and peritonitis. Hepatitis may also be noted.

TREATMENT

THERAPEUTIC GOALS

- Educate and inform owner.
- Stabilize patient.
- Treat patient and assess possible contact with other birds and people.
- With proper treatment, the patient should overcome infection.

ACUTE GENERAL TREATMENT

- Nursing care to stabilize patient
  - Administer warmed crystalloid fluids SC, IV, IO (50-150 mL/kg/d maintenance plus dehydration deficit factored in if needed) at a rate of 10-25 mL/kg over a 5-minute period or at a continuous rate of 100 mL/kg/q 24 h.

- Increase environmental temperature to 85°F-90°F (29°C-32°C).
- Provide a humidified environment by placing warm moist towels in the incubator.
- Nutritional support is required in most cases.

- Medication
  - Doxycycline
    - Medicated feed for budgerigars and cockatiels
      - Mix 1 part cracked steel oats and 3 parts hulled millet (measured by volume). Add 5 to 6 mL of sunflower oil/kg of the oat-seed mixture, and mix thoroughly to coat all seeds. Add 300 mg of doxycycline hyclate (from capsules)/kg of the oat-seed mixture and mix to evenly coat seed. Mix fresh daily. Feed as sole diet for 30 days.
    - Medicated water
      - Studies indicate that 200-400 mg of doxycycline hyclate/L drinking water (cockatiels), 400-600 mg/L for Goffin's cockatoos, and 800 mg/L for African grey parrots will maintain therapeutic concentrations. Empirical use of 400 mg/L drinking water appears to work for other psittacine species. Mix fresh daily.
    - Oral administration
      - 25-50 mg/kg PO q 12-24 h
    - Injectable
      - Vibravenös: 25-50 mg/kg IM q 5-7 d × 5-7 treatments
      - Doxycycline hyclate: 25-50 mg/kg slow bolus IV q 24 h × 3d
  - Oxytetracycline
    - LA 200: 50 mg/kg IM q 24 h × 5-7 d
  - Azithromycin
    - Zithromax: 50 mg/kg PO q 24 h × 30 d

CHRONIC TREATMENT

Prevent reexposure.

DRUG INTERACTIONS

Doxycycline: oral administration will chelate calcium

POSSIBLE COMPLICATIONS

- Do not use azithromycin if severe hepatic or renal disease.
- Muscle injection sites may become painful and damaged when long-acting doxycycline and oxytetracycline are used.
- Bone malformation due to calcium binding of doxycycline when used in young birds

RECOMMENDED MONITORING

Monitor treatment response through clinical reaction of patient and serial CBCs throughout long term treatment period.

PROGNOSIS AND OUTCOME

- When presented early in the disease process and treated properly, the prognosis is good.
- The prognosis degrades as the number of complications increases, and if the patient's condition is poor upon presentation.

PEARLS & CONSIDERATIONS

COMMENTS

- Owners should be aware of the zoonotic potential of avian chlamydiosis.
- Owners should know the signs of a sick bird and symptoms associated with psittacosis.
- Treatment compliance is essential when avian chlamydiosis cases are treated.

PREVENTION

- Restrict access to birds with unknown health history.
- Purchase birds from reputable aviaries.
- Quarantine for 30 days new birds and birds that have been to bird shows and fairs.

CLIENT EDUCATION

- All bird owners should be familiar with bird and human diseases caused by the *C. psittaci* organism.
- Bird owners who are suffering from flulike symptoms should always inform their physician that they own birds.

SUGGESTED READINGS

Compendium of measures to control *Chlamydophila psittaci* infection among humans (psittacosis) and pet birds (avian chlamydiosis), 2008. www.nasphv.org and www.avma.org.

Fudge AM: Avian chlamydiosis. In Rosskopf WJ, Jr, et al, editors: Diseases of cage and aviary birds, Baltimore, 1996, Williams & Wilkins, pp 572–585.

CROSS-REFERENCES TO OTHER SECTIONS

Conjunctivitis

AUTHOR: **MEGAN KIRCHGESSNER**

EDITOR: **THOMAS N. TULLY, JR.**

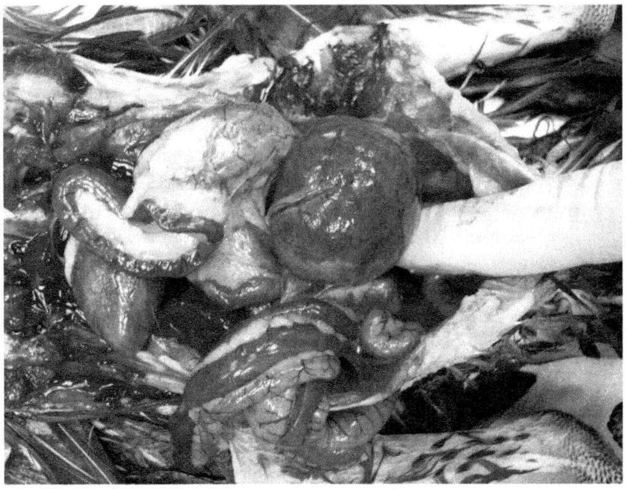

Chlamydophila psittaci Severe splenomegaly is commonly seen in cases infected with *Chlamydophila*. *(Photo courtesy Jörg Mayer, The University of Georgia, Athens.)*

BIRDS

Chronic Egg Laying

Client Education Sheet Available on Website

BASIC INFORMATION

DEFINITION

Chronic egg laying occurs when hens lay repeated clutches or produce larger than normal clutch sizes, regardless of the presence of a mate or appropriate breeding season. Chronic egg laying birds are often predisposed to the development or occurrence of egg binding, egg yolk coelomitis, salpingitis, metritis, nutritional depletion, and osteoporosis.

EPIDEMIOLOGY

SPECIES, AGE, SEX Reproductively active hens of all avian species may be affected, but commonly seen in gallinaceous species, waterfowl, finches, canaries, budgies, lovebirds, and cockatiels

RISK FACTORS Hens that are provided excellent nutritional diets and are comfortable with their surroundings

GEOGRAPHY AND SEASONALITY Canaries may have a winter predisposition to the condition because that is the time of year when they lay eggs. But depending on the light cycle where the cage is located, egg laying can occur at any time of year.

ASSOCIATED CONDITIONS AND DISORDERS Egg binding, egg yolk coelomitis, salpingitis, metritis, nutritional depletion, hypercholesterolemia leading to heart disease and possible cerebral infarcts, and osteoporosis

CLINICAL PRESENTATION

DISEASE FORMS/SUBTYPES Large numbers of infertile eggs laid or multiple clutches of eggs laid with or without a male present for fertilization

HISTORY, CHIEF COMPLAINT

- The history includes the production of a large number of eggs, with or without a pause between clutches.
- The presence of reproductively stimulating toys and objects in the bird's cage is frequently discovered, and a matelike relationship between the bird and a particular owner is often revealed.
- The history may include one or several episodes of egg binding.

PHYSICAL EXAM FINDINGS The bird may have poor body condition and, if actively laying an egg, it may be palpable in the caudal coelomic cavity.

ETIOLOGY AND PATHOPHYSIOLOGY

- This is a presentation of an overactive normally functioning reproduction cycle of the patient.
- Concern is focused on the predisposition of the patient to complicating illness and disease conditions, and on the immune compromised status of the animal, owing to high stress levels induced by the hyperactive reproductive cycle.

DIAGNOSIS

DIFFERENTIAL DIAGNOSIS

- Neoplasia
- Hormonal imbalance

INITIAL DATABASE

- Complete blood count: leukocytosis, heterophilia, and monocytosis due to chronic inflammation associated with the stresses of egg laying and possible secondary infection due to an immune compromised condition
- Plasma blood chemistry panel: may reveal hypercalcemia, hypercholesterolemia, and hyperglobulinemia, if the hen is ovulating. If the hen is calcium depleted secondary to the production of a large number of eggs, hypocalcemia may be observed.
- Radiographic images may reveal decreased bone density or polyostotic hyperostosis (increased density of the medullary cavities of the ulna and tibiotarsus) or an egg within the oviduct.

TREATMENT

THERAPEUTIC GOAL

Cessation of egg laying

ACUTE GENERAL TREATMENT

- Behavior modification: several behavioral and environmental modifications should be recommended before pharmacologic or surgical interventions are pursued
  - Decreasing the photoperiod to 8-10 hours of daylight per day and removing any reproductively stimulating toys from the cage may help to decrease the hen's drive to lay eggs.
  - Access to nesting environments and nesting material (e.g., boxes, dark spaces, shredded papers) should be restricted.
  - When eggs are laid by the hen, the owner may or may not want to remove the eggs from the cage. There does not seem to be any basis for leaving the eggs with or removing the eggs from the hen.
  - The hen should be deprived of any interaction with her perceived or actual mate, and any stimulatory petting of the pelvis, dorsum, or cloacal region should be avoided.
- Diet change: a diet change to a low-fat, reduced-caloric formulated feed appears to anecdotally reduce or stop chronic egg production.
- Therapeutic measures: little if any scientific foundation is known for the beneficial effects of the drugs listed in preventing avian species from laying eggs. Clinically, it does appear that leuprolide acetate has a positive effect in reducing egg laying in cockatiels. Scientific studies have shown that it has no effect on stopping pigeons from laying eggs. These drugs are not avian specific, and results vary between avian species and orders.
  - Leuprolide acetate: administer every 14 days; 3 doses are usually adequate
    - 700-800 μg/kg IM for birds weighing <300 g
    - 500 μg/kg IM for birds weighing >300 g
  - Tamoxifen: nonsteroidal antiinflammatory used to block estrogen; leukopenia most frequent side effect
    - 2 mg/kg PO q 24 h
  - Human chorionic gonadotropin: if second egg laid, repeat dose on day 3; if third egg laid, repeat dose on day 7. Not consistently effective and some birds refractory to treatment
    - 5000 IU/kg IM on days 1, 3, and 7 q 3-6 wk prn

CHRONIC TREATMENT

Surgery: salpingohysterectomy is the treatment of choice, but owners are often unwilling to subject their pet to surgical and anesthetic risks. Unfortunately, surgery is often pursued only when the condition becomes life threatening, at which point surgical and anesthetic risks dramatically increase. The ovary is not removed with this surgery, so the ovary may continue to ovulate, even though the oviduct has been removed, leading to internal ovulation of the follicle. In waterfowl, this is a common occurrence after removal of the oviduct.

POSSIBLE COMPLICATIONS

- Lack of response to treatment
- Internal ovulation with removal of the oviduct

RECOMMENDED MONITORING

- Continue to check for egg laying by the patient or reproductive behavior (e.g., clucking, nesting).
- If reproductive behavior is noticed before egg laying, retreatment with a therapeutic agent may be needed.

PROGNOSIS AND OUTCOME

Guarded for cessation of egg laying, except in cases where surgical removal of the oviduct has shown a successful response

PEARLS & CONSIDERATIONS

COMMENTS

- Behavior modification and diet may have a significant impact on cessation of egg laying in these patients.
- Therapeutic measures have yielded mixed results depending on the agent and the avian species being treated. Little scientific evidence supports the use of this therapy.
- Surgery to remove the oviduct is the only way to confidently stop chronic egg laying birds, but this is a risky surgical procedure and may lead to internal ovulation, especially in waterfowl species.

PREVENTION

Owners should be instructed to avoid petting the pelvis, dorsum, or cloacal region, and should be discouraged from kissing the bird's beak. This, in combination with the recommendation to have various people handle the bird, should prevent a matelike relationship from forming between the bird and any one particular member of the household. The cage and furniture should be cleaned and rotated periodically in an attempt to discourage territorial behavior.

CLIENT EDUCATION

See Comments and Prevention. Knowledge of this condition before purchase of a bird, in particular cockatiels and lovebirds, may contribute to the decision of a potential bird owner to purchase a male to circumvent this potential concern.

SUGGESTED READING

Bowles HL: Reproductive diseases of pet bird species, Vet Clin North Am Exotic Anim Pract 5:489–506, 2002.

AUTHOR: **MEGAN KIRCHGESSNER**

EDITOR: **THOMAS N. TULLY, JR.**

BIRDS

Cloacal Prolapse

BASIC INFORMATION

DEFINITION

A cloacal prolapse is a protrusion of cloacal mucosa through the cloacal sphincter. It may contain oviduct, ureter, phallus, intestines, or cloacal tissue or masses.

EPIDEMIOLOGY

SPECIES, AGE, SEX All avian species, ages, and sexes may be affected.

GENETICS AND BREED PREDISPOSITION High prevalence in cockatoos, cockatiels, and budgerigars

RISK FACTORS Chronic cloacal prolapse in cockatoos may be associated with sexual behavior or hormonal influence.

ASSOCIATED CONDITIONS AND DISORDERS

- Intestinal parasitism
- Enteritis
- Colitis
- Egg binding
- Constipation
- Foreign body
- Cloacitis
- Cloacal masses

CLINICAL PRESENTATION

DISEASE FORMS/SUBTYPES

- Prolapse of the cloacal tissue
- Prolapse of the cloacal tissue with intestines or oviduct that may include an egg

HISTORY, CHIEF COMPLAINT Intestine is coming out of the vent, or something is "sticking" out of the vent.

PHYSICAL EXAM FINDINGS

- Depression
- Reluctance to perch
- Fluffed feathers
- Protruding cloaca intestines or oviduct, which (with or without egg)

ETIOLOGY AND PATHOPHYSIOLOGY

Straining by the bird will cause a breakdown of the support structures of the cloacal and/or surrounding tissue, resulting in an external presentation of the internal mucosal surface of the caudal intestinal and/or urogenital structures. Sexual hormones in females might result in weakening of the supporting tissues.

DIAGNOSIS

DIFFERENTIAL DIAGNOSIS

- Intussusception: rule out by passing a probe between the mass and the vent (the probe should not penetrate more than 1-3 cm). If the probe passes 4-6 cm, suspect prolapsed intussusception.
- Oviductal prolapse: presence of an egg within the oviduct will confirm the diagnosis
- Papillomatosis: suspected papillomatous lesions may be identified with the aid of a 5% acetic acid solution (e.g., apple cider vinegar). When applied to papillomatous tissues, the surface will blanch to white from the normal pink color. Fine-needle aspiration and cytologic examination and/or biopsy with subsequent histopathologic examination may confirm the diagnosis.
- Phallus prolapse

INITIAL DATABASE

- Complete blood count: usually normal; inflammatory or stress leukogram may be present
- Intestinal parasite examination: fecal direct and flotation
- Fecal Gram stain
- Cloacal culture and sensitivity
- Plasma biochemistry panel: hypercalcemia, hypercholesterolemia in egg-laying birds

ADVANCED OR CONFIRMATORY TESTING

- Radiographic imaging: may demonstrate egg, foreign body
- Ultrasound: may demonstrate intussusception, egg, internal ovulation

- Cloacal endoscopy: may demonstrate cloacal mass, cloacitis

TREATMENT

THERAPEUTIC GOALS

- Prevent any permanent damage to prolapsed tissue.
- Replace prolapsed tissue.
- Have replaced tissue remain in place.
- Remove egg if oviduct is prolapsed.

ACUTE GENERAL TREATMENT

- Avoid further desiccation and contamination or trauma of the prolapsed tissue by flushing the prolapsed mucosa with warm saline; cover it with a sterile lubricating material.
- Administer a warmed crystalloid solution (e.g., Normosol) subcutaneously (100 mL/kg/d).
- Increase environmental temperature to 85°F-95°F (29°C-35°C).
- Nutritional support is required if the patient is not eating.
- After flushing the mucosa with warm saline, use a sterile swab to replace the tissues.
- Osmotic agents may help if severe swelling is present.

CHRONIC TREATMENT

- Two simple transverse stay sutures, one on each side and perpendicular to the vent, may be placed to physically prevent reprolapsing of the tissue.
- Cloacoplasty or cloacopexy may be necessary in recurrent cloacal prolapse.
- Papillomas may be surgically debulked.
- Clomipramine 1-3 mg/kg q 12 h for 6 weeks has been used successfully in cockatoos with idiopathic cloacal prolapse.
- Broad-spectrum antibiotics if suspected damage to the integrity of the mucosal surface of the prolapsed tissue
- Analgesic/antiinflammatory medication (meloxicam 0.5 mg/kg PO, IM q 12 h for psittacine and raptor species) if suspected pain and/or inflammation

POSSIBLE COMPLICATIONS

- Blockage of fecal material and subsequent toxicity due to an inability to void because of a constricted vent as a result of improper placement of stay sutures or purse-string suture
- Reprolapse after replacement of tissue
- Retention sutures are contraindicated when the prolapsed cloaca is caused by papillomas.

RECOMMENDED MONITORING

For at least a week after initial presentation, food intake, fecal output, and behavior should be monitored on a daily basis.

PROGNOSIS AND OUTCOME

- Good for simple prolapse where the cause has been identified and properly treated
- Guarded for undiagnosed prolapse
- Poor for prolapse associated with papillomatosis

PEARLS & CONSIDERATIONS

COMMENTS

- If at all possible, the underlying cause should be identified. If identified, the problem should be treated appropriately for best chance for resolution.
- Diagnosing the cause of cloacal prolapse can be very difficult. Knowledge of this difficulty by the owner is essential in reducing frustration and in maintaining confidence in the veterinarian's ability to treat the animal.
- Even if a diagnosis is made, resolution of the problem may not be achieved.

PREVENTION

- Address underlying cause.
- Leuprolide acetate 500-750 µg/kg IM q14 d to reduce short-term reproductive activity
- Deslorlin implant (4.7 mg) sc q 3-6 months
- Salpingohysterectomy is indicated if egg binding is associated with reproductive tract/oviductal pathology (e.g., neoplasia) or for definitive treatment to avoid reproductive activity.

CLIENT EDUCATION

Owners should be aware that some cases may be refractory to treatment.

SUGGESTED READINGS

Bennet RA, Harrison GJ: Soft tissue surgery. In Ritchie BW, et al, editors: Avian medicine: principles and applications, Brentwood, TN, 1994, HBD International Inc., pp 1125–1131.

Joyner KL: Theriogenology. In Ritchie BW, et al, editors: Avian medicine: principles and applications, Brentwood, TN, 1994, HBD International Inc., pp 748–804.

Zantop DW: Clomipramine hydrochloride for prolapsing cloaca, Exotic DVM 6:20, 2004.

AUTHOR: **DAVID SANCHEZ-MIGALLON GUZMAN**

EDITOR: **THOMAS N. TULLY, JR.**

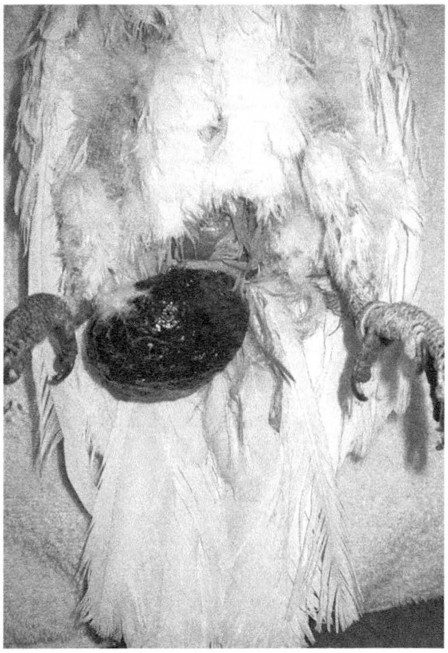

Cloacal prolapse Prolapsed oviduct in a cockatoo; often surgical intervention (spay, cloacopexy) is needed to improve the condition. *(Photo courtesy Jörg Mayer, The University of Georgia, Athens.)*

Conjunctivitis

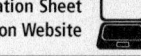

Client Education Sheet Available on Website

BASIC INFORMATION

DEFINITION

Irritation and inflammation of the conjunctiva

EPIDEMIOLOGY

SPECIES, AGE, SEX

- Finches are very susceptible to conjunctivitis caused by *Mycoplasma gallisepticum*. An epidemic occurred in the eastern house finch in 1994.
- A conjunctivitis for which no causative agent has been determined has been described in cockatiels, although *Chlamydophila psittaci* is commonly diagnosed in this species.
- Cryptosporidial conjunctivitis has been described in parakeets, ducks, and pheasants.

RISK FACTORS

- Cigarette smoke exposure
- Exposure to aerosolized toxins
- Exposure to chemical fumes
- High doses of UVB light exposure

CONTAGION AND ZOONOSIS

- *Chlamydophila psittaci* infection in poultry and pet birds has been linked to psittacosis in humans. This can result in clinical signs ranging from asymptomatic infection to influenza-like symptoms.
- Outbreaks have occurred among workers in turkey-processing plants.
- Mortalities have been reported among elderly and immune suppressed individuals.

GEOGRAPHY AND SEASONALITY

- May be noted in areas with low humidity and dusty environments
- May occur more often as the result of environmental exposure to dust in the hot dry months of the year

ASSOCIATED CONDITIONS AND DISORDERS

- Keratoconjunctivitis
- Blepharitis
- Infraorbital sinusitis
- Neoplasia
  - Lymphoma
  - Fibrosarcoma

CLINICAL PRESENTATION

DISEASE FORMS/SUBTYPES

- Localized irritation
- Orbital or periorbital disease
- Septicemia manifestation
- Conjunctival edema/hyperplasia

HISTORY, CHIEF COMPLAINT

- Reddened, inflamed conjunctiva
- Ocular discharge
- Ocular discomfort
- Conjunctival tissue extending beyond the lid margins

PHYSICAL EXAM FINDINGS

- Chemosis
- Hyperemia of the conjunctiva
- Blepharospasm
- Ocular discharge
  - Serous
  - Purulent
  - Mucopurulent
- Bird may exhibit concurrent respiratory symptoms, including nasal discharge or dyspnea.

ETIOLOGY AND PATHOPHYSIOLOGY

- Localized irritation
  - Trauma
  - Foreign body
  - Cigarette smoke exposure
  - Chemical fume exposure
  - Aerosolized toxins (Air freshener, cleaning solutions)
- Bacterial
  - *Chlamydophila psittaci* (see *Chlamydophila psittaci*)
  - *Mycoplasma* spp.
  - *Escherichia coli*
  - *Haemophilus* spp.
  - *Salmonella* spp.
  - *Mycobacterium avium*
  - *Actinobacillus suis*
- Parasitic
  - Protozoan
    - Cryptosporidiosis
    - *Encephalitozoon hellem*
  - Nematodes
    - *Oxyspirura mansoni*
    - *Thelazia* spp.
  - Trematodes
    - *Philophthalmus* spp.
- Viral
  - Herpesvirus
  - Avian influenza virus
  - Paramyxovirus 3
  - Reovirus
  - Goose parvovirus
  - Adenovirus: quail bronchitis
- Idiopathic
  - Cockatiel conjunctivitis

DIAGNOSIS

DIFFERENTIAL DIAGNOSIS

- Conjunctivitis as a primary cause must be distinguished from any lacrimal, orbital, eyelid, or systemic illness causing secondary conjunctivitis.
- Respiratory disease often accompanies conjunctivitis in birds.

INITIAL DATABASE

- Ophthalmic examination
- Schirmer tear test
- Fluorescein stain
- Tonometry
- Conjunctival culture and sensitivity
- Conjunctival cytologic examination
- Complete blood count
- Fecal examination

ADVANCED OR CONFIRMATORY TESTING

- Conjunctival biopsy
- Testing using PCR technology
- Serology

TREATMENT

THERAPEUTIC GOALS

- Remove inciting cause.
- Prevent secondary infection.
- Reduce inflammation.
- Remove exudates.
- Maintain surface moisture.

ACUTE GENERAL TREATMENT

- Remove foreign body if present.
- Broad-spectrum topical antibiotic therapy is indicated. Topical triple antibiotics, gentamicin, and ciprofloxacin are often used while definitive diagnosis and/or sensitivity panel is pending.
- Doxycycline (Vibravenös, not currently available in the United States) 50-100 mg/kg IM q7 d is suggested while definitive diagnosis is pending, to treat for possible *C. psittaci* and *Mycoplasma* spp. infections.
- Flurbiprofen ophthalmic drops to reduce pain and inflammation
- Artificial tears may be used to cleanse and maintain moisture of the eye.

CHRONIC TREATMENT

- Eliminate factors causing irritation to the bird's environment.
- *C. psittaci*
  - Doxycycline
    - Vibramycin 25 mg/kg PO q 12 h for 45 days
    - Vibravenös 50-100 mg/kg IM q 7 d for 6 injections
  - Oxytetracycline (LA-200 50 mg/kg IM q 24 h × 5-7 days) if doxycycline is unavailable
- *Mycoplasma* spp.
  - Doxycycline (Vibramycin 25 mg/kg PO q 12 h for 21 days)
  - Tylosin (Tylan 20-40 mg/kg IM q 8 h or 50 mg/L drinking water)

- Erythromycin (Erymycin 100 10-20 mg/kg PO q 12 h or 1500 mg/L drinking water)
- Nematodes
  - Fenbendazole (Panacur 15 mg/kg PO q 24 h for 5 days)
  - Ivermectin (Ivomec 0.2 mg/kg PO, SC, IM once)
- Trematodes
  - Praziquantel (Droncit 5-10 mg/kg PO, repeat after 2-4 weeks)
  - Flukes may be manually removed with forceps and flushing.
  - Addition of saltwater bowls for dabbling ducks may reduce parasite numbers.

DRUG INTERACTIONS

- Doxycycline is a calcium chelator; therefore caution must be used when administered orally to younger birds or birds on long-term treatment.
- Fenbendazole has been reported to cause immune suppression and septicemia in some birds.

POSSIBLE COMPLICATIONS

- Keratoconjunctivitis
- Underrunning of the conjunctiva
- Permanent opacity
- Rupture of the globe

RECOMMENDED MONITORING

- A thorough weekly ophthalmic exam is recommended while the conjunctivitis is being treated.
- It is important to monitor bird for signs of respiratory disease.

PROGNOSIS AND OUTCOME

Prognosis is good if a definitive diagnosis is obtained and the problem is correctly treated.

PEARLS & CONSIDERATIONS

COMMENTS

A thorough history is important, to determine whether the bird has been in the presence of irritating substances such as cigarette smoke or aerosolized air fresheners.

PREVENTION

- Elimination of risk factors
- Provide a clean, stress-free environment with minimal crowding.
- Maintenance of a clean dust-free environment

CLIENT EDUCATION

Cigarette smoke and harsh cleaners such as ammonia and bleach can be very irritating to a bird and can cause respiratory distress and signs of conjunctivitis.

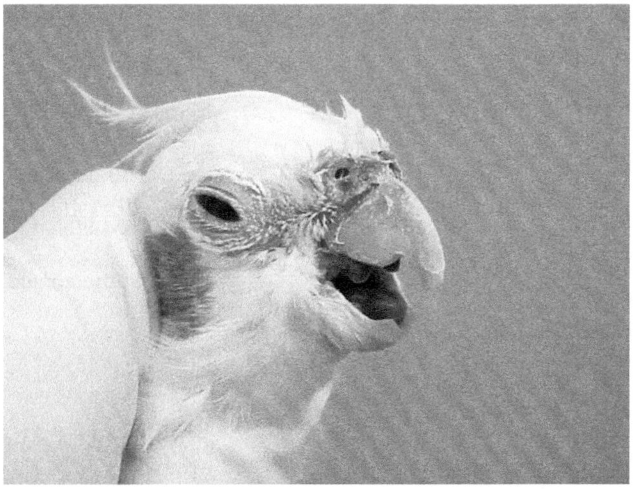

Conjunctivitis Conjunctival hyperemia and chemosis in a cockatiel *(Nymphicus hollandicus)* affected with conjunctivitis due to *Chalmydophila psittaci* infection. *(Photo courtesy Thomas N. Tully, Jr.)*

SUGGESTED READINGS

Dhondt KV, et al: Effects of route of inoculation on *Mycoplasma gallisepticum* infection in captive house finches, Avian Pathol 36:475–479, 2007.

Eidson M: Psittacosis/avian chlamydiosis, J Am Vet Med Assoc 221:12–13, 2002.

Farmer KL, et al: Susceptibility of a naive population of house finches to *Mycoplasma gallisepticum*, J Wildl Dis 38:282–286, 2002.

Gerlach H: Mollicutes (mycoplasma, acholeplasma, ureaplasma). In Harrison GJ, et al, editors: Clinical avian medicine and surgery, Philadelphia, 1986, Saunders, pp 454–456.

Jones A, et al: Diagnostic challenge, J Exotic Pet Med 16:122–125, 2007.

Kollias GV, et al: Experimental infection of house finches with *Mycoplasma gallisepticum*, J Wildl Dis 40:79–86, 2004.

Paulman A, et al: Outbreak of herpesviral conjunctivitis and respiratory disease in gouldian finches, Vet Pathol 43:963–970, 2006.

Phalen DN, et al: *Encephalitozoon hellem* infection as the cause of a unilateral chronic keratoconjunctivitis in an umbrella cockatoo *(Cacatua alba)*, Vet Ophthalmol 9:59–63, 2006.

Sareyyupoglu B, et al: *Chlamydophila psittaci* DNA detection in the faeces of cage birds, Zoonoses Public Health 54:6–7, 2007.

Tsai S, et al: Eye lesions in pet birds, Avian Pathol 22:95–112, 1993.

CROSS-REFERENCES TO OTHER SECTIONS

Chlamydophila psittaci
Sinusitis, Chronic

AUTHOR: **SHANNON N. SHAW**

EDITOR: **THOMAS N. TULLY, JR.**

BIRDS

Constipation (Ileus)

BASIC INFORMATION

DEFINITION

Constipation may be defined as infrequent or difficult evacuation of feces, usually characterized by the presence of hard dry fecal material.

SYNONYMS

Ileus, obstipation

EPIDEMIOLOGY

SPECIES, AGE, SEX All species and ages and both sexes of birds may be affected.

GENETICS AND BREED PREDISPOSITION
- Macaws, cockatoos, and conures are species commonly diagnosed with proventricular dilatation disease.
- Ostriches may present with impaction that leads to ileus.

RISK FACTORS
- Dehydration
- Dysbiosis
- Inappropriate environmental conditions
- Gastrointestinal disease

ASSOCIATED CONDITIONS AND DISORDERS
- Anorexia
- Depression
- Toxemia
- Septicemia

CLINICAL PRESENTATION

DISEASE FORMS/SUBTYPES Lack of fecal material is noticed in the cage, with the bird straining to defecate.

HISTORY, CHIEF COMPLAINT
- Nonspecific
- Depression
- Inappetence
- Lack of stool in the cage
- Straining and tail wagging at the bottom of the cage

PHYSICAL EXAM FINDINGS
- Weight loss
- Caked dried fecal material around vent
- Dried fecal material in distal intestinal tract and cloaca
- Distention of the caudal coelom

ETIOLOGY AND PATHOPHYSIOLOGY

Inability of fecal material to be evacuated from the intestinal tract due to a physical obstruction or lack of proper intestinal function

DIAGNOSIS

DIFFERENTIAL DIAGNOSIS

- Physical obstruction
  - Foreign body
  - Heavy parasite infection leading to blockage of the intestinal tract
  - Intestinal torsions, adhesions, or strictures
  - Neoplasia
  - Egg binding
  - Papillomatosis lesions
- Decreased peristaltism
  - Proventricular dilatation disease (PDD)
  - Peritonitis
  - Heavy metal toxicity
  - Thrombosis of splanchnic vessels

INITIAL DATABASE

- Complete blood count: if the animal is dehydrated, a relative increase in packed cell volume (PCV) and total protein values may be noted. A condition of dysbiosis associated with ileus may cause proliferation of pathogenic bacteria, resulting in an inflammatory leukogram.
- Plasma biochemistry panel: electrolytes should be checked because metabolic disturbances may occur owing to the movement of fluids between vascular and intestinal lumens
- Radiographic images: plain radiographic images may reveal a foreign body or tissue mass causing an obstruction within or to the intestinal tract

ADVANCED OR CONFIRMATORY TESTING

- Contrast radiography: barium sulfate may be used, at a dose of 5 mL/kg body weight administered via crop tube, or contrast may be placed directly in the lumen of the proventriculus through a urinary catheter. The immediate presence of contrast in the proventriculus allows assessment of the size of the proventriculus and is very helpful in the diagnosis of PDD. If a decreased rate of passage is suspected, barium contrast mixed with liquid food may be fed to the bird, and a series of conscious radiographs can be taken, with the animal in a small box equipped with a perch; lateral beam exposures are used. Radiographs may help to rule out the presence of extraintestinal compression.
- Ultrasound: use of ultrasound diagnostic testing for an extensive and detailed exam of the gastrointestinal tract is very difficult owing to the presence of air sacs within the coelomic cavity
- Endoscopy: proventricular and ventricular exploration can be performed by rigid endoscopy when a foreign body is suspected. Cloacal endoscopy may reveal the presence of papillomas. An otoscope must be used before endoscopic examination of the cloaca to flush and eliminate impacted fecal material. An exploratory coelomic endoscopic examination may help identify extraintestinal causes of obstruction, adhesions, strictures, or torsions.
- Biopsy: tissue biopsy may be used to evaluate suspect masses or growths. Crop biopsy is a diagnostic technique that may be used for suspect PDD cases. A blood vessel section must be included within the crop biopsy sample to ensure collection of a nerve.

TREATMENT

THERAPEUTIC GOALS

- Have the avian patient return to normal gastrointestinal function.
- For birds diagnosed with PDD, improve gastrointestinal function and ensure a better quality of life.

ACUTE GENERAL TREATMENT

- Treatment options can be divided in the resolution of specific causes and in nonspecific treatment, applicable to any presentation of constipation.
- Constipated patients may become dehydrated quickly owing to movement of fluids from the vascular compartment toward the intestinal lumen; electrolyte imbalances need to be considered (based on laboratory data) when a crystalloid solution is selected. Fluid should be administered through the intravenous or intraosseous route.
- Antibiotic therapy should be initiated with ticarcillin/clavulanic acid 100 mg/kg IM q 12 h, in combination with metronidazole for anaerobic florae 10-50 mg/kg PO q 12 h. Use of sulfonamides is contraindicated until dehydration status has been resolved.
- Cathartics: mineral oil can be used in combination with creamy peanut butter in a 2:1 mixture and administered at 5-10 mL/kg body weight
- Nonsteroidal antiinflammatory drugs (NSAIDs) can be used for any constipation presentation, but this class of drugs is specifically indicated in cases of PDD. The effectiveness of NSAIDs in treating PDD has not been scientifically established, but anecdotal reports have described varying responses depending on the avian species treated.
  - Meloxicam 0.2 mg/kg PO q 24 h
  - Celecoxib 10 mg/kg PO q 12-24 h
- Surgery is indicated if foreign bodies need to be removed.
- Intestinal surgery is performed when torsion, adhesion, or external pressure causes external pressure, blocking gastrointestinal motility.
- Excision of cloacal papillomas is indicated when a tissue mass is blocking the vent, thereby preventing the bird from defecating.
- To treat lead toxicity, one of the following drugs may be used:
  - Calcium EDTA 30-35 mg/kg IM q 12 h × 3-5 days, off 3-4 days, repeat prn
  - Dimercaptosuccinic acid (DMSA) 25-35 mg/kg PO q 12 h × 5 day/wk × 3-5 weeks
  - Penicillamine 30 mg/kg PO q 12 h × 7 days minimum

CHRONIC TREATMENT

NSAIDs listed in the acute treatment section may be used as long-term treatment for PDD.

POSSIBLE COMPLICATIONS

- Long-term NSAID use may cause renal and/or intestinal pathology. If NSAIDs are used, regular monitoring of the patient's blood and plasma chemistry values is required.
- Penicillamine is an oral chelating agent that is extremely unpalatable. Birds may have a very severe convulsive reaction when penicillamine is orally administered.

RECOMMENDED MONITORING

- Fecal/urine output
- Hydration status
- Appetite
- Weight

PROGNOSIS AND OUTCOME

- Prognosis is dependent on the underlying cause of constipation and the condition of the bird when presented.
- Extremely poor prognosis for birds diagnosed with PDD

PEARLS & CONSIDERATIONS

COMMENTS

- Birds need critical care when first presented with constipation.
- Resolution of impacted fecal material and removal of the foreign body are important considerations in cases in which these problems have been identified.
- No curative measures are known for patients diagnosed with PDD. The cause of PDD has not been identified, although a viral agent is suspected. Crop biopsies are extremely nonproductive in definitively diagnosing PDD. Fluoroscopic examination is the best way to determine gastrointestinal motility and to diagnose PDD at this time.

PREVENTION

- Proper husbandry and nutrition and maintenance of hydration
- Reduced exposure to cage toys that may be chewed and ingested or to lead objects

CLIENT EDUCATION

- If the bird is not producing fecal material, have the animal examined by a veterinarian as soon as possible.
- Use newspaper as a cage substrate so fecal material can be evaluated on a daily basis.
- Know normal fecal output and appearance.

SUGGESTED READINGS

Gelis S: Gastroenterology. In Harrison GJ, et al, editors: Clinical avian medicine, vol I, Palm Beach, FL, 2006, Spix Publishing Inc., pp 411–441.

Lumeij JT: Gastroenterology. In Ritchie BW, et al, editors: Avian medicine: principles and application, Lake Worth, FL, 1994, Wingers Publishing, pp 482–521.

AUTHOR: **ALBERTO RODRIGUEZ BARBON**

EDITOR: **THOMAS N. TULLY, JR.**

BIRDS

Crop Stasis

BASIC INFORMATION

DEFINITION

The reduction or cessation of gastrointestinal content flow from the crop into the proventriculus

SYNONYMS

Gut stasis, crop impaction, sour crop

EPIDEMIOLOGY

SPECIES, AGE, SEX Birds of any breed, age, or sex may experience crop stasis. Crop stasis is often a sign of illness in neonatal and juvenile birds.

GENETICS AND BREED PREDISPOSITION Primary crop stasis has been described in racing pigeons in Europe.

RISK FACTORS

- Dehydration
- Foreign body
- Improper formula temperature when feeding young birds
- Burns
- Impaction
- Overstretching of the crop
- Crop infection: bacterial, fungal, or parasitic cause
- Infections causing ileus: *Eimeria* spp., polyomavirus, psittacine beak and feather disease virus (circovirus), septicemia, *Sarcocystis* spp., bacterial/mycotic infection resulting in ingluvitis
- Hypothermia
- Toxicity: lead
- Proventricular dilation disease (Bornavirus or other etiology)

CONTAGION AND ZOONOSIS

- Although crop stasis itself is not contagious or zoonotic, infectious agents such as Gram-negative bacteria, *Chlamydophila psittaci*, yeast, and *Eimeria* spp. have been known to result in crop stasis.
- Some Gram-negative bacteria such as *Escherichia coli* and *Salmonella* spp. are infectious to humans through fecal-oral contact.

GEOGRAPHY AND SEASONALITY Crop stasis can be associated with dehydration so may be more common during seasons or locations of increased temperatures.

ASSOCIATED CONDITIONS AND DISORDERS See Risk Factors.

CLINICAL PRESENTATION

DISEASE FORMS/SUBTYPES

- Primary dysfunction of the crop
- Secondary dysfunction of the crop due to dysfunction of the distal gastrointestinal tract
- Gut stasis: stasis of the entire gastrointestinal tract

HISTORY, CHIEF COMPLAINT

- Full crop for prolonged length of time
- Regurgitation
- May have history of force-feeding, burns, or foreign body ingestion
- With coccidial infection, may have a history of diarrhea

PHYSICAL EXAM FINDINGS

- Full crop with palpable contents
- May have low body temperature
- With psittacine beak and feather disease: may see green or mucoid diarrhea, feather abnormalities, soft or elongated beak, or hyperkeratosis of the skin
- With polyomavirus: may see ascites, erythematous skin, subcutaneous hemorrhages, diarrhea, or delayed feathering
- May have "sour" smell to breath, caused by yeast overgrowth or fermenting of formula in the crop

ETIOLOGY AND PATHOPHYSIOLOGY

- Dependent on primary cause: see Risk Factors

- Cause of primary neuropathic crop stasis is unknown.
- With lead toxicity: studies have suggested that crop dysfunction is induced by the action of lead acting directly on smooth muscle or on neural elements in crop tissue

DIAGNOSIS

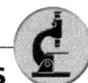

DIFFERENTIAL DIAGNOSIS

See Risk Factors.

INITIAL DATABASE

- Complete blood count
- Plasma chemistry panel
- Crop cytology
- Crop culture
- Cloacal culture
- Radiographs
- Contrast study with barium sulfate or iohexol

ADVANCED OR CONFIRMATORY TESTING

- Exploratory endoscopy procedure using a rigid or flexible endoscope
- Crop biopsy
- Ingluviotomy

TREATMENT

THERAPEUTIC GOALS

- Correct underlying cause.
- Remove fermented food material from crop via gavage tube. Flush crop with warm saline after food has been removed.
- Aid passage of easily digested food material and medication after old formula and food have been removed. Always initiate treatment with a small amount of nutritional supplementation.

ACUTE GENERAL TREATMENT

Instill a small amount of warm water into the crop with a red rubber feeding tube or a crop needle; massage gently, then remove food material.

CHRONIC TREATMENT

- Correct underlying cause.
- Treat for bacterial, fungal, or parasitic infection.
- Increase body temperature.
- Provide adequate hydration.

POSSIBLE COMPLICATIONS

- Aspiration of feed material into the trachea
- Overstretching of the crop may lead to recurrent stasis presentations.
- Hypoglycemia
- Dehydration
- Poor body condition and nutritional status if chronic

RECOMMENDED MONITORING

Palpation, ultrasound, and radiographs (plain and contrast films) may be used to assess the passage of crop contents.

PROGNOSIS AND OUTCOME

- Dependent on primary cause
- Primary crop stasis due to overstretching or neuropathy carries a poor prognosis.

PEARLS & CONSIDERATIONS

PREVENTION

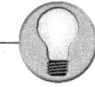

- Polyomavirus vaccination
- A crop bar made of a nonstick elastic material (e.g., Vet Wrap, 3M Inc., Minneapolis, MN); may help prevent overfilling of stretched crop tissue

CLIENT EDUCATION

- When crop feeding birds, make sure never to overfill crop, and feed formula at a proper temperature. Do not feed greater than 5% of body weight.
- Check temperature of formulas to avoid crop burns or to feed at a low temperature, predisposing the animal to bacterial and mycotic infections.
- Avoid housing birds around materials that may create foreign bodies.

SUGGESTED READINGS

Boyer I, et al: Lead induction of crop dysfunction in pigeons through a direct action on neural or smooth muscle components of crop tissue, J Pharm Exp Ther 234:607–615, 1985.
Flammer K, et al: Neonatology. In Ritchie BW, et al, editors: Avian medicine: principles and application, Lake Worth, FL, 1994, Wingers Publishing, pp 825–828.
Harper F, et al: Crop stasis and regurgitation in racing pigeons, Vet Rec 133:196, 1993.

AUTHOR: **SHANNON N. SHAW**

EDITOR: **THOMAS N. TULLY, JR.**

BIRDS

Dehydration

BASIC INFORMATION

DEFINITION

The physiologic state when the body loses more water than it takes in. A negative fluid balance is created; therefore, the circulating blood volume decreases, tissue fluids are reduced, and tissues become dehydrated.

EPIDEMIOLOGY

SPECIES, AGE, SEX All species, ages, and sexes can be affected.

RISK FACTORS

- Vomiting
- Burns
- Diarrhea
- Extensive skin wounds
- Anorexia
- Fever
- Renal failure
- Lack of water intake

GEOGRAPHY AND SEASONALITY Birds may be more susceptible to dehydration in hotter climates and seasons.

ASSOCIATED CONDITIONS AND DISORDERS See Risk Factors.

CLINICAL PRESENTATION

DISEASE FORMS/SUBTYPES

- Estimation of the degree of dehydration can be difficult but can be done using the following criteria:
  - 5%: most birds with a history of decreased food and water intake, prolonged skin tenting
  - 7%: basilic vein refill time greater than 1 to 2 seconds
  - 10%: sunken eyes, tacky mucous membranes (Cloaca)

HISTORY, CHIEF COMPLAINT

- Lethargy
- Depression
- Death
- May have history of anorexia, regurgitation, diarrhea, exposure to elevated temperature, or extensive skin wounds or burns

PHYSICAL EXAM FINDINGS

- Dry mucous membranes
- Prolonged skin tenting
- Sunken eyes
- Delayed refill time of basilic vein
- Delay in upper palpebral return to place when lifted

ETIOLOGY AND PATHOPHYSIOLOGY

Dehydration is caused by decreased water intake or increased water loss.

Decreased intake can occur from anorexia caused by illness or limited availability of water. Water loss can result from regurgitation, diarrhea, increased evaporation through tissue exposure due to burns or trauma, fever, direct sunlight exposure, and/or blood loss due to trauma or gastrointestinal parasites.

DIAGNOSIS

DIFFERENTIAL DIAGNOSIS

Dehydration may occur as a secondary consequence to many illnesses, therefore any generalized disease process should be considered as differential diagnoses.

INITIAL DATABASE

- Complete blood count: elevated packed cell volume and total solids support a diagnosis of dehydration
- Chemistry panel: uric acid and albumin will also be elevated with dehydration; electrolytes may show changes depending on cause of dehydration

ADVANCED OR CONFIRMATORY TESTING

- Additional testing to diagnose causes of dehydration can include the following:
  - Radiographs
  - Ultrasound
  - Fecal float
  - Gram staining
  - Crop culture
  - Bacterial or viral titers

TREATMENT

THERAPEUTIC GOAL

Replace fluid deficit to correct clinical signs and provide maintenance fluid requirements.

ACUTE GENERAL TREATMENT

- Calculate fluid deficit. This can be done by multiplying the bird's weight in kilograms by the % of estimated dehydration.
  - The fluid deficit can be replaced in 2 to 3 days. This should be added to the maintenance fluids.
  - The recommended maintenance rate for psittacines is 50-150 mL/kg/d depending on species of bird.
  - For most birds, the recommended daily maintenance fluid requirement is 100 mL/kg/d.
  - Baby birds have a maintenance rate 2 to 3 times higher.
- Fluids can be replaced through the intravenous, intraosseous, subcutaneous, or oral route.
  - An intravenous catheter provides the most reliable and fastest route for replacement fluid administration.
  - A common site for IV catheter placement is the jugular vein or the medial tarsal vein.
- Fluids should be warmed before replacement.
  - Fluid replacement may be performed with crystalloid products, but this treatment must be monitored closely in terms of patient response, and crystalloid products must be maintained because they rapidly leave the vasculature.
  - Colloidal products such as plasma and hetastarch can be used to maintain plasma oncotic pressure and to maintain circulatory volume.
  - The standard dose for hetastarch—10-15 mL/kg—can be given as an IV or IO bolus.
  - Crystalloid volume must be reduced by the volume of hetastarch used to avoid volume overload.

CHRONIC TREATMENT

- Subcutaneous and oral fluid therapy does not provide rapid replacement but can be used in stable patients. Common locations for subcutaneous administration include the axillary, inguinal, and subscapular areas.
- Oral administration of 5% dextrose is more effective than use of lactated Ringer's solution. Gatorade or Pedialyte can also be used. Oral fluids can be delivered with ball-tipped crop gavage needles or with red rubber tubes of appropriate size. Oral therapy is not recommended in birds that are having seizures, have gastrointestinal stasis, or are recumbent, all of which may predispose them to regurgitate.

DRUG INTERACTIONS

None described, but care must be observed to prevent overhydration and to provide appropriate fluid replacement therapy for the patient. This can be achieved by monitoring the electrolyte values of the patient and hydration status.

POSSIBLE COMPLICATIONS

- Severe dehydration can cause multiple-organ failure and death.
- Dehydration may exacerbate renal disease; thus dehydrated patients should be monitored closely with the use of electrolyte and plasma chemistry values.

RECOMMENDED MONITORING

- Birds receiving intensive fluid therapy should be monitored for signs of respiratory distress.
- Birds with cardiovascular disease should be treated with caution.
- Packed cell volume, total solids, and uric acid may be used to reassess hydration and kidney function during monitoring.

PROGNOSIS AND OUTCOME

- Dependent on severity of dehydration
- Renal involvement warrants a poorer prognosis.
- If the inciting factor can be removed and fluid volume restored, prognosis is good.

PEARLS & CONSIDERATIONS

PREVENTION

- Good health through proper diet and husbandry
- Disease prevention and access to clean water

CLIENT EDUCATION

Do not leave birds exposed to direct sunlight.

SUGGESTED READINGS

Lichtenberger M: Shock and cardiopulmonary-cerebral resuscitation in small mammals and birds, Vet Clin North Am Exot Anim Pract 10:275–291, 2007.

Pollock C: Diagnosis and treatment of avian renal disease, Vet Clin North Am Exot Anim Pract 9:107–128, 2006.

Tully T: Psittacine therapeutics, Vet Clin North Am Exot Anim Pract 3:59–90, 2000.

AUTHOR: **SHANNON N. SHAW**

EDITOR: **THOMAS N. TULLY, JR.**

Diarrhea

BASIC INFORMATION

DEFINITION

Abnormal frequency and liquidity of fecal discharge. Diarrhea may be defined as an undefined mass of fecal material and urine that is evacuated from the cloaca of a bird. Polyuria is defined as formed stool with a large quantity of urine surrounding the fecal material.

SYNONYM

Runny stool, pasty vent

EPIDEMIOLOGY

SPECIES, AGE, SEX All species and ages and both sexes

GENETICS AND BREED PREDISPOSITION No specific genetic/breed predisposition. Certain bird species (e.g., Lories) normally have a "loose" stool caused by dietary intake.

RISK FACTORS

- Hepatic disease: atoxoplasmosis
- Renal disease
- Pancreatic disease
- Bacterial infection: *Campylobacter* spp., *Chlamydophila psittaci, Escherichia coli, Pseudomonas* spp., *Aeromonas* spp., *Salmonella* spp., *Citrobacter* spp.
- Viral infection (see Viral Diseases): adenovirus, avian polyomavirus, herpesvirus, circovirus, proventricular dilatation disease (PDD) (see Proventricular Dilatation Disease), paramyxovirus
- Foods with elevated water content
- Ingested toxins: lead, zinc, pesticides
- Heavy metal toxicity
- Dietary changes
- Ingested foreign bodies (see Foreign Bodies)
- Intestinal parasitism: coccidiosis, *Cryptosporidia* spp., *Microsporidia* spp., *Giardia* spp., *Hexamita* spp.
- Stress and anorexia
- Septicemia
- Malabsorption syndrome

CONTAGION AND ZOONOSIS

- Diarrhea caused by the bacterial infection *C. psittaci* (see *Chlamydophila psittaci*); this organism is a zoonotic intracellular bacterium that can infect humans exposed to birds that are diagnosed with this disease.
- The intestinal parasite *Giardia* spp. may cause disease in humans. Although intermittently diagnosed in avian species, bird handlers should be aware of the possible zoonotic potential.

ASSOCIATED CONDITIONS AND DISORDERS

- Dehydration
- Anorexia
- Renal
- Cachexia
- Anemia
- Gastroenteritis
- Weakness

CLINICAL PRESENTATION

DISEASE FORMS/SUBTYPES

- Liquid (unformed) stool
- Discolored stool
- Whole seed/undigested food in stool

HISTORY, CHIEF COMPLAINT

- Abnormal (liquid/unformed) stool
- Abnormal consistency and coloration of stool
- Undigested food in stool
- Depression
- Anorexia
- Soiled vent feathers
- Polyuria/Polydipsia
- Vomiting

PHYSICAL EXAM FINDINGS

- Dehydration
- Cachexia
- Weakness
- Soiled vent feathers

ETIOLOGY AND PATHOPHYSIOLOGY

- Liquid unformed stool may be caused by physiologic abnormalities that include decreased intestinal transit time to malabsorption syndromes.
- Discolored stool that is liquid and unformed may be associated with gastrointestinal hemorrhage, bacterial and viral infections, dyes, and food items.
- Whole seed/undigested food in stool is usually an indication of abnormal digestive processes (e.g., pancreatitis, neoplasia, PDD) and/or hypermotility of the digestive tract (e.g., colibacillosis, salmonellosis, viral infection).

DIAGNOSIS

DIFFERENTIAL DIAGNOSIS

- Hepatic disease: atoxoplasmosis
- Renal disease
- Pancreatic disease
- Bacterial infection: *Campylobacter* spp., *C. psittaci, E. coli, Pseudomonas* spp., *Aeromonas* spp., *Salmonella* spp., *Citrobacter* spp.

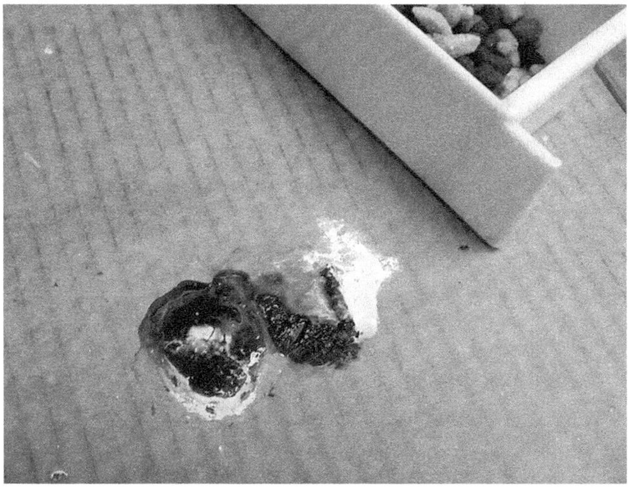

Diarrhea Diarrhea in birds is sometimes difficult to note. The feces are not formed and show a soft consistency; this is abnormal. *(Photo courtesy Thomas N. Tully, Jr.)*

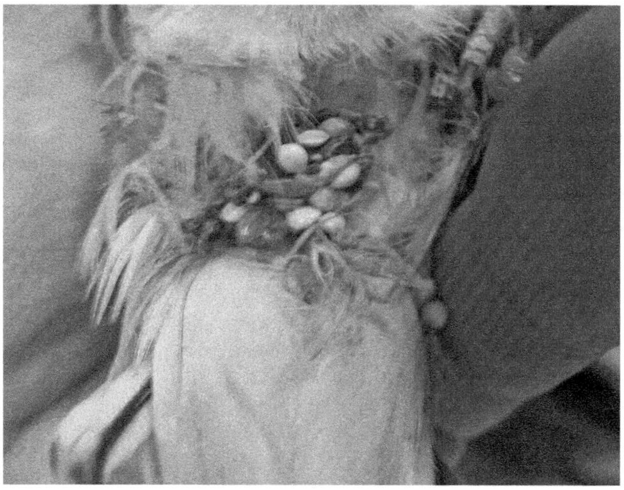

Diarrhea Soiled vent with seeds attached to moist diarrhea and matted feathers. *(Photo courtesy Thomas N. Tully, Jr.)*

- Viral infection: adenovirus, avian polyomavirus, herpesvirus, circovirus, PDD, paramyxovirus
- Foods with elevated water content
- Ingested toxins: lead, zinc, pesticides
- Heavy metal toxicity
- Dietary changes
- Ingested foreign bodies
- Intestinal parasitism: coccidiosis, *Cryptosporidia* spp., *Microsporidia* spp., *Giardia* spp., *Hexamita* spp.
- Stress and anorexia
- Septicemia
- Malabsorption syndrome

INITIAL DATABASE

- Cytologic examination of fecal, cloacal, crop, and/or proventricular lavage fluid. Retrieved fluid can be mixed with saline or counterstain to identify microorganisms.
- Gram stains of fecal, cloacal, crop, and/or proventricular swabs
- Fecal Gram stains: assessment of intestinal flora
- Direct fecal examination: protozoal parasite evaluation
- Fecal flotation: intestinal parasite examination
- Complete blood count (CBC): leukocytosis with concurrent heterophilia may be observed when gastroenteritis is present as a result of infectious processes involving bacterial organisms. Hypochromic regenerative anemia occurs in some cases of lead toxicity.
- Plasma biochemistry panel: amylase may be elevated in pancreatitis cases
- Culture and sensitivity of swab submitted from cloaca, crop, and/or proventriculus mucosa

ADVANCED OR CONFIRMATORY TESTING

- Imaging
  - Survey whole-body radiographs
  - Contrast studies to determine gastrointestinal motility
- Endoscopy
  - Upper gastrointestinal tract
  - Cloaca
  - Removal of foreign bodies
- Impression smears of abnormal masses
- Biopsy of abnormal tissue (e.g., renal, hepatic)
- Heavy metal–specific testing
  - Lead tissue concentrations in the liver, kidney, and brain of 3 to 6 ppm wet weight are suggestive of lead toxicosis; greater than 6 ppm is diagnostic. Blood levels for lead intoxication in birds, 0.25 ppm (significant when associated with clinical signs); >0.5 ppm is considered high.
  - Zinc concentrations in the pancreas of 26.11 µg/g on a dry weight basis were considered normal in cockatiels; concentrations of 312.4-2418 µg/g were considered toxic. In liver, subclinical birds are less than 40 ppm wet weight, and concentrations greater than 75 ppm were correlated with toxicosis. Normal zinc blood levels in parrots is <2.5 ppm. 2.6-3.4 is reported as above normal levels and 3.5-4.4 is high. Any zinc blood levels above 4.5 ppm is considered toxic. Normal zinc levels for waterfowl and poultry are slightly higher than those used for parrots.

TREATMENT

THERAPEUTIC GOALS

- Stabilize and improve patient's physical condition.
- Provide supportive therapy to control anorexia, dehydration, and gastroenteritis.
- Treat initiating cause of diarrhea and secondary disease processes that are diagnosed secondary to the primary cause.

ACUTE GENERAL TREATMENT

- All treatment is to be performed on a stable patient.
  - Nursing care
    - Administer warmed crystalloid fluids SC, IV, IO (50-150 mL/kg/d maintenance plus dehydration deficit factored in if needed) at a rate of 10-25 mL/kg over a 5-minute period or at a continuous rate of 100 mL/kg/q 24 h.
    - Increase environmental temperature to 85°F-90°F (29°C-32°C).
    - Provide a humidified environment by placing warm moist towels in the incubator.
    - Nutritional support is required in most cases.
- Surgical considerations: patient should be stabilized and on chelation therapy before any surgical procedure is attempted. Removal of heavy metal objects from the gastrointestinal tract of the stable patient should be attempted. Surgical procedures to remove objects from the gastrointestinal tract include the following:
  - Use of a small, very strong magnet, glued to the tip of an enteral feeding tube, to remove zinc-coated ferrous items
  - Endoscopic removal of foreign objects (e.g., string, cloth, leather, wood) or heavy metal particles or gastric lavage can be attempted in stable patients of sufficient size.
  - Occasionally, proventriculotomy or enterotomy procedures may be necessary if other attempts to remove foreign objects fail.
- Medications
  - Drugs of choice
    - Appropriate antimicrobial therapy based on culture and sensitivity and suitable diagnostic testing
    - Appropriate antiparasitic medication based on culture and sensitivity
    - Chelation therapy if needed (see Heavy Metal Toxicity)
  - Alternative drugs
    - Sucralfate 25 mg/kg PO q 8 h: esophageal, crop, and gastrointestinal protectant
    - Kaolin/pectin 2 mL/kg PO q 6-12 h: intestinal protectant, antidiarrheal
    - Bismuth subsalicylate 1-2 mL/kg PO q 12 h: intestinal protectant, antidiarrheal
    - Cimetidine 5 mg/kg PO, IM q 8-12 h: proventriculitis, gastric ulceration

CHRONIC TREATMENT

Celecoxib 10 mg/kg PO q 24 h × 6-24 weeks: PDD has been advocated as a treatment although clinical response of avian patients to this therapy has been universally disappointing.

POSSIBLE COMPLICATIONS

- D-Penicillamine: do not give if lead is present in the gastrointestinal tract (increases absorption of heavy metal particles)
- D-Penicillamine: extremely unpalatable even when mixed with liquid corn syrup. Birds may have severe reaction (e.g., retching, convulsions) when this drug is given orally.
- Cathartics may cause diarrhea and are contraindicated in birds that present with diarrhea, dehydration, and hypovolemia.

RECOMMENDED MONITORING

- Repeat CBC and plasma chemistry panel to monitor treatment response and recovery.
- Monitor hydration status on a daily basis.
- Monitor eating habits and stool volume, consistency, color, and odor as a response to treatment.
- If parasites and/or microorganisms are the primary cause of diarrhea, retest for treatment response and status of infection.
- Weight of patient should be assessed on a daily basis.

PROGNOSIS AND OUTCOME

- Acute cases that have a treatable cause have a good prognosis toward complete resolution.
- Chronic cases of diarrhea in which the patient is in poor physical condition

upon presentation have a more guarded prognosis.
- Disease processes that cause diarrhea that cannot be treated to resolution (e.g., circovirus, proventricular dilatation disease) have a grave prognosis over time. This is the case even though the disease condition may be stabilized for a period of time.

PEARLS & CONSIDERATIONS

COMMENTS

- A quick diagnosis of the primary cause of diarrhea in an avian patient often results in an effective treatment regimen.
- Diarrhea in avian patients has many causes.
- It is important to know the difference between diarrhea and polyuria.
- Stabilization of the avian patient that presents with diarrhea through appropriate hydration therapy will help restore the patient's overall physical condition.

PREVENTION

- Reduce stress within the bird's environment.
- Provide an appropriate diet.
- Quarantine all new birds and birds that have been exposed to other avian species at bird shows and bird fairs for 30 days.
- Owners must maintain immune competent animals.
- Provide clean water and discourage the use of untreated well water and automatic watering systems.

CLIENT EDUCATION

- Use paper as the substrate on the cage bottom so that the stool can be assessed.
- The most common cause of abnormal stool in birds is dietary change or provision of different food items—not disease.
- Know what the bird's normal stool looks like.

SUGGESTED READING

Bauck L: Abnormal droppings. In Olsen GH, et al, editors: Manual of avian medicine, St Louis, 2000, Mosby Inc., pp 62–70.

Jones MP, et al: Supportive care and shock. In Olsen GH, et al, editors: Manual of avian medicine, St Louis, 2000, Mosby Inc., pp 17–46.

Monks D: Gastrointestinal disease. In Harcourt-Brown N, et al, editors: BSAVA manual of psittacine birds, ed 2, Quedgeley, Gloucester, 2005, British Small Animal Veterinary Association Woodrow House, pp 180–190.

Pollock CG, et al: Birds. In Carpenter JW, editor: Exotic animal formulary, ed 3, St Louis, 2005, Elsevier/Saunders, pp 135–264.

Quesenberry KE, et al: Supportive care and emergency therapy. In Ritchie BW, et al, editors: Avian medicine: principles and applications, Brentwood, TN, 1994, HBD International Inc., pp 383–416.

CROSS-REFERENCES TO OTHER SECTIONS

Chlamydophila psittaci
Foreign Bodies
Heavy Metal Toxicity
Proventricular Dilatation Disease
Viral Diseases

AUTHOR & EDITOR: **THOMAS N. TULLY, JR.**

BIRDS

Dystocia

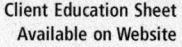

Client Education Sheet Available on Website

BASIC INFORMATION

DEFINITION

Failure of an egg to pass through the oviduct within a normal period of time. Most companion birds lay eggs at intervals of 48 hours; psittacine individual times may vary. Dystocia can be obstructive or nonobstructive.

SYNONYM

Egg binding

EPIDEMIOLOGY

SPECIES, AGE, SEX

- All species
- Reproductively active females

RISK FACTORS

- Stress
- Adverse environmental conditions (e.g., cold, dry)
- Inappropriate husbandry
- Ovarian anatomic abnormalities
- Endocrine disorders
- Neoplasia
- Nutritional deficiency (e.g., calcium [see Hypocalcemia], vitamin E)
- Obesity
- Malformed eggs (e.g., soft-shelled eggs)
- Abdominal hernia
- Oviductal disease (see Follicular Stasis)
- Systemic/Metabolic disease
- Chronic egg layer (see Chronic Egg Laying)
- First time laying an egg
- Young or old bird

GEOGRAPHY AND SEASONALITY

Depending on avian species affected, dry cold environmental conditions may predispose hens to this disease process.

ASSOCIATED CONDITIONS AND DISORDERS

- Anorexia
- Depression
- Weakness
- Dyspnea
- Nesting Behavior

CLINICAL PRESENTATION

DISEASE FORMS/SUBTYPES

- Egg with shell or soft shell within the reproductive tract
- Inability of egg to pass caused by egg of large size or adhesion of egg to oviductal mucosa
- Inability of egg to pass due to improper function of oviduct
- Prolapse of oviduct out of the vent with egg still in reproductive tract (see Cloacal Prolapse)

HISTORY, CHIEF COMPLAINT

- Nonspecific
- Depression
- Inappetence
- Abnormally wide stance
- Reluctance to fly or perch
- Drooped wings

PHYSICAL EXAM FINDINGS

- Distention or weakness of the caudal coelom
- Possible palpation of egg in caudal body cavity
- Egg present in oviduct that has prolapsed out of the vent

ETIOLOGY AND PATHOPHYSIOLOGY

- Abnormally prolonged presence of an egg in the oviduct causes a multitude of complications.
- An egg lodged in the pelvis may compress the pelvic vessels and kidneys, causing circulatory disorders and shock.
- An impacted egg may cause metabolic disturbances by interfering with normal defecation and micturition, inducing ileus and renal dysfunction (see Constipation [Ileus]).
- Pressure necrosis to all three layers of the oviductal wall may ultimately lead to rupture.

DIAGNOSIS

DIFFERENTIAL DIAGNOSIS

- Egg-related peritonitis
- Septicemia
- Caudal coelomic organomegaly

INITIAL DATABASE

- Complete blood count (CBC): leukocytosis with concurrent heterophilia may be present
- Plasma biochemistry panel: creatine kinase (CK) and aspartate aminotransferase (AST) may be elevated, indicating skeletal muscle enzyme leakage from tissue damage or catabolic state. Glucose levels may be decreased. Calcium levels are normally elevated in a laying hen. Calcium levels may be normal or decreased in a bird that has been provided a poor diet, or if the hen has laid excessive eggs.
- Cloacal culture

ADVANCED OR CONFIRMATORY TESTING

- Imaging: radiography and ultrasound will aid in evaluation of the position and characterization of the egg(s). Eggs with noncalcified shell may appear similar to a mass in the caudal coelomic cavity. Multiple eggs may be identified owing to an obstruction distally or secondary to motility disorders.
- Eggs could be within the oviduct or ectopic due to oviductal rupture or retroperistalsis.

TREATMENT

THERAPEUTIC GOALS

- Stabilize and improve patient's physical condition.
- Remove the egg in question through natural processes or medical intervention.
- Assess conditions that led to egg retention; address problems to prevent recurrence if possible.
- Keep bird as inpatient until delivery of all eggs and stable.
- Medical treatment is attempted first in nonobstructive cases of egg binding.
- If oviposition has not occurred within 2-12 hours, or there is indication of obstruction, surgical intervention should be considered.

ACUTE GENERAL TREATMENT

- All treatment is to be performed on a stable patient.
  - Nursing care
    - Administer warmed crystalloid fluids SC, IV, IO (50-150 mL/kg/d maintenance plus dehydration deficit factored in if needed) at a rate of 10-25 mL/kg over a 5-minute period or at a continuous rate of 100 mL/kg/q 24 h.
    - Increase environmental temperature to 85°F-90°F (29°C-32°C).
    - Provide a humidified environment by placing warm moist towels in the incubator.
    - Nutritional support is required in most cases.
- Manual delivery: with the bird anesthetized, the cloaca is lubricated with a water-soluble lubricant (e.g., K-Y Jelly). The egg is palpated through the abdominal wall, and constant lateral pressure is applied to move the egg caudally. Care must be taken to avoid breaking the egg or applying direct pressure over the kidneys.
- Ovocentesis: a 19- to 22-gauge needle is inserted into the egg through the abdominal wall or through the cloaca if the egg is visible. The contents of the egg are then aspirated. Soft shell eggs may be easily collapsed; firmer eggshells may need to be collapsed gently before removal. Eggshell pieces must be removed carefully because sharp pieces can cause uterine damage and serve as a source of infection.
- Surgical delivery: indicated in cases of uterine torsion, egg severely adherent to the oviductal wall, uterine rupture, and ectopic egg. Ventral or lateral laparotomy and possible salpingohysterectomy should be performed.
- Medications
  - Drugs of choice
    - Calcium gluconate 50-100 mg/kg IM or SC
    - Prostaglandin E_2 0.02-0.1 mg/kg applied topically to the uterovaginal sphincter; relaxes uterovaginal sphincter and increases uterine contraction
  - Alternative drug therapy
    - Oxytocin 5 IU/kg IM, may repeat q 30 min; not produced in birds; may help initiate oviductal contractions but may be ineffective if uterovaginal sphincter is contracted
    - Vitamin D_3 (Vital E-A+D): 10,000 IU vitamin A and 1000 IU vitamin D_3/300 g body weight

CHRONIC TREATMENT

- Leuprolide acetate 500-750 µg/kg q 14 d for 3 treatments: to prevent ovulation
- Salpingohysterectomy
- Deslorelin implant (4.7 mg) sc q 3-6 months depending on species
- Environmental modification: decrease hours of light per day to 8-10, decrease caloric intake, remove reproductive stimuli (e.g., nest, toys, cagemate, owner interactions)

DRUG INTERACTIONS

- Prostaglandin, oxytocin, and manual delivery contraindicated in cases of uterine constriction, torsion, rupture, ectopic eggs, or mechanical obstruction
- Prostaglandin E_2 should be administered by an individual wearing latex gloves—not by an owner. Women can be adversely affected by the hormonal effects of prostaglandin E_2 through transdermal absorption.

POSSIBLE COMPLICATIONS

- Potential for oviductal infection
- Oviductal injury
- Internal ovulation for patients in which a salpingohysterectomy has been performed
- Leuprolide acetate may not work to prevent ovulation and deslorelin.

RECOMMENDED MONITORING

- Repeat radiographs if suspected retained eggshells.
- Repeat CBC and plasma chemistry panel if oviductal infection or trauma is suspected.
- If oviductal tissue integrity is compromised, broad-spectrum antibiotics are recommended.
- Analgesic/antiinflammatory medication is required in cases of suspected pain and inflammation.
- Monitor appetite, fecal output, and behavior for 5 to 7 days post presentation for egg binding.

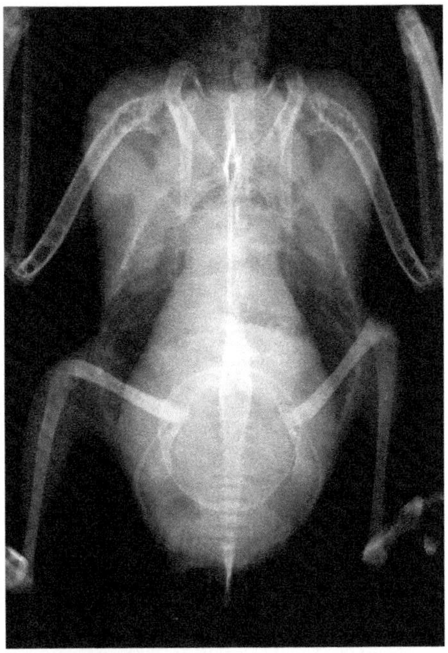

Dystocia Egg binding in a cockatiel. Before medical management is started, radiographic evaluation of the size and number of eggs is indicated. *(Photo courtesy Jörg Mayer, The University of Georgia, Athens.)*

PROGNOSIS AND OUTCOME

- Uncomplicated cases have a good prognosis.
- The prognosis degrades as the number of complications increases.

PEARLS & CONSIDERATIONS

COMMENTS

- Malnourished, old, and obese birds appear to be at increased risk for oviductal inertia.
- Medical management of egg binding cases often helps stabilize the patient by correcting physiologic deficits that may have been caused by dietary insufficiency or by the disease condition (e.g., calcium).
- Removal of the egg will greatly improve the patient's condition.

PREVENTION

- Address the underlying cause.
- Leuprolide acetate or dislorelin therapy (may not work).
- Environmental modifications (see Chronic Treatment).
- Salpingohysterectomy (risk for internal ovulation).

CLIENT EDUCATION

- Owners should be aware of the sex of their bird.
- Owners should know the signs of egg binding.

SUGGESTED READINGS

Bowles H: Evaluating and treating the reproductive system. In Harrison GJ, Lightfoot TL, editors: Clinical avian medicine, vol II, Florida, 2006, Spix Publishing, pp 519–539.

Crosta L, et al: Physiology, diagnostics, and diseases of the avian reproductive tract, Vet Clin North Am Exot Anim Pract 1:57–84, 2003.

Romagnano A: Avian obstetrics, Sem Avian Exot Pet Med 5:180–188, 1996.

Speer B: Disease of the urogenital system. In Altman RB, et al, editors: Avian medicine and surgery, Philadelphia, 1997, WB Saunders, pp 633–644.

CROSS-REFERENCES TO OTHER SECTIONS

Chronic Egg Laying
Cloacal Prolapse
Constipation (Ileus)
Follicular Stasis
Hypocalcemia

AUTHOR: **DAVID SANCHEZ-MIGALLON GUZMAN**

EDITOR: **THOMAS N. TULLY, JR.**

BIRDS

Ectoparasitism

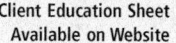

Client Education Sheet Available on Website

BASIC INFORMATION

DEFINITION

The presence of parasites on or within the epidermis/dermis of the body

EPIDEMIOLOGY

SPECIES, AGE, SEX All birds regardless of age and sex can be infected/infested. Older and younger birds may be more predisposed because of an immune compromised state.

GENETICS AND BREED PREDISPOSITION Budgerigars commonly present with *Knemidocoptes* spp. infestations. It appears these mites may be introduced to young birds through contact with their parents.

RISK FACTORS

- Immune suppressed individuals
- Contact with infested birds
- Poorly maintained facilities

CONTAGION AND ZOONOSIS The transmission of ectoparasites in facilitated by physical proximity, overcrowding and environmental conditions that contribute to the parasite presence. Many ectoparasites may act as vectors for other diseases transmissible to other avian species or humans.

ASSOCIATED CONDITIONS AND DISORDERS

- Anemia
- Hemoparasites

CLINICAL PRESENTATION

DISEASE FORMS/SUBTYPES

- Mites
  - *Knemidocoptes* spp. (scaly leg mite): more prevalent in budgerigars and passerines; usual locations for lesions are cere and featherless areas of the legs and vent. Infestations can be severe and chronic, leading to cere hyperkeratosis and beak malformations.
  - *Dermanyssus* spp. (roost or nocturnal mites): mites that feed on blood meals and are usually found on birds during the night. These mite infestations can be difficult to diagnose owing to night feeding. Direct visualization may be accomplished during the night or by placing a white sheet in the cage or enclosure overnight and may aid in identification and diagnosis.
  - *Ornithonyssus* spp. (northern fowl mite, tropical fowl mite): mites that feed on blood meals and may be found on birds at any time of day or night.
  - *Dermantonyssus* spp.: pathogenic
- Feather lice
  - Birds are susceptible to species of Mallophaga lice that feed on keratin (e.g., skin, feathers). Avian lice in general are not highly pathogenic. Extremely high numbers of lice on an avian patient are usually indicative of immune suppression or other disease conditions or poor hygiene.
- Ticks
  - Not a primary concern in most avian species. Serious reactions with death as a consequence have been reported in birds as a result of tick reactions due to unknown pathophysiologic processes.
- Flies
  - Hippoboscid flies in large numbers may cause anemia and have been reported to transmit West Nile virus and hemoparasites (e.g., *Haemoproteus* spp.). Black flies from the family Simuliidae also feed on blood meals and can transmit *Leucocytozoon* spp. hemoparasites.
- Mosquitoes
  - Will cause anemia and can transmit disease (e.g., West Nile virus, equine encephalitis viruses).

HISTORY, CHIEF COMPLAINT

- Observation of parasites on bird skin and/or feathers
- Areas of hyperkeratosis on the beak, featherless areas of the leg, or malformed beak
- Depression of the patient

PHYSICAL EXAM FINDINGS

- As above regarding history and chief complaint
- Skin may be hyperkeratotic and acanthotic, presenting with thickening, irregularity, and flaking.

ETIOLOGY AND PATHOPHYSIOLOGY

External parasites can be divided into two classifications:

- Dermal parasites that eat and affect the outer keratin layer of the skin
- Parasites that feed off blood meals from the host

DIAGNOSIS

DIFFERENTIAL DIAGNOSIS

Several conditions can cause cutaneous signs that should be differentiated from the exclusive presence of ectoparasites, including other infectious diseases caused by bacteria, fungus, virus (e.g., pox virus, circovirus, polyomavirus), nutritional deficits, self-trauma secondary to behavioral alterations, and neoplasia.

INITIAL DATABASE

- Complete blood count: observe for a generalized inflammatory response and anemia
- Direct visualization: direct detection of parasites in the skin and feathers. Lice eggs may be observed along the primary and secondary feathers; use of a light source against the plumage may facilitate the task.
- Adhesive tape: a piece of adhesive tape can be placed on the lesions and examined under the microscope.

ADVANCED OR CONFIRMATORY TESTING

- Feather digest
  - This technique is performed in quill infestations caused by mites.
  - The feather is placed in 10% solution of potassium hydroxide and centrifuged.
  - Microscopic examination is used to examine the material that is left after centrifugation.
- Skin scrape
  - Indicated for diagnosis of mites, although some species may require deep skin biopsy
  - A drop of oil on the microscope slide aids in examination: in the presence of very desquamative lesions, the use of 10% potassium hydroxide is indicated.
- Skin biopsy
  - Punch or excisional biopsies can be performed on avian species.
  - The anatomic area should be considered because damage to the primary or secondary feather follicle may occur, causing irreversible damage.
  - Taking a skin punch biopsy through a piece of transparent tape placed over the affected area prevents deformation of the sample and helps the pathologist visualize alignment of the epithelium.
  - Aseptic preparation is not recommended because this may interfere with the diagnosis.

TREATMENT

THERAPEUTIC GOAL

Clear the bird of external parasites, and prevent reinfestation.

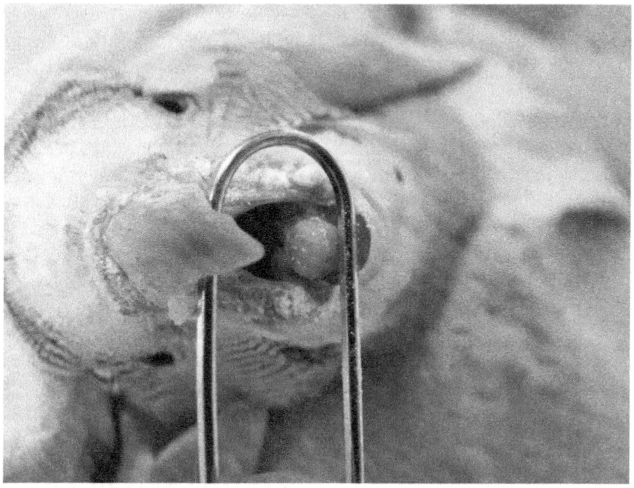

Ectoparasitism External parasites.

ACUTE GENERAL TREATMENT

- Mites
  - Ivermectin 0.2 mg/kg PO, SC, IM q14 d for a total of two treatments
- Lice and ticks
  - Pyrethrin dusting: 5% sevin dust, light dusting to plumage once, repeat as needed
  - Fipronil: spray skin in the axillary or inguinal area once and repeat in 30 days

CHRONIC TREATMENT

- Maintain the immune status of birds.
- Maintain good husbandry practices.
- Maintain a clean environment for the birds.
- Prevent exposure to wild birds that may carry external parasites.

DRUG INTERACTIONS

Parenteral use of ivermectin in small passerine and psittacine species may be toxic.

POSSIBLE COMPLICATIONS

- Propylene glycol–based Ivomec may cause severe respiratory tract irritation if aspirated during oral administration.
- The alcohol base of fipronil can damage feathers if feathers are exposed to the antiparasitic agent.

RECOMMENDED MONITORING

Monitor environment for reexposure, especially for *Dermanyssus* spp. and *Ornithonyssus* spp.

PROGNOSIS AND OUTCOME

- The prognosis is good if birds are not severely infested and if limited secondary conditions are associated with the external parasites.
- The prognosis is more guarded for avian patients that are severely infested and are suffering from secondary life-threatening complications (e.g., anemia) or other diseases.

PEARLS & CONSIDERATIONS

COMMENTS

- Pet avian species (e.g., passerine, psittacine) are rarely infested by external parasites, except for budgerigars and canaries with *Knemidokoptes* spp.
- Poultry are commonly infested with *Dermanyssus* spp. and *Ornithonyssus* spp.
- Pigeons, owls, and raptor species are commonly diagnosed with hippoboscid flies.

PREVENTION

- Maintain excellent husbandry within the loft, coop, or aviary.
- Prevent exposure to birds that are infested with external parasites.
- Keep the loft, coop, or aviary clean.
- Check birds on a regular basis for evidence of external parasites.

CLIENT EDUCATION

See above, and maintain a mosquito-free environment as much as possible.

SUGGESTED READINGS

Greiner EC: Parasitology. In Altman RB, et al, editors: Avian medicine and surgery, Philadelphia, 1997, WB Saunders, pp 332–349.

Greiner EC, et al: Parasites. In Ritchie BW, et al, editors: Avian medicine: principles and application, Lake Worth, FL, 1994, Wingers Publishing, pp 1007–1029.

AUTHOR: **ALBERTO RODRIGUEZ BARBON**

EDITOR: **THOMAS N. TULLY, JR.**

Edema, Soft Tissue

BASIC INFORMATION

DEFINITION

A collection of extracellular fluid within soft tissues

SYNONYMS

Soft tissue swelling, wing tip swelling (raptors), constrictive toe syndrome, pulmonary edema

EPIDEMIOLOGY

SPECIES, AGE, SEX All species and ages and both sexes

GENETICS AND BREED PREDISPOSITION Macaw and parrot species appear to be susceptible to constrictive toe syndrome that causes edematous swelling in the distal toe.

RISK FACTORS

- Trauma (see Trauma)
- Neoplasia
- Infectious disease
- Heart disease
- String foreign body around toe or wing tip

CONTAGION AND ZOONOSIS

- Infectious diseases, including avian influenza and fowl cholera, may be a cause of edematous wattles or combs in poultry (see Viral Diseases).
- Bands or jesses that are too tight on the bird's leg(s).

ASSOCIATED CONDITIONS AND DISORDERS

- Depression
- Inability to use affected limb
- Dyspnea
- Lameness

CLINICAL PRESENTATION

DISEASE FORMS/SUBTYPES

- Peripheral edema
- Pulmonary edema

HISTORY, CHIEF COMPLAINT

- Localized swelling
- Diffuse swelling along long bones
- Difficulty breathing
- Swollen toes

PHYSICAL EXAM FINDINGS

- Diffuse, localized, nodular or pedunculated swelling
- May be soft or firm
- Fractures
- Hematoma
- Dyspnea
- Cardiac arrhythmia
- Swollen toes distal to constrictive tissue band

ETIOLOGY AND PATHOPHYSIOLOGY

- Noninfectious causes: trauma (wing tip edema of raptors), fractures, feather cysts (especially in canaries)
- Iatrogenic: tight bandages, surgical trauma
- Coelomic mass effect: pulmonary edema
- Cardiac disease (see Cardiac Disease)
- Pulmonary edema: fluid overload, pulmonary disease, airborne toxins, obstruction of trachea, electrical shock
- Infectious causes: viral diseases in poultry often cause swelling of the comb or wattles
- Constrictive toe syndrome/constriction of toe by string foreign body: connective tissue circumferential bands restrict blood flow to distal toe, causing edema and swelling
- Vitamin C deficiency in Ptarmigan and grouse chicks <4 weeks old causing skeletal muscle edema.
- Neonatal edema Edematous chicks usually associated with high humidity, thick shell or inadequate ventilation during incubation; may result in external yolk sac upon hatch
- Postavian circovirus infection syndrome, in which transudate to modified transudate occurs in the coelomic cavity. No treatment and the birds usually die or are euthanized.

DIAGNOSIS

DIFFERENTIAL DIAGNOSIS

- Hematoma
- Granulomas and abscesses
- Neoplasia
- Parasitic cysts in the subcutis or muscle

INITIAL DATABASE

- Physical examination to include investigation of causes of iatrogenic swelling
- Radiographs if tumor, trauma, or bony involvement is suspected
- Complete blood count
- Plasma chemistry panel
- Cardiology evaluation

ADVANCED OR CONFIRMATORY TESTING

Fine-needle aspirate, biopsy (wedge or incisional), or surgical excision of nodular swellings with histopathologic analysis

TREATMENT

THERAPEUTIC GOALS

- Resolution of edema
- Treatment of underlying cause

ACUTE GENERAL TREATMENT

- Compression bandages may be used acutely to reduce localized areas of swelling, particularly of the distal limb or wing. Compression bandages should not be used on the keel because this may restrict keel movement, resulting in suffocation.
- Heat may improve circulation and reduce edema but often is not practical for birds because they are easily stressed.
- Wing tip edema may be treated with
  - Propentofylline 5 mg/kg po q 12 h for 20-40 days
  - Isoxsuprine 5-10 mg/kg po q 24 h for 20-40 days
- Pulmonary edema may be treated with
- Furosemide 0.15 mg/kg IM, if necessary
  - Surgical incision of constrictive tissue band on toes that are swollen, to restore blood flow
- General furosemide diuretic dose for birds 1-2.2 mg/kg po q 12-24 h
- Overdose may cause dehydration and electrolyte abnormalities
- Raptors and lories very sensitive to this drug

CHRONIC TREATMENT

Varies with the cause of swelling and may include surgical treatment, bandaging, chemotherapy, or radiation therapy.

POSSIBLE COMPLICATIONS

- When using furosemide: caution should be used so that the patient does not become dehydrated. Treatment generally is not indicated for mildly afflicted patients.
- May need to reincise constrictive tissue bands on birds that present with swollen toes if the initial treatment is ineffective.

RECOMMENDED MONITORING

- Monitor affected area and patient's general attitude.
- Monitor pulmonary edema
  - Respiratory rate
  - Character of respiration
  - Oxygenation of blood
    - Blood gases
- Monitor patient's ability to use affected area.
- Monitor toes of patients that have been treated with constrictive toe syndrome.

PROGNOSIS AND OUTCOME

- Prognosis varies based on underlying cause of fluid accumulation.
- Bandage-induced edema often carries a good prognosis if the constrictive material is removed.
- For constricted toe syndrome, the prognosis for saving an affected toe is dependent on ability to restore normal blood flow to the distal part of the extremity.

PEARLS & CONSIDERATIONS

COMMENTS

- Quick treatment of avian patients that present with edema reduces the chances of permanent pathologic changes to surrounding tissue.
- Medical therapy of pulmonary edema associated with coelomic masses or heart disease provides a temporary solution.
- Bandages should be placed carefully, especially when placed on the distal extremities of avian patients.

PREVENTION

- Proper bandage application is needed.
- Monitor distal extremities for swelling when bandage is applied.
- Proper caging can prevent wing tip trauma.

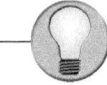

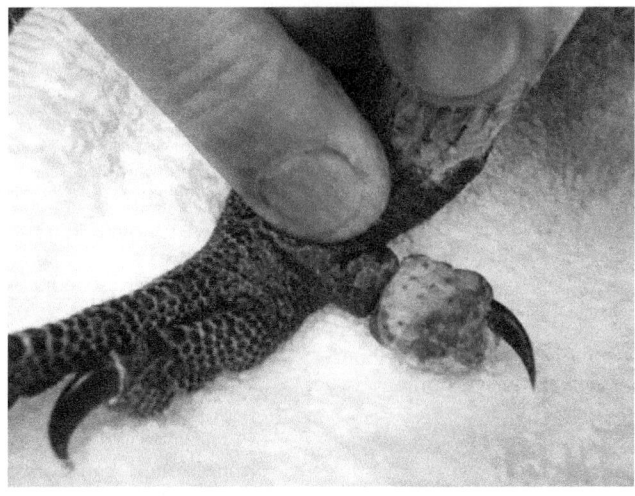

Edema, Soft Tissue Constricted toe syndrome in a blue and gold macaw due to vascular congestion distal to the connective tissue stricture. *(Photo courtesy Thomas N. Tully, Jr.)*

- Higher humidity in an avian nursery may help reduce the incidence of constricted toe syndrome.

CLIENT EDUCATION

See Prevention.

SUGGESTED READINGS

Bowles HL, et al: Surgical resolution of soft tissue disorders. In Harrison GJ, et al, editors: Clinical avian medicine, vol II, Palm Beach, FL, 2006, Spix Publishing Inc., pp 775–831.

Disorders of the musculoskeletal system. In Altman RB, et al, editors: Avian medicine and surgery. Philadelphia, 1996, WB Saunders, pp 523–539.

Dorrestein GM, et al: Clinical pathology and necropsy. In Harcourt-Brown N, et al, editors: BSAVA manual of psittacine birds, ed 2, Quedgeley, Gloucester, 2005, British Small Animal Veterinary Association Woodrow House, pp 80–86.

CROSS-REFERENCES TO OTHER SECTIONS

Cardiac Disease
Trauma
Viral Diseases

AUTHOR: **GWENDOLYN R. JANKOWSKI**

EDITOR: **THOMAS N. TULLY, JR.**

BIRDS

Emaciation

Client Education Sheet Available on Website

BASIC INFORMATION

DEFINITION

A state in which body mass is low owing to chronic energy deficiency (negative energy balance)

SYNONYMS

Poor body condition, cachexia, going light

EPIDEMIOLOGY

SPECIES, AGE, SEX All species and ages and both sexes

RISK FACTORS

- Malabsorptive and digestive disorders
- Musculoskeletal or neurologic disorders
- Infectious disease (e.g., proventricular dilatation disease [PDD], mycobacteriosis, megabacteriosis)
- Neoplasia
- Dietary change (transition from seed to pelleted diet)
- Lack of food
- Endoparasitism
- Ingested foreign body

CONTAGION AND ZOONOSIS Tuberculosis may be transmitted to people and other birds. Appropriate precautions should be taken with birds that may be infected.

ASSOCIATED CONDITIONS AND DISORDERS

- Dyspnea
- Diarrhea
- Crop stasis (see Crop Stasis)

CLINICAL PRESENTATION

DISEASE FORMS/SUBTYPES

- Primary (starvation)
- Secondary (disease related)

HISTORY, CHIEF COMPLAINT

- Weight loss of more than 10% within a week or 20% within a 2-4 week period
- It is important to distinguish between anorectic birds and chronic wasting in the face of normal appetite and nutrition.
- May have an inadequate diet

PHYSICAL EXAM FINDINGS

- Weight loss and/or poor growth
- Protruding keel bone
- Poor pectoral muscle mass
- Dehydration (see Dehydration)
- Regurgitation/vomiting or diarrhea (see Regurgitation/Vomiting)
- Undigested seed in the feces
- Soiled vent
- Generalized muscle atrophy and/or decreased liver size
- Decreased fat storage: evaluate by wetting feathers over caudal body, flank, thighs, neck to observe yellowish subcutaneous fat deposits
- Weight below species typical range (must evaluate on individual basis)

ETIOLOGY AND PATHOPHYSIOLOGY

- Inadequate caloric intake
- Proventricular dilatation disease/PDD
- Macrorhabdus ornithogaster (megabacteriosis)
- Reproductive disease

- May be secondary to increased metabolic demand from exercise, infectious or neoplastic disease
- In clinical practice, the most common causes of chronic wasting in the face of a normal appetite include neoplasia, PDD (bornavirus is a suspected cause), and megabacteriosis in budgerigars. Tuberculosis should be considered, along with other infectious agents and parasites.

DIAGNOSIS

DIFFERENTIAL DIAGNOSIS

- Starvation
- Inanition
- Tuberculosis
- PDD
- Endoparasitism
- Neurologic, respiratory, and gastrointestinal diseases (see Enteritis)
- Ingested foreign body

INITIAL DATABASE

- Physical examination to include observation of the bird eating
- Changes noted on CBC/plasma chemistry panel results vary depending upon etiology of the disease presentation. Abnormal results may include decreased marrow cell aplasia, decreased triglyceride, cholesterol, albumin, AST, and glucose levels in severe cases.
- Complete blood count
- Plasma chemistry panel
- Radiographs
- Fecal parasite examination

ADVANCED OR CONFIRMATORY TESTING

- Crop and/or cloacal cultures may be helpful if GI bacterial infection/overgrowth is suspected.
- Acid-fast stains on feces of tuberculosis suspects. Shedding is intermittent, so stains should be repeated daily.
- Liver biopsy for mycobacteriosis
- Viral testing
- Crop biopsy for possible confirmation of PDD (see Proventricular Dilatation Disease).

TREATMENT

THERAPEUTIC GOALS

- Weight gain or stabilization
- Resolution of the underlying problem
- Determination of an appropriate maintenance diet

ACUTE GENERAL TREATMENT

- May gavage feed 3%-5% of body weight q 6-12 h based on clinical condition of bird
- Treat the underlying problem.
- Nutritional, heat, and fluid support (see Anorexia)
- Diazepam 0.25-0.50 mg/kg IM q 24 h × 2-3 days may be used for raptors as an appetite stimulant.

CHRONIC TREATMENT

Treat the underlying problem.

POSSIBLE COMPLICATIONS

- Aspiration secondary to assist or gavage feeding (see Dehydration)
- Re-feeding syndrome: normally intracellular ions move into bloodstream with progressive emaciation and are excreted
- Avoid by supplementing high fat, low carbohydrate critical care formula with adequate concentrations of potassium, phosphate, magnesium: supplement electrolytes as needed.
- Clinical signs of re-feeding syndrome include profound consciousness and respiratory or cardiac arrest, and death
- Death

RECOMMENDED MONITORING

- Monitor weight on a daily basis.
- Monitor treatment response by patient.

PROGNOSIS AND OUTCOME

Varies depending on underlying cause and severity of weight loss

PEARLS & CONSIDERATIONS

COMMENTS

- When establishing a differential diagnosis, it is important to distinguish birds that are eating well and still losing weight from birds that are unable or unwilling to eat.
- Neoplasia, tuberculosis, and PDD are top differentials in a bird that is eating well and is losing weight.
- Megabacteriosis is a common cause of emaciation or "going light" in budgerigars (see Megabacteriosis).

PREVENTION

- Appropriate diet and husbandry
- Annual wellness exams

CLIENT EDUCATION

- Appropriate diet and husbandry
- Importance of regular exams
- Monitor bird's dietary intake.
- If switching a bird from a seed diet to a pellet diet, have the owner consult with the veterinarian.

SUGGESTED READINGS

Dorrestein GM: Nursing the sick bird. In Tully TN, et al, editors: Avian medicine, Oxford, UK, 2000, Butterworth-Heinemann, pp 74–112.
Pollock CG, et al: Birds. In Carpenter JW, editor: Exotic animal formulary, ed 3, St Louis, 2005, Elsevier/Saunders, pp 135–264.
Quesenberry KE, et al: Supportive care and emergency therapy. In Ritchie BW, et al, editors: Avian medicine: principles and applications, Brentwood, TN, 1994, HBD International Inc., pp 383–416.

CROSS-REFERENCES TO OTHER SECTIONS

Anorexia
Crop Stasis
Dehydration
Enteritis
Megabacteriosis
Proventricular Dilatation Disease
Regurgitation/Vomiting

AUTHOR: **GWENDOLYN R. JANKOWSKI**
EDITOR: **THOMAS N. TULLY, JR.**

BIRDS

Enteritis

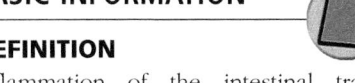

BASIC INFORMATION

DEFINITION

Inflammation of the intestinal tract, usually referring to the small intestine

EPIDEMIOLOGY

SPECIES, AGE, SEX

- Chickens, mynahs, toucans, pigeons, canaries, finches, and lories are most susceptible to coccidiosis.
- Cryptosporidiosis has been reported in chickens, turkeys, quail, psittacines, waterfowl, finches, and pheasants.
- Histomoniasis is mainly a disease of turkeys but has been reported in other birds.

- Circovirus causes enteritis in pigeons.
- Ulcerative enteritis is found in quails.
- Necrotizing typhlitis caused by spirochetes leads to severe disease in rheas.
- Herpesvirus causes disease in waterbirds, Amazon parrots, macawas, cockatoos, cockatiels, conures, and budgerigars.
- Enteritis due to adenovirus infection has been reported in turkeys, chickens, and African grey parrots.
- Newcastle disease has been reported in poultry and in wild and companion birds.
- Any species, age, or sex may be affected. Birds younger than 12 months of age may be more susceptible to some forms of enteritis.

GENETICS AND BREED PREDISPOSITION

All breeds are susceptible to enteritis. Genetic factors may exist.

RISK FACTORS

- Stress
- Travel
- Overcrowding
- Poor sanitation
- Nutritional deficiencies
- Introduction of novel animals to the flock

CONTAGION AND ZOONOSIS

- Many causative agents of avian enteritis are transmissible to humans. These include bacterial infections such as *Salmonella*, which is an important causative agent for foodborne gastroenteritis. Gastroenteritis in humans has also been associated with *Campylobacter* species from poultry.
- *Chlamydophila psittaci* is the causative agent for psittacosis in humans.
- Some bacteria such as *Serpulina pilosicoli* are found to colonize both avian and human intestinal tracts.
- *Yersinia pseudotuberculosis* has been reported to cause appendicitis in humans.
- Newcastle disease has been reported to cause transient conjunctivitis in exposed humans.

GEOGRAPHY AND SEASONALITY

- Pacheco's disease was first reported in Brazil and initial outbreaks in the United States were associated with birds imported from South America. The virus is now found worldwide.
- Duck virus enteritis is enzootic in North America. It has been reported in Europe, India, Thailand, and Vietnam.
- Outbreaks of Eastern equine encephalitis have been reported in the United States, especially along the Atlantic Coast and in the upper Midwest.
- Rotavirus has been reported to be more prevalent during seasons with lower humidity.
- Spirochetosis has been reported most commonly in rheas in the summer and fall (in the United States).

CLINICAL PRESENTATION

DISEASE FORMS/SUBTYPES

- Necrotic enteritis
- Ulcerative enteritis
- Hemorrhagic enteritis
- Catarrhal enteritis

HISTORY, CHIEF COMPLAINT

- Diarrhea
- Anorexia
- Depression
- Weight loss

PHYSICAL EXAM FINDINGS

- Diarrhea
- "Soiled vent": caked feces around cloaca
- Lethargy
- Dehydration
- Chronic cases may show emaciation and reduced growth.

ETIOLOGY AND PATHOPHYSIOLOGY

- Irritation of the intestinal mucosa results in hypermotility and enhanced secretion in the gastrointestinal tract. This can result in severe fluid and electrolyte loss.
- Bacterial: salmonellosis, *Pasteurella multocida, Campylobacter* spp., spirochetosis, *Clostridium colinum, Clostridium perfringens, Clostridium difficile,* mycobacteriosis, *Yersinia pseudotuberculosis,* avian chlamydiosis, *Aeromonas hydrophila, Pasteurella anatipestifer, Escherichia coli*
- Viral: coronavirus, paramyxovirus: Newcastle disease; adenovirus: inclusion body hepatitis, hemorrhagic enteritis, Marek's disease; orthomyxovirus: avian influenza; arbovirus: Eastern equine encephalitis, Western equine encephalitis, Highland J virus; herpesvirus: Pacheco's disease, duck virus enteritis; and pigeon circovirus, avian polyomavirus, rotavirus, and astrovirus
- Parasitic: protozoan: coccidiosis, cryptosporidiosis, histomoniasis; trematode: *Sphaeridiotrema globulus*; nematode: *Ascarida galli, Heterakis gallinarum, Capillaria* spp.; cestodes: *Raillietina* spp., *Choanotaenia* spp., *Davainea* spp., *Amoebotaenia* spp., *Hymenolepis* spp.; acanthocephalans

DIAGNOSIS

DIFFERENTIAL DIAGNOSIS

- Toxin
- Foreign body
- Obstruction
- Hepatic disease
- Renal disease
- Pancreatitis
- Dietary indiscretion
- Dietary change
- Antibiotic use

INITIAL DATABASE

- Fecal flotation
- Fecal direct smear
- Fecal Gram stain
- Fecal culture
- Complete blood count
- Chemistry panel
- Radiographs

ADVANCED OR CONFIRMATORY TESTING

- Ultrasound
- Intestinal biopsy
- Polymerase chain reaction
- Serology: ELISA, hemagglutination and hemagglutination inhibition tests, virus neutralization tests, plaque neutralization tests, agar gel precipitation tests, complement fixation
- Virus isolation
- Immunohistochemistry

TREATMENT

THERAPEUTIC GOALS

- Eliminate underlying cause.
- Correct dehydration.
- Prevent emaciation.

ACUTE GENERAL TREATMENT

- Dependent on etiologic agent
- Bacterial enteritis: antibiotics. Choice should be based on culture and sensitivity results. Possible choices include the following:
  - Doxycycline 25 mg/kg PO q 12 h
  - Amoxicillin 100 mg/kg PO q 8 h
  - Enrofloxacin 15 mg/kg PO q 12 h
  - Trimethoprim/sulfamethoxazole 20 mg/kg PO q 8-12 h (psittacine species)
  - Streptomycin 30 mg/kg IM q 24 h
  - Erythromycin 10-20 mg/kg PO q 12 h
- Viral enteritis: no effective treatment Provide supportive therapy.
- Parasitic enteritis
  - Coccidiosis
    - Sulfadimethoxine 25 mg/kg PO q 12 h × 5 days
    - Toltrazuril 10 mg/kg q 48 h × 3 treatments (raptors) or 25 mg/L drinking water × 2 days, repeat in 14-21 days
  - *Cryptosporidium*: no effective treatment
  - *Histomonas*
    - Ipronidazole (not available in the United States) 130 mg/L drinking water × 7 days
    - Metronidazole 200-400 mg/kg feed (chickens, use with caution as may cause reduced weight gain)
  - *Capillaria*
    - Fenbendazole 20-100 mg/kg PO once
    - Ivermectin 0.2 mg/kg PO, SC, IM once, repeat in 2 weeks

- Ascarids
  - Pyrantel pamoate 7 mg/kg PO, repeat in 2 weeks
  - Levamisole 10-20 mg/kg SC once
- Cestodes and trematodes:
  - Praziquantel 7.5 mg/kg SC, IM, repeat in 2-4 weeks most species, except finches
- Correct dehydration. See Dehydration.

CHRONIC TREATMENT

Crop feeding may be initiated for birds that are anorectic or severely emaciated.

DRUG INTERACTIONS

- Fenbendazole has been reported to cause immune suppression and septicemia in some birds.
- Levamisole has a narrow margin of safety, use with caution as deaths have been reported.

POSSIBLE COMPLICATIONS

- Severe dehydration and/or electrolyte imbalances can occur with prolonged diarrhea.
- Emaciation and severe debilitation can result from chronic enteritis.

RECOMMENDED MONITORING

- It is recommended to monitor hydration status and electrolytes of the bird.
- A fecal Gram stain can be performed to monitor response to therapy if bacteria are the causative agents of the enteritis.
- A fecal float and/or direct smear should be rechecked 2 weeks after treating for parasites. Three negative fecals are recommended before treatment is discontinued.

PROGNOSIS AND OUTCOME

- Dependent on duration of clinical signs and severity of diarrhea and electrolyte imbalances
- Prognosis is good if cause can be determined and eliminated.
- Septic birds have a poor prognosis.

PEARLS & CONSIDERATIONS

COMMENTS

- It is recommended to initiate therapy with a broad-spectrum antibiotic with bactericidal activity against Gram-negative organisms before a definitive diagnosis is determined.
- Use of parasitic medications should be based on fecal analysis to discourage parasite resistance.

PREVENTION

- Yearly fecal analysis is recommended for all birds, especially in a flock situation.
- All new birds should be quarantined for a period of 30 days with three negative fecals obtained before introduction to the rest of the flock.
- Vaccines are available for some enteric pathogens, including salmonellosis, *Cryptosporidium* spp., *Eimeria* spp., polyomavirus, spirochetosis (not in United States), and Newcastle disease.
- Tick and mosquito control is important for prevention of spirochetosis.

CLIENT EDUCATION

- Birds are less likely to suffer from enteritis if they are free of stress, overcrowding, and unsanitary conditions. Most enteric pathogens are transmitted by the fecal-oral route.
- Practice good hygiene when handling birds to avoid cross-contamination and zoonotic infection.

SUGGESTED READINGS

Bonar C, et al: Suspected fenbendazole toxicosis in 2 vulture species *(Gyps africanus, Torgos tracheliotus)* and marabou storks *(Leptoptilos crumeniferus)*, J Avian Med Surg 17:16–19, 2003.

Buckles EL, et al: Cases of spirochete-associated necrotizing typhlitis in captive common rheas *(Rhea Americana)*, Avian Dis 41:144–148, 1997.

Circella E, et al: Coronavirus associated with an enteric syndrome on a quail farm, Avian Pathol 36:251–258, 2007.

Droual R, et al: Inclusion body hepatitis and hemorrhagic enteritis in two African grey parrots *(Psittacus erithacus)* associated with adenovirus, J Vet Diagn Invest 7:150–154, 1995.

Farkas T, et al: Rapid and simultaneous detection of avian influenza and Newcastle disease viruses by duplex polymerase chain reaction assay, Zoonoses Pub Health 54:38–43, 2007.

Ijaz MK, et al: Seasonality and prevalence of rotavirus in Al-Ain, United Arab Emirates, Clin Diagn Virol 2:323–329,1994.

Lamps LW, et al: The role of *Yersinia enterocolitica* and *Yersinia pseudotuberculosis* in granulomatous appendicitis: a histologic and molecular study, Am J Surg Pathol 25:508–515, 2001.

Lillehoj EP, et al: Vaccines against the avian enteropathogens *Eimeria, Cryptosporidium* and *Salmonella*, Anim Health Res Rev 1:47–65, 2000.

McOrist S, et al: Parasitic enteritis in superb lyrebirds *(Menura novaehollandiae)*, J Wildl Dis 25:420–421, 1989.

Nelson CB, et al: An outbreak of conjunctivitis due to Newcastle disease virus (NDV) occurring in poultry workers, Am J Public Health Nations Health 42:672–678,1952.

Ng J, et al: Identification of novel *Cryptosporidium* genotypes from avian hosts, Appl Environ Microbiol 72:7548–7553, 2006.

O'Toole D, et al: Clostridial enteritis in red lories *(Eos bornea)*, J Vet Diagn Invest 5:111–113, 1993.

Panigrahy B, et al: Bacterial septicemias in two psittacine birds, J Am Vet Med Assoc 186:983–984, 1985.

Pantin-Jackwood MJ, et al: Periodic monitoring of commercial turkeys for enteric viruses indicates continuous presence of astrovirus and rotavirus on the farms, Avian Dis 51:674–680, 2007.

Pizarro M, et al: Ulcerative enteritis (quail disease) in lories, Avian Dis 49:606–608, 2005.

Prattis SM, et al: A retrospective study of disease and mortality in zebra finches, Lab Anim Sci 40:402–405, 1990.

Roscoe DE, et al: Trematode *(Sphaeridiotrema globulus)*-induced ulcerative hemorrhagic enteritis in wild mute swans *(Cygnus olor)*, Avian Dis 26:214–224, 1982.

Sacco RE, et al: Experimental infection of C3H mice with avian, porcine, or human isolates of *Serpulina pilosicoli*, Infect Immun 65:5349–5353, 1997.

Sanchez S, et al: Animal sources of salmonellosis in humans, J Am Vet Med Assoc 221:492–497, 2002.

Shirley MW, et al: Challenges in the successful control of the avian coccidian, Vaccine 25:5540–5547, 2007.

Teixeira MC, et al: Detection of turkey coronavirus in commercial turkey poults in Brazil, Avian Pathol 36:29–33, 2007.

Ward MP, et al: Outbreak of salmonellosis in a zoologic collection of lorikeets and lories (*Trichoglossus* spp., *Lorius* spp., and *Eos* spp.), Avian Dis 47:493–498, 2003.

Williams RB: Tracing the emergence of drug-resistance in coccidia (*Eimeria* spp.) of commercial broiler flocks medicated with decoquinate for the first time in the United Kingdom, Vet Parasitol 135:1–14, 2006.

CROSS-REFERENCES TO OTHER SECTIONS

Dehydration

AUTHOR: **SHANNON N. SHAW**

EDITOR: **THOMAS N. TULLY, JR.**

BIRDS

Feather Picking

Client Education Sheet Available on Website

BASIC INFORMATION

DEFINITION

A condition thought to be due to the desire to perform a natural behavior and the inability to do so that is manifested by the bird pulling off its own feathers with its beak.

SYNONYMS

Feather plucking, feather trauma

EPIDEMIOLOGY

SPECIES, AGE, SEX Macaws, Amazon parrots, cockatoos, cockatiels, Quaker parrots, and African grey parrots are most often represented, although many other companion avian species have been diagnosed with this condition.

GENETICS AND BREED PREDISPOSITION Genetic factors are thought to be involved with the development of feather picking because of the species predilection of patients diagnosed with this disease.

RISK FACTORS

- Behavioral
  - Boredom
  - Crowding
  - Environmental change
  - Reproductive frustration
  - Psychological disturbance
  - Dominance
  - Hypersensitivity reaction
- Medical conditions that affect the skin
  - Parasites
  - Malnutrition
  - Neoplasia
  - Toxin exposure
  - Trauma
  - Endocrine disease
  - Viral disease
  - Bacterial disease
  - Fungal disease

CONTAGION AND ZOONOSIS Complications due to *Chlamydophila psittaci* infection may result in feather damage or loss.

ASSOCIATED CONDITIONS AND DISORDERS

- Hypovitaminosis A
- Hypocalcemia
- Giardiasis in cockatiels
- Hypothyroidism
- Psittacine beak and feather disease (circovirus)
- Pox virus
- Hormone deficiency
- Polyomavirus

CLINICAL PRESENTATION

DISEASE FORMS/SUBTYPES The disease can vary in severity from mild and localized feather picking to severe and generalized with self-mutilation.

HISTORY, CHIEF COMPLAINT

- Bird observed picking at its feathers
- Featherless areas of the skin are observed.

PHYSICAL EXAM FINDINGS

- Featherless areas of the skin or mutilated feathers
- Healthy feathers will be observed on the head with damage to areas that are accessible to the bird's beak.

ETIOLOGY AND PATHOPHYSIOLOGY

- Underlying disease must be ruled out because it is thought that abnormal behaviors can be acquired through trauma, infection, or toxicity.
- Viral infections such as circovirus and polyomavirus have been associated with feather picking, abnormal feather growth, and feather loss. They are thought to be due to changes in the central nervous system or to inflammation and irritation of the feather follicles or skin.
- Stereotypic behaviors such as feather picking are thought to arise from psychological causes, wherein the inability to perform a natural behavior causes a redirected behavior in the form of feather trauma or picking. This conflict can arise from inappropriate environment or management. Examples of conflict include inability to perform normal social behavior, competition from other birds or animals, and lack of predictability and controllability of the environment. If the item causing conflict is not removed, the inappropriate behavior eventually will increase in frequency and will appear in situations out of context.
- It is thought that experiences early in a companion bird's life may contribute to a patient's predisposition to feather pick. Chicks that are captive bred and incubator hatched may be inadequately socialized, which may lead to an inability to psychologically adapt to a captive pet environment, leading to feather picking.
- Although little information on the pathophysiology of feather picking is available, biochemical and neuropathologic changes are assumed to occur in affected birds. Stereotypic behaviors may be influenced by increased dopaminergic activity.

DIAGNOSIS

DIFFERENTIAL DIAGNOSIS

- Feather picking should be distinguished from normal grooming behavior, cagemate trauma, and sexual picking, where a bird will pick feathers to prepare a brood patch.
- Before the diagnosis of feather picking as a primary behavioral disorder can be made, the presence of underlying disease must be ruled out. See Associated Conditions and Disorders.

INITIAL DATABASE

- Complete blood count (CBC): abnormalities may be noted as heterophilia and monocytosis
- Plasma chemistry panel: creatine kinase values may be elevated
- Fecal examination
- Whole-body radiographs
- Cytologic examination of skin lesions
- Culture and sensitivity of skin lesions

ADVANCED OR CONFIRMATORY TESTING

- Biopsy of lesion(s)
- Psittacine beak and feather disease (circovirus): polymerase chain reaction PCR-based testing
- Polyomavirus: PCR-based technology
- Heavy metal toxicology tests

TREATMENT

THERAPEUTIC GOALS

- Correct underlying cause.
- Treat medical disease if present.
- Remove items causing conflict

ACUTE GENERAL TREATMENT

- If the situation is life threatening, mechanical barriers and or/Elizabethan collars can be used; however, these are ineffective and can cause additional psychological stress.
- Treat with antibiotics if significant skin mutilation is present.
- Treat with fluid therapy and/or blood transfusions if blood loss due to self-mutilation is significant.

CHRONIC TREATMENT

- Try to identify and remove conflict causing the destructive behavior.
- Modify environment. Increase the size of the bird's enclosure. Offer the bird time outdoors when temperatures are not extreme. Provide toys and enrichment to occupy the bird's time.
- Desensitization and counter-conditioning may be necessary. The bird may be exposed to the stimulus at low levels, so feather picking is not induced. Praise should be offered when the stimulus is present. The bird will begin to associate the originally

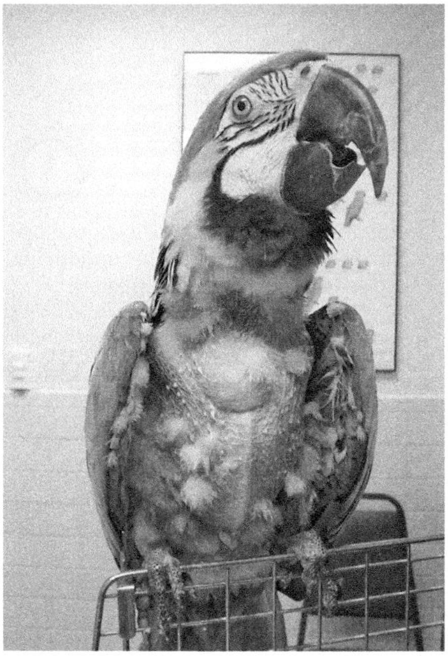

Feather Picking Typical appearance of a feather picker; all feathers that can be reached with the beak are mutilated (feather destructive behavior). Self-induced complete removal of feathers on the body by a macaw. *(Photo courtesy Jörg Mayer, The University of Georgia, Athens.)*

unpleasant stimulus with a positive experience.

- Drug therapy: this should not be the first and only treatment for feather picking but may be an option for certain case presentations
  - Dopamine antagonists and opiate receptor blockade: haloperidol, naloxone, hydrocodone
  - Tricyclic antidepressants: doxepin, clomipramine
  - Benzodiazepines: diazepam, lorazepam, alprazolam, clonazepam
  - Anxiolytics: buspirone
  - Hormone therapy: may be effective with breeding birds or birds that are actively laying eggs: lupron

DRUG INTERACTIONS

Tricyclic antidepressants may cause increased gastrointestinal transit times.

POSSIBLE COMPLICATIONS

- Advanced feather picking may lead to immune suppression and thus increased susceptibility to disease.
- Blood loss
- Infection

RECOMMENDED MONITORING

- It is suggested for the owner to keep a log and document when the feather picking occurs and the activities that are associated with it.
- It is recommended to recheck the extent of feather picking at least once a month after the initial presentation—sooner if the condition is extremely problematic. CBC may be used to assess blood loss and/or systemic inflammatory response.

PROGNOSIS AND OUTCOME

Feather picking is a challenging condition to treat; prognosis is guarded at best.

PEARLS & CONSIDERATIONS

PREVENTION

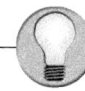

It has been noted that birds are less likely to develop stereotypic activities if they have received behavior training.

CLIENT EDUCATION

- Provide the bird with an appropriate nutrition and environment. The stress-free environment should be large enough for the bird to display normal behavior.
- The bird should be provided with enrichment that allows him to display natural behaviors such as tearing papers, foraging for food items or other objects, or eating time-consuming foods.

SUGGESTED READINGS

Jenkins J: Feather picking and self-mutilation in psittacine birds, Vet Clin North Am Exotic Anim Pract 4:651–668, 2001.
Juarbe-Diaz S: Animal behavior case of the month, J Am Vet Med Assoc 216:1562–1564, 2000.
Rosenthal K, et al: Cytologic, histologic, and microbiologic characterization of the feather pulp and follicles of feather-picking psittacine birds: a preliminary study, J Avian Med Surg 18:103–106, 2004.
Seibert LM, et al: Placebo-controlled clomipramine trial for the treatment of feather picking disorder in cockatoos, J Am Anim Hosp Assoc 40:261–269, 2004.

AUTHOR: **SHANNON N. SHAW**

EDITOR: **THOMAS N. TULLY, JR.**

BIRDS

Follicular Stasis

BASIC INFORMATION

DEFINITION

The formation of mature follicles on the ovary, but the follicles never ovulate into the oviduct

SYNONYMS

Cystic ovarian disease, preovulatory egg binding

EPIDEMIOLOGY

SPECIES, AGE, SEX All species, reproductively active females

RISK FACTORS

- Diet very rich in energy
- Excessive number of daylight hours
- Inappropriate husbandry
- Ovarian anatomic abnormalities
- Endocrine disorders
- Ovarian neoplasias

ASSOCIATED CONDITIONS AND DISORDERS

- Anorexia
- Depression
- Increased serum calcium levels
- Nesting behavior

CLINICAL PRESENTATION

DISEASE FORMS/SUBTYPES Large nonovulated follicles on the ovary

HISTORY, CHIEF COMPLAINT

- Nonspecific
- Depression
- Inappetence

PHYSICAL EXAM FINDINGS

- Weight loss
- Distention of the caudal coelom

ETIOLOGY AND PATHOPHYSIOLOGY

Inability of the follicle to ovulate as a result of any number of physiologic and/or disease conditions

DIAGNOSIS

DIFFERENTIAL DIAGNOSIS

- Ovarian cystoadenoma
- Cystoadenocarcinoma
- Ovarian anatomic abnormalities
- Endocrine disorders

INITIAL DATABASE

- Complete blood count: leukocytosis may be present with neutrophilia in the differential count, especially if secondary coelomitis is present

- Plasma biochemistry panel: hypercalcemia and hypercholesterolemia are common findings caused by the chronic action of reproductive hormones in the mobilization of calcium and fat

ADVANCED OR CONFIRMATORY TESTING

Diagnostic imaging

- Radiographs
  - Polyostotic hyperostosis is commonly observed owing to continuous mobilization of calcium.
  - Soft tissue density can be observed cranially to the kidney, correspondent with gonad enlargement.
  - Hepatomegaly may be present as a result of hepatic lipidosis due to the constant mobilization of fat, with subsequent displacement of viscera.
  - Presence of fluid in the body cavity is a common finding.
- Ultrasound
  - The patient may show cysts filled with fluid in the ovarian area.
  - The presence of free fluid in the coelomic cavity may be noted.
- Endoscopy
  - A left lateral approach, between seventh and eighth ribs, allows a very clear view of the ovary, revealing different cystic structures of varying size filled with a pale yellow fluid. Aspiration of the fluid may be attempted as a diagnostic and treatment measure, although the risk of leaking in the air sacs should be considered.
  - If the ovary appears abnormal, biopsy is indicated.
  - Cytology: aspiration of cystic fluid often reveals a low number of cells

TREATMENT

THERAPEUTIC GOALS

- Treat the nonovulating hen through removal of nonovulated follicles, or remove the oviduct.
- Prevent the nonovulatory condition from recurring.

ACUTE GENERAL TREATMENT

- Husbandry modifications
- Change to appropriate diet
- Behavior modification
- Change in the number of hours of light
- Antibiotic treatment for cases of secondary bacterial infection or possible exposure
- Antiinflammatory medication

CHRONIC TREATMENT

- Surgery
  - Aspiration of cysts
  - Salpingohysterectomy and partial ovariectomy are indicated to achieve complete resolution.
- Medications
  - Deslorelin subcutaneous implants 4.7 mg have been used in the treatment of this condition, although there are no studies about the longevity of their action or effectivity.
  - Leuprolide acetate: administer every 14 days; 3 doses are usually adequate
    - 700-800 μg/kg IM for birds weighing <300 g
    - 500 μg/kg IM for birds weighing >300 g
  - Tamoxifen: nonsteroidal antiinflammatory used to block estrogen; leukopenia most frequent side effect
    - 2 mg/kg PO q 24 h
  - Human chorionic gonadotropin: If second egg laid, repeat dose on day 3. If third egg laid, repeat dose on day 7. Not consistently effective, and some birds refractory to treatment
    - 250-500 IU/kg IM on days 1, 3, and 7

POSSIBLE COMPLICATIONS

None noted, other than possible coelomitis associated with chronic inflammation or primary neoplastic disease

RECOMMENDED MONITORING

General condition of patient

PROGNOSIS AND OUTCOME

Prognosis is guarded for reduction in the nonovulatory follicle development of affected hens if the underlying cause is not identified and treated.

PEARLS & CONSIDERATIONS

COMMENTS

Follicular stasis can be treated, but the condition, regardless of the treatment used, does not promote good reproductive status within a breeding aviary. Often very little return is seen in birds in this condition.

PREVENTION

- Proper diet
- Proper husbandry
- Routine checkups by veterinarian
- Examination by veterinarian for baseline medical information and periodic physical examination

CLIENT EDUCATION

As above.

SUGGESTED READINGS

Bowles HL: Evaluating and treating the reproductive system. In Harrison GJ, et al, editors: Clinical avian medicine, vol II, Palm Beach, FL, 2006, Spix Publishing, pp 519–540.

Bowles HL: Reproductive diseases of pet bird species, Vet Clin North Am Exotic Anim Pract 5:489–506, 2002.

AUTHOR: **ALBERTO RODRIGUEZ BARBON**

EDITOR: **THOMAS N. TULLY, JR.**

BIRDS

Foreign Bodies

BASIC INFORMATION

DEFINITION

A foreign body is an inanimate object that is abnormally located in a tissue, duct (e.g., gastrointestinal tract), airway, or cavity of the avian patient.

EPIDEMIOLOGY

SPECIES, AGE, SEX All species and ages and both sexes are possible candidates to present with foreign bodies.

RISK FACTORS

- Tracheal foreign bodies
  - Anatomic characteristics of birds may make them more prone to tracheal foreign bodies: lack of an epiglottis, increased tracheal diameter, increased tidal volume, and narrowing of the distal trachea as it nears the syrinx
  - Millet seed inhalation into the trachea in smaller companion avian species in which this seed is a major part of the diet (e.g., cockatiels, budgerigars)
- Gastrointestinal (GI) foreign bodies
  - Juvenile psittacine species are vigorous feeders before fledgling; they are very curious and frequently ingest foreign bodies such as feeding tubes, cage substrate, toys, or whole seeds.
  - GI foreign bodies are most commonly located in the crop, proventriculus, and ventriculus.

- Ingestion of grit and bedding materials may lead to impaction of the ventriculus.
- Pica may also occur secondary to proventricular disorders (e.g., gastritis, proventricular dilatation disease [PDD]).

ASSOCIATED CONDITIONS AND DISORDERS

- Anorexia
- Depression
- Lack of fecal material
- Grinding of beak
- Open beak breathing
- Dyspnea
- Open distended glottis
- Nonhealing tissue wound

CLINICAL PRESENTATION

DISEASE FORMS/SUBTYPES

- Respiratory
- GI
- Embedded in tissue

HISTORY, CHIEF COMPLAINT

- Nonspecific
- Depression
- Inappetence
- Lack of fecal material
- Nonhealing wound
- Extreme dyspnea
- The bird usually presents with an acute onset of clinical signs, but presentation may be chronic in cases of partial or intermittent obstruction.
- Anorexia can result from a foreign body located in beak/oral tissue. Neurologic signs may be present when heavy metals (e.g., lead) have been ingested.
- Penetrating foreign bodies can be encountered in the tongue, the mouth, the beak, and the skin.

PHYSICAL EXAM FINDINGS

- GI foreign bodies may cause vomiting and/or regurgitation, hemorrhagic enteritis, anorexia, crop stasis, weight loss, and lethargy.
- In cases of perforation (e.g., wire, sewing needle), the bird may be presented with signs of shock or severe depression.
- Open beak breathing
- Distended glottis
- Dehydration
- Nasal, conjunctival, or aural foreign bodies cause an acute, unilateral discharge and/or discomfort.
- Caudoventral displacement of the ventriculus can be palpated when the proventriculus is enlarged.
- Birds with tracheal foreign bodies exhibit voice changes, dyspnea, tail-bobbing, coughing, respiratory distress, open-mouth breathing, and neck extension.

ETIOLOGY AND PATHOPHYSIOLOGY

The foreign body can partially block the respiratory tract or can partially/fully block the GI tract. In either case, the function of the respective body systems will be impaired. If a foreign body perforates the GI tract, the septic condition will adversely affect the health of the animal, in many cases resulting in death.

DIAGNOSIS

DIFFERENTIAL DIAGNOSIS

- Tracheal foreign body
  - Tracheitis: fungal (e.g., *Aspergillus* spp.), bacterial (e.g., Gram negative, *Chlamydophila psittaci*), viral (e.g., Amazon viral tracheitis, parakeet herpes virus, poxvirus, influenza)
  - *Aspergillus* spp.: granuloma of the syrinx, other types of syringeal granulomas
  - Tracheal trauma
  - Glottis, periglottal lesions (e.g., internal papillomatosis)
  - Squamous metaplasia of epithelial surfaces of trachea and syrinx due to hypovitaminosis A
  - Parasites: *Syngamus trachea* (rare in companion birds), *Sternostoma tracheacolum* in passerines
  - Postincubation tracheal stenosis, tracheal xanthogranuloma
  - Neoplasia (e.g., tracheal, syringeal)
  - Respiratory allergy, hypersensitivity (e.g., macaws, Amazon parrots)
  - Airsacculitis, pneumonitis
  - Toxin inhalation (e.g., Teflon [PTFE], cigarette smoke, other pyrrolysis products, ammonia)
  - External compression of the trachea (e.g., goiter, thyroid neoplasia)
  - Extrarespiratory dyspnea due to marked organomegaly or ascites
- GI foreign bodies
  - With complete or partial obstruction
    - Neoplasia (e.g., papilloma, carcinoma, sarcoma)
    - Stricture
    - Intussusception
    - Abscess, granulomas
    - Extraluminal obstruction (e.g., compressing neoplastic mass, egg binding)
    - Impaction (e.g., parasitism, ingestion of excess fine grit)
    - Koilin dysplasia with detachment
  - Without obstruction
    - Proventriculitis: fungal (e.g., *Candida* spp., *Macrorhabdus ornithogaster*), bacterial (e.g., *Chlamydophila psittaci, Mycobacterium* spp., Gram-negative bacteria)
    - PDD
    - Proventricular ulceration with perforation
    - Volvulus
    - Hemorrhagic enteritis, enteritis
    - Lead toxicosis (acute, chronic)
    - Systemic disease leading to GI stasis
- Other locations
  - Nostrils: rhinitis, sinusitis, rhinolith (nasal granuloma located at the level of the nares), choanal atresia
  - Surface epithelium (skin): ulcerative dermatitis, feather picking, trauma

INITIAL DATABASE

- Direct visualization or transillumination of the trachea may reveal a foreign body.
- Wheezing can be heard on auscultation.
- Complete blood count: inconsistent findings. A slight heterophilic leukocytosis may be present because of stress. If a perforation occurs, peritonitis can cause high elevation of heterophils. Chronic disease results in hypoproteinemia, depression anemia (nonregenerative anemia), and sometimes monocytosis.
- Blood gases: on ionogram and venous blood gas, findings are consistent with respiratory acidosis caused by hypoventilation with tracheal obstruction and metabolic alkalosis in cases of vomition
- Microbiologic examination/cytologic examination: can help rule out bacterial, fungal, and neoplastic causes
- Radiography: this imaging technique may be useful in visualizing radiopaque foreign bodies, especially if they contain metal. For GI foreign bodies, a functional ileus is often present with dilatation of the proventriculus and intestinal loops, depending on location. For tracheal foreign bodies, hyperinflation of air sacs is frequently observed.

ADVANCED OR CONFIRMATORY TESTING

- Tissue biopsy for histopathologic examination of suspect mass
- Contrast radiography: contrast radiography may delineate a foreign body in the GI tract with an intraluminal filling defect. Contrast fluoroscopy can also be performed to confirm and further delineate the functional defect. Contrast radiography of the trachea (tracheobronchogram) may be useful in localizing foreign bodies; however, pulmonary edema caused by contrast medium irritation should be a matter of concern.
- Endoscopy is an invaluable tool in diagnosing foreign bodies. Tracheoscopy can be performed using a sheathed 3.5-mm rigid endoscope, an unsheathed 2.7-mm rigid endoscope, a 1.9-mm rigid endoscope, or a 1.2-mm semirigid endoscope, depending on the size of the patient. GI endoscopy can be performed using rigid endoscopy through an ingluviotomy incision or flexible endoscopy. Coelioscopy

can also be used to evaluate the lungs and air sac system.

- Exploratory surgery: an exploratory coeliotomy may be performed to visualize intestinal loops

TREATMENT

THERAPEUTIC GOALS

- Stabilize patient.
- Remove foreign body to regain normal function of affected body system.
- Treat secondary conditions associated with foreign body.

ACUTE GENERAL TREATMENT

- Tracheal foreign bodies
  - Limit stress and place the patient in a critical care unit with supplemental oxygen 10 minutes before an intervention.
  - Air sac cannulation is a necessity.
  - Endoscopically guided removal using grasping forceps may be possible.
  - Suction with a urinary catheter in the smaller bird is another acute treatment option. A needle can be passed through the trachea distal to the foreign body to prevent it from migrating downward.
  - Insertion of a needle below the foreign body to dislodge and expulse via the glottis using a syringe has also been described.
  - Pushing the foreign body into bronchi or an air sac must be considered as a final option for deep foreign bodies.
  - Tracheotomy can be performed in an attempt to retrieve the foreign body. Surgical approach at the level of the thoracic inlet is useful in cases of syringeal obstruction.
  - Tracheostomy should be considered as a final surgical option.
- GI foreign bodies
  - Fluid replacement is mandatory, given that birds with GI foreign bodies are frequently dehydrated.
  - Proventricular lavage can be tried. The bird must be intubated during this procedure.
  - Removal using endoscopy can be attempted, but care should be taken not to lacerate the upper GI tract.
  - Some foreign bodies may be manipulated from the crop to the oral cavity in young birds.
  - A strong magnet glued to the end of a red rubber tube may be used to remove magnetic metal foreign bodies from the crop, proventriculus, and ventriculus.
  - Medications
    - GI motility depressors may be used to relieve GI hypermotility and abdominal discomfort associated with obstruction.
      - Loperamide 0.2 mg/kg IM, IV q 12 h
      - Butylscopolamine 0.4 mg/kg IM, IV q 12 h
    - Gastrokinetics should be avoided in cases where a GI foreign body may be involved.
    - When regurgitation and vomiting are noticed, antiemetic medications that are not gastrokinetic may be given.
      - Metopimazine 0.5-1 mg/kg IM q 24 h
      - Maropitant 1 mg/kg IM q 24 h
    - Gastric protectors are a valuable adjunct for gastric foreign bodies
      - Sucralfate 25 mg/kg PO q 8 h
      - Aluminum hydroxide 30-90 mg/kg PO q 12 h
    - Mineral oil may be tried to help lubricate and pass a foreign body.
    - Chelation therapy should be started when metal objects are discovered and should be continued until blood levels for zinc and lead have been evaluated.
- Other locations (e.g., tissue, coelomic cavity)
  - Removal of the foreign body is followed by débridement, cleaning, and wound care.

CHRONIC TREATMENT

- Tracheal foreign body
  - Tracheal resection and anastomosis may be performed depending on the location and severity of tracheal lesions. Removal of a maximum of five tracheal rings or approximately 10% of the trachea is acceptable.
- GI foreign bodies
  - Ingluviotomy: for foreign bodies also located in the posterior esophagus: An incision is made through the skin overlying the left lateral area of the crop. An incision is made through the crop wall in an avascular area. After the foreign body is removed, the crop incision is closed using a two-layer inverting pattern or one layer of simple continuous sutures followed by an inverting pattern. The skin is closed as a separate layer using a simple interrupted pattern.
  - Proventriculotomy: A left lateral coeliotomy should be performed to visualize the proventriculus. The

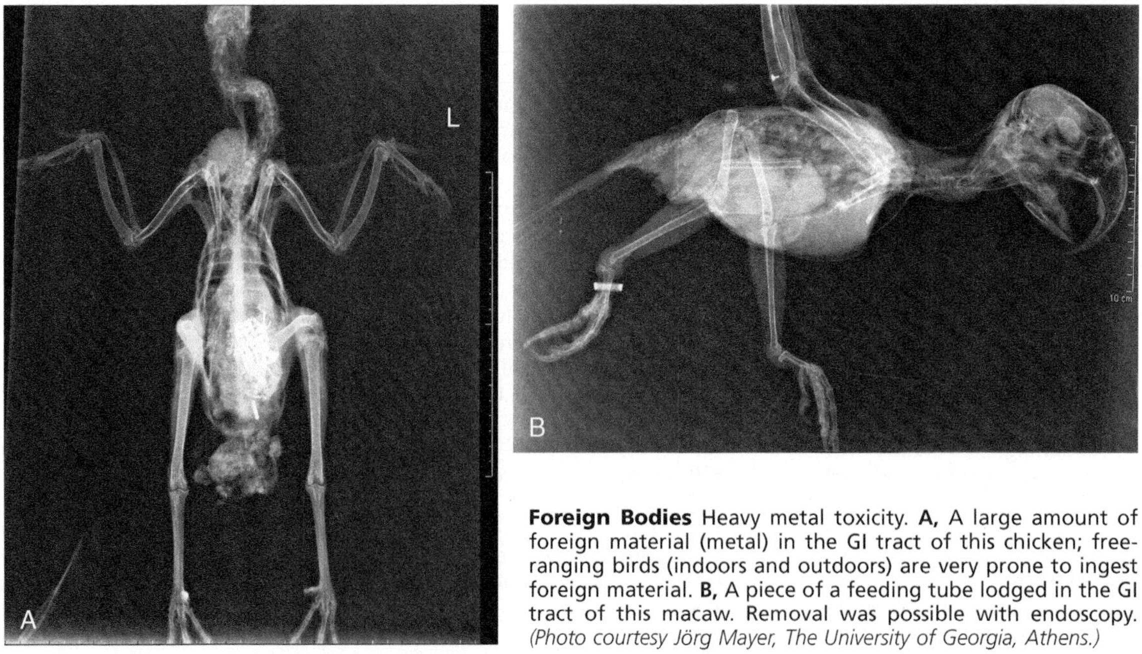

Foreign Bodies Heavy metal toxicity. **A,** A large amount of foreign material (metal) in the GI tract of this chicken; free-ranging birds (indoors and outdoors) are very prone to ingest foreign material. **B,** A piece of a feeding tube lodged in the GI tract of this macaw. Removal was possible with endoscopy. *(Photo courtesy Jörg Mayer, The University of Georgia, Athens.)*

proventriculus is identified, and two stay sutures are placed in this structure. The coelomic cavity is then packed with moistened gauze sponges. The proventriculus is incised underneath the liver for removal of the foreign body. The proventriculus incision is closed in two layers (one simple continuous and the second inverted). The liver is then placed over the incision to promote healing.
- Enterotomy: Microsurgical techniques are required when performing enterotomy surgeries due to the thin and delicate nature of the avian intestines. The enterotomy procedures are required for intestinal foreign body removal.

POSSIBLE COMPLICATIONS

- Pressure necrosis of the tissue where the foreign body lodges
- Septicemia if the foreign body perforates the GI tract
- Heavy metal toxicosis associated with lead, copper, and zinc foreign body ingestion

RECOMMENDED MONITORING

- Surgical sites
- Respiratory function post removal
- GI function post removal

PROGNOSIS AND OUTCOME

- In most cases, the prognosis is good if secondary complications are minor and the foreign body is completely removed.
- Management of tracheal foreign bodies in small psittacines (e.g., cockatiels, budgerigars) and syringeal granulomas in medium-sized parrots (e.g., African grey) and macaws is challenging, and these conditions may carry a poor prognosis.

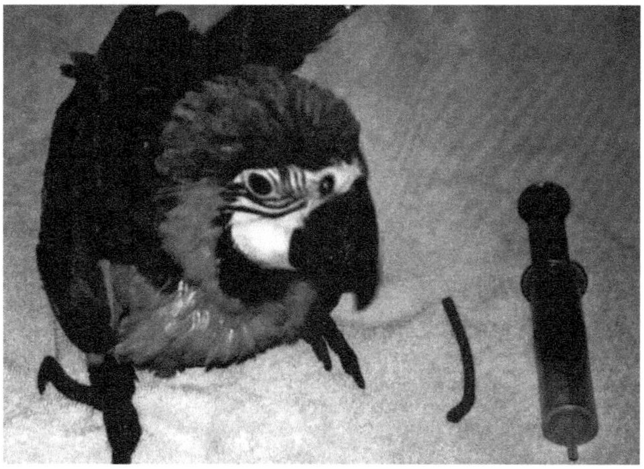

Foreign Bodies Foreign body (tube) removed from macaw.

PEARLS & CONSIDERATIONS

COMMENTS

- A quick presentation of an avian patient suffering from foreign body ingestion or inhalation will usually increase the chance for treatment success.
- Pet bird owners should be aware of clinical signs associated with foreign body disease.
- New pet bird owners should purchase only domestically raised, weaned companion psittacine species.

PREVENTION

- Proper feeding and careful supervision of young companion avian species are recommended.
- Unweaned birds should be hand-fed only by experienced personnel.
- Cage toys and furniture appropriate for the size of the bird in question should be purchased.
- Prevent access to heavy metals (e.g., lead).

CLIENT EDUCATION

See above.

SUGGESTED READINGS

Bennett RA, et al: Soft tissue surgery. In Ritchie BW, et al, editors: Avian medicine: principles and application, Lake Worth, FL, 1994, Wingers Publishing, pp 1096–1136.
Clayton LA, et al: Endoscopic-assisted removal of a tracheal seed foreign body in a cockatiel *(Nymphicus hollandicus)*, J Avian Med Surg 19:14–18, 2005.
Ford S: Tracheal foreign body removal in small birds, Proc Annu Conf Assoc Avian Vet 49–53, 2007.
Hadley TL: Disorders of the psittacine gastrointestinal tract, Vet Clin North Am Exotic Anim Pract 8:329–349, 2005.
Lumeij J: Gastroenterology. In Ritchie BW, et al, editors: Avian medicine: principles and application, Lake Worth, FL, 1994, Wingers Publishing, pp 482–521.
Tully TN, et al: Pneumonology. In Ritchie BW, et al, editors: Avian medicine: principles and application, Lake Worth, FL, 1994, Wingers Publishing, pp 556–581.
Westerhof I: Treatment of tracheal obstruction in psittacines using a suction technique: a retrospective study of 19 birds, J Avian Med Surg 9:45–49, 1995.

AUTHORS: **HUGUES BEAUFRÈRE AND W. MICHAEL TAYLOR**

EDITOR: **THOMAS N. TULLY, JR.**

BIRDS

Fractures

BASIC INFORMATION

DEFINITION

A break in a bone

SYNONYM

Broken bone

EPIDEMIOLOGY

SPECIES, AGE, SEX All species and ages and both sexes

RISK FACTORS

- Trauma
- Calcium deficiency resulting in pathologic fractures
- Hens that are prolific egg layers that have no calcium supplementation
- Pellets from a gun
- Improper handling
- A bird that is frightened when restrained
- Crushing injury

ASSOCIATED CONDITIONS AND DISORDERS

- Neurologic disorders
- Anorexia
- Lameness
- Inability to fly
- Septicemia
- Weakness

CLINICAL PRESENTATION

DISEASE FORMS/SUBTYPES

- Closed fracture
- Open fracture
- Pathologic fracture
- Amputation

HISTORY, CHIEF COMPLAINT

- Lameness
- Depression
- Inappetence
- Paralysis
- Inability to fly
- Bleeding from area on affected limb
- Broken beak

PHYSICAL EXAM FINDINGS

- Laxity in long bones of affected limb
- Beak fracture and trauma
- Weakness
- Lameness
- Paralysis/paresis
- Subcutaneous emphysema if pneumatic bones fractured (e.g., humerus)

ETIOLOGY AND PATHOPHYSIOLOGY

- Stress on the cortical bone can result in a break of the cortex. A complete break of the cortex that penetrates the skin is called an *open fracture.* A complete closed fracture does not penetrate the skin. When only one radiographic cortex is broken, this is called an *incomplete* or *greenstick fracture.* Fractures can occur transverse across the cortex or at an oblique angle. Multiple bone fragments constitute a compound fracture.
- Pathologic fractures occur as the result of weakened cortices caused by resorption of calcium secondary to nutritional imbalance or preexisting disease processes such as osteomyelitis and neoplasia.
- Amputation consists of complete fracture and removal of the distal extremity tissue, including bone. Nonelective amputation in avian species usually occurs as the result of a predator attack and bite wounds.

DIAGNOSIS

DIFFERENTIAL DIAGNOSIS

- Soft-tissue trauma
- Joint luxation
- Generalized toxicity
- Neoplasia
- Neurologic disease
- Organophosphate toxicity

INITIAL DATABASE

- Complete blood cout (CBC)
- Plasma biochemistry panel
- Fecal parasite examination

ADVANCED OR CONFIRMATORY TESTING

Imaging: radiographs—two planes

TREATMENT

THERAPEUTIC GOALS

- Stabilize and improve patient's physical condition.
- Stabilize fracture(s).
- Treat any secondary disease processes.
- Promote fracture healing to maintain a good quality of life.
- If fracture caused by nutritional deficiencies, appropriately adjust the diet.
- If amputation occurs owing to a bite wound, treat the patient to prevent secondary bacterial septicemia.

ACUTE GENERAL TREATMENT

- All treatment is to be performed on a stable patient.
  - Nursing care
    - Administer warmed crystalloid fluids SC, IV, IO (50-150 mL/kg/d maintenance plus dehydration deficit factored in if needed) at a rate of 10-25 mL/kg over a 5-minute period or at a continuous rate of 100 mL/kg/q 24 h.
    - Increase environmental temperature to 85°F-90°F (29°C-32°C).
    - Provide a humidified environment by placing warm moist towels in the incubator.
    - Nutritional support is required in most cases.
- Fractures involving the bones of the distal limb can often be splinted or placed in a coaptation bandage (e.g., figure-of-eight, syringe case splint).
- Fractures of the femur and humerus require open fixation. In extremely small and light birds (e.g., budgerigar), a femur fracture will heal with cage rest.
- Surgical considerations: the patient should be stabilized and placed on pain management before any surgery procedure is attempted.
  - Surgical methods used in mammalian patients can be applied to avian fractures.
  - Because of the very strong thin cortical bone, plates that have screws are often difficult to use owing to the relatively small area of bone for the screw to gain purchase.
- Medications
  - Drugs of choice
    - Pain management
      - Butorphanol 0.5-4 mg/kg IM, IV q 1-4 h
      - Meloxicam 0.2 mg/kg PO, IM, q 24 h
    - Antibiotics: usually a third-generation cephalosporin is a good choice
      - Cefotaxime 75-100 mg/kg IM, IV q 4-8 h
      - Ceftazidime 50-100 mg/kg IM, IV q 4-8 h

RECOMMENDED MONITORING

- Repeat radiographs to determine healing progress and growing stability of fracture.
- Repeat CBC and plasma chemistry panel to monitor treatment response and recovery.
- Monitor appetite, fecal output, and behavior during treatment period.

PROGNOSIS AND OUTCOME

- Acute cases have a good prognosis, especially if surrounding tissue and blood supply are intact.
- Closed fractures have a better prognosis than open fractures.
- Simple fractures have a better healing prognosis than compound fractures.
- Maxillary and mandibular beak fractures are difficult to heal. Complete fractures of the maxillary or mandibular part of the beak will not heal.
- Pathologic fractures due to nutritional deficiencies will heal once the dietary insufficiencies are resolved. If significant changes to the bone structure do not occur, the prognosis for an acceptable recovery is good.

PEARLS & CONSIDERATIONS

COMMENTS

- The cortices of avian bone are strong but brittle.
- The cortices of avian bone offer less holding power for orthopedic devices, and the cortices will shatter easily when pressure is applied.
- It is difficult to find enough cancellous bone for grafting; therefore, this procedure is rarely performed on avian patients.
- Birds have pneumatic bones in which the medullary cavity directly communicates with the air sac system. Know which bones are pneumatic (e.g., humerus).
- Avian bones easily penetrate the surface epithelium when fractured owing to lack of surrounding soft tissue.

PREVENTION

- Prevent trauma (see Trauma).
- Prevent nutritional deficiencies.

- Provide an appropriate diet, especially to reproductively active hens.

CLIENT EDUCATION

See Prevention.

SUGGESTED READINGS

Harcourt-Brown N: Orthopaedic and beak surgery. In Harcourt-Brown N, et al, editors: BSAVA manual of psittacine birds, ed 2, Quedgeley, Gloucester, 2005, British Small Animal Veterinary Association Woodrow House, pp 120–135.

Olsen GH, et al: Limb dysfunction. In Olsen GH, et al, editors: Manual of avian medicine, St Louis, 2000, Mosby Inc., pp 493–526.

Pollock CG, et al: Birds. In Carpenter JW, editor: Exotic animal formulary, ed 3, St Louis, 2005, Elsevier/Saunders, pp 135–264.

Tully TN: Orthopedics, Vet Clin North Am Exotic Anim Pract 5:1–96, 2002.

CROSS-REFERENCES TO OTHER SECTIONS

Trauma

AUTHOR & EDITOR: **THOMAS N. TULLY, JR.**

BIRDS

Gout

BASIC INFORMATION

DEFINITION

Gout is defined as abnormal accumulation of uric acid in the bloodstream and consequent deposition of uric acid on and within visceral tissues and articular surfaces. Uric acid is the end product of nitrogen metabolism in birds, and it is produced in the liver. Gout is classified as visceral or articular; both disease presentations may occasionally occur in the same patient.

SYNONYMS

Articular gout, visceral gout

EPIDEMIOLOGY

SPECIES, AGE, SEX All species, regardless of age and sex, are susceptible to this disease condition.

GENETICS AND BREED PREDISPOSITION Budgerigars appear to be predisposed to articular gout.

RISK FACTORS

- Older birds
- Dehydration
- All-seed diet or improper nutritional intake

ASSOCIATED CONDITIONS AND DISORDERS

- Lameness
- Depression
- Anorexia
- Organ failure (e.g., renal)
- Fluffed feathers (hypothermia)

CLINICAL PRESENTATION

DISEASE FORMS/SUBTYPES

- Articular gout: uric acid deposits within synovial capsules and tendon sheaths of joints, in particular, the metatarsal and phalangeal joints
- Visceral gout: uric acid deposits on and within the tissue of major organs

HISTORY, CHIEF COMPLAINT

- Birds suffering from the effects of articular gout generally present with signs of shifting leg lameness, an inability to flex and extend certain joints, and joint swelling.
- Birds affected by visceral gout usually display nonspecific clinical signs (e.g., lethargy, anorexia, dehydration).

PHYSICAL EXAM FINDINGS

- White raised nodules on the feet and lower legs
- Polyuria and polydipsia, especially in larger parrots
- Nonspecific depression, anorexia, and depression

ETIOLOGY AND PATHOPHYSIOLOGY

Renal disease, increased protein ingestion, prolonged dehydration, or reduced renal excretion of urates can result in decreased uric acid elimination and consequent elevation in blood uric acid levels. Blood level increases in uric acid due to renal insufficiency eventually will lead to the ability of the animal to adequately maintain the solubility of sodium urate in plasma, resulting in monosodium urate crystal precipitation in tissues.

DIAGNOSIS

DIFFERENTIAL DIAGNOSIS

- Multiple septic joints
- Severe immune-mediated polyarthropathy
- Other systemic illness causing nonspecific clinical signs (e.g., infectious, metabolic, neoplastic disease)

INITIAL DATABASE

- Complete blood count (CBC): may reveal a nonregenerative anemia, secondary to decreased secretion of erythropoietin in severe, prolonged cases of renal disease
- Plasma biochemistry panel: biochemical analysis of plasma typically reveals a pronounced elevation in uric acid and may also reveal an inverse calcium-to-phosphorus ratio
- Radiographic imaging: radiographs may reveal radiopaque opacities on articular and visceral surfaces
- Cytologic smears of raised white nodules on the feet: Gram's stain of the white chalky material harvested from raised white nodules on the feet of an affected bird will show Gram-positive uric acid crystals

ADVANCED OR CONFIRMATORY TESTING

- Ultrasound of internal organs: although difficult to perform in avian species because of the extensive coelomic air sac system, hyperechoic areas within the kidneys may be indicative of uric acid crystal deposits in renal tissue.
- Gross necropsy/histopathologic examination: visceral gout is characterized by precipitation of urate crystals in the kidneys or on the serosal surfaces of heart, liver, mesenteries, air sacs, and/or peritoneum. Articular gout is characterized by deposits of urate crystals (also known as *tophi*) on both intraarticular and periarticular tissues (e.g., synovial capsules, tendon sheaths). Urate deposits in both articular and visceral gout appear grossly as a chalky, white covering. Uric acid crystals have been observed histologically within the lamina propria of the proventriculus, ventriculus, intestines, and kidney. Periodic renal biopsies will facilitate assessment of renal pathology.

TREATMENT

THERAPEUTIC GOALS

- Pain management
- Antiinflammatory medication
- Supportive care
- Medication used for treatment of increased uric acid blood levels to reduce the incidence of tissue and articular deposition of uric acid crystals has uniformly been disappointing when birds diagnosed with articular and/or visceral gout are treated.

ACUTE GENERAL TREATMENT

- Hyperuricemia is treated with aggressive diuresis with intravenous or intrasosseous fluid therapy.

- Appropriate diet modifications are made (to decrease protein ingestion).
- Prolonged subcutaneous fluid administration is often recommended upon discharge from the hospital.

CHRONIC TREATMENT

- Although clinical response to treatment is poor to nonexistent and no scientific evidence indicates that therapeutic measures used to treat uricemia are successful, clinicians try to use drugs to combat this condition with awareness that no other options are available.
  - Allopurinol 10 mg/kg PO q 4-12 h
  - Colchicine 0.04 mg/kg PO q 12-24 h
  - Vitamin A 33,000 IU/kg (10,000 IU/300 g) IM q 7 d (Aquasol)
  - Omega-3 fatty acid 0.1-0.2 mL/kg of flaxseed oil to corn oil mixed at a ratio of 1:4 PO or added to food; ratio of omega-6/omega-3 is 4-5:1

DRUG INTERACTIONS

Dehydration and renal disease associated with visceral gout may result in adverse responses to nonsteroidal antiinflammatory medications, especially cyclooxygenase (COX) inhibitory products (e.g., meloxicam).

POSSIBLE COMPLICATIONS

- Internal organ failure
- Death
- Non–weight-bearing lameness

RECOMMENDED MONITORING

- Hydration status
- Body condition
- Uric acid levels
- Liver enzyme levels

PROGNOSIS AND OUTCOME

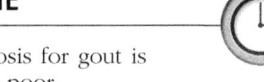

The prognosis for gout is guarded to poor.

PEARLS & CONSIDERATIONS

COMMENTS

- Proper diet and consistent water availability are the best measures to prevent onset of gout in birds.
- Once the disease process has begun, it is very difficult if not impossible to treat an avian patient.

PREVENTION

Yearly health maintenance visits to the veterinarian and consequent yearly biochemistry analyses allow for early detection of slight increases in uric acid levels and initiation of prophylactic subcutaneous fluid administration.

CLIENT EDUCATION

See above.

SUGGESTED READING

Echols MS: Evaluating and treating the kidneys. In Harrison GJ, et al, editors: Clinical avian medicine, vol II, Palm Beach, FL, 2006, Spix Publishing, pp 451–492.

AUTHOR: **MEGAN KIRCHGESSNER**

EDITOR: **THOMAS N. TULLY, JR.**

BIRDS

Heavy Metal Toxicity

Client Education Sheet Available on Website

BASIC INFORMATION

DEFINITION

Intoxication due to acute or chronic exposure to some form of heavy metal, most commonly lead, zinc, and copper (less commonly, mercury and iron). Heparinized whole-blood lead concentrations greater than 20 µg/dL (0.2 ppm) are suggestive and levels greater than 50 µg/dL (0.5 ppm) are diagnostic in most psittacine birds when accompanied by clinical signs. Blood zinc levels greater than 200 µg/dL (2.0 ppm) are suggestive of zinc toxicosis.

SYNONYM

Plumbism for lead toxicity

EPIDEMIOLOGY

SPECIES, AGE, SEX Most commonly reported in psittacines, waterfowl, and raptors fed with gunshot prey

RISK FACTORS

- Potential sources of lead include weights (curtains, fishing and diving, sailing and boating accessories, wheel balances), bells with lead clappers, batteries, solder, lead pellets from shotgun shells, lead-based paints, lead-free paints with leaded drying agents, galvanized wire, glazed ceramics, costume jewelry, contaminated cuttlefish bone, seeds for planting (coated with lead arsenate), and mirror backs.
- Potential sources of zinc include galvanized containers, galvanized mesh, hardware cloth, staples, galvanized nails, fertilizers, some paints, zinc pyrithione shampoos, zinc oxide, zinc undecylenate (Desenex cream), and pennies (post 1982).

CLINICAL PRESENTATION

HISTORY, CHIEF COMPLAINT Ingestion of particles containing lead, zinc, or copper; gunshot pellets affecting joints

PHYSICAL EXAM FINDINGS

- Depression
- Weakness
- Vomiting
- Diarrhea
- Polyuria
- Polydipsia
- Anorexia
- Ataxia
- Seizures
- Hemoglobinuria: lead toxicity

ETIOLOGY AND PATHOPHYSIOLOGY

- Lead is absorbed in the gastrointestinal tract; it is retained by soft tissues and stored in bone.
- Lead is slowly excreted by the kidneys and appears to affect major organs, as seen in direct effects of necrosis in gastrointestinal tract epithelium, damage to red blood cells (increased fragility), depression of bone marrow, liver degeneration and necrosis, and central nervous system (CNS) edema.
- Zinc is absorbed in the gastrointestinal tract and distributes to various tissues (e.g., liver, kidney, reproductive), but the pancreas is the target organ. Zinc is not stored in bone.

DIAGNOSIS

DIFFERENTIAL DIAGNOSIS

- Infectious encephalopathy
- Proventricular dilatation disease
- Infectious enteritis and hepatitis

INITIAL DATABASE

- Complete blood count (CBC)/Biochemistry

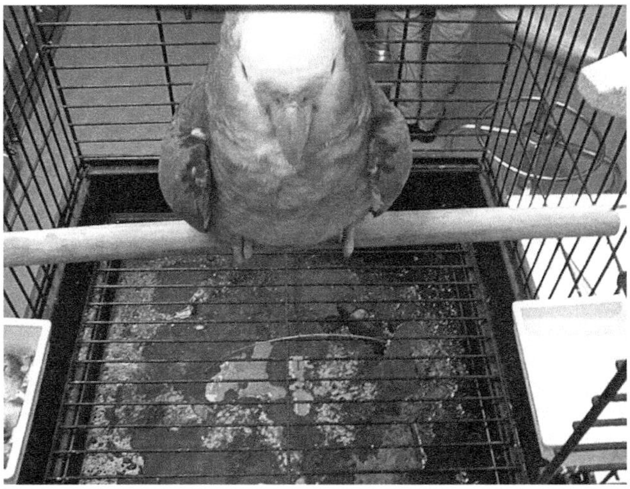

Heavy Metal Toxicity Yellow-headed Amazon parrot with hemoglobinuria caused by lead toxicity. *(Photo courtesy Jörg Mayer, The University of Georgia, Athens.)*

- Leukocytosis in most heavy metal toxicosis
- Hypochromic regenerative anemia occurs in some affected birds.
- Elevation of lactate dehydrogenase (LDH), aspartate aminotransferase (AST), bile acids, and creatine phosphokinase (CPK)
- Lipase and amylase may be elevated in zinc toxicity.

ADVANCED OR CONFIRMATORY TESTING

- Lead tissue concentrations (liver, kidney, brain) of 3 to 6 ppm wet weight are suggestive of lead toxicosis; concentrations greater than 6 ppm are diagnostic.
- Zinc tissue concentrations in the pancreas of 26.11 μg/g on a dry weight basis were considered normal in cockatiels; concentrations of 312.4-2418 μg/g were considered toxic. In liver, asymptomatic birds are less than 40 ppm wet weight, and concentrations greater than 75 ppm were correlated with toxicosis.
- Imaging: radiopaque metal density material may be noted in the gastrointestinal tract; not diagnostic

TREATMENT

ACUTE GENERAL TREATMENT

- Appropriate health care
  - Inpatient
    - First course of chelation, depending on severity of clinical signs
    - Supportive therapy is directed at controlling seizures, anemia, immune suppression, and anorexia.
  - Nursing care
    - Administer warmed crystalloids SC (50 mL/kg) or IV or IO (10-25 mL/kg over 5 minutes), at bolus 24 h to d or continuous rate (100 mL/kg/24 h).
    - Increase environmental temperature to 85°F-95°F (29°C-35°C).
    - Nutritional support is required in most cases.
- Surgical considerations
  - The need for surgery is not urgent as long as the bird is given chelation and is improving.
  - Removal of heavy metal objects from the gastrointestinal tract or affected joints
  - Use of a magnet attached to an enteral tube is useful in ferrous items that are zinc coated. Endoscopic removal of heavy metal particles or gastric lavage can be attempted in stable patients that are of sufficient size. Occasionally, proventriculotomy or enterotomy may be necessary if other attempts to remove metal particles fail.
- Medications
  - Drugs of choice
    - Midazolam or diazepam 0.5-2 mg/kg IV or IM for controlling seizures. Diazepam has poor IM absorption compared with midazolam. Repeat if necessary.
    - Fluid therapy with crystalloids SC, IV, or IO 100 mL/kg/24 h to d.
    - Calcium disodiumversenate ($CaNa_2EDTA$) 35 mg/kg IM or SC q 12 h for 5 days, then off for 3 days, then repeat as needed
    - Bulk diets and cathartics (e.g., grit, metamucil, peanut butter) to evacuate particles from the gastrointestinal tract
    - Antibiotics and antifungals may be indicated because lead can be immune suppressive.
    - Nutritional support is required in most cases.

DRUG INTERACTIONS

- Possible interactions
  - Depletion of zinc, iron, and manganese with long-term chelation therapy
- Alternative drugs
  - D-Penicillamine 30-55 mg/kg PO q 12 h
  - Dimercaptosuccinic acid (DMSA) 25-35 mg/kg PO q 12 h; preferred oral chelator
  - D-Penicillamine: do not give if lead or zinc is present in the gastrointestinal tract (increases absorption)
  - Cathartics may cause diarrhea and are contraindicated in dehydrated and hypovolemic birds.

RECOMMENDED MONITORING

- Blood heavy metal should be assessed after chelation of therapy.
- Repeat CBC and chemistry panel to monitor progress.

PROGNOSIS AND OUTCOME

Permanent neurologic signs (e.g., blindness) possible

PEARLS & CONSIDERATIONS

COMMENTS

- Signs should dramatically improve within 24-48 hours after chelation therapy is begun.
- Severe cases with chronic exposure may have permanent damage.

PREVENTION

Determine source of heavy metals and remove them from the patient's environment.

SUGGESTED READINGS

Dumonceaus G, et al: Toxins. In Ritchie BW, et al, editors: Avian medicine: principles and applications, Brentwood, TN, 1994, HBD International Inc., pp 1030–1052.

LaBonde J: Toxicity in pet avian patients, Sem Avian Exotic Pet Med 4:23–31, 1995.

Puschner B, Poppenga RH: Lead and zinc intoxication in companion birds, Compend Contin Educ Vet 31(1):El–12, 2009.

Samour J: Lead toxicosis in falcons: a method for lead retrieval, Semin Avian Exotic Pet Med 14:143–148, 2005.

AUTHOR: **DAVID SANCHEZ-MIGALLON GUZMAN**

EDITOR: **THOMAS N. TULLY, JR.**

BIRDS

Hepatic Lipidosis

BASIC INFORMATION

DEFINITION

Hepatopathy induced by metabolic changes that lead to an excessive accumulation of triglycerides in liver tissue, with resulting cholestasis and hepatic dysfunction

SYNONYMS

Fatty liver syndrome, hepatic steatosis, fatty infiltration of the liver

EPIDEMIOLOGY

SPECIES, AGE, SEX All species and ages and both sexes

GENETICS AND BREED PREDISPOSITION Amazon parrots, galah cockatoos, cockatoos, budgerigars, lorikeets

RISK FACTORS Given the complexity of lipid metabolism (avian lipid metabolism pathways and regulation are not fully understood), a multitude of factors may predispose a bird to hepatic lipidosis.

- High-fat, low-protein diet
- Overfeeding of neonates (cockatoos, macaws) using a high-energy ration
- Multinutrient-deficient diet, especially essential fatty acids (linoleic acid), essential and sulfur amino acids (choline, methionine, cysteine), lipotrophic factors that promote metabolism of fat (L-carnitine), and vitamins such as biotin, vitamin E, vitamins B_1, B_2, B_6, and B_{12}, and folic acid
  - o Impaired fatty acid beta-oxidation
  - o Impaired synthesis and secretion of very low-density lipoproteins (VLDLs) essential for normal hepatic lipid metabolism and transport
  - o Impaired lipolysis, excessive hepatic lipogenesis
- Restricted exercise, sedentary lifestyle
- Hereditary factors
- Increased lipogenesis such as estrogen-induced lipogenesis during active egg laying, increased activity of hormone-sensitive lipase with diabetes mellitus, stress-associated hepatic lipogenesis and peripheral lipolysis (promoted by catecholamines, corticosteroids, and thyroxine), and estrogenic-like action of pesticides
- Thyroid dysfunction
- Acute release of fatty acids from adipose stores in an overweight and anorectic bird does not seem to promote fatty liver syndrome as observed in cats.

ASSOCIATED CONDITIONS AND DISORDERS

- Obesity
- Atherosclerosis
- Neurologic signs
- Fat emboli in brain tissue
- Dyspnea
- Weakness

CLINICAL PRESENTATION

DISEASE FORMS/SUBTYPES Hepatic lipidosis with resulting cholestasis and hepatic dysfunction

HISTORY, CHIEF COMPLAINT The bird may be presented for anorexia, dyspnea, nonspecific sickness, green stools, regurgitation, or polyuria-polydipsia. History frequently points out an improper nutritional background. Upon physical examination, the bird is often noted to be obese or slightly overweight.

PHYSICAL EXAM FINDINGS

- Lethargy, weakness, weight loss
- Dehydration
- Hepatic enlargement that may be palpable or visible through the skin
- Dyspnea due to hepatic enlargement and/or intracoelomic fat accumulation
- Abdominal distention due to hepatic enlargement and/or ascites (usually with concurrent heart disease)
- Biliverdinuria (increased renal excretion of biliverdin) due to cholestasis
- Poor feather condition: pigment changes, stress bars
- Neurologic signs due to hepatic encephalopathy (rare)
- Polyuria, diarrhea, regurgitation, and/or vomiting
- Melena, bloody droppings in case of coagulopathy (final stage)
- Some integument conditions of poorly understood pathogenesis are occasionally associated with lipid hepatopathy:
  - o Overgrown rhinotheca with abnormal “woody” or “punky” keratin (especially budgerigars) (see Overgrown Beak and Claws)
  - o Feather picking
  - o Abnormal nail keratin consistency and color

ETIOLOGY AND PATHOPHYSIOLOGY

The general disease signs are various but consistent with hepatic failure, enlargement, or insufficiency. The course of the disease is generally chronic, but clinical illness may appear acute. Concurrent conditions associated with poor nutrition may also be present. The laying hen may die acutely of fatty liver hemorrhagic syndrome resulting from rupture of hepatic blood vessels during egg laying. It should be stressed that other forms of lipid deposition (e.g., atherosclerosis; fat deposition in kidneys, skin, abdomen, lungs, and spleen) that lead to other physical findings can be found concurrently with hepatic lipidosis.

DIAGNOSIS

DIFFERENTIAL DIAGNOSIS

Any hepatobiliary disease, particularly if chronic and noninfectious, that could induce hepatomegaly

- Hepatic congestion, portal hypertension
- Hepatic fibrosis, cirrhosis
- Hepatotoxins: mycotoxins (e.g., aflatoxins produced by *Aspergillus* spp., ochratoxins), plants, drugs (e.g., antifungals, volatile anesthetics, some antibiotics, steroids), pesticides, heavy metals, environmental toxins, vitamin A
- Hepatic neoplasia or metastasis to liver
- Amyloidosis (rarely reported in psittacines)
- Iron storage disease, especially in lorikeets, Sturnidae, and Ramphastidae
- Infectious hepatitis: bacterial (*Chlamydophila psittaci*, *Mycobacteria*

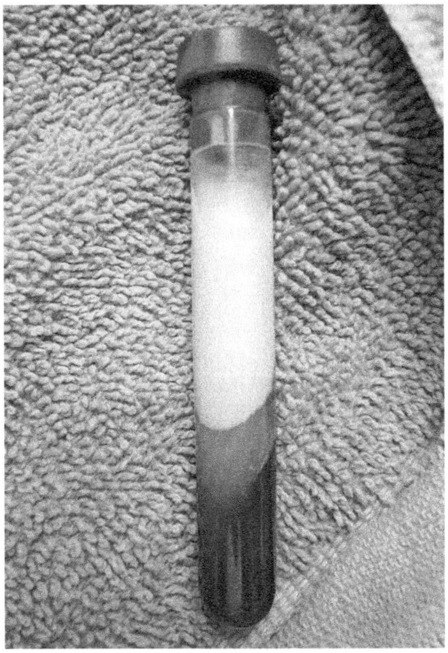

Hepatic Lipidosis Severe hypercholesterolemia in a bird. This can often be seen in birds on a high-fat diet. *(Photo courtesy Jörg Mayer, The University of Georgia, Athens.)*

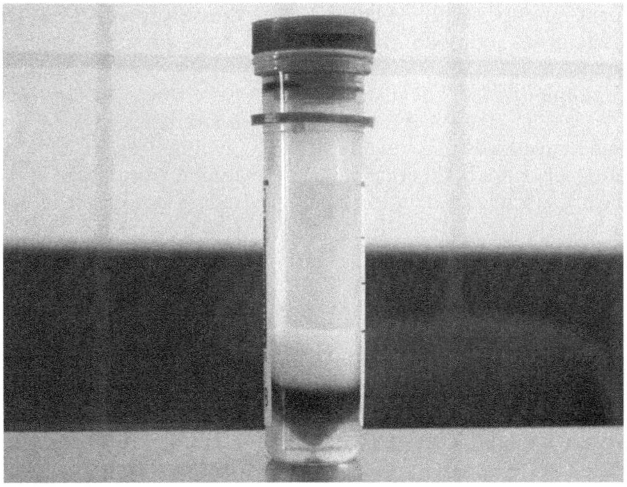

Hepatic Lipidosis Severely lipemic serum from a cockatiel diagnosed with hepatic lipidosis; such lipemia interferes strongly with biochemistry. *(Courtesy Hugues Beaufrère and Clinique Vétérinaire Brasseur.)*

spp., Gram-negative hepatitis), viral (polyomavirus, herpesvirus, adenovirus, reovirus), and parasitic (trematodes, protozoa)
  - Conditions causing extra-respiratory dyspnea
- Other organomegaly, intraabdominal masses

INITIAL DATABASE

Complete blood count (CBC) often shows a mild nonregenerative anemia and mild leukocytosis or leukopenia. CBC helps to rule out inflammatory hepatopathies.

- Clinical pathologic examination should target and evaluate recent hepatocellular damage, hepatic function, lipid metabolism, and electrolytes.
- Aspartate aminotransferase (AST): high sensitivity but low specificity should always be interpreted with creatine kinase (CK) values. Plasma activities may be normal in very advanced cases and are not consistently increased in hepatic lipidosis.
- Glutamate dehydrogenase (GLDH): mitochondrial enzyme, low sensitivity but high specificity, accurate elevation in cases of severe hepatocellular damage
- Bile acids: high sensitivity and high specificity, test hepatic function, moderate to high elevation
- Total protein (TP), albumin, coagulation factors, uric acid: decreased with impairment of hepatic production
- Hypoglycemia may be seen because of impaired gluconeogenesis, starvation, or chronic disease; elevation in cases of diabetes mellitus
- Lipemic serum and hyperlipidemia are common with elevation in triglycerides and cholesterol due to impaired lipid metabolism. Lipemic serum can strongly interfere with some biochemical tests.
- Hypokalemia could also be present if the bird has regurgitated, has vomited, or is polyuric.

ADVANCED OR CONFIRMATORY TESTING

- Imaging
  - Radiographs frequently reveal an enlarged liver with compression of coelomic air sacs and concomitant overinflation of axillary diverticuli of interclavicular air sacs. Ascites may be present but is rarely important without concurrent heart disease. Cardiomegaly should be ruled out.
  - Ultrasonographic examination of the liver in affected birds shows an enlarged liver with rounded margins and diffuse alteration of parenchyma, which is hyperechoic. Ascites may be confirmed as well. Ultrasound examination is especially useful to rule out liver congestion, in which biopsy could lead to a fatal hemorrhage.
  - Endoscopy allows visualization of the liver via a lateral approach, through entry into the ventral hepatic peritoneal cavity from the left or right caudal thoracic air sacs, or by a direct approach, via the ventral midline. Livers exhibiting lipidosis are enlarged with pale or mottled yellow parenchyma and rounded margins.
- Histopathologic examination
  - Definitive diagnosis of hepatic lipidosis requires a liver biopsy that may be taken using endoscopy, ultrasound, or surgery. Histologically, hepatic lipidosis is characterized by vacuolation and degeneration of hepatocytes. A prognosis may be determined by assessing the degree of degeneration, vacuolation, and inflammation present in the sample.
  - Birds with severe hepatic lipidosis are in metabolic crisis, and anesthesia for collection of a liver biopsy is inappropriate until the patient is stabilized.

TREATMENT

THERAPEUTIC GOALS

- Stabilize and improve patient's physical condition.
- Improve nutritional status of patient.
- Treat secondary conditions that may be leading to patient's poor physical health.
- Develop a plan for gradual weight loss and improved nutritional offerings.
- Improve status of liver function.
- Increase patient exercise if appropriate, to consume energy and to stimulate enteric motility.
- Limit stress, which may promote storage of triglycerides in the liver.

ACUTE GENERAL TREATMENT

- Supportive care
  - Fluid replacement is important because dehydration compromises hepatic circulation. Avoid lactated fluids because a bird with severe hepatic lipidosis could present lactate intolerance. Avoid excessive glucose or dextrose infusion, which is thought to potentiate triglyceride accumulation by inhibiting beta-oxidation of fatty acids.

- Supplement fluids with water-soluble vitamins, and with potassium if hypokalemic.
- Consider administration of vitamin K_1.
- Hypoproteinemic birds may require the addition of colloids (hetastarch, oxyglobin) 10-15 mL/kg/d IV or a 5 mL/kg bolus.
- Ascitic fluid should not be removed by abdominocentesis because this would deplete protein stores, except if the bird is severely dyspneic. Just remove as needed for diagnostic purposes.
- Place the bird in an incubator with oxygen if very depressed or dyspneic.

- Other considerations
  - Hepatic encephalopathy, if present, may be managed with lactulose 150-650 mg/kg q 12 h. Supplementation with proteins should be limited.
  - Ascites should be controlled with furosemide 1-2 mg/kg as needed, generally once to twice daily.
  - Vomiting, regurgitation, and nausea can be addressed with antiemetic drugs: metoclopramide 0.5 mg/kg q 6 h, metopimazine 0.5-1 mg/kg q 24 h.
  - Chronic egg laying or reproductive status should be suppressed with leuprolide acetate 500-1000 mcg/kg q 14 d or hCG 500-1000 IU q 3-5 wk.
  - Ursodeoxycholic acid has been shown to have cytoprotective, anti-inflammatory, antioxidant, and anti-fibrotic effects on hepatocytes, and to increase the production of glutathione. This drug is used in human medicine for cholestasis and attenuation of hepatotoxicity, and in feline medicine for cholangiohepatitis. However, no real benefit has been demonstrated in feline or human medicine in triglyceride accumulation disorders. Dosage: 15 mg/kg q 24 h

CHRONIC TREATMENT

- Nutritional considerations
  - Providing a well-balanced diet free of toxins is the single most important treatment in hepatic lipidosis; formulated diets with correct quantities of fresh fruits and vegetables are highly suggested.
  - Supplement proteins to reduce lipid accumulation in the liver unless hepatic encephalopathy is a concern. Several recovery or neonatal psittacine formulas have a high content of proteins and should be used for nutritional support in birds suffering from hepatic lipidosis (e.g., Recovery Formula, Harrison Bird Food, crude protein 35%; Exact, Kaytee, crude protein 22%; A21, Nutribird, Versele-laga, crude protein 21%; Neonate formula, Harrison Bird Food, crude protein 26%).
  - Avoid excessive energy intake.
  - Inhibit peripheral lipolysis by providing at least the resting energy requirement for ideal body weight.
  - Carbohydrate supplementation is contraindicated because it inhibits beta-oxidation of fatty acids.
  - Gavage feed the bird if anorectic as many times as necessary to ensure intake of the correct balance and quantity of food. Vitamins may be added to the feeding as required.
  - Medications
- Supporting lipid metabolism with dietary supplementation
  - Supplementation with vitamins (especially B complex, biotin, E, and vitamin K_1) and essential amino acids
  - Supplementation in lipotrophic factors: choline and methionine 40-50 mg/kg q 24 h
  - L-Carnitine 100-250 mg/kg q 24 h could be helpful in that it is an important component of the mitochrondrial membrane, and it transports fatty acid in the matrix, where beta-oxidation occurs. This agent is regularly used in the management of feline lipidosis, even though its use is controversial because carnitine deficiency has not been demonstrated in cats with hepatic lipidosis.
  - Other antioxidant agents could be tried such as silymarin 50/75 mg/kg q 12 h.
  - *N*-acetylcysteine (NAC) and *S*-adenosyl-methionine (SAMe) 15-20 mg/kg q 24 h may help to prevent oxidative stress and stabilize hepatocellular membranes. Both are glutathione precursors and contain sulfur amino acids. NAC and SAMe may assist in lipid metabolism and other aspects of metabolism of the liver. SAMe is also a precursor of L-carnitine.

POSSIBLE COMPLICATIONS

- Use furosemide with caution in hypokalemic birds.
- Anabolic steroids (stanozolol) should be avoided because they can inhibit bile flow and seem to increase the risk of hepatic lipidosis in cats. Anabolic steroids and glucocorticoids also have an inhibitory influence on beta-oxidation.
- Tetracyclines (e.g., doxycycline) have lipogenic effects on hepatocytes in many mammals and consequently should be used with caution in birds suffering from hepatic lipidosis.

RECOMMENDED MONITORING

- Control weight; an obese bird should lose weight gradually.
- Reassess liver damage and function at regular intervals using hepatic biochemistry and by monitoring clinical improvement.
- A recheck liver biopsy may be indicated after completion of therapy.
- Assess the progress of diet conversion as well as body weight at regular rechecks until stable.

PROGNOSIS AND OUTCOME

- Prognosis is usually guarded in cases of avian hepatic lipidosis because of the chronic nature of the disease.
- Outcome is dependent on the severity of the presenting illness and the ability of the owner to adjust the patient's lifestyle and maintain a proper diet.

PEARLS & CONSIDERATIONS

COMMENTS

- Certain bird species are susceptible to hepatic lipidosis; owners of these species should be aware of the bird's chances of developing this disease.
- Owners with young obese birds should have the animals monitored on a regular basis for subclinical signs of hepatic lipidosis through blood testing.
- The condition may take time to reverse.

PREVENTION

- Start birds on a proper diet.
- Allow birds to exercise.
- Provide an adequate pelletized diet with correct quantities of fresh vegetables and fruits.
- Avoid high-fat, multinutrient-deficient diets (all-seed diets).
- Carefully monitor signs of hepatic disturbance.

CLIENT EDUCATION

- Inform the owner that hepatic lipidosis is usually of nutritional origin.
- Inform the owner that despite the acute presentation, hepatic lipidosis is a chronic disease that likely has been progressing for months.
- Provide basic advice for converting the bird to a balanced diet.

SUGGESTED READINGS

Center SA: Feline hepatic lipidosis. Vet Clin North Am (Small Anim Pract) 35:225–269, 2006.

Fudge AM: Testing the liver and the gastro-intestinal function. In Fudge AM, editor:

Laboratory medicine: avian and exotic pets, Philadelphia, 2000, WB Saunders, pp 47–55.
Lumeij J, Hepatology. In Ritchie BW, et al, editors: Avian medicine: principles and application, Lake Worth, FL, 1994, Wingers Publishing, pp 522–537.
Scherk MA, et al: Toxic, metabolic, infectious, and neoplastic liver diseases. In Ettinger SJ, et al, editors: Textbook of veterinary internal medicine, vol 2, ed 6, St Louis, 2005, Elsevier/Saunders, pp 1464–1477.

CROSS-REFERENCES TO OTHER SECTIONS

Overgrown Beak and Claws

AUTHORS: **HUGUES BEAUFRÈRE AND W. MICHAEL TAYLOR**

EDITOR: **THOMAS N. TULLY, JR.**

BIRDS

Hypocalcemia

BASIC INFORMATION

DEFINITION

A demonstrable serum calcium level below the established reference range

EPIDEMIOLOGY

SPECIES, AGE, SEX

- Any species of bird may suffer from hypocalcemia. It is frequently reported in African grey parrots.
- Birds between 2 and 5 years may show increased susceptibility.
- Hypocalcemia is more common in egg-laying females

GENETICS AND BREED PREDISPOSITION

- African grey parrots
- Excessive egg-laying hens (e.g., cockatiels)

RISK FACTORS

- Low-calcium diet
- Vitamin D–deficient diet
- Excessive dietary vitamins A and E
- Excessive dietary phosphorus
- Indoor birds in an ultraviolet (UV)-deficient environment
- High–egg-producing birds

ASSOCIATED CONDITIONS AND DISORDERS

- Nutritional secondary hyperparathyroidism
- Fibrous osteodystrophy
- Rickets
- Osteoporosis
- Pathologic fractures
- Chronic egg laying

CLINICAL PRESENTATION

DISEASE FORMS/SUBTYPES

- Hypocalcemia of African grey parrots
- Nutritional hypocalcemia

HISTORY, CHIEF COMPLAINT

- Seizures
- Lethargy
- Weakness
- Production of noncalcified eggs
- Fractures

PHYSICAL EXAM FINDINGS

- Seizures
- Weakness
- Ataxia
- Poor feather condition
- Bone deformities
- Fractures

ETIOLOGY AND PATHOPHYSIOLOGY

- Calcium is an abundant body mineral, most of which is found in the bones. Ionized calcium, the metabolically active form, functions in coagulation, calcification of egg shells, muscle and nerve conduction, and parathyroid hormone regulation.
- Vitamin D_3 aids calcium absorption from the gastrointestinal tract through the synthesis of calcium-binding proteins. UVB light is necessary for conversion of vitamin D into the metabolically active form of vitamin D_3 (cholecalciferol). Studies have shown that when a D_3-deficient diet is fed, excessive quantities of vitamins A and E in the diet affect the utilization of vitamin D_3 negatively.

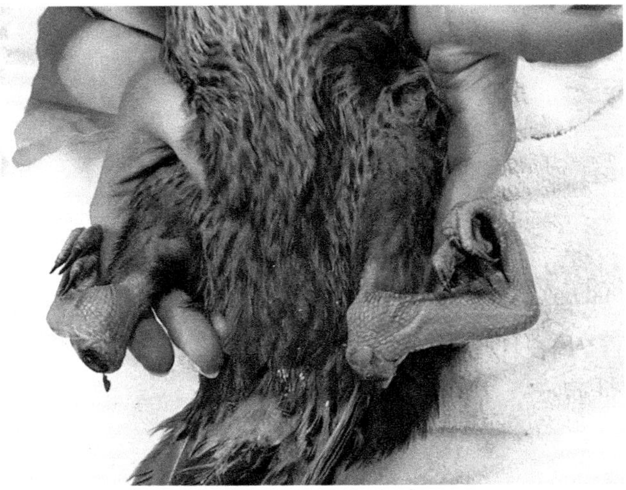

Hypocalcemia Skeletal leg deformities caused by a nutritional calcium deficiency.

- A fall in plasma calcium stimulates the production of parathyroid hormone, a major function of which is to increase osteoclastic activity, thus mobilizing calcium from the bones and increasing blood plasma concentration. Nutritional secondary hyperparathyroidism leads to excessive mobilization of calcium. This resorbed bone is replaced by fibrous connective tissue, which can lead to deformities and pathologic fractures. Parathyroid hormone also increases the resorption of calcium in the kidneys, thereby decreasing urinary loss.

DIAGNOSIS

DIFFERENTIAL DIAGNOSIS

- Hypoglycemia
- Neoplasia
- Heavy metal toxicity
- Organophosphate toxicity
- Infectious disease (viral, bacterial, fungal, or parasitic)
- Hepatic disease
- Renal disease

INITIAL DATABASE

- Plasma chemistry panel: serum calcium is species specific, and reference ranges should be provided by the laboratory used. Reference ranges for African grey parrots of between 2.0 and 3.0 mmol/L have been observed in birds exhibiting clinical signs of hypocalcemia.
- Ionized calcium: sample reference ranges for African grey parrots are between 0.96 and 1.22 mmol/L.
- Whole-body radiographs can detect lack of cortical bone density.

ADVANCED OR CONFIRMATORY TESTING

- 25-Hydroxycholecalciferol
- 1,25-Dihydroxycholecalciferol
- Parathyroid hormone

TREATMENT

THERAPEUTIC GOALS

- Correct clinical signs.
- Correct any husbandry issues contributing to hypocalcemia.

ACUTE GENERAL TREATMENT

- Calcium gluconate 10-100 mg/kg IM q 12 h prn
- Vitamin A, D, and E supplementation may be given if deficiencies are suspected.
  - Vital E-A + D (Schering Plough): 3300 IU/kg (1000 IU/300 g/BW) IM q 7 d prn
- Fluid therapy
- Stabilize pathologic fractures if present.

CHRONIC TREATMENT

- Oral calcium glubionate: 25 mg/kg q 24 h prn
- UVB supplementation
- Dietary changes
- Manage excessive egg laying.
  - Salpingectomy
  - Hormone therapy (see leuprolide acetate)

DRUG INTERACTIONS

- Animals with cardiac or renal disease should be carefully monitored while receiving calcium therapy.
- Excessive amounts of vitamins A and D may cause hypercalcemia owing to increased mobilization of calcium from bones and gastrointestinal absorption.

POSSIBLE COMPLICATIONS

- Seizures
  - Regurgitation and aspiration
- Pathological fractures: birds with hypocalcemia should be handled cautiously
- Coma
- Death

RECOMMENDED MONITORING

Total calcium and ionized calcium

PROGNOSIS AND OUTCOME

Dependent on severity of clinical signs. Prognosis is poor if extensive remodeling of bones has taken place.

PEARLS & CONSIDERATIONS

COMMENTS

Chronic cases of hypocalcemia may achieve a normal plasma calcium concentration through compensating mechanisms. It is recommended to treat for hypocalcemia if clinical signs and history are strongly suggestive, despite a normal plasma calcium concentration.

PREVENTION

- Birds should be fed a good quality pelleted diet without excessive vitamin A and E supplementation.
- Birds that are provided a source of UVB light may be at lower risk for development of hypocalcemia.

CLIENT EDUCATION

See Prevention.

SUGGESTED READINGS

Aburto A, et al: Effects of different levels of vitamins A and E on the utilization of cholecalciferol by broiler chickens, Poult Sci 77:570–577, 1998.

de Matos R: Calcium metabolism in birds, Vet Clin North Am Exot Anim Pract 11:59–82, 2008.

Elaroussi MA, et al: Calcium homeostasis in the laying hen. 1. Age and dietary calcium effects, Poult Sci 73:1581–1589, 1994.

Stanford M: Clinical pathology of hypocalcaemia in adult grey parrots *(Psittacus e erithacus)*, Vet Rec 161:456-457, 2007.

Stanford M: Effects of UVB radiation on calcium metabolism in psittacine birds, Vet Rec 159:236–241, 2006.

Stanford M: Measurement of 25-hydroxycholecalciferol in captive grey parrots *(Psittacus e erithacus)*, Vet Rec 153:58–59, 2003.

Stevens VI, et al: Dietary level of fat, calcium, and vitamins A and D3 as contributory factors to rickets in poults, Poult Sci 62: 2073–2082, 1983.

Toyoda T, et al: Nutritional secondary hyperparathyroidism and osteodystrophia fibrosa in a Hodgson's hawk-eagle *(Spizaetus nipalensis)*, Avian Pathol 33:9–12, 2004.

AUTHOR: **SHANNON N. SHAW**

EDITOR: **THOMAS N. TULLY, JR.**

Hypovitaminosis

Client Education Sheet and Additional Images Available on Website

BASIC INFORMATION

DEFINITION

Disease conditions that result from improper dietary vitamin supplementation

SYNONYMS

Vitamin A deficiency, white muscle disease (vitamin E)

EPIDEMIOLOGY

SPECIES, AGE, SEX All species and ages and both sexes

RISK FACTORS

- Improper dietary offerings (vitamins A, D, E)
- Diets high in rancid fats, such as liquid lorikeet diets (vitamin E)
- Malabsorption syndromes (vitamins A, D, E)
- Calcium deficiency (vitamin D)
- Little exposure to ultraviolet (UV) light (vitamin D)
- Liver or renal disease (vitamin D)

ASSOCIATED CONDITIONS AND DISORDERS

- Immune suppression may predispose to infectious disease, particularly aspergillosis.
- Squamous metaplasia predisposes these patients to pododermatitis (see Pododermatitis).
- *Giardia* spp. infections may result in poor absorption of vitamins A and E.
- Hypocalcemia (vitamin D) (see Hypocalcemia)
- Nutritional secondary hyperparathyroidism (vitamin D)

CLINICAL PRESENTATION

DISEASE FORMS/SUBTYPES

- Primary/Nutritional
- Secondary

HISTORY, CHIEF COMPLAINT

- Vitamin A
  - All-seed diet is a common finding.
  - None: often owners are unaware of early clinical signs that may be detected on physical examination
  - Poor egg laying, decreased sexual activity
  - White caseous material or pustules around or in the mouth and sinuses
  - Head, neck, or facial dermatitis and feather loss
  - Lethargy and anorexia (see Anorexia) (due to secondary infection)
- Vitamin E
  - Muscle dysfunction/weakness
  - Splayed legs
  - Neurologic signs (see Neurologic Disease)
- Vitamin D
  - Thin-shelled, soft eggs
  - Increased rate of early embryonic death
  - Mandibular malformation

PHYSICAL EXAM FINDINGS

- Vitamin A deficiency
  - Blunted choanal papillae (early sign)
  - White pustules in the upper gastrointestinal (GI) tract
  - Caseous material that may occlude the infraorbital sinuses or salivary glands; accumulates under the eyelids or blocks the syrinx
  - Muted feather coloration
  - Poor egg/sperm production
  - Polyuria/Polydipsia (due to gout or renal failure)
  - Hyperkeratosis of the plantar surface of the feet
  - Infectious diseases such as pneumonia or GI bacterial overgrowth secondary to immune suppression
- Vitamin E deficiency
  - Splayed legs
  - Weakness
  - Undigested seed in the droppings from ventricular weakness
  - Neurologic signs: ataxia, torticollis
  - Pain
  - Rhabdomyolysis
- Vitamin D deficiency
  - Soft-shelled eggs
  - Soft or rubbery bones
  - Pathologic fractures (see Fractures)

ETIOLOGY AND PATHOPHYSIOLOGY

- Vitamin A
  - Vitamin A is required for mucopolysaccharide synthesis, which is involved in appropriate development and function of epithelial surfaces, vision, immune response, and red or yellow pigments in the feathers.
  - Diseases resulting in poor absorption, such as giardiasis, may lead to hypovitaminosis.
  - Most clinical signs are a result of abnormal epithelium (squamous metaplasia).
- Vitamin E
  - Vitamin E is an antioxidant essential for proper function of epithelial tissue, the nervous system, immune function, and muscle function.

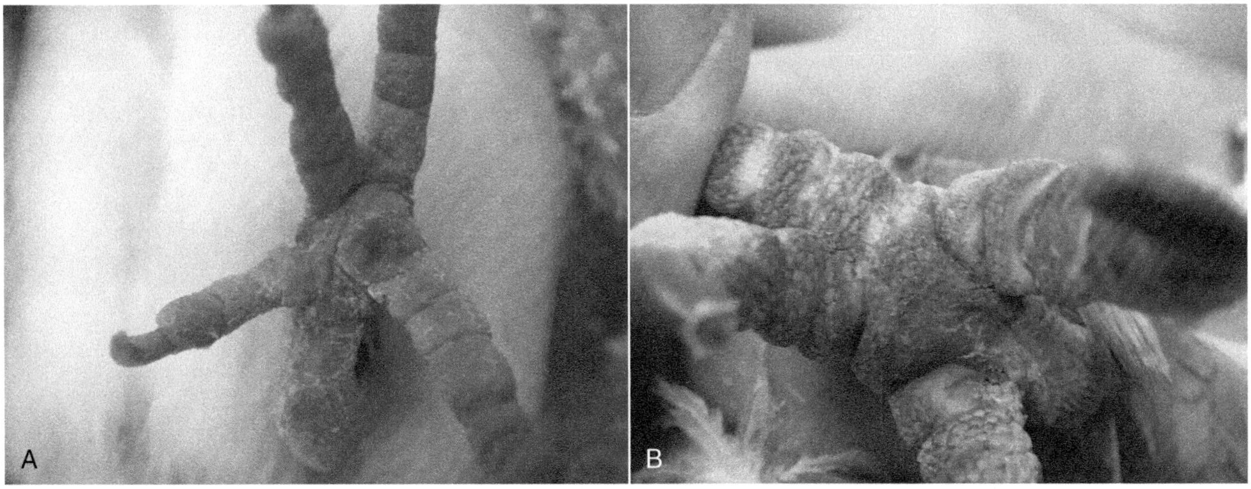

Hypovitaminosis Hyperkeratosis and peeling of plantar surface epithelium in a parrot suffering from vitamin A deficiency.

- Vitamin D
  - Vitamin D along with PTH is required for absorption of calcium in the intestinal tract, mobilization of calcium from bone, and reabsorption of calcium in the renal tubules.

DIAGNOSIS

DIFFERENTIAL DIAGNOSIS

- Vitamin A
  - Hyperkeratosis: pododermatitis
  - Oral plaques: *Candida, Trypanosoma*
  - Periosteal proliferation: reproductive female, tuberculosis, nutritional imbalances (oversupplementation with vitamin D)
- Vitamin E
  - Toxicities: lead, zinc, organophosphates are most common
  - Infectious disease: proventricular dilatation disease, paramyxovirus
  - GI parasitism
  - Trauma
  - Hypocalcemia
- Vitamin D
  - Calcium deficiency
  - Primary hyperparathyroidism (rare)
  - Renal secondary hyperparathyroidism (rare)

INITIAL DATABASE

- Physical examination
- Nutritional evaluation of diet
- Complete blood cell count
- Plasma chemistry panel
- Fecal examination (float and direct)

ADVANCED OR CONFIRMATORY TESTING

- Serum vitamin A concentrations should be interpreted with caution as they may not appropriately represent whole body vitamin A levels. Liver biopsy may be considered to confirm diagnosis, but response to treatment is generally adequate.
- Muscle biopsy for possible vitamin E deficiency
- Imaging studies such as radiographs or endoscopy may be required to fully characterize lesions, particularly with secondary diseases such as pneumonia.

TREATMENT

THERAPEUTIC GOALS

- Resolve clinical signs of hypovitaminosis.
- Make appropriate husbandry changes to prevent recurrence.

ACUTE GENERAL TREATMENT

- Treat for underlying problems such as GI parasites.
- Parenteral administration of vitamin A initially: 10,000 IU/300 g body weight IM q 7 d
- Parenteral administration of vitamin E 0.06 mg/kg IM q 7 d in psittacine and raptor species; piscivorous species: vitamin E demands vary by species
- Treat any underlying disorders (e.g., parasitism).
- Parenteral administration of vitamin D 1000 IU/300 g body weight IM q 7 d
- Parenteral administration of calcium 50-100 mg/kg IM calcium gluconate 10% once, then oral administration 25 mg/kg calcium glubionate PO q 24 h

CHRONIC TREATMENT

- Dietary changes such as including pellets in the diet
- Resolve GI causes of poor absorption.
- Dietary modification to include sources of calcium and vitamin D
- Exposure to UVB light

POSSIBLE COMPLICATIONS

- Hypervitaminosis A: signs include weight loss (see Emaciation), dermatitis, hemorrhage, decreased bone strength
- Hypervitaminosis E is rare; more than 100 times the normal vitamin E requirement is needed to reach toxic levels
- Hypervitaminosis D
  - Hypercalcemia
  - Soft-tissue mineralization
  - Nephrocalcinosis
  - Polydipsia

RECOMMENDED MONITORING

Monitor for clinical signs of hypervitaminosis after administering parenteral treatment.

PROGNOSIS AND OUTCOME

Good with treatment and dietary changes

PEARLS & CONSIDERATIONS

COMMENTS

- Adequate diet will prevent disease conditions caused by vitamin deficiencies.
- Windows filter out UVB light, so exposure to sunlight through windows will not increase UVB exposure.

PREVENTION

- Appropriate diet for the species
- Yearly physical exams are a good way to screen for early signs of vitamin deficiency such as blunted choanal papillae.

CLIENT EDUCATION

Importance of husbandry and nutrition

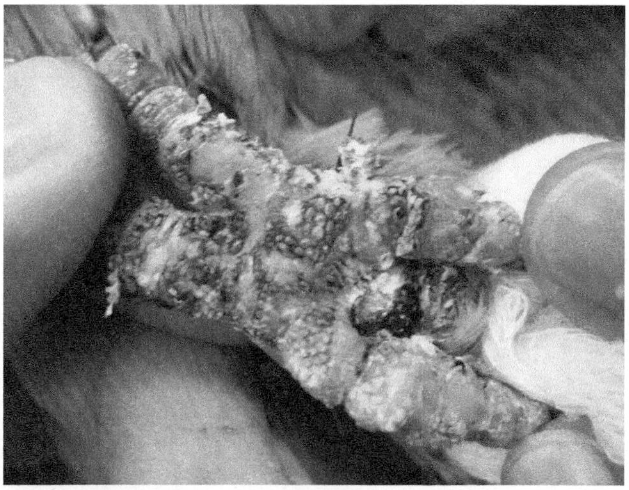

Hypovitaminosis Plantar surface focal pressure necrosis lesion that was attributed to complications arising from vitamin A deficiency and improper perches in the bird's environment.

SUGGESTED READINGS

Harrison GJ, et al: Nutritional disorders. In Lightfoot T, et al, editors: Clinical avian medicine, vol I, Palm Beach, FL, 2006, Spix Publishing, pp 108–140.

McDonald D: Section I, Nutrition and dietary supplementation. In Lightfoot T, et al, editors: Clinical avian medicine, vol I, Palm Beach, FL, 2006, Spix Publishing, pp 86–107.

Hypocalcemia
Neurologic Disease
Pododermatitis

AUTHOR: **GWENDOLYN R. JANKOWSKI**

EDITOR: **THOMAS N. TULLY, JR.**

BIRDS

Liver Disease

Client Education Sheet Available on Website

BASIC INFORMATION

DEFINITION

Loss of adequate hepatic function due to acute or chronic damage. The liver has high regenerative capacity and functional reserve, so only when most of the hepatic parenchyma is affected will signs of hepatic failure become evident.

EPIDEMIOLOGY

SPECIES, AGE, SEX Common condition seen in birds with poor diets or in birds exposed to infectious agents that can cause destruction of the hepatic parenchyma

CLINICAL PRESENTATION

PHYSICAL EXAM FINDINGS

- We can separate the clinical signs in nonspecific disease from signs usually associated with liver disease.
- Among the nonspecific signs, we find anorexia, lethargy, weight loss, polyuria and polydipsia, poor feather condition, and dyspnea.
- Signs usually associated with liver disease include green or yellow droppings caused by excessive biliverdin or bilirubin, abdominal swelling due to hepatomegaly or ascites secondary to hypoalbuminemia, coagulopathies, melena, abnormal beak and nails, and abnormal color in the feathers caused by lack of pigment synthesis.

ETIOLOGY AND PATHOPHYSIOLOGY

- Hepatic lipidosis: known also as *fatty liver syndrome,* occurs if the deposition of fat within hepatocytes, due to an increased use of fat by liver. Dietary causes are the main etiology, such as insectivorous raptors (e.g., merlins) fed on pinkies or psittacines fed on oily seeds. Other causes of lipidosis include mobilization of fat reserves in prolonged periods of anorexia or in females during egg-laying as a result of estrogen-controlled lipogenesis.
- Visceral gout: accumulation of uric acid crystals in different organs, including the liver; usually the course of the disease is very fast, and animals tend to die before signs of liver failure are noted.
- Amyloidosis: secondary amyloidosis is seen in chronic infection situations or in prolonged stress situations; continuous deposition of proteins in the hepatic parenchyma causes necrosis by pressure.
- Lipofuscinosis: lipofuscin is a pigment that accumulates in hepatocytes secondary to diseases in which an increase in biological oxidation is present. Vitamin E deficiency may be causative because of its antioxidant role.
- Nutritional
  - Microhepatica: although small livers are a common finding in psittacines, reduced size of the liver can be linked with fibrosis secondary to diet-rich seeds.
  - Hemochromatosis: although included as nutritional disease, the cause of this disease remains unclear; several authors have reported that the cause of the disease is nutritional; other studies suggest genetic causes. Hemochromatosis is described as iron accumulation associated with deleterious effects for the body. This condition is described in birds from the following families: Sturnidae, Paradisaeidae, Bucerotidae, and Ramphastidae.
  - Hypervitaminosis D_3: due to oral oversupplementation; this condition can cause mineralization of soft tissues, including the liver.
- Toxins: several drugs, including antibiotics and antifungal drugs, are considered potentially hepatotoxic for birds; therefore, liver function should be assessed regularly in birds exposed to these drugs for prolonged periods, in the same way that some plants and fruits like avocado, or environmental substances like lead and zinc, are reported to be hepatotoxic.
- Infectious diseases: several parasitic, bacterial, and viral diseases can cause liver failure
  - Protozoa
    - Atoxoplasma: generally affects young birds, between 2 and 9 months old
    - Toxoplasma: can cause hepatomegaly
    - Sarcocystis: Old World avian species are more sensitive to this parasite, which, on top of pulmonary lesions, causes hepatomegaly and splenomegaly
    - Cryptosporidium: affects epithelial cells in biliary tract
    - Plasmodium: common cause of hepatosplenomegaly; certain species of the orders Strigiformes and Sphenisciformes are more susceptible
    - *Leucocytozoon:* can cause necrosis by its presence; usually no inflammatory reaction is associated
    - *Haemoproteus*: schizonts can be found in the liver, although generally this condition is nonpathogenic
    - *Histomonas*: can cause severe local hepatocellular necrosis; has been reported commonly in poultry; known as *blackhead.*
    - *Trichomonas*: although this pathogenic effect is limited to the gastrointestinal tract, if it is not treated, it can invade the liver, causing necrosis
  - Trematodes: some species from the family Dicrocoelidae have been reported in birds, causing liver damage as the result of migration, pressure necrosis, biliary stasis, and hyperplasia of bile ducts

   - Nematodes: different intestinal nematodes can penetrate intestinal mucosa and travel to the liver, causing a major inflammatory reaction with secondary fibrosis
   - Bacteria: several bacteria have been associated with liver failure as primary agents or secondary to other conditions such as viral disease
      - Gram-positive bacteria: usually cause hepatitis secondary to septicemia or with infection of the lungs or air sacs due to proximity to the liver. *Staphylococcus*, *Streptococcus*, and *Clostridium* are common Gram-positive bacteria isolated in abscess in hepatic parenchyma
      - Gram-negative bacteria: *Salmonella*, *Escherichia coli*, *Pseudomonas*, and *Yersinia* are isolated frequently, causing multifocal necrosis and a major inflammatory response.
      - *Mycobacterium*: usually with chronic presentation, endoscopy may reveal areas of necrosis and caseous material in liver parenchyma
      - *Chlamydophila*: very common in psittacines; causes different degrees of hepatic necrosis; generally respiratory or gastrointestinal signs are observed.
      - *Bacillus piliformis*: very rare in birds, as other bacteria tend to cause necrosis of the liver. Because *Chlamydophila* is an obligate intracellular bacterium that can be seen in hepatocytes, cytoplasm is accompanied by a strong inflammatory response.
   - Fungal: *Aspergillus* is the most common fungus isolated in cases of liver failure, although other fungi, such as *Candida*, have been isolated. Although *Aspergillus* is not a common primary pathogen in the liver, the aflatoxins that the fungus produces are highly hepatotoxic.
   - Virus
      - Herpesvirus: usually the presentation is peracute or acute, making diagnosis and treatment very difficult. In some situations, isolation of viral antigens from cloacal mucosa is possible; the presence of cloacal papillomas may suggest that the liver is affected by herpesvirus.
      - Polyomavirus: very commonly reported in psittacines, affecting young birds, younger than 12 months of age
      - Adenovirus: has been reported as a cause of hepatitis, mainly in psittacines and poultry, although cases in waterfowl, raptors, and pigeons have been described
      - Circovirus: liver damage is usually present in young birds, which are more susceptible, causing severe necrosis
      - Reovirus: reported in psittacines as acute systemic disease, causing focal hepatic necrosis with minimal inflammation
      - Hepadnavirus: causes hepatitis in ducks
- Neoplasia: bile duct carcinoma or adenoma, lymphoid leukosis, fibrosarcoma, hemangioma

DIAGNOSIS

DIFFERENTIAL DIAGNOSIS

- Hepatomegaly can occur secondary to congestive heart failure; these conditions share some clinical signs. Obesity in neonates can result in hepatomegaly.
- Microhepatica can be related to portosystemic shunts in young animals.

INITIAL DATABASE

Complete blood count. Biochemistry

- Leukocytosis is common when the cause is a bacterial or fungal infection; leukopenia will be present if a viral infection or toxicosis is responsible.
- Examination of the blood smear may reveal the presence of hemoprotozoa.
- The increase in bile acids offers the best combination of specificity and sensitivity when evaluating hepatic pathologies.
- Low levels of uric acid may be linked to hepatic disease because synthesis takes place in the liver.
- Hyperuricemia can be linked to lipemia, so high levels of uric acid may be present in cases of hepatic lipidosis.
- Increased enzymes are not specific to liver failure in birds. The most specific enzyme is aspartate aminotransferase (AST), although in birds, it is present in muscular tissue, too. Usually levels of creatine kinase (CK) and AST can be evaluated together. If only AST is elevated, this is more likely to be related to a liver problem, although the clinician should keep in mind that an increase in CK may be noted, especially if the blood sample has been taken in a conscious bird under heavy physical restraint.

ADVANCED OR CONFIRMATORY TESTING

- Clearance tests
   - Clearance tests of indocyanine green, bromsulphalein, and galactose are very sensitive to small losses in liver function.
- Imaging
   - Radiography
      - Changes in the size of the liver can be detected on radiographs, although on some occasions, the use of radiographic contrast is necessary in the proventriculus and ventriculus to delimit liver contour and position more accurately.
      - The shadow of the liver in a dorsoventral view should be noted between two lines drawn from the shoulder to the hip joints.
   - Ultrasound
      - Provides information about the size and structure of the liver
      - Ultrasound can be used to perform fine-needle aspirations; a 22-gauge needle attached to a 2-mL syringe can be used for multiple penetrations in liver parenchyma with application of gentle suction to avoid hemodilution of the sample.
   - Endoscopy
      - Can provide extra information regarding the extent and type of lesions noted in hepatic parenchyma, although in term of collecting, biopsy can be preferable a surgical approach because of the high risk of coagulopathy.
      - One important contraindication for endoscopy in case of liver failure would be the presence of ascites, especially if the approach requires going through the air sacs.
   - Biopsy and histopathology
   - Fine-needle aspirations provide a low number of hepatocytes, but the sample can be useful in assessing the presence of vacuolation in hepatic lipidosis or hemosiderin pigment in hemochromatosis; however, iron stores seen histologically do not prove that hemochromatosis is the cause of the problem.
   - Percutaneous needle biopsies can be taken, although risks of hemorrhage after the procedure make this technique not ideal.
   - Midline or lateral laparotomy is a fast procedure involving easy access to the liver; complications can be corrected more easily.
   - Biopsies can provide useful information when we want to isolate the infectious agent causing the hepatic dysfunction, or when we suspect a possible neoplasia.
   - In cases of chronic hepatitis, it can be difficult to isolate the original cause because severe histologic changes are noted.
   - Hepatic biopsies can be useful in assessing the potential toxicity of different substances or in assessing levels of certain enzymes like

cytochrome P450 1A in birds exposed to petroleum products.
- Bacteriology
  - Swabs from the surface of the liver rarely reveal the pathogen causing the disease; biopsy can be more helpful in attempts to isolate the infectious agents.
- Fecal exam
  - Flotation and stain of fecal material may reveal the presence of different parasites affecting the liver.
- Other diagnostic tests
  - Specific serologic tests, immunoassays, and PCR are used to isolate specific infectious agents.

TREATMENT

ACUTE GENERAL TREATMENT

- Hospitalization
- Birds should be kept in a low-stress area; if an infectious agent is suspected, isolation should be considered.
- Oxygen therapy may be required if dyspnea is present.
- Fluid therapy
  - Selection of fluids should be based on biochemistry and should be devoid of lactate.
  - Administration of colloids may be useful if hypoalbuminemia is present, although clotting times should be monitored.
- Nutritional support
  - Gavage feeding should be established in anorectic and weight loss patients.
- Treatment of clinical signs
  - Hepatic encephalopathy
    - Objective of treatment would be to restore normal neurologic function. Use of lactulose to decrease levels of ammonia in the blood and to increase osmotic pressure in the gastrointestinal tract helps to reduce ascites.
  - Ascites
    - Removal of large volume of coelomic fluid can cause massive protein loss; this would be indicated in cases of severe respiratory compromise.
    - Use of diuretics such as furosemide 0.1- 2 mg/kg PO, SC, IM, IV q 6-24 h is indicated to reduce the fluid load.
  - Coagulopathies
    - Cholestasis can decrease the production of coagulation factors and antithrombin III and can alter the absorption of vitamin K.
    - Petechiae and melena can be observed as consequences.
    - Vitamin K can be administered in a dose of 2.5-10 mg/kg IM q 12-24 h to compensate for decreased absorption.
    - If melena is present, suggesting gastrointestinal ulceration, H2 blockers such as ranitidine and famotidine can be used; sucralfate at a dose of 25 mg/kg PO q 8 h can be used to enhance ulcer healing.
- Treatment of specific conditions
  - Nutrition
    - Low-fat diets should be introduced in birds with hepatic lipidosis. L-Carnitine supplementation can reduce lipids levels in blood, although this has been reported only in budgerigars.
    - Addition of tea to the diet can reduce uptake of iron owing to high content in tannins; in cases of hemochromatosis, food items rich in vitamin C should be avoided because ascorbic acid has the opposite effect.
  - Antibiotics and antifungal therapy
    - Broad-spectrum antibiotics and antifungals can be used to treat patients with infectious agents affecting the liver.
  - Colchicine
    - Used in cases of visceral gout and amyloidosis, or in any case with cirrhosis and fibrosis of the liver, because of its antiinflammatory properties; although it can promote gout formation, this agent can be used at a very low dose of 0.04 mg/kg PO q 12-24 h and increased gradually.
  - Chelating agents
    - Edetate calcium disodium can be used in cases of heavy metal toxicity at a dose of 10-40 mg/kg IM q 12 h.
    - Deferoxamine can be used as a chelating agent in cases of hemochromatosis at a dose of 20 mg/kg PO q 4 h until recovery.
  - Milk thistle *(Silybum marianum)*
    - Extract from milk thistle seeds has antioxidant and antiinflammatory effects. It has been used in combination with lactulose in cases of liver failure.
  - Vitamin E
    - Has been used successfully in the treatment of hepatic lipidosis in turkeys and Strigiformes.
  - Ursodeoxycholic acid (Ursodiol)
    - This hydrophilic bile acid inhibits absorption of hydrophobic bile acids; it is suspected to reduce liver injury at a cellular level and to decrease fibrosis, but no studies with birds have been performed. It can potentiate cholestasis.

AUTHOR: **ALBERTO RODRIGUEZ BARBON**

EDITOR: **THOMAS N. TULLY, JR.**

BIRDS

Megabacteriosis

BASIC INFORMATION

DEFINITION

A condition affecting birds that is caused by gastric colonization of the organism *Macrorhabdus ornithogaster.*

SYNONYM

Avian gastric yeast

EPIDEMIOLOGY

SPECIES, AGE, SEX Megabacteriosis has been described in both wild and companion birds. It has been associated with lymphoplasmacytic gastritis in poultry. It is widespread in budgerigars and causes a progressive wasting condition. It has also been described in parrotlets, lovebirds, canaries, finches, ostrich, and chickens.

GENETICS AND BREED PREDISPOSITION Genetic factors are thought to be involved.

RISK FACTORS
- Megabacteriosis-positive parents
- Stress: may be associated with molting, breeding, or overcrowding
- Poor nutrition

CONTAGION AND ZOONOSIS
- Although the transmission of megabacteriosis still is not largely understood, contagion between birds is likely.
- Megabacteriosis is not zoonotic.

GEOGRAPHY AND SEASONALITY Megabacteriosis is a common cause of illness in budgerigars in the United Kingdom.

CLINICAL PRESENTATION

DISEASE FORMS/SUBTYPES
- Proventricular/ventricular disease
- Asymptomatic infection

HISTORY, CHIEF COMPLAINT
- Severe weight loss
- Dysphagia
- Vomiting
- Regurgitation
- Diarrhea
- Death

PHYSICAL EXAM FINDINGS
- Poor body condition
- Lethargy
- Beak grinding or signs of pain

ETIOLOGY AND PATHOPHYSIOLOGY
- Megabacteriosis is caused by the organism *Macrohabdus ornithogaster.*
  - This organism is a filamentous to rod-shaped Gram-positive ascomycetous yeast.
  - This organism colonizes the isthmus of the proventriculus and ventriculus.
  - Transmission remains largely unclear. The organism is shed in the feces of diseased birds but has also been isolated from clinically healthy birds. Immune suppression is likely to play a role in the establishment of disease.

DIAGNOSIS

INITIAL DATABASE
- Direct fecal smear: Gram staining or a quick stain may be useful. Not all birds shed the organism in their feces, however.
- Complete blood count: may see a leukocytosis, heterophilia, and/or anemia

ADVANCED OR CONFIRMATORY TESTING
Ventricular scrapings and histopathologic examination can be used for postmortem evaluation.

TREATMENT

THERAPEUTIC GOALS
- Eliminate organism.
- Eliminate shedding.
- Reduce clinical signs.

ACUTE GENERAL TREATMENT
- Amphotericin B: give 100-109 mg/kg by gavage twice a day for 30 days
- Clean and disinfect environment.

PROGNOSIS AND OUTCOME
Guarded

PEARLS & CONSIDERATIONS

PREVENTION
It has been shown experimentally to reduce infection among chicks if the eggs are pulled from the parents and are cleaned and if contact is prevented between chicks and adult birds or the eggs.

CLIENT EDUCATION
- Hand-rearing of chicks is a time-consuming process but may result in reduced prevalence of megabacteriosis.
- Quarantine and analyze multiple fecal samples for all newly acquired birds for a minimum of 30 days before introducing them to other birds.

SUGGESTED READINGS

Baker J: Megabacteria in diseased and healthy budgerigars, Vet Rec 140:627, 1997.

Hannafusa Y, et al: Growth and metabolic characterization of *Macrorhabdus ornithogaster,* J Vet Diagn Invest 19:256–265, 2007.

Henderson G, et al: Haematological findings in budgerigars with megabacterium and *Trichomonas* infections associated with "going light," Vet Rec 123:492–494, 1988.

Marlier D, et al: Increasing incidence of megabacteriosis in canaries *(Serinus canaries domesticus),* Vet J 172:549–552, 2006.

Moore R, et al: A method of preventing transmission of so-called "megabacteria" in budgerigars *(Melopsittacus undulates),* J Avian Med Surg 15:283–287, 2001.

Phalen D: Diagnosis and management of *Macrorhabdus ornithogaster* (formerly megabacteria), Vet Clin North Am Exot Anim Pract 8:299–306, 2005.

Tomaszewski E, et al: Phylogenetic analysis identifies the "megabacterium" of birds as a novel anamorphic ascomycetous yeast, *Macrorhabdus ornithogaster* gen. *nov.,* sp. *nov.,* Int J Syst Evol Microbiol 53:1201–1205, 2003.

AUTHOR: **SHANNON N. SHAW**

EDITOR: **THOMAS N. TULLY, JR.**

BIRDS

Mycoses

BASIC INFORMATION

DEFINITION
Infections resulting from fungal growth within host tissues

SYNONYM
Fungal disease

EPIDEMIOLOGY

SPECIES, AGE, SEX
- Young birds are more susceptible to certain fungal infections, such as candidiasis.
- All species and sexes of birds are susceptible to fungal infections.
- African grey parrots and *Pionus* parrots have increased susceptibility to aspergillosis.
- Cryptococcosis has been reported in macaws, African grey parrots, pigeons, canaries, and cockatoos.
- Cutaneous mycoses are not commonly reported in avian species.

RISK FACTORS
- Immune suppression
- Prolonged antibiotic therapy
- Stress or corticosteroid therapy
- Malnutrition
- Unsanitary environment

CONTAGION AND ZOONOSIS
- Many fungal organisms such as *Aspergillus* and *Candida* are commonly found in the environment. Infection usually takes place through inhalation. Infection is usually linked to immune suppression. *Aspergillus* species present an infection risk to granulocytopenic humans and chemotherapeutic patients.
- Cryptococcosis is a zoonotic fungal disease. It is a leading cause of mortality due to fungal disease in AIDS patients. Inhalation of droppings of infected birds can be a mode of transmission.
- Poultry workers suffering from skin lesions known as "chicken poison disease" have possibly been linked to *Candida* organisms.
- *Histoplasma* species may cause pneumonitis progressing to reticuloendothelial disease in humans.
- *Trichophyton gallinae* causes pruritus of the scalp in humans.

GEOGRAPHY AND SEASONALITY
Most fungal organisms are ubiquitous.

ASSOCIATED CONDITIONS AND DISORDERS
- Cutaneous *Staphylococcus*
- Pneumonia
- Air sacculitis
- Crop stasis (see Crop Stasis)
- Newcastle disease virus
- Herpesvirus
- Adenovirus
- Reovirus
- Circovirus
- Polyomavirus
- Feather picking (see Feather Picking)

CLINICAL PRESENTATION

DISEASE FORMS/SUBTYPES
- Superficial mycoses: result from fungal growth within the skin
- Deep mycoses: fungal elements invade deeper body tissues or become systemic

HISTORY, CHIEF COMPLAINT
- For all systemic mycoses: deaths in flock, poor growth, lethargy, depression
- *Aspergillus*: respiratory signs such as open-mouth breathing
- Candidiasis: regurgitation, vomiting

PHYSICAL EXAM FINDINGS
- Systemic mycoses can produce very nonspecific clinical signs such as lethargy or a ruffled appearance.
- Aspergillosis
  - Open-mouth breathing
  - Increased respiratory rate
  - Head bob, tail bob
  - Oculonasal discharge
  - Emaciation
  - Weakness
  - Biliverdinuria
- Candidiasis: may have white patches in throat and esophagus; comb infections in chickens present as crusty white patches or diffuse lesions
- Superficial mycoses can present as a crusty dermatitis with pruritus and feather loss.

ETIOLOGY AND PATHOPHYSIOLOGY
- Systemic mycoses
  - *Aspergillus* sp., most commonly *Aspergillus fumigatus:* a ubiquitous organism colonizes the avian respiratory system but may be found in other organ systems.
  - *Candida* sp., most commonly *Candida albicans:* involves a normal inhabitant of the avian gastrointestinal tract. Disruption in the composition of normal bacterial organisms or the gastrointestinal mucosa may predispose a bird to infection.
  - *Cryptococcus neoformans:* this yeast has been isolated from the droppings of pigeons; produces a granulomatous disease of internal organs. Much remains unknown about the pathophysiology and transmission.
  - *Histoplasma capsulatum* causes infection of the reticuloendothelial system; not commonly reported
- Superficial mycoses: rarely reported in avian species; have been implicated as causes for feather picking
  - *Trichophyton gallinae*
  - *Microsporum gypseum*
  - *Microsporum ripariae*
  - *Trichosporon asahii*
  - *Fusarium oxysporum*
  - *Rhodotorula* species
  - *Mucor* species
  - *Malassezia*
  - *Cladosporium herbarum* has been reported to cause a secondary infection in a house sparrow with cutaneous staphylococcosis.

DIAGNOSIS

DIFFERENTIAL DIAGNOSIS
- Aspergillosis (signs of respiratory illness)
  - Disseminated neoplasia B
  - Mycobacteriosis
  - Coligranulomas caused by *Escherichia coli*
  - Foreign body granulomas
  - Aerosolized toxicosis
- Candidiasis (signs of regurgitation)
  - Crop burn
  - Foreign body
  - Neoplasia
  - Ingluvitis (bacterial)
  - Over feeding
  - Improper formula temperature in neonates
- Dermatophytes
  - Bacterial dermatitis
  - External parasites
  - Feather picking
  - Nutritional deficiencies
  - Psittacine beak and feather disease
  - Endocrine disease

INITIAL DATABASE
- Cytology: crop swab, tracheal wash, fecal swab, or throat lesions
- Fungal culture: crop, tracheal wash, granulomas, skin lesions
- Complete blood count (CBC): may see inflammatory response (leukocytosis, monocytosis, heterophilia)
- Radiographs: with aspergillosis, may see air sacculitis and bronchopneumonia with mixed bronchial and interstitial patterns, as well as splenomegaly

ADVANCED OR CONFIRMATORY TESTING
- Biopsy and histopathologic examination of lesions
- Necropsy may be used to confirm or reach a definitive diagnosis in a flock situation. Birds with candidiasis may have a "Turkish towel" appearance to the crop.

TREATMENT

THERAPEUTIC GOALS
- Eliminate mycotic infection.
- Determine and eliminate factors contributing to stress and/or immune suppression.

ACUTE GENERAL TREATMENT
- Amphotericin B (1.5 mg/kg iv q 8 h × 3-7 days; 1 mg/kg intratracheal q 8-12 h, dilute to 1 mL with sterile water for aspergillosis) is a macrolide fungicidal agent that binds to ergosterol in the fungal cell membrane; this alters membrane permeability and causes cell death. It has activity against *Aspergillus, Candida, Histoplasma,* and *Mucor* species.
- Nystatin (300,000-600,000 U/kg PO q 8-12 h × 7-14 days, psittacines) is a polyene antifungal agent with similar action to amphotericin B. However, it is not absorbed systemically. It is used to treat gastrointestinal candidiasis. Nyotran is a formulation with liposomal encapsulation that may prove less toxic and is currently undergoing clinical trials.
- Fluoropyrimidines (e.g., flucytosine [50-75 mg/kg PO q 8 h]): inhibit fungal DNA and RNA synthesis
- Azoles (itraconazole [10-20 mg/kg PO q 12-24 h], fluconazole [10-20 mg/kg PO q 12 h], voriconazole [12.5 mg/kg PO q 12 h]): fungistatic agents; voriconazole is considered fungicidal against *Aspergillus* sp. but is more expensive than other azole agents; mechanism of action is through inhibition of cytochrome P450–dependent ergosterol synthesis; activity against *Aspergillus, Cryptococcus,* and *Candida* species.
- Allylamines (terbinafine [10-15 mg/kg PO q 12-24 h): fungicidal and fungistatic; inhibits biosynthesis of ergosterol and creates accumulation of toxic sterols; potential use for azole-sensitive birds with aspergillosis; usually prescribed for treatment of dermatophytes in humans
- Topical treatment with antifungal creams may be used for superficial mycoses.

CHRONIC TREATMENT
Fluid therapy and crop feeding may be necessary for severely debilitated birds (see Denydration).

DRUG INTERACTIONS
- Amphotericin B: renal toxicity
- Nystatin is more toxic than amphotericin B and should not be given if gastrointestinal epithelium is not

intact as systemic absorption may occur.
- Fluoropyrimidines: drug resistance has been demonstrated with *Candida, Cryptococcus*, and *Aspergillus* species. These drugs should be used only in combination with other antifungal agents.
- Azoles: severe hepatitis can develop; fluconazole has been associated with anorexia in African grey parrots; voriconazole is reported to have fewer side effects than other azoles. Side effects can include visual disturbances, gastrointestinal irritation, skin rashes, and hepatic abnormalities.
- Allylamines: caution in patients with hepatic and renal disease

POSSIBLE COMPLICATIONS

- Anorexia
- Cachexia
- Dehydration
- Self-mutilation

RECOMMENDED MONITORING

CBC can be used to monitor the inflammatory response during treatment for systemic fungal diseases.

PROGNOSIS AND OUTCOME

- If factors related to immune suppression and stress can be identified and removed, a better prognosis is the result.
- Prognosis is poor if fungal hyphae are seen on fecal cytology.
- Aspergillosis is difficult to treat and carries a poor prognosis.

PEARLS & CONSIDERATIONS

COMMENTS

- Clinical signs of aspergillosis develop late in the course of disease, making treatment difficult.
- Candidiasis is frequently a secondary infection; efforts should be made to detect any underlying illness.
- Fungal resistance is becoming increasingly common; care should be exercised when an antifungal regimen is prescribed.

PREVENTION

Environmental sanitation is an important measure to be taken because most fungal infections are transmitted from the environment.

CLIENT EDUCATION

- Proper diet and husbandry should be maintained to eliminate these factors as causes for immune suppression.
- Birds should be provided with a high-quality pelleted diet to ensure that they receive all vitamins and minerals that they need.
- They should be maintained at an appropriate species-specific temperature and provided adequate ventilation.

SUGGESTED READINGS

Cermeno JR, et al: *Cryptococcus neoformans* and *Histoplasma capsulatum* in dove's (*Columba livia*) excreta in Bolivar state, Venezuela, Rev Latinoam Microbiol 48:6–9, 2006.

Coles BH: Prescribing for exotic birds. In Bishop Y, editor: The veterinary formulary, ed 5, London, 2001, Pharmaceutical Press, pp 99–105.

Dahlhausen B, et al: The use of terbinafine hydrochloride in the treatment of avian fungal disease, Proc Annu Conf Assoc Avian Vet 307–311, 2000.

Dallwig RK, et al: What is your diagnosis? Aspergillosis, J Am Vet Med Assoc 231: 205–206, 2007.

Drummond ED, et al: [Behaviour azole fungicide and fluconazole in *Cryptococcus neoformans* clinical and environmental isolates], Rev Soc Bras Med Trop 40:209–211, 2007.

Efuntoye MO, et al: Occurrence of keratinophilic fungi and dermatophytes on domestic birds in Nigeria, Mycopathologia 153:87–89, 2002.

Femenia F, et al: Clinical, mycological and pathological findings in turkeys experimentally infected by *Aspergillus fumigatus*, Avian Pathol 36:213–219, 2007

Flammer K, et al: An overview of antifungal therapy in birds, Proc Annu Conf Assoc Avian Vet 1–4, 1993.

Flammer K, et al: Pharmacokinetics of fluconazole after oral administration of single and multiple doses in African grey parrots, Am J Vet Res 67:417–422, 2006.

Flammer K, et al: Pharmacokinetics of voriconazole after oral administration of single and multiple doses in African grey parrots (*Psittacus erithacus timneh*), Am J Vet Res 69:114–121, 2008.

Grunder S, et al: Mycological examinations on the fungal flora of the chicken comb, Mycoses 48:114–119, 2005.

Hubalek Z: Cutaneous staphylococcosis and secondary infection of house sparrow with the fungus *Cladosporium herbarum*, Folia Parasitol (Praha) 21:59–66, 1974.

Hubalek Z, et al: A dermatophyte from birds: *Microsporum ripariae* sp. *nov*., Sabouraudia 11:287–292, 1973.

Moellering RC Jr, et al: Antimicrobial resistance prevention initiative—an update: proceedings of an expert panel on resistance, Am J Infect Control 35:S1–S23, 2007.

Nielsen K, et al: *Cryptococcus neoformans* mates on pigeon guano: implications for the realized ecological niche and globalization, Eukaryot Cell 6:949–959, 2007.

Orosz SE: Antifungal drug therapy in avian species, Vet Clin North Am Exot Anim Pract 6:337–350, 2003.

Osorio C, et al: Comb candidiasis affecting roosters in a broiler breeder flock, Avian Dis 51:618–622, 2007.

Pfaller MA, et al: In vitro activities of voriconazole, fluconazole, and itraconazole against 566 clinical isolates of *Cryptococcus neoformans* from the United States and Africa, Antimicrob Agents Chemother 43:169–171, 1999.

Preziosi DE, et al: Distribution of *Malassezia* organisms on the skin of unaffected psittacine birds and psittacine birds with feather-destructive behavior, J Am Vet Med Assoc 228:216–221, 2006.

Redig P: Infectious diseases; fungal diseases. In Samour J, editor: Avian medicine, London, 2000, Harcourt, pp 275–291.

Richard JL, et al: Advances in veterinary mycology, J Med Vet Mycol 32(Suppl 1):169–187, 1994.

Schmidt V, et al: Plasma concentrations of voriconazole in falcons, Vet Rec 161:265–268, 2007.

Tsai SS, et al: Isolation of *Candida albicans* and their sensitivity to antifungal agents, Zhonghua Min Guo Wei Sheng Wu Ji Mian Yi Xue Za Zhi 15:38–45, 1982.

Ustimenko AN, et al: Prevention of aspergillosis in ducklings, Veterinariia (2):60, 1980.

CROSS-REFERENCES TO OTHER SECTIONS

Crop Stasis
Dehydration
Feather Picking

AUTHOR: **SHANNON N. SHAW**

EDITOR: **THOMAS N. TULLY, JR.**

BIRDS

Neurologic Disease

BASIC INFORMATION

DEFINITION

Neurologic disease may affect the central nervous system (CNS), which includes the brain, spinal cord, and peripheral nervous system, the latter of which consists of the cranial nerves, spinal cord roots, spinal nerves, peripheral nerve branches, and the neuromuscular junction.

SYNONYMS

Neurologic deficits, seizure

EPIDEMIOLOGY

SPECIES, AGE, SEX All species and ages and both sexes of avian species may be affected.

RISK FACTORS

- Stress
- Nutritional deficiencies (e.g., hypocalcemia [see Hypocalcemia], hypomagnesemia)
- Trauma
- Environmental toxins (e.g., Teflon, plug-in air fresheners)
- Neoplasias
- Viral, bacterial, or fungal disease affecting brain and/or spinal cord

GEOGRAPHY AND SEASONALITY Depending on avian species affected, dry, cold environmental conditions may predispose hens to this disease process.

ASSOCIATED CONDITIONS AND DISORDERS

- Seizure activity
- Impaired function of the wings and/or legs
- Weakness

CLINICAL PRESENTATION

DISEASE FORMS/SUBTYPES

- Young birds are usually ill as a result of nutritional deficiencies.
- Wild birds are most often affected by traumatic, infectious, or toxic disorders.
- Old birds are most commonly affected by neoplastic or degenerative disorders.
- African greys are often presented with seizures caused by hypocalcemia.

HISTORY, CHIEF COMPLAINT Any one or more of the following may be described as part of the history regarding the presenting patient:

- Seizure activity
- Paralysis
- Paresis
- Proprioceptive deficits
- Ataxia
- Tremors
- Dysmetria
- Head tilt
- Circling
- Nystagmus
- Visual defects

PHYSICAL EXAM FINDINGS

- The physical examination may confirm the clinical signs noted by the owner when the history was being taken.
- Over and above the complete physical exam, a more complete neurologic examination is required.
  - The neurologic exam includes observation (e.g., mentation, posture, movement), palpation (e.g., integument, muscles, skeleton), functional assessment of the cranial nerves, evaluation of proprioceptive deficits and spinal reflexes, and sensory evaluation.
    - The cranial nerves can be evaluated by the menace response (II and V), the papillary light reflex (II and III), strabismus (III, IV, and VI), the palpebral reflex (V), jaw tone (V, VII), and the oculocephalic reflex (III, IV, VI, VIII).
    - Postural reactions that can be tested include proprioceptive positioning, hopping, drop and flap reaction, extensor postural thrust reaction, and placing reactions.
    - Spinal reflexes examined include wing withdrawal reflex, leg withdrawal reflex, crossed extensor, patellar reflex, and vent tone.
    - Birds do not have a cutaneous trunci muscle, so a panniculus response cannot be used to help localize a spinal lesion.

ETIOLOGY AND PATHOPHYSIOLOGY

- Seizures can result from primary or secondary disorders of the brain that cause spontaneous depolarization of cerebral neurosis.
- Seizures have three components: aura, ictus, and postictal phase.
- Ataxia results from disorders that interfere with recognition or coordination of position changes involving the head, trunk, or limbs.
- Ataxia is divided into three categories: sensory, vestibular, and cerebellar.
- Paralysis and paresis result from disorders that cause motor deficits.
  - Paresis may be presented with upper motor neuron clinical signs (e.g., loss of voluntary function, loss of reflexes, weakness, muscle atrophy) when affecting peripheral nerves.
  - Head tilt, circling, or nystagmus can be caused by central (brainstem) or peripheral (middle or inner ear) vestibular disease.
  - Peripheral lesions cause head tilt toward the side of the lesion; usually the bird falls or circles toward the side of the lesion.
  - Central lesions may cause head tilt or circling in the opposite direction.

DIAGNOSIS

DIFFERENTIAL DIAGNOSIS

- Generalized weakness
- Severe illness

INITIAL DATABASE

- Complete blood count: may show leukocytosis in patients with inflammatory, infectious, neoplastic, and/or toxic disorders
- Plasma biochemistry panel: may show abnormalities in metabolic and toxic disorders
- Imaging
  - Radiography: lateral and ventrodorsal views are recommended, with the beam centered in the area of interest (e.g., cervical, thoracic lumbar, synsacrum). The junction of the synsacrum with the thoracolumbar spine is a location susceptible to mechanical stress and vertebral subluxation. The axial skeleton of the birds should be extended, and the spine should be parallel to the cassette. Normal skull radiographs do not rule out involvement of tympanic bullae.

ADVANCED OR CONFIRMATORY TESTING

- Imaging
  - CT scan/MRI: CT can be useful when evaluating skeletal soft tissue structures, better enhanced with iodinated contrast intravenously at 0.45 mg/kg, in cross-sectional images. Images can be reformatted by computer software to obtain three-dimensional images. MRI is the imaging modality of choice for the CNS because it is useful in evaluating soft tissue contrast with increased detail when compared with CT. MRI is characterized by blurring with physiologic organ movement and incurs a higher cost than CT.

- Myelography: diagnostic format useful in identifying, localizing, and characterizing spinal cord lesions. The region of injection is found by placing the thumb and middle finger on the bony prominences of the iliac crest, with the index finger used to palpate to the first indentation cranial to the synsacrum. Iohexol 240 mg/mL at 0.88 mL/kg is injected using a 27-gauge needle at 0.5 mL/min. With duck, goose, and swan skeletal structures, thoracic and lumbar vertebrae have overlapping plates of bone that would prevent positioning of a needle in the subarachnoid space.
- Scintigraphy: imaging technique useful in providing functional information when used with a digital image processor. Scintigraphy involves intravenous administration of a small amount of a gamma-emitting radionuclide. Brain scan may allow identification of a damaged blood-brain barrier and focal lesions of the brain, but it is not particularly accurate in diagnosing degenerative disease or diffuse inflammatory processes. Bone scan identifies metastatic bone lesions, avascular necrosis, osteomyelitis, osteoarthritis, and other processes that affect bone turnover. Scintigraphy is particularly useful in identifying spinal abnormalities in birds.
- Electromyography: diagnostic test that is useful in evaluation of peripheral nerve or muscle disease; performed by inserting an electrode into the muscle and recording the electrical activity produced. In normal resting muscle, no electrical activity is observable once electrode placement is stabilized, and no audible signal is created.

TREATMENT

THERAPEUTIC GOALS

- Depending on severity of clinical signs and progression of neurologic disease:
  - Outpatient treatment for isolated seizures, mild ataxia, and head tilt
  - Inpatient treatment for cluster seizures (more than 3 seizures /24 h); status epilepticus; moderate to severe head tilt, paresis, and paralysis
- Determine cause of seizure activity or neurologic signs, and treat.
- Stop or reduce seizure activity or neurologic signs to gain good quality of life for the patient.

ACUTE GENERAL TREATMENT

- When patient presents with seizure activity, all perches and cage furniture should be removed from the enclosure. In the hospital cage, use soft bedding and provide shallow food and water bowls, or spread the bird's food on the cage floor if necessary. Lixit-type water bottles may be used to prevent the bird from spilling the water or drowning. The patient should be constantly supervised. When patient presents with paresis/paralysis, provide soft bedding to prevent sternal ulcers; check and frequently clean. With head trauma cases, place the bird in a dark, quiet area at an environmental temperature of 23°C (73.4°F).
- With a seizuring patient, administration of diazepam 0.5-1 mg/kg IV or IO q 1-4 h should be considered.
- Anesthetize patients in status epilepticus that fail to respond to intravenous diazepam and phenobarbital. Antiepileptic activity of propofol is superior to that of pentobarbital.
- With head trauma cases, treatment recommendations include mannitol 0.25-0.5 mg/kg IV slowly, together with crystalloid fluid therapy IV 25-75 mL/kg/d.
- In head tilt cases in which otitis media or interna is a result of suspected bacterial infection, consider long-term systemic antibiotic treatment with enrofloxacin 15 mg/kg IM/PO q 12 h until culture and sensitivity results are available.
- With CNS presentations with a bacterial origin, consider administration of antibiotics (e.g., enrofloxacin) that cross the blood-brain barrier.
- Treat other disorders according to the primary cause.
- The underlying cause of the seizure activity should be identified and treated accordingly (e.g., nutritional [hypocalcemia in African grey parrots, hypoglycemia in neonates], toxic [heavy metal type {see Heavy Metal Toxicity}, infectious]).

CHRONIC TREATMENT

For long-term therapy in idiopathic cases, phenobarbital 1-10 mg/kg PO q 12 h may be used.

DRUG INTERACTIONS

- Phenobarbital is highly protein bound and is metabolized in the liver. In patients with hypoalbuminemia or liver disease, lower the dose and closely monitor dose levels.
- Use of corticosteroid therapy in birds is controversial; this treatment should be used only when necessary.

POSSIBLE COMPLICATIONS

- Ineffective treatment to reduce seizure activity
- Arrhythmias, aspiration pneumonia, cardiovascular collapse, and death with status epilepticus
- Permanent neurologic deficits may follow severe status epilepticus, regardless of the cause.
- Aspiration pneumonia with moderate to severe paresis or paralysis of the legs due to inability to stand up and facilitate crop emptying; with generalized lower motor neuron signs, swallowing reflex may be affected.

RECOMMENDED MONITORING

- Inpatients with seizure history should be under constant supervision and monitored for recurrence.
- Inpatients should undergo neurologic exam daily to monitor status.

PROGNOSIS AND OUTCOME

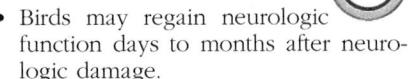

- Birds may regain neurologic function days to months after neurologic damage.
- Patients with paralysis and loss of deep pain perception have a poor prognosis for recovery.
- Paralysis associated with fracture of the leg is usually reversible; when associated with coelomic neoplasia, it is usually irreversible.

PEARLS & CONSIDERATIONS

COMMENTS

- With the seizuring patient, emphasize to the client that antiepileptic treatment in such cases treats only the clinical signs. Diagnostic testing is needed to identify the primary cause of the ultimate resolution if possible.
- Prognosis for vestibular disorders (e.g., head tilt) and paralysis is usually poorer than for peripheral disorders.
- Withhold food until the patient can swallow.
- A correct diet should be provided if nutritional deficiencies are suspected.

PREVENTION

- Provide proper diet.
- Prevent exposure to lead.
- Do not use plug-in air fresheners or scented candles around birds.
- Provide an environment that reduces traumatic incidences.

CLIENT EDUCATION

See previous discussion.

SUGGESTED READINGS

Bennet RA: Neurology. In Ritchie BW, et al, editors: Avian medicine: principles and applications, Brentwood, TN, 1994, HBD International Inc., pp 723–747.

Clippinger TL, et al: The avian neurologic examination and ancillary neurodiagnostic

techniques, J Avian Med Surg 10:221–247, 1996.
Rosenthal K: Disorders of the avian nervous system. In Altman RB, et al, editors: Avian medicine and surgery, Philadelphia, 1997, WB Saunders, pp 461–488.

AUTHOR: **DAVID SANCHEZ-MIGALLON GUZMAN**

EDITOR: **THOMAS N. TULLY, JR.**

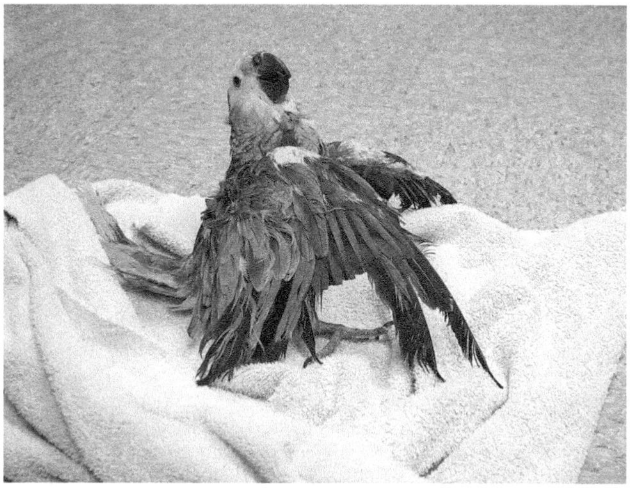

Neurologic Disease The amazon shows severe CNS signs and inability to balance. Full neurologic examination, including adequate imaging (CT or MRI), should be performed. *(Photo courtesy Jörg Mayer, The University of Georgia, Athens.)*

BIRDS

Ocular Lesions

Additional Images Available on Website

BASIC INFORMATION

DEFINITION

Lesion affecting the ocular globe and its adnexa (eyelids, glands, conjunctiva)

SYNONYMS

Eye lesions, ophthalmologic lesions

EPIDEMIOLOGY

SPECIES, AGE, SEX All species and ages and both sexes

GENETICS AND BREED PREDISPOSITION

- Birds of prey are frequently presented with ocular lesions secondary to trauma.
- Genetic factors predisposing birds to some congenital (reported palpebral malformation, ectropion, microphthalmia, corneal dermoid, cataracts, retinal dysplasia, colobomas) and acquired ocular lesions are unknown but suspected. Cataract development through heredity may be encountered in some canary breeds (e.g., Norwich, Yorkshire).
- Some species are more susceptible than others to virus-induced ocular lesions.
- Passerines and budgerigars are more commonly affected by facial cnemidocoptes mange.
- Species-specific idiopathic causes, such as mynah keratitis, have been reported.
- Color mutation variants of several species (e.g., cockatiels, budgerigars, lovebirds) are commonly presented for conjunctivitis.
- Budgerigar acute blindness is frequently caused by brain or pituitary neoplasms.

RISK FACTORS

- Affection of the periocular tissues (e.g., infraorbital sinus, skin over the skull)
- Nutritional deficiencies: hypovitaminosis A, in particular, can cause squamous metaplasia of the lacrimal glands and epithelial hyperplasia
- Trauma, dehydration (decreased tear production)
- Environmental factors such as constant darkness, light, or visual field occlusion have been shown to cause myopia and hyperopia in chickens.

CONTAGION AND ZOONOSIS

- Bacterial agents affecting the eyes can potentially be zoonotic in immune compromised people: *Chlamydophila psittaci, Mycobacterium* spp., *Mycoplasma* spp. Newcastle disease (paramyxovirus I) can cause ophthalmic lesions in birds as part of a systemic syndrome and is reported to cause conjunctivitis in immune deficient people.
- Viral and bacterial ophthalmologic affection should be considered contagious.

GEOGRAPHY AND SEASONALITY Ocular lesions that are caused by mosquito-borne viral infection (e.g., West Nile virus, chorioretinitis, poxvirus blepharitis) are more prevalent during spring and summer.

ASSOCIATED CONDITIONS AND DISORDERS

- Trauma (see Trauma)
- Some systemic bacterial, parasitic, and viral infections (see Viral Diseases) can lead to ocular lesions.
- Blindness or decreased visual acuity may result in a decreased appetite and reluctance to fly.
- Severe ocular infection (panophthalmitis) may spread, and neoplasms may metastasize.

CLINICAL PRESENTATION

DISEASE FORMS/SUBTYPES Depend on the ophthalmologic anatomic structures affected (eyelids, conjunctiva, lens, uvea, retina) and the nature (infectious, degenerative, developmental, neoplastic) and extent of the lesion.

HISTORY, CHIEF COMPLAINT

- Blindness
- Behavioral and appetite changes (due to decreased vision or discomfort)
- Cosmetic appearance of ocular lesions
- Ocular discharge (epiphora)
- Trauma (birds of prey)

PHYSICAL EXAM FINDINGS

- Blindness; decreased or absent palpebral, corneal, and pupillary reflexes; asymmetry of the eyes (e.g., exophthalmia, anisocoria, asymmetric palpebral opening); blepharospasm
- Evidence of trauma (e.g., hemorrhage in auricular canals, wounds, lesions of anterior eye segment, eyelids)
- Various abnormal physical findings if ocular lesions are part of generalized disease

ETIOLOGY AND PATHOPHYSIOLOGY

- Congenital: color mutations; canary and finch breeds
- Foreign bodies, feathers
- Viral: poxvirus (passerines, birds of prey, ratites, Amazon parrots), herpesvirus (psittaciformes, gouldian finches, birds of prey), papillomavirus (African grey parrots), adenovirus (quails, anseriformes, psittaciformes), flavivirus (birds of prey), paramyxovirus (psittaciformes, galliformes, anseriformes), orthomyxovirus (psittaciformes, galliformes, anseriformes), reovirus (psittaciformes)
- Bacterial: *Chlamydophila psittaci* (see *Chlamydophila psittaci*), *Mycoplasma* spp., *Mycobacterium avium* and *tuberculosis, Salmonella* spp., *Staphylococcus* spp., *Streptococcus* spp., *Escherichia coli*
- Parasitic: protozoa *(Toxoplasma gondii)*, helminths (*Oxyspirura* spp., *Thelazia* spp., *Filaria* spp.), arthropods (*Cnemidocoptes* spp.)
- Fungal: *Candida* spp., *Cryptococcus neoformans, Aspergillus* spp.
- Metabolic: hypovitaminosis A
- Trauma: birds of prey
- Toxic: cigarette smoke, chemical fumes, dust, photosensitization
- Neoplasm: extraocular (brain tumor, pituitary adenoma, retrobulbar neoplasms, eyelid and conjunctival neoplasms), intraocular (sarcoma, carcinoma, lymphoma, melanoma)
- Idiopathic

DIAGNOSIS

DIFFERENTIAL DIAGNOSIS

- Periocular lesions
- Central neurologic diseases

INITIAL DATABASE

- Complete blood count and plasma biochemistry profile: unremarkable for primary eye lesions; vary depending on the origin when part of a systemic process
- Ophthalmologic examination: ocular lesions can be visualized and localized on specific ocular anatomic structures using a slit lamp and a direct or indirect ophthalmoscope. For enhanced visualization of the fundus, several mydriatic methods have been described in birds: isoflurane anesthesia, isoflurane air sac perfusion, D-tubocurarine intracameral injection, and topical administration of a combination of atropine, phenylephrine, and vecuronium. Common lesions in birds comprise eyelid injuries, blepharitis, conjunctivitis, corneal ulceration, uveitis, hyphema or intravitreal hemorrhage, cataract, chorioretinitis, retinal detachment, and lesions of the pecten oculi. Other, less commonly reported lesions include glaucoma, lens luxation, asteroid hyalosis, and neoplasms. Chorioretinal scarring is common and must be distinguished from active lesions.
- Ancillary ophthalmologic tests: fluorescein staining is positive for corneal ulceration, electroretinography might differentiate retinopathies from central blindness, and tear production (Schirmer tear test or phenol red thread tear test) may be decreased (predisposing cause) or increased (reflex tear production) in corneal ulceration
- Radiography: exophthalmia and fracture of the scleral ring may be visualized

ADVANCED OR CONFIRMATORY TESTING

- Ultrasound examination of the eyes: may further define intraocular neoplasms, lens luxation, retinal detachment, pecten oculi tearing. Color Doppler may reveal decreased pecten blood flow.
- Advanced imaging: CT and MRI have been used to further evaluate avian eyes.
- Cytologic examination of conjunctiva or cornea: may reveal inflammatory and epithelial cells, bacteria, *Chlamydophila psittaci* elementary or reticulated bodies, poxvirus Bollinger bodies (fine-needle aspirate [FNA] from cutaneous lesions), or fungal organisms
- Specific molecular testing: may be positive when specific viruses (e.g., herpesviruses) or bacteria (e.g., *Chlamydophila psittaci*) are suspected
- Culture: may reveal the presence of Gram-negative or -positive bacteria. Results are difficult to interpret and might reflect a secondary infection. *Mycoplasma* spp. and *Chlamydophila psittaci* do not grow when routine bacteriologic methods are used.
- Histopathologic examination: indicated for mass, granuloma, and conjunctival hyperplasia, and after enucleation

TREATMENT

THERAPEUTIC GOALS

- Reverse or stabilize lesions.
- Treat potential infection.
- Manage ocular pain and inflammation.
- Address a potential systemic process.

ACUTE GENERAL TREATMENT

- Depends on the nature and extent of ocular lesions: treatment should follow the same approach as for small animals but with anatomic peculiarities of the avian eye in mind. Treatments for common avian ophthalmologic problems are presented.
- Diseases of the eyelids
    - Congenital or acquired malformations are treated surgically when possible. Blepharoplasty has been reported in psittacines.
    - Eyelid laceration: surgical reconstruction should be attempted. In case of important disruption of the upper or lower eyelids, compensation by the third eyelid is expected. Loss of the third eyelid will lead to chronic keratitis.
    - Blepharitis should be treated with local antibiotics and with local or systemic nonsteroidal antiinflammatory medication.
    - Cnemidocoptes mite infestations can be treated with topical ivermectin (0.01%) associated with systemic treatment (transcutaneous or intramuscular). Treatment is usually repeated weekly for three treatments.

- Vitamin A might help if a deficiency is suspected.
- Therapy for poxvirus lesions is directed toward treatment of secondary bacterial infection.

• Conjunctivitis
- Topical antibiotics: depend on suspected causative agent; tetracyclines, chloramphenicol (chloromycetin opththalmic solution, 1 drop topical q 6-8 h), and quinolones (ciprofloxacin HCl [0.3%] 1 drop topical q 6-8 h) are the preferred choices
- Local nonsteroidal antiinflammatories: diclofenac, flurbiprofen
- Systemic nonsteroidal antiinflammatories: if important blepharitis or chemosis is present
- When avian chlamydiosis or mycoplasmosis is suspected, systemic doxycycline (25-50 mg/kg, orally, q 12-24 h) or azithromycin (45 mg/kg PO q 24 h) and topical tetracyclines or azithromycin can be used.
- Other initiating or perpetuating causes, including foreign body removal, feather misorientation, and affection of the eyelids and tear film, should be addressed.

• Corneal ulceration
- Local antibiotics: fusidic acid, chloramphenicol, quinolones, tobramycin bacitracin-neomycin-polymixin B 3 to 4 times daily. In case of nonhealing, epitheliotoxic antibiotics should be avoided. If possible, antibiotic selection should be based on culture and sensitivity.
- Fungal keratitis must be treated with topical antimycotic medication.
- Severe infected corneal ulcers should be treated hourly.
- Artificial tears should be given 2 to 4 times daily.
- Topical corticosteroids and anesthetics are contraindicated.
- Atropine is not an effective cycloplegic in birds.
- Pain can be managed with systemic nonsteroidal antiinflammatory drugs.
- Temporary tarsorrhaphy may be an option in hard-to-treat birds and with slow-healing noninfected ulcers but prevents further topical treatment. Third eyelid flaps are not recommended owing to the powerful associated muscles.
- E-collar placement is necessary if the bird is scratching.

• Uveitis
- When an infectious cause is suspected, local antibiotics that penetrate the cornea (e.g., quinolones, gentamicin [gentamicin sulfate, 1 drop topical q 4-8 h], chloramphenicol) and systemic antibiotics can be used.
- Local and systemic antiinflammatory medication: corticosteroid eye therapy should be used with caution in birds
- Intracameral injection of D-tubocurarine (0.01-0.03 mL 0.3% solution) (for mydriasis) might prevent the development of synechiae and provide long-lasting cycloplegia.

• Eye trauma
- Eyelid injuries, corneal ulcerations, and uveitis (anterior and/or posterior) should be treated accordingly.
- Local and systemic nonsteroidal antiinflammatories
- Recombinant tissue-plasminogen activator (rTPA): intracameral and intravitreal injections have been reported in birds and may facilitate blood clot resorption and prevent formation of synechiae. For intravitreal hemorrhage (through the scleral ossicles), care should be taken not to puncture the more concave avian lens.
- Enucleation or evisceration should be considered in cases of severe injury, infection, or neoplasia.

• Cataracts
- Local nonsteroidal antiinflammatories can be used to limit associated low-grade uveitis.
- Phacoexeresis should be considered in cases of advanced cataracts. Lens removal by phacoemulsification is the recommended technique in birds. Lens prosthesis placement has been reported in owls.

• Chorioretinitis
- Systemic antibiotic or antiparasitic medications may be given.
- No treatment is currently available for viral lesions.

CHRONIC TREATMENT

Most lesions take weeks to months to resolve.

POSSIBLE COMPLICATIONS

- Spread of infection
- Loss of the eye or vision, phthisis bulbi
- Glaucoma may be a complication of untreated intraocular inflammation and lens luxation.
- Retinal detachment may be a complication of intravitreal hemorrhage, asteroid hyalosis.
- Laceration and subsequent hypovascularization of the pecten oculi might reduce its main role of nutritive function of the vitreal body and avascular retina (accomplished by frequent low-amplitude oscillatory motions of the globe). This has otherwise never been documented.

RECOMMENDED MONITORING

Recheck ophthalmologic examinations should be performed on a regular basis to assess response to the treatment and the evolution of lesions.

PROGNOSIS AND OUTCOME

- The prognosis is fair for uncomplicated blepharitis, conjunctivitis, and corneal ulcers.
- Some cases of avian conjunctivitis (e.g., cockatiels) can be frustrating to treat.
- Avian lenses allow a wide range of accommodation by anterior motion and deformation. Thus, removal is associated with significantly decreased visual acuity.
- Prognosis for retinal lesions depends on the extent, progression, and location. Affection of the foveae significantly decreases vision.
- Intraocular hemorrhage may take time to resolve without treatment. Hyphema may take weeks, and intravitreal hemorrhage months.

PEARLS & CONSIDERATIONS

COMMENTS

- Avian eye anatomy and physiology are very different from those of mammals, and birds are extremely visual animals. Therefore, thorough knowledge of avian ophthalmology and its peculiarities is mandatory when one is dealing with birds.
- A rigorous and complete ophthalmologic examination should be conducted in case of any suspicion of eye lesions.
- Fundus examination should be performed in every bird of prey presented because of the extremely high incidence of posterior eye segment lesions in the absence of external or anterior eye segment lesions.
- Overall health check should be performed because eye lesions can reflect a systemic disease.

PREVENTION

- Trauma prevention
- Good prophylactic methods for infectious ocular diseases
- Adequate "visual environment" that should take into consideration fundamental differences in light perception of avian eyes: flicker-free and full-spectrum types of light are recommended.

CLIENT EDUCATION

Ocular lesions should be evaluated and treated as soon as possible to prevent complications.

SUGGESTED READINGS

Kern TJ: Exotic animal ophthalmology (birds). In Gelatt KN, editor: Veterinary ophthalmology, ed 4, Boston, 2007, Blackwell Publishing, pp 1381–1389.

Murphy CJ: Raptor ophthalmology. Compendium of Continuing Education for the Practicing Veterinarian 9:241–260, 1987.

Williams D: Ophthalmology. In Ritchie BW, et al, editors: Avian medicine: principles and applications, Lake Worth, FL, 1994, Wingers Publishing, pp 673–694.

Maureen: Cite Maggs exotic chapter as ref. #4

CROSS-REFERENCES TO OTHER SECTIONS

Chlamydophila psittaci
Trauma
Viral Diseases

AUTHORS: **HUGUES BEAUFRÉRE AND CHANTALE L. PINARD**

EDITOR: **THOMAS N. TULLY, JR.**

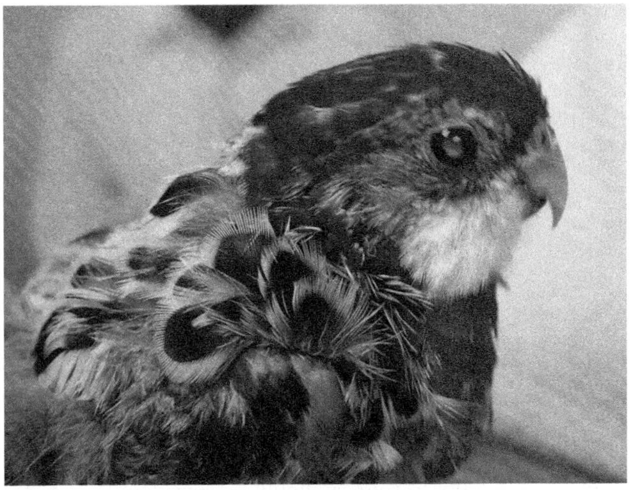

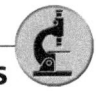

Ocular Lesions Mature cataracts are common finings in older birds. Surgical removal (phacoemulsification) is an option if the animal is large enough. *(Photo courtesy Jörg Mayer, The University of Georgia, Athens.)*

BIRDS

Organophosphate Toxicity

BASIC INFORMATION

DEFINITION

Exposure to organophosphates (OPs) that has resulted in pathology owing to inhibition of acetylcholinesterase

SYNONYM

Paralysis

EPIDEMIOLOGY

SPECIES, AGE, SEX All species and ages and both sexes

RISK FACTORS Exposure to fertilizers or insecticides

ASSOCIATED CONDITIONS AND DISORDERS

- Bilateral rear limb paralysis
- Inability to fly
- Salivation
- Lacrimation
- Polyuria

CLINICAL PRESENTATION

DISEASE FORMS/SUBTYPES Neurologic and muscle dysfunction

HISTORY, CHIEF COMPLAINT

- May not have known history of exposure to compounds containing OPs
- Acute onset of neurologic signs (e.g., bilateral rear limb lameness) (see Neurologic Disease)

PHYSICAL EXAM FINDINGS

- Ataxia
- Seizures
- Tremors
- Paralysis
- Anorexia
- Crop stasis
- Diarrhea

ETIOLOGY AND PATHOPHYSIOLOGY

OPs bind acetylcholinesterase permanently, resulting in excessive acetylcholine at the nerve endplates. This results in an inability of the bird to stop muscle activity, leading to clinical disease signs such as tremors and eventually paralysis.

DIAGNOSIS

DIFFERENTIAL DIAGNOSIS

- Lead or zinc toxicity
- Botulism (*Clostridium botulinum* toxin)
- Infectious disease such as West Nile virus, influenza virus, paramyxovirus, and proventricular dilatation disease (see Viral Diseases)
- Hypocalcemia

INITIAL DATABASE

- Complete blood count
- Plasma chemistry panel

ADVANCED OR CONFIRMATORY TESTING

- OP analysis (acetylcholinesterase levels)
- Whole blood for lead analysis
- Blood work to include serum samples for zinc levels (see Heavy Metal Toxicity)
- Radiographs

TREATMENT

THERAPEUTIC GOAL

Restore normal neurologic function through supportive care (see Trauma) and prevention of further OP binding.

ACUTE GENERAL TREATMENT

- Atropine 0.2-0.5 mg/kg IM q 3-4 h until signs have resolved
- Pralidoxime chloride (2-PAM) can be given at 10-100 mg/kg q 24-48 h or repeat once q 6 h, in conjunction with atropine. Best to administer within 24-36 hours of suspected OP toxicity with lower doses of 2-PAM being used in combination with atropine.

DRUG INTERACTIONS

2-PAM may reduce the protective effects of atropine.

RECOMMENDED MONITORING

- Monitor patient's response to treatment.
- Continue supportive therapy (e.g., fluid therapy, nutritional support) during treatment period.

PROGNOSIS AND OUTCOME

The prognosis is good if the bird is quickly treated after the onset of clinical signs.

PEARLS & CONSIDERATIONS

COMMENTS

OP toxicity is unusual in psittacines unless the owner has allowed the bird access to treated plants outdoors or is treating a plant near the bird's cage.

PREVENTION

Prevent exposure to OP insecticides.

CLIENT EDUCATION

Educate client on the dangers of bird exposure to OP insecticides.

SUGGESTED READING

Lightfoot TL, et al: Pet bird toxicity and related environmental concerns, Vet Clin Exot Anim 11:229–259, 2008.

CROSS-REFERENCES TO OTHER SECTIONS

Heavy Metal Toxicity
Neurologic Disease
Trauma
Viral Diseases

AUTHOR: **GWENDOLYN R. JANKOWSKI**

EDITOR: **THOMAS N. TULLY, JR.**

BIRDS

Overgrown Beak and Claws

BASIC INFORMATION

DEFINITION

Overgrowth of the beak and nails so as to make daily life functions such as perching or eating difficult. Sharp claws make handling of the bird uncomfortable for the owner; therefore, the owner may be reluctant to interact with this companion animal. Birds have claws with an epithelial covering, causing many people to incorrectly call them nails. Trimming a bird's claws often results in traumatizing the underlying germinal epithelium and vascular layer, causing bleeding.

EPIDEMIOLOGY

SPECIES, AGE, SEX Any avian species and age or sex of bird may be affected.

RISK FACTORS

- Poor diet
- Beak malformation
- Inadequate sunlight
- Lack of materials to chew on and/or rough surfaces
- Poor husbandry in cage or flight environment

CONTAGION AND ZOONOSIS Although overgrowth of the beak and nails (claws) is not contagious as a primary cause, several secondary causes such as mites and viral infections (e.g., circovirus) may be contagious between birds. These secondary conditions will lead to beak and claw overgrowth through their effects on underlying germinal tissue.

ASSOCIATED CONDITIONS AND DISORDERS

- *Knemidokoptes* spp.
- Vitamin deficiencies
- Chronic liver disease
- Psittacine beak and feather disease (circovirus infection)
- Trauma

CLINICAL PRESENTATION

DISEASE FORMS/SUBTYPES

- Primary
  - It is very rare for a bird in good health that receives proper husbandry and care to experience overgrown beak and claws.
- Secondary
  - Overgrown beak and claws are usually caused by a nutritional deficiency, poor husbandry conditions within the bird's environment, or underlying disease.
  - In budgerigars, liver disease has been implicated as a possible cause of beak overgrowth, but no specific pathophysiologic cause has been determined.

HISTORY, CHIEF COMPLAINT

- Overgrown beak
  - The beak is long and misshapen.
  - The bird may experience difficulty eating.
  - Trauma may occur to the thoracic inlet area of the body if the beak is extremely overgrown.
  - With circovirus infection, necrosis may affect the beak in combination with overgrowth.
- Overgrown claws
  - The nails are sharp, pointed, and are painful to the client when handling the bird.
  - Elongated claws may curve and catch on cage bars, causing the bird to pull the epithelial sheath off of the claw. Severely overgrown claws may curl around and damage the toe pad.

PHYSICAL EXAM FINDINGS

- Sharp and/or elongated beak extending past mandible, possibly extending to the thoracic inlet
- Long, pointed or curved nails

ETIOLOGY AND PATHOPHYSIOLOGY

- Beak tissue is produced by the epidermis and has underlying vascular germinal tissue. Trimming should not be necessary if the bird is maintained in the proper environment with adequate nutrition.
- If normal occlusion of the upper and lower beak is not maintained, the beak will show abnormal growth.
- Normal wear through perching and activity is required for the nails to sustain a normal growth pattern.
- A correlation may be noted between abnormal liver function and overgrowth of beak tissue, but the mechanism has not been described.
- Elongation of beak and nails due to viral irritation of the germinal epithelial layer caused by circovirus infection.

DIAGNOSIS

DIFFERENTIAL DIAGNOSIS

No differential diagnoses to overgrowth of the beak and claws other than primary causes previously described (see Etiology and Pathophysiology).

INITIAL DATABASE

- Complete blood count and plasma chemistry profile (especially review liver enzyme values), bile acid for liver function
- Testing is based on history and clinical signs.

ADVANCED OR CONFIRMATORY TESTING

- Diagnostics can be used to rule out an underlying condition
  - Dermatology workup, including skin (beak) scraping to look for ectoparasites
  - PCR-based diagnostic testing or feather follicle biopsy testing for psittacine beak and feather disease

TREATMENT

THERAPEUTIC GOALS

- Trim claws and/or beak to a length that is comfortable for the bird and the owner within the parameters of what is normal for the species being treated.
- There is no treatment for circoviral infections.
- Treat Knemidocoptic mite infestations with ivermectin, and trim abnormal beak tissue as much as the bird will allow, leading to normal growth once medicated. Nonaffected birds in the cage do not need to be treated.
- If elongated beak growth occurs as the result of malocclusion, correction of the malocclusion will reduce the likelihood of recurrence (e.g., scissors beak, prognathism).

ACUTE GENERAL TREATMENT

Some birds may require sedation for trimming of beak and nails because this can be a very stressful procedure.

- Claws
  - Claws should be trimmed to the level of the distal digital pad when the toe is fully extended. If claws are trimmed to the level of the distal digital pad, the vascular supply to the distal claw will be compromised in most cases. A hemostatic agent (e.g., silver nitrate stick) should be close at hand for use in case of bleeding.
  - Canine and feline nail trimmers may be used.
  - A dremel may be used to trim the claws in birds weighing over 150 grams.
  - Chemical cautery such as silver nitrate may be useful if bleeding occurs.
  - The toe should be squeezed after the claw is trimmed, to increase blood pressure to the distal trimmed tip. This will ensure that adequate hemostasis has been achieved.
  - Electrocautery can be used to trim a bird's claws if it weighs less than 150 grams.
- Beak
  - The beak can be trimmed with the use of a dremel.
  - Both upper and lower beaks should be included in routine trimming.
  - Chemical cautery, electrocautery, and tissue glue can be used if bleeding occurs. Caution must be used when tissue glue is used to stop beak bleeding, to prevent gluing the tongue to the beak. The flow of blood from a beak tip is fast and voluminous; therefore, electrocautery works well to stop bleeding.
  - Most beaks need to be smoothed out to remove excess beak surface tissue that has not sloughed. Care should be taken to not abrade down into the vascular germinal tissue layer. The hard outer surface of the beak tissue is very thin.
  - Mineral oil may be applied to give the beak a smooth appearance, especially after removal of excess surface epithelium.

CHRONIC TREATMENT

- Correct nutritional deficiencies.
- Provide bird with wood to chew.
- Treat underlying illnesses.
- Treat trauma or correct malocclusion.

POSSIBLE COMPLICATIONS

- A severely overgrown beak may lead to difficulty prehending food and thus to malnutrition.
- Severely overgrown claws may eventually curl around, causing trauma to the toes. This may result in infection or feet deformities.

PROGNOSIS AND OUTCOME

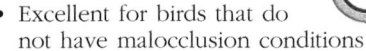

- Excellent for birds that do not have malocclusion conditions
- If the beak is damaged or is significantly removed for a malocclusion, the beak will have to be trimmed on a routine basis on the unaffected areas.

PEARLS & CONSIDERATIONS

PREVENTION

- Provide bird with adequate perches, nutrition, sunlight exposure, and bathing time.
- Cement stones can be used to help wear the nails, but the feet must be checked for the development of pododermatitis on the plantar surface of the foot. Abrasive surface perches used to reduce nail growth provide the majority of contact with the plantar weight-bearing surface of the foot, not the claw.

CLIENT EDUCATION

- See preventive measures above.
- All bird owners should have their companion animals treated and groomed by a veterinarian. This ensures that a professional overview of the procedure is being performed and recommendations for revisits discussed.

SUGGESTED READINGS

Harrison GJ, et al: Clinical practice. In Harrison GJ, et al, editors: Clinical avian medicine, vol 1, Palm Beach, FL, 2006, Spix Publishing, pp 12–17.

Perry RA: The avian patient. In Ritchie BW, et al, editors: Avian medicine: principles and application, Lake Worth, FL, 1994, Wingers Publishing, pp 40–42.

AUTHOR: **SHANNON N. SHAW**

EDITOR: **THOMAS N. TULLY, JR.**

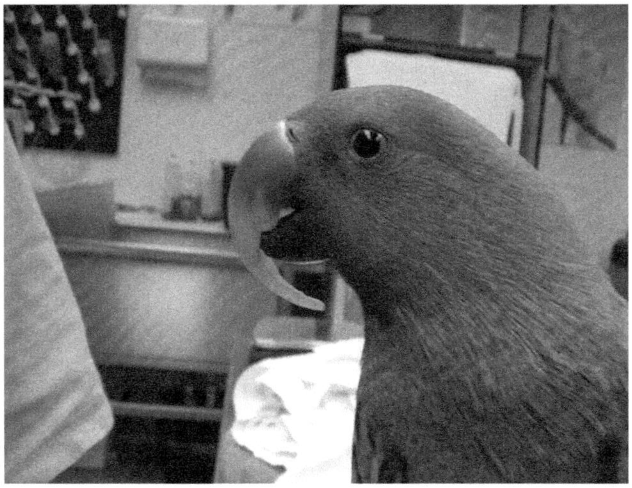

Overgrown Beak and Claws Elongated beak that needs trimming on a male eclectus parrot. This is a rare presentation.

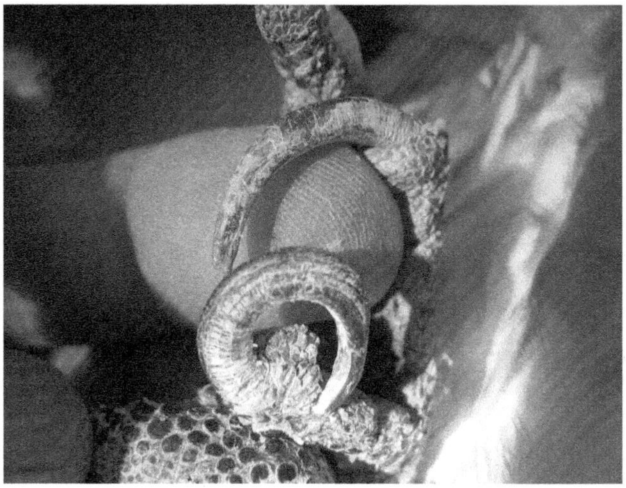

Overgrown Beak and Claws Long claws on a cockatoo presented for trimming.

BIRDS

Papillomas

BASIC INFORMATION

DEFINITION

A benign tumor with characteristic histopathology of epithelial hyperplasia; it may arise from the skin, mucous membranes, or glandular ducts

SYNONYM

Papillomatosis

EPIDEMIOLOGY

SPECIES, AGE, SEX

- Internal papillomas have been reported in several species of parrots, including conures, Amazon parrots, macaws, and hawk-headed parrots.
- Cloacal papillomas are found most commonly in macaws and Amazon parrots.
- Oral papillomas are found most commonly in macaws.
- Cutaneous papillomas are found most commonly in African grey parrots.

RISK FACTORS

- Chronic local irritation
- Immune suppression
- Exposure to other birds with clinical signs consistent with papillomatosis

CONTAGION AND ZOONOSIS

- An infectious origin has been suggested for both cutaneous (papillomavirus) and internal forms of papillomatosis (herpesvirus); however, studies have remained inconclusive. Much remains unknown regarding the epidemiology of this disease.
- No zoonosis has been reported for avian papillomas.

ASSOCIATED CONDITIONS AND DISORDERS Papillomas may be associated with development of squamous cell carcinoma, as well as biliary, hepatic, intestinal, and pancreatic carcinomas.

CLINICAL PRESENTATION

DISEASE FORMS/SUBTYPES

- Internal/cloacal papillomas (oral, respiratory, cloacal mucosa)
- Cutaneous papillomas: papillomas are found on the head and legs of birds

HISTORY, CHIEF COMPLAINT

- Circumscribed irregular proliferative growths present on birds legs, mouth, skin, or cloaca. These growths may be interfering with normal functions of the bird such as prehending food or perching.
- Birds with internal papillomatosis may have poor reproductive performance, weight loss, regurgitation, tenesmus, melena, or a soiled vent.

PHYSICAL EXAM FINDINGS

- Raised irregular proliferative lesions present on a bird's head, legs, cloaca, choana, or mouth; lesions may be crusty and ulcerative; they may bleed profusely when traumatized
- Cloacal papillomas may present as a cloacal prolapse.
- With internal papillomatosis, bird may be emaciated and/or dehydrated.

ETIOLOGY AND PATHOPHYSIOLOGY

- Cutaneous papillomas are caused by a papillomavirus in the family Papovaviridae.
- Papillomas have been found in the crop, esophagus, conjunctiva, proventriculus, ventriculus, choana, and cloaca, and may be caused by a herpesvirus.

DIAGNOSIS

DIFFERENTIAL DIAGNOSIS

- Cloacal prolapse (see Cloacal Prolapse)
- Dystocia
- Breeding behavior
- Hypocalcemia
- Cloacal mass
- Bacterial cloacitis
- Tenesmus due to enteritis, or enteric parasite infection
- Carcinoma
- For chronic regurgitation/diarrhea/ill thrift
  - Foreign body
  - Obstruction
  - Neoplasia
  - Infectious: bacterial, fungal, parasitic
  - Metabolic disease: liver disease, kidney disease
  - Enteritis (see Enteritis)
  - Pancreatitis
  - Food allergy

INITIAL DATABASE

- Histopathologic examination is necessary to establish a definitive diagnosis of a papilloma. The typical appearance consists of epithelial hyperplasia with monomorphic epithelial cells with large nuclei.

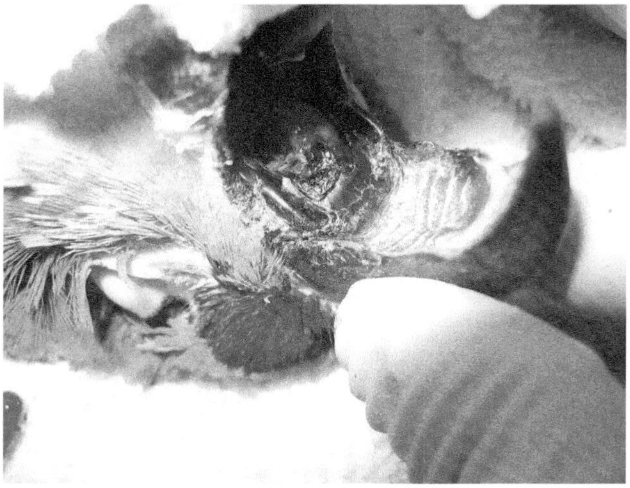

Papillomas Choanal papilloma.

- Complete blood count (CBC)
- Plasma chemistry panel
- Radiographs
- Fecal examination for parasites

ADVANCED OR CONFIRMATORY TESTING

- Endoscopy and biopsy
- Exploratory laparotomy with biopsy
- Electron microscopy
- PCR-based technology testing

TREATMENT

THERAPEUTIC GOALS

- Remove lesions that interfere with normal functioning of the bird and prevent transmission.
- Prevent secondary infection.

ACUTE GENERAL TREATMENT

- Removal of external lesions:
  - Surgically
  - By electrocautery
  - Through cryosurgery
- Broad-spectrum antibiotics are recommended to treat for secondary infection.

CHRONIC TREATMENT

- Supportive therapy (fluids, crop feeding) may be necessary for severely debilitated birds.
- See Dehydration.

POSSIBLE COMPLICATIONS

- In nestlings
  - Poor development
  - Beak abnormalities
  - Death
- Immune suppression
- Secondary infection
- Birds with cloacal papillomatosis have reportedly suffered from malignant tumors of the pancreas subsequently.
- Scarring can occur following removal of cloacal tumors. This can result in incontinence or stricture formation.

RECOMMENDED MONITORING

CBC may be used to monitor the bird's inflammatory response before and after removal of papillomas.

PROGNOSIS AND OUTCOME

Birds suffering from internal papillomas have a poor prognosis, and life expectancy is decreased.

PEARLS & CONSIDERATIONS

COMMENTS

- The cloaca of psittacines should be evaluated routinely for the presence of papillomas. A cotton-tipped applicator can be used to gently evert the cloaca. Also, papillomas that are present may grossly resemble a cloacal prolapse upon initial presentation. Use of acetic acid (vinegar) on a cotton-tipped swab and applied to suspect tissue will turn that tissue white if the integrity of said tissue is compromised by papillomatous growth.
- Removal of papillomas is palliative, and tumors often recur. Spontaneous regression has been reported.

PREVENTION

- Quarantine all birds for at least 30 days before introducing them to the flock until further information regarding transmission of papillomas becomes available.
- Autogenous vaccines have not proved effective for avian papillomatosis.

CLIENT EDUCATION

As above

SUGGESTED READINGS

Gallagher A, et al: Internal papilloma disease in green-winged macaws *(Ara chloroptera)*, Aust Vet J 75:9, 1997.

Gibbons PM, et al: Internal papillomatosis with intrahepatic cholangiocarcinoma and gastrointestinal adenocarcinoma in a peach-fronted conure *(Aratinga aurea)*, Avian Dis 46:1062–1069, 2002.

Johne R, et al: Herpesviral, but no papovaviral sequences, are detected in cloacal papillomas of parrots, Arch Virol 147:1869–1880, 2002.

Latimer KS, et al: Investigation of parrot papillomavirus in cloacal and oral papillomas of psittacine birds, Vet Clin Pathol 26:158–163, 1997.

Pennycott TW: Scaly leg, papillomas and pox in wild birds, Vet Rec 152:14, 2003.

Styles DK, et al: A novel psittacid herpesvirus found in African grey parrots *(Psittacus erithacus erithacus)*, Avian Pathol 34:150–154, 2005.

Sundberg JP, et al: Cloacal papillomas in psittacines, Am J Vet Res 47:928–932, 1986.

Youl JM, et al: Multidrug-resistant bacterial ingluvitis associated with squamous cell carcinoma in a budgerigar *(Melopsittacus undulatus)*, Vet Clin North Am Exot Anim Pract 9:557–562, 2006.

CROSS-REFERENCES TO OTHER SECTIONS

Cloacal Prolapse
Dehydration
Enteritis

AUTHOR: **SHANNON N. SHAW**

EDITOR: **THOMAS N. TULLY, JR.**

Pneumonia

BASIC INFORMATION

DEFINITION

Inflammation of pulmonary parenchyma, with accumulation of inflammatory fluid causing a reduction in gaseous exchange

SYNONYM

Lower respiratory disease

EPIDEMIOLOGY

SPECIES, AGE, SEX All species and ages and both sexes

RISK FACTORS

- Stress/immune suppression
- Adverse environmental conditions
- Inappropriate husbandry
- Cardiac disease (see Cardiac Disease)
- Aspiration
- Septicemia
- Dusty environments
- Exposure to dry hay/grass/nest box litter
- Nutritional deficiencies (e.g., vitamin A)
- Environmental exposure to irritants (e.g., cigarette smoke)

ASSOCIATED CONDITIONS AND DISORDERS

- Anorexia
- Depression
- Dyspnea
- Weakness

CLINICAL PRESENTATION

DISEASE FORMS/SUBTYPES

- Cardiac disease induced owing to inefficient heart function
- Aspiration of food material, water, or medication
- Primary bacterial or fungal pulmonary infection

HISTORY, CHIEF COMPLAINT

- Nonspecific
- Depression
- Inappetence
- Abnormally wide stance
- Reluctance to fly or perch
- Drooped wings
- Tail bobbing
- Loss of voice
- Exercise intolerance
- Dyspnea

PHYSICAL EXAM FINDINGS

- Weight loss
- Dyspnea
- Fluffed feathers
- Depression
- Moist sneeze/cough
- Moist audible breathing sounds

ETIOLOGY AND PATHOPHYSIOLOGY

- Predisposing factors (e.g., immune suppression, environmental conditions, bacterial/fungal infection) lead to disease processes that affect the ability of lung tissue to properly function.
  - Viral
    - Paramyxovirus
    - Adenovirus
    - Orthomyxovirus
  - Bacterial
    - Gram-positive organisms: *Streptococcus* spp., *Staphylococcus* spp.
    - Gram-negative organisms: *Escherichia coli, Yersina* spp., *Klebsiella* spp., *Salmonella* spp., *Pasteurella* spp.
    - *Chlamydophila psittaci* (see *Chlamydophila psittaci*)
    - *Mycobacterium* spp.
  - Fungal
    - *Aspergillus* spp. (see *Aspergillosis*), *Trichosporon* spp., *Absidia* spp., *Nocardia* spp., *Cryptococcus* spp., *Candida* spp.
  - Parasites
    - *Atoxoplasma* spp., *Sarcocystis* spp.
  - Environmental toxins
    - Polytetrafluoroethylene (PTFE) gas is released when nonstick cookware (e.g., Teflon) is heated to excessive temperatures; also present on and in other substances
    - Cigarette smoke
    - Paint fumes
  - Aspiration pneumonia: especially hand-fed birds, sick birds being treated with medication and being fed critical care diet
  - Immune mediated/unknown: hypersensitivity syndrome

DIAGNOSIS

DIFFERENTIAL DIAGNOSIS

- Air sacculitis
- Generalized septicemia
- Coelomic organomegly
- Tracheitis
- Glottis abscess
- Oral trauma

INITIAL DATABASE

- Lung auscultation: changes in respiratory noises in avian species are more subtle than in mammals owing to the position and minor movement of the lung parenchyma
- Complete blood count (CBC): leukocytosis is linked with inflammatory reaction possibly related to bacterial and/or fungal infection. Leukopenia may be noted with a severe septic condition or viral infection. Monocytosis is often present when chronic bacterial infections (e.g., avian chlamydiosis, mycobacteriosis) are present.

ADVANCED OR CONFIRMATORY TESTING

- Imaging: normal avian lungs appear to have a honeycomb structure when viewed on radiographic images. Lateral and ventrodorsal views should be taken to assess the pulmonary parenchyma. Lateral and dorsal aspects of the lungs can appear more radiopaque in the healthy bird owing to the summation of muscle tissue. Inspiration and expiration do not affect the radiographic appearance of the pulmonary parenchyma owing to reduced movement of the lung tissue in avian species. Acute pneumonia is noted as an increased parabronchial pattern in the midportion of the lungs. In chronic conditions, lung changes extend to the caudal portions of the lung fields
- Endoscopy: normal appearance of the lung on endoscopy shows a pale pink color with a spongy texture. An endoscopic approach through the caudal thoracic air sac allows for visualization of the septal aspect of the lung. The intercostal approach to exploration of the costal aspect of the lung is difficult in avian species because of the small pleural space and limited movement of the endoscope. An alternative approach for visualization of the lungs is through the thoracic inlet; again, this insertion site is not very practical because of the limited surface of the lung that can be observed. Changes in color and tissue texture should be evaluated. Reddish coloration is indicative of congestion or inflammation; white or grey surface color may suggest edema. Swabs for bacterial/fungal culture and sensitivity may be taken during the endoscopic procedure.
- Tissue biopsy: biopsy samples may be collected during the endoscopic procedure. A surgical approach to collection of lung biopsy samples has been described as gaining access through the fifth intercostal space, allowing excellent visualization of lung tissue.

- Transtracheal lavage: lavage fluid from normal patients should reveal a low number of cells. This procedure is performed by flushing (0.5-1 mL/kg body weight) sterile saline into the upper respiratory tract and immediately aspirating the fluid back into the syringe. The presence of erythrocytes may suggest congestion, and the presence of inflammatory cells usually is related to infectious pneumonia. If food or nonpathogenic fungus organisms are noted in the sample, aspiration should be considered as a possible cause of the disease condition.
- Culture and sensitivity: microbial culture and sensitivity testing should be performed when a bacterial or fungal infection is suspected. Samples can be collected during an endoscopic examination or when fluid is collected from a transtracheal lavage. Gram stains can be used to identify involvement of bacteria before bacterial culture results are received from the laboratory.

TREATMENT

THERAPEUTIC GOALS

- Stabilize and improve patient's physical condition.
- Assess patient and determine disease problem.
- Treat disease condition(s).
- Confirm disease condition and follow through with appropriate treatment.
- Determine origin to prevent or reduce recurrence.
- Restore patient to good health.

ACUTE GENERAL TREATMENT

- Oxygen therapy: oxygen therapy may be needed if severe respiratory distress is present, or if stabilization of the patient is necessary for assessment of the patient's condition.
- Antibiotic medication: this is required for primary and secondary bacterial infections that may be associated with the disease condition. Culture and sensitivity is necessary to confirm that the appropriate treatment is being administered.
- Antifungal medication: because of the number of adverse effects associated with fungal medication, a confirmed diagnosis is recommended before long-term treatment with these therapeutic agents is provided.
- Nebulization: this is an extremely useful therapeutic measure in medicating avian respiratory disease; with nebulization, medication is directly administered to respiratory tissue
- Medications used for nebulization:
  - Amikacin
    - 5-6 mg/mL sterile water or saline × 15 min q 8-12 h
    - 6 mg/mL sterile water and 1 mL acetylcysteine (20%) until dissipated q 8 h
  - Aminophylline
    - 3 mg/mL sterile water or saline × 15 min
  - Amphotericin B
    - 7-10 mg/mL sterile water × 15 min
  - Cefotaxime
    - 10 mg/mL saline × 10-30 min q 6-12 h
  - Enilconazole
    - 0.2 mg/5 mL saline q 12 h × 21 days
  - Enrofloxacin
    - 10 mg/mL saline × 15 min q 12 h
- It is recommended that particles emitted from the nebulizer measure <5 μm to allow for optimal dispersion throughout the patient's respiratory system. Another advantage of nebulization therapy is that it allows the use of drugs that are potentially toxic when administered parenterally or orally (e.g., gentamicin). During nebulization therapy, the respiratory tract is humidified, aiding the elimination of excess mucus. Although some medications (e.g., oil-based drugs) are not suitable to be nebulized, a wide range of antibiotics and antifungal medications are acceptable. Nebulization of antihistamines and steroids has been used to control presentation of respiratory distress in cases of hypersensitivity syndrome
- In case of pulmonary edema, a diuretic should be used to clear fluids out of the airways
  - Furosemide at 0.05 mg/300 g IM 12 q h
  - Mannitol at 0.5 mg/kg IV slowly

CHRONIC TREATMENT

Antifungal therapy may have to be administered on a long-term basis.

DRUG INTERACTIONS

Certain species of birds are sensitive to many therapeutic agents (e.g., African grey parrots are sensitive to itraconazole). It is imperative that veterinarians are knowledgeable about any medication risk involved for the avian species they are treating, especially if long-term administration of the product is required.

POSSIBLE COMPLICATIONS

- Lack of treatment response
- Adverse reaction to medication
- Tissue damage too severe for adequate respiratory function even if disease is treated

RECOMMENDED MONITORING

- Repeat radiographs to assess lung tissue.
- Repeat CBC and plasma chemistry panel to assess treatment response.
- Repeat endoscopic examinations to assess treatment response and lung tissue.
- Analgesic/antiinflammatory medication is required in cases of suspected pain and inflammation.
- Monitor appetite, fecal output, and behavior during the treatment period.

PROGNOSIS AND OUTCOME

- Uncomplicated cases have a good prognosis.
- The prognosis is poor for cases that involve respiratory toxins (e.g., PTFE) and severe fungal infection.

PEARLS & CONSIDERATIONS

COMMENTS

- PTFE toxicity is usually a fatal presentation.
- Pneumonia can be treated in avian patients with a successful outcome.

PREVENTION

- Purchase weaned birds.
- When administering oral medication or critical care diet, do so before placing in the cage or incubator—the last procedure.
- Provide proper husbandry care and nutritional offerings.
- Reduce stress.
- Prevent exposure to airborne toxins or irritants.

CLIENT EDUCATION

See Prevention.

SUGGESTED READINGS

Carpenter JW, editor: Exotic animal formulary, ed 3, St Louis, 2005, Elsevier/Saunders, pp 223–225.

Girling SJ: Respiratory disease. In Harcourt-Brown N, et al, editors: BSAVA manual of psittacine birds, ed 2, Gloucester, UK, 2005, British Small Animal Veterinary Association, pp 170–179.

Tully TN, et al: Pneumonology. In Ritchie BW, et al, editors: Avian medicine: principles and application, Lake Worth, FL, 1994, Wingers Publishing, pp 556–581.

CROSS-REFERENCES TO OTHER SECTIONS

Aspergillosis
Cardiac Disease
Chlamydophila psittaci

AUTHOR: **ALBERTO RODRIGUEZ BARBON**

EDITOR: **THOMAS N. TULLY, JR.**

Pododermatitis

Client Education Sheet Available on Website

BASIC INFORMATION

DEFINITION

Pododermatitis is a general term for any inflammatory or degenerative condition of the avian foot; it may range from very mild redness or swelling to chronic, infiltrative abscesses and osteomyelitis.

SYNONYMS

Bumblefoot, infectious pododermatitis

EPIDEMIOLOGY

SPECIES, AGE, SEX

- Captive raptors, including those of the family Falconidae
- Can affect any avian species of any age and sex

GENETICS AND BREED PREDISPOSITION Falcon species, eagles, ospreys, red-tailed hawks

RISK FACTORS

- Especially affects overweight birds
- Birds that lack exercise
- Birds that are supplied improper perches or do not have multiple perch types or surfaces
- Overgrown talons
- Unilateral damage to one foot or leg, causing increased weight bearing to the contralateral limb
- Traumatic puncture/bite wounds to the feet
- Poor sanitation and husbandry
- Inadequate nutrition
- Severe poxvirus infection
- Frostbite
- Trap injury
- Thermal and electrical burns/wounds

ASSOCIATED CONDITIONS AND DISORDERS

- Dermatitis around wound area
- Osteomyelitis
- Tendonitis
- Septic arthritis
- Depression
- Anorexia

CLINICAL PRESENTATION

DISEASE FORMS/SUBTYPES

- Grade 1: early insult or lesion of a prominent plantar area with no apparent underlying infection
  - Associated clinical signs: hyperemia, early ischemia, or hyperkeratotic reaction
- Grade 2: infection of underlying tissues in direct contact with the surface lesion with no gross swelling
  - Associated clinical signs: puncture (with localized infection), local ischemic necrosis
- Grade 3: infection with gross pedal inflammatory swelling
  - Associated clinical signs: serous or caseous fluid draining from fibrotic lesion
- Grade 4: infection with swelling of underlying tissues involving deep vital structures
  - Associated clinical signs: chronic wound, producing tenosynovitis, arthritis, and/or osteomyelitis
- Grade 5: crippling deformity and loss of function

HISTORY, CHIEF COMPLAINT

- Foot or leg injury
- Depending on severity, mild lameness to non–weight-bearing lameness of the affected limb

PHYSICAL EXAM FINDINGS

- Grade 1: associated clinical signs: hyperemia, early ischemia or hyperkeratotic reaction
- Grade 2: associated clinical signs: puncture (with localized infection), local ischemic necrosis
- Grade 3: associated clinical signs: serous or caseous fluid draining from fibrotic lesion
- Grade 4: associated clinical signs: chronic wound, producing tenosynovitis, arthritis, and/or osteomyelitis
- Grade 5: crippling deformity and loss of function

ETIOLOGY AND PATHOPHYSIOLOGY

- Constant pressure in the plantar aspect of the foot caused by improper perch material, an overweight bird, and/or lack of exercise results in disruption of epithelial integrity of the skin over the metatarsal pad, and occasionally over the digital pads. Resulting pressure necrosis in the focal area of affected skin compromises the barrier protecting underlying tissue from exposure to bacterial organisms.
- The organism(s) (e.g., *Staphylococcus aureus*) often thrives in the tissue environment of an avian foot.
- As mentioned earlier, other factors can seed bacteria into the bird's foot tissue, but a wound caused by pressure necrosis is the most common scenario.
- Complications associated with the infectious process reduce the already meager blood supply to the foot. Reduced blood supply leads to failure of the bird's immune system to neutralize pathogens, resulting in the development of a chronic granulomatous disease. In addition to reducing the blood supply, the granuloma formation further isolates pathogens from systemic antibiotics and immune factors.
- The disease becomes progressive and degenerative.
- Rupture of the flexor tendons, osteomyelitis, and septic arthritis of the tarsometatarsal phalangeal joints will occur in severe cases.

DIAGNOSIS

DIFFERENTIAL DIAGNOSIS

- Acute foot injuries
- Trauma
- Abrasive perch surfaces
- Nutritional deficiencies
- Neoplasia

INITIAL DATABASE

- Complete blood count: often unremarkable; may see leukocytosis, characterized by heterophilia and monocytosis in more severe chronic cases
- Plasma chemistry panel: creatine kinase may be elevated in more severe cases
- Culture and sensitivity of affected area
- Radiographic images may reveal periosteal reaction in cases of osteomyelitis or septic arthritis with soft tissue swelling.

ADVANCED OR CONFIRMATORY TESTING

Testing used to gain information for the initial database can also be used to evaluate treatment response.

TREATMENT

THERAPEUTIC GOALS

- Treat infection.
- Treat to reduce complications of healing that may affect use of the foot.
- Healing will reduce the possibility of rapid recurrence.

ACUTE GENERAL TREATMENT

- Bandaging to remove weight from the plantar surface of the foot
  - Interdigitating foot bandages are the recommended types for mild cases.
  - Donut-type bandages for severe cases, especially where surgical débridement is needed
  - Bandages should be changed daily until condition improves; then use can be prolonged to 2-3 days, with small increases as the condition resolves.

- Bandages should be applied to both feet to avoid development of bumblefoot in the other foot as the result of shifts in weight bearing.
- Surgical débridement
  - Bumblefoot of grade 3 and higher requires aggressive surgical débridement, followed by flushing with warm saline.
  - Surgery debulks the antigen load and inflammatory debris and allows for vascular perfusion with delivery of immune factors and systemic antibiotics to affected tissues.
  - If secondary healing by granulation is intended, the injury should be managed as an open wound.
  - If first-intention healing is deemed appropriate, consider the use of antibiotic impregnated beads followed by closing of the wound.
- Medication
  - Preparation H applied topically with massage of the affected area in mild cases to improve blood supply
  - Dexamethasone, dimethyl sulfoxide (DMSO), and antibiotics such as piperacillin/tazobactam (Zosyn) create an effective combination for topical application in acute cases with severe inflammation.
  - Formula for topical medication for bumblefoot lesions described above:
    - Piperacillin/tazobactam 2 g
    - Dexamethasone 4 mg
    - DMSO qs up to 10 mL
    - This formulation should be kept refrigerated for 7 days.
- Antibiotic-impregnated beads, following aggressive surgical débridement, offers an effective method for delivery of antibiotics to an infected ischemic site.
  - Footpad toughening products applied topically are recommended during advanced stage of healing, where they may strengthen the pink, tender skin that has regenerated on the planter surface.
  - Systemic antibiotics are recommended in grade 2 and higher bumblefoot.
  - Production of antibiotic-impregnated PMMA beads
    - Antibiotic concentration of beads: use powdered form of antibiotic only
      - Ratio of aminoglycoside to bone cement: Simplex P (Stryker Howmedica Osteonics, Mahwah, NJ): 3 g antibiotic/40 g packet bone cement
      - Ratio of penicillin to bone cement: 8 g antibiotic/40 g packet bone cement
      - Ratio of fluoroquinolones to bone cement: 7 g antibiotic/40 g packet bone cement
      - Ratio of clindamycin to bone cement: 6 g antibiotic/40 g packet bone cement
    - Bead production
      - Mix antibiotic powder with cement polymer powder.
      - Mix the powder compound, vigorously shaking for 2 minutes.
      - Separate mixed compound into 1 g aliquots.
      - Place liquid monomer into evaporation-proof container, and chill to 0°C (32°F) in the freezer.
      - Quickly mix 0.7 mL of the chilled polymer with a 1 g aliquot of the powder compound to a homogenous "loose batter" consistency, and load into a 3 mL syringe.
      - Immediately expel the liquid dough in a line onto a sterile surface.
      - With a gloved hand, scoop tiny pieces of dough from the line and roll them between the index finger and the palm of the hand into tiny smooth beads.
      - Beads are sterilized using ethylene oxide or gamma radiation.
      - If ethylene oxide is used, beads must be aerated for 24 hours to allow for dissipation of gas.
      - PMMA beads need to be remove after 2-4 weeks. Alternatively use antibiotic impregnated calcium sulfate hemihydrate beads, which are biodegradable and should be absorbed over time.

CHRONIC TREATMENT

- Chronic bumblefoot is a slow healing condition that may require 2-6 months to heal; periodic reevaluations should be performed.
- Grade 3 and higher bumblefoot lesions may require aggressive surgical débridement, followed by flushing with warm saline.
  - Surgery to debulk the proliferative infected granulation tissue allows for vascular perfusion, enabling the delivery of immune factors and systemic antibiotics to affected tissues.
  - If secondary-intention healing is preferred, the lesion should be managed as an open wound.
  - If primary-intention healing is the treatment of choice, one should consider the use of antibiotic-impregnated methylmethacrylate beads, followed by closing of the wound. The beads should be removed once healing has occurred.

POSSIBLE COMPLICATIONS

- No response to treatment
- Bacterial septicemia
- Dermal loss that will delay healing time or prevent primary closure of the wound once infection has been treated

RECOMMENDED MONITORING

- Regular monitoring—daily in severe cases—of foot lesions should take place to observe for treatment response.
- Chronic bumblefoot lesions are often slow to heal, possibly requiring 2-6 months depending on severity and treatment response.

PROGNOSIS AND OUTCOME

- Good for grade 1-3 bumblefoot lesions if underlying structures are not affected and treatment response is quick
- Guarded to poor for grade 4-5 bumblefoot lesions when osteomyelitis and septic arthritis are complicating factors

PEARLS & CONSIDERATIONS

COMMENTS

- Knowledge by owners and/or keepers of the causes of bumblefoot is needed to prevent development of lesions, or treatment should be sought at early onset.
- Some avian species and individual birds are more susceptible to bumblefoot lesions; considerations regarding maintenance of these individuals in captivity should be evaluated if recurrence of this disease process is continual.

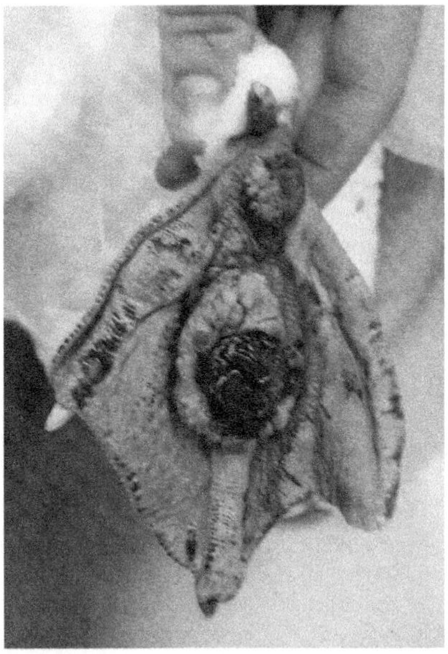

Pododermatitis A severe bumblefoot lesion in a duck. These lesions are common in waterfowl kept on hard and solid surfaces (e.g., concrete). *(Photo courtesy Jörg Mayer, The University of Georgia, Athens.)*

PREVENTION

- Correct husbandry practices, including various perch types and materials in the enclosure for the bird to select
- Maintenance of proper or lower weight of the bird in captivity
- Increased exercise or flying time
- A nutritious balanced diet or a proper diet for the species in question
- Periodic evaluation of the feet to identify early bumblefoot lesions

CLIENT EDUCATION

See Prevention.

SUGGESTED READINGS

Harcourt-Brown NH: Foot and leg problems. In Beynon PH, et al, editors: Manual of raptors, pigeons and waterfowl, Cheltenham, UK, 1996, BSAVA Ltd, pp 163–168.

Remple JD: A multifaceted approach to the treatment of bumblefoot in raptors, J Exot Pet Med 15:49–55, 2006.

Remple JD, et al: Antibiotic-impregnated polymethyl methacrylate beads in the treatment in the treatment of bumblefoot in raptors. In Lumeij JT, et al, editors: Raptor biomedicine III, Lake Worth, FL, 2000, Zoological Education Network, Inc., pp 255–265.

AUTHOR: **DAVID SANCHEZ-MIGALLON GUZMAN**

EDITOR: **THOMAS N. TULLY, JR.**

BIRDS

Polytetrafluoroethylene (Teflon) Toxicity

BASIC INFORMATION

DEFINITION

Pathology from inhalation of fluorinated gases present in the air as the result of heating of polytetrafluoroethylene (PTFE) to above 240°C (464°F). At 240°C (464°F) PTFE gives off toxic particulates while there is significant decomposition of the compound at 340°C (680°F).

SYNONYMS

Teflon toxicity, polymer fume fever

EPIDEMIOLOGY

SPECIES, AGE, SEX All species and ages and both sexes

RISK FACTORS Proximity to areas in which nonstick cookware, irons, ironing boards, heat lamps, or other appliances with a nonstick surface are in use

ASSOCIATED CONDITIONS AND DISORDERS
- Dyspnea
- Depression

CLINICAL PRESENTATION

DISEASE FORMS/SUBTYPES
- Sudden death
- Respiratory/neurologic

HISTORY, CHIEF COMPLAINT
- Most common presenting complaint is sudden death.
- Dyspnea
- Incoordination
- Coma

PHYSICAL EXAM FINDINGS
- Dyspnea
- Pulmonary edema, hemorrhage, and necrosis
- Weakness and incoordination
- Seizures

ETIOLOGY AND PATHOPHYSIOLOGY

- Vaporization of fluorinated gases occurs owing to degradation of PTFE at temperatures above 240°C (464°F); gases are inhaled by birds in the vicinity.
- Respiratory epithelium is exposed to inhaled acidic gases, causing hemorrhage and congestion.

DIAGNOSIS

DIFFERENTIAL DIAGNOSIS

- Cardiovascular disease
- Pulmonary thromboembolism

INITIAL DATABASE

- Stabilize the patient before beginning diagnostics.
- Oxygen therapy before physical examination may be beneficial.

ADVANCED OR CONFIRMATORY TESTING

Radiographs if the bird is stable, to assess pulmonary edema

TREATMENT

THERAPEUTIC GOALS

- Reestablish appropriate ventilation and oxygen saturation (Spo_2).
- Prevent secondary infection (pneumonia).

ACUTE GENERAL TREATMENT

- Oxygen therapy: oxygen may be provided at 40%-50% initially; however, prolonged exposure to high levels may be associated with toxicity
- Bronchodilators: terbutaline 0.1 mg/kg PO q 12-24 h; theophylline 2 mg/kg PO q 12 h
- Diuretics: furosemide 0.15 mg/kg IM up to every 8 hours as needed, or 1-2 mg/kg PO once daily as needed. May be required for symptomatic therapy with pulmonary edema; however, use caution, particularly in dehydrated patients
- Antiinflammatories: meloxicam 0.2 mg/kg PO q 12 h
- Antimicrobials: should be broad spectrum such as amoxicillin or, for severely debilitated birds, enrofloxacin
- Heat: most debilitated birds are hypothermic and should be placed in an incubator for warmth

CHRONIC TREATMENT

Supportive care

POSSIBLE COMPLICATIONS

Secondary bacterial/mycotic infection (pneumonia)

RECOMMENDED MONITORING

- Repeat auscultation at least daily to assess results of therapy.
- Monitoring of pulmonary edema may be possible radiographically as well if the patient is stable; however, this is not usually the case.

PROGNOSIS AND OUTCOME

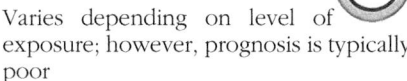

Varies depending on level of exposure; however, prognosis is typically poor

PEARLS & CONSIDERATIONS

PREVENTION

Birds' respiratory systems are extraordinarily sensitive to inhaled toxins. When gases are present in the home or near the aviary, birds should be removed or windows opened for ventilation.

CLIENT EDUCATION

Clients should be informed early and reminded frequently, preferably at annual examinations, about potential hazards of Teflon cookware for their birds.

SUGGESTED READING

Lightfoot TL, et al: Pet bird toxicity and related environmental concerns, Vet Clin North Am Exot Anim Pract 11:229–259, 2008.

AUTHOR: **GWENDOLYN R. JANKOWSKI**

EDITOR: **THOMAS N. TULLY, JR.**

BIRDS

Proventricular Dilatation Disease

Client Education Sheet Available on Website

BASIC INFORMATION

DEFINITION

A viral progressive and frequently fatal disease affecting the neural system, especially the autonomic portion of the gastrointestinal (GI) tract (myenteric plexus) and attributed to avian bornaviruses

SYNONYMS

Macaw wasting disease, proventricular dilatation syndrome, neuropathic gastric dilatation, myenteric ganglioneuritis, lymphoplasmacytic encephalomyelitis, avian bornaviruses

EPIDEMIOLOGY

SPECIES, AGE, SEX All species and ages and both sexes

GENETICS AND BREED PREDISPOSITION Although proventricular dilatation disease (PDD) is diagnosed most commonly in macaws, African grey parrots, cockatoos, eclectus, and conures, it can be seen in any psittacine bird and in some other species (e.g., Canada goose, canary, toucan, duck, falcon, chicken, quail) at any age. Budgerigars seem to be resistant to the disease.

CONTAGION AND ZOONOSIS Oral-fecal transmission from bird to bird has been suggested.

ASSOCIATED CONDITIONS AND DISORDERS

- Neurologic conditions (e.g., seizure activity, ataxia)
- Polyphagia
- Diarrhea (see Diarrhea)
- Anemia
- Gastroenteritis
- Weakness

CLINICAL PRESENTATION

DISEASE FORMS/SUBTYPES

- Dilatation of the proventriculus
- Paralytic ileus, diarrhea
- Nonspecific neurologic signs

HISTORY, CHIEF COMPLAINT

- Neurologic signs (see Neurologic Disease)
- Depression
- Polyphagia
- Paralysis
- Diarrhea
- Extreme weight loss
- Vomiting

PHYSICAL EXAM FINDINGS Any bird with digestive or neurologic signs or a combination of the two should be suspected of having PDD. Clinical signs are variable, and no general picture can be drawn for a bird affected by PDD. Some birds develop an acute form of the disease; others develop a more chronic form that may persist for years. Birds affected by the digestive form of the disease frequently exhibit maldigestion (undigested food in the stools), diarrhea, regurgitation, and/or weight loss. Subtle behavioral changes, mild ataxia, wasting despite a good appetite, or peripheral neuritis may be the only clinical sign. Other signs that have been noted concurrently with PDD include feather picking, blindness, and cardiac conduction abnormalities.

ETIOLOGY AND PATHOPHYSIOLOGY

- Although the pathophysiology of the disease is unclear, recently discovered avian bornaviruses have been proven to be the etiologic agents of the disease. Recent biomolecular investigations (Kisler, 2008) have significantly linked avian bornaviruses to the disease. The disease has been experimentally induced in cockatiels using brain homogenates. Experiments fulfilling Kock's postulate were performed in Patagonian conures and cockatiels.
- Several genotypes (ABV 1-6) with various pathogenicities have been described.
- Avian bornaviruses have been reported to be present in many tissues from infected birds, including the gonads and the eyes.
- Variable incubation period: 3 weeks to 3 months has been suggested. A state of chronic infection may exist. Recent experimental infection studies report incubation periods of about 80-110 days in cockatiels and 66 days in Patagonian conures.
- An autoimmune reaction of the avian host following infection with the virus has been suggested as the cause of the lesions observed in autonomic ganglia.
- Secondary colonization or overgrowth by bacteria and fungi may occur in the poorly motile GI tract.
- Microscopic lesions are segmental and are randomly distributed. Disruption of coordination and control of the myenteric plexus of the ingluvies, esophagus, proventriculus, ventriculus, and/or duodenum will cause atrophy of the muscular layer with dilatation and focal disturbances in contractility that range from minor to catastrophic. The main pacemaker for the gastroduodenal cycle seems to be located near the isthmus. Segmental damage at this site is hypothesized to cause severe proventricular dilatation.

DIAGNOSIS

DIFFERENTIAL DIAGNOSIS

- Diseases that can cause dilatation of the proventriculus
  - Physiologic dilatation of the proventriculus of young psittacines or fruit/nectar-eating species, some Eclectus parrots
  - Chronic lead toxicosis
  - Proventriculitis (fungal, bacterial) and/or ventriculitis (fungal)
  - Myoventricular dysgenesis, koilin dysgenesis
  - Obstruction: foreign body, neoplasia, stricture, parasitism (e.g., cestodes, nematodes)
- Conditions that lead to a paralytic ileus, diarrhea (including those listed above)
  - Enteritis: bacterial, viral, or parasitic
  - Upper digestive tract disease (crop and esophagus): bacterial, viral (especially polyomavirus in young birds, papillomatosis), fungal, or parasitic
  - Organopathy: hepatitis, pancreatitis
  - Intoxication
  - Dietary changes
- Diffuse neurologic conditions should be considered with neurologic presentations of the disease:
  - Vascular: atherosclerosis, ischemic infarction, cerebrovascular accident
  - Infectious: viral (see Viral Diseases) (viral encephalitis, paramyxoviruses, polyomavirus, reovirus, avian viral serositis), bacterial (*Chlamydophila psittaci, Mycobacterium* spp., *Listeria monocytogenes, Salmonella* spp.), fungal (*Aspergillus* spp., *Candida* spp.) parasites (*Baylisascaris procyonis, Toxoplasma, Sarcocystis*)
  - Traumatic: head trauma, cranial hypertension
  - Toxic: heavy metals, primarily chronic lead poisoning, insecticides, botulism
  - Metabolic: hypocalcemia (e.g., African greys), hypoglycemia, hepatic encephalopathy, other electrolyte imbalances (e.g., salt toxicity, magnesium)
  - Idiopathic epilepsy, idiopathic tremors
  - Neoplasms of the nervous system
  - Degenerative diseases
  - Nutritional deficiencies: vitamins E, B_1, B_6, selenium

INITIAL DATABASE

- Complete blood count (CBC): plasma biochemistry panel
  - Inconsistent but helpful to assess the patient's health status and rule out other diseases. In rare, acute cases of PDD, a primary heterophilia may be seen. More often, the patient has a nearly reference range hemogram. Occasionally, slight lymphocytosis and monocytosis may be observed, as well as an increase in creatine kinase (CK) levels. Hypoproteinemia, primarily hypoalbuminemia, depression, anemia, and hypoglycemia are frequently noted in advanced cases and are associated with a decompensating patient. Many birds with abnormal duodenal motility exhibit increased plasma amylase and/or lipase levels.
- Crop: fecal cytologic examination and/or bacteriologic examination
  - The main purpose of a cytologic exam is to determine whether a secondary fungal (usually *Candida* spp.) and/or bacterial overgrowth is present. Bacterial culture and sensitivity will help in establishing appropriate antimicrobial treatment.

ADVANCED OR CONFIRMATORY TESTING

- Imaging
  - On plain radiographs, a dilated, gas-filled proventriculus or an elevated dorsal border of the proventriculus may be seen in advanced cases with predominantly GI signs, but this finding is not pathognomonic for PDD. Contrast radiographs using barium sulfate will effectively highlight GI morphology and may demonstrate increased transit times. They should be exposed without anesthesia so as not to further impair GI motility. Barium contrast fluoroscopy is the most useful technique for demonstrating the motility and structural abnormalities associated with the disease. Focal hypomotility or dysmotility of the esophagus, crop, proventriculus, ventriculus, and duodenum may be detected. The normal gastroduodenal cycle of the turkey was described by Duke (Denbow, 2000). We have observed similar contraction sequences in a variety of parrot species, except that ventricular contractions and retroperistaltic waves of the duodenum occur more frequently. Fluoroscopic studies in normal Amazon parrots have been published. The complex coordination and interaction of proventricular, ventricular, and duodenal contractions seem especially prone to disruption during PDD infection. In the normal parrot, the ventriculus will complete 3-6 contraction cycles per minute.
  - In a PDD-positive bird, the following findings may be observed on contrast fluoroscopy:
    - Decrease of 50% to 100% in proventricular, ventricular, and/or duodenal contractions
    - Incoordination of peristalsis, retroperistalsis, and gastric contractions
    - Dilatation of the ingluvies, esophagus, proventriculus, ventriculus, and/or duodenum
- Endoscopy
  - Endoscopy can be used to evaluate the outer surfaces of the proventriculus and the ventriculus and to magnify pathologic changes (e.g., serosal inflammation, thickness evaluation). Gastroscopy could help to rule out pyloric obstruction but is seldom useful in PDD owing to gastric filling and poor emptying leading to inadequate visualization.
- Histopathologic examination
  - A definitive diagnosis of PDD cannot currently be made without a diagnostic biopsy or necropsy of the myenteric plexus that demonstrates accumulation of lymphocytes and plasmacytes within ganglia. Infiltrates in other peripheral nerves (e.g., brachial, sciatic) or in the central nervous system are also characteristic of the disease.
    - Crop biopsy remains the safest tool at this time to accurately diagnose PDD despite a false-negative rate of approximately 40%. To maximize the value of any given sample, we suggest the following:
      - Perform a full-thickness biopsy of the crop wall.
      - Center the biopsy upon a branch of the ingluvial artery to ensure collection of nerve tissue.
      - Collect a large biopsy specimen (0.5-1 cm) or take multiple biopsy specimens if possible.
  - Patient discomfort and iatrogenic damage to the crop are minimal if good technique is followed. Other possible sites for myenteric plexus biopsy (e.g., esophagus, proventriculus, ventriculus, duodenum) are much less favorable owing to greater morbidity or lack of access. Adrenal biopsies have been described but are invasive and less specific and may be associated with a higher risk of complications in an already depressed bird. A negative biopsy does not rule out the disease. Immunohistochemistry can also be used.
  - It should be noted that an uncommon viral disease caused by a togavirus, avian viral serositis, may cause similar histopathologic lesions in the myenteric ganglia.
- Serology
  - Serology for avian bornaviruses using Western blot assay has been used in several research settings but is not commercially available.
- Molecular diagnostics
  - Since the discovery of avian bornaviruses and some advanced molecular investigations, primers are now available for PCR testing. A few laboratories currently offer this test on blood and oral-fecal swabs. PCR can also be performed on a piece of crop tissue sampled during a crop biopsy procedure and stored in the freezer. It should be stressed that subclinical carriers are common

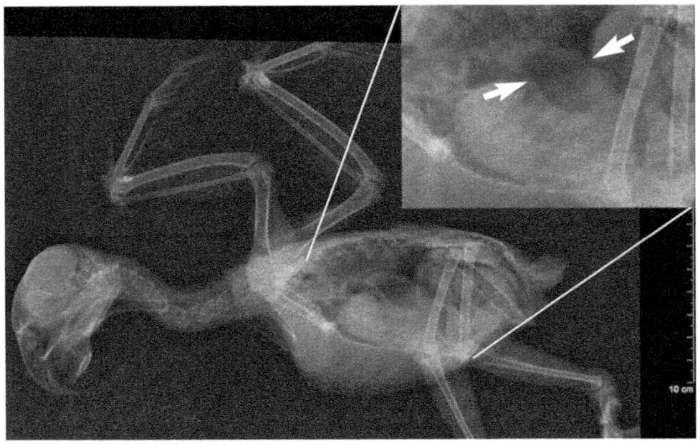

Proventricular Dilatation Disease Proventricular dilatation disease (PDD) with arrows: radiographic appearance of PDD. Note the air in the proventriculus and the distention. Diagnosis was made via crop biopsy in this case. *(Photo courtesy Jörg Mayer, The University of Georgia, Athens.)*

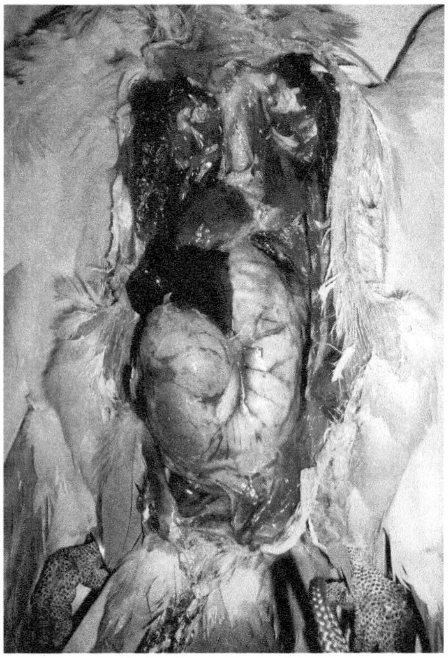

Proventricular Dilatation Disease Necropsy of a blue and gold macaw presented for tremors and imbalance. Note the enlarged, seed-filled, and thin-walled proventriculus. *(Courtesy Hugues Beaufrère and Clinique Vétérinaire, Brasseur, Belgium.)*

and that recovery of avian bornavirus nucleic acids from a bird does not necessarily imply the presence of the disease but is rather supporting evidence. PCR testing can also be performed on tissue biopsy specimens.

- Necropsy
  - Postmortem examination and histopathologic examination of the ingluvies, proventriculus, ventriculus, adrenal glands, heart, and peripheral and central nervous systems are mandatory to confirm a diagnosis of PDD because lesions are segmental and randomly distributed. Macroscopic lesions include poor body condition; proventricular, ventricular, and/or duodenal distention; multifocal ulcerations of the proventricular and ventricular mucosa; thinning of the proventricular and ventricular wall; and the presence of undigested food in the intestinal tract. Immunohistochemistry can also be used.

TREATMENT

THERAPEUTIC GOALS

- Stabilize and improve patient's physical condition.
- Provide an easily digestible high-energy diet.
- Provide supportive therapy to control seizures, anemia, immune suppression, dehydration, and gastroenteritis.
- Stabilize inflammatory neurologic condition.
- Treat for good quality of life if the owner wants to maintain the bird after a definitive diagnosis is obtained.

ACUTE GENERAL TREATMENT

- All treatment is to be performed on a stable patient.
  - Nursing care
    - Administer warmed crystalloid fluids SC, IV, IO (50-150 mL/kg/d maintenance plus dehydration deficit factored in if needed) at a rate of 10-25 mL/kg over a 5-minute period or at a continuous rate of 100 mL/kg/q 24 h.
    - Increase environmental temperature to 29°C to 35°C (85°F-90°F).
    - Nutritional support is required in most cases.
      - Highly digestible and well-balanced food should be provided because ingluvial, proventricular, and ventricular functions are affected. Pellets, especially extruded products, are easier to digest than seeds.
      - Pancreatic enzymes (e.g., Avian Enzyme, Harrison Bird Food) can be added to food to facilitate the digestive process.
      - A semiliquid diet can be offered or gavage fed to severely affected birds.
      - Probiotics can also be used to compete with pathogens.
- Palliative treatment
  - Nonsteroidal antiinflammatory drugs (NSAIDs), especially cyclooxygenase (COX)-2 selective inhibitors (celecoxib 10 mg/kg q 12-24 h, meloxicam 0.3-1 mg/kg q 12-24 h), have been proven to reduce and sometimes reverse clinical signs and to slow progression of the disease. Response to NSAID treatment can be poor, however.
  - Antimicrobial drugs may be essential with secondary fungal or bacterial overgrowth or opportunistic infection.
  - Gastrokinetic drugs have been suggested as an adjunct to treatment; however, demonstrable effects have yet to be experimentally proven. Metoclopramide 0.5 mg/kg q 8-12 h (higher doses than 0.5 mg/kg are frequently associated with dopaminergic side effects, especially in birds with neurologic involvement), cisapride 1 mg/kg q 8-12 h.
  - Seizures or tremors may be managed with diazepam 0.5-1 mg/kg, phenobarbital 1-10 mg/kg q 12 h, or levetiracetam 50 mg/kg q 8 h.
  - Simethicone 30-100 mg/kg × 2-3 treatments may be useful in reducing gas distention.
  - Amantadine, an antiviral with anti-bornaviral properties, can be attempted at a dose of 10-20 mg/kg q 12-24 h and has been associated with improved outcomes in some cases. A dose of 1 mg/kg did not reduce shedding in African grey parrots.
  - Ribavirin, an antiviral with anti-bornaviral properties, can also be tried at 15-20 mg/kg. It was ineffective in reducing shedding in African grey parrots.
  - Interferon can be tried with recombinant omega interferon of feline origin (Virbagen Omega) 1,000,000 units/bird q 1-7 d, or with gamma interferon of poultry origin 1,000,000 units/bird q 1-7 d. However, no scientific data support their use in the management of PDD so far.

CHRONIC TREATMENT

See Palliative treatment (above). PDD is a chronic disease with no curative treatment.

POSSIBLE COMPLICATIONS

Palliative treatment may not have any effect at all on the disease process.

RECOMMENDED MONITORING

- Repeat radiographs if monitoring passage of food and progression of the disease.
- Repeat CBC and plasma chemistry panel to monitor treatment response if any.
- Monitor appetite, fecal output, and behavior during treatment.
- Monitor body weight and general health status.
- Screen regularly for secondary infection.
- Contrast radiographs or fluoroscopy can be repeated to assess GI morphology and motility. Diet changes should be considered when radiographs are interpreted.

PROGNOSIS AND OUTCOME

At this time, the prognosis is grave for birds with a confirmed case of PDD. Outcomes are uniformly fatal over time. Fluoroscopic evaluation of GI motility can refine the prognosis.

PEARLS & CONSIDERATIONS

COMMENTS

- Owner must be prepared that the prognosis is guarded to poor and that death may be inevitable, especially if the central nervous system is affected.

- Because a PDD outbreak can be devastating in an aviary, a parrot collection, or a flock, any affected bird should be placed in strict isolation with no direct or indirect contact with other birds.
- An aviary or home visit by a veterinarian is usually warranted.
- Review basic cage and food and water bowl hygiene. Current epidemiologic evidence suggests that the fecal-oral route is the predominant mode of transmission. Avian bornaviruses have also been reported to be shed from ocular, nasal, and respiratory secretions and from feather dust; the virus can be detected in the air of an infected aviary.
- Review proper use of recommended cleaning and disinfection solutions.
- Review and encourage proper cage security. Are there any frequent "escape artists" in this collection of birds? PCR testing of birds to determine their ABV status may be warranted.
- Avian bornaviruses and PDD pathogenesis are currently areas of intense research, and the reader may be aware that more information about this disease will be available over the next few years.

PREVENTION

Become knowledgeable about the disease, and purchase ABV-negative birds only from aviaries in which there is no known history of PDD. This will not prevent the disease but may reduce the risk of purchasing a bird with PDD.

CLIENT EDUCATION

See comments above.

SUGGESTED READINGS

Denbow DM: Gastrointestinal anatomy and physiology. In Whittow GC, editor: Sturkie's avian physiology, San Diego, 2000, Academic Press.

Gancz AY, et al: Experimental induction of proventricular dilatation disease in cockatiels *(Nymphicus hollandicus)* inoculated with brain homogenates containing avian bornavirus 4, Viro J 6:100, 2009.

Hoppes S, et al: The isolation, diagnosis, transmission, and control of avian bornavirus and proventricular dilatation disease, Vet Clin North Am Exot Anim Pract 13:495–508, 2010.

Kisler AL, et al: Recovery of divergent avian bornaviruses from cases of proventricular dilatation disease: identification of a candidate etiologic agent, Viro J 5:88, 2008.

Rinder M, et al: Broad tissue and cell tropism of avian bornavirus in parrots with proventricular dilatation disease, J Virol 83:5401–5407, 2009.

Ritchie BW, editor: Avian viruses: function and control, Lake Worth, FL, 1995, Wingers Publishing, pp 439–448.

CROSS-REFERENCES TO OTHER SECTIONS

Diarrhea
Neurologic Disease
Viral Diseases

AUTHORS: **HUGUES BEAUFRÈRE AND W. MICHAEL TAYLOR**

EDITOR: **THOMAS N. TULLY, JR.**

BIRDS

Regurgitation/Vomiting

BASIC INFORMATION

DEFINITION

Regurgitation is an involuntary or voluntary expulsion, generally passive, of materials from the esophagus and/or the crop. Vomiting is a forceful, involuntary ejection of materials from the stomach and may be differentiated by the pH (generally <5) and the content (bile, bile-stained food materials) of the vomitus. It is not always clinically possible to separate regurgitation from vomiting; they may occur together.

SYNONYM

Nausea

EPIDEMIOLOGY

SPECIES, AGE, SEX All species and ages and both sexes

RISK FACTORS

- Regurgitation is a clinical sign that may be seen in disorders of the gastrointestinal (GI) tract, especially of the esophagus and the crop, that lead to dysmotility, hypomotility, or hypermotility of the esophageal and/or ingluvial and/or proventricular and/or ventricular musculature.
- Any intraluminal or extraluminal obstruction, compression, or impaction can induce regurgitation.
- Many systemic and extra-GI diseases can account for regurgitation or vomiting.
- In baby psittacines, crop dysmotility can result from improper feeding methods or infectious disease.
- Chronic regurgitation with loss of normal ingesta throughout may lead to progressive loss of intestinal epithelium replacement that may be enhanced by malnutrition.

ASSOCIATED CONDITIONS AND DISORDERS

- Neurologic conditions
- Anorexia
- Depression
- Hepatitis
- Gastroenteritis
- Weakness

CLINICAL PRESENTATION

DISEASE FORMS/SUBTYPES

- Extra-GI conditions
  - Behavioral regurgitation can be seen in several contexts such as excitement, weaning, and courtship. No alteration in general health status and no weight loss should occur.
  - Stress, motion sickness, recovery from inhalant anesthesia
  - Intoxication: iatrogenic causes (itraconazole, trimethoprim/sulfadiazine, doxycycline), plants, heavy metals (see Heavy Metal Toxicity) pesticides
  - Compression or extraluminal obstruction: goiter in budgerigars, organomegaly, ascites, neoplasia along the upper GI tract, egg binding, clavicular air sac infection, coracoid callus, Elizabethan collar
  - Systemic disease (e.g., aspergillosis, hepatic failure, renal failure, heart failure, peritonitis, pancreatitis, sepsis, psittacine beak and feather disease [PBFD]), end-stage chronic disease
- Primary GI conditions
  - Viral diseases: proventricular dilatation disease, Pacheco's disease, polyomavirus, avian viral serositis, poxvirus, papillomatosis
  - Bacterial ingluvitis, overgrowth
  - Fungal diseases (see Mycoses): candidiasis, *Macrorhabdus*
  - Parasitism: trichomoniasis, capillariasis
  - Obstruction: foreign body, stricture, stenosis, neoplasia, impaction, ingluvioliths, sequel to severe esophageal and ingluvial infections
  - Proventriculitis, generalized enteritis (avian chlamydiosis, clostridiosis, Gram-negative bacteria), gastric ulceration
  - Paralytic ileus

- Food allergies, nutritional problems
- Crop necrosis, burns, fistula: overheated formula, caustic materials
- Traumatic lacerations of ingluvial and chest areas, bite wounds, coracoid fractures, trauma secondary to tube feeding

- Common causes of crop stasis in nonweaned psittacines
  - Crop infections: yeast, Gram-negative or -positive bacterial overgrowth
  - Viral diseases: polyomavirus, proventricular dilatation disease, Pacheco's disease
  - Overstretching of the crop, atonic crop
  - Crop burns, overheated feeding mixture (e.g., microwaved food)
  - Low formula temperature, excessively thin formula
  - Crop impaction by food, too thick formula
  - Rupture of crop wall caused by feeding tube
  - Foreign body, substrate ingestion
  - Paralytic ileus due to generalized disease, hypothermia, hypoglycemia

HISTORY, CHIEF COMPLAINT

- Neurologic signs
- Depression
- Inappetence
- Diarrhea (see Diarrhea)
- Regurgitation
- Vomiting
- Sour crop/crop stasis

PHYSICAL EXAM FINDINGS

- Matted feathers around head
- Weakness
- Poor body condition
- Observation of vomiting/regurgitation

ETIOLOGY AND PATHOPHYSIOLOGY

See Disease Forms/Subtypes.

DIAGNOSIS

DIFFERENTIAL DIAGNOSIS

- Regurgitation can be seen in every bird but is common in unweaned psittacines with crop stasis (i.e., "sour crop"). Vomiting is frequently associated with endogenous (e.g., hyperuricemia) or exogenous (e.g., lead) intoxication.
- Regurgitation is a clinical sign, not a disease. A bird will often shake its head when regurgitating, thus depositing materials on the face, feathers, and head and in the cage. Upon physical examination, crop stasis, which can be a sign of generalized GI stasis, may be noted. The crop should be palpated and transilluminated for foreign bodies or impaction, and the ingluvial wall inspected for evidence of erythema, inflammation, laceration, or necrosis. The mouth should be examined because many of the diseases affecting the oral cavity also affect the esophagus and the crop.

INITIAL DATABASE

- Cytologic examination of the upper alimentary tract/crop wash/proventricular wash
  - An attempt to differentiate regurgitation from vomiting can be based on material pH and content. With regurgitation, food does not seem to be digested and pH is neutral (6.8-7.5), whereas vomitus is partially digested and the pH is generally 2-3 or less (pH of proventricular hydrochloric acid).
  - Cytologic examination of a crop wash or a swab can give valuable information.
  - Wet mounts
    - Examination for flagellates, other motile protozoa: *Trichomonas* spp.
    - Examination for *Macrorhabdus ornithogaster*
  - Stained smears: Gram, Hemacolor, Diff-Quik
    - Bacterial overgrowth or infection if a large number of monomorphic bacteria are observed
    - Yeast infection, candidiasis if many budding yeasts and/or hyphae are present; it should be noted that some food may contain nonbudding yeast
    - Cornified squamous epithelial cells in large numbers and aggregates suggest hypovitaminosis A.
    - Inflammatory cells are not seen in acute infection but are evident in more chronic problems.
    - *Capillaria* spp. ova: double operculated
    - Normal findings: squamous epithelial cells, background debris, varying quantities of bacteria represented by a variety of morphologic types; some yeasts at low number
  - Centrifugation and microscopic examination of the sediment
    - *Capillaria* spp. ova
    - *Candida* spp.
  - Culture and sensitivity should be performed with suspicion of an infection.
- Fecal examination
  - A fecal flotation could be performed to check for parasite ova that may indicate a nematode or trematode infestation.
- Complete blood count (CBC)/biochemistry panel
  - CBC and biochemistry panel should be performed as a minimum database to look for metabolic or systemic disease and to assess patient health status and electrolyte balance. A regurgitating bird may show hypokalemia and metabolic alkalosis.

ADVANCED OR CONFIRMATORY TESTING

- Ancillary diagnostic tests
  - Laboratory tests, including blood lead level, *Chlamydophila psittaci* testing (PCR, serology), and polyomavirus PCR, must be considered.
- Imaging
  - The crop should be emptied before radiographs are taken, to prevent aspiration. Radiographs are useful for foreign bodies, metal particles, and proventricular dilatation and for evaluation of internal organs. Administration of contrast media helps to evaluate morphology, transit times, and sometimes intraluminal or extraluminal lesions. Fluoroscopy may be used to assess motility and morphology.
  - GI endoscopy may be used for further examination of the upper digestive tract and for collection of samples. The proventriculus and the ventriculus are best visualized with flexible scopes. Coeloscopy is extremely useful for examination and sampling of internal organs. Care should be taken when scoping a neonate or adult bird with gastric dilatation because of the reduced air sac space.
  - Ultrasound examination can be used to evaluate the liver, the ventriculus, the heart, and masses or organ enlargement.

TREATMENT

THERAPEUTIC GOALS

- Stabilize and improve the patient's physical condition.
- Provide supportive therapy to control vomiting/regurgitation, anorexia, dehydration, and gastroenteritis.
- Resolve the problem causing vomiting/regurgitation.

ACUTE GENERAL TREATMENT

- All treatment is to be performed on a stable patient.
  - Nursing care
    - Administer warmed crystalloid fluids SC, IV, IO (50-150 mL/kg/d maintenance plus dehydration deficit factored in if needed) at a rate of 10-25 mL/kg over a 5-minute period or at a continuous rate of 100 mL/kg/q 24 h.
    - Increase environmental temperature to 29°C to 35°C (85°F-90°F).
    - Provide a humidified environment by placing warm moist towels in the incubator.

- Correction of electrolytes and acid-base balance: venous blood gas and ionogram can help to assess metabolic disturbances and enable correction using IV or IO therapy. Regurgitation or vomiting can lead to hypokalemia and metabolic alkalosis.
- Place the bird in an incubator with supplemental heat and oxygen.
- Empty the crop as needed to prevent further regurgitation and microbial proliferation. It may be flushed as well twice a day.
- Reduce stress.
- Nutritional support is considered depending on the frequency of regurgitation and the general condition of the patient. Supplemental vitamins may be added as necessary. An esophagostomy feeding tube can be passed from the esophagus into the proventriculus to feed the bird while the esophagus and the crop are healing.
- Massage crop content every hour with added warm saline.
- Feed small but frequent volumes.
- Crop bra can be used in neonates to elevate a distended or atonic crop and to facilitate emptying.

- Relief of obstruction or impaction
  - Flush and empty the crop regularly.
  - Endoscopy of the crop can be used to remove foreign bodies, substrate materials.
  - Some foreign bodies localized in the crop can be removed by manipulation using a hemostat.
  - Ingluviotomy, proventriculotomy (see later)
- Surgery considerations
  - Ingluviotomy may be needed to remove foreign bodies, ingluvioliths, or impacted food and to allow access to the proventriculus and the ventriculus with a rigid endoscope (see Foreign Bodies).
  - Treatment of crop burns and fistulas: edges of the fistula must be cleaned and excised. The crop and the skin should be separated and then closed in two layers. In the acute phase of burns, the extent of devitalized tissue may be difficult to assess, and surgery must be delayed until a clear demarcation occurs.
  - Proventriculotomy may be needed to remove foreign bodies or heavy metal materials; however, proventriculoscopy is less traumatic (see Foreign Bodies).
- Medications
  - Antimicrobials
    - Broad-spectrum antibiotics
      - Clavamox 125 mg/kg PO q 12 h: beta-lactamase inhibitors are safe
      - Metronidazole 10-30 mg/kg IM q 24 h × 2 d: extremely useful for anaerobes
      - Ciprofloxacin 10 mg/kg PO q 12 h: fluoroquinolones are safe but are ineffective against anaerobes
    - Antifungal drug
      - Nystatin 300 000-600 000 IU/kg PO q 8-12 h
    - Mild crop burns (with no fistula or subcutaneous food pocket) can be treated with antibiotics and topical triple antibiotic ointment.
- Other considerations
  - Antiemetic and gastrokinetic drugs are used as needed:
    - Metoclopramide 0.5-1 mg/kg PO IM q 8-12 h
    - Cisapride 0.5-1 mg/kg PO q 8-12 h
  - Antiulcerogenic drugs may be helpful when an ulcer or erosion is suspected:
    - Sucralfate 25 mg/kg PO q 8 h
    - Cimetidine 5 mg/kg PO IM q 8-12 h
    - Omeprazole 0.5-1 mg/kg PO q 24 h
  - When clinical signs or history is consistent with a toxic condition, antitoxins may be used:
    - Penicillamine 30 mg/kg PO q 12 h × 7 d (may cause emesis)
    - Ca-EDTA 30-40 mg/kg PO IM q 12 h for lead poisoning
    - Activated charcoal 2-8 g/kg PO
  - Probiotics may be used to compete with pathogens and improve environmental conditions within the GI tract.

CHRONIC TREATMENT

Celecoxib 10 mg/kg PO q 24 h × 6-24 wk for birds with proventricular dilatation disease

POSSIBLE COMPLICATIONS

- Sulfonamide antibiotics should be avoided because of their emetic effect.
- If the bird is regurgitating/vomiting, oral medications are not recommended in most cases.

RECOMMENDED MONITORING

- Repeat radiographs to monitor general condition of GI tract and determine function.
- Repeat CBC and plasma chemistry panel to monitor treatment response and recovery.
- Repeat culture/sensitivity of crop during treatment to assess treatment efficacy.
- Monitor appetite, fecal output, and behavior during treatment period.
- Monitor weight, attitude, and appetite of patient to determine treatment response.

PROGNOSIS AND OUTCOME

- Dependent on cause of regurgitation and condition of patient when presented
- Most patients with bacterial/fungal ingluvitis, if treated promptly and with the correct medication, have a good prognosis if the patient is not too debilitated.

PEARLS & CONSIDERATIONS

COMMENTS

- Inform that crop stasis in neonates is a common condition of multifactorial but frequently husbandry origin.
- Warn the owner that crop stasis could reflect a generalized GI stasis.

PREVENTION

- Provide basic nutritional and management advice for hand-feeding (e.g., digital temperature measurement of formula).
- Prevent ingestion of foreign bodies.
- An unweaned bird should not be sold except to a person competent in hand-feeding.
- Screen birds for infectious diseases: psittacine beak and feather disease, polyomavirus, *Chlamydophila psittaci*
- Polyomavirus vaccination is also an option.

CLIENT EDUCATION

- Inform owners of cage toys that may cause GI blockage and of appropriate toys for the species of bird that they own.
- See Prevention.

SUGGESTED READINGS

Hoefer HL, et al: The gastrointestinal tract. In Altman RB, et al, editors: Avian medicine and surgery, Philadelphia, 1997, WB Saunders, pp 412–453.

Lumeij JT: Gastroenterology. In Ritchie BW, et al, editors: Avian medicine: principles and application, Lake Worth, FL, 1994, Wingers Publishing, pp 482–521.

CROSS-REFERENCES TO OTHER SECTIONS

Diarrhea
Foreign Bodies
Heavy Metal Toxicity
Mycoses

AUTHORS: **HUGUES BEAUFRÈRE AND W. MICHAEL TAYLOR**

EDITOR: **THOMAS N. TULLY, JR.**

BIRDS

Renal Disease

Client Education Sheet Available on Website

BASIC INFORMATION

DEFINITION

Disease of renal tissue that may result from progressive destructive pathophysiologic processes (chronic renal failure) or from rapid, severe, and often reversible conditions (acute renal failure)

SYNONYMS

Renal failure, kidney failure, renal compromise

EPIDEMIOLOGY

SPECIES, AGE, SEX All species and ages and both sexes

GENETICS AND BREED PREDISPOSITION Budgerigars: renal adenocarcinoma

RISK FACTORS

- Infectious disease
- Dehydration
- Improper nutrition
- Toxicity
- Neoplasia
- Shock
- Older birds
- Systemic/metabolic disease

GEOGRAPHY AND SEASONALITY Hot, dry environmental conditions may predispose birds to dehydration that can lead to renal disease.

ASSOCIATED CONDITIONS AND DISORDERS

- Anorexia
- Depression
- Dyspnea
- Polyuria/polydipsia
- Weakness
- Hypertension

CLINICAL PRESENTATION

DISEASE FORMS/SUBTYPES

- Acute renal disease
- Chronic renal disease
- Renal failure

HISTORY, CHIEF COMPLAINT

- Nonspecific
- Depression
- Inappetence
- Polyuria
- Polydipsia
- Weight loss
- Anuria
- Oliguria

PHYSICAL EXAM FINDINGS

- Weight loss
- Distention of the caudal coelom
- Dehydration
- Articular gout
- Abdominal mass (see Tumors)
- Ascites
- Dyspnea
- In larger birds, the caudal renal division can be palpated with a lubricated gloved finger via the cloaca.

ETIOLOGY AND PATHOPHYSIOLOGY

- Congenital
- Infectious disease
  - Bacterial: Gram-negative, Gram-positive bacteria
  - Parasitic: *Isospora* spp., *Cryptosporidium* spp., *Microsporidium* spp.
  - Viral (see Viral Diseases): adenovirus, herpesvirus, paramyxovirus, polyomavirus, retrovirus, togavirus
  - Fungal: *Aspergillus* spp.
- Nutritional: hypercalcemia, hypervitaminosis D, hypovitaminosis A, high-protein diet, high-cholesterol diet
- Toxic: lead, zinc, mycotoxins, ethylene glycol, antibiotic medication (e.g., aminoglycoside, sulfonamide), allopurinol, nonsteroidal antiinflammatory drugs (NSAIDs)
- Neoplastic: renal adenocarcinoma, adenoma, nephroblastoma, lymphosarcoma
- Metabolic: amyloidosis, diabetes mellitus, lipidosis
- Vascular: dehydration, shock
- Other: urolithiasis and ureteral obstructive disease, renal hemorrhage

DIAGNOSIS

DIFFERENTIAL DIAGNOSIS

- Dehydration
- Septicemia
- Caudal coelomic organomegaly

INITIAL DATABASE

- Complete blood count (CBC): may indicate dehydration, anemia, or inflammation
- Plasma biochemistry panel: elevated uric acid levels may occur when glomerular filtration decreases by more than 70% to 80% (i.e., severely dehydrated birds), or when a large number of renal tubules have been damaged. In carnivorous birds, significant elevations of blood uric acid occur physiologically after a high-protein meal: thus 24-hour fasting before sampling is needed. Renal disease may be present when uric acid levels are within the normal range (e.g., anorexia, concurrent liver disease, polyuria/polydipsia [PU/PD]). Urea and creatinine are considered to have little value in the detection of renal disease. Increased plasma urea concentrations may be seen in dehydrated birds. In carnivorous birds, significant elevations of blood urea nitrogen (BUN) occur physiologically after a high-protein meal. Albumin may be decreased in protein-losing nephropathies (e.g., amyloidosis). Elevations of phosphorus and potassium may or may not occur with renal disease and are very dependent on treatment of samples after collection.
- Urinalysis is not diagnostic for renal disease in birds owing to fecal contamination. The presence of casts may indicate renal pathology. All other parameters included with a urinalysis are suspect owing to likely fecal contamination of the "urine" sample.

ADVANCED OR CONFIRMATORY TESTING

- Imaging
  - Radiography: useful in assessing the size, location, and radiopacity of the kidneys. Kidneys are best assessed when a lateral angle is viewed. Renal enlargement is noted as obliteration of air space around the kidneys (psittacine species), ventral displacement of the abdominal viscera beneath the kidneys, or enlargement of the kidneys. Increased opacity may occur as a result of dehydration and renal gout.
  - Ultrasound: useful in assessing the size, location, and density of the kidneys. Sonographic imaging of the normal kidneys is considered very difficult owing to the presence of surrounding air sacs. Fluid accumulation in the coelomic cavity and organomegaly may compress the air sacs, allowing ultrasonographic imaging of the kidneys.
  - Intravenous excretory urography: should not be used in birds with severe renal compromise (i.e., when plasma chemistry indicates renal impairment) but can be used when only morphologic changes are present
- Diagnostic procedures
  - Water deprivation test: useful to rule out unknown causes of PU/PD, including central and nephrogenic diabetes insipidus and psychogenic polydipsia. Birds with diabetes insipidus become dehydrated but maintain diluted urine (increased osmolality and specific gravity). Birds with psychogenic

polydipsia should tolerate the water deprivation test well and should develop more concentrated urine.
  - Glomerular filtration rate: limited practical use; can be calculated by measuring the clearance of a marker substance (e.g., H-inulin). Urine flow rate is calculated from ureteral urine.
  - Biopsy: indicated to definitively diagnose renal disease and specific pathologic tissue damage. Rarely, histopathologic lesions are pathognomonic of disease. Endoscopically guided biopsy is the most common method of collecting renal tissue samples for microscopic evaluation. Renal biopsy is contraindicated if coagulopathies are present.

TREATMENT

THERAPEUTIC GOALS

- Stabilize and improve patient's physical condition.
- Treat underlying cause of renal disease.
- Patients with compensatory chronic renal failure may be managed as outpatients; patients with hyperuricemic crisis should be managed as inpatients.

ACUTE GENERAL TREATMENT

- Normuric and polyuric birds should be administered warmed crystalloid solution SC (50-150 mL/kg/d). IV or IO boluses (10-25 mL/kg over 5 min) can be given or administration can occur at a continuous rate (50-100 mL/kg/d). Anuric or oliguric birds should be monitored carefully during fluid therapy until urine flow is normalized.
- Medications
  - Allopurinol 10-30 mg/kg PO, q 12 h: reported use for reduction of plasma uric acid concentrations is controversial. Allopurinol has been reported to be toxic in red-tailed hawks but appears to be relatively safe in galliformes, psittacine species, and columbiformes.
  - Urate oxidase 100-200 IU/kg PO, q 12 h: considered a safer and more effective alternative to allopurinol
  - Cochicine 0.04 mg/kg PO, q 12-24 h: used in cases of hyperuricemia and renal fibrosis
  - NSAIDs: use of low-dose aspirin (0.5-1 mg/kg PO, q 12-24 h) has been reported, but the beneficial effects of low-dose or specific NSAID therapy have not been studied in birds with renal disease.
  - Antibiotic therapy: used in cases of suspect or confirmed bacterial nephritis; recommended course of 6 weeks minimum. Avoid the use of antibiotics that could cause or aggravate renal disease (e.g., aminoglycosides, sulfonamides).

CHRONIC TREATMENT

Supportive care

DRUG INTERACTIONS

Avoid nephrotoxic drugs.

POSSIBLE COMPLICATIONS

Lack of treatment response

RECOMMENDED MONITORING

- Repeat CBC and plasma chemistry panel to evaluate treatment response or disease progress.
- Assess hydration status.
- Note how much water the patient drinks.

PROGNOSIS AND OUTCOME

- Acute renal disease depends on severity and cause of disease.
- Long-term renal disease carries a guarded to poor prognosis.
- Chronic renal disease is often progressive over months to years.

PEARLS & CONSIDERATIONS

COMMENTS

- Owners should be aware that chronic renal disease is progressive and often leads to renal failure.
- Owners should know that many cases of renal disease are difficult to diagnose and treat.
- Renal disease may lead to feather picking.

PREVENTION

- Good husbandry
- Proper diet
- Prevent access to toxins.

SUGGESTED READINGS

Echols MS: Evaluating and treating the kidneys. In Harrison GJ, et al, editors: Clinical avian medicine, vol II, Palm Beach, FL, 2006, Spix Publishing, Inc., pp 451–492.

Lierz M: Avian renal disease: pathogenesis, diagnosis and therapy, Vet Clin Exot Anim 6:29–55, 2003.

Lumeij JT: Pathophysiology, diagnosis and treatment of renal disease of birds of prey. In Lumeij JT, et al, editors: Raptor biomedicine III, Lake Worth, FL, 2000, Zoological Education Network, Inc., pp 169–178.

CROSS-REFERENCES TO OTHER SECTIONS

Viral Diseases
Bacterial Diseases
Tumors

AUTHOR: **DAVID SANCHEZ-MIGALLON GUZMAN**

EDITOR: **THOMAS N. TULLY, JR.**

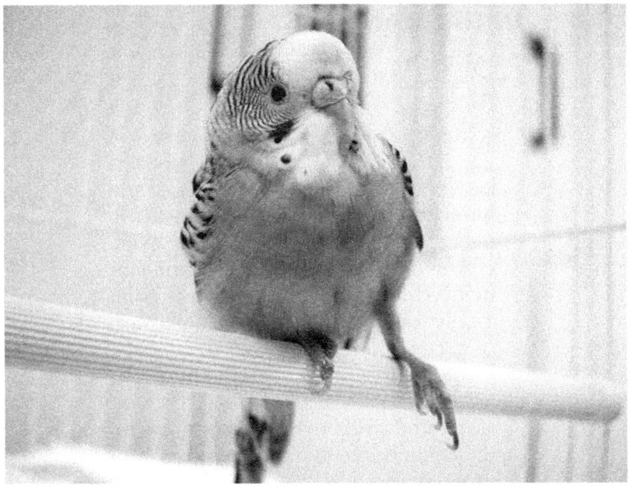

Renal Disease A parakeet with a renal tumor. Note the extended leg. The leg is often paralyzed owing to compression of the sciatic nerve by the tumor. *(Photo courtesy Jörg Mayer, The University of Georgia, Athens.)*

BIRDS

Sinusitis, Chronic

BASIC INFORMATION

DEFINITION

Chronic sinusitis may be defined in avian species as long-term, recurrent, and/or nonresponsive irritation and inflammation of the upper respiratory system of the avian patient, including the infraorbital sinus and all of its diverticula.

SYNONYMS

Runny nose, "cold," flu

EPIDEMIOLOGY

SPECIES, AGE, SEX Any avian species of both sexes, regardless of age

RISK FACTORS

- Immune suppression
- Dietary deficiency (e.g., vitamin A)
- Chronic irritation to the respiratory mucosa
- Trauma to the upper respiratory system

CONTAGION AND ZOONOSIS If *Chlamydophila psittaci* is diagnosed, it is a potential zoonotic agent.

ASSOCIATED CONDITIONS AND DISORDERS

- Dyspnea
- Nasal discharge
- Sneezing
- Exophthalmos
- Epiphora
- Anorexia
- Depression

CLINICAL PRESENTATION

DISEASE FORMS/SUBTYPES

- Choanal atresia
- Atrophic rhinitis
- Nasal granuloma
- Bacterial/fungal sinusitis

HISTORY, CHIEF COMPLAINT

- Head shaking
- Periorbital swelling
- Nasal and/or ocular discharge (e.g., purulent, serous)
- Facial swelling
- Anorexia
- Dyspnea
- Sneezing
- Nasal and/or ocular discharge and dyspnea may be present to the owner for several weeks to several years.

PHYSICAL EXAM FINDINGS

- Periorbital swelling
- Nasal/ocular discharge
- Facial swelling
- Occluded nares
- Dyspnea
- Poor body condition
- Depression
- Ruffled feathers
- Sneezing
- Choanal papilloma
- Irritation and feather loss on and around head due to self-trauma

ETIOLOGY AND PATHOPHYSIOLOGY

Chronic sinusitis may be classified as long-term irritation of the upper respiratory system that may be attributed to primary infection by resistant pathogens or to the presence of a mass or granuloma that acts as a nidus for the inflammatory process.

DIAGNOSIS

DIFFERENTIAL DIAGNOSIS

- Gram-negative bacteria: *Escherichia coli, Haemophilus* spp., *Klebsiella* spp., *Pasteurella* spp., *Pseudomonas* spp., *Salmonella* spp., *Yersinia* spp., *Mycobacterium avium*
- Opportunistic Gram-positive bacteria: *Streptococcus* spp., *Staphylococcus aureus*
- Intracellular bacteria: *Chlamydophila psittaci, Mycoplasma* spp.
- Fungal infections: *Aspergillus* spp., *Candida albicans, Cryptococcus* spp.
- Viral infections: Amazon tracheitis, Pacheco's disease, poxvirus, infectious laryngotracheitis, avian influenza, reovirus
- Allergic or hypersensitivity reactions
- Neoplasia: papilloma, lymphoma, adenocarcinoma
- Nutritional deficiency: hypovitaminosis A
- Trauma: foreign body
- Developmental: choanal atresia

INITIAL DATABASE

- Complete blood count: leukocytosis is typically present in the face of chronic sinusitis. A regenerative left shift is often observed in cases of chronic bacterial and fungal sinusitis and neoplasia. Toxic heterophils and monocytosis are typically observed in patients with severe bacterial avian chlamydiosis or viral or aspergillosis-induced sinusitis. Monocytosis is commonly observed with chronic fungal or bacterial infections (e.g., avian chlamydiosis, mycobacterial infection) and tissue necrosis. Leukopenia has been associated with overwhelming bacterial or viral infection, chlamydiosis, or aspergillosis.
- Culture of the infraorbital sinus: bacterial and fungal nasal cultures should always be collected before initiation of any therapeutic measures.
- Cytologic examination of infraorbital sinus samples: a sample for nasal sinus cytology is typically obtained via nasal flush or infraorbital sinus aspiration. Normal cytology of the avian sinus usually demonstrates few cells and no intracellular bacteria. Squamous epithelial cells observed in low numbers and a small number of nonbudding yeasts are typically considered normal findings. Increased numbers of inflammatory cells are indicative of sinusitis. Samples should be evaluated utilizing the Gram stain technique. Normal bacterial flora of the avian infraorbital sinus consists of greater than 90% Gram-positive rods and cocci.
- Radiographic imaging: radiographs of the skull and cervical area, including the infraorbital sinus and its diverticula, may reveal soft tissue densities consistent with exudate or a soft tissue, a space-occupying mass within the sinus, and/or osteolysis or proliferation of surrounding bone.

ADVANCED OR CONFIRMATORY TESTING

- Contrast radiography: iohexol can be injected into the external nares to highlight sinus masses or to determine the patency of the sinus from the nares to the choanal slit. Contrast radiography is very helpful in diagnosing birds that have choanal atresia.
- CT: has been used to better assess changes in bony structures surrounding the nasal sinuses
- MRI: has been used to better evaluate the nature of soft tissue densities detected on skull radiographs. The next most appropriate therapeutic measure, surgery versus continuation of medical therapy, can be determined based on these results.

TREATMENT

THERAPEUTIC GOALS

- With chronic sinusitis, the goal is to determine the underlying cause of the problem. This is often complicated by pathologic changes to the infraorbital sinus and possibly to surrounding tissue and bone. Informing an owner of the infraorbital anatomy and complications caused by the long-term inflammatory process is essential for treatment compliance and for an understanding of slow but progressive treatment response.

- Treatment for chronic sinusitis in the avian patient is a long-term proposition. Often aggressive treatment procedures (e.g., flushing) are needed with diminishing frequency as the patient recovers. It is not unusual for treatment time to equal the duration of illness before diagnosis.
- Ultimate therapeutic goal involves quality of life and resolution of the problem of chronic sinusitis. Treatment can be effective only if excessive mucus or cellular debris is removed from the infraorbital sinus. Suction using human infant nasal suction bulbs is effective in removal of significant amounts of mucus from the nares.
- Speer's Super Sinus Flush
  - Base solution: add 3.5 mg neomycin, 124.5 mg trypsin, 10 mg amphotericin B to a 30-mL water-soluble diluent.
  - Add 0.1-0.4 mL of base solution to 10-20 mL of saline; shake well.
  - Directly flush through the nares once a day until easy uniform flow is noted out of the choanal slit from both sides with equal resistance.

ACUTE GENERAL TREATMENT

- Treatment with appropriate oral and parenteral antimicrobial drugs through culture and sensitivity may be initiated upon presentation and modified if necessary once results of the laboratory test have been obtained.
- Broad-spectrum antibiotics may be initiated while waiting for culture results.
  - Ciprofloxacin 15-20 mg/kg PO, IM q 12 h
  - Ticarcillin/clavulanic acid 100 mg/kg IM q 12 h
  - Trimethoprim/sulfamethoxazole 20 mg/kg PO q 8-12 h for psittacines
- Nebulization with antibiotics may be initiated in the hospital, and warm water nebulization via a humidifier may be continued at home. Once the patient is stable, nasal flushes with dilute chlorhexidine or saline should be instituted.
  - Nebulization drugs
    - Amphotericin B 100 mg in 15 mL saline
    - Gentamicin 50 mg in 10 mL saline
    - Amikacin 50 mg in 10 mL saline
    - Enrofloxacin 100 mg in 10 mL saline
- If hypersensitivity is suspected as the cause of the sinusitis, therapy with diphenhydramine (2-4 mg/kg PO q 12 h) or a bronchodilator (aminophylline 4 mg/kg PO q 6-12 h) may be initiated.

CHRONIC TREATMENT

- The precise location of a discrete sinus mass can often be determined through contrast radiology, CT, or MRI. The mass can be surgically removed via sinusotomy. Temporary drains are frequently sutured in the infraorbital sinus postoperatively to assist with administration of topical medications.
- If choanal atresia is diagnosed, a red rubber tube can be applied through the nares and infraorbital sinus out of the choanal slit to enlarge the constricted opening.
- Nursing care: depending on the clinical state of the patient, hospitalization may be recommended or needed. Intraosseous or intravenous fluids, heat, nebulization of saline and antibiotics, oxygen therapy, and parenteral antibiotics may be warranted.

POSSIBLE COMPLICATIONS

Surgical procedures involving the infraorbital sinus and surrounding structures result in significant blood loss. This complicates exposure of targeted tissue during surgery and for many companion avian species is life threatening owing to blood loss.

RECOMMENDED MONITORING

Frequent evaluation of treatment response via the assessment of clinical signs and the improvement of affected tissue

PROGNOSIS AND OUTCOME

- Prognosis is guarded for all cases of chronic sinusitis diagnosed in avian patients owing to the complexity of the infraorbital sinus. The infraorbital sinus with its many diverticula makes treatment difficult, and over time, pathology associated with the disease process becomes a common complicating factor.
- With a multiple-treatment approach and frequent veterinary visits, the patient's quality of life is improved even without complete resolution of the problem.

PEARLS & CONSIDERATIONS

COMMENTS

- The underlying cause of chronic sinusitis is difficult to diagnose because of secondary infectious processes and pathology from long-term irritation associated with the disease.
- Owners must be informed of the importance of determining the extent of the pathology and the need to properly diagnose conditions that are causing the problem(s).
- Owner compliance with treatment and veterinary care are essential for any success that may be achieved.

PREVENTION

- Owners should be warned of the extremely sensitive nature of the avian respiratory tract.
- Smokers should be advised to discontinue smoking in the vicinity of the bird and to wash their hands before handling the bird.
- Owners should be informed of the risk of injury to the avian respiratory system from perfumes, incense, candles, plug-in air fresheners, and burned cooking or baking utensils. Owners should be made aware that any of these respiratory irritants can cause a primary sinusitis or may predispose a bird to secondary bacterial or fungal sinus infection.

CLIENT EDUCATION

See previous discussion.

SUGGESTED READINGS

Phalen DN: Respiratory medicine of cage and aviary birds, Vet Clin North Am Exot Anim Pract 3:423–452, 2000.

Tully TN, et al: Pneumonology. In Ritchie BW, et al, editors: Avian medicine: principles and application, Lake Worth, FL, 1994, Wingers Publishing, pp 556–581.

AUTHOR: **MEGAN KIRCHGESSNER**

EDITOR: **THOMAS N. TULLY, JR.**

BIRDS

Trauma

BASIC INFORMATION

DEFINITION

A wound or injury

SYNONYMS

Injury, wound, contusion, abrasion

EPIDEMIOLOGY

SPECIES, AGE, SEX All species and ages and both sexes

GENETICS AND BREED PREDISPOSITION

- Cockatoos may self-mutilate.
- Male cockatoos may attack their female mate.
- Female eclectus parrots may attack their male mate.

RISK FACTORS

- Firearms
- Flying into stationary object
- Cagemate injury due to fighting
- Vehicular collision
- Electrical shock
- Falling on hard surfaces
- Ceiling fans, sliding glass doors

ASSOCIATED CONDITIONS AND DISORDERS

- Behavioral disorders
- Hemorrhage
- Edema
- Infection
- Fractures (see Fractures)
- Ocular disorders
- Contusion
- Lacerations
- Abrasions
- Neurologic disorders

CLINICAL PRESENTATION

DISEASE FORMS/SUBTYPES

- Blunt trauma
- Biting trauma
- Electrical trauma

HISTORY, CHIEF COMPLAINT

- Bleeding wound
- Disuse or malposition of limb
- Lameness
- Depression

PHYSICAL EXAM FINDINGS

- Wounds
- Hemorrhage
- Shock
- Dehydration
- Fracture(s)
- Lethargy
- Anorexia
- Recumbency

ETIOLOGY AND PATHOPHYSIOLOGY

- Edema and subcutaneous hemorrhage may be present from electrical shock wounds.
- Laceration or excessive force resulting in injury to the body of the avian patient

DIAGNOSIS

DIFFERENTIAL DIAGNOSIS

- Coagulopathies
- Self-mutilation
- Dermatopathy
- Nutritional deficiencies
- Infection
- Systemic disease
- Neoplasia

INITIAL DATABASE

- Evaluate for dehydration and shock: the patient should be stabilized before diagnostic testing is begun
- Radiographs if fracture, luxation, or visceral damage is suspected. Ultrasound or CT may also be required.
- Complete blood count (CBC) and/or chemistry may be indicated with hemorrhage, dehydration, or visceral trauma. Only 1% of the bird's weight in grams may be taken for blood work (1 mL of blood for every 100 g body weight). If the bird has already lost blood or is suspected of having a clotting disorder, CBC and chemistry may be contraindicated.

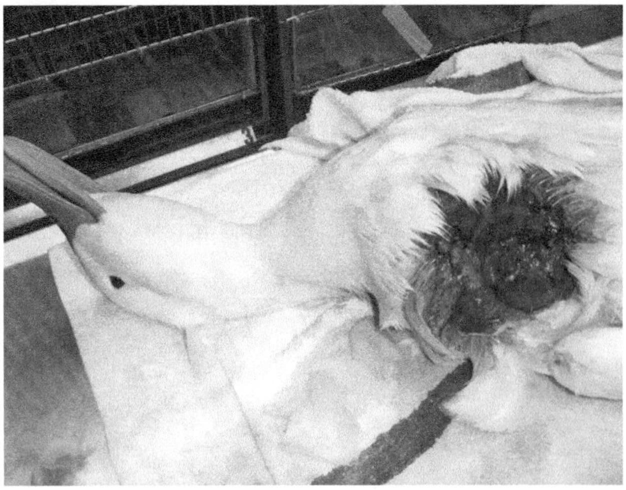

Trauma Severe trauma due to dog attack involving the pectoral area of the duck. *(Courtesy Thomas N. Tully, Jr.)*

TREATMENT

THERAPEUTIC GOALS

- Stabilize the patient. Stop active hemorrhage, correct dehydration and negative energy balance.
- Stabilize fractures.
- Stop self-mutilation behaviors.

ACUTE GENERAL TREATMENT

- Care must be taken not to stress the bird because this may kill a debilitated patient.
- Heat: most sick or traumatized birds are hypothermic and should be hospitalized in a warm, humid environment; 30°C (86°F) with 70% humidity is preferred. An incubator works well and may also be used to administer oxygen if necessary. Birds with suspected head trauma should not be placed in heat but should be placed in a quiet dark enclosure. Patients with respiratory disease may be sensitive to heat. Consequently, these birds should be monitored closely or placed in critical care units that are regulated at slightly cooler temperatures.
- Oxygen: dyspneic birds should receive oxygen therapy before handling. An enclosed space such as an incubator, which may be connected to oxygen to achieve a concentration of 40% to 50%, is preferable. Oxygen toxicity from prolonged exposure at 50% has been documented and should be avoided. In cases of tracheal or syringeal obstruction, placement of an air sac tube is required. This is done by placing the bird in right lateral recumbency with the dorsal leg pulled caudally. The eighth rib should be palpated and a small incision made in the lateral body wall just caudal to that rib. Dissect through soft tissue using mosquito forceps, and place the tube into the air sac. Be careful not to damage other organs by inserting the tube too

far or with too much force. A feather may be held over the opening of the tube to observe air flow with respiration. Air sac tubes will not help lower respiratory tract disease or dyspnea secondary to toxicity or compression.

- Fluid therapy: mildly dehydrated birds may be rehydrated by administration of oral fluids; 30 mL/kg by mouth every 6-8 hours has been suggested. Moderately dehydrated birds should receive subcutaneous fluids along with oral fluid therapy. Fluids may be administered in the axillary area, the intrascapular area, or the flank. Replacement values should be estimated along with maintenance amounts (100 mL/kg/d) to determine appropriate volumes. It should be stated that avian fluid maintenance requirements vary from 60-150 ml/kg/d depending on species being treated. Smaller avian species are generally considered to have a higher range of daily fluid requirements. For severely dehydrated birds, IV or IO fluid administration is required and may be used in conjunction with subcutaneous fluid administration. These birds are at high risk for death from handling stress associated with catheter placement, so appropriate judgment is essential in these situations. Catheters may be placed in the basilic or median metatarsal veins. IO catheters should be placed in the distal ulna or the proximal tibia. Hypoproteinemic patients, those with fewer than 2 total solids, should be given hetastarch; 10-15 mL/kg q 8 h for up to 4 treatments is recommended.
- Stop hemorrhage: compression may be used to stop active hemorrhage and should be attempted first. Bandaging with a pressure wrap may aid in compression but should not be attempted around the keel region because this may result in suffocation. Silver nitrate sticks may be used on nail beds but should not be used on feather follicles. Cautery or application of ferric subsulfate may be attempted if bleeding persists. Once bleeding stops, allow the bird to calm down before investigating the wound further, as stress and elevations in blood pressure may result in clot removal and recurrence of bleeding. Birds produce blood cells in about half the time mammals take (about 2 weeks) and therefore recover from anemia more quickly with appropriate supportive care (see Anemia).
- Nutritional support: birds that are not eating and/or drinking should be given oral nutritional supplementation in the form of a liquid diet, which may be gavage-fed. Crop capacity is approximately 5% body weight in grams in adult birds and is slightly higher in juveniles. Sick birds are more prone to regurgitation, which should be avoided. Proper administration and watching for signs of fluid in the back of the throat are essential during gavage feeding. A large gavage tube should be used (and palpated in the esophagus) to avoid the risk of placing the tube into the trachea. Total parenteral nutrition may be indicated in cases of severe head trauma or digestive disorders. TPN is not frequently used in birds and should be administered through an IV catheter only if required. Bacterial contamination is a likely complication.
- Prevent self-mutilation: placement of an E-collar will prevent the bird from exacerbating wounds by picking. A circular collar may be made from old radiographs. The edges should be covered with padding or tape to prevent pressure sores from the collar. The collar may be placed so that the large "cone" portion is directed cranially or caudally.
- Wound care: similar to that provided for other species. Bite or scratch wounds should not be closed unless they are large, or unless this is required for function. Wounds should be treated immediately with four-quadrant antibiotic therapy (within 12 hours). Many of these (bite/scratch) wounds may not be visible to the naked eye, so if trauma is suspected, therapy should be instituted.
- Stabilize fractures: fractures should be stabilized with splints and/or figure-eight bandages immediately and then evaluated for the best long-term treatment (surgical, splinting, etc.). Open fractures and those that will require surgical fixation are indications for beginning antibiotic therapy.
- Corticosteroids: dexamethasone sodium phosphate (2 mg/kg IM once) may be used in cases of severe trauma, including head trauma, shock, or toxicity. They should not be used for cases in which immune suppression, fungal disease, or organophosphate toxicity is suspected. Prednisolone sodium succinate is preferred in other species for neurologic emergencies. Doses of 0.5-1.0 mg/kg IM given once have been effective in birds.
- Replacing blood volume: transfusions are indicated when the packed cell volume (PCV) drops acutely below 20% and should be homologous (from the same species) whenever possible. Calculated blood volume is 8% of the patient's body weight; 10% of the calculated blood volume should be supplied in a transfusion. If oxyglobin is available, it may be used to increase the oxygen-carrying capacity of the blood and is given at 30 mL/kg IV slowly once. Aggressive fluid therapy with colloids and crystalloids is essential for supporting the cardiovascular system when significant blood loss has occurred.
- Pain management: analgesics such as butorphanol are indicated for severe injuries such as fractures. Certain species of birds have been shown to have a higher abundance of kappa receptors in the brain; therefore, butorphanol is often considered the drug of choice for management of severe pain. Meloxicam should be used in conjunction with butorphanol, particularly when a strong inflammatory response is present. Meloxicam may be used alone for mildly to moderately painful wounds or for other causes of inflammation.

CHRONIC TREATMENT

These cases often require long-term follow-up and chronic wound management.

RECOMMENDED MONITORING

- Monitor the wound.
- Monitor patient's response to supportive therapy.
- Monitor fracture healing, if injury is present.

PROGNOSIS AND OUTCOME

Variable: debilitated birds upon admission have a poor prognosis; however, those that receive appropriate therapy early and are relatively stable often have a good prognosis.

PEARLS & CONSIDERATIONS

COMMENTS

It is often difficult to take a "hands-off" approach to medicine; however, debilitated birds benefit from heat and oxygen therapy before physical examination or handling. These patients may tolerate fluid and nutritional support with empirical treatment if given some time in an incubator with oxygen support and in a quiet environment before or between treatments. Minimizing stress is essential.

PREVENTION

- Know birds and species that are housed together to prevent cagemate trauma.
- Provide proper enclosures for birds to help reduce traumatic injury due to inappropriate housing.
- Clip a bird's wing feathers to reduce trauma due to flying into walls, ceiling fans, sliding glass doors, etc.

- Participate in wildlife education for the general public.

CLIENT EDUCATION

- The owner should be made aware that a debilitated bird may die at any time, particularly when stressed, and that although every attempt will be made to minimize stress, some treatments are stressful but are necessary to attempt to save the bird's life.
- See Prevention.

SUGGESTED READINGS

Dorrestein GM: Nursing the sick bird. In Tully TN, et al, editors: Avian medicine, Oxford, UK, 2000, Butterworth-Heinemann, pp 74–112.

Harrison GJ, et al: Emergency and critical care. In Harrison GJ, et al, editors: Clinical avian medicine, vol I, Palm Beach, FL, 2006, Spix Publishing, Inc., pp 213–232.

Pollock CG, et al: Birds. In Carpenter JW, editor: Exotic animal formulary, ed 3, St Louis, 2005, Elsevier/Saunders, pp 135–264.

Quesenberry KE, et al: Supportive care and emergency therapy. In Ritchie BW, et al, editors: Avian medicine: principles and applications, Brentwood, TN, 1994, HBD International, Inc., pp 383–416.

CROSS-REFERENCES TO OTHER SECTIONS

Anemia
Fractures

AUTHOR: **GWENDOLYN R. JANKOWSKI**

EDITOR: **THOMAS N. TULLY, JR.**

BIRDS

Tumors

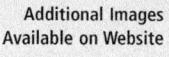

Additional Images Available on Website

BASIC INFORMATION

DEFINITION

New growths of tissue in which cell multiplication is out of control and progressive

EPIDEMIOLOGY

SPECIES, AGE, SEX

- Prolonged exposure to sunlight has been described as a cause of predisposition in some integument neoplasias; long-term therapies with steroids have been linked to the development of tumors.
- Some specific tumors such as papillomas and hemangiomas have been related to virus infections, herpesvirus, and avian hemangioma virus, respectively.

CLINICAL PRESENTATION

PHYSICAL EXAM FINDINGS A large range of clinical signs vary with the organs affected, but signs related to the paraneoplastic syndrome such as weight loss are common to a large number of tumors.

ETIOLOGY AND PATHOPHYSIOLOGY

- Integument neoplasias
  - Basal cell tumor (feather folliculoma)
    - Benign neoplasm that appears as a firm mass containing yellow keratinaceous material
    - Must be differentiated from feather cysts
    - Surgical removal has been performed successfully.
  - Basal cell carcinoma
    - Undifferentiated epithelial skin tumor with variable malignancy; appears as a broad-based mass that has been described in the margin of the third eyelid and the cervical and ingluvial regions
    - Surgical removal has been performed, but reappearance is common.
  - Fibroma and fibrosarcoma
    - Neoplasm from fibrous connective tissue
    - Fibrosarcomas are locally invasive, presenting irregular and indistinct borders, and are frequently ulcerated with skin attached to the mass; the malignant version is more commonly reported. They have been most frequently diagnosed in integument areas around the cere and beak, wings, and legs but have been described in other areas too.
    - Surgical removal, radiation treatment, and intratumoral cisplatin have been attempted in avian species.
  - Hemangioma
    - This is a benign tumor of vascular endothelium. Macroscopically, it can be observed as a circumscribed, soft, and red to black swelling in the skin of the feet, inguinal area, cloaca, neck, and wings, but it has been described in the spleen too.
    - It has been detected frequently in budgerigars, with no age predisposition. It should be differentiated from malignant melanoma, vascular malformation (arteriovenous fistula and aneurysm), hematoma, and highly vascular granulation tissue.
    - Complete surgical removal is curative.
  - Hemangiosarcoma (or hemangioendothelioma or angiosarcoma)
    - This tumor tends to be locally invasive and multicentric; when found in the skin, inflammation and necrosis can be observed. Hemangiosarcoma has been described in a wide range of psittaciformes, with no sex predisposition.
    - Treatment involves complete surgical removal in combination with radiation and chemotherapy.
  - Lipoma
    - This is a benign tumor of adipose tissue.
    - It is soft, pale yellow, encapsulated, and lobulated in the subcutis in the sternum area, although it has been described in the abdomen and the thighs less commonly. It has been reported in different psittacines but very commonly in budgerigars.
    - Birds may show abnormal perching positions to keep balance when the tumor reaches a large size.
    - Surgical removal in combination with L-carnitine modified diets can be curative.
    - Recurrence is common if incomplete removal is performed.
    - A possible relation with abnormal thyroid gland has been described.
  - Liposarcoma
    - This appears as a yellow to grey mass in the subcutis; it is firmer, more infiltrative, and more vascular than a lipoma.
    - It occurs rarely in psittacines.
  - Myelolipoma
    - This benign tumor is composed of fat and hematopoietic cells. Areas of mineralization can appear.

- This tumor has been reported in wings, thighs, thorax, spleen, and liver.
- Complete surgical removal is curative.
- Hemangiolipoma
  - Adipose tissue tumor with vascular structures; it has been described in ovary and subcutaneous tissue.
  - Cutaneous pseudolymphoma
  - Large nodular lymphocytic proliferation infiltrating the dermis
- Malignant melanoma
  - Abnormal growth of melanocytes, located usually in the beak and the face
  - Shows dark coloration with irregular borders and infiltrating surrounding tissues
  - Appearance is similar to hemangioma and hemangiosarcoma.
- Cutaneous papilloma
  - Virally induced; presented in face and feet
- Squamous cell carcinoma
  - Appears as a proliferative, irregular, broad-based mass or ulcerated area
  - Commonly found in the integument and the upper digestive tract
- Xanthoma
  - Mass including macrophages, multinucleated giant cells, and cholesterol
  - Most common presentation is skin, although described in internal organs; appears as yellow to orange area and is locally invasive

- Tumors described in the uropygial gland
  - Squamous cell carcinomas, adenocarcinomas, and adenomas have been diagnosed as affecting this exocrine gland. Metaplasia due to hypovitaminosis A should be considered as a differential diagnosis.
- Gastrointestinal neoplasias
  - Leiomyosarcoma
    - Malignant tumor; very vascular, involving smooth muscle
    - Usually appears as a large mass in the coelomic cavity
  - Papilloma
    - Proliferative, grey-white growth on mucous membranes, usually diagnosed in the mouth and cloaca
    - Herpesviruses are suspected to induce the formation of this tumor.
    - It affects primarily New World psittacines.
    - Growth shows cyclic behavior with regression and recurrence usually related to the immune status of the patient.
  - Squamous cell carcinoma
    - Affects the upper gastrointestinal tract, causing lesions with poorly defined borders, hemorrhage, and necrosis in surrounding tissues
    - Depending on the location, signs may vary and include dysphagia, regurgitation, and dyspnea.
  - Proventricular and ventricular adenocarcinoma
    - Usually affects proventriculus and gastric isthmus
    - Causes thickening and irregularity of the proventriculus wall with variable amounts of blood loss and necrosis
    - Metastasis to lungs and pancreas has been described.
  - Cholangiocarcinoma
    - Locally invasive, can metastasize
  - Pancreatic tumor
    - Adenoma, adenocarcinoma, and carcinoma
    - Pancreas appears diffusely enlarged with increased consistency.
- Hemolymphatic system neoplasias
  - Thymoma
    - Tumor can appear cystic and hemorrhagic, involving surrounding tissues along the neck; no metastasis
  - Lymphosarcoma
    - Multicentric lymphoma is the most common neoplasia in psittaciformes and passerines of all ages.
    - Animals affected can present a wide range of clinical signs depending on the organs involved, but liver, kidneys, and spleen are most commonly involved, appearing enlarged and pale.
    - Anemia is a common finding, and a leukemic profile is uncommon.
    - The cutaneous form of lymphosarcoma is usually reported, affecting the head and neck.
    - Chemotherapy protocols have been tried in birds but not very successfully.
- Muskuloskeletal neoplasias
  - Chondroma and chondrosarcoma
    - Chondroma has been described in the skull, causing head tilt, although there is no predilection for location.
  - Osteoma and osteosarcoma
    - Osteoma: a benign growth in the surface of the bone; has been described in the skull
    - Osteosarcoma: reported in long bones; amputation and treatment with doxorubricin have been described as treatment
  - Rhabdomyoma and rhabdomyosarcoma
    - The benign form presents a reddish coloration resembling normal muscle; the malignant version has irregular borders and the coloration tends to be darker.
  - Synovial cell carcinoma
    - Rare in birds; a proliferative mass that causes destruction of joint and bone
- Endocrine neoplasias
  - Adrenal gland
    - Nonfunctional and functional cases have been reported; metastases are commonly observed.
    - Have been reported in budgerigars and macaws
  - Pituitary tumor
    - Adenocarcinomas, carcinomas, and chromophobe pituitary tumors have been described.
    - Exophthalmia is a common finding due to invasion of neoplastic cells along the optic nerve.
    - Different neurologic and endocrine signs have been described as polyuria, cere color changes, circling, and blindness.
  - Thyroid gland tumors
    - Carcinomas and adenomas can affect the thyroid gland.
    - Commonly reported in budegerigars and cockatiels but described in amazons too
    - Clinical signs observed, such as respiratory noises and regurgitation, are related to upper respiratory and gastrointestinal tracts.
- Reproductive neoplasias
  - Ovarian/oviductal neoplasms
    - Adenocarcinomas, carcinomas, cystadenocarcinomas, and granulosa cell tumors have been diagnosed in the ovary.
    - Have been reported in cockatiels and budgerigars
    - Clinical signs include egg retention, persistent breeding behavior, and distention of coelomic cavity.
  - Cystadenoma and cystadenocarcinoma
    - Large, yellow masses with multiple cystic spaces
    - Can cause left-sided lameness due to pressure over the lumbar plexus and muscle wasting
    - Surgical removal is the indicated treatment, although complete resection is difficult to achieve.
  - Testicular tumor
    - Uncommon; a few cases have been reported in budgerigars and cockatiels
    - Seminomas are commonly bilateral.
    - Sertoli cell tumors: nodular firm masses; these tumors can cause hyperostosis and different changes in the hemogram
    - Interstitial cell tumors tend to be cystic and hemorrhagic.
- Respiratory system neoplasias
  - Nasal/sinus carcinoma or adenocarcinoma

    - Grey coloration growths from mucosa or glandular epithelium; can be quite large causing deformation of the skull
  - Lung carcinoma
    - Appears as multiple grey nodules in lung parenchyma; may extend into air sacs
  - Air sac carcinoma
    - Rare; have been described in large psittacines
    - Lesions include nodules filled with fluid and polypoid masses. Pneumatized bones can be involved.
- Urinary system neoplasias
  - Renal tumors
    - Different tumors, including nephromas, adenocarcinomas, carcinomas, and adenomas, have been described. Appearance is variable; metastases are rare.
    - Very common in budgerigars
    - Unilateral lameness due to pressure on the lumbar plexus is a very indicative clinical sign.

DIAGNOSIS

INITIAL DATABASE

- Complete blood count/Biochemistry
  - Anemia, a common finding, could be linked to chronic blood loss due to ulceration or related to the paraneoplastic syndrome.
  - Depending on the organ affected and the degree of invasion, different changes in biochemistry can be observed; increases in uric acid are described in cases of kidney involvement.

ADVANCED OR CONFIRMATORY TESTING

- Radiographs
  - Contrast radiographs can be very useful in the diagnosis of gastrointestinal tumors.
- Ultrasound
  - Ultrasound can prove useful in the diagnosis of some tumors located in the coelomic cavity, although the presence of air sacs limits its use.
- Endoscopy
  - Endoscopy of the gastrointestinal and respiratory tracts can prove very useful in examination of closely neoplastic lesions and in collection of samples for histopathologic examination.
- Magnetic resonance
- Computed tomography
  - Useful in the diagnosis of bone tumors
- Cytology
  - Fine-needle aspirations are very easily performed; can be useful in the diagnosis of tumors such as lipoma, lymphoma, and melanoma
- Biopsy
  - Samples must be taken from between healthy and abnormal tissue, unless a bone tumor is being tested.
  - Electrosurgery should be avoided because the extreme heat can cause deformation of the tissue architecture.
  - Punch biopsies are indicated for tumors in the oral cavity and skin, but they do not provide a deep sample.
  - Surface biting instruments are very useful in the use of endoscopy to collect samples; one problem with this technique is the small size of the samples.
  - Needle biopsies: require small samples but easily performed; do not require much equipment
- Culture and sensitivity
  - Indicated in skin tumors due secondary bacterial infection

TREATMENT

ACUTE GENERAL TREATMENT

- Diet modification
  - Supplementation with L-carnitine at a dose of 1000 mg/kg has proved to reduce the volume of lipomas in budgerigars; this reduction can facilitate excision of the tumor.
- Steroids
  - Due to serious immune suppression that steroids can cause in birds, use of these drugs should be considered very carefully; broad-spectrum antibiotics and antifungals are indicated.
- Nonsteroidal antiinflammatory drugs (NSAIDs)
  - Owing to antitumoral effects demonstrated in small animal species, NSAIDs may be a therapeutic option.
- Intralesional chemotherapy
  - The main advantage of this technique is the higher therapeutic effect compared with systemic chemotherapy.
  - Use of cisplatin has been described in birds in this therapeutic mode at doses of 1 mg/cm^3 of tissue. Cisplatin does not diffuse more than 4 mm so with larger lesions, several injections may be required.
  - Use of intralesional chemotherapy generally requires anesthesia because of the accuracy required.
  - It can cause local side effects like inflammation.
  - If secondary bacterial or fungal infections are present, these problems should be resolved before this therapeutic measure is applied.
  - Combinations with other local techniques such as hyperthermia or radiotherapy have been described.
- Systemic chemotherapy
  - If vascular access is required, the election would be the right jugular; the ulnar vein predisposition to from hematomas makes it undesirable for administration of chemotherapeutics.
  - Cisplatin and carboplatin have been used in psittacines, and pharmacokinetic values have been established.
- Radiotherapy
  - Indicated in the treatment of local tumors, its use is not reported very frequently in avian species and tends to be unsuccessful unless aggressive therapies are used. Birds appear to be very resistant to radiation.
- Immune therapy
  - Immune stimulating drugs like acemannan have been used in the treatment of a fibrosarcoma in a cockatoo, in combination with surgery.
- Surgery
  - Surgery is the most extended therapeutic measure in the treatment of neoplasia.
  - Electrocautery and carbon dioxide laser are especially useful in the resection of tumors to provide good hemostasis; this is of capital importance in small birds, in which any small blood loss is significant.
  - Submission for histopathologic examination after excision is recommended to assess the margins of the tumor.

AUTHOR: **ALBERTO RODRIGUEZ BARBON**

EDITOR: **THOMAS N. TULLY, JR.**

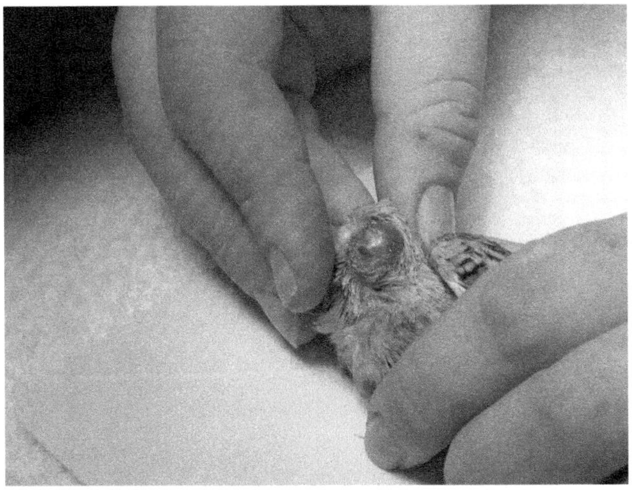

Tumors Neoplasia on the face of a budgerigar.

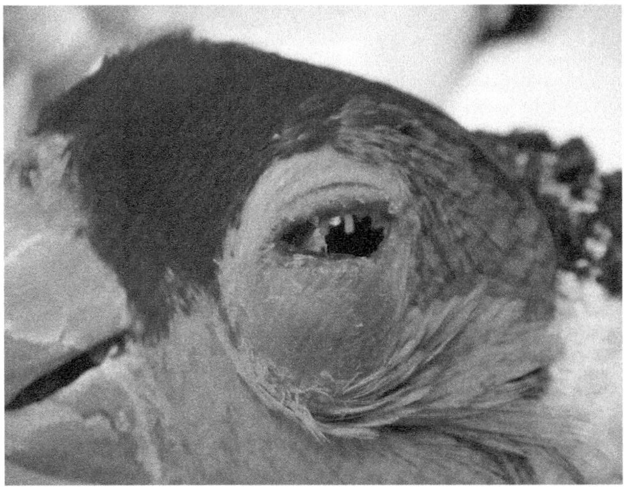

Tumors Round cell sarcoma under the ventral lid margin of an Amazon parrot.

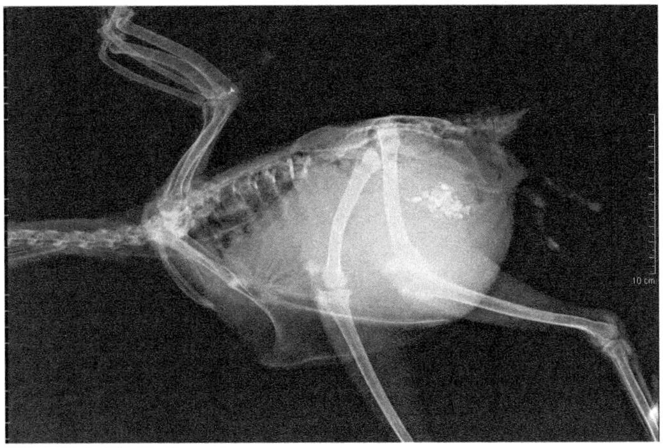

Tumors A large renal carcinoma in a rooster; note the lack of details in the coelomic cavity without notable distention of the coelom. *(Photo courtesy Jörg Mayer, The University of Georgia, Athens.)*

BIRDS

Uropygial Gland Disease Conditions

BASIC INFORMATION

DEFINITION

Disease conditions that affect the uropygial gland, a bilobed secretory gland located on the uropygium

The uropygial area is located dorsally over the pygostyle, on the midline, at the base of the tail. Secretions of this gland are an important component in maintaining feathers' condition.

SYNONYMS

Preen gland, oil gland

EPIDEMIOLOGY

SPECIES, AGE, SEX All species that have a uropygial gland and all ages and both sexes can be affected by uropygial gland disease presentations.

GENETICS AND BREED PREDISPOSITION None specific, but certain avian species (e.g., Amazon parrots, hyacinth macaws) do not have a uropygial gland; therefore, they would not be susceptible to disease conditions associated with this gland.

RISK FACTORS
- Trauma to uropygial gland
- Self-mutilation/feather/picking around the gland
- Impaction of the gland
- Infectious cause (e.g., bacterial)
- Glandular or ductular neoplasia
- Nutritional deficiencies (e.g., vitamin A)

ASSOCIATED CONDITIONS AND DISORDERS
- Poor feather condition
- Inability of feathers to become water resistant
- Self-trauma and/or mutilation to the uropygial gland area

CLINICAL PRESENTATION

DISEASE FORMS/SUBTYPES
- Trauma to the gland
- Neoplasia of glandular and/or ductal tissue
- Impaction of the gland
- Granuloma/abscess of the gland

HISTORY, CHIEF COMPLAINT
- Nonspecific

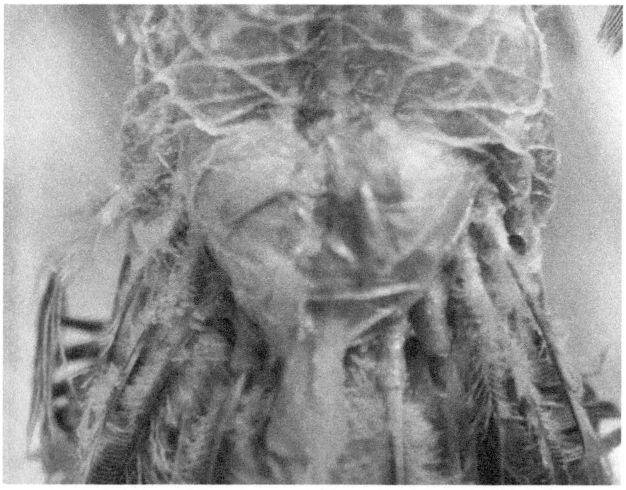

Uropygial Gland Disease Conditions Normal appearance of the bilobed uropygial gland on this feather-picking parrot.

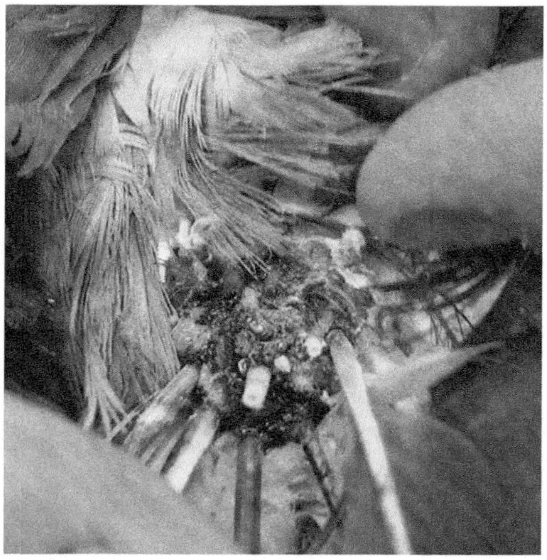

Uropygial Gland Disease Conditions Large tumor of the uropygial gland in a parakeet. Surgical excision often is incomplete and recurrence is common; aggressive radiation offers a good follow-up option after removal of the bulk of the mass.

- Excessive preening over the caudal dorsal surface of the back
- Poor feather quality
- Water birds unable to maintain their bodies at proper level on the water surface
- Bleeding in area around uropygial gland
- Large mass in area around uropygial gland

PHYSICAL EXAM FINDINGS

- Asymmetric lobes of the uropygial gland
- Large mass incorporating all or part of the uropygial gland
- Necrotic tissue of the uropygial gland
- Feather loss and blood around the area of the uropygial gland
- Observation of the patient compulsively irritating and traumatizing the uropygial gland

ETIOLOGY AND PATHOPHYSIOLOGY

- The uropygial gland, often referred to as the *oil* or *preen gland*, is an epidermal holocrine gland localized on the uropygium of most birds. It is composed of two lobes separated by an interlobular septum and covered by an external capsule. A dorsocaudally oriented papilla contains one, two, or multiple ducts and a tuft of down feathers at the openings. The nerve supply of the gland has both a medullar and a sympathetic origin. The gland is vascularized by branches of the caudal artery.
- Composition of avian uropygial gland secretions is very complex and may vary with species, gender, season, diet, and hormonal regulation. The secretion is a complex mixture of ester waxes, fatty acids, lipids, and wax alcohols. Secretions are spread among the plumage by preening. Contact of the beak with the papilla induces a flow of secretion.
- Possible roles of uropygial gland secretions:
  - Antimicrobial activity against feather-degrading bacteria and fungi
  - Antiabrasive effects to prevent feather barbules from breaking and to maintain plumage in good condition when the feathers are drawn through the bill during preening
  - As protection against feather-degrading ectoparasites such as feather lice
  - Hydrophobic properties, which have a role in plumage waterproofing in some species
  - Conversion of provitamin D to vitamin D by ultraviolet light and ingestion by further preening
  - Sex-linked changes in the ultraviolet appearance of the plumage
  - Production of pheromones
  - Excretory functions of several pesticides and pollutants
  - The fact that some bird species lack a preen gland suggests that preen oil is not universally important, or that they may use alternative strategies for feather maintenance.

DIAGNOSIS

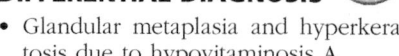

DIFFERENTIAL DIAGNOSIS

- Glandular metaplasia and hyperkeratosis due to hypovitaminosis A
- Neoplasia: adenoma, adenocarcinoma, squamous cell carcinoma, papilloma
- Abscessation, adenitis
- Impaction
- Granulomas: fungi, foreign bodies
- Trauma, rupture of the gland, chronic ulcerative dermatitis of the uropygial and periuropygial area

INITIAL DATABASE

- Complete blood count (CBC): in most cases unremarkable; slight leukocytosis or monocytosis may be observed in cases with inflammation or secondary infection
- Plasma biochemistry panel: no specific biochemistry abnormalities noted
- Cytologic examination/cultures: Cytologic examination can be performed on gland secretions or ulcerations. The main purpose is to determine whether an infection is present with inflammatory cells and bacteria (monomorphic intracellular) or neoplasia (neoplastic cells present). Culture and sensitivity should be performed as appropriate.

ADVANCED OR CONFIRMATORY TESTING

Histopathologic examination: tissue biopsy is essential to confirm neoplasia and to characterize the tumor type (see Tumors). Biopsy is useful to differentiate neoplasia from infectious or granulomatous processes.

TREATMENT

THERAPEUTIC GOAL

Resolution of the disease condition and return of normal function of the uropygial gland

ACUTE GENERAL TREATMENT

- Treatment of a uropygial gland problem will depend on the diagnosis.

- Nursing care
  - Digital pressure in cases of impacted, abscessed, or metaplastic glands may be helpful in exuding the contents. Application of hot compresses may help in liquefying the content before expulsion.
  - Wound care and cleaning are necessary if ulceration or erosion is noted. Adherent dressings (e.g., 3M Tegaderm, 3M Tegaderm-Foam-Adhesive-Dressing, 3M Tegaderm-Hydrocolloid-Thin-Dressing [3M, St Paul, Minn]) should be considered whenever possible with an infected or extensive wound in this area. Treatments that can be used alone or in combination with surgery are described later.
- For impacted uropygial glands, an incision over the affected lobe(s) with subsequent removal of the impacted material; the incision should be left to heal by secondary intention

CHRONIC TREATMENT

- Systemic chemotherapy
- Topical chemotherapy (e.g., 5-fluorouracil application)
- Intratumoral chemotherapy (e.g., carboplatin, cisplatin)
- Radiation therapy involves administration of ionizing radiation to tumor cells. Strontium 90 ophthalmic applicator therapy has been used to apply 100 Gy in the treatment of uropygial tumors.
- Cryotherapy has several advantages: minimal systemic effects, minimal postoperative bleeding, and safe repeat treatments.

DRUG INTERACTIONS

- Any chemotherapy and radiation therapy should be administered by a trained oncology specialist. Chemotherapeutic and radiation therapeutic agents present a serious health hazard for people around the patient during treatment application.
- If chemotherapeutic and radiation therapy is not administered correctly and at the proper dose, the patient may die or suffer permanent injury.

POSSIBLE COMPLICATIONS

- Death from blood loss during surgery to remove the uropygial gland
- Lack of treatment response
- Recurrence of uropygial disease condition
- Death or permanent injury due to selected treatment protocol

RECOMMENDED MONITORING

- Monitor diseased uropygial gland for treatment response.
- Repeat CBC and plasma chemistry panel when radiation or chemotherapy is being used.
- Analgesic/antiinflammatory medication is required in cases of suspected pain and inflammation.
- Monitor appetite, fecal output, and behavior during treatment period, until the disease condition has resolved.

PROGNOSIS AND OUTCOME

- Uncomplicated cases have a good prognosis.
- The prognosis degrades as the number of complications increases, especially in cases in which neoplasia has been diagnosed or severe trauma to the gland has occurred.

PEARLS & CONSIDERATIONS

COMMENTS

- Some avian species (e.g., some macaw species, Amazon parrots) do not have a uropygial gland.
- With many avian species, the uropygial gland may be removed without adverse consequences.
- The uropygial gland is very important for water birds to maintain the health and condition of their feathers while swimming.
- The uropygial gland is vascular; care should be taken when excising the gland to reduce hemorrhage associated with removal.
- A definitive diagnosis is necessary to establish a proper treatment protocol for the patient.

PREVENTION

- Routinely check the uropygial gland as part of the physical examination.
- Provide a well-balanced diet.

CLIENT EDUCATION

- Inform the owner of the location and function of the uropygial gland.
- Discuss that it is normal for birds to preen and rub their head in the area of the gland.
- Bleeding, loss of feathers, and gross enlargement of the gland or areas around the gland are abnormal.

SUGGESTED READINGS

Altman RB: Soft tissue surgical procedures. In Altman RB, et al, editors: Avian medicine and surgery, Philadelphia, 1997, WB Saunders, pp 704–732.
Filippich LJ: Tumor control in birds, Semin Avian Exotic Pet Med 13:25–43, 2004.
Lucas AM, et al: Avian anatomy: integument, part II, agriculture handbook 362, Washington DC, 1972, U.S. Government Printing Office, pp 613–626.
Nemetz LP, et al: Strontium-90 therapy for uropygial neoplasia, Proc Conf Assoc Avian Vet 25:15–20, 2004.

CROSS-REFERENCES TO OTHER SECTIONS

Tumors

AUTHORS: **HUGUES BEAUFRÉRE AND W. MICHAEL TAYLOR**

EDITOR: **THOMAS N. TULLY, JR.**

BIRDS

Viral Diseases

BASIC INFORMATION

DEFINITION

Diseases caused directly or indirectly by the pathogenic action of a virus

SYNONYM

Viral infection

EPIDEMIOLOGY

SPECIES, AGE, SEX All species and ages and both sexes. Some are more prevalent in youngsters (circovirus, polyomavirus).

GENETICS AND BREED PREDISPOSITION

- Species have various susceptibilities to specific viral diseases:
  - Psittaciformes are more prone to herpesvirus (type 1, 2, or 3; Pacheco, Amazon tracheitis virus, internal papillomatosis), proventricular dilatation disease (see Proventricular Dilatation Disease) (PDD; bornaviruses), circovirus (psittacine beak and feather disease [PBFD]),

polyomavirus, reovirus, adenovirus, paramyxovirus, togavirus.
- Falconiformes and strigiformes are most commonly infected with poxvirus, adenovirus (falcon adenovirus), herpesvirus (falcon herpesvirus, eagle herpesvirus, owl herpesvirus), paramyxovirus, influenzavirus, flavivirus (West Nile virus).
- Passeriformes are most often affected by poxvirus, herpesvirus, polyomavirus, paramyxovirus, cytomegalovirus, and circovirus.
- Columbiformes are mainly diagnosed with circovirus, adenovirus, herpesvirus, poxvirus, and paramyxovirus.
- Anseriformes are more susceptible to herpesvirus (duck plague virus), picornavirus (duck viral hepatitis), parvovirus (goose parvovirus infection), paramyxovirus (type I), and orthomyxovirus (influenzavirus).
- Galliformes are principally susceptible to retrovirus (avian leukosis, reticuloendotheliosis virus), adenovirus (egg drop syndrome, marble spleen disease), herpesvirus (infectious laryngotracheitis, Marek's disease), birnavirus (Gumboro disease), influenzavirus, paramyxovirus (Newcastle disease), and adenovirus.

RISK FACTORS
- Stress-associated immune depression (e.g., importation, poor nutrition, captive conditions)
- Mixing of species from various origins, large groups of birds
- Contact with latently or chronically infected birds
- Lack of prophylaxis, hygiene, quarantine

CONTAGION AND ZOONOSIS
- All viral diseases are contagious, but contagiosity depends on the virulence and the mode of transmission. Contagion from one species to another depends on the host range of the virus. Mosquito-borne viral diseases are less contagious from one bird to another.
- Avian viruses reported to be zoonotic are avian influenza, Newcastle disease, West Nile virus, and other mosquito-borne encephalitis.

GEOGRAPHY AND SEASONALITY
- Mosquito-borne viral infections (poxvirus, viral encephalitis viruses) are more prevalent during spring and summer.
- Polyomavirus and PBFD seem to be more commonly diagnosed in pet psittacines in Europe than in North America. PBFD is also endemic in Australia.
- Avian viral serositis and other types of avian encephalitis are restricted to particular geographic regions of the United States.

ASSOCIATED CONDITIONS AND DISORDERS
- Systemic infection is common with viral outbreaks and with some specific avian viruses: circovirus (PBFD), polyomavirus (in particular, in budgerigar, lovebirds, lories, and cockatoos), influenzavirus (galliformes), and paramyxovirus (galliformes) are especially known for their devastating effects.
- Immune deficiencies associated with circovirus infection (psittacines, pigeons, canaries, geese) might predispose to a variety of secondary diseases. Multiple viral infections (PBFD, polyomavirus, pigeon circovirus, and adenovirus) are not uncommon.
- Feather abnormalities are common with PBFD and polyomavirus and have been reported with West Nile virus and herpesvirus.
- Skin and mucocutaneous conditions are documented with poxvirus, herpesvirus (cloacal papillomatosis, foot lesions in macaws and cockatoos), and papillomavirus in African grey parrots.
- Hepatitis (see Liver Disease): herpesvirus, adenovirus, reovirus, polyomavirus
- Gastroenteritis: PDD, herpesvirus, poxvirus (diphtheric and systemic forms), picornavirus, reovirus, paramyxovirus, adenovirus
- Cardiac disease: West Nile virus, polyomavirus, PDD, togavirus
- Neurologic disorders: paramyxovirus (PVM1 in all birds, PVM3 in *Neophema* spp. and passerines), influenzavirus, PDD, togavirus, flavivirus, adenovirus
- Nephritis: polyomavirus, adenovirus, herpesvirus, retrovirus
- Ascites: polyomavirus, avian viral serositis (togavirus), systemic viral infection

CLINICAL PRESENTATION

DISEASE FORMS/SUBTYPES
- Acute infection and presentation
- Chronic infection
- Latent infection

HISTORY, CHIEF COMPLAINT
- Lethargy, anorexia, fluffy at the bottom of the cage
- Labored breathing
- Regurgitation, vomiting, change in droppings
- Ascites, abdominal distention
- Polyuria-polydipsia
- Neurologic signs (see Neurologic Disease)

PHYSICAL EXAM FINDINGS
- Clinical signs or lesions are often nonspecific or pathognomonic for any viral diseases and may affect all organ systems.
- Neoplasia and masses are reported for herpesviruses (internal papillomatosis, Marek's disease), retroviruses (avian leukosis), poxviruses, and papillomavirus (African grey parrots).

ETIOLOGY AND PATHOPHYSIOLOGY
- Results of entry and replication of a virus within host cells: cytolysis, immune system stimulation or depression, oncogenicity, and latency
- Transmission: oral-fecal route (adenovirus, herpesvirus, orthomyxovirus, paramyxovirus, polyomavirus, circovirus, reovirus, PDD), respiratory secretions (herpesvirus, orthomyxovirus, paramyxovirus, polyomavirus, PDD), vectors (poxvirus, togavirus, flavivirus), direct contact with wounds or feather dust (poxvirus, circovirus, polyomavirus, PDD), contamination of eggs
- Incubation period: short for most diseases (3-12 days). Some viruses may take months to years to induce clinical disease (PDD, Marek's disease, herpesviruses causing internal papillomatosis, circovirus). Herpesviruses are well known for latent infections.
- Clinical disease will depend on species susceptibility, the bird's immune system, the presence of stressors, viral load, and the virulence of the agent.

DIAGNOSIS

DIFFERENTIAL DIAGNOSIS
- Bacterial, fungal, and parasitic infections
- Other causes of gastroenteritis, hepatitis, neurologic symptoms, and systemic diseases

INITIAL DATABASE
- Complete blood count (CBC): normal to moderate heterophilic leukocytosis, lymphocytosis, monocytosis. Anemia and leukopenia are occasionally observed with some viral infections, in particular PBFD in African grey parrots. Reactive lymphocytes are occasionally observed on the blood smear.
- Plasma biochemistry panel: depends on the organ affected. Dramatic increase in hepatic enzymes can be seen with acute viral hepatitis. Hyperglobulinemia is an occasional finding.
- Radiographs may show organomegaly (nephromegaly, splenomegaly, hepatomegaly, proventriculus enlargement) and some fluid accumulation in pericardial, hepato-peritoneal, and intestino-peritoneal cavities.
- Cytologic examination may be useful: fine-needle aspirates from poxvirus nodular lesions frequently show intracytoplasmic inclusion bodies (Bollinger bodies).

ADVANCED OR CONFIRMATORY TESTING

- Serology: low sensitivity for peracute and acute infections; few serologic assays are validated for pet birds
  - Enzyme-linked immunosorbent assay (ELISA) may be useful but has variable sensitivity depending on cross-reactivity between species of birds and chicken or availability of species-specific antibodies. ELISA is commonly used for poultry viral diseases.
  - Virus neutralization assay is seldom an option for the veterinary practitioner because of prolonged turnaround time and technical difficulties. It is available for a few of the major psittacine viruses.
  - Hemagglutination inhibition assay (HIA) is applicable only to viruses able to aggregate avian red blood cells; this test is commonly used in paramyxovirus, influenzavirus, and West Nile virus detection and typing.
  - Complement fixation assay may be useful, but such assays lack validation in avian species.
- Immunofluorescent assay (IFA) necessitates that conjugates are available for pet bird species viruses. This test is offered, for instance, for reovirus and Pacheco's disease.
- Electron microscopy is relatively nonsensitive and nonspecific and is not readily available. It may still be valuable for detection of viruses in fixed tissues for which no other tests are available.
- Virus isolation techniques are expensive and time-consuming. Therefore, their value is limited in clinical situations.
- PCR detects nucleic acid fragments, has generally good sensibility and specificity, and is more readily commercially available for virus detection. Accessibility depends on the availability of specific primers. It should be kept in mind that viral nucleic acids detected from different sites have different diagnostic values. PCR is currently offered for PBFD, Pacheco's disease, general herpesvirus, polyomavirus, West Nile virus, and avian bornaviruses.
- Histopathologic examination is invaluable in detecting lesions induced by the virus, visualizing inclusion bodies, and explaining clinical signs. Many viruses induce specific microscopic lesions. Targeted biopsies obtained by endoscopy are the preferred choices. Immunohistochemistry can be used when specific antibodies are available. In situ DNA hybridization is also valuable to confirm the presence of specific viral DNA in tissues. Antemortem viral infection diagnosis by histopathologic examination remains the preferred technique for many viruses, including poxvirus, papillomavirus, adenovirus, reovirus, and PDD.

TREATMENT

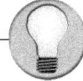

THERAPEUTIC GOALS

- Stabilize and improve patient's physical condition.
- Limit systemic and local inflammatory reactions.
- Affect the virus replication cycle.
- Limit viral transmission.
- Treat any secondary bacterial infections.
- Provide symptomatic treatment.

ACUTE GENERAL TREATMENT

- Provide supportive care: supplemental heat, humidity, oxygen, fluid replacement, force-feeding
- Medications
  - Broad-spectrum antibiotics: TMS 60 mg/kg PO q 12 h, enrofloxacin 15 mg/kg PO q 12 h, amoxicillin/clavulanate 125 mg/kg PO q 12 h
  - Nonsteroidal antiinflammatories: meloxicam 0.3-1.0 mg/kg PO q 12-24 h
  - Antivirals: acyclovir is useful in herpesvirus outbreak and active infection but seems ineffective in internal papillomatosis. Other antivirals against specific viral families may be tried, but data on their clinical effectiveness are lacking.
  - Interferons activate cells' natural protection against virus infection: recombinant omega interferon (1,000,000 IU IM q 7 d for 3 wk), poultry gamma interferon

CHRONIC TREATMENT

Chronic infection and latent infection may be challenging to treat; therapy is most often limited to symptomatic treatment.

POSSIBLE COMPLICATIONS

Complications are related to progression of the infection and include death, latency, chronic infection, and development of neoplasia. It is to be noted that internal papillomatosis seems to be associated with pancreatic and bile duct carcinomas in the long term.

RECOMMENDED MONITORING

- General health monitoring should be performed with regular physical examination, CBC, and biochemistry panels.
- During the course of the disease, a bird should be retested. A positive bird may become negative and may be considered cured, and a negative bird may become positive if a previous sample was taken during the incubation period. Two positive tests several months apart may indicate a permanently infected bird.

PROGNOSIS AND OUTCOME

Depends on the course of the disease, the susceptibility of the species, and the bird's immune response but may be death, recovery, latent infection, or chronic infection

PEARLS & CONSIDERATIONS

COMMENTS

It should be kept in mind that many viral infections remain subclinical in birds, and some may be persistently infected.

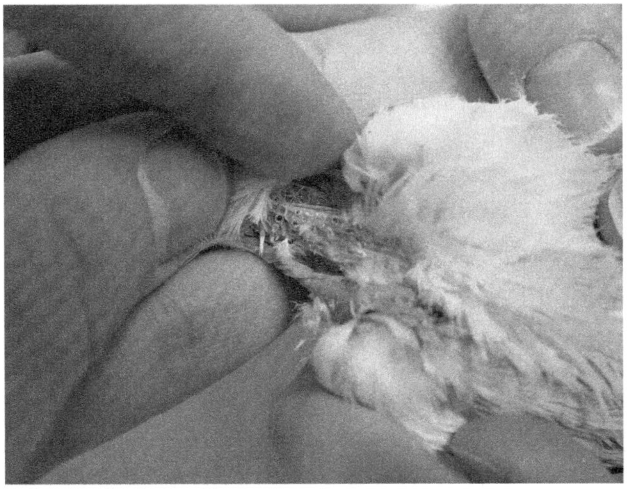

Viral Diseases Necropic feather stumps can be a sign of psittacine beak and feather disease. A biopsy of the affected area including the feather follicle should be performed. *(Photo courtesy Jörg Mayer, The University of Georgia, Athens.)*

PREVENTION

- The goals of prevention are to limit viral exposure and transmission and to detect subclinical infection.
- Birds should be maintained in an adequate environment and should be properly fed.
- A good hygiene protocol is mandatory in pet stores, collections, aviaries, or breeding facilities. Facilities and equipment should be cleaned and disinfected regularly.
- In and out should be controlled: visitors, objects, animals; contact with wild animals should be minimized
- Any new bird should be quarantined for at least 1 month and tested for the common viruses. Sick birds should be isolated. Health monitoring and disease screening can also be performed.
- Vaccines currently available for pet birds include polyomavirus, psittacine herpesvirus, canary poxvirus, and West Nile virus, but effectiveness may be inconsistent among species. Some other vaccines for major psittacine viral diseases are in development.

CLIENT EDUCATION

See Prevention.

SUGGESTED READINGS

Greenacre C: General concepts of virology, Vet Clin North Am Exotic Pet Pract 8:1–6, 2005.

Phalen DN: Avian viral diagnostics. In Fudge AM, editor: Laboratory medicine: avian and exotic pets, Philadelphia, 2000, WB Saunders, pp 111–124.

Ritchie BW: Avian viruses, function and control, Lake Worth, FL, 1995, Wingers Publishing.

CROSS-REFERENCES TO OTHER SECTIONS

Proventricular Dilatation Disease
Polyomavirus
Liver Disease
Neurologic Disease

AUTHOR: **HUGUES BEAUFRÈRE**

EDITOR: **THOMAS N. TULLY, JR.**

SMALL MAMMALS: RATS

Chromodacryorrhea

BASIC INFORMATION

DEFINITION

Porphyrin-pigmented tears secreted by the harderian glands of rats. Chromodacryorrhea literally means "excessive production of colored tears" (*chromo* Gk = color; *dacryo* Gk = gland; *rhea* = to pour out).

SYNONYM

Red tears

EPIDEMIOLOGY

SPECIES, AGE, SEX Besides rats, red-pigmented harderian gland secretions are seen in certain strains of inbred mice (e.g., C3H, A, I, JK, C57 mice), Syrian hamsters, Chinese hamsters *(Cricetulus griseus),* and deer mice *(Peromyscus leucopus).* Old and sick rats are most commonly affected.

RISK FACTORS

- Stress
- Overcrowding
- Poor husbandry

CONTAGION AND ZOONOSIS Sialodacryoadenitis virus (SDAV) can directly affect the harderian glands.

ASSOCIATED CONDITIONS AND DISORDERS Pain, stress, systemic infection (*Mycoplasma pneumoniae,* SDAV). Any disease that leads to depression and reduced grooming. Chronic physiological stress in rats is likely to cause chromodacryorrhea.

CLINICAL PRESENTATION

HISTORY, CHIEF COMPLAINT

- Sudden onset of red staining around the eyes and nostrils
- Labored breathing
- Reduced appetite
- Lethargy
- Recent purchase from a pet store

PHYSICAL EXAM FINDINGS

- Red staining around the eyes and nostrils, and occasionally the forepaws (from wiping the nares)
- Usually clinical signs are associated with nutritional deficiencies, chronic physiologic stress (e.g., disease), chronic light exposure, or dacryoadenitis.

ETIOLOGY AND PATHOPHYSIOLOGY

- Any disease or condition that results in chronic stress will result in chromodacryorrhea.
- Harderian glands of rodents with "red tears" exhibit a variety of histological autofluorescence patterns. In addition, their secretions are also affected by protoporphyrin binding to lipids, affecting fluorescence.
  - Inflammation of the harderian gland (i.e., dacroadenitis) causes an increase in secretions. The most common cause is infection with SDAV, a coronavirus of rats.
  - The tears are secreted via activation of the parasympathetic nervous system via muscarinic receptors. Anticholinergic drugs have been shown to block secretions.
  - Harderian glands' secretions predominantly contain lipids that act as pheromones. The presence of porphyrins in Harderian gland secretions is more the exception than the rule when describing these secretions in rodents. Generally, porphyrins give color to secretions.

DIAGNOSIS

DIFFERENTIAL DIAGNOSIS

- Epistaxis
- Conjunctivitis

INITIAL DATABASE

- Wood's lamp examination reveals bright orange-red fluorescence; allows differentiation from dried blood
- Further diagnostics will dependent on the clinical signs and suspected primary underlying disease, such as respiratory tract disease (see Respiratory Tract Disease, Acute, and Respiratory Tract Disease, Chronic).

TREATMENT

THERAPEUTIC GOAL

Address specific underlying cause if known.

ACUTE GENERAL TREATMENT

- Depends on the underlying primary cause (e.g., nutritional deficiency, respiratory disease)
- If due to SDAV, clinical signs will persist for 1 week, then will resolve spontaneously. Mortality is low.

CHRONIC TREATMENT

- Maintain proper husbandry.

- Ensure proper diet.
- Minimize stress.

RECOMMENDED MONITORING

If clinical signs persist longer than 1 week and no specific underlying cause can be identified, recommend recheck appointment for further diagnostics.

PROGNOSIS AND OUTCOME

Prognosis depends on underlying cause. If clinical signs are due to stress or husbandry, the prognosis is excellent if properly addressed. For other causes, the prognosis will vary from poor to good.

PEARLS & CONSIDERATIONS

COMMENTS

Many clients will present in distress because their pet is "bleeding from the eyes." They will be relieved to know that their pet is not actually bleeding but will need to understand that this clinical sign can be an indicator of a greater underlying disease that warrants investigation.

CLIENT EDUCATION

Chromodacryorrhea is not an actual disease in most cases but an indicator for an underlying problem or stress.

SUGGESTED READING

Donnelly TM: What's your diagnosis? Blood-caked staining around the eyes in Sprague-Dawley rats, Lab Anim Sci 26(1):17–18, 1997.
Harkness JE, et al: Chromodacryorrhea in laboratory rats *(Rattus norvegicus)*: etiologic considerations. Lab Anim Sci 30:841–844, 1980.

CROSS-REFERENCES TO OTHER SECTIONS

Respiratory Tract Disease, Acute
Respiratory Tract Disease, Chronic

AUTHOR: **BRIAN A. EVANS AND THOMAS M. DONNELLY**

EDITOR: **CHRISTOPH MANS**

SMALL MAMMALS: RATS

Mammary and Pituitary Tumors

Client Education Sheet Available on Website

BASIC INFORMATION

DEFINITION

Mammary gland tumors are the most frequently occurring tumors in female rats. Histologically, most are mammary fibroadenomas, although adenocarcinomas are also seen.

SPECIAL SPECIES CONSIDERATION

Rats have 12 mammary glands along the mammary chain, which extends from the cervical region to the tail base. Mammary tumors can arise in any of these locations.

EPIDEMIOLOGY

SPECIES, AGE, SEX

- Older animals are most frequently affected (>1 year of age).
- Females are at higher risk than males; an incidence of 2% to 16% has been reported experimentally in male rats.

GENETICS AND BREED PREDISPOSITION In inbred rat strains susceptible to mammary tumors expression levels of several prolactin-regulated genes are significantly elevated (e.g., messenger RNA's encoding prolactin and its cell surface receptor are amplified) indicating the presence of increased prolactin signaling in the mammary glands of mammary tumor susceptible rat strains.

RISK FACTORS

- Sex: females at higher risk than males
- Age: higher risk at greater than 2 years of age
- Nutrition: increased incidence with high-fat diets, reduced incidence with food restriction
- Prolactin-secreting pituitary tumors: increased risk of mammary tumors
- Neuter status: decreased risk if ovariectomized by 90 days of age; suspected to also have decreased risk even if ovariectomized after 90 days of age, but this has not been proven.
- The frequency of mammary tumors and pituitary tumors is significantly lower in 18- to 24-month-old ovariectomized (4%) versus sexually intact (mammary tumors, 49%; pituitary tumors, 59%) rats. Therefore, the decreased frequency of mammary tumor development could be related to the decreased frequency of prolactin-secreting pituitary tumors.

ASSOCIATED CONDITIONS AND DISORDERS Prolactin-secreting pituitary tumors (see Risk Factors)

CLINICAL PRESENTATION

HISTORY, CHIEF COMPLAINT

- Rapidly growing mass in region of mammary gland tissue
- Bleeding and/or odor if secondarily infected or ulcerated

PHYSICAL EXAM FINDINGS

- Circumscribed, movable, firm, subcutaneous mass in the region of the mammary glands, which extends from the cervical region to the tail base.
- The overlying skin may be ulcerated or infected if the mass is large, or if the surface has been traumatized.

ETIOLOGY AND PATHOPHYSIOLOGY

- As with other species, most mammary gland development occurs during puberty primarily under influence of estrogen and pregnancy under the influence of progesterone and prolactin.
- Neutering sexually immature females removes estrogen influence during mammary growth and prevents mammary epithelial ductal elongation, bifurcation, and extension throughout the fat pad. Inhibition of ductal morphogenesis significantly reduces the risk of mammary tumors by limiting the amount of mammary tissue that develops.
- Estrogen is an important stimulator of prolactin secretion that acts directly on pituitary lactotrophs and via the hypothalamus. Experimentally prolactinomas can be induced in rats by chronic estrogen administration. In the mammary gland, prolactin stimulates alveolar epithelial proliferation with its fibrous connective tissue support structure.
- Aging female rats exhibit changes in estrous cycle and reproductive patterns. At 10-12 months of age, the once-regular ovulatory cycles gradually become lengthened and irregular and eventually develop into a prolonged period of constant estrus characterized by ovaries containing big follicles that secrete large quantities of estrogen. Neutering sexually mature females removes constant estrogen secretion and decreases prolactin secretion so benign mammary tumors either do not develop or do not increase in size.
- Female rats with benign mammary tumors have 27 times higher plasma levels of prolactin than 6-month-old virgin rats, and prolactin levels similar

to that of rats on the seventh day postpartum. Because of this, rats with prolactin-secreting pituitary tumors are at increased risk of mammary tumor development.
- In aging rats, prolactin secretion is increased and is reflected in the high blood prolactin level in both sexes. This change is due to a reduction of hypothalamic dopamine activity. The escape from hypothalamic inhibitory control leads to lactotroph hyperplasia and a high incidence of prolactin cell adenomas in old rats.
- Gene expression of spontaneous fibroadenomas and adenocarcinomas compared to a normal rat mammary gland in the same developmental state has shown that fibroadenomas do not progress to adenocarcinoma.
- Adenocarcinomas arise de-novo (i.e., without prior adenoma stage) and represent fewer than 10% of mammary tumors in pet rats.
- Fibroadenomas can reach 8-10 cm in diameter and do metastasize.

DIAGNOSIS

DIFFERENTIAL DIAGNOSIS

- Dermal/subcutaneous abscess (e.g., from bite wounds, foreign body penetration)
- Neoplasia (e.g., lymphoma)
- Mastitis

INITIAL DATABASE

- Fine-needle aspirate: caution during interpretation because large mammary tumors may be necrotic and can be difficult to differentiate from an abscess on cytology
- Blood work: complete blood count and serum biochemistry screening as a preoperative workup
- Thoracic radiographs/CT: preoperative workup if underlying respiratory disease is suspected

ADVANCED OR CONFIRMATORY TESTING

Histopathologic examination

TREATMENT

THERAPEUTIC GOALS

- Stabilization of the patient if septic or has suffered blood loss
- Complete surgical removal of the tumor (mastectomy) and prevention of recurrence

ACUTE GENERAL TREATMENT

- If necessary, stabilization of the patient if mammary tumor is infected/sepsis is present, or if blood loss has ensued from ulceration of the mass.
- Complete surgical removal of the tumor and any ulcerated/infected skin or tissue is the treatment of choice.
  - Because tumors may be quite large, closure of dead space is important to prevent seroma formation.
  - Some masses are difficult to remove if they are in close association with the vulva.
- Concurrent ovariectomy is recommended if patient is stable.

CHRONIC TREATMENT

Because recurrence of mammary tumors at different locations can frequently occur, repeated surgical removal might be necessary.

POSSIBLE COMPLICATIONS

Rats are notorious for mutilation of surgical sites, so appropriate pain medication with monitoring is compulsory. Use of an E-collar is necessary in some cases to prevent mutilation.

RECOMMENDED MONITORING

Tumors are likely to recur in other mammary glands in both male and female rats, especially if ovariectomy is not performed at the same time. Constant monitoring and palpation of the mammary glands are important.

PROGNOSIS AND OUTCOME

- In general, survival following mastectomy is good.
- Quality of life is improved post mastectomy; however, controversy continues over whether tumor removal actually prolongs survival time.
- Death can occur with sepsis or blood loss if the mammary mass is not surgically removed and becomes ulcerated or infected.

CONTROVERSY

- To date, the only proven treatment and prevention of mammary tumor development consists of surgical removal of the tumor and ovariectomy. Other treatments have been discussed but have not proven to be effective in preventing recurrence of spontaneous tumors or in decreasing their size once present.
- Cabergoline is a prolactin inhibitor that suppresses pituitary prolactin secretion and can be given orally. It has been successfully used in the palliative treatment of a pituitary adenoma in a rat at a dose of 0.6 mg/kg PO q 72 h, and thus may be helpful in rats that have mammary tumor development secondary to prolactin-secreting pituitary tumors and in those unable to undergo ovariectomy.
- Gonadotropin-releasing hormone (GnRH) agonists
  - Deslorelin implants (4.7 mg) have been used experimentally to suppress estrus in rats for 1 year and may be useful in rats that cannot be ovariectomized.
  - Leuprolide acetate has been experimentally shown to suppress the ability of the pituitary-gonadal system to secrete gonadotropin and testosterone for over 5 weeks; similar to deslorelin because it may be useful in rats that cannot undergo ovariectomy
- Melatonin induces apoptosis of rat prolactin-secreting tumors. Experimentally, SC melatonin administration in experimentally induced tumor-bearing rats significantly increased survival time and reduced prolactin levels but did not change the mammary tumor growth rate.
- Tamoxifen: antiestrogen used in the treatment of human breast cancer. This agent would be useful only in mammary adenocarcinomas that are estrogen receptor positive. This drug is NOT recommended, given the low incidence of adenocarcinoma in rats and the fact that it has been shown to induce hepatic cancer and proliferation of the rat uterus.

PEARLS & CONSIDERATIONS

COMMENTS

Histopathologic examination of removed tumors should be performed because spontaneous mammary adenocarcinoma has a 5%-10% incidence. Individual genetic variability and environmental factors such as nutrition and maternal effects in utero and during lactation most likely affect quantitative trait loci (QTL) that control susceptibility to mammary adenocarcinoma. However, the individual genetic traits and QTL that influence gene function have not yet been elucidated.

PREVENTION

- Ovariectomy of female rats by 90 days of age
- Treatment of prolactin-secreting pituitary tumors

CLIENT EDUCATION

- All clients who own female rats should be educated about the importance of ovariectomy before 90 days of age.
- Additionally, clients should be educated on the importance of early detection and removal of tumors before they become too large to be safely removed surgically.

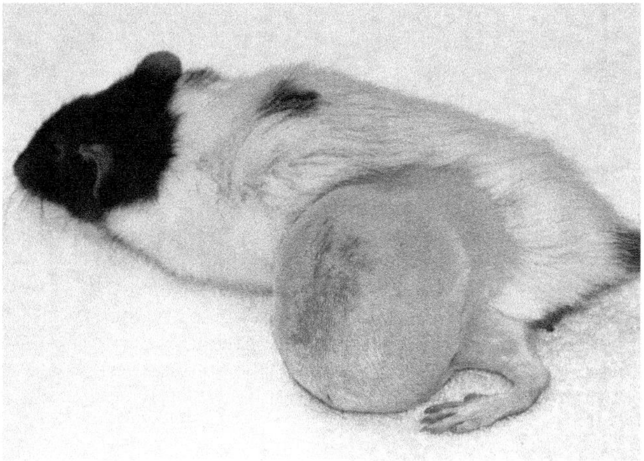

Mammary and Pituitary Tumors Large mammary fibroadenoma on a female rat. Note the close proximity to the left hind leg which impeded normal ambulation.

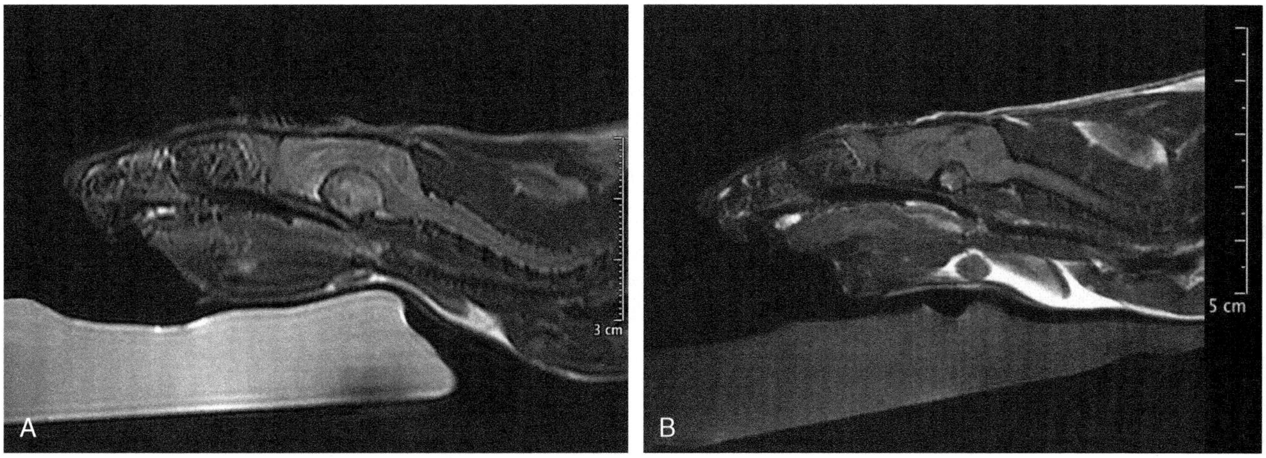

Mammary and Pituitary Tumors A, An MRI scan of the head of a 3-year-old rat showing a large pituitary tumor within the brain. **B,** An MRI scan of the same rat shown in A eight weeks after treatment with cabergoline. Note the significant shrinking of the tumor. *(Photo courtesy Jörg Mayer, The University of Georgia, Athens.)*

SUGGESTED READINGS

Alkis I, et al: Long term suppression of oestrus and prevention of pregnancy by deslorelin implant in rats, Bull Vet Inst Pulawy 55:237–240, 2011.

Hotchkiss C, et al: Effect of surgical removal of subcutaneous tumors on survival of rats, J Am Vet Med Assoc 206:1575–1579, 1995.

Marxfeld H, et al: Gene expression in fibroadenomas of the rat mammary gland in contrast to spontaneous adenocarcinomas and normal mammary gland, Exp Toxicol Pathol 58:145–150, 2006.

Mayer J, et al: Extralabel use of cabergoline in the treatment of a pituitary adenoma in a rat, J Am Vet Med Assoc 239:656–660, 2011.

Saez MC, et al: Melatonin increases the survival time of animals with untreated mammary tumours: neuroendocrine stabilization, Mol Cell Biochem 278:15–20, 2005.

AUTHOR: **NICOLE R. WYRE AND THOMAS M. DONNELLY**

EDITOR: **CHRISTOPH MANS**

SMALL MAMMALS: RATS

Renal Disease

BASIC INFORMATION

DEFINITION

Kidney or *renal disease* is a general term that describes any damage that reduces the functioning of the kidney.

SYNONYMS

- Kidney disease: renal disease, kidney disease, kidney failure, chronic renal failure, nephropathy, suppurative pyelonephritis, suppurative nephritis
- Chronic progressive nephrosis in rats: progressive renal disease in rats, progressive glomerulonephrosis, old rat nephropathy, glomerulosclerosis
- Nephrocalcinosis: renal tubular mineralization

EPIDEMIOLOGY

SPECIES, AGE, SEX

- Male rats develop a more severe form of chronic progressive nephrosis, usually earlier in life than females; lesions are more severe in rats over 12 months of age.
- Nephrocalcinosis is more common in females and can be found in animals as young as 7 weeks of age. Blood estrogen levels may play a role in that the disease can be prevented by ovariectomy and is induced in castrated male and female rats by estrogen administration.

GENETICS AND BREED PREDISPOSITION A significantly higher prevalence of chronic progressive nephrosis is seen in the Sprague-Dawley strain of rat. Osborne-Mendel and Buffalo strains are relatively insusceptible. Elevated prolactin levels are suspected of contributing to more severe disease.

RISK FACTORS

- Chronic progressive nephrosis: high-protein diets designed for superior body growth result in earlier onset of more severe disease
- Nephrocalcinosis: may be the result of a number of dietary factors, including magnesium deficiency, elevated dietary phosphorus or calcium, and diet preparations with a low calcium-to-phosphorus ratio
- Suppurative pyelonephritis/nephritis: isosthenuria, urolithiasis, and lower urinary tract infections

CLINICAL PRESENTATION

DISEASE FORMS/SUBTYPES

- Chronic progressive nephrosis
- Nephrocalcinosis
- Suppurative pyelonephritis/nephritis

HISTORY, CHIEF COMPLAINT

- Clinical signs vary with severity of kidney pathology:
  - Polydipsia and polyuria
  - Anorexia
  - Weight loss
  - Lethargy

PHYSICAL EXAM FINDINGS

- In any rat with renal disease, morbidity may vary from slight to none to significant, depending on the progression and severity of disease.
  - Lethargy
  - Weight loss
  - Cachexia
  - Dehydration
  - Poor fur quality
  - Abdominal pain
  - Diarrhea
  - Hypertension

ETIOLOGY AND PATHOPHYSIOLOGY

- Chronic progressive nephrosis
  - A high protein diet may acutely increase the glomerular filtration rate, possibly causing intraglomerular hypertension, which would lead to progressive loss of renal function.
  - Albuminuria not only serves as a marker of glomerular injury but is also associated with tubulointerstitial injury.
- Nephrocalcinosis
  - In rats, no single mechanism has been identified that explains the association between all dietary factors that have been related to the prevalence of nephrocalcinosis.
  - Nutritional studies have shown that diets high in phosphorus or low in calcium, with a net Ca : P molar ratio of less than 1.0, contribute to the development of nephrocalcinosis lesions. Increasing the calcium and phosphorus content and the Ca : P ratio to greater than 1.0 and closer to 1.3 markedly decreased the incidence and severity or prevented the occurrence of nephrocalcinosis lesions.
- Suppurative pyelonephritis/nephritis
  - Caused by various predominantly gram-negative bacterial organisms (e.g., *Pseudomonas, Escherichia coli, Proteus mirabilis*), which usually ascend to renal pelvis from lower urinary tract.
  - Chronic pyelonephritis is more common and frequently is clinically inapparent.

DIAGNOSIS

DIFFERENTIAL DIAGNOSIS

- Hydronephrosis
- Neoplasia
- Polycystic kidney disease
- Calculi-associated obstructive disease
- Toxic nephrosis
- Ischemic injury

INITIAL DATABASE

- Urinalysis
  - Isosthenuria (normal specific gravity, 1.022-1.050)
  - Proteinuria (mild proteinuria is normal in rats)
  - Hematuria
  - Sediment analysis: casts, crystals, inflammatory or neoplastic cells, bacteria
- Urine culture
- Complete blood count: may be normal
  - Nonregenerative anemia
  - Leukocytosis
- Serum biochemistry profile
  - BUN elevation
  - Creatinine elevation
  - Hyperphosphatemia
  - Hypocalcemia or hypercalcemia
  - Hypokalemia or hyerpkalemia
  - Hypercholesterolemia
  - Hypoproteinemia
- Diagnostic imaging
  - Radiography: assess for increases or decreases in kidney size, radiopaque calculi within the urinary tract, abdominal masses associated with the urinary tract, and bladder distention.
  - Ultrasonography: discern size, contour, and texture of the kidneys, allowing for differentiation of focal versus diffuse disease

ADVANCED OR CONFIRMATORY TESTING

- Perform ultrasound-guided fine-needle aspiration for cytology
- Contrast urography
- Histopathologic examination

TREATMENT

THERAPEUTIC GOALS

- Delay progression of renal disease.
- Preserve overall patient well-being and quality of life.
- Promote diuresis and diminish the consequences of azotemia.
- Treat underlying or concurrent urinary tract infection,

ACUTE GENERAL TREATMENT

- Discontinue any potentially nephrotoxic drugs.
- Identify and treat any prerenal or postrenal abnormalities.
- Identify any treatable conditions such as urolithiasis or pyelonephritis.
- Fluid therapy
  - To induce diuresis and correct azotemia, electrolyte, and acid-base imbalances
  - Use of isotonic crystalloids
  - Subcutaneous administration: 60-100 mL/kg/d
  - Intravenous fluid therapy
    - Use lateral coccygeal or cephalic vein.
    - Maintenance fluids are 3-4 mL/kg/h.
  - Potassium supplementation of fluids based on blood potassium measurement
- Antibiotic therapy
  - Indicated for cases of suppurative pyelonephritis/nephritis and cystitis
  - Antibiotic selection should be based on culture and susceptibility whenever possible.
  - For empirical treatment, or for cases with negative urine culture, despite clinical suspicion, use antibiotics, which are effective against Gram-negative organisms and are renally excreted, to reach high tissue concentrations.
  - Amoxicillin/clavulanic acid 15-20 mg/kg PO q 8-12 h
  - Trimethoprim-sulfa 15-30 mg/kg PO q 12 h

 - Enrofloxacin 10-20 mg/kg PO q 12-24 h
- If hyperphosphatemic, alter diet and initiate enteric phosphate binders:
  - Aluminum hydroxide 30-90 mg/kg/d, divided and administered with food
- Treat increased gastric acidity with H2 blockers:
  - Famotidine 0.5 mg/kg PO, SC q 24 h
  - Ranitidine 1-2 mg/kg PO, SC q 12 h
- Multivitamin supplementation is recommended because the excessive amount of urine produced by failing kidneys commonly results in loss of water-soluble vitamins.

CHRONIC TREATMENT

- Maintain long-term dialysis with maintenance subcutaneous fluid therapy (owners can be taught to do this at home): 60-100 mL/kg/d SC.
- Antibiotic therapy for chronic pyelonephritis should be at least 4-6 weeks.
- Dietary management: high protein appears to be the major cause of severe nephropathy, and the term *protein-overload nephropathy* is often used. Changing the source of protein to one such as soy protein, restricting caloric intake, or modifying the diet to decrease protein consumption could decrease the severity of nephropathy. Changing the diet so that the Ca:P ratio is greater than 1.0 and is closer to 1.3 may decrease the incidence and severity of nephrocalcinosis in rats.
- The hyperphosphatemia that occurs in chronic renal failure is closely related to dietary protein intake because protein-rich diets are also high in phosphorus.
- Consider use of omega-3 fatty acid supplements based on studies showing their beneficial effects in other species.

POSSIBLE COMPLICATIONS

- Anorexia
- Gastrointestinal ulceration
- Hyperphosphatemia
- Acidosis
- Anemia

RECOMMENDED MONITORING

- Overall condition and clinical response to therapy should be assessed in all patients with renal disease. Frequency of follow-up assessments varies with initial diagnosis and severity of disease. Periodic assessments for azotemia, anemia and phosphorus, and potassium and protein imbalances are recommended.
- Monitor body weight and condition, and adjust nutrition accordingly.
- Urinalysis and urine culture in patients being treated for pyelonephritis

PROGNOSIS AND OUTCOME

- With any diagnosis of renal insufficiency or failure, prognosis varies with severity of clinical pathologic findings, duration of disease, and severity of primary renal failure. If secondary to infection or obstructive disease, prognosis is determined by duration of the disease process and success in treatment—medical or surgical—of the underlying condition of secondary renal insufficiency.
- Depending on initial diagnosis, disease severity, and response to therapy, quality of life issues and euthanasia should be discussed with the owner in terms of any patient with renal disease.

CONTROVERSY

Hematology, clinical chemistry, and urinalysis values may vary significantly with strain or breed of animal, nutritional status, sex, sampling site or frequency, time of day, stressors, age, health status, drug exposure, and environment. Therefore, normal values are broad; these variables should be kept in mind when interpreting individual animal values.

PEARLS & CONSIDERATIONS

- Many different terms are used to describe renal function and its deterioration.
  - *Azotemia* refers to increased concentrations of urea nitrogen and creatinine and other nonproteinaceous nitrogenous waste products in the blood. *Renal azotemia* denotes azotemia caused by renal parenchymal changes.
  - Uremia is the presence of all urine constituents in the blood. Usually a toxic condition, it may occur secondary to renal failure or postrenal disorders, including urethral blockage.
  - Renal reserve may be thought of as the percentage of "extra" nephrons—those not necessary to maintain normal renal function. Although it probably varies from animal to animal, this value is greater than 50% in most mammals.
  - Renal insufficiency begins when the renal reserve is lost. Animals with renal insufficiency outwardly appear normal, but have a reduced capacity to compensate for stresses such as infection or dehydration and have lost urine concentrating ability.
  - Renal failure is a state of decreased renal function that allows persistent abnormalities (azotemia and inability to concentrate urine) to exist; it refers to a level of organ function rather than a specific disease entity. Acute renal failure generally refers to cases of sudden decline of glomerular filtration rate resulting in an accumulation of nitrogenous waste products and inability to maintain normal fluid balance. Chronic renal failure generally refers to an insidious onset with slow progression (usually months to years) of azotemia and inadequately concentrated urine.
- It is important to realize that most of the renal diseases discussed can manifest as varying stages of compromise in renal reserve, renal insufficiency, or renal failure. If or when the disease process progresses depends on variables such as the specific disease in question, environmental factors, and the individual animal itself.

COMMENTS

- NTP-2000 open formula is one diet available in laboratory medicine that is low in protein (14.0%) and has a Ca:P ratio approximating 1.3:1; it has been found to decrease the incidence of nephrocalcinosis in rats.
- Another laboratory rat diet, AIN-93G, has a lower phosphorus content (0.3%) and a higher Ca:P ratio and has been shown to lower the incidence of nephrocalcinosis.
- Dietary salt content has been found to have an effect on hypertension associated with hydronephrosis in rats. Hydronephrosis as a result of partial ureteral blockage led to increased blood pressure, which worsened significantly on a high-salt diet versus a low-salt diet.
- High levels of dietary soy isoflavones induced nephrocalcinosis formation, depending on the strain of laboratory rat.

CLIENT EDUCATION

Chronic renal failure requires continuous treatment and monitoring. Unless a specific underlying cause is diagnosed and treated successfully, treatment in many cases will be lifelong.

SUGGESTED READINGS

Fisher PG: Exotic mammal renal disease: causes and clinical presentation, Vet Clin North Am Exotic Anim Pract 9:33–67, 2006.
Fisher PG: Exotic mammal renal disease: diagnosis and treatment, Vet Clin North Am Exotic Anim Pract 9:69–96, 2006.
Rao GN: Diet and kidney diseases in rats, Toxicol Pathol 30:651–656, 2002.

AUTHOR: **PETER G. FISHER**

EDITOR: **CHRISTOPH MANS**

SMALL MAMMALS: RATS

Respiratory Tract Disease, Acute

BASIC INFORMATION

DEFINITION

Acute bacterial pneumonia in rats is caused by subclinical infection with *Streptococcus pneumoniae* and/or *Corynebacterium kutscheri,* which develops into clinical pneumonia and/or septicemia secondary concurrent infection or immunosuppression.

SYNONYMS

- Pseudotuberculosis *(Corynebacterium kutscheri)*
- Pneumococcal infection *(Streptococcus pneumoniae)*
- Diplococcal infection *(Streptococcus pneumoniae)*

EPIDEMIOLOGY

SPECIES, AGE, SEX Older animals are at increased risk for *C. kutscheri.* Younger animals are at increased risk for *S. pneumoniae.*

RISK FACTORS
- Concurrent infection with *Mycobacterium pulmonis* or CAR bacillus
- Immune suppression

CONTAGION AND ZOONOSIS
- *Corynebacterium kutscheri*
  - Gram-positive bacillus bacteria
  - Transmission probably occurs through direct contact or oronasal exposure
- *Streptococcus pneumoniae*
  - Alpha-hemolytic Gram-positive diplococcal bacteria
  - Transmission probably occurs through direct contact or oronasal exposure
  - Zoonotic potential

ASSOCIATED CONDITIONS AND DISORDERS Chronic respiratory disease (murine respiratory mycoplasmosis)

CLINICAL PRESENTATION

DISEASE FORMS/SUBTYPES With both of these bacterial infections, animals can have no apparent clinical signs or can have severe respiratory disease and/or acute death.

HISTORY, CHIEF COMPLAINT
- Acute death
- Labored breathing
- Sneezing
- Oculonasal discharge
- Lethargy
- Lameness
- Head tilt

PHYSICAL EXAM FINDINGS
- Dyspnea
- Tachypnea
- Cyanosis
- Rales
- Porphyrin epiphora (chromodacryorrhea)
- Nasal discharge—with or without porphyrin staining
- Muffled heart sounds
- Collapse, tachycardia, poor peripheral pulses if septic shock
- Torticollis and/or nystagmus if otitis media present
- Arthralgia if arthritis present

ETIOLOGY AND PATHOPHYSIOLOGY

- Both *S. pneumoniae* and *C. kutscheri* colonize the upper respiratory tract (nasopharynx and tympanic bulla with *S. pneumoniae* and oropharynx, cervical, and submandibular lymph nodes with *C. kutcheri*) and can remain subclinical in the absence of concurrent disease.
- Concurrent infection with other pathogens (see Respiratory Tract Disease, Chronic) and confounding stressors lead to immune suppression, triggering a latent infection to become clinical.
- Suppurative inflammation of the upper respiratory tract is followed by infection of the lower respiratory tract, leading to bronchopneumonia and pleuritis.
- Bacteremia can lead to infection in other organs such as arthritis, meningitis, pericarditis, hepatitis, splenitis, and peritonitis or acute death.

DIAGNOSIS

DIFFERENTIAL DIAGNOSIS

- Respiratory signs
  - Congestive heart failure
  - Chronic respiratory disease (if owners have not been aware of respiratory disease)
- Acute death
  - Sepsis from other bacterial infections (e.g., salmonellosis)
- Otitis media
  - Extension of otitis externa

INITIAL DATABASE

- Thoracic radiographs/CT: findings consistent with pulmonary consolidation and/or pleural effusion
- Skull radiographs/CT/MRI: tympanic bullae sclerosis or effusion if otitis media is present
- Serologic testing: *C. kutscheri* (ELISA)
- Complete blood count: neutrophilia, neutropenia if septic
- Serum biochemistry: hypoglycemia if septic
- Brochoalveolar lavage:
  - Cytology, Gram stain
    - *S. pneumoniae*: encapsulated Gram-positive diplococci
    - *C. kutscheri*: slightly curved Gram-positive rods
  - Aerobic culture and sensitivity
- Submandibular lymph node aerobic culture for *C. kutscheri*: caution as nonclinical animals can harbor bacteria in these lymph nodes

ADVANCED OR CONFIRMATORY TESTING

- Histopathologic examination
- *C. kutscheri*: necrotizing and suppurative pulmonary lesions, fibrinopurulent fibrosis with intralesional bacterial colonies that are pathognomonic (diphtheroid appearance of the bacilli with "Chinese letter" configurations)

TREATMENT

THERAPEUTIC GOALS

- Stabilization of the septic patient
- Eradication of the bacterial infection
- Management of concurrent disease (see Respiratory Tract Disease, Chronic)

ACUTE GENERAL TREATMENT

- Oxygen therapy if patient is dyspneic and/or cyanotic
- Fluid therapy: may require intraosseous administration if patient is severely compromised
- Antibiotic therapy should be based on aerobic culture and sensitivity results:
  - *S. pneumoniae*: highly resistant strains are found in humans, so appropriate antibiotic use is extremely important
    - Amoxicillin/clavulanic acid 15-20 mg/kg PO, SC q 12 h
    - Azithromycin 15-30 mg/kg PO q 12 h
  - *C. kutscheri*
    - Amoxicillin/clavulanic acid 15-20 mg/kg PO, SC q 12 h
    - Ampicillin 20-50 mg/kg PO, SC, IM q 12 h
    - Chloramphenicol 30-50 mg/kg PO, SC, IM q 8-12 h
    - Doxycycline 5-10 mg/kg PO q 12 h

CHRONIC TREATMENT

See Respiratory Tract Disease, Chronic.

POSSIBLE COMPLICATIONS

Oral doxycycline should not be given with any dairy products or other products containing calcium because this will decrease its bioavailability.

RECOMMENDED MONITORING

- Patients with severe disease should be hospitalized until they are able to go home on oral medications.
- Patients should be closely monitored for signs of chronic respiratory disease.

PROGNOSIS AND OUTCOME

Little is known about the prognosis of pure acute bacterial pneumonia because co-infection with other respiratory pathogens is common, as are subclinical infections.

PEARLS & CONSIDERATIONS

PREVENTION

Because both of these bacteria can be present without causing clinical disease, preventive measures are focused on decreasing stress, avoiding immune suppressive drugs, and maintaining appropriate diet/husbandry to avoid conversion to clinical disease.

CLIENT EDUCATION

All clients owning rats should understand the frequency of respiratory disease in rats and the importance of proper housing (good ventilation, avoidance of crowding, avoidance of dusty bedding such as wood shavings) and close observation for any signs of respiratory disease, so that treatment can be administered as soon as possible.

SUGGESTED READINGS

Amao H, et al: Natural and subclinical Corynebacterium kutscheri infection in rats, Lab Anim Sci 45:11–14, 1995.

Barthold SW, et al: The effect of selected viruses on Corynebacterium kutscheri infection in rats, Lab Anim Sci 38:580–583, 1988.

Borkowski GL, et al: Diagnostic exercise: pneumonia and pleuritis in a rat [Streptococcus pneumoniae], Lab Anim Sci 40:323–325, 1990.

Corning BF, et al: Group G streptococcal lymphadenitis in rats, J Clin Microbiol 29: 2720–2723, 1991.

CROSS-REFERENCES TO OTHER SECTIONS

Respiratory Tract Disease, Chronic

AUTHOR: **NICOLE R. WYRE**

EDITOR: **CHRISTOPH MANS**

SMALL MAMMALS: RATS

Respiratory Tract Disease, Chronic

Client Education Sheet Available on Website

BASIC INFORMATION

DEFINITION

Chronic respiratory disease (CRD) in rats is a multifactorial respiratory tract infection caused primarily by *Mycoplasma pulmonis*, commonly in association with other concurrent infections, resulting in chronic bronchitis and bronchiectasis.

SYNONYMS

CRD, murine respiratory mycoplasmosis (MRM)

EPIDEMIOLOGY

SPECIES, AGE, SEX Older animals are at increased risk.

RISK FACTORS

- Immune status (e.g., age, genotype of certain rats)
- Concurrent diseases (e.g., diabetes mellitus, neoplasia)
- General ventilation of housing
- Ammonia levels in bedding
- Nutritional status (e.g., deficiency of vitamin A or E)
- Obesity

CONTAGION AND ZOONOSIS

- This disease complex is due to the synergism of several pathogens transmitted directly, through aerosol or in utero. The major pathogen is *Mycoplasma pulmonis*, but other pathogens involved in establishing infection include the following:
  - Cilia-associated respiratory bacillus (CAR bacillus, Gram-negative filamentous bacterium)
  - Sendai virus (paramyxovirus)
  - Sialodacryoadenitis virus (coronavirus)

ASSOCIATED CONDITIONS AND DISORDERS

- Otitis media and torticollis (secondary to *M. pulmonis* middle ear infection)
- Reduced fertility (secondary to *M. pulmonis* oophoritis and salpingitis infection)

CLINICAL PRESENTATION

HISTORY, CHIEF COMPLAINT

- Nasal discharge
- Sneezing
- Labored breathing
- Lethargy
- Head tilt

PHYSICAL EXAM FINDINGS

- Porphyrin epiphora (chromodacryorrhea)
- Nasal discharge—with or without porphyrin staining
- Dyspnea
- Tachypnea
- Rales
- Cyanosis
- Muffled heart sounds
- Torticollis and/or nystagmus with otitis media

ETIOLOGY AND PATHOPHYSIOLOGY

- *M. pulmonis* colonizes the epithelial cells of the respiratory tract, middle ear, and epithelia of female genital tract.
- Although *M. pulmonis* causes upper and lower respiratory system lesions, the primary lesion is subacute chronic bronchitis that resembles chronic obstructive respiratory disease in humans.
- CRD in rats is a chronic inflammatory condition resulting in the hypersecretion and impaired clearance of mucus in which elevated levels and activation of macrophages and neutrophils play an important role.
- Once established in the lower respiratory tract, chronic bronchitis and bronchiolitis develop and progress to bronchiectasis and bronchiolectasis. Collections of mucus, leukocytes, and cellular debris accumulate in the lumen due to ciliostasis. There may be rupture of the bronchiolar walls, releasing inflammatory cells, mucus, and debris into the adjacent parenchyma, and developing pulmonary abscessation.
- As the airways become filled with mucus, bronchiolar lumen diameter decreases and a biofilm develops over bronchiolar epithelium, protecting secondary bacterial invaders from immune defenses and most antibiotics.
- *M. pulmonis* also causes an atrophic rhinitis in which the nasal turbinates become inflamed with a mixed pyogranulomatous infiltrate. The rhinitis accounts for the upper respiratory signs seen in CRD of rats. Because rats are obligate nose breathers, rhinitis results in open mouth breathing, hypoxia, and its associated metabolic disorders such as respiratory acidosis and myocyte irritability.

DIAGNOSIS

DIFFERENTIAL DIAGNOSIS

- Respiratory signs
  - Neoplasia (primary pulmonary or metastatic)
  - Acute bacterial pneumonia (see Respiratory Tract Disease, Acute)
  - Congestive heart failure
- Otitis media
  - Extension of otitis externa

INITIAL DATABASE

- Thoracic radiographs/CT: findings are consistent with bronchopneumonia, bronchitis, and/or atelectasis
- Skull radiographs/CT/MRI: tympanic bullae sclerosis or effusion if otitis media is present
- Complete blood count: may be normal or consistent with chronic inflammation (neutrophilia, monocytosis)
- Serologic testing: *M. pulmonis*, CAR bacillus, Sendai virus
- Bronchoalveolar lavage for PCR testing *(M. pulmonis)* and aerobic culture (for secondary bacterial pathogens). Culture for *M. pulmonis* requires special mycoplasma media.

ADVANCED OR CONFIRMATORY TESTING

- Histopathologic examination
  - Silver-impregnation staining needed to diagnose CAR bacillus co-infection

TREATMENT

THERAPEUTIC GOAL

Elimination of the disease is impossible. The goal of therapy is to improve the rat's quality of life by controlling secondary bacterial infections and preventing acute dyspneic episodes.

ACUTE GENERAL TREATMENT

- Oxygen therapy
- Fluid support if presence of secondary dehydration

CHRONIC TREATMENT

- Antibiotic therapy will not eliminate the pathogen. Antibiotic selection ideally is based on culture and sensitivity results.
- Doxycycline 5-10 mg/kg PO q 12 h: preferred antibiotic because it has additional antiinflammatory properties and is secreted by respiratory epithelial cells
- Enrofloxacin 10-20 mg/kg PO, IM, SC q 24 h: CAUTION with SC or IM injection as can cause severe pain and tissue necrosis. Dilute with sterile saline before injection.
- Tylosin 10 mg/kg PO, SC IM q 12-24 h: not recommended as use in drinking water because it may reduce water consumption
- Azithromycin 15-30 mg/kg PO q 24 h
- Nutritional support as animals may lose weight with chronic disease

DRUG INTERACTIONS

Oral doxycycline should not be given with any dairy or other products containing calcium because this will decrease its bioavailability.

RECOMMENDED MONITORING

- Respiratory rate and effort
- Body weight/condition
- Appetite

PROGNOSIS AND OUTCOME

Because many factors contribute to rat respiratory issues, the disease cannot be eliminated, but clinical signs may be ameliorated with antibiotics and supportive care.

CONTROVERSY

- Use of corticosteroids as anti-inflammatory agents has been recommended to decrease the inflammation. Most (experimental) studies in rats have found steroids do not affect signs, function, and indices of inflammation. There is also significant concern that corticosteroid efficacy will be accompanied by consequential impairment of the rat's immune defenses leading to fatal pulmonary abscessation and/or pneumonia.
- Use of bronchodilators (both oral and inhaled) has been recommended because these agents are helpful in humans with chronic bronchitis. Specific studies with bronchodilators have not been performed in rats with chronic respiratory disease, but they may be helpful.
- Nebulized hypertonic saline solution (7%) has been used successfully in humans with cystic fibrosis as a mucolytic agent. It breaks down the mucous biofilm and gives relief for ~8 hours.
- Concurrent nebulization with bronchodialators and/or antibiotics has been recommended to directly deliver medications. Specific studies using these nebulizations have not been performed in rats with chronic respiratory disease but may be helpful.

PEARLS & CONSIDERATIONS

PREVENTION

This disease complex *(M. pulmonis)* is thought to be ubiquitous in pet rats; thus prevention of infection is nearly impossible. Preventing contributing factors such as proper ventilation, bedding, and diet and decreasing stress can be helpful.

CLIENT EDUCATION

All clients who own rats should be educated about the ubiquitous nature of *M. pulmonis* and the importance of ventilation, low cage ammonia levels, avoidance of dusty bedding such as wood shavings, and appropriate nutrition in decreasing the potential severity of chronic respiratory disease in rats.

SUGGESTED READING

Deeb B: Respiratory disease in pet rats, Exotic DVM 7:31–33, 2005.

Donnelly TM: Application of laboratory animal immunoassays to exotic pet practice, Exotic DVM 8:19–26, 2006.

Rempe S, et al: Tetracyclines and pulmonary inflammation, Endocr Metab Immune Disord Drug Targets 7:232–236, 2007.

Schoeb TR, et al: Effects of viral and mycoplasmal infections, ammonia exposure, vitamin A deficiency, host age, and organism strain on adherence of *Mycoplasma pulmonis* in cultured rat tracheas, Lab Anim Sci 43:417–424, 1993.

Wark P, et al: Nebulised hypertonic saline for cystic fibrosis, Cochrane Database Syst Rev CD001506, 2009.

CROSS-REFERENCES TO OTHER SECTIONS

Respiratory Tract Disease, Acute

AUTHOR: **NICOLE R. WYRE**

EDITOR: **CHRISTOPH MANS**

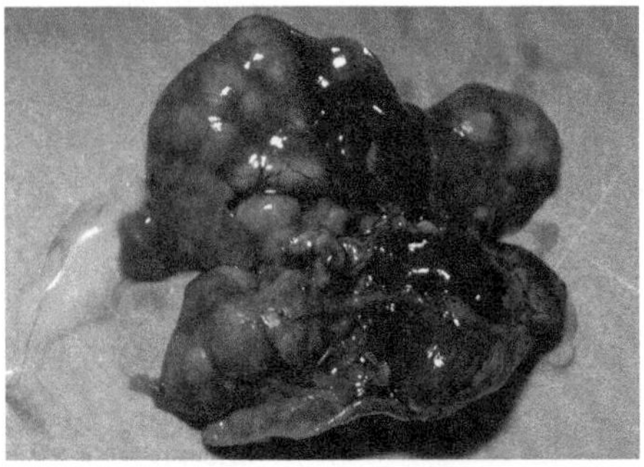

Respiratory Tract Disease, Chronic Rat lungs, abscesses secondary to chronic infection.

Skin Diseases

BASIC INFORMATION

DEFINITION

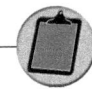

Infectious and noninfectious diseases of the integument

SYNONYMS

Dermatitis, pyoderma, ulcerative dermatitis, ringworm, dermatophytosis, acariasis, ring tail, abscesses, bite wounds

EPIDEMIOLOGY

RISK FACTORS Inappropriate bedding (e.g., cedar, pine) can cause contact dermatitis.

CONTAGION AND ZOONOSIS

- Dermatophytes are potentially zoonotic.
- *Ornithonyssus bacoti* (tropical rat mite) is a zoonotic parasite.

ASSOCIATED CONDITIONS AND DISORDERS

- Conspecific trauma
- Nutritional deficiencies
- Chronic renal insufficiency

CLINICAL PRESENTATION

DISEASE FORMS/SUBTYPES

- Ectoparasitosis
- Bacterial dermatitis/ulcerative dermatitis
- Abscesses
- Dermatophytosis
- Ringtail
- Neoplasia

HISTORY, CHIEF COMPLAINT

- Skin wounds
- Rough hair coat
- Pruritus
- Hair loss
- Weight loss
- Lethargy
- Swellings on body
- Tail tip lesion

PHYSICAL EXAM FINDINGS Will vary depending on cause:

- Alopecia
- Pruritus
- Localized erythema
- Abrasions, excoriations, ulcerations
- Scaling, crusting
- Lichenification
- Cutaneous or subcutaneous masses

ETIOLOGY AND PATHOPHYSIOLOGY

- Bacterial dermatitis/ulcerative dermatitis
  - *Staphylococcus* spp.
  - Usually secondary to self-trauma due to pruritus from mites or pruritus/pain over skin of salivary glands during sialodacryoadenitis (SDA) virus infection; dermatophytosis, fight wounds
- Abscesses
  - *Staphylococcus aureus, Streptococcus* spp., *Pasteurella pneumotropica, Actinomyces bovis*
  - Often secondary to conspecific trauma
- Parasites
  - All ectoparasitic infections can be complicated by secondary infections and self-mutilation. These secondary complications need to be identified and treated.
  - Rat fur mite *(Radfordia ensifera)*: common; mild infestation produces few ill effects, but heavy infestation causes pruritus, leading to self-traumatization, and ulcerative dermatitis. Transmission is by direct contact.
  - Sarcoptic mites (e.g., *Sarcoptes scabiei, Sarcoptes anacanthos, Trixacarus diversus*): less common. Transmission is by direct contact. Leads to pruritus, crusting, and hyperkeratosis. Animals with clinical signs are often immune compromised.
  - *Notoedres muris*: causes typical papulous lesions on ear pinnae
  - Tropical rat mite *(Ornithonyssus bacoti)*: Blood sucking mite; opportunistic ectoparasite. It spends a relatively short time on a host (usually at night) and penetrates the skin for feeding only. Cause severe pruritus. Animals appear nervous, particular in evening hours and at night. Severe infestations can cause anemia, debilitation, and death.
  - Demodectic mites *(Demodex ratti, Demodex norvegicus, Demodex ratticola)*: rare
  - Lice *(Polyplax serrata, Polyplax spinulosa)*: Common; blood sucking lice. Located mainly at neck, at shoulders, and over back; poor fur condition and pruritus, which leads to self-mutilation
  - Pinworms *(Syphacia obvelata)*: perianal pruritus and tail base mutilation
- Dermatophytosis
  - *Microsporum* spp., *Trichophyton mentagrophytes*
  - Clinical signs vary: alopecia, erythema, dandruff formation. Animals usually are not pruritic, unless secondary bacterial infection present.
  - Immune deficiency or stress may be underlying cause in chronic cases.
- Neoplasia: fibroadenoma of the mammary glands (most common), mammary adenocarcinoma, lymphoma, etc. (see Mammary and Pituitary Tumors)
- Ringtail
  - Occurs in young rats (7-19 days) and is characterized by dry skin and formation of annular constrictions, which might progress to swelling, and tissue necrosis. Autoamputation might occur.
  - Low environmental relative humidity (less than 20%-40%) appears to be the cause; it is more often seen in rats housed in hanging cages and is rarely seen in pet rats.

DIAGNOSIS

DIFFERENTIAL DIAGNOSIS

- Alopecia: trauma, dermatophytosis, chronic kidney disease, nutritional deficiency (low protein), neoplasia, barbering (behavorial)
- Ulcerative and crusting lesions: self-trauma, due to mites, secondary bacterial infections, fight wounds, neoplasia
- Pruritus: mites, secondary bacterial infections
- Crusting or flaking of skin: dermatophytosis, mites, nutritional deficiencies
- Cutaneous masses: neoplasia, inflammation, abscesses
- Localized erythema or pododermatitis: contact allergy, contact irritation (cleaners), trauma from bedding/cage material

INITIAL DATABASE

- Full dietary history
- Dermatologic examination
  - Skin scraping (sedation or general anesthesia may be required)
  - Acetate tape preparation
  - Impression smears
- Fine-needle aspirate and cytology of cutaneous and subcutaneous masses
- Dermatophyte culture
- Bacterial culture and sensitivity

ADVANCED OR CONFIRMATORY TESTING

- Serum biochemistry: if underlying organ disease is suspected
- Radiographs: to rule out underlying skeletal abnormalities (e.g., osteoarthritis; osteomyelitis) in cases of pododermatitis
- Biopsy and histopathologic examination of skin lesion

TREATMENT

THERAPEUTIC GOALS

- Eliminate pruritus and discomfort.

- Treat primary and secondary infections.
- Promote healing of skin lesions.

ACUTE GENERAL TREATMENT

- If animal is self-mutilating: shorten and blunt nail tips. In severe case, temporarily apply bandages to hindfeet. Apply E-collar to prevent removal of bandages.
- Ectoparasites
  - Ivermectin 0.2-0.4 mg/kg SC, PO q 7-14 d
  - Selamectin 10-25 mg/kg topically q 21-28 d
  - Treat until clinical signs are resolved and no more parasites are found on the animals.
  - Treat in-contact animals.
  - Treat the environment to prevent reinfection: regular bedding changes and cage cleaning. Discard cage furnishing that cannot be disinfected (e.g., wood-based furnishing).
- Bacterial dermatitis/ulcerative dermatitis
  - If indicated, provide systemic antibiotic therapy based on culture and sensitivity whenever possible
  - Start empirical treatment pending culture and sensitivity:
    - Cephalexin 30 mg/kg PO q 12 h
    - Amoxicillin/clavulanic acid 15-20 mg/kg PO q 12 h
    - Trimethoprim-sulfa 15-30 mg/kg PO q 12 h
    - Chloramphenicol 30-50 mg/kg PO q 8-12 h
    - Enrofloxacin 10-20 mg/kg PO, q 12-24 h
- Skin abscesses
  - Lance, débride, and flush or remove in toto if possible.
  - If indicated, provide systemic antibiotic therapy based on culture and sensitivity whenever possible.
- Dermatophytosis
  - Systemic antifungal therapy
    - Terbinafine 20-30 mg/kg PO q 24 h
    - Itraconazole 5-10 mg/kg PO q 24 h
  - Topical antifungal therapy
    - Enilconazole (1:50, emulsion as spray or moist wipe)
    - Miconazole/chlorhexidine shampoos
    - Lime sulfur dips (1:40, q 7 d)
    - Used alone or in combination with systemic therapy
    - Used preferably in cases of suspected dermatophytosis, while dermatophyte culture results are awaited
  - Environmental decontamination: frequent damp mopping of hard surfaces rather than sweeping can reduce environmental spread of spores; 1:10 bleach solution can be used to clean environment. Contact time: 10 minutes
- Monitoring: once-weekly dermatophyte test medium (DTM) cultures. Discontinue treatment when two consecutive negative cultures are obtained.
- Antihistamines
  - Diphenhydramine 1-2 mg/kg PO q 12 h
  - Hydroxyzine 2 mg/kg PO q 8-12 h
- Antiinflammatory drugs: meloxicam 0.3-0.5 mg/kg PO, SC q 12-24 h
- Neoplasia: surgical mass removal (see Mammary and Pituitary Tumors)
- Nutritional deficiency: improve diet; provide access to commercial pelleted diet

CHRONIC TREATMENT

Dermatophytosis will often require long-term therapy.

RECOMMENDED MONITORING

- Resolution of clinical signs
- Repeated evaluation for presence of ectoparasites
- Weekly DTM cultures for dermatophytosis cases

PROGNOSIS AND OUTCOME

Good to fair

PEARLS & CONSIDERATIONS

PREVENTION

- Provision of a commercial diet
- Quarantine all new incoming animals for a minimum of 30 days before allowing contact with other animals.

CLIENT EDUCATION

Dermatophytes are contagious; clients should seek medical advice if lesions are found on humans in the household.

SUGGESTED READINGS

Agren MS, et al: Effect of topical zinc oxide on bacterial growth and inflammation in full-thickness skin wounds in normal and diabetic rats, Eur J Surg 157:97–101, 1991.

Galler JR, et al: Ulcerative dermatitis in rats with over fifteen generations of protein malnutrition, Br J Nutr 41:611–618, 1979.

Honma M, et al: Plantar decubitus ulcers in rats and rabbits, Jikken Dobutsu 38:253–258, 1989.

Taylor DK, et al: Lanolin as a treatment option for ringtail in transgenic rats, J Am Assoc Lab Anim Sci 45:83–87, 2006.

CROSS-REFERENCES TO OTHER SECTIONS

Mammary and Pituitary Tumors

AUTHOR: **CHRISTOPH MANS**

EDITOR: **THOMAS M. DONNELLY**

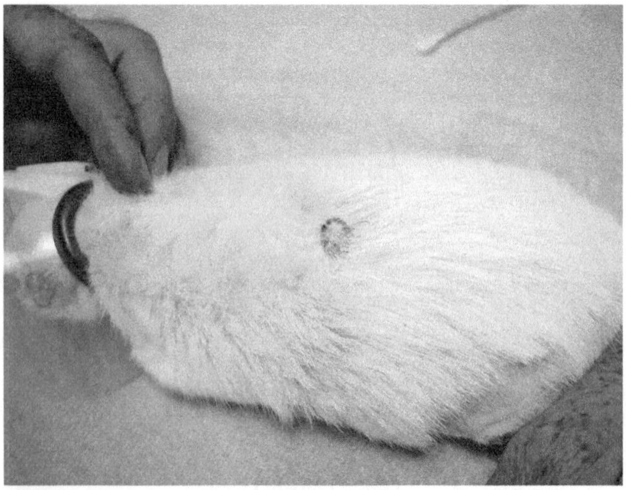

Skin Disease This skin lesion in a rat was caused by a subcutaneous injection of enrofloxacin; always dilute the drug if it needs to be injected SC or IM. *(Photo courtesy Jörg Mayer, The University of Georgia, Athens.)*

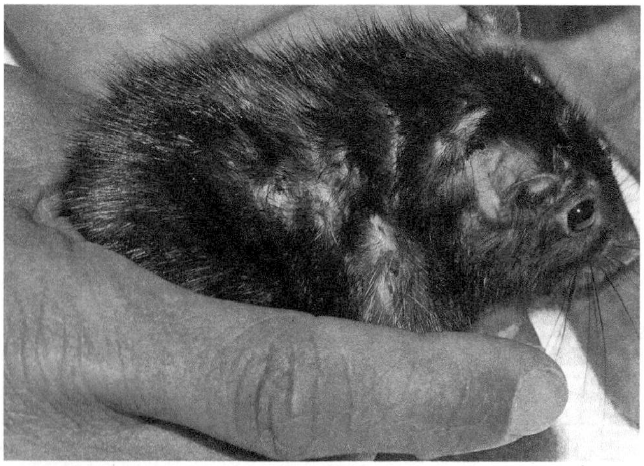

Skin Disease Skin lesions located over the shoulder and neck area, which were induced by fighting with cage mates. Isolation of the rat led to complete resolution of the skin lesions. Self-trauma, secondary to ectoparasite induced pruritus, can present in similar fashion.

Anorexia

BASIC INFORMATION

DEFINITION

Anorexia is a symptom defined by the lack of spontaneous feeding behavior for an abnormal period of time. Weight loss is usually a consequence of lack of nutrients when associated with anorexia.

SYNONYMS

Dysorexia, inappetence, poor appetite, weight loss, cachexia, underweight, reduced body condition

SPECIAL SPECIES CONSIDERATIONS

- Any condition that can lead to pain or that causes discomfort can alter the feeding behavior of guinea pigs.
- Guinea pigs are grazing animals; therefore, high-quality grass hay should always be offered free-choice.
- Guinea pigs digest fibers more efficiently than rabbits and tend to eat more slowly.
- Guinea pigs lack the enzyme L-gluconolactone oxidase that is needed to synthesize vitamin C. Therefore, vegetables rich in vitamin C should be included in the diet.
- Temporary anorexia occurs 12-24 h before parturition in pregnant guinea pigs.

EPIDEMIOLOGY

SPECIES, AGE, SEX

- An apparent wasting syndrome characterized by anorexia, weight loss, and death in 3-4-week-old guinea pigs due to an enteric coronavirus infection has been reported.
- Older female guinea pigs are prone to ovarian cysts, which can lead to anorexia due to abdominal distension and compression of the gastrointestinal (GI) tract.
- Adult guinea pigs fed an inappropriate diet are possibly predisposed to develop acquired dental disease.

GENETICS AND BREED PREDISPOSITION Peruvian and long hair breeds may be predisposed to gastric trichobezoars.

RISK FACTORS

- Vitamin C–deficient diet
- Fiber-deficient diet
- Pregnancy

ASSOCIATED CONDITIONS AND DISORDERS

- Dermatologic conditions (pododermatitis [see Pododermatitis], poor fur condition)
- Dental disease (see Dental Disease)
- Ovarian cysts (see Ovarian Cysts)
- Hyperthyroidism (see Hyperthyroidism)
- Neoplasia

CLINICAL PRESENTATION

HISTORY, CHIEF COMPLAINT

- Reduced appetite
- Weight loss
- Lethargy

PHYSICAL EXAM FINDINGS

- Dehydration
- Cachexia
- Poor fur quality, bilateral alopecia
- Cheek teeth malocclusion
- Incisor malocclusion
- Absence of food in the oral cavity
- Pain during jaw manipulation
- Tachypnea
- Cervical, facial, or abdominal mass
- Abdominal distention
- Abdominal tympany
- Abdominal pain

ETIOLOGY AND PATHOPHYSIOLOGY

- Any stressful or painful condition can prevent normal feeding behavior.
  - Digestive/dietary causes:
    - Dental disease
    - Hypovitaminosis C (see Hypovitaminosis C)
    - GI ileus
    - GI tympany (see Intestinal Disorders)
    - Gastric dilatation and volvulus (see Gastric Dilatation and Volvulus)
    - GI obstruction (e.g., foreign body, neoplasia)
    - Enteritis/dysbacteriosis
  - Nondigestive causes:
    - Dehydration
    - Physical or emotional stress
    - Pain (i.e., arthritis, urolithiasis, otitis media)
    - Urinary disorders (e.g., renal insufficiency, urolithiasis)
    - Respiratory disorders (see Respiratory Tract Disease)
    - Metabolic disorder: ketoacidosis, hepatic lipidosis
    - Neoplasia (e.g., thyroid neoplasia, lymphoma)
    - Infectious causes (e.g., lymphadenitis)
    - Pregnancy

DIAGNOSIS

INITIAL DATABASE

- Full dietary history
- Full environment history
- Full toxin exposure history
- Complete intraoral examination under general anesthesia, preferably endoscopy-guided
- Whole body radiographs: evaluate for disorders of the GI and urinary tracts.
- Urine analysis: hematuria and/or pyuria can occur in patients with hepatic lipidosis, diabetic ketonuria, or aciduria.
- Complete blood count: usually normal, but leukocytosis, anemia, and hemoconcentration may be seen.
- Serum biochemistry: azotemia, increased liver enzymes, hypoglycemia, hyperglycemia, hypoproteinemia, hypoalbuminemia, hyperbilirubinemia may be seen.

ADVANCED OR CONFIRMATORY TESTING

- Abdominal ultrasound to assess:
  - GI tract (gut motility, obstruction)
  - Reproductive and urinary tracts (e.g., ovarian cysts, uterine disease, urolithiasis)
  - Liver
- Hormonal panel: thyroid hormones

TREATMENT

THERAPEUTIC GOALS

- Correct dehydration.
- Alleviate pain.
- Restore gut motility.
- Treat primary underlying disorder (e.g., dental disease, organ disease, neoplasia).
- Restore normal appetite.
- Restore normal body weight and condition.

ACUTE GENERAL TREATMENT

- Fluid therapy
- Nutritional support (unless obstruction is suspected)
  - Syringe feeding
  - Nasogastric tube placement: allow emptying of the air out of the stomach in case of gastric dilatation; always empty air out of stomach before providing enteral nutrition.
- Pain relief
  - Buprenorphine 0.03-0.05 mg/kg SC q 6-12 h
  - Meloxicam 0.3-0.5 mg/kg PO, SC q 24 h (contraindications: dehydration, kidney disease)
- Antibiotics
  - Enrofloxacin 10-20 mg/kg PO, IM, SC, q 12-24 h

- Chloramphenicol 30-50 mg/kg PO, SC, IM q 8 h
    - Trimethoprim-sulfa 30 mg/kg PO SC q 12 h
    - Metronidazole 20 mg/kg PO q 12 h
- Prokinetics (contraindications: intestinal obstruction or perforation)
    - Rehydration and nutritional support will resolve hypomotility in most cases. The use and possible benefits of prokinetic drugs in guinea pigs are controversial.
    - Metoclopramide 0.2-1 mg/kg PO, SC, IV q 4-6 h
    - Cisapride 0.5 mg/kg PO q 12 h
    - Trimebutine 1.5 mg/kg PO q 8 h
    - Ranitidine: 2-4 mg/kg PO, IM, SC, IV q 8-12 h
- Antifoaming agents
    - Simethicone 70 mg/kg q 1 h × 2-3 treatments
- Vitamin C 50-100 mg/kg PO, SC q 24 h for treatment of deficiencies, 10-30 mg/kg PO for maintenance

CHRONIC TREATMENT

- Treatment of dental disease
- Nonsteroidal antiinflammatory drugs for chronic pain
- Dietary correction
- Vitamin C supplementation

DRUG INTERACTIONS

It has been suggested that administration of cisapride and ranitidine together results in enhanced intestinal contractility. The clinical efficacy of this combined treatment in guinea pigs is unknown.

POSSIBLE COMPLICATIONS

- Hepatic lipidosis
- Hypovitaminosis C
- Sepsis

RECOMMENDED MONITORING

- Activity level
- Appetite
- Fecal output
- Urine output
- Body weight

PROGNOSIS AND OUTCOME

Prognosis is fair to poor depending on the origin.

CONTROVERSY

- The use of prokinetic drugs is controversial, as the clinical efficacy of any of the recommended drugs has not been demonstrated in guinea pigs. The dosages and dosing frequency used are extrapolated from other species. Most guinea pigs with GI stasis will respond to appropriate supportive care, including fluid therapy, analgesia, and nutritional support alone, making the use of prokinetic drugs discretionary.
- Probiotics are sometimes included in the treatment plan.

PEARLS & CONSIDERATIONS

COMMENTS

- After stabilization of the patient and restoration of GI motility, the goal should be to identify and treat the primary underlying cause of anorexia. This will improve the case outcome and reduce the risk of recurrence of clinical signs.
- Experimentally, audiovestibular system diseases (e.g., otitis media, otitis interna) in guinea pigs result in anorexia that has been attributed to central nervous system leptin (an adipocyte peptide involved in regulation of food intake) disturbance.

PREVENTION

- Provide high-quality grass hay.
- Ensure appropriate dietary vitamin C intake.

CLIENT EDUCATION

Discuss the importance of an appropriate diet.

SUGGESTED READINGS

Horner KC, et al: Receptors for leptin in the otic labyrinth and the cochlear-vestibular nerve of guinea pig are modified in hormone-induced anorexia, Hear Res 270:48–55, 2010.

Jaax GP, et al: Coronavirus-like virions associated with a wasting syndrome in guinea pigs, Lab Anim Sci 40:375–378, 1990.

Theus M, et al: Successful treatment of gastric trichobezoar in a Peruvian guinea pig *(Cavia aperea porcellus)*, J Exotic Pet Med 17:2, 2008.

CROSS-REFERENCES TO OTHER SECTIONS

Cheilitis
Dental Disease
Gastric Dilatation and Volvulus
Hyperthyroidism
Hypovitaminosis C
Intestinal Disorders
Ovarian Cysts
Pododermatitis
Respiratory Tract Disease

AUTHOR: **HUYNH MINH**

EDITOR: **CHRISTOPH MANS**

SMALL MAMMALS: GUINEA PIGS

Cheilitis

BASIC INFORMATION

DEFINITION

Cheilitis or inflammation of the lips is a disorder described in guinea pigs. It presents as inflammation and hyperkeratosis of the mucocutaneous junction of the lips.

SYNONYMS

Scabs around the mouth, lip sores

EPIDEMIOLOGY

SPECIES, AGE, SEX

- The disease appears to be specific to guinea pigs.
- There is no sex predilection.
- Affected animals are usually 1 to 5 years of age.

CONTAGION AND ZOONOSIS Guinea pig cheilitis has been suggested to be contagious.

CLINICAL PRESENTATION

HISTORY, CHIEF COMPLAINT

- Nonhealing scabs and ulcers around the mouth of one or more guinea pigs
- Lesions tend to wax and wane over several weeks but never completely resolve.
- Despite the presence of these lesions, affected guinea pigs continue to eat normally in most cases.

PHYSICAL EXAM FINDINGS

- In the early stage of the disease, crusts aggregate at the lip commissures, then eventually spread along the lips and the philtrum.
- Mild form
    - Multiple scabs, particularly on the corners of the lips
    - The guinea pig is still in good health and is eating normally at this stage.
- Severe form
    - Generalized inflammation and scabbing of the lips
    - Lesions may involve the oral mucosa and affect food intake
    - Reduced body condition

ETIOLOGY AND PATHOPHYSIOLOGY

- Etiology unknown, but likely multifactorial
- Coarse, fibrous hay or sharp pieces of pelleted feed may cause trauma to the corners of the mouth, allowing bacteria and fungi to gain entry opportunistically via abrasions.
- Common opportunistic organisms isolated from cheilitis lesions include *Staphylococcus* spp. and *Candida albicans*, among others.
- Nutritional deficiencies have been suggested: vitamins A, B, and C (see Hypovitaminosis C); fatty acid, protein; mineral and trace elements (Mg, Zn, Mn).

DIAGNOSIS

DIFFERENTIAL DIAGNOSIS

- Trauma
- Ringworm
- *Trixacarus caviae*
- Allergic dermatitis

INITIAL DATABASE

- Cytology
  - Impression smears
  - Tape preparations
  - Hair plucks
  - Skin scrapings

ADVANCED OR CONFIRMATORY TESTING

- Histopathologic examination
  - Large colonies of bacteria are often seen in association with the lesions.
  - Infiltration with neutrophils, lymphocytes, and macrophages may be seen.
  - Thickened, hyperkeratotic epidermis
  - Segmental erosions and ulcers
- If clinical signs are mild, histopathologic examination may not be required.

TREATMENT

THERAPEUTIC GOAL

Resolution of lip lesions

ACUTE GENERAL TREATMENT

- Topical therapy
  - 10% povidone-iodine or 0.125% chlorhexidine solution will reduce bacterial and fungal components and improve oral hygiene. Lesions should be gently cleansed twice daily.
    - Crusty exudates should be manually removed from the mucocutaneous junction.
  - Topical ointment
    - Consider wound healing ointments that contain zinc and vitamin A.
    - Consider ointments containing antibiotics and antifungal drugs.
    - Do not use ointment containing bacitracin (e.g., BNP ointment) because it will cause potentially fatal dysbacteriosis.
  - Continue topical therapy (antiseptic cleansing and topical ointment) for 7 days after visual resolution of the lesions. Systemic antibiotics are not necessary in most cases.
- Analgesia: meloxicam 0.3 mg/kg PO q 24 h
- Nutrition and supportive care
  - Ensure adequate vitamin C (100 mg/kg PO q 24 h).
  - Reduce stress and provide a clean, quiet, and comfortable environment.
- Husbandry
  - All food bowls and drinkers should be disinfected. Washing the items in a dishwasher or soaking for 10 minutes in a dilute chlorine solution can achieve this.
  - Wired hutches should be scrubbed with a suitable disinfectant.

CHRONIC TREATMENT

If the guinea pig presents with the severe form of cheilitis, treatment may be required for 3-4 weeks and lesions may recur.

POSSIBLE COMPLICATIONS

- Self-mutilation, subsequent bleeding, and secondary infection of lesions can be avoided by
  - Trimming nails
  - Avoiding coarse hays and other abrasive foods, which may rub against the lip lesions during prehension.

RECOMMENDED MONITORING

- Return for an examination 1 week after initial diagnosis and then again 1 week after resolution of clinical signs.
- If lesions are not responding to therapy, a biopsy should be obtained for histopathologic examination and tissue submitted for bacterial and fungal culture and sensitivity.
- The clinician should warn owners that recurrence of the lesions is possible.

PROGNOSIS AND OUTCOME

Guinea pig cheilitis has a low mortality rate. If the owner focuses on oral hygiene, the prognosis for the affected guinea pig is excellent. Generally, after the appropriate treatment plan is begun, healing of lesions occurs within 2-3 weeks.

SUGGESTED READINGS

Richardson V: Diseases of domestic guinea pigs, Oxford, 2000, Blackwell Publishing, pp 78–79.
Smith M: Staphylococcal cheilitis in the guinea-pig, J Small Anim Pract 18:47–50, 1977.

CROSS-REFERENCES TO OTHER SECTIONS

Hypovitaminosis C

AUTHOR: **GRETTA HOWARD**

EDITOR: **CHRISTOPH MANS**

SMALL MAMMALS: GUINEA PIGS

Dental Disease

BASIC INFORMATION

DEFINITION

Disorders affecting the dentition and associated structures

SPECIAL SPECIES CONSIDERATIONS

- Dental formula: 2(I1C0P1M3) = 20
- Incisor teeth and cheek teeth grow continuously throughout life (elodont).
- Incisor teeth and cheek teeth have a long crown (hypsodont) and no anatomic root (aradicular).
- Each tooth can be divided into a *clinical crown* (above the gingival sulcus)

and the *reserve crown* (subgingival part).
- Incisor teeth in guinea pigs are white.
- The ratio of mandibular to maxillary incisor teeth length is 3:1.
- Premolar and molar cheek teeth are anatomically identical in guinea pigs and therefore can be referred to as *cheek teeth 1-4* (CT1-4).
- Guinea pigs have curved cheek teeth, resulting in oblique occlusal planes of about 30 degrees to the horizontal plane.
- The occlusal surface of each cheek tooth is roughened owing to the presence of enamel ridges.
- The presence of food material in the oral cavity is normal in guinea pigs and needs to be distinguished from pathologic food impaction or retention secondary to dental disease.

EPIDEMIOLOGY

SPECIES, AGE, SEX Acquired dental disease is more common in guinea pigs >2 years of age.

GENETICS AND BREED PREDISPOSITION Suspected, but not proven

RISK FACTORS
- Low-fiber diets leading to insufficient wear of continuously growing teeth
- Trauma
- Vitamin C deficiency

ASSOCIATED CONDITIONS AND DISORDERS Exophthalmos, facial abscesses, hepatic lipidosis, diarrhea, weight loss

CLINICAL PRESENTATION

DISEASE FORMS/SUBTYPES
- Incisor teeth disorders
- Cheek teeth disorders
- Periapical abscesses

HISTORY, CHIEF COMPLAINT
- Reduced food intake
- Reduced fecal output
- Weight loss
- Poor coat condition
- Lethargy
- Diarrhea
- Wet or stained fur around the mouth

PHYSICAL EXAM FINDINGS
- General loss of condition
- Poor coat condition
- Lethargy
- Tympany
- Diarrhea
- Small and irregular fecal pellet
- Malocclusion of incisor teeth
- Fractured incisor teeth
- Soiled or wet fur around mouth
- Cheilitis
- Facial abscesses
- Exophthalmia
- Intraoral examination (general anesthesia required)
  - Coronal elongation of cheek teeth (CT)
  - Tongue entrapment secondary to coronal elongation of mandibular CT1-CT2
  - Sharp enamel points or spurs leading to buccal and lingual mucosal erosions and discomfort
  - Change in occlusal surface plane
  - Food impaction

ETIOLOGY AND PATHOPHYSIOLOGY

- Incisor teeth disorders
  - Incisor malocclusion occurs commonly secondary to cheek teeth malocclusion.
  - Trauma (e.g., excessive chewing on cage bars or cage furnishings, iatrogenic)
- Cheek teeth disorders
  - Malocclusion, coronal elongation, and sharp enamel spur formation are currently believed to occur secondary to insufficient tooth wear because of feeding of inappropriate diets.
  - In captivity, diets are often significantly lower in fiber compared with diets of wild guinea pigs. Ingestion of less abrasive food requires less mastication, resulting in less dietary abrasion of the cheek teeth and consequent elongation of clinical and reserve crowns.
  - Other nutritional causes such as abnormal calcium and/or vitamin D metabolism have been suggested but not proven in guinea pigs.
- Periapical abscesses
  - Infections involving the apex will often result in formation of abscesses.
  - Periapical abscesses can become evident as facial swelling or as exophthalmos if infection involves the maxillary cheek teeth (see Intestinal Disorders).

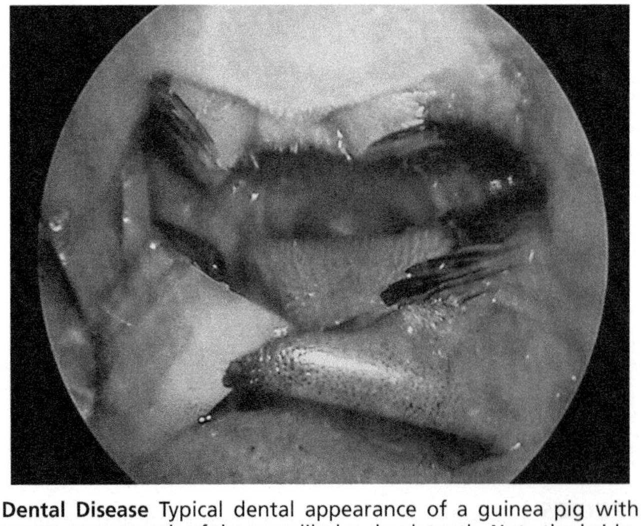

Dental Disease Typical dental appearance of a guinea pig with severe overgrowth of the mandibular cheek teeth. Note the bridging effect, which traps the tongue underneath. Also, note the approximate 30-degree angle of the occlusal surfaces, which is normal in guinea pigs. Oral assessment with an endoscope facilitates the exam significantly.

DIAGNOSIS

DIFFERENTIAL DIAGNOSIS

- Weight loss
  - Systemic disease (i.e., metabolic, infectious, organ failure)
  - Gastrointestinal disease (see Intestinal Disorders)
  - Hypovitaminosis C (see Hypovitaminosis C)
  - Hyperthyroidism
- Diarrhea
  - Gastrointestinal disease
- Anorexia (see Anorexia)
  - Systemic disease (i.e., metabolic, infectious, organ failure)
  - Hypovitaminosis C
  - Pain
- Poor coat condition
  - Ectoparasites
  - Hypovitaminosis C
  - Endocrine disorders (i.e., ovarian cysts, hyperthyroidism)
- Exophthalmia (see Ocular Disorders)
  - Buphthalmia
  - Retrobulbar cyst or neoplasia
- Facial swelling
  - Neoplasia
  - Foreign body–induced abscess

INITIAL DATABASE

- Complete intraoral examination under general anesthesia
  - Endoscopic guided intraoral examination (stomatoscopy) is preferred for a complete intraoral examination.
  - Use magnification and focal illumination if stomatoscopy cannot be performed.

- Imaging
  - Skull radiographs (five views: lateral, left and right oblique, ventrodorsal, rostrocaudal)
- CT scan of head: preferred over skull radiographs
- Fine-needle aspiration and cytologic examination of facial swellings. Aerobic bacterial culture and sensitivity if purulent material is revealed.
- Complete blood count and biochemistry profile may be normal. Rule out concurrent diseases that will affect the prognosis.

TREATMENT

THERAPEUTIC GOALS

- Resolve intraoral soft tissue trauma and associated pain.
- Restore normal occlusion if possible.
- Recover the animal's ability to eat unaided.

ACUTE GENERAL TREATMENT

- Provide supportive care as needed:
  - Fluid therapy 60-100 mL/kg/d SC, PO, IV
  - Nutritional support: syringe-feed with high-fiber diet for herbivores (e.g., Oxbow Critical Care for Herbivores, 50-80 mL/kg PO q 24 h, divide into 4-5 feedings) or with crushed and soaked pellets
  - Analgesia
    - Buprenorphine 0.02-0.05 mg/kg SC q 6-8 h
    - Meloxicam 0.3-0.5 mg/kg PO or SC q 24 h once adequately hydrated
- Treatment of cheek teeth malocclusion
  - General anesthesia required
  - Specialized equipment required
    - Use low-speed dental drill, a diamond burr, cheek dilators, and a mouth gag.
    - Use appropriate magnification and illumination; preferably, a rigid endoscope or otoscope is used.
  - Avoid iatrogenic damage to soft tissue during dental procedures.
  - Shorten elongated clinical crowns:
    - Remove sharp enamel spurs, which lead to soft tissue trauma buccally and lingually. Maxillary cheek teeth form spurs buccally; mandibular cheek teeth overgrowth often leads to tongue entrapment in guinea pigs.
    - Restore the physiologic oblique occlusal plane, which is about 30 degrees to the horizontal plane, slanting from buccal to lingual.
    - Do not attempt to extract cheek teeth unless severely diseased and severely mobile, secondary to periodontal infection or fracture. Cheek teeth extraction in guinea pigs is technically challenging and often is not feasible clinically.
- Treatment of incisor teeth malocclusion
  - Sedation or general anesthesia required
  - Specialized equipment required
    - Use a low-speed diamond or carbon cutting blade or a high-speed dental drill.
  - Avoid iatrogenic damage to the soft tissue during incisor teeth trimming.
    - Use a tongue depressor or spatula to protect the lips and tongue during trimming.
    - Do not use nail clippers or scissors to trim incisor teeth.
    - Avoid excessive shortening of the clinical crowns because this will lead to temporary functional loss of the incisor teeth. The normal ratio of the length of mandibular to maxillary incisor teeth is 3:1.
- Antibiotic therapy
  - Indicated only if evidence of periodontal or periapical infection exists
  - Periodontal and periapical infections are mixed anaerobic-aerobic infections normally caused by the physiologic oral bacterial flora.
  - Ensure appropriate coverage against anaerobic bacteria.
  - Trimethoprim-sulfa 30 mg/kg PO q 12 h. Combine with metronidazole for improved anaerobic coverage
  - Enrofloxacin 10-20 mg/kg PO q 12-24 h. Combine with metronidazole for anaerobic coverage
  - Metronidazole 20-30 mg/kg PO q 12 h. Combine with trimethoprim-sulfa or enrofloxacin for aerobic coverage
  - Chloramphenicol 30-50 mg/kg PO q 12 h
  - Azithromycin 30 mg/kg PO q 24 h

CHRONIC TREATMENT

- Repeated corrections of cheek teeth and incisor teeth malocclusion under general anesthesia
- Tooth extraction (fractured or severely diseased teeth)
  - Rarely indicated in guinea pigs and technically very challenging
  - Consider referral to a specialist if extractions might be indicated.
- Periapical abscess treatment
  - Several techniques have been reported.
  - Consider referral to a specialist if periapical abscess treatment is necessary.
- Nutritional support
  - Nutritional support: syringe-feed with high-fiber diet for herbivores (e.g., Oxbow Critical Care for Herbivores, 50-80 mL/kg PO q 24 h, divided into 4-5 feedings) or crushed and soaked guinea pig pellets until the animal is eating sufficient amounts of food unaided
- Vitamin C 50-100 mg/kg PO, SC q 24 h for treatment of deficiencies; 10-30 mg/kg PO for maintenance
- Analgesia
- Antibiotic therapy

DRUG INTERACTIONS

- Do not administer cephalosporins, penicillins, erythromycin, or clindamycin orally.
- Do not administer meloxicam to dehydrated animals.

POSSIBLE COMPLICATIONS

- Incomplete extraction of elodont teeth may result in regrowth if germinative

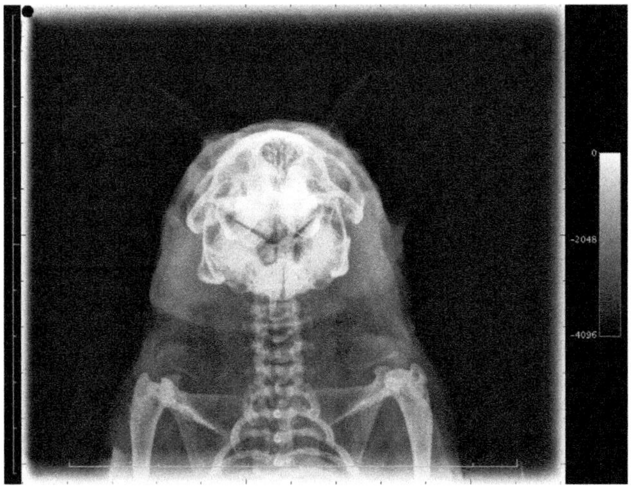

Dental Disease Rostrocaudal view of a normal guinea pig skull. Note the distinct occlusal plane of visible molar teeth; with overgrown cheek teeth, this line disappears. *(Photo courtesy Jörg Mayer, The University of Georgia, Athens.)*

tissue is not completely removed during extraction.
- Iatrogenic damage to the teeth, tongue, or buccal mucosa

RECOMMENDED MONITORING

- Food intake
- Fecal output
- Body weight

PROGNOSIS AND OUTCOME

- Good to fair for animal with no secondary complications and if client is compliant with recommended treatment
- Guarded for periapical abscesses, dependent on location, extent of disease, and animal's general condition
- Poor if animal is in poor body condition or is suffering from systemic disease, or if client is not compliant with recommended treatments

PEARLS & CONSIDERATIONS

COMMENTS

Congenital dental disease is rare in rodents; most dental disease is acquired.

PREVENTION

Provision of an appropriate diet that is high in fiber and allows for appropriate wear of the cheek teeth

CLIENT EDUCATION

- Educate owners about appropriate dietary requirements of guinea pigs.
- Owners must be informed that repeated and often lifelong treatment of dental malocclusion under general anesthesia is required.

SUGGESTED READINGS

Capello V, et al: Small mammal dentistry. In Carpenter JW, et al, editors: Ferrets, rabbits and rodents: clinical medicine and surgery, ed 3, St Louis, 2012, WB Saunders, pp 452–471.

Jekl V, et al: Quantitative and qualitative assessments of intraoral lesions in 180 small herbivorous mammals, Vet Rec 162:442–449, 2008.

CROSS-REFERENCES TO OTHER SECTIONS

Anorexia
Hypovitaminosis C
Intestinal Disorders
Ocular Disorders

AUTHOR: **CHRISTOPH MANS**

EDITOR: **THOMAS M. DONNELLY**

SMALL MAMMALS: GUINEA PIGS

Gastric Dilatation and Volvulus

BASIC INFORMATION

DEFINITION

Acute and generally fatal syndrome in which the stomach fills with gas and fluid, followed by rotation on its mesenteric axis

SYNONYMS

Bloat, gastric tympany, gastric torsion

EPIDEMIOLOGY

SPECIES, AGE, SEX No age or sex association has been reported.

GENETICS AND BREED PREDISPOSITION No breed or genetic association has been identified.

RISK FACTORS Risk factors are unknown. Sudden diet changes and diets high in concentrate (e.g., pelleted diets), as well as gastrointestinal stasis and painful conditions, have been presumed to be possible risk factors.

ASSOCIATED CONDITIONS AND DISORDERS Gastrointestinal stasis, any cause of pain

CLINICAL PRESENTATION

DISEASE FORMS/SUBTYPES Gastric tympany without volvulus

HISTORY, CHIEF COMPLAINT

- Acute onset of depression
- Sudden death
- Reluctance to move
- Abdominal distention
- Inappetence

PHYSICAL EXAM FINDINGS

- Depression
- Painful body posture
- Gas-filled, tympanic cranial abdomen
- Pain may be noted on abdominal palpation.
- Dyspnea
- Cyanotic or pale mucous membrane
- Signs consistent with hypovolemic shock: tachycardia, weak pulses, pale mucous membranes, dyspnea, hypothermia

ETIOLOGY AND PATHOPHYSIOLOGY

- The cause of gastric dilatation/volvulus (GDV) in guinea pigs is not fully understood. Gastrointestinal stasis, pain, or a sudden change in the diet may contribute to development of the syndrome.
- Guinea pigs cannot vomit owing to a well-developed cardiac sphincter. With mechanical or physical outflow obstruction from the stomach, swallowed saliva and gastric fluids quickly accumulate. Fermentation of the stomach content produces a large amount of gas.
- Gastric gas accumulation usually precedes volvulus in guinea pigs.
  - In cases of gastric volvulus, rotation of the stomach on its mesenteric axis from 180 to 540 degrees has been reported.
- Distention of the stomach leads to reduced venous return to the heart by compression of the vena cava and portal veins. The consequences of reduced venous return are decreased cardiac output, decreased arterial blood pressure, and myocardial ischemia. Hypovolemic shock and cardiovascular failure are common consequences.
- Ischemia of the stomach wall due to reduced perfusion predisposes to gastric necrosis and perforation.
- Pressure on the diaphragm leads to reduced ventilation. Reduced cardiac output leads to reduced lung perfusion. Both mechanisms lead to tissue hypoxia.
- Cardiovascular shock can also be caused by endotoxemia.

DIAGNOSIS

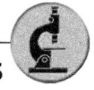

DIFFERENTIAL DIAGNOSIS

- Patients with advanced gastrointestinal stasis can mimic clinical signs of GDV.
- Gastric tympany and dilatation without volvulus

- Gastrointestinal obstruction
- Any painful condition can cause depression and reluctance to move. Common painful conditions in guinea pigs are dental disease (see Dental Disease), trauma, urinary calculi (see Urolithiasis), and disorders secondary to hypovitaminosis C (see Hypovitaminosis C).
- Common causes of dyspnea and tachypnea in guinea pigs include pneumonia (see Respiratory Tract Disease), pleural effusion, pulmonary edema, and metabolic acidosis.
- Cardiovascular shock can be caused by hypovolemia, sepsis, or endotoxemia.

INITIAL DATABASE

- Provide supportive care before diagnostic testing if patient is hypovolemic or in shock.
- Abdominal radiographs: large, gas-filled stomach silhouette positioned on the right side of the cranial abdomen. The distended stomach can occupy a large portion of the abdomen. In some cases, the stomach may be displaced caudally with intestines visible cranial to the stomach. Generally, little gas accumulation is noted in the intestine distal to the stomach. Free abdominal gas suggests gastric perforation.
- Complete blood count/biochemistry abnormalities vary with the degree of shock and secondary metabolic and systemic disorders.

ADVANCED OR CONFIRMATORY TESTING

Confirmation of GDV is made by surgical exploration. Because of the poor prognosis associated with GDV in guinea pigs, a thorough discussion with clients should occur before proceeding.

TREATMENT

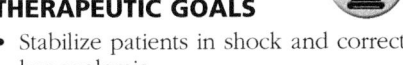

THERAPEUTIC GOALS

- Stabilize patients in shock and correct hypovolemia.
- Provide analgesia.
- Perform decompression of the stomach and correction of volvulus.
- To date, no successful treatment of GDV in guinea pigs has been reported, and because of the poor prognosis, euthanasia should be discussed with the client.

ACUTE GENERAL TREATMENT

- Place an intravenous or intraosseous catheter. Administer isotonic crystalloids (60 mL/kg/h; 90 mL/kg/h if in shock) to correct hypovolemia. Monitor patient closely during fluid administration.
- Provide oxygen if patient is hypoxemic.
- Opioids are recommended for mediation of visceral pain: buprenorphine (0.03-0.05 mg/kg SC, IM, IV, IO q 6-12 h), hydromorphone (0.1 mg/kg SC, IV, IO q 8 h), and fentanyl (0.5 μg/kg/h CRI IV, IO).
- Gastric decompression can be attempted by orogastric tube or by percutaneous trocarization. Both procedures carry risks. Use a well-lubricated open-ended flexible rubber tube for orogastric intubation. If a tube cannot be passed successfully into the stomach, percutaneous trocarization with a hypodermic needle can be attempted. Percutaneous trocarization carries the risk of stomach rupture.
- Upon patient stabilization and gastric decompression, surgical intervention is indicated. The patient needs to be placed in dorsal recumbence with the cranial part of his body elevated to decrease the pressure of the stomach on the lungs. The volvulus is reduced, and the integrity of the stomach is assessed. In cases of necrosis of the stomach, a gastrectomy could be attempted. To prevent recurrence, a gastropexy is performed by suturing the serosa of the stomach to the abdominal wall. No successful outcome after surgical treatment of GDV in guinea pigs has been reported.

CHRONIC TREATMENT

- Pain management
- Fluid and nutritional support

DRUG INTERACTIONS

- Gastric motility agents (e.g., metoclopramide) are contraindicated in cases of uncorrected GDV but might be indicated after surgical correction.
- Nonsteroidal antiinflammatory drugs (NSAIDs) should be avoided in hypovolemic patients, especially in patients in shock.

POSSIBLE COMPLICATIONS

- Metabolic and electrolyte abnormalities
- Cardiac arrhythmias
- Necrosis of the stomach due to ischemia
- Gastric ulceration
- Gastrointestinal ileus
- Anorexia

RECOMMENDED MONITORING

- Behavior consistent with pain
- Appetite
- Fecal output

PROGNOSIS AND OUTCOME

- The prognosis is poor.
- No reports have described successful treatment of guinea pigs diagnosed with GDV.

CONTROVERSY

In many cases of GDV, guinea pigs die with no prior clinical signs.

PEARLS & CONSIDERATIONS

COMMENTS

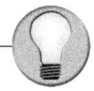

- Sudden death and collapse due to cardiovascular failure are common in guinea pigs diagnosed with GDV. Therefore, initial stabilization is critical.
- Correction of hypovolemia should be performed before abdominal radiographs are taken.

CLIENT EDUCATION

Avoid sudden diet changes, as well as diets high in simple carbohydrates and starch.

SUGGESTED READINGS

Dudley ES, et al: Gastric volvulus in guinea pigs: comparison with other species, J Am Assoc Lab Anim Sci 50:526–530, 2011.

Mitchell EB, et al: Gastric dilatation-volvulus in a guinea pig *(Cavia porcellus)*, J Am Anim Hosp Assoc 46:174–180, 2010.

Pignon C, et al: Diagnostic challenge: gastric dilatation and volvulus in a guinea pig, J Exotic Pet Med 19:189, 2010.

CROSS-REFERENCES TO OTHER SECTIONS

Dental Disease
Hypovitaminosis C
Respiratory Tract Disease
Urolithiasis

AUTHOR: **CHARLY PIGNON**

EDITOR: **CHRISTOPH MANS**

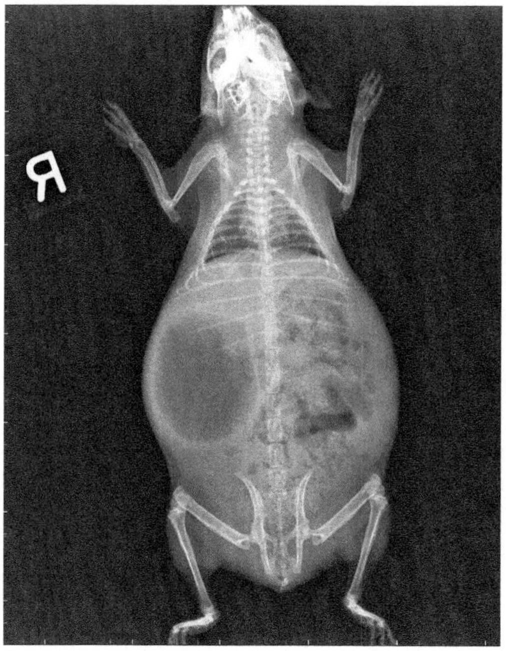

Gastric Dilatation and Volvulus Guinea pig gastric dilatation and volvulus.

SMALL MAMMALS: GUINEA PIGS

Hyperthyroidism

BASIC INFORMATION

DEFINITION

A clinical syndrome characterized by continued excessive secretion of thyroid hormones by the thyroid gland

SYNONYM

Thyrotoxicosis

EPIDEMIOLOGY

SPECIES, AGE, SEX

- Guinea pigs of all ages can be affected, but most cases are seen in patients older than 3 years.
- No sex predilection is known.
- The prevalence of thyroid pathology in guinea pigs in one study was 4.6%.

CLINICAL PRESENTATION

HISTORY, CHIEF COMPLAINT

- Weight loss
- Reduced body condition
- Normal or increased appetite
- Polydipsia and polyuria
- Hyperactivity, nervousness
- Soft feces or diarrhea
- Alopecia

PHYSICAL EXAM FINDINGS

- Poor body condition
- Poor fur condition and alopecia over the dorsum and inguinal area
- Palpable thyroid gland(s)
- Tachycardia, heart murmur, arrhythmia
- Hyperesthesia
- Soft feces or diarrhea

ETIOLOGY AND PATHOPHYSIOLOGY

- Excessive thyroid hormone (thyroxine and triiodothyronine) production and secretion can be caused by thyroid hyperplasia, adenoma, and carcinoma. In one retrospective study, 55% of all thyroid pathologies were adenocarcinomas.
- Excessive circulating thyroid hormones lead to an increase in metabolic rate and exacerbate effects on the sympathetic nervous system.

DIAGNOSIS

DIFFERENTIAL DIAGNOSIS

- Endoparasites can cause weight loss and abnormal soft feces.
- Renal disease can cause polydipsia and polyuria and weight loss.
- Ovarian cysts can cause alopecia and weight loss (see Ovarian Cysts).
- Dental disease can cause weight loss.

INITIAL DATABASE

- Serum biochemistry profile: rule out renal disease
- Serum thyroxine (T_4) measurement: reference range, 1.1-5.2 µg/dL (14.2-66.9 nmol/L)
- Ultrasound examination of the thyroid can be performed to detect any anatomic changes in the gland. Because the location is very superficial, high-frequency transducers (at least 10 MHz) should be used.
- Fine-needle aspiration and cytologic examination of palpable thyroid masses is performed under ultrasound guidance.

ADVANCED OR CONFIRMATORY TESTING

- Nuclear scintigraphy appears to be the most precise diagnostic tool that can be used to document the function of a potentially abnormal thyroid gland.
- Trial therapy of methimazole can be attempted because response to medical treatment is usually very fast and obvious (weight gain, behavioral changes within 48 hours).

TREATMENT

THERAPEUTIC GOAL

Restore normal thyroid hormone levels and eliminate clinical signs.

ACUTE GENERAL TREATMENT

- Hyperthyroidism is a chronic disease. Therefore, urgent acute treatment usually is not required.
- Medical treatment
  - Methimazole 0.5-2 mg/kg PO q 12-24 h: most cases respond to q 24 h dosing
  - Carbimazole 1-2 mg/kg PO q 24 h
  - These drug dosages are extrapolated from feline doses and have been successful in anecdotal cases. The appropriate dose has to be determined by repeat assays of thyroid hormone level and by following the clinical signs.
  - Therapy is expected to be lifelong.
- Surgical treatment
  - Thyroidectomy is potentially curative if the neoplastic thyroid gland is not invading surrounding tissues. Surgery remains technically difficult, and risk of removing the parathyroid glands during the procedure is a concern.
  - Ectopic thyroid tissue may not be removed during thyroidectomy unless radionuclide imaging has allowed presurgical identification.
  - Medical treatment should be initiated several weeks before thyroidectomy is performed.
- Radioactive treatment
  - Iodine-131 (I-131) 1 mCi/animal SC once
  - I-131 is considered the best treatment option in other species for long-term control and possible cure of hyperthyroidism.
  - Special handling facilities and post-therapy isolation for several days to weeks are required.

CHRONIC TREATMENT

Medical treatment required is lifelong, and dose and frequency need to be adjusted depending on clinical signs and thyroid hormone levels.

POSSIBLE COMPLICATIONS

- Malignant thyroid neoplasm invades the tissues locally and in other species can lead to metastasis in the lungs.
- Methimazole has been described to induce side effects in cats and dogs such as vomiting, anorexia (see Anorexia), depression, eosinophilia, leukopenia, and lymphocytosis. To date, no side effects have been described in guinea pigs.

RECOMMENDED MONITORING

Recheck of the patient, including physical examination and measurement of blood levels of T_4 hormones, should be performed every 2 weeks until clinical signs are improving and/or thyroid hormone levels are within the reported reference range. Then rechecks should be performed every 3 months.

PROGNOSIS AND OUTCOME

- If no signs of malignancy (invasion of local tissue or lung metastasis) are noted, the prognosis is good.
- Medical therapy is not curative, and discontinuation of medical therapy will result in relapse of clinical signs.

CONTROVERSY

Percutaneous ethanol ablation of thyroid tumors has been reported in guinea pigs but is not recommended.

PEARLS & CONSIDERATIONS

COMMENTS

Hyperthyroidism is an uncommon syndrome in guinea pigs. However, it might be currently underdiagnosed owing to the limited amount of available literature.

CLIENT EDUCATION

It is important to weigh the guinea pig on a regular basis. In some breeds such as Peruvian, it is difficult for the owner to monitor the body condition.

SUGGESTED READINGS

Mayer J, et al: Advanced diagnostic approaches and current management of thyroid pathologies in guinea pig, Vet Clin North Am Exot Anim Pract 13:509–523, 2010.

Mayer J, et al: Thyroid scintigraphy in a guinea pig with suspected hyperthyroidism, Exot DVM 11:25, 2009.

Muller K, et al: Serum thyroxine concentrations in clinically healthy pet guinea pigs *(Cavia porcellus)*, Vet Clin Pathol 38:507–510, 2009.

CROSS-REFERENCES TO OTHER SECTIONS

Anorexia
Ovarian Cysts

AUTHOR: **CHARLY PIGNON**

EDITOR: **CHRISTOPH MANS**

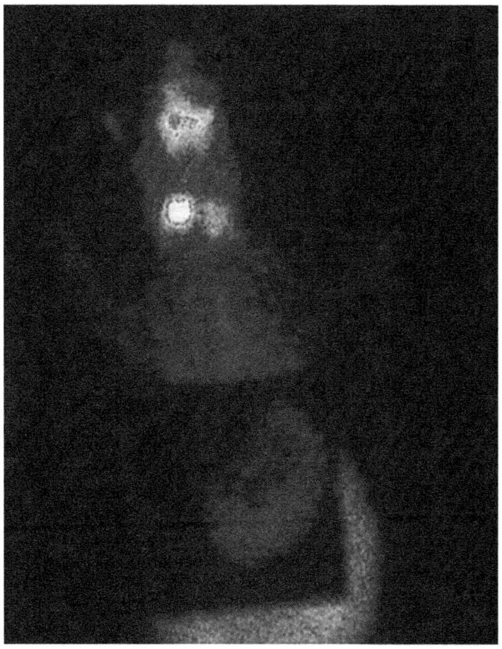

Hyperthyroidism Scintigraphy in a guinea pig with hyperthyroidism. Note the increased pattern of uptake of the right thyroid (*white spot on the left*).

SMALL MAMMALS: GUINEA PIGS

Hypovitaminosis C

BASIC INFORMATION

DEFINITION

Clinical disease resulting from vitamin C (ascorbic acid) deficiency. Subclinical vitamin C deficiency will lower the guinea pig's resistance to many other disease processes.

SYNONYMS

Scurvy, scorbutus, hypovitaminosis C

SPECIAL SPECIES CONSIDERATIONS

Guinea pigs, like humans, lack the enzyme L-gulonolactone oxidase, which is required in the synthesis of ascorbic acid from glucose. Guinea pigs therefore have an absolute requirement for vitamin C in their diet.

EPIDEMIOLOGY

SPECIES, AGE, SEX Guinea pigs of all breeds and age are affected. Guinea pigs need approximately 10 mg vitamin C/kg body weight daily for maintenance and 30 mg vitamin C/kg body weight daily for pregnancy. The vitamin C requirement for sick, or convalescent guinea pigs is higher.

ASSOCIATED CONDITIONS AND DISORDERS

- Vitamin C deficiency will reduce the guinea pig's resistance to disease and will predispose to and cause a variety of disorders:
  - Dental disease
  - Swollen joints (knee joints)
  - Lameness
  - Poor fur condition
  - Secondary bacterial infection
  - Delayed wound healing
- Sub-clinical scurvy (vitamin C at 0.5 mg/kg BW for 16 weeks) causes a marked increase in serum cholesterol, LDL-cholesterol, VLDL-cholesterol, triglycerides, and total lipids.
- If the guinea pig has concurrent vitamin E deficiency it will exhibit a progressive paralysis, probably caused by oxidative injury in the central nervous system.

CLINICAL PRESENTATION

DISEASE FORMS/SUBTYPES

- Acute or subclinical
- Subclinical vitamin C deficiency is more common and generally underdiagnosed

HISTORY, CHIEF COMPLAINT

- Anorexia
- Weight loss
- Lethargy
- Diarrhea
- Poor fur quality
- Lameness
- Teeth grinding
- Vocalization from pain

PHYSICAL EXAM FINDINGS

- Cachexia
- Inability to move jaw freely
- Dental malocclusion
- Swollen knee joints, lameness
- Hypersalivation
- Gingival bleeding
- Hematoma formation
- Poor hair coat
- Diarrhea
- Chronic nonhealing skin wounds
- Elevated resting body temperature
- Hematuria

ETIOLOGY AND PATHOPHYSIOLOGY

- Guinea pigs have an absolute dietary requirement for vitamin C.
- Vitamin C is necessary for collagen synthesis. Lack of dietary vitamin C intake will lead to defective type IV collagen, laminin, and elastin synthesis, which compromises blood vessel integrity and results in gingival and joint hemorrhage. An impaired clotting mechanism, as indicated by increased prothrombin time, also contributes to hemorrhage.
- Periodontal ligament integrity is also compromised by defective collagen synthesis, which leads to loose teeth and progressive malocclusion.
- Vitamin C deficiency lowers the delayed type hypersensitivity response, decreases T-lymphocytes, and impairs leukocyte chemotaxis and bactericidal activity.
- Vitamin C-deficient guinea pigs usually die within 3-4 weeks from anemia and widespread hemorrhages or from secondary bacterial infections. Affected animals begin to lose weight after ~10 d. Loss of weight continues until death.

DIAGNOSIS

DIFFERENTIAL DIAGNOSIS

Depending on predominant clinical signs, vitamin C deficiency is a differential for many commonly seen disorders in guinea pigs, such as anorexia, weight loss, dental disease, skin and fur disorders, and secondary bacterial infection.

INITIAL DATABASE

- Radiographs will show enlarged costochondral junctions of the ribs and epiphyses of the long bones.
- Total lipids may be elevated (serum cholesterolemia > 60 mg/dL and serum triglycerides > 30 mg/dL).
- Patient may be anemic.
- Serum levels of ascorbic acid can be measured but are rarely used clinically.

TREATMENT

THERAPEUTIC GOALS

- Correct the vitamin C deficiency.
- Treat secondary complications.

ACUTE GENERAL TREATMENT

- The daily requirement of vitamin C for healthy guinea pigs is 10 mg/kg although some references suggest 15-25 mg/kg. Guinea pigs diagnosed with vitamin C deficiency can receive 50-100 mg/kg daily. No risk of overdose is present because any excess is excreted via the kidneys.
- Nutritional support for anorexic patients
- Analgesia if arthralgia present
  - Meloxicam 0.3-0.5 mg/kg PO, SC q 24 h
- Secondary infections should be treated appropriately.

CHRONIC TREATMENT

- Long-term vitamin C supplementation
  - Via the drinking water at a concentration of 200-400 mg/L: water should be changed daily because aqueous solutions may lose up to 50% of vitamin C in 24 hours. Aqueous solutions of vitamin C will more rapidly deteriorate in metal, hard water, or heat and are more stable in neutral to alkaline solutions.
  - Vitamin C as tablet or liquid.
  - Fresh red and green pepper, cabbage, kale, and oranges are high in vitamin C and should be offered daily.
  - Commercial guinea pig pellets contain fortified levels of vitamin C that exceed maintenance requirements. The stability of vitamin C in diets varies with composition of the diet, storage temperature, and humidity. The feed content of vitamin C is reduced by dampness,

heat, and light. In fortified diets approximately one-half of the initial vitamin C may be oxidized and lost 90 days after the diet has been mixed and stored above 22°C.

PROGNOSIS AND OUTCOME

- Poor if the main presenting signs are anorexia, salivation, and inability to move the jaw
- Better for lameness and reluctance to move
- Good for conditions arising from subclinical deficiency

CONTROVERSY

Supplementation should be provided with vitamin C only, not with a multivitamin. Using a multivitamin preparation at the correct rate for vitamin C may result in accidental overdose of other vitamins.

PEARLS & CONSIDERATIONS

COMMENTS

Vitamin C supplementation should be considered for any diseased guinea pig.

PREVENTION

Ensure adequate dietary vitamin C intake.

CLIENT EDUCATION

- Do not use commercial guinea pig diets older than 3 months after date of milling/production.
- Clients should not rely on dry feed mixes that include vitamin C; a fresh food source of vitamin C must be given daily.
- Offer small quantities of vitamin C–rich fresh vegetables and fruits daily.
- Soluble vitamin C can be added to the drinking water daily; this is particularly useful over winter and during times of stress.
- Vitamin C should be given to any sick or convalescent guinea pig.

SUGGESTED READINGS

Burk RF, et al: A combined deficiency of vitamins E and C causes severe central nervous system damage in guinea pigs, J Nutr 136: 1576–1581, 2006.

Clarke GL, et al: Subclinical scurvy in the guinea pig, Vet Pathol 17:40–44, 1980.

Hickman DL, et al: Morbidity and mortality in a group of young guinea pigs. Subclinical hypovitaminosis C, Lab Anim (NY) 32:23–25, 2003.

Meredith A: Hypovitaminosis C in the guinea pig (Cavia porcellus), Companion Anim 11: 81–82, 2006.

National Research Council (US), Subcommittee on Laboratory Animal Nutrition. Nutrient Requirements of Guinea Pigs. In Nutrient requirements of laboratory animals, ed 4, Washington, DC, 1995, National Academy of Sciences, pp 103–124.

AUTHOR: **VIRGINIA C.G. RICHARDSON**

EDITOR: **CHRISTOPH MANS**

SMALL MAMMALS: GUINEA PIGS

Intestinal Disorders

BASIC INFORMATION

DEFINITION

Common disorders affecting the intestine of guinea pigs that can be classified as having primary noninfectious and infectious causes.

SYNONYMS

Diarrhea, tympany, bloat, dysbacteriosis, dysbiosis, gastroenteritis, enteritis

SPECIAL SPECIES CONSIDERATIONS

- Guinea pigs are herbivorous hindgut fermenters and are coprophagic. Ingestion of cecotrophs from the anus occurs several times daily.
- The digestive tract of guinea pigs allows digestion of a dry, high-fiber diet. Digestion of fiber occurs in the voluminous cecum and in the sacculated ascending colon. The volume of the cecum accounts for up to 65% of the volume of the entire gastrointestinal tract.
- Normal intestinal flora consists predominantly of Gram-positive coccoid bacteria, anaerobic bacteria, and lactobacilli. Any disturbance in the normal intestinal microflora can lead to overgrowth of opportunistic pathogens, which can result in septicemia endotoxemia and enterotoxemia.
- Guinea pigs, like humans, lack the enzyme L-gulonolactone oxidase, which is required in the synthesis of ascorbic acid from glucose. Guinea pigs therefore have an absolute requirement for vitamin C in their diet.
- Guinea pigs should be fed predominantly high-quality grass hay. Supplemental commercial guinea pig pellets should be offered. Vitamin C should be supplemented daily in the form of fresh vegetables (e.g., red pepper). Treats such as dried or fresh fruits and vegetables should be offered only occasionally; preference should be given to items low in carbohydrates. Fresh water must be available at all times.

EPIDEMIOLOGY

RISK FACTORS

- Inappropriate diet
- Vitamin C–deficient diet
- Sudden diet changes
- Dental disease
- Inappropriate oral antibiotic therapy
- Systemic disease
- Stress
- Pain
- Poor sanitation

CONTAGION AND ZOONOSIS

- *Salmonella* spp.
- *Rodentolepis nana*
- *Giardia duodenalis*
- *Cryptosporidium wrairi*

ASSOCIATED CONDITIONS AND DISORDERS

- Dental disease
- Hypovitaminosis C
- Septicemia, endotoxemia

CLINICAL PRESENTATION

DISEASE FORMS/SUBTYPES

- Enteritis/Diarrhea
- Tympany

HISTORY, CHIEF COMPLAINT

- Any systemic disease or painful or stressful condition may result in secondary gastrointestinal problems with nonspecific clinical signs, such as anorexia, lack of fecal output, and lethargy.
- General complaints may include the following:
  - Anorexia (see Anorexia)
  - Lethargy
  - Depression
  - Weight loss
  - Poor general condition
  - Poor coat condition
  - Teeth grinding
  - Sunken eyes

- Enteritis/diarrhea
  - Soft feces or diarrhea
  - Fecal staining around anus
  - Distended abdomen
  - Rapid breathing
- Tympany
  - Distended abdomen
  - Hunched body posture
  - Rapid breathing

PHYSICAL EXAM FINDINGS

- Unspecific findings can include the following:
  - Depression and lethargy
  - Dehydration
  - Cachexia
  - Poor coat condition
  - Perianal staining
  - Hunched body posture
- Enteritis/diarrhea
  - Perianal fecal soiling
  - Malodorous, soft fecal material
  - Tympanic intestine on abdominal palpation
  - In severe cases, animals can become endotoxemic, septicemic, and/or suffer from metabolic disturbances; therefore, animals may become increasingly depressed and might progress into shock.
- Tympany
  - Severity of clinical signs changes with progression and degree of tympany.
  - Distended and tense abdomen
  - Hunched body posture or lateral recumbence in advanced cases
  - If animal is in shock (hypovolemic, septic), clinical findings can include hypothermia, tachypnea, tachycardia, severe depression, and pale mucous membranes.

ETIOLOGY AND PATHOPHYSIOLOGY

- Gastrointestinal disease can have a variety of infectious and noninfectious causes.
- Dysbacteriosis is defined as a condition caused by an imbalance of the normal flora of the gastrointestinal tract. Dysbacteriosis is present in most cases of gastrointestinal disease in guinea pigs.
- Enteritis/dysbacteriosis/diarrhea
  - Dietary causes are considered more common in guinea pigs: overfeeding of fresh green feed or items high in simple carbohydrates (treats, grains); sudden changes in diet, etc.
  - Iatrogenic: antibiotic-induced dysbacteriosis secondary to oral administration of inappropriate antibiotics or ingestion of topical antibiotic, such as ointments used for topical wound management (e.g., triple antibiotic ointment), is also common in guinea pigs. Antibiotics such as cephalosporins, penicillins, clindamycin, and erythromycin should not be administered orally because of their predominant Gram-positive spectrum, which will lead to disturbance of the normal intestinal flora, followed by dysbacteriosis, septicemia, endotoxemia, enterotoxemia, and usually death.
  - Dental disease: dental malocclusion and intraoral pain can lead to improper chewing and selective food intake, with preference given to food items for which less chewing activity is necessary and that consequently are lower in fiber content; this may lead to dysbacteriosis and diarrhea
  - Primary gastrointestinal infections in guinea pigs are rare. Secondary infections with opportunistic pathogens are common and develop secondary to an initial disturbance of the intestinal flora, leading to dysbacteriosis and overgrowth of opportunistic pathogenic bacterial, parasitic, or fungal organisms.
  - Bacterial
    - *Escherichia coli, Pseudomonas aeruginosa, Listeria monocytogenes, Citrobacter freundii, Clostridium difficile, Clostridium perfringens*: overgrowth secondary to these organisms leads to enteritis, septicemia and endotoxemia, or enterotoxemia and is frequently fatal. Infection occurs usually by contaminated food; immune suppression and poor sanitation contribute to the development of clinical disease.
    - *Salmonella typhimurium, Salmonella enteritidis*: uncommon infection usually caused by contaminated feed; high mortality; immune suppression predisposed to development of clinical signs, including diarrhea, depression, and abortion
  - Parasitic
    - *Eimeria caviae*: strictly host specific; asymptomatic infection common, but immune suppression and poor sanitation can lead to clinical disease. Recently weaned guinea pigs are commonly affected. Clinical signs include watery diarrhea.
    - *Balantidium caviae, Entamoeba muris, Trichomonas caviae, Giardia duodenalis*: considered nonpathogenic but can cause enteritis in rare cases, if the guinea pig is immune compromised or is suffering from dysbacteriosis (i.e., secondary to dental disease). Organisms in low numbers may be seen during routine fecal examination of healthy animals.
    - *Cryptosporidium wrairi*: can cause cachexia and diarrhea, poor coat condition, and death in young or immune compromised guinea pigs by causing small intestinal enteritis; infection via ingestion of oocysts. Immune competent animals develop immunity and recover from infection within 4 weeks.
    - *Nematodes*: *Paraspidodera uncinata*: pinworm that resides in the large intestine and usually does not cause clinical symptoms. Due to its direct life cycle, heavy infections can occur if sanitation is poor and if the guinea pig is immune compromised
    - *Cestodes*: *Rodentolepis nana* (previously *Hymenolepis nana*) is rare in guinea pigs and is often asymptomatic. It does not require an intermediate host; therefore, large numbers of parasites can reside in the host, causing disease. Heavy infection will result in anorexia, diarrhea, weight loss, poor fur condition, and possible death.
  - Fungal
    - *Cyniclomyces guttulatus* (previously *Saccharomycopsis guttulata*): this yeast organism is part of the normal gastrointestinal flora. Overgrowth and diarrhea can be seen in cases of dysbacteriosis due to another (primary) cause, such as sudden diet change. Overgrowth is always considered a secondary problem; therefore, the primary cause should be identified.
- Tympany (see Gastric Dilatation Disease)
  - Secondary to dysbacteriosis, intestinal obstruction, or torsion
  - Severity of clinical signs changes with progression and degree of tympany.
  - Distended and tense abdomen
  - Hunched body posture or lateral recumbence in advanced cases
  - If animal is in shock (hypovolemic, septic), clinical findings can include hypothermia, tachypnea, tachycardia, severe depression, and pale mucous membranes.

DIAGNOSIS

DIFFERENTIAL DIAGNOSIS

Chronic diarrhea, weight loss, and poor coat condition: dental disease, hyperthyroidism (see Hyperthyroidism) and hypovitaminosis C (see Hypovitaminosis C)

INITIAL DATABASE

- Full dietary history
- Full husbandry history
- Consider the following tests based on clinical presentation:
  - Fecal flotation

- Fecal wet mount
- Fecal cytologic examination
- Whole-body radiographs
- Biochemistry profile: may be normal. Hyperglycemia, dehydration, and azotemia may be evident. Rule out concurrent diseases that will affect the prognosis (e.g., hepatic lipidosis, ketoacidosis, renal insufficiency).
- Complete blood count: hemoconcentration, anemia, leukocytosis, or leukopenia
- Urine analysis: ketonuria, low pH (normal urine pH 8-9), glucosuria

ADVANCED OR CONFIRMATORY TESTING

- Dental examination: rule out intraoral lesions (see Dental Disease)
- Fecal culture for enteric opportunistic pathogens (e.g., *Escherichia coli*, *Salmonella* spp.): interpretation may be difficult
- *Cryptosporidium* antigen ELISA

TREATMENT

THERAPEUTIC GOALS

- Rehydration and relief of discomfort
- Restoration of gastrointestinal motility and normal appetite
- Treatment of secondary infections and complications
- Treatment of primary underlying causes if possible

ACUTE GENERAL TREATMENT

- If animal is anorexic, dehydrated, or in discomfort, provide supportive care as needed:
  - Fluid therapy
    - Maintenance fluid rate: 60-100 mL/kg/d SC, PO, IV, IO
    - Replace fluid deficits and maintain normovolemia.
  - Nutritional support
    - Syringe-feed with high-fiber diet for herbivores (e.g., Oxbow Critical Care for Herbivores, 50-80 mL/kg PO q 24 h, divided into 4-5 feedings) or crushed and soaked pellets.
    - Vitamin C (50-100 mg/kg PO, SC q 24 h) for treatment of deficiencies; 10-30 mg/kg PO for maintenance
  - Analgesia: buprenorphine 0.02-0.05 mg/kg SC q 6-8 h
  - Antibiotic therapy
    - Not necessary if guinea pig is in stable condition, bright, alert, and is still eating
    - Consider antibiotics for treatment of predominantly Gram-negative opportunistic pathogens in guinea pigs with severe dysbacteriosis, and when an infectious cause is suspected but unconfirmed and the animal is in a compromised general condition.
    - Give antibiotics by injection (SC, IM, IV) and avoid the oral route in debilitated patients, patients with impaired gastrointestinal function, and in animals suspected to be septicemic.
    - Trimethoprim-sulfa 30 mg/kg PO q 12 h
    - Chloramphenicol 30-50 mg/kg PO, SC, IM, IV q 8 h
    - Metronidazole 20-30 mg/kg PO, IV q 12 h
    - Enrofloxacin 10-20 mg/kg SC, PO q 12-24 h
  - Antiparasitic therapy
    - Treat in-contact animals.
    - Clean and disinfect the environment to prevent reinfection: regular bedding changes and cage cleaning; discard cage furnishings that cannot be disinfected (e.g., wood-based furnishing)
    - Metronidazole 20-30 mg/kg PO q 12-24 h for 5 days for treatment of *Trichomonas*, *Entamoeba*, etc.
    - Fenbendazole 20-50 mg/kg PO q 24 h for 5 days for treatment of nematodes, as well as *Trichomonas*, *Entamoeba*, etc.
    - Trimethoprim-sulfa 30 mg/kg PO q 12-24 h for 5-10 days for treatment of *Eimeria*
    - Toltrazuril 10 mg/kg PO q 24 h for 3 days for treatment of *Eimeria*
    - Praziquantel 5-10 mg/kg SC, PO q 10 d for treatment of cestodes
    - No specific and effective treatment is available for *Cryptosporidium wrairi*.
  - Antifungal therapy
    - Nystatin 100,000 IU/kg PO q 8 h for 5 days if *C. guttulatus* overgrowth is high, or if no response to treatment of primary cause with dietary changes is seen
  - Tympany
    - Depends on degree of tympany: mild cases should be treated with supportive care (see earlier). Severe cases require aggressive cardiovascular support: oxygen, intravenous/intraosseous fluid therapy, and parenteral antibiotic therapy. After patient is stabilized, diagnose and treat the underlying cause.
    - Decompression via an orogastric tube placed under sedation. Trocarization carries risks that might outweigh the possible benefits
    - Antifoaming drugs such as simethicone 70 mg/kg q 1 h × 2-3 treatments have been recommended. Clinical efficacy is questionable, particularly in advanced cases of tympany.

CHRONIC TREATMENT

- Vitamin C 10-30 mg/kg PO for maintenance
- Dietary correction

POSSIBLE COMPLICATIONS

- Hepatic lipidosis
- Hypovitaminosis C
- Endotoxemia, enterotoxemia
- Sepsis

RECOMMENDED MONITORING

- Activity level
- Appetite
- Fecal output
- Urine output
- Body weight

PROGNOSIS AND OUTCOME

- Prognosis is generally better if an underlying primary cause can be identified and successfully treated.
- Good-fair: acute diarrhea if animal is still eating and is in good body condition, and if no inappropriate antibiotics have been administered orally
- Fair-poor: if animal is suffering from systemic disease or is cachexic, depressed, and dehydrated

CONTROVERSY

Use of prokinetic drugs in guinea pigs is controversial; clinical efficacy has not been demonstrated for any of the recommended drugs. Prokinetic drugs are contraindicated in cases in which an infectious process or an obstruction cannot be ruled out. Most guinea pigs with suspected underlying gastrointestinal hypomotility will respond to appropriate supportive care alone, including fluid therapy, analgesia, and nutritional support, making use of prokinetic drugs unnecessary.

PEARLS & CONSIDERATIONS

COMMENTS

After stabilization of the patient and restoration of normal gastrointestinal motility, the goal should be to identify and treat the primary underlying cause to improve the case outcome and reduce the risk of recurrence of clinical signs.

PREVENTION

- Most gastrointestinal disorders in guinea pigs are directly or indirectly husbandry and diet related. Adequate client education regarding nutritional needs and basic quarantine actions for newly acquired guinea pigs, including examination of feces and regular health checks, will prevent most gastrointestinal disorders in guinea pigs.

- Do not administer oral antibiotics such as cephalosporins, penicillins, erythromycin, and clindamycin. Do not use topical ointments that contain bacitracin (e.g., triple antibiotic ointment) because of risk of ingestion by chinchillas. Oral administration or accidental ingestion of these antibiotics can lead to dysbacteriosis, endotoxemia, enterotoxemia, and death.

CLIENT EDUCATION

Guinea pigs should be fed predominantly high-quality grass hay. Supplemental commercial guinea pig pellets should be offered. Vitamin C should be supplemented daily in the form of fresh vegetables (e.g., red pepper). Treats such as dried or fresh fruits and vegetables should be offered only occasionally; preference should be given to items low in carbohydrates. Fresh water must be available at all times.

SUGGESTED READINGS

Hawkins MG, et al: Disease problems of guinea pigs. In Carpenter JW, et al, editors: Ferrets, rabbits and rodents: clinical medicine and surgery, ed 3, St Louis, 2012, WB Saunders, pp 295–310.

Ward M: Rodents: digestive system disorders. In Keeble E, et al, editors: BSAVA manual of rodents and ferrets, Gloucester, UK, 2009, British Small Animal Veterinary Association, pp 123–141.

CROSS-REFERENCES TO OTHER SECTIONS

Anorexia
Dental Disease
Gastric Dilatation Disease
Hyperthyroidism
Hypovitaminosis C

AUTHOR: **CHRISTOPH MANS**

EDITOR: **THOMAS M. DONNELLY**

SMALL MAMMALS: GUINEA PIGS

Neurologic Disorders

BASIC INFORMATION

DEFINITION

Neurologic disorders are a group of symptoms related to abnormalities of the neurologic system, including the central and peripheral nervous system, characterized by mechanical noncoordination of the patient.

SYNONYMS

Ataxia, head tilt, torticollis, vestibular syndrome, paresis, paralysis, incoordination, seizure, fits, tremor, epilepsy, twitching

EPIDEMIOLOGY

SPECIES, AGE, SEX

- Recently introduced young individuals are prone to sarcoptic mange.
- Hypocalcemia can occur in females 1 week before or after parturition.
- Newborns that have suffered a difficult birth can exhibit brain damage.

CONTAGION AND ZOONOSIS

- *Streptococcus pneumoniae, Streptococcus zooepidemicus,* and *Bordetella bronchiseptica* are frequently isolated from the inner ear of guinea pigs.
- Lymphocytic choriomeningitis (LCM) (see Lymphocytic Choriomeningitis Virus, Sec. VI), a zoonotic virus transmitted by contaminated feces, through urine, or from a bite. Mice are the main reservoirs; this virus rarely causes clinical disease in pet guinea pigs.

ASSOCIATED CONDITIONS AND DISORDERS

- Hypovitaminosis C (see Hypovitaminosis C)
- Trauma

CLINICAL PRESENTATION

DISEASE FORMS/SUBTYPES

- Seizures
- Head tilt
- Leg paresis/paralysis

HISTORY, CHIEF COMPLAINT

- Seizures
  - Spontaneous cluster of seizures
  - Scratching
  - Tremor
  - Polypnea
- Head tilt
  - Torticollis
  - Nystagmus
  - Falling on side
  - Rolling over
- Leg paresis/paralysis
  - Lameness of one or both legs
  - Pododermatitis
  - History of trauma

PHYSICAL EXAM FINDINGS

- Head tilt
- Nystagmus (rare in vestibular guinea pigs)
- Normal consciousness or depression
- Painful response upon palpation of the limbs
- Painful response upon palpation of the spine
- Proprioceptive deficits (proprioceptive test can be difficult to perform in stressed guinea pigs)
- Abnormal withdrawal reflex
- Lack of deep pain

ETIOLOGY AND PATHOPHYSIOLOGY

- Seizurelike crisis can be caused by sarcoptic mange in guinea pigs.
- Seizures can be caused by a metabolic disease or an intracranial disease.
- Insulinomas and hypoglycemia have been repeatedly reported as the cause for seizures in guinea pigs.
- Head tilt is commonly caused by middle ear infection that has progressed to the inner ear.
- Paralysis may be secondary to hypovitaminosis C due to intramuscular hemorrhage.
- Chronic median and ulnar nerve compression at the level of the metacarpals can lead to forelimb paresis and weakness.
- LCM virus is an Arenavirus transmitted transplacentally, by inhalation, by ingestion, or through direct contact with urine, saliva, or feces. The major hosts are mice.

DIAGNOSIS

DIFFERENTIAL DIAGNOSIS

- Seizures
  - Infectious: sarcoptic mange *(Trixacarus caviae)*, toxemia, sepsis, LCM virus
  - Metabolic: insulinoma, liver failure, renal failure, ketosis, hypocalcemia, hypoglycemia
  - Toxic
  - Traumatic
  - Neoplastic
- Vestibular syndrome
  - Otitis media and interna
  - Parasitic *(Encephalitozoon cuniculi)*
- Paralysis
  - Trauma
  - Vitamin C deficiency
  - Median and ulnar neuropathy
  - Infectious (LCM virus)

INITIAL DATABASE

- Full dietary history
- Full history for potential exposure to toxins or mice (natural LCM virus reservoir)
- Skin scraping/skin cytologic exam: rule out sarcoptic mange
- Skull radiographs: assess for soft tissue opacity within the tympanic bullae or bony changes in the wall of the tympanic bullae, which are suggestive of otitis media
- Complete blood count: leukocytosis
- Biochemistry: hypoglycemia, hyperglycemia, hypocalcemia, increased liver enzymes and/or total bilirubin, azotemia

ADVANCED OR CONFIRMATORY TESTING

- MRI or CT scan: tympanic bulla abnormalities, intracranial lesions, anatomic/congenital defects
- If hypoglycemic: measure serum insulin levels to rule out insulinoma
- Cerebrospinal fluid (CSF) tap: cytology, bacterial culture
- LCM virus PCR (serum, CSF, biopsy and necropsy specimens), serology (IFA: serum, CSF)
- Electromyography (EMG): spontaneous activity potential, slow nerve conduction

TREATMENT

THERAPEUTIC GOALS

- Alleviate neurologic symptoms until recovery.
- Provide supportive care.

ACUTE GENERAL TREATMENT

- For seizures or head tilt: stop the cluster of seizures and restore balance
  - Benzodiazepines: midazolam 0.5-2 mg/kg SC, IM; diazepam 0.5-3 mg/kg IV or intrarectal. Repeat administration, if no effect.
  - Dextrose 50% 1-2 mL/kg IV, IO, PO. Dilute for IV/IO administration.
  - Calcium gluconate 50-100 mg/kg, IM (diluted), slow IV, or IO
  - Meclizine 12.5-25 mg/kg PO q 12 h in case of vestibular disease
- Antibiotic therapy
  - Trimethoprim-sulfa 30 mg/kg PO, IM q 12 h
  - Enrofloxacin 10-20 mg/kg IM, SC, PO, IV q 12-24 h
  - Chloramphenicol 30-50 mg/kg PO, SC, IM, IV q 8 h
- Trauma or painful condition
  - Buprenorphine 0.02-0.05 mg/kg SC, IM, or IV q 6-8 h
  - Meloxicam 0.3-0.5 mg/kg SC, IM, or IV q 24 h
- Nutritional support: critical care formula for herbivores: 50-80 mL/kg/d
- Fluid therapy: 100 mL/kg/d SC, IV, IO
- Hypovitaminosis C: vitamin C 100 mg/kg PO, SC, IM
- Sarcoptic mange
  - Ivermectin 0.2-0.5 mg/kg SC, PO q 7-14 d
  - Selamectin 15-30 mg/kg spot-on q 14-28 d

CHRONIC TREATMENT

- Vitamin C supplementation: 50-100 mg/kg PO q 24 h
- Nutritional support: critical care formula for herbivores: 50-80 mL/kg/d
- Fenbendazole 20 mg/kg PO for 28 days, in cases of positive *E. cuniculi* serologic testing
- Prolonged antibiotic therapy
- Seizure management: phenobarbital
- Pain management
- Surgery to relieve compression of median and ulnar nerves. Lesion occurs under the transverse cartilaginous bar, which supports the footpad.

POSSIBLE COMPLICATIONS

- Anorexia
- Hypovitaminosis C secondary to anorexia
- Decubitus wounds

RECOMMENDED MONITORING

- Neurologic status
- Fecal output

PROGNOSIS AND OUTCOME

Fair to poor depending on the cause

CONTROVERSY

Use of steroids is controversial.

PEARLS & CONSIDERATIONS

CLIENT EDUCATION

Although mice are the main hosts of LCM virus, guinea pigs are susceptible to LCM virus, and strict hygiene rules should be followed.

SUGGESTED READINGS

Anderson MH, et al: Changes in the forearm associated with median nerve compression at the wrist in the guinea-pig, J Neurol Neurosurg Psychiatry 33:70–79, 1970.

Boot R, et al: Otitis media in guinea pigs: pathology and bacteriology, Lab Anim 20: 242–248, 1986.

Burk RF, et al: A combined deficiency of vitamins e and c causes severe central nervous system damage in guinea pigs, J Nutr 136: 1576–1581, 2006.

Vannevel JY, et al: Insulinoma in 2 guinea pigs *(Cavia porcellus)*, Can Vet J 46:339–341, 2005.

CROSS-REFERENCES TO OTHER SECTIONS

Hypovitaminosis C

Lymphocytic Choriomeningitis Virus (Section VI)

AUTHOR: **HUYNH MINH**

EDITOR: **CHRISTOPH MANS**

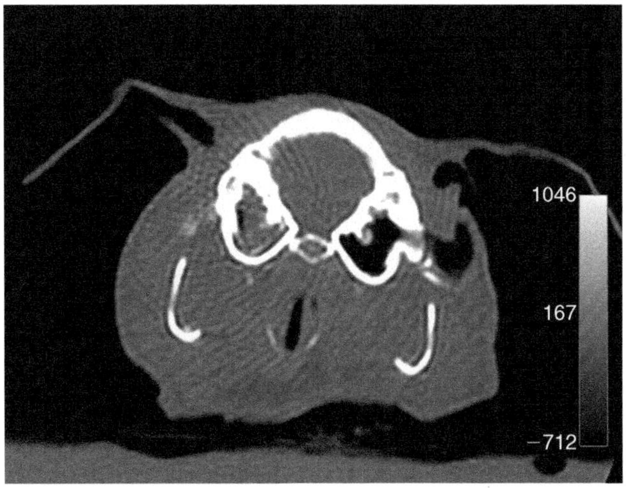

Neurologic Disorders Guinea pig neuro-otitis. Computed tomography image of the head of a guinea pig, which presented with left-sided head tilt. Note the soft tissue opacity within the left middle ear (arrow) consistent with otitis media. Compare the left middle ear with the black, air-filled appearance of the right middle ear.

SMALL MAMMALS: GUINEA PIGS

Ocular Disorders

BASIC INFORMATION

DEFINITION

Ocular disorders are characterized by any morphologic or anatomic abnormalities of the globe, including lesions of the eye itself, as well as of adjacent structures.

SYNONYMS

Corneal ulcer, eye discharge, epiphora, eye redness, conjunctivitis, uveitis, cataract, exophthalmos, fatty eye

SPECIAL SPECIES CONSIDERATIONS

- The menace reflex cannot be assessed in guinea pigs because they will not blink.
- Guinea pigs have a limited tear film, a rudimentary nictitating membrane, and a paurangiotic retina.

EPIDEMIOLOGY

SPECIES, AGE, SEX

- Cataracts can occur in animals as young as 9-10 months.
- Young animals from 1-4 weeks of age are most commonly affected by *Chlamydophila caviae.*
- Old animals frequently have an intraocular ectopic bone formation called *osseous choristoma.*

GENETICS AND BREED PREDISPOSITION

- *Listeria* spp. keratitis has been reported in hairless guinea pigs.
- "Fatty eye," a conjunctival lipid deposition, is more common in Self White, Black, Cream, and Rex breeds.
- Congenital defects (anophthalmos, cataracts) have been reported in Roan x Roan guinea pigs, and microphthalmia may be associated with all white-coated animals.
- Lens luxation secondary to cataracts has been described in Abyssinian guinea pigs.
- Corneal ulceration can occur by distichiasis and entropion in Texel guinea pigs.

RISK FACTORS

- Straw beddings and sharp pieces of plant material can traumatize the eye or can serve as foreign bodies.
- Inappropriate nutrition enhances the risk of dental malocclusion.

CONTAGION AND ZOONOSIS

- Conjunctivitis can be caused by *Chlamydophila caviae* and is contagious.
- Healthy carrier animals of *C. caviae* are common, and all in-contact animals of the collection should be treated.
- *C. caviae* is considered specific to guinea pigs; to date, the zoonotic potential is unknown and no cases in humans have been reported.

ASSOCIATED CONDITIONS AND DISORDERS

- Dental disease
- Hypovitaminosis C (see Hypovitaminosis C)
- Otitis media

CLINICAL PRESENTATION

DISEASE FORMS/SUBTYPES

- Corneal ulcer
- Eye discharge
- Conjunctivitis
- Exophthalmos

HISTORY, CHIEF COMPLAINT

- Eye discharge
- Abnormal white spot in the eye
- Sticky eye
- Blepharospasm
- Redness
- Third eyelid prolapse

PHYSICAL EXAM FINDINGS

- External aspect
  - Blepharospasm
  - Eye discharge
  - Exophthalmos
- Cornea
  - Opacity of the corneal surface
  - Ulceration
  - Foreign body
- Conjunctiva
  - Chemosis
  - Lipid deposit in the conjunctiva
- Intraocular
  - Mineral deposit on iris
  - Lens opacity (senile or diabetogenic cataracts)
- Assess the blinking response (palpebral and corneal reflexes).
- Assess the retropulsion of the globe.

ETIOLOGY AND PATHOPHYSIOLOGY

- *C. caviae* is a Gram-negative organism that replicates in the epithelial cells of the conjunctiva in guinea pigs. The infection is usually self-limiting.
- Osseous choristoma or heterotopic bone formation can occur in older animals, corresponding to mineralization of the ciliary body. The cause remains unknown.
- Exophthalmos is most commonly associated with periapical tooth abscess of the maxillary cheek teeth.

DIAGNOSIS

DIFFERENTIAL DIAGNOSIS

- Blepharitis
  - Dermatophytes *(Trichophyton mentagrophytes),* mainly in young animals
  - Hypovitaminosis C
- Eye discharge
  - Infectious (see Conjunctivitis)
  - Lacrimal duct obstruction
  - "Pea eye" protrusion of portions of the lacrimal glands
  - Dental disease
  - Hypovitaminosis C
- Corneal ulcer
  - External irritation
    - Foreign body
    - Trichiasis
    - Entropion
  - Tears deficiency
    - Keratoconjunctivitis sicca
    - Facial paralysis (secondary to otitis media)
    - Anesthesia
- Corneal abnormalities
  - Corneal edema
  - Corneal dermoid
  - Lymphosarcoma
  - Lipid or mineral deposit
- Conjunctivitis
  - Vitamin C deficiency
  - Infectious disease
    - *C. caviae*
    - *Streptococcus* spp.
    - *Bordetella bronchiseptica*
    - *Candida albicans*
  - Allergic conjunctivitis
  - "Fatty eye" (conjunctival lipid deposit)
- Intraocular abnormalities
  - Cataract
  - Osseous choristoma
- Exophthalmos
  - Periapical abscess of maxillary cheek teeth
  - Trauma
  - Neoplasia

INITIAL DATABASE

- Full husbandry and dietary history
- Ophthalmic exam (including fundus examination)
  - Schirmer test (3.8 ± 1.3 mm/min)
  - Fluorescein test
  - Intraocular eye pressure (normal value, 16.5 ± 3.2 mm Hg)
- Conjunctival cytologic exam: intracytoplasmic inclusion body may be seen in epithelial cells infected by *C. caviae,* if stained with Macchiavello or Giemsa stain

- Skull radiographs
- Dental examination (under general anesthesia, preferably endoscopy-guided)

ADVANCED OR CONFIRMATORY TESTING

- *Chlamydophila* PCR from conjunctival swab
- CT/MRI scan: screening for retrobulbar mass effect, sinusitis, lacrimal duct obstruction
- Complete blood count: leukocytosis
- Biochemistry: hyperglycemia
- Occular ultrasound: screening for retrobulbar mass

TREATMENT

THERAPEUTIC GOALS

- Protect the integrity of the eye surface.
- Limit and stabilize intraocular damage.

ACUTE GENERAL TREATMENT

- Eye lubricant
- Topical antibiotic
  - Ciprofloxacin ophthalmic drops/ointment q 4-12 h
  - (Oxy-) tetracycline ophthalmic drops/ointment q 4-6 h
  - Tobramycin ophthalmic drops q 4-6 h (ineffective against *Chlamydophila*)
  - Gentamicin ophthalmic drops/ointment q 4-6 h (ineffective against *Chlamydophila*)
- Topical analgesia
  - Flurbiprofen drops q 4-6 h
  - Diclofenac drops q 4-6 h
  - Atropine drops/ointment (0.5%-1%) q 4-6 h
- Systemic analgesia
  - Buprenorphine 0.02-0.05 mg/kg SC q 6-8 h
  - Meloxicam 0.3-0.5 mg/kg PO, SC q 24 h
- Anticollagenase therapy in cases of deep corneal ulcer
  - *N*-Acetylcysteine topical drops q 2-6 h
  - Autologous serum eye drops q 4-6 h
- Steroidal therapy in cases of suspected allergic conjunctivitis without corneal ulceration
  - Prednisolone ophthalmic drops q 4-6 h
- Blepharitis secondary to dermatophytosis
  - Systemic antifungal therapy
    - Terbinafine 20-30 mg/kg PO q 24 h
    - Itraconazole 5-10 mg/kg PO q 24 h
  - Topical antifungal therapy
    - Enilconazole (1:40 emulsions as spray or moist wipe)

CHRONIC TREATMENT

- Antibiotic treatment
  - Enrofloxacin 20 mg/kg PO q 12-24 h
  - Metronidazole 20-30 mg/kg PO q 12 h
- Nonsteroidal antiinflammatory
  - Meloxicam 0.3-0.5 mg/kg q 24 h PO
- Dental procedure in cases of tooth root involvement; enucleation is often required in cases of retrobulbar abscesses.
- Provide vitamin C 100 mg/kg PO q 24 h.
- Keratectomy in cases of recurrent ulcer
- Enucleation

DRUG INTERACTIONS

Topical drops should not be mixed and should be given at least at 20-minute intervals.

POSSIBLE COMPLICATIONS

- Panophthalmia
- Corneal perforation

RECOMMENDED MONITORING

- Corneal edema and ulceration
- Exophthalmos

PROGNOSIS AND OUTCOME

Excellent to poor according to the cause

CONTROVERSY

Schirmer tear test values are controversial in this species; normal values ranging from 0.36 ± 1.1 mm/min to 3.8 ± 1.3 mm/min have been published in various studies.

PEARLS & CONSIDERATIONS

PREVENTION

- Provide soft and dust-free bedding.
- Provide food rich in vitamin C.

SUGGESTED READING

Coster ME, et al: Results of diagnostic ophthalmic testing in healthy guinea pigs, J Am Vet Med Assoc 232:1825–1833, 2008.
Williams D, et al: Ocular disease in the guinea pig *(Cavia porcellus)*: a survey of 1000 animals, Vet Ophthalmol 13(Suppl):54–62, 2010.

CROSS-REFERENCES TO OTHER SECTIONS

Conjunctivitis
Hypovitaminosis C

AUTHOR: **HUYNH MINH**

EDITOR: **CHRISTOPH MANS**

SMALL MAMMALS: GUINEA PIGS

Ovarian Cysts

Client Education Sheet and Additional Images Available on Website

BASIC INFORMATION

DEFINITION

Ovarian cysts may be unilateral or bilateral, may contain clear serous fluid, and may grow up to 2-4 cm in diameter.

SYNONYM

Cystic ovaries

SPECIAL SPECIES CONSIDERATIONS

Multiple ovarian cysts are usually present on the ovaries of female guinea pigs older than 1 year. As female guinea pigs age they develop more and bigger cysts. Although no statistically significant correlation has been noted between reproductive history and the prevalence of cysts, breeding records may indicate reduced fertility in affected females older than 15 months.

EPIDEMIOLOGY

GENETICS AND BREED PREDISPOSITION Ovarian serous cysts are a normal component of the cyclic guinea pig ovary. Alterations in the inhibin-follicle–stimulating hormone system appear to modulate the development and incidence of serous cysts.

RISK FACTORS

- The presence of ovarian cysts is associated with a higher incidence of cystic endometrial hyperplasia, mucometra, endometritis, and fibroleiomyoma.

ASSOCIATED CONDITIONS AND DISORDERS Uterine leiomyomas are often seen in conjunction with serous cysts.

CLINICAL PRESENTATION

HISTORY, CHIEF COMPLAINT Owners may see anorexia (see Anorexia), alopecia, depression, and signs related to the urinary tract, such as dysuria, anuria, and occasionally hematuria.

PHYSICAL EXAM FINDINGS

- Clinical examination generally reveals palpable abdominal masses.
- Alopecia in guinea pigs with ovarian cysts is rare; the reported incidence is <5% (see Skin Diseases).

ETIOLOGY AND PATHOPHYSIOLOGY

- In guinea pigs, three types of ovarian cysts are observed:
  - Serous cysts (cystic rete ovarii)
  - Follicular cysts
  - Parovarian cysts
- These cysts can be differentiated only histologically.
- The most common ovarian cysts are serous cysts. In one study, serous cysts were present throughout the estrous cycle, with an overall incidence of 64%.
  - Serous cysts are cystic rete ovarii. Serous cysts are lined with a simple cuboidal-to-columnar epithelium composed of cells bearing solitary cilia or tufts of cilia. Cells of these cysts do not have the ultrastructural characteristics of steroid-synthesizing cells, nor do they possess 3β-hydroxysteroid dehydrogenase activity. Thus, serous cysts appear incapable of steroidogenesis and do respond to surges of luteinizing hormone, similar to a follicular cyst.
- Follicular cysts occurred in 22% of guinea pigs in one study. Follicular cysts always coincide with serous cysts but are less common during diestrus.
  - Follicular cysts are derived from preovulatory follicles that fail to ovulate. The aberrant follicular structure reaches ovulatory size, fails to ovulate, and alters normal ovarian cyclicity. Traditionally, follicular cysts (in cattle and horses) are considered as large anovulatory, follicular structures that lack a functional corpus luteum. The wall is lined by flattened granulosa cells separated from thecal cells.
- Parovarian cysts are rare
  - A parovarian cyst is a cyst of the epoophoron or parovarium, a vestigial structure associated with the ovary, consisting of a cranial group of mesonephric tubules and a corresponding portion of the mesonephric duct.

DIAGNOSIS

DIFFERENTIAL DIAGNOSIS

Other causes of abdominal masses in guinea pigs include splenic hematoma, splenic and uterine hemangiomas, uterine fibroma, and ovarian teratoma.

INITIAL DATABASE

- Complete blood count and biochemistry profile: usually unremarkable
- Imaging
  - Diagnosis of ovarian cysts by plain radiography is difficult because of the similar opacity of ovarian cysts and abdominal neoplasms.
  - Ultrasonography allows imaging of the inner structure of the masses. Ultrasonographic features of fluid-filled cysts >2 cm in diameter include compartmentalization and connection to the ovary.

ADVANCED OR CONFIRMATORY TESTING

Always perform histopathologic examination on excised ovarian cysts to evaluate for the presence of ovarian neoplasia.

TREATMENT

THERAPEUTIC GOALS

The usual treatment of choice for cystic ovaries in guinea pigs is surgical removal of the reproductive tract. In certain cases, surgery might not be a suitable option owing to the high anesthetic risk status of the patient. Ultrasound-guided aspiration of the cyst provides an adequate temporary solution in these cases. However, aspiration usually needs to be followed by medical and/or surgical treatment to prevent rapid reaccumulation of fluid.

ACUTE GENERAL TREATMENT

- A diagnosis of ovarian cyst does not indicate the type of ovarian cyst. Although surgery is the definitive treatment, hormonal therapy may be attempted when ovarian follicular cysts are present. If cysts fail to shrink in response to treatment, they were not follicular cysts, and surgery becomes the preferred method of treatment.
- Follicular cysts
  - Human chorionic gonadotropin (hCG) at a dose of 1000 IU/guinea pig IM repeated in 7-10 days can be used to treat follicular ovarian cysts in guinea pigs. However, at this dosage, the volume is approximately 1 mL, which is a large volume to be given to a guinea pig. Furthermore, hCG will stimulate an antibody response, making the second and third doses potentially less effective, and possibly stimulating an allergic reaction following subsequent injections. In humans, hCG injection can cause local irritation, edema, and pain.
  - An alternative drug that may be used to treat follicular ovarian cysts is gonadotropin-releasing hormone (GnRH). Veterinary uses of GnRH typically include treating ovarian cysts in cattle and inducing estrus in cats. GnRH is a neuropeptide, so it does not stimulate an immune response. A dose of 25 μg/animal q 2 wk for 2 injections is effective. The commercially available form of GnRH (Cystorelin, Merial) is available in a multidose vial for injection at a concentration of 50 μg/mL. The 0.5-mL volume of the injection is significantly less than that recommended for hCG, making it tolerable for the small patient.
- Serous and parovarian cysts
  - Perform surgery.

DRUG INTERACTIONS

- GnRH is used for the treatment of ovarian follicular cysts in dairy cattle. Preparations of hCG, luteinizing hormone (LH), and progesterone are used to treat ovarian follicular cysts in cattle, but treatment outcomes are highly variable.
- Ovarian follicular cysts are nonovulated follicles with incomplete luteinization. Historically, cystic ovaries in cattle and horses have responded to an exogenous source of LH such as hCG. GnRH initiates release of normal physiologic levels of endogenous LH to cause luteinization of the follicular cyst wall. It then degenerates as a corpus luteum (i.e., goes to corpus albicans and then atresia).
- Ovulation of a follicular cyst in response to GnRH treatment usually does not occur. However, luteinization of follicular cysts following GnRH treatment does occur.

RECOMMENDED MONITORING

If hCG or GnRH fails to cause degeneration of the ovarian cyst, the guinea pig probably has serous cysts (cystic rete ovarii) or may even have a parovarian cyst. Surgical removal of the reproductive tract then becomes the de facto treatment of choice.

PROGNOSIS AND OUTCOME

- Good
- Advanced age, ovarian-hypophyseal imbalance, and ovarian cysts appear to favor development of ovarian

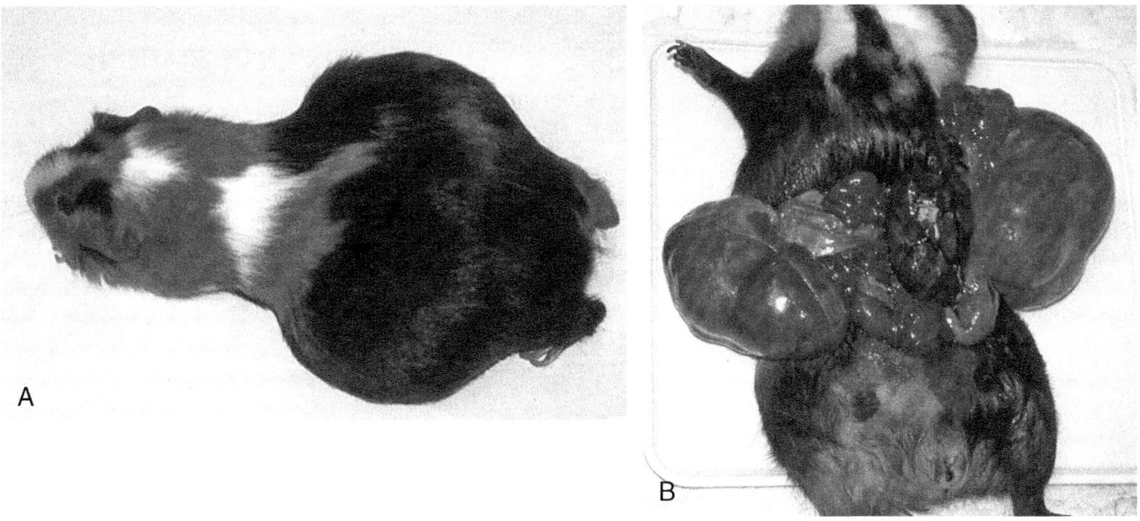

Ovarian Cysts A, Female guinea pig with bilateral abdominal swellings caused by ovarian cysts. **B,** Image of the same guinea pig in **A** showing large fluid-filled cysts on both ovaries. *(Courtesy Virginia C.G. Richardson.)*

neoplasia. Limited reports have described ovarian neoplasms in guinea pigs; most tumors are ovarian teratomas or granulosa cell tumors. These tumors do not appear to metastasize.

PEARLS & CONSIDERATIONS

COMMENTS

Guinea pig gonadotrophin-releasing hormone (gpGnRH) has a lower biological activity compared with other mammalian species' GnRH due to its unique two amino acid substitutions. This structural change is accompanied by affinity changes in the gpGnRH receptor. Consequently, treatment with GnRH agonists (e.g., deslorelin) that selectively bind to and activate other mammalian species GnRH receptors, may not cause GnRH stimulation in guinea pigs. To date, one report describes no reduction in ovarian cyst size with deslorelin implants.

PREVENTION

Early neutering of female guinea pigs will prevent ovarian cysts and uterine disorders, including neoplasia.

SUGGESTED READINGS

Beregi A, et al: Ultrasonic diagnosis of ovarian cysts in ten guinea pigs, Vet Radiol Ultrasound 40:74–76, 1999.

Field KJ, et al: Spontaneous reproductive tract leiomyomas in aged guinea-pigs, J Comp Pathol 101:287–294, 1989.

Mayer J: The use of GnRH to treat cystic ovaries in guinea pig, Exotic DVM 5:36, 2003.

Nielsen TD, et al: Ovarian cysts in guinea pigs: influence of age and reproductive status on prevalence and size, J Small Anim Pract 44:257–260, 2003.

Schuetzenhofer G, et al: Effects of deslorelin implants on ovarian cysts in guinea pigs, Schweiz Arch Tierheilkd 153:416–417, 2011.

Shi FX, et al: Serous cysts are a benign component of the cyclic ovary in the guinea pig with an incidence dependent upon inhibin bioactivity, J Vet Med Sci 64:129–135, 2002.

CROSS-REFERENCES TO OTHER SECTIONS

Anorexia
Skin Diseases

AUTHORS: **THOMAS M. DONNELLY AND VIRGINIA C.G. RICHARDSON**

EDITOR: **CHRISTOPH MANS**

SMALL MAMMALS: GUINEA PIGS

Perineal Sac Impaction or Rectal Impaction

BASIC INFORMATION

DEFINITION

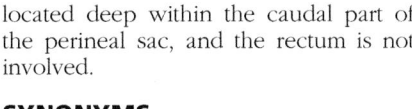

Fecal matter and a thick sebaceous secretion accumulate in the perineal sac especially of older male guinea pigs. Whether this accumulation is normal or abnormal is debated. However, in older, obese male guinea pigs, the accumulation is excessive, and owners object to the smell. Sometimes the perineal sac becomes inflamed. The result is known as *perineal sac impaction,* although older texts incorrectly call the condition *rectal impaction.* The latter term is incorrect because the anus is located deep within the caudal part of the perineal sac, and the rectum is not involved.

SYNONYMS

- Perineal sac: circumanal skin fold(s)
- Perineal sac impaction: anal fold dermatitis

SPECIAL SPECIES CONSIDERATIONS

- In the guinea pig, two distinct scent-producing areas—the prominent sebaceous gland located mid-dorsally above the caudal vertebrae and the perineal gland located within the perineal sac (circumanal skin fold)—are known. Both gland areas are much more highly developed in males than in females.
- Material from the perineal gland is deposited during the perineal drag—a behavior pattern in which an animal moves its perineal region across a surface. This behavior deposits olfactory communicants and is a form of scent marking. Both male and female guinea pigs engage in this behavior, but it is more common in males.

- Males scent mark when the environment is altered, during male–male aggressive encounters, and during courtship activities.
- Perineal dragging is most common when the environment is changed because the chemicals (pheromones) deposited during scent marking serve to familiarize a new environment and to mark the home range or territory. Scent marking may repel other males, may attract females, or may serve both functions.
- Urine and bacteria are responsible for components of biologically significant odors of guinea pig perineal scent marks.

EPIDEMIOLOGY

SPECIES, AGE, SEX

- The perineal scent gland is testosterone dependent. The perineal sac is much less developed in females and castrated males.
- Perineal scent gland sebum production increases dramatically at 4-5 weeks, when circulating testosterone levels are increasing.
- Sebum production is dependent on rank—dominant males produce more sebum.

RISK FACTORS

- Obesity, improper feeding, coarse straw bedding, and unsanitary conditions are often associated with perineal sac impaction.
- When guinea pigs are group housed, the condition is seen more frequently in the dominant male guinea pig.

ASSOCIATED CONDITIONS AND DISORDERS Balanoposthitis (inflammation of the penis and prepuce) due to impaction of sebaceous secretions and hairs within the prepuce is often seen in male guinea pigs with perineal sac impaction.

CLINICAL PRESENTATION

HISTORY, CHIEF COMPLAINT Many owners object to the odor and dropping of malodorous fecal pellets and discharge.

PHYSICAL EXAM FINDINGS

- In the deep part of this mucocutaneous area are many sebaceous scent glands that produce a thick, oily malodorous secretion that mixes with keratin and feces.
- Perineal pruritus and discharge may be seen.

ETIOLOGY AND PATHOPHYSIOLOGY

- Feces and sebaceous material accumulate in the perineal sac.
- Foreign objects such as bedding (e.g., straw, hay, wood shavings) and the animal's hairs can accumulate in the perineal sac, hardening the contents and causing true impaction.
- Inflammation and pruritus follow.

DIAGNOSIS

DIFFERENTIAL DIAGNOSIS

- Perineal abscessation
- Perineal neoplasia

INITIAL DATABASE

Examination of perineal sac and contents is usually diagnostic.

TREATMENT

THERAPEUTIC GOAL

Prevent chronic accumulation of perineal sac contents.

ACUTE GENERAL TREATMENT

- Normal check and cleaning of this area, as well as proper husbandry, are enough to prevent or correct this problem.
- Gentle removal of perineal sac contents and regular cleaning with a cotton-tipped applicator and oil are sufficient to keep the area clean.
- If the perineal sac is inflamed, careful cleaning with diluted chlorhexidine solution and application of silver sulfadiazine cream is recommended.
- Correct sanitary problems if guinea pig husbandry is poor.
- Advise owners to avoid coarse bedding (e.g., straw, hay, wood shavings).

CHRONIC TREATMENT

Castration (see Castration, Sec. II) will reduce the size of the perineal sac and will reduce the quantities of sebaceous secretions.

POSSIBLE COMPLICATIONS

Risk of scrotal panniculitis.

PROGNOSIS AND OUTCOME

With regular cleaning of perineal sac and good husbandry, prognosis is excellent.

PEARLS & CONSIDERATIONS

COMMENTS

Whether the perineal sac is impacted or whether accumulation of feces and sebaceous secretions has occurred in the boar is not well established. The important aspect of this condition is that owners object to the smell and to scent marking, which leaves impacted feces smeared on the perineal area of the boar.

PREVENTION

- Weekly cleaning of perineal sac with cotton-tipped applicator and oil
- Good husbandry

CLIENT EDUCATION

Material from the perineal glands is placed on the substrate during the perineal drag. The guinea pig squats and pulls its hindquarters forward, dragging the perineum across the ground. When males "rump" (lift one or rarely both hind legs over the back or rump of a female), material from the perineal gland is placed on the female.

SUGGESTED READINGS

Beauchamp GK: The perineal scent gland and social dominance in the male guinea pig, Physiol Behav 13:669–673, 1974.

Donnelly TM, et al: Guinea pig and chinchilla care and husbandry, Vet Clin North Am Exot Anim Pract 7:351–373, 2004.

Multiple authors: Discussion thread on guinea pig cloaca (male guinea pig anal fold), February 18, 2006, Exotic DVM Professional Forum, Website at ExoticDVM@yahoogroups.com.

CROSS-REFERENCES TO OTHER SECTIONS

Castration (Section II)

AUTHOR: **THOMAS M. DONNELLY**

EDITOR: **CHRISTOPH MANS**

Pododermatitis

Client Education Sheet and Additional Images Available on Website

BASIC INFORMATION

DEFINITION

Pododermatitis is a chronic inflammation of the palmar or plantar footpads. In simple cases, it involves ulceration of the footpad; in complex cases, cellulitis, synovitis, tendonitis, and osteomyelitis of footpad structures may be noted.

SYNONYM

Bumblefoot, sore hocks

EPIDEMIOLOGY

RISK FACTORS Pododermatitis is a common condition seen in obese guinea pigs housed on wire or abrasive floors. Poor sanitation is a predisposing factor and contributes to pododermatitis in guinea pigs not housed on abrasive or wire floors.

CONTAGION AND ZOONOSIS

- *Staphylococcus aureus* is frequently involved in the disease process and probably enters the foot through a cutaneous wound from wire or abrasive flooring.
- Awns and straw in the bedding can cause foot punctures.
- Inflammation can progress to osteoarthritis and systemic amyloidosis secondary to chronic staphylococcal infection.

ASSOCIATED CONDITIONS AND DISORDERS Inflammation of associated footpad structures, including tendonitis, synovitis, and osteomyelitis

CLINICAL PRESENTATION

DISEASE FORMS/SUBTYPES

- Ulcers are often graded according to severity:
  - Grade I lesions affect the epidermis and the superficial dermis.
  - Grade II lesions extend to the subcutis. Ulcer edges are often undermined.
  - Grade III lesions extend to the deep fascia.
  - Grade IV lesions involve the underlying bone.

HISTORY, CHIEF COMPLAINT

- The owner may notice swollen paws, lameness, and reluctance to move.
- Poor cage cleaning, housing of patient in wire-bottomed cage or cage with traumatic, rough surfaces
- Coarse straw bedding can also cause abrasion and penetrating footpad injuries.

PHYSICAL EXAM FINDINGS

- Patients are often obese and sedentary.
- Wide range of clinical signs:
  - Nonspecific findings such as anorexia, depression, or weight loss
  - Specific findings such as lameness of affected limb(s)
  - No overt clinical signs; ulceration may be an incidental finding on clinical examination
- Affected footpads show erythema (mild), blistering (moderate), and ulceration (severe); ulcerated lesions are covered by dry scab.

ETIOLOGY AND PATHOPHYSIOLOGY

Pressure-induced ischemia and inflammation from a variety of factors such as obesity, coarse bedding, penetrating footpad injury, and chronic wet bedding from poor husbandry produce abnormally thickened footpad epithelium and/or a footpad wound. Prolonged pressure compresses capillary circulation, causing tissue damage or necrosis and producing an ulcer. Chronic active inflammation (granulomatous cellulitis) spreads in the footpad and the paw.

DIAGNOSIS

DIFFERENTIAL DIAGNOSIS

Lesions of bumblefoot are unique and should not be confused with other conditions.

INITIAL DATABASE

- Complete blood count (CBC)/Biochemistry
  - Often unremarkable; the main purpose of the CBC is to determine whether an infectious process is occurring. Leukocytosis, typically characterized by lymphocytosis, may be seen. Long-standing cases of chronic pododermatitis can develop systemic amyloidosis secondary to chronic staphylococcal infection. In such animals, kidney and liver parameters may be abnormal.

ADVANCED OR CONFIRMATORY TESTING

- Histopathologic examination
  - Interpretation of biopsies from a footpad with pododermatitis may be misleading to pathologists who do not routinely examine rodent tissues.
  - The exuberant nature of the chronic-active inflammation may cause it to be mistaken for a fibrosarcoma.
- Bacteriology
  - Swab cultures do not effectively reveal the infecting organism because they collect only surface-contaminating organisms.
  - Tissue biopsy and culture, fluid aspiration cultures, and bone biopsy may be better alternatives for culturing the infecting organism.
- Imaging
  - Untreated chronic pododermatitis can progress to osteoarthritis and rarely to osteomyelitis. Radiographs of the affected paw (two views) are useful in revealing the extent of inflammation before treatment, during monitoring of treatment, and when a prognosis is needed. Osteoarthritic and osteomyelitic footpads have poorer prognoses.

TREATMENT

THERAPEUTIC GOALS

- Resolution of inflammation and infection in the paw
- Reepithelialization of the footpad

ACUTE GENERAL TREATMENT

- Surgery
  - Surgical treatment is often unsuccessful because an abscess to be excised or drained is rarely present. The lesion is a diffuse cellulitis that infiltrates surrounding tissue.
  - Cutting the tissue generally results in severe bleeding.

CHRONIC TREATMENT

- Nursing care
  - Good management of the ulcer is critical for healing. However, treatment is prolonged (may take 3-6 months) and is labor-intensive. Healing requires dedication by the owner to commit time in caring for the ulcer.
- Wound cleansing
  - Weigh benefits of cleaning against trauma to the tissue bed caused by cleaning. The affected paw should be soaked in a warm saline solution before the wound dressing is applied.
  - In the initial phases of treatment when the footpad ulcer can be considered an infected chronic wound, it is appropriate to use cleansers and disinfectants until the infection has resolved.
  - Most wound disinfectants may slow wound healing because they are cytotoxic to fibroblasts, reduce

WBC viability, and decrease phagocytic efficiency. Therefore, only use wound disinfectants (e.g., chlorhexidine, povidone iodine) in infected wounds.
- Wound dressing
  - Apply a hydrogel or hydrocolloidal wound dressing over the entire ulcer.
  - Hydrogel wound covers (e.g., gauze, sheet) are preferable initially compared with hydrogel wound filler because hydrogel wound covers do not have to be changed every day. In addition, hydrogel wound fillers contain large amounts of propylene glycol, which can sting when applied to raw tissue.
  - Use hydrogels on wounds with minimal or no exudate; use hydrocolloids on wounds that are draining low to moderate amounts of exudate.
  - Unless the wound is obviously infected, do not apply a topical antimicrobial.
  - Protective padding should be applied over primary wound dressing.
  - The combined wound dressing, padding, and adhesive bandage should not be so thick that the patient cannot use its leg.
  - In early stages of wound dressing, daily assessment and redressing of the wound may be required.
  - Redressing of the wound may be adjusted to twice weekly or once weekly once the patient has adapted to the wound dressing.
- Antibiotics
  - Long-term antibiotic administration throughout the course of treatment is essential. Treatment may be required for as long as 2-6 months. Enrofloxacin 10-20 mg/kg PO q 12-24 h and ciprofloxacin 10-20 mg/kg PO q 12-24 h are safe and effective antibiotics in guinea pigs.
  - Antibiotics may have to be reassessed for efficacy during the course of treatment.
- Analgesia
  - Analgesia is essential. Any swelling in the footpad is extremely painful.
    - Meloxicam 0.3-0.5 mg/kg PO, SC q 24 h
    - Buprenorphine 0.03-0.05 mg/kg SC q 6-12 h

RECOMMENDED MONITORING

- Regularly review wound management and reassess the choice of dressings.
- Measure and record the diameter of the ulcer at each dressing to assess progress. Consider using a digital camera to take pictures that can be used to assess progress.

PROGNOSIS AND OUTCOME

With time, ulcerated lesions generally heal and reepithelialize; however, some healed lesions are predisposed to ulcerate again. Often, affected paws remain swollen after healing. These guinea pigs may need to wear a permanent soft boot on the affected paw.

CONTROVERSY

- Use of laser therapy (phototherapy)
  - Some clinicians recommend the use of low-level laser therapy to accelerate healing. The efficacy of such treatment has not yet been proved.

PEARLS & CONSIDERATIONS

COMMENTS

- Most hydrocolloids react with wound exudate to form a gel-like covering that protects the wound bed and maintains a moist wound environment.
- The clinician should focus on a wound dressing material that is able to hydrate dry wounds without macerating the skin around the wound, and that can, if necessary, actively pull (as opposed to absorb passively) exudate from exuding wounds.

PREVENTION

- Reduce weight of obese guinea pigs.
- Remove wire or abrasive flooring.
- Remove straw or hay bedding.
- Clean animals' living quarters daily. Guinea pigs will defecate and urinate in their living quarters. Unless their housing is cleaned daily, guinea pigs will stand in wet, fecal contaminated bedding.

CLIENT EDUCATION

- Warn owners that chronic pododermatitis is a slow healing condition that may require 2-6 months to heal.
- Clients need to revisit their veterinarian regularly for reassessment and redressing of the wound. Even with

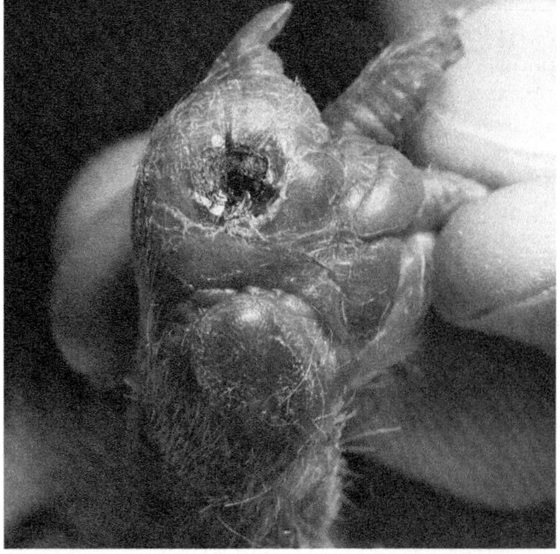

Pododermatitis Grade 3 pododermatitis of the palmar aspect of the left fore limb in a guinea pig. Note the deep ulceration and the marked soft tissue swelling.

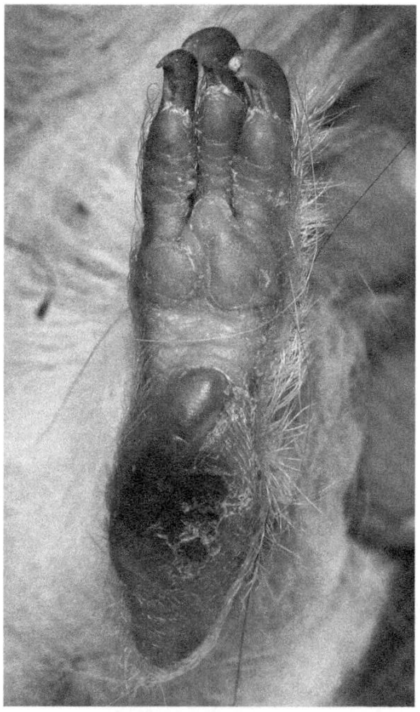

Pododermatitis Grade 1 pododermatitis of the plantar aspect of the left hind limb in a guinea pig.

experienced clients, do not let the revisit period exceed 2 weeks.
- Most clients cannot reassess and redress the wound suitably. Redressing requires at least two experienced persons.
- If the guinea pig is overweight, encourage the client to reduce the pet's weight.

SUGGESTED READINGS

Bohmer E, et al: Osteolysis of the second and third toe [German], Tierarztl Prax Ausg K Kleintiere Heimtiere 25:468–470, 1997.
Brown C, et al: Treatment of pododermatitis in the guinea pig, Lab Anim NY 37:156–157, 2008.
Taylor JL, et al: Chronic pododermatitis in guinea pigs: a case report, Lab Anim Sci 21:944–945, 1971.

AUTHORS: **CYNTHIA BROWN AND THOMAS M. DONNELLY**

EDITOR: **CHRISTOPH MANS**

SMALL MAMMALS: GUINEA PIGS

Pregnancy and Parturient Disorders

BASIC INFORMATION

DEFINITION

Diseases associated with pregnancy and the postpregnancy period

SYNONYMS

Dystocia, pregnancy toxemia

SPECIAL SPECIES CONSIDERATIONS

- Guinea pigs have a bicornuate uterus with a short uterine body (12 mm long), a single cervix, and a vaginal closure membrane that seals the vaginal orifice but is absent during estrus and at parturition.
- Females are sexually mature by 1-2 months.
- Guinea pigs are nonseasonally polyestric, and the duration of each estrus cycle is 15-17 days. Estrus lasts for about 6-11 hours, and ovulation is spontaneous.
- Gestation period averages 68 days (59-72 days), and litter size ranges from 1-13, but most litters consist of 2-4 pups.

EPIDEMIOLOGY

SPECIES, AGE, SEX Female guinea pigs of any age

RISK FACTORS
- First breeding after 7 months of age
- Poor husbandry
- Obesity
- Poor nutrition

CLINICAL PRESENTATION

DISEASE FORMS/SUBTYPES
- Dystocia
- Pregnancy toxemia
- Uterine torsion

HISTORY, CHIEF COMPLAINT
- Lethargy
- Inappetence
- Difficult or prolonged pregnancy or birthing

PHYSICAL EXAM FINDINGS
- Vaginal discharge
- Partially birthed fetus
- Prolapsed vagina/uterus
- Animals suffering from pregnancy toxemia stop eating and initially are depressed, then become comatose and usually die within 5-6 days if the condition is not recognized early.
- In cases of uterine torsion, one may find signs of shock, lateral recumbence, dyspnea, and/or seizures.

ETIOLOGY AND PATHOPHYSIOLOGY

- Dystocia
  - Guinea pigs have a high perinatal mortality.
  - Dystocia and stillbirths are related to large fetuses, subclinical ketosis, and fusion of the symphysis pubis.
  - If females are bred after 7 months of age, the symphysis pubis often fuses and does not separate during parturition.
- Pregnancy toxemia
  - Although clinical signs are similar, two forms of pregnancy toxemia have been recognized: the fasting/metabolic form and the circulatory or preeclampsia form. Both occur in late pregnancy.
  - Metabolic pregnancy toxemia occurs in obese sows, especially females in their first or second pregnancy. The disease is caused by increased energy demands due to fetal growth, leading to a negative energy imbalance and increased fat mobilization. Changes in feeding routine, obesity, and stress may be predisposing factors.
  - The circulatory or preeclampsia form is due to uteroplacental ischemia. The gravid uterus compresses uterine and other blood vessels, resulting in significant reduction of blood to the uterine vessels. Placental necrosis, hemorrhage, ketosis, and death follow. If suspected, emergency cesarean section and/or ovariohysterectomy is required to save the sow's life.

DIAGNOSIS

DIFFERENTIAL DIAGNOSIS

- Pyometra
- Endometritis (see Uterine and Vaginal Disorders)
- Cystic ovaries (see Ovarian Cysts)
- Other causes of shock, including hypovolemic or endotoxemic or septic shock
- Rectal prolapse
- Mammary gland neoplasia

INITIAL DATABASE

- If a female strains continually for longer than 20 minutes or fails to produce pups after 2 hours of intermittent straining, consider dystocia.
- Careful examination is performed to assess how much separation of the symphysis pubis is present. At least the width of the index finger is needed to permit passage of the fetus.
- Abdominal radiographs
- Abdominal ultrasound
- Complete blood count, biochemistry panel, urinalysis

TREATMENT

THERAPEUTIC GOAL

- Stabilization of the patient
- Resolution of dystocia

ACUTE GENERAL TREATMENT

- If animal is anorexic (see Anorexia), dehydrated, or in discomfort, provide supportive care as needed:
  - Fluid therapy
    - Maintenance fluid rate: 60-100 mL/kg/d SC, PO, IV, IO
    - Replace fluid deficits and maintain normovolemia.
    - For cases of constipation, use the enteral (oral) route to rehydrate intestinal contents.
  - Nutritional support
    - Syringe-feed with high-fiber diet for herbivores (e.g., Oxbow

Critical Care for Herbivores, 50-80 mL/kg/d PO divided into 4-5 feedings) or crushed and soaked pellets.
  - Vitamin C 50-100 mg/kg PO, SC q 24 h for treatment of deficiencies, 10-30 mg/kg PO for maintenance
- Analgesia
  - Buprenorphine 0.02-0.05 mg/kg SC q 6-8 h
  - Meloxicam 0.3-0.5 mg/kg PO q 24 h
- Dystocia
  - If adequate separation of the pubic symphysis has occurred, oxytocin injection (1-2 units IM) can be given. If the fetus is stuck, application of a water-based lubricant in the vagina might aid in pup removal. If conservative treatments fail to resolve dystocia within a reasonable amount of time, a cesarean section is necessary. The uterus should be opened close to the bifurcation of the horns.
  - If the patient presents in shock, stabilize patient before treatment of dystocia is initiated.
- Pregnancy toxemia
  - Treatment is rarely successful in advanced cases. Aggressive treatment is necessary and involves administration of IV/IO fluids and dextrose, nutritional supplementation, and emergency cesarean section if patient is hypertensive, from compression of blood vessels by gravid uterus.

POSSIBLE COMPLICATIONS

- Endometritis
- Pyometra
- Shock

RECOMMENDED MONITORING

- Vaginal discharge
- Appetite
- Fecal output
- Urine ketones

PROGNOSIS AND OUTCOME

- Uncomplicated dystocias have a good prognosis for recovery.
- Pregnancy toxemia and uterine torsion have a poor prognosis for recovery.

PEARLS & CONSIDERATIONS

COMMENTS

Breeding guinea pigs necessitates frequent check-ups, as in any other species. Inform the client regarding the need for prefarrowing testing, including radiographs and ultrasound, to assess the number and viability of the litter. These exams are also important for assessing the body condition and discussing diet choices.

PREVENTION

- Appropriate diet and avoidance of obesity
- First breeding by 3-5 months of age is recommended to avoid fusion of the pelvic symphysis before the first parturition. Fusion of the pelvic symphysis occurs in nulliparous guinea pigs by 7-8 months of age.

CLIENT EDUCATION

- Breeding guinea pigs necessitates frequent check-ups, as in any other species.
- Appropriate diet and prevention of obesity will reduce the risk of pregnancy toxemia.

SUGGESTED READINGS

Ganaway JR, et al: Obesity predisposes to pregnancy toxemia (ketosis) of guinea pigs, Lab Anim Sci 21:40–44, 1971.
Seidl DC, et al: True pregnancy toxemia (preeclampsia) in the guinea pig (Cavia porcellus), Lab Anim Sci 29:472–478, 1979.
Wahl LM, et al: Effect of hormones on collagen metabolism and collagenase activity in the pubic symphysis ligament of the guinea pig, Endocrinology 100:571–579, 1977.

CROSS-REFERENCES TO OTHER SECTIONS

Anorexia
Ovarian Cysts
Uterine and Vaginal Disorders

AUTHOR: **BRIAN A. EVANS**

EDITOR: **CHRISTOPH MANS**

SMALL MAMMALS: GUINEA PIGS

Respiratory Tract Disease

BASIC INFORMATION

DEFINITION

Pneumonia in guinea pigs is caused by two main bacterial pathogens: *Bordetella bronchiseptica* and *Streptococcus pneumoniae*, as well as by guinea pig adenovirus (GPAdV).

SPECIAL SPECIES CONSIDERATIONS

Guinea pigs are obligate nasal breathers; therefore, even upper respiratory disease alone can cause significant dyspnea.

EPIDEMIOLOGY

SPECIES, AGE, SEX

- *S. pneumoniae* is more common in young or pregnant guinea pigs.
- *B. bronchiseptica* is more common in young guinea pigs.

RISK FACTORS

- All pathogens
  - Stress (overcrowding, transport, pregnancy)
  - Inappropriate ventilation and bedding
  - Hypovitaminosis C (see Hypovitaminosis C)
- *B. bronchiseptica*
  - Being housed with rabbits that naturally carry this bacteria as part of their normal respiratory flora

CONTAGION AND ZOONOSIS

- *S. pneumoniae*
  - Alpha-hemolytic *Streptococcus*—Gram-positive diplococcus
  - Capsular types 4 and 19 found in guinea pigs
  - Transmission may occur via respiratory aerosol, by direct contact, or during birth.
  - Can be carried in >50% of nonclinical animals
  - *S. pneumoniae* isolates of guinea pigs appear to be a specialized clone/serotype for this species. Human pneumococcal isolates do not appear to infect guinea pigs, and guinea pig isolates do not appear to infect humans.
- *B. bronchiseptica*
  - Transmission is via respiratory aerosol, direct contact, and fomites.
  - Short Gram-negative rod or coccobacillus
  - Incubation 5-7 days
  - Can be carried in >20% of nonclinical animals

- Guinea pig adenovirus
  - DNA virus
  - Transmitted via respiratory aerosol or direct contact
  - Incubation period 5-10 days

GEOGRAPHY AND SEASONALITY
Pneumonia epizootics in winter months have been described in research settings.

CLINICAL PRESENTATION

DISEASE FORMS/SUBTYPES

- With both *S. pneumoniae* and *B. bronchiseptica*, animals can have no apparent clinical signs or can have severe respiratory disease and/or acute death.
- The dominant pattern of GPAdV infection appears to be transient but clinically silent with mild lesion development. Guinea pigs with clinical respiratory signs, including pneumonia and death, may represent a more obvious but less common expression of age-related susceptibility or lowered resistance due to as yet uncharacterized stressors or variables (e.g., immunosuppression, viral strain variance and anesthetic gas irritation).

HISTORY, CHIEF COMPLAINT

- Labored breathing
- Nasal discharge
- Sneezing
- Lethargy
- Decreased appetite
- Acute death
- Abortion
- Lameness
- History of newly introduced guinea pig into household or contact with rabbits

PHYSICAL EXAM FINDINGS

- Dyspnea
- Tachypnea
- Cyanosis
- Rales
- Oculonasal discharge
- Collapse, tachycardia, poor peripheral pulses if in septic shock
- Torticollis and/or nystagmus if otitis media present
- Arthralgia if arthritis present

ETIOLOGY AND PATHOPHYSIOLOGY

- Because both *B. bronchiseptica* and *S. pneumoniae* can be carried in subclinical animals, other factors such as stress, immune suppression, and hypovitaminosis C are necessary for development of clinical disease.
- *B. bronchiseptica*
  - Bacteria attach to ciliated respiratory epithelial cells, causing ciliostasis and inflammation leading to decreased clearance of other organisms and particulate matter.
  - Can lead to middle ear and uterine infection as well
- *S. pneumoniae*
  - Initially, this bacterium becomes established in the upper respiratory tract, where it is protected from phagocytosis by a polysaccharide capsule.
  - Once established, the bacterium activates an alternate complement pathway, leading to pathologic changes in the respiratory epithelium.
  - Bacteremia can lead to septic arthritis if concurrent hypovitaminosis C is present.
  - Can lead to middle ear infection
- Guinea pig adenovirus
  - GPAdV enters the tracheal and bronchial epithelial cells, leading to cell damage and epithelial erosions resulting in inflammation and obstruction of the airways. The incubation period is about 5-10 days followed by transient virus shedding (in nonfatal cases) of about 10-12 days after which the virus is eliminated from the host.

DIAGNOSIS

DIFFERENTIAL DIAGNOSIS

- Respiratory signs
  - Neoplasia (primary pulmonary or metastatic)
  - Congestive heart failure
- Otitis media
  - Extension of otitis externa
  - Streptococcal lymphadenitis due to *S. zooepidemicus* (see Guinea Pigs: *Streptococcus zooepidemicus*)

INITIAL DATABASE

- Thoracic radiographs/CT: findings consistent with bronchopneumonia, pleural effusion, and pulmonary consolidation
- Skull radiographs/CT/MRI: tympanic bullae sclerosis or effusion if otitis media is present
- Complete blood count: neutrophilia, neutropenia if septic
- Serum biochemistry: hypoglycemia if septic
- Transtracheal lavage
  - Aerobic culture and sensitivity and Gram stain
  - Interpret culture and sensitivity with caution because both *B. bronchiseptica* and *S. pneumoniae* can be cultured from clinically normal guinea pigs
  - Cytologic examination
- Serologic testing
  - ELISA and indirect immunofluorescence (IIF) for *B. bronchiseptica*.
  - ELISA and indirect fluorescent antibody (IFA) for GPAdV. Polymerase chain reaction (PCR) is also available.

ADVANCED OR CONFIRMATORY TESTING

- Histopathologic examination
  - GPAdV: intranuclear inclusion bodies in respiratory epithelium and consolidation of cranial lung lobes. PCR on formalin-fixed tissue is also available.

TREATMENT

THERAPEUTIC GOALS

- Stabilization of the septic patient
- Eradication of the bacterial infection. This can be difficult because carrier states can develop.
- Correction of underlying disease, especially hypovitaminosis C
- Assist feeding to avoid GI stasis.

ACUTE GENERAL TREATMENT

- Oxygen therapy if patient is dyspneic or cyanotic
- Fluid therapy: may require intravenous or intraosseous administration in severely compromised patients
- Antibiotic therapy should be based on aerobic culture and sensitivity results:
  - *S. pneumoniae*: Highly resistant strains to penicillins, macrolides, and fluoroquinolones have been reported in humans, so appropriate antibiotic use, based on culture and sensitivity, is extremely important.
  - *B. bronchiseptica* possesses a β-lactamase and is resistant to many penicillins and cephalosporins and mostly resistant to trimethoprim-sulfamethoxazole. Most isolates are sensitive to fluoroquinolones.
  - GPAdV: no direct treatment but some antibiotics are used for control of secondary bacterial infection
    - Chloramphenicol 30-50 mg/kg PO, SC, IM, IV q 8 h
    - Enrofloxacin 10-20 mg/kg PO, SC, IM, IV q 24 h: CAUTION with SC or IM injection as can cause severe pain and tissue necrosis. Dilute with sterile saline before injection.
    - Trimethoprim-sulfa 30 mg/kg PO, SC q 12 h
- Vitamin C 50-100 mg/kg PO, SC q 24 h for treatment of deficiencies, 10-30 mg/kg PO for maintenance
- Nutritional support: syringe feeding with high-fiber diet for herbivores (e.g., Oxbow Critical Care for Herbivores) or crushed and soaked pellets

RECOMMENDED MONITORING

- Patients with severe disease should be hospitalized until able to go home on oral medications.
- Respiratory rate and effort, body weight/condition, and appetite should

be monitored in the hospital and at home by the client.

PROGNOSIS AND OUTCOME

- Outcome depends on concurrent disease, severity of infection, and promptness of antibiotic treatment (for bacterial infection).
- Because no cure for adenoviral pneumonia is known, outcome depends on prevention/treatment of secondary bacterial infection and supportive care of the patient.
- Eradication of the disease may prove difficult because carrier states can be present.

CONTROVERSY

Nebulization with normal saline, hypertonic saline, bronchodilators, and/or antibiotics has been recommended to hydrate the respiratory tract and directly deliver medications. Specific studies with these nebulizations have not been performed in guinea pigs with pneumonia.

PEARLS & CONSIDERATIONS

PREVENTION

- All pathogens
    - Reduction/elimination of stressors (e.g., transport, overcrowding, pregnancy)
        - Appropriate housing with adequate ventilation, low ammonia levels, and low dust/debris
        - Adequate vitamin C supplementation to avoid hypovitaminosis C
        - Isolation of any new guinea pigs
- *B. bronchiseptica*
    - Vaccination with canine *Bordetella* bacterin reported to be safe and efficacious in guinea pigs but is not widely used. Vaccination can cause a localized upper respiratory infection.
    - Separation from dogs and rabbits that may carry/be infected with *B. bronchiseptica*

CLIENT EDUCATION

- Guinea pigs are sensitive prey animals that can easily become stressed. Adequate housing that enables them to hide and have adequate ventilation is important.
- Bedding such as wood shavings should be avoided because its use can lead to dust and contact irritation of the mucous membranes.
- Vitamin C supplementation is important to avoid hypovitaminosis C.
- Guinea pigs should not be housed with rabbits because they can carry *B. bronchiseptica*.

SUGGESTED READINGS

Boot R, et al: Otitis media in guinea pigs: pathology and bacteriology, Lab Anim 20: 242–248, 1986.

D'Amore E, et al: An outbreak of bacterial pneumonia in a group of guinea pigs: All Glass Impinger as a method to isolate the pathogens from the environment, Anim Technol 51:9–12, 2000.

van der Linden M, et al: Molecular characterization of pneumococcal isolates from pets and laboratory animals, PLoS ONE December:e8286, 2009.

Smith T: Some bacteriological and environmental factors in the pneumonias of lower animals with special reference to the guinea-pig, J Med Res 29:291–325, 1913.

Weisbroth SH: Guinea pig adenovirus: Homotypic serologic reagents for detection of antibodies in guinea pig sera, Animal Health Matters. Hudson, NY, 2006, Taconic, webpage disease review. http://www.taconic.com/wmspage.cfm?parm1=281.

Witt WM, et al: Streptococcus pneumoniae arthritis and osteomyelitis with vitamin C deficiency in guinea pigs, Lab Anim Sci 38:192–194, 1988.

CROSS-REFERENCES TO OTHER SECTIONS

Hypovitaminosis C
Streptococcus zooepidemicus

AUTHORS: **NICOLE R. WYRE AND THOMAS M. DONNELLY**

EDITOR: **CHRISTOPH MANS**

SMALL MAMMALS: GUINEA PIGS

Skin Diseases

BASIC INFORMATION

DEFINITION

Infectious and noninfectious diseases of the integument

SYNONYMS

Alopecia, dermatitis, pyoderma, ringworm, dermatophytosis, acariasis, *Trixacarus caviae,* scabies, abscesses, neoplasia, pododermatitis

EPIDEMIOLOGY

RISK FACTORS

- For pododermatitis: obesity, lack of exercise, poor hygiene, inappropriate bedding, arthritis, age, and trauma
- Symptomatic ectoparasitism and dermatophytosis: immune suppression, poor sanitation

CONTAGION AND ZOONOSIS

- *Trixacarus caviae* is potentially zoonotic.
- Dermatophytes are potentially zoonotic.

ASSOCIATED CONDITIONS AND DISORDERS

- Conspecific trauma
- Ovarian cysts
- Cervical lymphadenopathy
- Cheilitis
- Hypovitaminosis C
- Chronic renal insufficiency
- Hyperthyroidism
- Hyperadrenocorticism

CLINICAL PRESENTATION

DISEASE FORMS/SUBTYPES

- Ectoparasitosis
- Dermatophytosis
- Bacterial dermatitis
- Abscesses
- Pododermatitis
- Alopecia (nonpruritic)
- Neoplasia

HISTORY, CHIEF COMPLAINT

- Hair loss
- Rough hair coat
- Pruritus
- Weight loss
- Lethargy
- Swellings or wounds on body

PHYSICAL EXAM FINDINGS

- Will vary depending on cause
    - Alopecia
    - Pruritus
    - Localized erythema
    - Scaling, crusting
    - Lichenification
    - Cutaneous masses
    - Abrasions, excoriations, ulcerations

ETIOLOGY AND PATHOPHYSIOLOGY

- Parasites
    - All ectoparasitic infections can become complicated by secondary infection and self-mutilation.

- Direct contact is the predominant route of transmission:
  - Sarcoptic mange *(Trixacarus caviae)*
    - Pruritus: in severe cases, pruritus can provoke seizure-like episodes (see Neurologic Disease).
    - Crusting and hyperkeratosis
    - Animals with clinical signs are often immune compromised. Asymptomatic carriers possible
  - Demodicosis *(Demodex caviae)*: rarely causes clinical signs. Alopecia, erythema, scabs on head and forefeet. Pruritus, secondary bacterial infection possible. Healthy carriers, immune compromised animals show clinical signs.
  - Fur mites *(Chirodiscoides caviae)*: nonburrowing mite. Entire life cycle on host. Asymptomatic infection common. Pruritus, alopecia, erythema, and scabs can be seen in clinical cases.
  - Lice *(Gliricola porcelli, Gliricola ovalis)*: poor coat. Parasites localized mainly around ear, eyes, and neck. Can lead to pruritus, anemia, nervousness, loss of body condition; seizure-like episodes possible in severe cases, secondary to intense pruritus
- Dermatophytosis
  - Predominantly *Trichophyton mentagrophytes*, rarely *Microsporum gypseum*.
  - Ubiquitous organisms; subclinical carriers common; young or immune compromised animals will develop clinical signs
  - Transmission is by direct contact or by fomites, such as bedding.
  - Focal alopecia and scaling. Predilected areas include face, feet, and dorsum, but condition can be diffuse and generalized. Animals usually are not pruritic, unless secondary bacterial infection is present.
  - Immune deficiency and stress may be underlying causes in chronic cases.
- Bacterial dermatitis/ulcerative dermatitis
  - *Staphylococcus* spp.
  - Usually secondary to self-trauma due to pruritus from mites; dermatophytosis; fight wounds from chronic wetting due to hypersalivation
- Abscesses
  - *Staphylococcus aureus, Streptococcus* spp.
  - Cervical lymphadenitis caused by *Streptococcus zooepidemicus* (see *Streptococcus zooepidemicus*); soft subcutaneous swellings in ventral neck
- Pododermatitis
  - Obesity, lack of exercise, hypovitaminosis C, poor hygiene, inappropriate bedding, arthritis, age, and trauma have been suggested as predisposing factors.
  - Initial stage: erythema, crusting, inflammation, progressing to ulcerative lesions and, in severe cases, affecting underlying bone and tendons
  - Painful condition
  - *S. aureus* commonly isolated
  - Amyloidosis of the kidney, liver, spleen, adrenal glands, and pancreas has been linked to chronic pododermatitis.
- Alopecia (nonpruritic)
  - Ovarian cysts can cause bilateral symmetric flank alopecia.
  - May be seen during advanced pregnancy and early lactation
  - Hyperthyroidism (see Hyperthyroidism)
  - Hyperadrenocorticism
- Poor coat condition without pruritus
  - Increased shedding and thin or roughened coat, poor coat condition, and dandruff have been associated with stress and underlying disease (e.g., chronic renal insufficiency, dental disease, hypovitaminosis C).
- Neoplasia
  - Trichofolliculoma (most common): benign; discharge from central pore possible
  - Squamous cell carcinoma, liposarcoma, sebaceous gland adenoma, and others reported
  - Mammary tumors are usually malignant; male guinea pigs are more commonly affected.

DIAGNOSIS

DIFFERENTIAL DIAGNOSIS

- Alopecia: trauma, dermatophytosis, ovarian cysts, hyperthyroidism, hyperadrenocorticism, vitamin C deficiency, barbering, neoplasia
- Abscesses: neoplasia (e.g., lymphoma), lymphadenopathy
- Crusting or ulcerative lesions, hyperkeratosis: mites, secondary bacterial infection, cheilitis (see Cheilitis)
- Pruritus: mites, lice, secondary bacterial infection
- Crusting or flaking of skin: dermatophytosis, mites, lice, vitamin C deficiency
- Cutaneous masses: neoplasia, abscesses
- Localized erythema or pododermatitis: contact allergy, contact irritation (cleaners), trauma from bedding/cage material

INITIAL DATABASE

- Full dietary history
- Full husbandry history
- Dermatologic examination
  - Direct visualization (lice)
  - Acetate tape preparation
  - Skin scraping
  - Impression smears
- Dermatophyte culture
- Fine-needle aspirate and cytologic examination of cutaneous masses
- Bacterial culture and sensitivity

ADVANCED OR CONFIRMATORY TESTING

- Abdominal ultrasound: rule out ovarian cysts
- Radiographs: rule out underlying skeletal abnormalities (e.g., osteoarthritis; osteomyelitis) in cases of pododermatitis
- Serum biochemistry: if underlying organ disease is suspected
- Serum thyroxine (T_4) measurement
- Adrenocorticotropic hormone (ACTH) stimulation test and cortisol measurement in saliva
- Biopsy and histopathologic examination of skin lesion

TREATMENT

THERAPEUTIC GOALS

- Eliminate pruritus and discomfort.
- Treat primary and secondary infections.
- Promote healing of skin lesions.

ACUTE GENERAL TREATMENT

- Ectoparasites
  - Ivermectin 0.2-0.5 mg/kg SC, PO q 7-14 d
  - Selamectin 15-30 mg/kg topically q 14-28 d (q 14 d for demodex, but q 21-28 d for other ectoparasites).
  - Treat until clinical signs have resolved and no more parasites are found on animals.
  - Treat in-contact animals.
  - Treat the environment to prevent reinfection: regular bedding changes and cage cleaning. Discard cage furnishings that cannot be disinfected (e.g., wood-based furnishings).
- Bacterial infection
  - If indicated, provide systemic antibiotic therapy based on culture and sensitivity whenever possible.
  - Start empirical treatment pending culture and sensitivity:
    - Trimethoprim-sulfa 30 mg/kg PO q 12 h
    - Chloramphenicol 30-50 mg/kg PO q 8 h

- Enrofloxacin 10-20 mg/kg PO q 12-24 h
- Skin abscesses
  - Lance, débride, and flush or remove in toto if possible.
  - If indicated, provide systemic antibiotic therapy based on culture and sensitivity whenever possible.
- Cervical lymphadenitis: see *Streptococcus zooepidemicus*
- Pododermatitis
  - Depending on severity of disease
  - Mild: soaking in mild antiseptic solution, provision of soft bedding, reduction of body weight, increased exercise
  - Moderate cases: systemic therapy
  - Severe cases: surgical débridement, open wound management, regular bandage changes
  - Systemic antibiotic therapy based on culture and sensitivity, whenever possible
  - Analgesia: meloxicam 0.3-0.5 mg/kg PO, SC q 24 h, buprenorphine 0.03-0.05 mg/kg SC q 6-8 h
- Dermatophytosis
  - Systemic antifungal therapy
    - Terbinafine 20-30 mg/kg PO q 24 h
    - Itraconazole 5-10 mg/kg PO q 24 h
  - Topical antifungal therapy
    - Enilconazole 1:50 emulsion as spray or moist wipe
    - Miconazole/chlorhexidine shampoos
    - Lime sulfur dips (1:40, q 7 d)
    - Used alone or in combination with systemic therapy
    - Use preferably in cases of suspected dermatophytosis while awaiting dermatophyte culture results
  - Environmental decontamination: frequent damp mopping of hard surfaces rather than sweeping can reduce environmental spread of spores; 1:10 bleach solution can be used to clean environment: contact time 10 minutes
  - Monitoring: once-weekly dermatophyte test medium (DTM) cultures. Discontinue treatment once two consecutive negative cultures are obtained.
- Vitamin C deficiency: vitamin C 50-100 mg/kg PO, SC q 24 h for treatment of deficiencies, 10-30 mg/kg PO for maintenance. See Hypovitaminosis C.

CHRONIC TREATMENT

- Improve sanitary conditions in the animal's environment.
- Dermatophytosis will often require long-term therapy.

RECOMMENDED MONITORING

- Resolution of clinical signs
- Repeated evaluation for presence of ectoparasites
- Weekly DTM cultures in cases of dermatophytosis

PROGNOSIS AND OUTCOME

- Good to fair
- Poor: severe pododermatitis

PEARLS & CONSIDERATIONS

COMMENTS

Guinea pigs infected with *T. caviae* can present with a history of seizures due to severe pruritus (see Neurologic Disease).

PREVENTION

- Provision of a commercial diet
- Good sanitation
- Minimization of stress
- Quarantine of all new incoming animals for a minimum of 30 days before contact with other animals is allowed

CLIENT EDUCATION

Dermatophytes and *T. caviae* are contagious to humans; medical advice should be sought if lesions are found on humans in the household.

SUGGESTED READINGS

Donnelly TM, et al: Ringworm in small exotic pets, Sem Avian Exot Pet Med 9:82–93, 2000.

White SD, et al: Dermatologic problems in guinea pigs, Comp Cont Educ Pract Vet 25:690–697, 2003.

CROSS-REFERENCES TO OTHER SECTIONS

Cheilitis
Hyperthyroidism
Hypovitaminosis C
Neurologic Disease
Pododermatitis
Streptococcus zooepidemicus

AUTHOR: **CHRISTOPH MANS**

EDITOR: **THOMAS M. DONNELLY**

SMALL MAMMALS: GUINEA PIGS

Streptococcus zooepidemicus (Cervical Lymphadenitis)

BASIC INFORMATION

DEFINITION

Streptococcal lymphadenitis is a bacterial infection of the cervical lymph nodes caused by a commensal bacterium, *Streptococcus zooepidemicus,* which invades abraded mucosa. Rarely, an acute systemic form can occur in younger guinea pigs, leading to respiratory disease and sepsis.

SYNONYMS

Cervical lymphadenitis, lumps

Significant taxonomic and nomenclature changes in the genus Streptococci have resulted in the expansion from 4 phenotypically easy-to-differentiate species to 34 species. Difficulties between taxonomists and clinicians regarding appropriate nomenclature resulted in the introduction of subspecies. *Streptococcus zooepidemicus* was renamed *Streptococcus equi* subspecies *zooepidemicus.* However, many laboratories report the subspecies name only (e.g., the isolation of *S. zooepidemicus*) as it is easy to understand for clinicians.

SPECIAL SPECIES CONSIDERATION

Streptococcus zooepidemicus is a frequently isolated opportunist pathogen of horses and a cause of hemorrhagic pneumonia in dogs. A normal mucosal commensal of horses, it causes purulent respiratory infections of weanling and yearling horses and uterine infections in elderly mares. *Streptococcus* subspecies *equi* causes "strangles," a highly contagious upper respiratory infection in horses.

EPIDEMIOLOGY

SPECIES, AGE, SEX Females have been shown to be more susceptible to disease than males.

RISK FACTORS Any condition that results in oral mucosal abrasions such as dental disease, use of inappropriate toys or water bottles with sharp edges or sticks/foreign objects in hay.

CONTAGION AND ZOONOSIS *Streptococcus zooepidemicus* is a Gram-positive encapsulated beta-hemolytic streptococcus and is traditionally classified as a Group C streptococcus. In humans, it is associated with nephritis outbreaks and other infections (meningitis, endocarditis, and pneumonia) often traced back to the consumption of contaminated dairy products.

CLINICAL PRESENTATION

DISEASE FORMS/SUBTYPES

- Localized form
  - Bilateral or unilateral enlargement of cervical lymph nodes
  - Otitis media
- Acute systemic form
  - More common in younger guinea pigs
  - Sepsis, fibrinopurulent bronchopneumonia, pleuritis, and pericarditis

HISTORY, CHIEF COMPLAINT

- Localized form
  - Cervical swelling(s)
  - Torticollis
- Acute systemic form
  - Labored breathing
  - Anorexia, depression

PHYSICAL EXAM FINDINGS

- Localized form
  - Bilateral or unilateral cervical lymphadenopathy, which can be painful upon palpation
  - Torticollis or nystagmus if otitis media is present
- Acute systemic form
  - Dyspnea
  - Tachypnea
  - Cyanosis
  - Rales or muffled heart sounds
  - Collapse, tachycardia, poor peripheral pulses if in septic shock

ETIOLOGY AND PATHOPHYSIOLOGY

- *S. zooepidemicus* is a commensal organism in the nasopharynx and conjunctiva of guinea pigs.
- Disease occurs when the organism is able to invade via abrasions in the oral mucosa (most common), skin, or female genitalia. Invasion via respiratory aerosol is also reported.
- After invasion of underlying tissues, bacteria are spread via the lymphatics to draining lymph nodes, where replication and secondary inflammation occur.
- In adults, the disease usually remains localized in the lymph nodes, but in young guinea pigs, septicemia can occur, leading to death or respiratory disease.

DIAGNOSIS

DIFFERENTIAL DIAGNOSIS

- Cervical lymphadenopathy
  - Lymphoma
  - Sialocele
  - *Streptobacillus moniliformis* infection (see Rat Bite Fever)
  - Other causes of abscesses: periodontal, fungal, bite wounds, foreign body
- Otitis media
  - Extension of otitis externa
- Septicemia/respiratory disease
  - *Bordetella bronchiseptica*
  - *Streptococcus pneumoniae*
  - Guinea pig adenovirus (GPAdV)

INITIAL DATABASE

- Localized form
  - Aerobic culture and sensitivity from lymph node aspirates. An initial tentative diagnosis can often be made from Gram stain results revealing pure Gram-positive cocci.
  - Skull radiographs/CT: tympanic bullae, sclerosis, or effusion if otitis media is present
- Acute systemic form
  - Complete blood count: neutrophilia, neutropenia if septic
  - Serum biochemistry: hypoglycemia if septic
  - Thoracic radiographs/CT: findings consistent with bronchopneumonia

TREATMENT

THERAPEUTIC GOALS

- Localized form
  - Eradication of bacteria causing disease: because *S. zooepidemicus* is a commensal, complete eradication is not the treatment goal.
  - Identification and elimination of underlying causes of mucosal abrasions
- Acute systemic form
  - Stabilization of the septic patient

ACUTE GENERAL TREATMENT

- Localized form
  - Complete surgical removal of the abscessed lymph node, including its capsule
  - Antibiotic therapy: should be based on culture and sensitivity results
    - Chloramphenicol 20-50 mg/kg PO, SC, IM, IV q 8 h
    - Enrofloxacin 10-20 mg/kg PO, SC, IM, IV q 24 h; caution with SC or IM injection as can cause severe pain and tissue necrosis. Dilute with sterile saline before injection.
    - Trimethoprim-sulfa (30 mg/kg PO, SC q 12 h)
- Acute systemic form
  - Oxygen therapy
  - Fluid support: may require intravenous or intraosseous administration
  - Antibiotic therapy (see earlier): use parental route of administration
  - Nutritional support to prevent GI stasis: syringe feeding of high-fiber diet for herbivores (e.g., Oxbow Critical Care for Herbivores) or crushed and soaked pellets

POSSIBLE COMPLICATIONS

Depending on the size of the abscessed lymph node, surgical removal may be

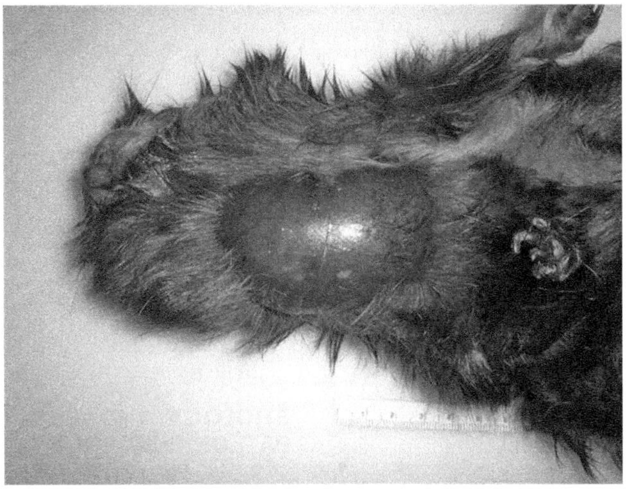

Streptococcus zooepidemicus Cervical lymphadenitits in a guinea pig. Pure growth of *Streptococcus zooepidemicus* was cultured from a cervical lymph node aspirate. *(Photo courtesy Jörg Mayer, The University of Georgia, Athens.)*

difficult because lesions can be near the trachea, jugular veins, and/or recurrent laryngeal nerve.

RECOMMENDED MONITORING

Cervical palpation for recurrence of infection if entire abscess and capsule could not be removed

PROGNOSIS AND OUTCOME

- Localized form
  - Good if able to surgically remove the entire infected lymph node
  - Incomplete resolution of signs if unable to surgically remove lymph node and capsule and/or if antibiotics alone are used
- Acute systemic form
  - Guarded to poor

PEARLS & CONSIDERATIONS

PREVENTION

- Treatment of any dental disease that could lead to mucosal abrasions
- Avoidance of toys, food, or water bottles that can cause mucosal abrasions

CLIENT EDUCATION

- Ensure that hay does not have foreign bodies or sharp plant material that may cause oral trauma.
- Water bottles used for guinea pigs should have a smooth ball tip; avoid those with metal levers that could cause oral trauma during drinking.
- Guinea pigs should not be allowed to play with toys that have metal or abrasive edges that could cause oral trauma.

SUGGESTED READING

Murphy JC, et al: Cervical lymphadenitis in guinea pigs: infection via intact ocular and nasal mucosa by *Streptococcus zooepidemicus,* Lab Anim Sci 41:251–254, 1991.

CROSS-REFERENCES TO OTHER SECTIONS

Rat Bite Fever

AUTHOR: **NICOLE R. WYRE**

EDITOR: **CHRISTOPH MANS**

SMALL MAMMALS: GUINEA PIGS

Urolithiasis

Client Education Sheet Available on Website

BASIC INFORMATION

DEFINITION

Urolithiasis describes calculi in any part of the urinary tract. Calculi in guinea pigs are found frequently in the urinary bladder or the urethra. Most uroliths in guinea pigs are calcium based.

SYNONYMS

Bladder stones, kidney stones, urinary calculus/calculi

SPECIAL SPECIES CONSIDERATIONS

- Unlike cats and dogs that have calculi composed of different materials (e.g., struvite, calcium oxalate, calcium phosphate, cysteine, urate), guinea pigs have calculi typically made up of calcium carbonate or calcium phosphate; calculi can also be composed of calcium oxalate, but this is rare. Consequently, guinea pig calculi are radiopaque.
- In female guinea pigs the external urethral opening is not located within the floor the vagina, but instead on the urinary papilla, which is located cranial to the vaginal opening.

EPIDEMIOLOGY

SPECIES, AGE, SEX Urolithiasis is a common problem in older guinea pigs (>4 years), especially in females (75%).

GENETICS AND BREED PREDISPOSITION Surveys of pet and laboratory guinea pigs suggest an overall 10% incidence.

RISK FACTORS Hypercalciuria from too much calcium in the diet is often due to feeding only alfalfa, a calcium-rich hay.

CONTAGION AND ZOONOSIS In one large survey, the incidence of bacteria associated with urolithiasis in guinea pigs was 3%.

ASSOCIATED CONDITIONS AND DISORDERS

- Recurrent bacterial cystitis
- Pyuria

CLINICAL PRESENTATION

HISTORY, CHIEF COMPLAINT

- Stranguria
- Dysuria
- Hematuria
- Anuria
- Polyuria
- Anorexia
- Abdominal pain (hunched posture)
- Vocalization during urination

PHYSICAL EXAM FINDINGS

- Palpation of cystic calculi in the urinary bladder
- Palpation of an enlarged, nonexpressible urinary bladder if urethral obstruction is present
- Small calculi and hematuria may be visualized during evaluation of urethral orifices.

ETIOLOGY AND PATHOPHYSIOLOGY

- The cause of urolithiasis in guinea pigs is unknown.
- Calcium carbonate is the predominant stone type isolated through composition analysis.
- Bacteria commonly cultured include *E. coli, Streptococcus pyogenes, Proteus mirabilis,* and *C. renale.*

DIAGNOSIS

DIFFERENTIAL DIAGNOSIS

- Hematuria, stranguria, dysuria
  - Bacterial cystitis
  - Renal disease (pyelonephritis, interstitial nephritis)
  - Rule out by identification of abnormal discharge from the vaginal opening vs. hematuria observed from the external urethral orifice.

INITIAL DATABASE

- Urinalysis
- Urine culture
- Abdominal radiographs: pay attention to coccygeal area and stretch hind limbs away from body because calculi are often lodged in the urethra and may be missed.
- If hind limbs are not stretched out, the femur may obscure a urethral calculus. It is easy to mistake patellar ossicles for a calculus in the urethra of males.
- Abdominal ultrasound to confirm calculi location and to evaluate the urinary and reproductive tract.

ADVANCED OR CONFIRMATORY TESTING

Cystocentesis for urine culture and sensitivity

TREATMENT

THERAPEUTIC GOALS

- Resolution of urinary outflow obstructions
- Removal of stones that present risk of causing urinary obstruction
- Resolution of bacterial cystitis
- Diet modification to reduce calcium-dense roughage and subsequent urinary calcium excretion
- Increased diuresis through increased water intake

ACUTE GENERAL TREATMENT

- Minimally invasive stone removal
  - For very small stone sediments, a urinary catheter can be passed to flush stones out by way of the urethra.
  - In females, cystoscopic stone removal has been reported. This technique is feasible only for stones that are not larger in diameter than the urethra.
- Surgical management
  - Routine cystotomy can be performed to remove large urinary bladder calculi.
- Treatment for suspected concurrent bacterial cystitis
  - Trimethoprim sulfonamide 30 mg/kg PO q 12 h pending urine culture results
- Urethral obstruction
  - Therapeutic management of obstructive postrenal azotemia
    - IV catheterization for fluid therapy
    - Urinary catheter placement and quantification of urine output
    - Nutritional support to delay gastrointestinal stasis
- Pain management
  - Buprenorphine 0.02-0.05 mg/kg SC q 6-8 h
  - Meloxicam 0.3-0.5 mg/kg PO, SC q 24 h
  - Tramadol 2.5-5.0 mg/kg PO q 12 h

CHRONIC TREATMENT

- Diet modification is thought to be helpful in managing severe calciuria. Avoid large quantities of alfalfa and alfalfa-based pellets and fresh greens, which contain large amounts of calcium (e.g., parsley).
- Increasing diuresis by increased water consumption. Provide multiple sources of fresh water. Flavor water with small amounts of unsweetened fruit juice. Offer a variety of fresh leafy greens.

POSSIBLE COMPLICATIONS

- Stone recurrence
- Urethral tears can occur with aggressive advancement of urinary catheters.
- Postoperative serosal adhesions can occur commonly in rodents that undergo any abdominal surgery.
- Suture reactions within the bladder wall or at the abdominal incision site

RECOMMENDED MONITORING

- Repeat chemistry screen should be performed to confirm resolution of azotemia.
- Repeated radiographs or focal urogenital tract ultrasounds can be recommended to screen for recurrence.

PROGNOSIS AND OUTCOME

- Prognosis is guarded because stone formation commonly recurs.
- Repeated surgical interventions can increase overall morbidity and mortality of affected patients.

PEARLS & CONSIDERATIONS

COMMENTS

- Guinea pigs have large urethral diameters relative to their size. Sterile red rubber urinary catheters (3.5-5 Fr) can be easily advanced into the urethra and bladder in both sexes. Therapeutic bladder flushes can be administered routinely to relieve severe calciuria. Urethral flushing can be performed to retropulse urethral stones back into the bladder for surgical removal.
- In male guinea pigs during urethral catheterization, the external urethral opening should not be confused with the opening of the intromittent sac, which is located ventral to the urethral opening (see figure).

PREVENTION

Because of the unknown cause of urinary calculi in guinea pigs, no effective method of prevention has been reported. However, foods high in calcium should not be offered to mature animals. Alfa-Alfa–based pellets and hay should be limited to growing, pregnant, or lactating animals.

CLIENT EDUCATION

- Avoid calcium-rich food items. Avoid Alfalfa–based pellets and hay.
- Increase water consumption. Provide multiple sources of fresh water. Consider flavoring water with small amounts of unsweetened fruit juice. Offer a variety of fresh leafy greens.
- Recurrence of urinary calculi is common. By reducing risk factors such as high dietary calcium intake and low water intake, recurrence may be only delayed.

SUGGESTED READINGS

Brown C, et al: Urethral catheterization of the male guinea pig *(Cavia porcellus)*, Lab Anim (NY) 36:20–21, 2007.
Hawkins MG, et al: Composition and characteristic of urinary calculi from guinea pigs, J Am Vet Med Assoc 234:214–220, 2009.

AUTHORS: **LA'TOYA LATNEY AND THOMAS M. DONNELLY**

EDITOR: **CHRISTOPH MANS**

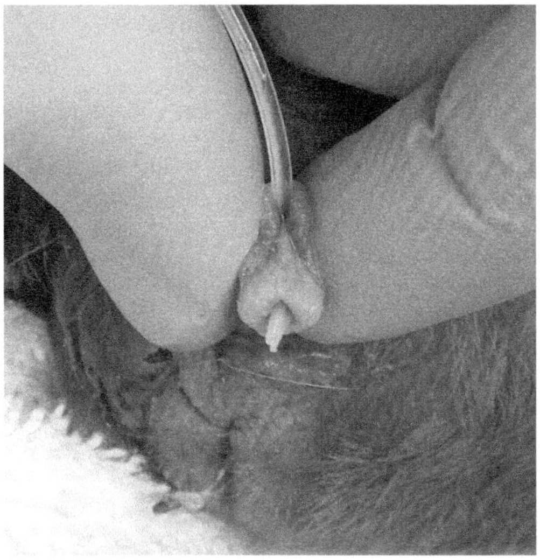

Urolithiasis Urethral catheterization in a male guinea pig. Note the partially everted intromittent sac (arrow; nb the two penile styles protruding from the intromittent sac), located ventral to the urethra, within the glans penis. Accidental catheterization of this blind sac can occur, if the opening of the intromittent sac is confused with the external urethral opening on the tip of the glans penis. The catheter is inserted into the urethra.

SMALL MAMMALS: GUINEA PIGS

Uterine and Vaginal Disorders

BASIC INFORMATION

DEFINITION

Diseases of the uterus, cervix, vagina, and vulva

SPECIAL SPECIES CONSIDERATIONS

- Guinea pigs have bicornuate uterus with a short uterine body (12 mm long), a single cervix, and a vaginal closure membrane that seals the vaginal orifice but is absent during estrus and during parturition.
- The urethral opening is not located within the vagina but on the urinary papilla cranial to the vaginal opening.

EPIDEMIOLOGY

SPECIES, AGE, SEX Female guinea pigs of any age

RISK FACTORS Poor husbandry, neoplasia, immune suppression, recent pregnancy (see Pregnancy and Parturient Disorders)

ASSOCIATED CONDITIONS AND DISORDERS Ovarian cysts (see Ovarian Cysts) can be associated with endometrial hyperplasia and endometritis. Vaginal/uterine prolapse may be associated with a recent parturition.

CLINICAL PRESENTATION

DISEASE FORMS/SUBTYPES

- Vaginitis
- Endometritis and pyometra
- Uterine/vaginal prolapse
- Uterine torsion

HISTORY, CHIEF COMPLAINT Based on the underlying disease process, the chief complaint may include vaginal discharge, inability to urinate, lethargy, or inappetence.

PHYSICAL EXAM FINDINGS On physical exam, one may find vaginal discharge with or without blood, an abdominal mass, perivulvar and vulvar inflammation, and/or a prolapsed vagina/uterus.

ETIOLOGY AND PATHOPHYSIOLOGY

- Vaginitis can be induced by soiled bedding and dirty cage conditions.
- Pyometra endometritis can be induced from ovarian cysts and/or normal ovulatory activity.
- Vaginal/uterine prolapse is most commonly seen in the parturient and periparturient periods.
- Uterine torsion is rare and is seen in gravid guinea pigs, usually after 30 days of gestation.

DIAGNOSIS

DIFFERENTIAL DIAGNOSIS

- Vaginitis
- Endometritis
- Pyometra
- Neoplasia
- Vaginal or uterine prolapse
- Uterine torsion

INITIAL DATABASE

- Bacterial culture and sensitivity and cytologic examination for cases presented with vaginal discharge
- Abdominal radiographs: assess for urolithiasis (see Urolithiasis), pyometra, neoplasia, and pregnancy
- Abdominal ultrasound
- Complete blood count, biochemistry panel, and urine analysis

ADVANCED OR CONFIRMATORY TESTING

- Exploratory laparotomy
- Histopathologic examination

TREATMENT

THERAPEUTIC GOAL

Resolution of underlying disease process

ACUTE GENERAL TREATMENT

- Vaginitis
  - Empirical systemic antibiotic therapy while bacterial culture and sensitivity is pending. Adjust treatment as indicated.
    - Trimethoprim-sulfa 30 mg/kg PO q 12 h
    - Chloramphenicol 30-50 mg/kg PO, SC, IM, IV q 8 h
    - Enrofloxacin 10-20 mg/kg SC, PO q 12-24 h
  - Careful lavage of the vaginal vestibule with diluted chlorhexidine
  - Improvement of husbandry practices
  - For pyometra, endometritis, neoplasia, and prolapsed vagina/uterus:
    - Ovariohysterectomy is indicated after animal has been stabilized.
- If animal is anorexic (see Anorexia), dehydrated, or in discomfort, provide supportive care as needed:
  - Fluid therapy
    - Maintenance fluid rate: 60-100 mL/kg/d SC, PO, IV, IO
    - Replace fluid deficits and maintain normovolemia.
  - Nutritional support
    - Syringe-feed with high-fiber diet for herbivores (e.g., Oxbow Critical Care for Herbivores, 50-80 mL/kg/d PO, divided into 4-5 feedings) or crushed and soaked pellets
    - Vitamin C 50-100 mg/kg PO, SC q 24 h for treatment of deficiencies, 10-30 mg/kg PO for maintenance
  - Analgesia
    - Buprenorphine 0.02-0.05 mg/kg SC q 6-8 h
    - Meloxicam 0.3-0.5 mg/kg PO, SC q 24 h

RECOMMENDED MONITORING

- Vaginal discharge
- Appetite
- Fecal output

PROGNOSIS AND OUTCOME

- Prognosis is good with vaginitis.
- Diseases requiring surgery carry a guarded prognosis.
- Animals presenting with uterine torsion are generally in shock and require emergency stabilization and surgery. The prognosis is guarded if animals can be stabilized.

PEARLS & CONSIDERATIONS

COMMENTS

- Because guinea pigs do not tolerate well postsurgical pain due to laparotomy, epidural anesthesia should be considered as part of the anesthetic and analgesic managment.
- Diagnostic testing is the key to uterine and vaginal disorders. Symptomatic therapy instead of diagnostic testing can lead to poorer outcomes if conditions requiring surgical intervention are not recognized.

PREVENTION

Good sanitation will help to avoid vaginitis.

CLIENT EDUCATION

- Surgery and anesthesia always carry risk and must be discussed with owners before the procedure is performed.
- Laparotomy in guinea pigs carries higher postsurgical risks compared with other rodent species.

SUGGESTED READINGS

Bodri MS, et al: What is your diagnosis? Poor intra- and retroperitoneal contrast suggestive of emaciation and alimentary visceral displacement consistent with bladder or uterine mass. Pyometra in a guinea pig, J Am Vet Med Assoc 202:654–655, 1993.

Kunstyr I: Torsion of the uterus and the stomach in guinea pigs, Z Versuchstierkd 23:67–69, 1981.

Okewole PA, et al: Uterine involvement in guinea pig salmonellosis, Lab Anim 23:275–277, 1989.

CROSS-REFERENCES TO OTHER SECTIONS

Anorexia
Ovarian Cysts
Pregnancy and Parturient Disorders
Urolithiasis

AUTHOR: **BRIAN A. EVANS**

EDITOR: **CHRISTOPH MANS**

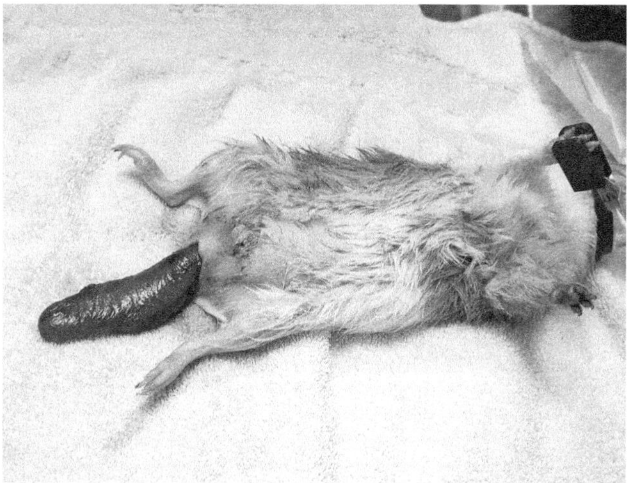

Uterine and Vaginal Disorders Prolapsed uterus of a female guinea pig after delivery. If the tissue is fresh, it can be cleared and replaced. If the prolapse is old, an ovariohysterectomy is indicated.

SMALL MAMMALS: HAMSTERS

Abdominal Distention

BASIC INFORMATION

DEFINITION

Swelling of the abdomen; nonspecific clinical sign associated with a number of disorders

EPIDEMIOLOGY

SPECIES, AGE, SEX

- Geriatric hamsters may be more predisposed to abdominal distention caused by neoplasia or organ failure.
- Young hamsters are more likely to develop signs secondary to bacterial enteritis.

CONTAGION AND ZOONOSIS See Intestinal Disorders

ASSOCIATED CONDITIONS AND DISORDERS

- Congestive heart failure
- Renal failure
- Hepatic failure
- Bacterial enteritis
- Amyloidosis
- Polycystic disease

CLINICAL PRESENTATION

HISTORY, CHIEF COMPLAINT

- Acute or chronic abdominal swelling
- Anorexia
- Polydipsia/polyuria
- Diarrhea
- Lethargy
- Vaginal discharge
- Recent parturition
- Irritability, hunched posture suggesting abdominal discomfort
- Respiratory distress
- Sudden death

PHYSICAL EXAM FINDINGS

- Depression
- Dehydration
- Cachexia
- Abdominal distention
- Palpable abdominal mass effects
- Diarrhea; wet perineum
- Vaginal discharge

ETIOLOGY AND PATHOPHYSIOLOGY

- Ileus
  - Inappropriate diet (e.g., low in fiber)
  - Dehydration
  - Often secondary to another condition
- Bacterial or antibiotic-associated enteritis (see Intestinal Disorders)
  - Proliferative ileitis may be associated with palpable abdominal masses:
    - Thickened ileum
    - Intussusception
    - Enlarged mesenteric lymph nodes
- Ascites
  - Secondary to renal failure
    - Amyloidosis has been associated with nephrotic syndrome in Syrian hamsters.
      - Amyloid deposited in kidney, liver, spleen, and adrenals
      - Incidence higher in female hamsters
    - Arteriolar nephrosclerosis (hamster nephrosis)

        - Incidence higher in female hamsters
        - May be coincident with amyloidosis
      - Pyelonephritis
    - Secondary to cardiac disease (see Cardiac Disease)
    - Secondary to neoplastic process
- Discrete abdominal masses
    - Neoplasia
        - Ovarian: usually benign
        - Uterine: usually malignant
            - Aged Chinese hamsters have a high incidence of uterine adenocarcinoma.
        - Lymphoma
            - Hamster polyomavirus can cause epizootic form of lymphoma with abdominal lymph node enlargement.
                - Young hamsters predisposed
    - Polycystic disease
        - Can affect many internal organs, but liver is most commonly affected
            - Hepatic cysts up to 3 cm in diameter have been noted.
        - Ovarian cysts
    - Pyometra
    - Pregnancy; ectopic pregnancy

DIAGNOSIS

DIFFERENTIAL DIAGNOSIS

- Obesity
- Vaginal discharge
    - Mucoid, musky-smelling discharge normal in females in estrus (every 4-7 days)
- Pregnancy
    - Russian hamsters may be predisposed to ectopic pregnancies.
    - Gestation period
        - Syrian hamster: 15-18 days
        - Russian (dwarf) hamster: 18-22 days
        - Chinese hamster: 21 days

INITIAL DATABASE

- Fecal analyses (flotation, direct smear, cytologic examination)
- Urinalysis
    - Isosthenuria may be noted in renal disease.
    - Urine specific gravity reference range: 1.040-1.060
- Cytologic examination of vaginal discharge
- Radiographs
- Abdominal ultrasound (small size of patient, presence of gas may make examination unrewarding)
- Routine complete blood count and biochemistry panel: may be limited to an estimated white cell count, packed cell volume, and selected tests in Syrian hamsters; may not be feasible in Russian (dwarf) hamsters
    - Nephrotic syndrome associated with hypoalbuminemia, hyperlipidemia, elevated creatinine

ADVANCED OR CONFIRMATORY TESTING

- Abdominocentesis (under general anesthesia; preferably ultrasound-guided)
    - Abdominal fluid analysis (cytologic examination, chemistry, culture)
- Echocardiography (see Cardiac Disease)
- Abdominal exploratory surgery
    - Histopathologic examination and/or culture of samples obtained
- Necropsy

TREATMENT

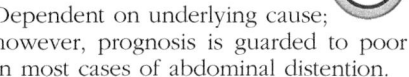

THERAPEUTIC GOALS

- Reduce distress and discomfort.
- Restore hydration and nutritional status.
- Treat underlying cause if feasible.

ACUTE GENERAL TREATMENT

- General supportive care
    - Calm, quiet environment to reduce stress
    - Warm incubator
    - Supplemental oxygen for patients in respiratory distress
    - Warmed fluids
        - Maintenance rate: 60-100 mL/kg/d
        - LRS, Normosol R SC; IO route may be considered if in shock and hamster is large enough (femur and tibia preferred sites)
    - Analgesia
        - Buprenorphine 0.05-0.1 mg/kg SC q 6-12 h
        - Meloxicam 0.3-0.5 mg/kg PO, SC q 24 h
            - Caution in dehydrated patients
            - Do not use if renal disease is suspected.
- Diuresis: furosemide 2-10 mg/kg IM, SC, PO q 4-12 h, if cardiac disease suspected (see Cardiac Disease)
- Abdominocentesis
    - May be therapeutic and diagnostic in acute cases if abdominal distention is causing respiratory distress; however, should not be considered a long-term therapy option
- Aspiration of ovarian or hepatic cysts may provide temporary resolution of distention:
    - Cysts will refill.
    - Must be performed under general anesthesia, preferably with ultrasound guidance
- Euthanasia in severe cases

CHRONIC TREATMENT

- Nutritional support once hamster is stable
- Renal failure
    - Fluid support may be continued with daily subcutaneous fluid administration.
    - Reduced protein diet may be of some limited usefulness.
- Cardiac failure
    - See Cardiac Disease
- Polycystic disease
    - Repeat ultrasound-guided aspiration under general anesthesia may be considered but is only palliative.
    - Ovarian cysts
        - Treatment of choice: ovariectomy or ovariohysterectomy
- Pyometra
    - Ovariohysterectomy
- Neoplasia
    - Surgical removal of affected organ may be attempted.

RECOMMENDED MONITORING

Recheck 1 week after discharge to monitor response to therapy and follow-up if patient has had surgery.

PROGNOSIS AND OUTCOME

Dependent on underlying cause; however, prognosis is guarded to poor in most cases of abdominal distention.

CONTROVERSY

Gonadotropin-releasing hormone agonists (i.e., leuprolide acetate, deslorelin) have been used as palliative therapy for ovarian cysts in guinea pigs; however, no literature is available to support this use in hamsters.

PEARLS & CONSIDERATIONS

COMMENTS

In many cases of abdominal distention, premortem diagnosis may be difficult to obtain.

PREVENTION

- Pregnancy can be prevented by separating hamsters by the age of sexual maturity:
    - Syrian and Russian (dwarf) hamsters: 6-8 weeks
    - Chinese hamsters: 7-14 weeks
- Avoid use of antibiotics, which can predispose to GI dysbiosis and antibiotic-associated enteritis (see Intestinal Disorders).

CLIENT EDUCATION

Ensure that owners are aware of the short gestation period in hamsters.

SUGGESTED READINGS

Buckley P, et al: A high incidence of abdominal pregnancy in the Djungarian hamster

(*Phodopus sungorus*), J Reprod Fertil 56: 679–682, 1979.
Fiskett RM: Lawsonia intracellularis infection in hamsters (*Mesocricetus auratus*), J Exotic Pet Med 20:277–283, 2011.
Murphy JC, et al: Nephrotic syndrome associated with renal amyloidosis in a colony of Syrian hamsters, J Am Vet Med Assoc 185: 1359–1362, 1984.
Schmidt RE, et al: Cardiovascular disease in hamsters: review and retrospective study, J Exotic Pet Med 16:49–51, 2007.
Simmons JH, et al: Hamster polyomavirus infection in a pet Syrian hamster (*Mesocricetus auratus*), Vet Pathol 38:441–446, 2001.
Somvanshi R, et al: Polycystic liver disease in golden hamsters, J Comp Pathol 97:615–618, 1987.

CROSS-REFERENCES TO OTHER SECTIONS

Cardiac Disease
Intestinal Disorders

AUTHOR: **DOMINIQUE L. KELLER**

EDITOR: **CHRISTOPH MANS**

SMALL MAMMALS: HAMSTERS

Cardiac Disease

BASIC INFORMATION

DEFINITION

Disease of the cardiovascular system, including atrial thrombosis and cardiomyopathy

EPIDEMIOLOGY

SPECIES, AGE, SEX

- Cardiac disease is common in the Syrian hamster (*Mesocricetus auratus*).
- Reports have also described disease in the Chinese hamster (*Cricetulus griseus*).

GENETICS AND BREED PREDISPOSITION Dilated cardiomyopathy is inherited in certain inbred laboratory hamster strains.

RISK FACTORS

- Aged hamsters (>1.5 years) are predisposed to cardiovascular disease.
- Female and neutered male hamsters develop cardiac disease earlier (13.5 months) than intact males (21.5 months).

CONTAGION AND ZOONOSIS Encephalomyocarditis virus is zoonotic.

ASSOCIATED CONDITIONS AND DISORDERS

- Cardiomyopathy may lead to development of atrial thrombosis.
- Disseminated intravascular coagulation (DIC) has been found in conjunction with cases of atrial thrombosis.

CLINICAL PRESENTATION

HISTORY, CHIEF COMPLAINT

- Anorexia
- Weight loss
- Lethargy
- Exercise intolerance
- Labored breathing
- Abdominal swelling
- Sudden death

PHYSICAL EXAM FINDINGS

- Affected hamsters show the following signs for up to 1 week before death:
  - Hyperpnea
  - Tachycardia (normal heart rate 250-500 bpm)
  - Cyanosis
- Other clinical signs may include the following:
  - Hypothermia; cold distal extremities
  - Tachypnea (normal respiratory rate: 35-135 bpm)
  - Dyspnea
  - Muffled heart sounds
  - Heart murmur
  - Ascites

ETIOLOGY AND PATHOPHYSIOLOGY

- Cardiomyopathy in Syrian hamsters may have a genetic component; however, the cause is unclear.
- Atrial thrombosis appears to be a consequence of heart failure. Bilateral ventricular hypertrophy is found in thrombosed hearts. The left atrium is most commonly affected and associated with disseminated intravascular coagulopathy. The cause is unknown.
- Heart failure and associated conditions in the Syrian hamster appear to be related to cardiovascular autonomic dysregulation.

DIAGNOSIS

DIFFERENTIAL DIAGNOSIS

- Neoplasia: lymphoma, hemangioma
- Metabolic disease
- Encephalomyocarditis virus (rare; primarily in laboratory models)

INITIAL DATABASE

- Full-body radiographs (lateral and dorsoventral views). Possible findings include the following:
  - Cardiac enlargement
  - Pulmonary edema
  - Pleural effusion
  - Hepatomegaly
  - Ascites
- Biochemistry: usually normal, but in severe cases, prerenal azotemia and hyponatremia may be revealed
- Complete blood count: usually normal

ADVANCED OR CONFIRMATORY TESTING

- Echocardiography is the diagnostic modality of choice in the diagnosis of cardiomyopathies.
- Reference ranges are available for echocardiographic parameters in Syrian hamsters under pentobarbital anesthesia:
  - Left ventricular internal diameter (LVID) in diastole: 3.7-4.5 mm; LVID in systole: 1.9-2.7 mm; left ventricular posterior wall in diastole (LVPWd): 0.9-1.1 mm; internal ventricular septum (IVS) in diastole: 0.9-1.1 mm, fractional shortening 44.7% ± 6.6%
- ECG: no reference ranges published for hamsters

TREATMENT

THERAPEUTIC GOALS

- Improve oxygenation status.
- Reduce pleural effusion or pulmonary edema.
- Improve cardiac output.
- Minimize length of hospitalization.

ACUTE GENERAL TREATMENT

Medication dosages are often extrapolations from other domestic species.

- General guidelines
  - Oxygen therapy
  - Warm incubator
  - Supplemental feeding for debilitated animals
  - Pleural and/or abdominal tap if indicated (sedation or general anesthesia recommended)
- Diuretics such as injectable furosemide are most useful initially in hospitalized patients. Oral furosemide should be considered for outpatients.

- Furosemide 2-10 mg/kg IM, SC, PO q 4-12 h
- Enalapril 0.5-1.0 mg/kg PO q 24 h
- Pimobendan 0.2-0.4 mg/kg PO q 12 h
- Digoxin 0.05-0.1 mg/kg PO q 12-24 h

CHRONIC TREATMENT

- Furosemide dose should be reduced to a lower maintenance dose once the fluid overload is corrected.
- Enalapril may be combined with pimobendan for long-term therapy.

DRUG INTERACTIONS

Effects of pimobendan may be attenuated if used concurrently with diltiazem, verapamil, propranolol, or other calcium antagonists or beta antagonists.

POSSIBLE COMPLICATIONS

- Atrial thrombosis
- DIC
- Sudden death

RECOMMENDED MONITORING

Recheck in 7 days from initial presentation, then in 30 days if animal continues to do well.

PROGNOSIS AND OUTCOME

- Poor: atrial thrombosis; cardiomyopathy usually progresses to atrial thrombosis and/or DIC
- Sudden death may occur even with treatment.

PEARLS & CONSIDERATIONS

PREVENTION

Little to no information is available on the efficacy of using prophylactic anticoagulant therapy in Syrian hamsters to prevent or reduce the severity of atrial thrombosis.

SUGGESTED READINGS

Heatley JJ: Cardiovascular anatomy, physiology, and disease of rodents and small exotic mammals, Vet Clin North Am Exot Anim Pract 12:99–113, 2009.
Schmidt RE, et al: Cardiovascular disease in hamsters: review and retrospective study, J Exotic Pet Med 16:49, 2007.
Salem VMC, et al: Reference values for M-mode and Doppler echocardiography for normal Syrian hamsters, Eur J Echocardiogr 6:41, 2005.

AUTHOR: **DOMINIQUE L. KELLER**

EDITOR: **CHRISTOPH MANS**

SMALL MAMMALS: HAMSTERS

Cheek Pouch Disorder

BASIC INFORMATION

DEFINITION

Disorders affecting the cheek pouches. Cheek pouch eversions and impactions occur most frequently.

SYNONYMS

Cheek pouch eversion, cheek pouch prolapse, cheek pouch impaction

SPECIAL SPECIES CONSIDERATIONS

- Cheek pouches are distensible evaginations of the lateral buccal wall.
- Cheek pouches are used to store and transport food and bedding material.
- Occasionally, a female hamster may place her young in her pouches.
- In Syrian hamsters *(Mesocricetus auratus)*, the cheek pouches can be 30-40 mm long and up to 20 mm wide when distended with material.

EPIDEMIOLOGY

SPECIES, AGE, SEX

- Hamsters of any age and species are susceptible.
- Russian dwarf hamsters *(Phodopus spp.)* may be predisposed to pouch eversion due to overfeeding.

RISK FACTORS

- Overfeeding; feeding of inappropriate food (e.g., sticky substances)
- Dental disease

ASSOCIATED CONDITIONS AND DISORDERS

- Neoplasia can occasionally be associated with cheek pouch eversion.
- Secondary trauma to prolapsed pouch tissue

CLINICAL PRESENTATION

DISEASE FORMS/SUBTYPES

- Cheek pouch impaction
- Cheek pouch eversion

HISTORY, CHIEF COMPLAINT

- Cheek pouch impaction:
  - Persistent swelling in facial or cervical region
  - Inability to completely evacuate cheek pouch
  - Frequent pawing at face or cheeks
  - Halitosis
- Cheek pouch eversion
  - Protrusion of material from oral cavity

PHYSICAL EXAM FINDINGS

- Cheek pouch impaction
  - Firm to semifirm swelling on the lateral head and neck
  - Food or debris may be present at pouch entrance and in pouch.
- Cheek pouch eversion
  - Tissue prolapsed or protruding from oral cavity
  - Prolapsed tissue may exhibit signs of abscessation, ulceration, and/or necrosis.
- Oral examination may reveal evidence of dental disease.
- Weight loss

ETIOLOGY AND PATHOPHYSIOLOGY

- Overfeeding can cause hamsters to "cache" food in their cheek pouches; this material may become adhered to the mucosal surface, making it difficult for the hamster to remove it on its own. The adhered material may also cause the cheek pouches to evert.
- Dental disease may predispose to abscess formation with spread from the oral cavity to the cheek pouch.
- Trauma to the cheek pouch mucosa from rough bedding, food, or bite wounds may lead to abscessation.
- Spontaneous squamous cell carcinoma of the cheek pouch with subsequent eversion has been reported in Djungarian hamsters *(Phodopus sungorus)*.

DIAGNOSIS

DIFFERENTIAL DIAGNOSIS

- Cheek pouch impaction
  - Lymphadenopathy (e.g., lymphoma)
  - Periodontal abscess
  - Neoplasia, not associated with the cheek pouches
- Cheek pouch eversion
  - Neoplasia of the oral cavity

INITIAL DATABASE

- Radiographs/CT of the skull may be indicated to determine whether underlying bony involvement is present and to evaluate the extent of dental disease.
- Endoscopy-guided intraoral examination for evaluation of the cheek pouches and oral cavity
- Fine-needle aspirate/cytologic examination

ADVANCED OR CONFIRMATORY TESTING

- Culture and sensitivity of cheek pouch abscesses
- Biopsy with histopathologic examination

TREATMENT

THERAPEUTIC GOALS

- Preserve the ability to prehend food normally.
- Restore healthy cheek pouch tissue.

ACUTE GENERAL TREATMENT

- Cheek pouch impaction
  - Manual removal of material under sedation or general anesthesia. Caution not to damage oral mucosa during procedure. Flush or swab the mucosa with sterile saline following removal of material.
- Cheek pouch eversion and prolapse
  - Manual reduction of the prolapse if the tissue is viable under sedation or general anesthesia. Nonviable tissue should be removed. One or more percutaneous, full-thickness single sutures (i.e., 3-0 to 4-0 nylon) should be placed to tack the everted tissue in correct anatomic position. Suture(s) should be removed in 10-14 days.
  - Abscesses, necrosis, or ulceration of the cheek pouches requires wound débridement, antimicrobial therapy, and possible amputation.
  - Antimicrobial therapy
    - Trimethoprim-sulfa 30 mg/kg PO q 12 h
    - Enrofloxacin 10-20 mg/kg PO, SC q 12-24 h; Caution with SC injection because it can cause severe pain and tissue necrosis. Dilute with sterile saline before injection.
    - Doxycycline 2.5-5 mg/kg PO q 12 h
    - Chloramphenicol 30-50 mg/kg PO q 8 h
- Pain management
  - Buprenorphine 0.05-0.1 mg/kg SC q 8-12 h
  - Meloxicam 0.3-0.5 mg/kg PO, SC q 24 h

CHRONIC TREATMENT

- Based on histopathologic examination results, surgery may be indicated to remove neoplastic tissue.
- Prolapse may recur, especially if tacking sutures are not placed, necessitating additional procedures.
- Amputation of the prolapsed cheek pouch tissue may be necessary if the tissue is necrotic or if prolapse is recurring despite initiated treatment.

POSSIBLE COMPLICATIONS

- Recurrent cheek pouch prolapse
- Necrosis of part or the entire cheek pouch, which requires amputation of affected tissue
- Untreated dental disease can cause anorexia and chronic infection.

RECOMMENDED MONITORING

Recheck appointment in 7-14 days or sooner if complications are noted.

PROGNOSIS AND OUTCOME

- Good to guarded for impaction, eversion, or cheek pouch abscesses if treated early
- Variable for neoplastic disease depending on size, location, and type of underlying tumor

PEARLS & CONSIDERATIONS

COMMENTS

Clients may present a hamster for cheek pouch disorders, which are actually normal storage of foodstuffs. Ensure that food material is not impacted, and advise owners to feed a small amount frequently to ensure that food does not become adhered to the underlying mucosa.

PREVENTION

- Small meals frequently
- Ensure a proper diet.
- Avoid bedding with potential to traumatize cheek pouch mucosa.
- Prevent overcrowding.

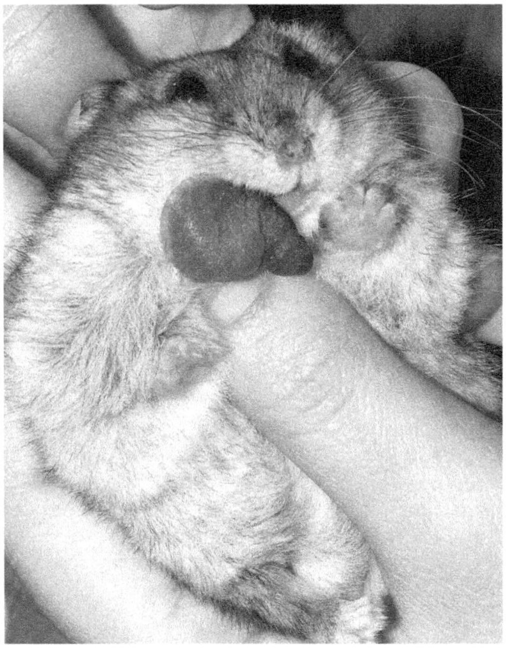

Cheek Pouch Disorder Russian dwarf hamster with partial prolapse of the right cheek pouch.

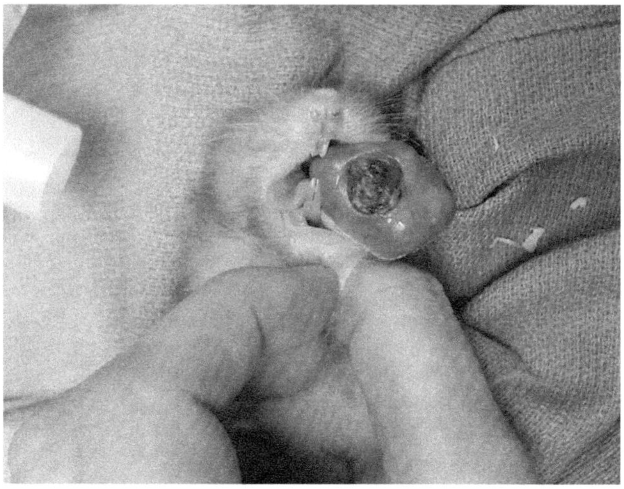

Cheek Pouch Disorder An everted check pouch with an abscess in a hamster. *(Photo courtesy Jörg Mayer, The University of Georgia, Athens.)*

SUGGESTED READING

Capello V: Surgical techniques in pet hamsters, Exotic DVM 5:32–37, 2005.

Martorell J, et al: Spontaneous squamous cell carcinoma of the cheek pouch in two dwarf hamsters *(Phodopus sungorus)*, Vet Rec 156:650–651, 2005.

AUTHORS: **BRIAN A. EVANS AND DOMINIQUE L. KELLER**

EDITOR: **CHRISTOPH MANS**

SMALL MAMMALS: HAMSTERS

Dental Disease

BASIC INFORMATION

DEFINITION

Disorders affecting the dentition

SPECIAL SPECIES CONSIDERATIONS

- Dental formula: 2(I1C0P0M3)
- Incisor teeth are erupted at birth; incisors have a long crown (hypsodont), have no anatomic root (aradicular), and therefore grow continuously (elodont).
- Cheek teeth have anatomic roots, erupt shortly after birth, and do not continue to erupt.

EPIDEMIOLOGY

SPECIES, AGE, SEX Hamsters of all ages and species are susceptible to dental disease.

CLINICAL PRESENTATION

HISTORY, CHIEF COMPLAINT

- Change in feed preference (i.e., interested only in eating treats)
- Anorexia
- Weight loss
- Ptyalism
- Lethargy

PHYSICAL EXAM FINDINGS

- Full oral examination will require sedation or general anesthesia and should be performed endoscopy-guided.
- Unkempt coat
- Cachexia
- Ptyalism
- Halitosis
- Maxillary or mandibular swelling(s)
- Draining tract on face
- Exophthalmos
- Overgrown, worn, maloccluded, or fractured incisors
- Fractured or mobile cheek teeth
- Soft tissue lesions secondary to malocclusion

ETIOLOGY AND PATHOPHYSIOLOGY

- Incisor teeth disorders
  - Incisor malocclusion
    - Trauma leading to fracture
    - Iatrogenic: attempts to trim teeth using inappropriate equipment
    - Excessive chewing on cage bars or cage furnishings
    - Congenital
  - Incisor elongation
    - Inappropriate diet
    - Lack of provision of hard chewing material
- Cheek teeth disorders
  - Malocclusion or fracture secondary
    - Trauma
  - Caries
    - Inappropriate diet (excessive carbohydrates such as sugary treats)
- Exophthalmia
  - Secondary to periapical abscesses of the maxillary cheek teeth
- Hamster parvovirus (HaPV)
- Naturally infected fetal and neonatal Syrian hamsters show discoloration, malformation, and loss of incisor teeth.

DIAGNOSIS

DIFFERENTIAL DIAGNOSIS

- Weight loss
  - Systemic disease
  - Neoplasia
- Ptyalism
  - Cheek pouch impaction or infection
  - Trauma
  - Foreign body in oral cavity
- Exophthalmia: see Ocular Disorders
- Facial swelling
  - Trauma
  - Abscess
  - Neoplasia
  - Cheek pouch disorders (see Cheek Pouch Disorders)
    - Normal filling of pouch with food or other material
    - Impacted cheek pouch

INITIAL DATABASE

- Skull radiographs (dental imaging equipment ideal for this procedure)
  - Views should include lateral, left and right 45° oblique lateral, and ventrodorsal; rostrocaudal views may also be useful for examining cheek teeth occlusal surfaces.
- Endoscopy-guided dental examination is necessary for a complete intraoral examination.
- Fine-needle aspirate and cytologic examination of facial swellings
- Cytologic examination and bacterial culture of draining tracts

ADVANCED OR CONFIRMATORY TESTING

- Skull CT scan (resolution of some scanners may limit their use) will require deep sedation or general anesthesia.
- Serology for parvovirus (HaPV cross-reacts with mouse parvovirus) when significant morbidity and mortality among suckling and weanling Syrian hamsters characterized by tooth loss or discoloration.

TREATMENT

THERAPEUTIC GOALS

- Treat underlying cause.
- Restore occlusion if possible.

ACUTE GENERAL TREATMENT

- General supportive care
  - Warmed fluids if dehydrated
    - Maintenance rate: 60-100 mL/kg/d
  - Analgesia
    - Buprenorphine 0.05-0.1 mg/kg SC or transmucosal q 8-12 h
    - Meloxicam 0.3-0.5 mg/kg PO, SC q 24 h once adequately hydrated
- Trim maloccluded teeth with a dental burr; cheek teeth treatment (e.g., periodontal procedures, extractions) will require endoscopic visualization.
- Appropriate antibiosis if a periapical or periodontal infection is present. Ensure appropriate coverage against anaerobic bacteria:
  - Metronidazole 20 mg/kg PO q 12 h
  - Penicillin G benzathine 50000 IU/kg SC q 3-7 d
  - Doxycycline 2.5-5 mg/kg PO q 12 h
  - Enrofloxacin 10-20 mg/kg PO q 12-24 h: combine with metronidazole for anaerobic coverage
  - Trimethoprim-sulfa 30 mg/kg PO q 12 h: combine with metronidazole for anaerobic coverage
  - Chloramphenicol 30-50 mg/kg PO q 8 h

- Euthanasia may be appropriate for severe cases.
- Stop all breeding for 12 weeks in Syrian hamsters if HaPV outbreak detected. Euthanize affected pups as stunted growth, ataxia, and death follow initial dental signs.

CHRONIC TREATMENT

- Tooth extraction (fractured or carious teeth)
  - Incisor teeth can be extracted by loosening the periodontal ligament using small-gauge hypodermic needles.
    - Iatrogenic fracture of the incisors or mandible is possible.
  - Cheek teeth may be difficult to extract.
    - Periapical abscesses may become very large before they are noted by owners.
      - Surgical management of cases that have progressed to osteomyelitis is challenging.
- Nutritional support
  - Force feeding
    - Appropriate critical care diet or blended mixture of hamster pellets until hamster is able to feed itself
  - Oral electrolyte support

DRUG INTERACTIONS

Do not use NSAIDs in a dehydrated animal.

POSSIBLE COMPLICATIONS

- Iatrogenic fracture of teeth, mandible, or, more rarely, maxilla is a possible complication of tooth trims or extractions.
- Extraction of elodont incisors may result in regrowth if germinative tissue is not completely removed during extraction.
- Elongated incisors may grow into and perforate the hard palate, leading to oronasal fistulas.
- Periapical infection may lead to osteomyelitis.
- Hamsters are very sensitive to antibiotic-associated dysbiosis: avoid oral administration of antibiotics with a Gram-positive spectrum (e.g., cephalosporins, penicillins, clindamycin).

RECOMMENDED MONITORING

- Maloccluded incisors may need trimming as frequently as every 2 weeks.
- Recheck in 1 week following discharge if tooth was extracted.

PROGNOSIS AND OUTCOME

- Fair to guarded for incisor malocclusion
- Fair to poor for other dental conditions

CONTROVERSY

Do not use nail trimmers to cut incisor teeth.

PEARLS & CONSIDERATIONS

COMMENTS

- Congenital dental disease is rare in rodents; most dental disease is acquired.
- The crown length ratio of upper to lower incisors should be about 1:3.
- Some degree of movement between mandibular incisors is normal owing to incomplete fusion of the mandibular symphysis.
- Normal hamster dental enamel is yellowish-orange.

PREVENTION

- Provision of a commercial pelleted diet and appropriate cage furniture (food grade wood, cardboard, etc.) is important.
- Sugary treats should be avoided as caries and periodontal disease develop in Syrian hamsters.

CLIENT EDUCATION

- Educate owners as to appropriate hamster dietary requirements.
- Show owners how to monitor incisor length in cases of chronic incisor malocclusion requiring frequent tooth trims.
- Owners must be informed that treatment of chronic dental disease often is only palliative.

SUGGESTED READINGS

Besselsen DG, et al: Natural and experimentally induced infection of Syrian hamsters with a newly recognized parvovirus, Lab Anim Sci 49:308–312, 1999.
Campbell RG, et al: Effect of certain dietary sugars on hamster caries, J Nutr 100:11–20, 1970.
Capello V: Diagnosis and treatment of dental disease in pet rodents, J Exotic Pet Med 17:114–123, 2008.

CROSS-REFERENCES TO OTHER SECTIONS

Cheek Pouch Disorders
Intestinal Disorders
Ocular Disorders

AUTHOR: **DOMINIQUE L. KELLER**

EDITOR: **CHRISTOPH MANS**

SMALL MAMMALS: HAMSTERS

Intestinal Disorders

Client Education Sheet Available on Website

BASIC INFORMATION

DEFINITION

Diseases of the lower gastrointestinal tract, which are frequently associated with increased frequency of defecation and loose feces or diarrhea

SYNONYMS

Wet tail, transmissible ileal hyperplasia, proliferative ileitis, Tyzzer's disease, antibiotic-associated enterocolitis, hamster enteritis

SPECIAL SPECIES CONSIDERATIONS

Hamsters can store large amounts of food in their cages; these stores can become sources of contaminated food if not cleaned out regularly.

EPIDEMIOLOGY

SPECIES, AGE, SEX Hamsters <5 weeks of age most susceptible to *Lawsonia intracellularis, Clostridium piliforme.*

RISK FACTORS

- Contaminated feed
- Stress
- Overcrowding

CONTAGION AND ZOONOSIS *Campylobacter fetus* spp. *jejuni, Salmonella* spp., *Clostridium difficile*, and *Rodentolepis nana* (prev *Hymenolepis nana*) are zoonotic.

CLINICAL PRESENTATION

HISTORY, CHIEF COMPLAINT

- Recent acquisition or transport
- Dietary change
- Increase in stress

- Anorexia
- Diarrhea
- Lethargy
- Soiled perineum, tail area ("wet tail")
- Irritability, hunched posture suggesting abdominal discomfort
- Sudden death

PHYSICAL EXAM FINDINGS

- Clinical signs very similar for the major causative agents
  - Diarrhea
  - Wet or soiled perineum
  - Depression
  - Dehydration
  - Cachexia
  - Weight loss
  - Abdominal distention
  - Palpable abdominal masses
  - Intestinal prolapse (especially in association with *L. intracellularis*)

ETIOLOGY AND PATHOPHYSIOLOGY

- Proliferative ileitis
  - *Lawsonia intracellularis*
  - Obligate gram-negative intracellular bacterium
  - Young hamsters (3-10 wk) most affected; after 12 weeks of age, appear to develop resistance
  - *Campylobacter fetus* spp. *jejuni* may also be associated with this syndrome in affected adult hamsters
- Tyzzer's disease
  - *Clostridium piliforme* (prev. *Bacillus piliforme*)
  - Gram-negative anaerobe, spore-forming intracellular bacterium
  - Weanlings (3-5 wk) most affected
- Antibiotic-associated enterocolitis
  - *Clostridium difficile*
  - Gram-positive anaerobe
  - Usually seen 2-10 days after oral administration of antibiotics with Gram-positive spectrum: lincosamides (lincomycin, clindamycin), beta-lactams (penicillin and cephalosporin derivatives), macrolides (erythromycin)
  - Occasional infection in hamsters with no antibiotic exposure
  - Incorrect use of oral antibiotics, which can eradicate physiologic Gram-positive population (especially *Lactobacillus, Bacteroides*), leading to overgrowth and toxin production of *C. difficile* and enterobacteria (e.g., *Escherichia coli*)
    - Intestinal impaction can occasionally be caused by heavy cestode (*R. nana*) infection.

DIAGNOSIS

DIFFERENTIAL DIAGNOSIS

- If weanlings affected, consider
  - *L. intracellularis, C. piliforme, E. coli, Salmonella* spp.
- Association with recent oral antibiotic administration
  - *C. difficile*
- Protozoa
  - *Giardia muris*
  - *Tritrichomonas muris*
  - *Spironucleus muris*
  - *Cryptosporidium* spp.
- Nematodes (rarely cause clinical disease, unless heavy infection)
  - Pinworms: *Syphacia obvelata, S. mesocriceti*
- Cestodes (rarely cause clinical disease unless heavy infection)
  - *R. nana* (dwarf tapeworm), *Hymenolepis diminuta* (rat tapeworm)
- Diet change: increase in fresh vegetable ration; change in pelleted ration
- Intestinal neoplasia (polyps, adenocarcinoma, lymphoma)
- Toxin exposure
- Mycotic (e.g., *Candida*) infections of the intestinal tract are rare in hamsters.

INITIAL DATABASE

- Fecal flotation and wet mount
- Fecal cytologic examination
- Acetate tape preparation for pinworms
- Radiographs
- Fecal culture and sensitivity (aerobic and anaerobic may be required): interpretation of culture results may be difficult

ADVANCED OR CONFIRMATORY TESTING

- PCR: *L. intracellularis, C. piliforme*
- *Giardia* antigen testing
- Abdominal ultrasound: small size of animal and possible intestinal tympany can limit the diagnostic value
- Necropsy

TREATMENT

THERAPEUTIC GOALS

- Restore hydration and nutritional status.
- Treat the underlying primary cause of intestinal disease.

ACUTE GENERAL TREATMENT

- General supportive care
  - Warm incubator
  - Fluid therapy
    - Fluids should be warmed to body temperature before administration.
    - Maintenance rate: 100 mL/kg/d
    - Subcutaneous administration is least stressful.
    - Shock doses of LRS or Normosol-R SC at 60-90 mL/kg; partial dose can be given IP in the left lower abdominal quadrant. IO route may be considered if hamster is large enough (femur and tibia preferred sites).
  - Quiet environment to reduce stress
  - Probiotics containing *Lactobacillus* spp. may be helpful based on anecdotal reports.
  - Nutritional and oral electrolyte support
- Analgesia
  - Buprenorphine 0.05-0.1 mg/kg SC q 6-12 h

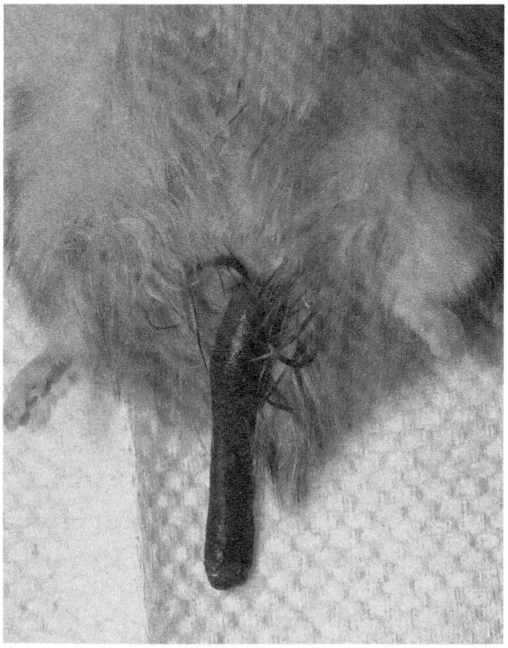

Intestinal Disorders Intestinal prolapse in a Syrian hamster.

- Antimicrobial therapy
  - *E. coli* infection: antibiotic therapy may worsen disease
  - *L. intracellularis*
    - Metronidazole 20 mg/kg PO q 12 h
    - Doxycycline 2.5-5 mg/kg PO q 12 h
    - Chloramphenicol 30-50 mg/kg PO q 12 h
    - Enrofloxacin 10 mg/kg PO, SC q 12 h: CAUTION with SC injection as it can cause tissue necrosis. Dilute with sterile saline before injection.
- Antibiotic-induced enteritis *(C. difficile)*
  - Discontinue use of inappropriate antibiotic.
  - Initiate treatment with appropriate antibiotic.
    - Metronidazole 20 mg/kg PO q 12 h
    - Trimethoprim-sulfa 30 mg/kg PO q 12 h
  - Supplemental vitamin B complex administration may be helpful (0.02-0.2 mL/kg SC; based 0.1 mg/mL/B_{12})
- Rectal/intestinal prolapse may be amenable to surgical correction but consider underlying cause before suggesting surgery to owners.
- Protozoa
  - Metronidazole 20 mg/kg PO q 12 h
  - *Cryptosporidium*: no effective treatment
- Nematodes
  - Ivermectin 0.2-0.4 mg/kg SC, PO, or topical; q 7-14 d for 3-4 doses
  - Fenbendazole 20 mg/kg PO q 24 h for 5 days
- Cestodes
  - Praziquantel 6-10 mg/kg PO, SC; repeat in 10 days

POSSIBLE COMPLICATIONS

- Rectal prolapse, intestinal obstruction, intussusception
- Infection with *L. intracellularis* may recur once therapy is discontinued.
- Bacterial enteritis may predispose to overgrowth of commensal protozoal fauna.

RECOMMENDED MONITORING

- Recheck in 1 week following discharge.
- Recheck fecal in 1 month following treatment for intestinal parasitism.

PROGNOSIS AND OUTCOME

Dependent on underlying cause

- Poor: *C. difficile, Salmonella* spp., *L. intracellularis*
- Fair: other causes of intestinal disease
- Fair to good: intestinal parasitism

PEARLS & CONSIDERATIONS

PREVENTION

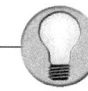

- Hamster food should be stored in an airtight container to prevent spoilage and contamination.
- Regular cage cleaning and removal of stored, potentially spoiled food

CLIENT EDUCATION

Educate clients as to the importance of minimum 30 day quarantine for new animals.

SUGGESTED READINGS

Cunnane SC, et al: Intussusception in the Syrian golden hamster, Br J Nutr 63:231–237, 1990.

Fiskett RM: Lawsonia intracellularis infection in hamsters (*Mesocricetus auratus*), J Exotic Pet Med 20:277–283, 2011.

Franklin CL, et al: Tyzzer's infection: host specificity of *Clostridium piliforme* isolates, Lab Anim Sci 44:568–572, 1994.

Hart M, et al: Multiple peracute deaths in a colony of Syrian hamsters (*Mesocricetus auratus*), Lab Anim (NY) 39:99–102, 2010.

Sambol SP, et al: Colonization for the prevention of *Clostridium difficile* disease in hamsters, J Infect Dis 186:1781–1789, 2002.

AUTHOR: **DOMINIQUE L. KELLER**

EDITOR: **CHRISTOPH MANS**

SMALL MAMMALS: HAMSTERS

Ocular Disorders

BASIC INFORMATION

DEFINITION

Abnormalities of the eyes and surrounding structures

SPECIAL SPECIES CONSIDERATIONS

Eyelid separation occurs at 15 days of age in Syrian hamsters *(Mesocricetus auratus)* and at 10-14 days in Russian (dwarf) hamsters (*Phodopus* spp.)

EPIDEMIOLOGY

SPECIES, AGE, SEX All species of hamsters can be affected.

GENETICS AND BREED PREDISPOSITION

- Certain species of Russian (dwarf) hamsters have a genetic predisposition to ocular disorders.
- Siberian hamsters (*Phodopus sungorus*) may develop diabetes mellitus with secondary cataracts.
- Djungarian hamsters (*Phodopus campbelli*) may be born with microphthalmia; they may also develop glaucoma.

RISK FACTORS

- Poor environmental hygiene and inappropriate bedding (stemmy hay, pine or cedar chips) can lead to ocular disease.
- Overcrowding can predispose to conspecific trauma.

ASSOCIATED CONDITIONS AND DISORDERS

- Allergies
- Dental disease
- Diabetes mellitus
- Trauma
- Cytomegalovirus infection

CLINICAL PRESENTATION

HISTORY, CHIEF COMPLAINT Will vary depending on underlying cause:

- Eye discharge
- Crusting around eyes
- Swelling of one or both eyes
- Ocular prolapse
- Behavior suggestive of visual impairment
- Anorexia
- Difficulty eating
- Weight loss
- Pawing at face

PHYSICAL EXAM FINDINGS Ocular changes may be unilateral or bilateral depending on cause:

- Blepharospasm
- Ocular discharge
- Conjunctivitis
- Corneal edema
- Corneal ulceration
- Hyphema or hypopyon
- Ocular foreign body
- Exophthalmos/buphthalmos
- Ocular proptosis
- Cataract (mydriatics may be necessary to identify)
- Facial swelling
- Dental disease

ETIOLOGY AND PATHOPHYSIOLOGY

- Infectious keratoconjunctivitis
  - *Pasteurella spp.*
  - *Streptococcus spp.*
  - Other bacteria
- Glaucoma may be genetic in Djungarian hamsters.
- Proptosis: can be caused by excessive manual restraint

DIAGNOSIS

DIFFERENTIAL DIAGNOSIS

- Exophthalmos/buphthalmos: retrobulbar abscess, dental disease, glaucoma, trauma, neoplasia
- Proptosis: trauma, retrobulbar abscess, dental disease
- Keratoconjunctivitis: allergies, trauma, poor environmental hygiene, use of irritating bedding
- Corneal injury: trauma, foreign body, chemical injury (caustic cleaners)
- Hyphema: trauma, uveitis, coagulopathy, neoplasia, glaucoma

INITIAL DATABASE

- Complete ocular examination (sedation or anesthesia may be necessary)
  - Slit lamp examination
  - Fluorescein staining
  - Tonometry (may not be feasible in Russian [dwarf] hamsters)
  - Fundic examination following mydriasis with tropicamide may be attempted, but small size of the eye may make examination difficult. Some rodents require additional mydriasis (i.e., 10% phenylephrine).
- Cytology: conjunctival and/or corneal scrapings
- Culture and sensitivity in cases of conjunctivitis

ADVANCED OR CONFIRMATORY TESTING

- Sedated or anesthetized (endoscopy-guided) intraoral examination
- Blood glucose to rule out diabetes
- Radiography/CT scan of skull: rule out dental disease and retrobulbar process
- Histopathologic examination of conjunctival biopsy specimens or enucleated globe

TREATMENT

THERAPEUTIC GOALS

Vary with underlying cause of disease

- Resolve bacterial infections.
- Salvage globe if feasible.
- Reduce risk of further injury to globe.
- Manage ocular pain.
- Identify and treat underlying disease (e.g., dental disease, glaucoma).

ACUTE GENERAL TREATMENT

- General guidelines
  - Cleanse affected eye with sterile eye wash.
  - Systemic analgesia if indicated
    - Meloxicam 0.3-0.5 mg/kg PO, SC q 24 h
    - Buprenorphine 0.05-0.1 mg/kg SC q 6-12 h
  - Topical antiinflammatory drugs, if indicated
    - Flurbiprofen drops 0.03% q 6-12 h
  - Topical antibiotic ointment if indicated
    - Gentamicin drops or ointment (0.3%)
    - Ciprofloxacin drops (0.3%): use only for confirmed Gram-negative infections
  - Topical lubrication (ointment or drops) if indicated
- Conjunctivitis and keratitis: varies depending on cause
  - Flush eye with sterile eye wash
  - Remove any foreign bodies
  - Topical antibiotics
- Exophthalmos/buphthalmos
  - Dental disease
    - Correction for dental malocclusion
    - Treatment of periodontal infection
  - Retrobulbar abscess
    - Abscess drainage and flushing; usually requires enucleation
    - Systemic antimicrobial therapy covering for anaerobic bacteria
      - Metronidazole 20 mg/kg PO q 12 h
      - Chloramphenicol 30-50 mg/kg PO q 8 h
      - Trimethoprim-sulfa 30 mg/kg PO q 12 h: does not provide anaerobic coverage and should be given in combination with, for example, metronidazole
      - Enrofloxacin 10-20 mg/kg PO q 12-24 h: does not provide anaerobic coverage and should be given in combination with, for example, metronidazole
    - Retrobulbar neoplasia
      - Enucleation and mass removal: complete removal often not possible
    - Glaucoma
      - Definitive diagnosis may be challenging.
      - Little information is available on acute or long-term medical treatment of glaucoma in hamsters.
- Proptosis
  - Gently cleanse affected eye with sterile eye wash to determine extent of damage.
  - Frequent lubrication for proptosed globe until eye can be removed or replaced
  - Temporary tarsorrhaphy if feasible
  - Enucleation
  - Treatment of underlying cause

CHRONIC TREATMENT

- Systemic analgesia as needed for chronic conditions
- Treat underlying systemic disease if present.
- Routine dental care may be needed.
- Eliminate underlying environmental causes.
- Chronic lubrication in cases of suspected idiopathic keratitis sicca

DRUG INTERACTIONS

Avoid topical antibiotics, which, if ingested, could lead to dysbacteriosis (lincosamides, cephalosporins, oral penicillins, macrolides).

POSSIBLE COMPLICATIONS

A chronic buphthalmic eye may eventually prolapse or rupture, requiring medical management or surgical intervention.

RECOMMENDED MONITORING

- Recheck 7-10 days post enucleation.
- Recheck examinations q 2-3 months for chronic conditions.
- Regular dental evaluations if dental disease has been diagnosed

PROGNOSIS AND OUTCOME

- Fair to good: enucleation following simple proptosis, conjunctivitis, corneal ulcers, uveitis
- Poor to fair: chronic buphthalmos depending on underlying condition; neoplasia; severe dental disease

PEARLS & CONSIDERATIONS

COMMENTS

Anesthesia or sedation is recommended for a full ophthalmic examination because this will reduce the degree of manual restraint needed.

PREVENTION

- Avoid beddings that release irritating volatile oils such as pine or cedar.
- Avoid housing adult Syrian hamsters in groups as this can lead to aggression.
- Overcrowding in dwarf hamster groups can also lead to aggression and trauma.

CLIENT EDUCATION

Avoid breeding hamsters with cataracts or suspected glaucoma because these may be heritable conditions.

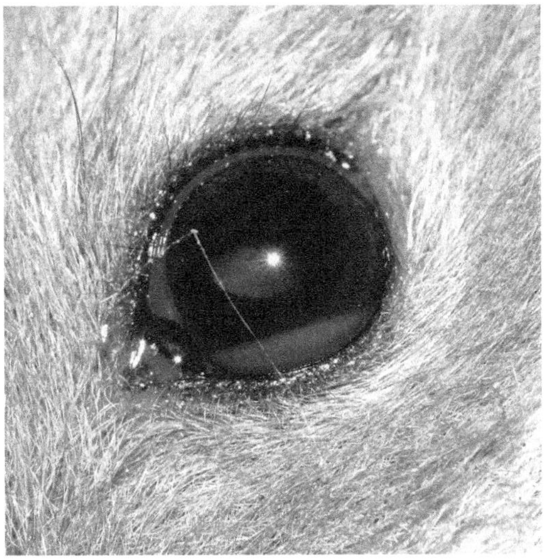

Ocular Disorders Hyphema (blood in the anterior chamber) in the ventral aspect of the left eye.

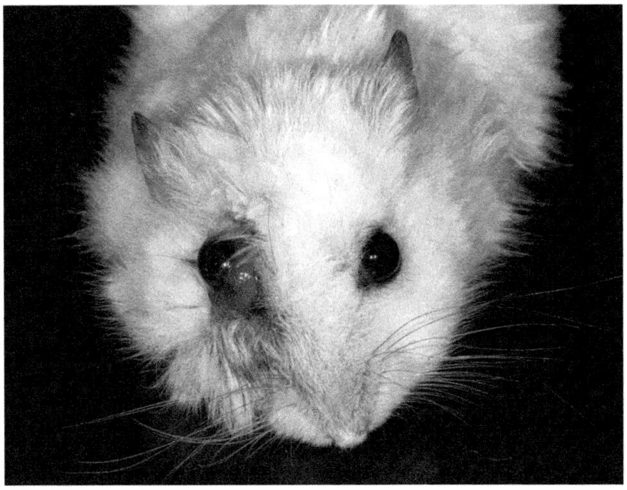

Ocular Disorders Proptosis of the right eye in a dwarf hamster.

SUGGESTED READINGS

Atkinson M: Suspected keratitis sicca in a Syrian hamster, Vet Rec 146:680, 2000.

Ekesten B, et al: Spontaneous buphthalmos in the Djungarian hamster *(Phodopus sungorus campbelli)*, Vet Ophthalmol 2:251–254, 1999.

AUTHOR: **DOMINIQUE L. KELLER**

EDITOR: **CHRISTOPH MANS**

SMALL MAMMALS: HAMSTERS

Renal Disease

BASIC INFORMATION

DEFINITION

Kidney or renal disease is a general term that describes any damage that reduces the functioning of the kidney.

SYNONYMS

- Kidney disease: renal disease, kidney failure, chronic renal failure, nephropathy, suppurative pyelonephritis, suppurative nephritis, polycystic kidney disease
- Amyloidosis in the hamster: protein-losing nephropathy
- Arteriolar nephrosclerosis in the hamster: hamster glomerulonephropathy

EPIDEMIOLOGY

SPECIES, AGE, SEX

- Amyloidosis in the hamster occurs earlier in females and more frequently in certain strains.
- Arteriolar nephrosclerosis in Syrian hamsters is associated with aging and is more frequent in females.

GENETICS AND BREED PREDISPOSITION Amyloidosis is a common geriatric disease in Syrian hamsters for which the exact pathogenesis is poorly understood.

RISK FACTORS Arteriolar nephrosclerosis: associations with excess dietary protein, underlying chronic viral infection, and renovascular hypertension have been made.

ASSOCIATED CONDITIONS AND DISORDERS Arteriolar nephrosclerosis and amyloidosis may be concurrent.

CLINICAL PRESENTATION

DISEASE FORMS/SUBTYPES

- Amyloidosis
- Arteriolar nephrosclerosis

HISTORY, CHIEF COMPLAINT Clinical signs vary with severity of kidney pathology:

- Polydipsia and polyuria
- Anorexia
- Weight loss
- Lethargy
- Abdominal distention

PHYSICAL EXAM FINDINGS

- In any hamster with renal disease, morbidity may vary from slight to none to significant depending on the progression of disease and the severity of disease.
- Lethargy
- Weight loss
- Cachexia
- Dehydration
- Poor fur quality
- Abdominal pain
- Abdominal distention
- Ascites
- Dyspnea
- Generalized edema
- Diarrhea

ETIOLOGY AND PATHOPHYSIOLOGY

- Amyloidosis
  - Amyloid is an insoluble pathologic proteinaceous substance deposited between cells in various tissues and organs of the body. Systemic amyloidosis can be classified as primary (AL or amyloid light chain), secondary (AA or amyloid associated), or familial. Secondary amyloidosis is more commonly described in animals and may be a reaction to diverse inflammatory stimuli.
  - Nephrotic syndrome is frequently associated with renal amyloidosis in hamsters and reflects amyloid deposition along the glomerular basement membranes. The resulting glomerulopathy causes severe loss of protein via the urine and a subsequent nephrotic syndrome characterized by malaise, fluid retention (edema, ascites, hydrothorax), hypoalbuminemia, hyperlipidemia, and eventual cachexia.
- Arteriolar nephrosclerosis
  - The cause and pathogenesis of the disease are poorly understood but have been interpreted to be

similar to those of progressive glomerulonephropathy in rats. Associations with excess dietary protein, underlying chronic viral infection, and renovascular hypertension have been made. Amyloidosis may be concurrent.

DIAGNOSIS

DIFFERENTIAL DIAGNOSIS

- Amyloidosis
- Arteriolar nephrosclerosis
- Polycystic disease (see Abdominal Distention)
- Suppurative pyelonephritis/nephritis
- Neoplasia (i.e., multicentric lymphoma)
- Congestive heart failure (see Cardiac Disease)

INITIAL DATABASE

- Urinalysis
  - Isosthenuria (normal specific gravity: 1.034-1.060)
  - Proteinuria
  - Hematuria
  - Sediment analysis: casts, crystals, inflammatory or neoplastic cells, bacteria
- Urine culture
- Serum biochemistry profile
  - Blood urea nitrogen (BUN) elevation
  - Creatinine elevation
  - Hypoalbuminemia
  - Hyperlipidemia
  - Hyperphosphatemia
  - Hypocalcemia or hypercalcemia
  - Hypokalemia or hyperkalemia
- Complete blood count: may be normal
  - Nonregenerative anemia
- Diagnostic imaging
  - Radiography: assess for increases or decreases in kidney size, radiopaque calculi within the urinary tract, abdominal masses associated with the urinary tract, and bladder distention.
  - Ultrasonography
    - Differentiate between ascites and polycystic disease.
    - Discern size, contour, and texture of the kidneys, allowing for differentiation of focal versus diffuse disease.

ADVANCED OR CONFIRMATORY TESTING

- Ultrasound-guided fine-needle aspiration for cytologic examination
- Histopathologic examination

TREATMENT

THERAPEUTIC GOALS

- Delay progression of renal disease.
- Preserve overall patient well-being and quality of life.
- Promote diuresis and diminish the consequences of azotemia.
- Treat underlying or concurrent urinary tract infection.

ACUTE GENERAL TREATMENT

- Discontinue any potentially nephrotoxic drugs.
- Identify and treat any prerenal or postrenal abnormalities.
- Identify any treatable conditions such as urolithiasis or pyelonephritis.
- Fluid therapy
  - To induce diuresis and correct azotemia and electrolyte and acid-base imbalances
  - Use of isotonic crystalloids
  - Subcutaneous administration: 60-100 mL/kg/d
  - Potassium supplementation of fluids based on blood potassium measurement
- If hyperphosphatemic, alter diet and initiate enteric phosphate binders
  - Aluminum hydroxide 30-90 mg/kg/d, divided and administered with food
- Treat increased gastric acidity with H2 blockers.
  - Famotidine 0.5 mg/kg PO, SC q 24 h
  - Ranitidine 1-2 mg/kg PO, SC q 12 h
- Multivitamin supplementation is recommended because the excessive amount of urine produced by failing kidneys commonly results in loss of water-soluble vitamins.
- Abdominal distention
  - Remove fluid from abdomen. This is a palliative treatment, and reaccumulation of fluid usually occurs within a few days. Removing fluid might improve the animal's comfort and improve dyspnea, if present.
- Antibiotic therapy
  - Indicated for cases of suppurative pyelonephritis/nephritis and cystitis
  - Antibiotic selection should be based on culture and susceptibility whenever possible.
  - For empirical treatment and for cases with negative urine culture, despite clinical suspicion, use antibiotics that are effective against Gram-negative organisms and are renally excreted to reach high tissue concentrations.
  - Trimethoprim-sulfa 15-30 mg/kg PO q 12 h
  - Enrofloxacin 10-20 mg/kg PO q 12-24 h

CHRONIC TREATMENT

- Maintain long-term dialysis with maintenance subcutaneous fluid therapy (owners can be taught to do this at home): 60-100 mL/kg/d SC
- Antibiotic therapy for chronic pyelonephritis should be given for at least 4-6 weeks.
- Dietary management: high protein appears to be the major cause of severe nephropathy; the term *protein overload nephropathy* is often used. Changing the source of protein to one such as soy protein, restricting caloric intake, or modifying the diet to decrease protein consumption could decrease the severity of nephropathy.
- Hyperphosphatemia that occurs in chronic renal failure is closely related to dietary protein intake because protein-rich diets are also high in phosphorus.
- Consider use of omega-3 fatty acid supplements based on studies showing their beneficial effects in other species.

POSSIBLE COMPLICATIONS

Anorexia, GI ulceration, hyperphosphatemia, acidosis, anemia, pulmonary edema, death

RECOMMENDED MONITORING

- Overall condition and clinical response to therapy should be assessed in all patients with renal disease. Frequency of follow-up assessments varies with initial diagnosis and severity of disease. Periodic assessments for azotemia, anemia, and phosphorus, potassium, and protein imbalances are recommended.
- Monitor body weight and condition, and adjust nutrition accordingly.
- Urinalysis and urine culture in patients being treated for pyelonephritis.

PROGNOSIS AND OUTCOME

- With any diagnosis of renal insufficiency or failure, prognosis varies with severity of clinical pathologic findings, duration of disease, and severity of primary renal failure. If secondary to infection or obstructive disease, prognosis is determined by duration of the disease process and success in treatment—medical or surgical—of the underlying condition of secondary renal insufficiency.
- Depending on initial diagnosis, disease severity, and response to therapy, quality of life issues and euthanasia should be discussed with the owner of any patient with renal failure.

CONTROVERSY

Hematologic, clinical chemistry, and urinalysis values may vary significantly with strain or breed of animal, nutritional status, sex, sampling site or frequency, time of day, stressors, age, health status, drug exposure, and environment. Therefore, normal values are broad, and these variables should be kept in mind when interpreting individual animal values.

PEARLS & CONSIDERATIONS

COMMENTS

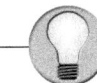

- *Renal failure* is a state of decreased renal function that allows persistent abnormalities (azotemia and inability to concentrate urine) to exist; this term refers to a level of organ function rather than to a specific disease entity. Acute renal failure generally refers to cases of sudden decline of glomerular filtration rate resulting in accumulation of nitrogenous waste products and inability to maintain normal fluid balance. *Chronic renal failure* generally refers to an insidious onset with slow progression (usually months to years) of azotemia and inadequately concentrated urine.
- Most of the renal diseases discussed can manifest as varying stages of compromise in renal reserve, renal insufficiency, or renal failure. If/when the disease process progresses depends on variables such as the specific disease in question, environmental factors, and the individual animal itself.

CLIENT EDUCATION

Chronic renal failure requires continuous treatment and monitoring. Unless a specific underlying cause is diagnosed and the patient is treated successfully, treatment in many cases will be lifelong.

SUGGESTED READINGS

Fisher PG: Exotic mammal renal disease: causes and clinical presentation, Vet Clin North Am Exot Anim Pract 9:33–67, 2006.

Fisher PG: Exotic mammal renal disease: diagnosis and treatment, Vet Clin North Am Exot Anim Pract 9:69–96, 2006.

CROSS-REFERENCES TO OTHER SECTIONS

Abdominal Distention
Cardiac Disease

AUTHOR: **PETER G. FISHER**

EDITOR: **CHRISTOPH MANS**

SMALL MAMMALS: HAMSTERS

Skin Diseases

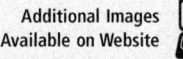

Additional Images Available on Website

BASIC INFORMATION

DEFINITION

Infectious and noninfectious diseases of the integument

SPECIAL SPECIES CONSIDERATIONS

- Syrian (golden) *(Mesocricetus auratus)* hamsters have bilateral sebaceous flank glands, which often are darkly pigmented and more prominent in males. Scent glands are used for marking. Scent glands should not be mistaken for neoplasia.
- Dwarf hamsters (*Phodopus* spp.) have a single ventral abdominal scent gland.

EPIDEMIOLOGY

SPECIES, AGE, SEX Hamster polyomavirus affects juvenile and adult Syrian hamsters differently. The cutaneous form of the disease is more common in adult hamsters.

GENETICS AND BREED PREDISPOSITION Syrian hamsters with two "satin" gene copies are predisposed to a thin or patchy hair coat.

RISK FACTORS

- Inappropriate bedding (e.g., cedar, pine) can cause contact dermatitis.
- Inappropriate nutrition

CONTAGION AND ZOONOSIS

- Dermatophytes are potentially zoonotic.
- *Ornithonyssus bacoti* (tropical rat mite) is a zoonotic parasite.

ASSOCIATED CONDITIONS AND DISORDERS

- Hyperadrenocorticism
- Amyloidosis
- Chronic renal insufficiency
- *Malassezia* dermatitis, often secondary to bacterial pyoderma or ectoparasite-induced dermatitis
- Conspecific trauma, often secondary to overcrowding
- Dental disease leading to reduced ability to groom
- Nutritional deficiencies

CLINICAL PRESENTATION

HISTORY, CHIEF COMPLAINT

- Rough hair coat
- Pruritus
- Hair loss
- Weight loss
- Lethargy
- Swellings on body

PHYSICAL EXAM FINDINGS Will vary depending on cause

- Alopecia
- Pruritus
- Localized erythema
- Abrasions, excoriations
- Scaling, crusting
- Lichenification
- Hyperpigmentation
- Cutaneous masses
- Pododermatitis

ETIOLOGY AND PATHOPHYSIOLOGY

- Abscesses
  - *Staphylococcus aureus, Streptococcus* spp., *Pasteurella pneumotropica, Actinomyces bovis*
  - Often secondary to conspecific trauma
- Hamster polyomavirus (HaPV; papovavirus)
  - Transmitted via urine
  - Hamsters infected as juveniles develop mesenteric lymphoma with metastasis to the liver, kidney, and thymus
  - Hamsters infected as adults develop epitheliomas, especially on the head and dorsum
- Dermatophytosis
  - *Microsporum* spp., *Trichophyton mentagrophytes*
  - Spontaneous occurring dermatophytosis is rare in Syrian hamsters. Infections cause dry, scaly lesions; encrustations with broken hair; or no clinical signs.
  - Immune deficiency or stress may be an underlying cause.
- Ectoparasites
  - Demodectic mites: *Demodex criceti, Demodex aurati*; clinical signs usually indicate underlying immune suppression
  - Sarcoptic mites: *Notoedres notoedres, Notoedres cati*
  - *Ornithonyssus bacoti*: blood-sucking mite; causes severe pruritus
- Allergic dermatitis: volatile components of bedding can be irritating to skin

- Pyoderma
  - *Staphylococcus* spp. secondary to self-trauma and pruritus from mites, dermatophytosis, neoplasia
- Pododermatitis: contact irritants, trauma, underlying osteoarthritis or osteomyelitis
- Hyperadrenocorticism (adrenal adenoma/carcinoma): can lead to thin skin, alopecia, and hyperpigmentation, in addition to more classic signs of polyuria and polyphagia
- Neoplasia, including lymphoma, hemangiosarcoma, melanoma, especially of the lateral flank glands in Syrian hamsters; epithelioma (HaPV), sebaceous gland adenoma, squamous cell carcinoma, cutaneous mastocytoma of the head in dwarf hamsters

DIAGNOSIS

DIFFERENTIAL DIAGNOSIS

- Alopecia: trauma, hyperadrenocorticism, dermatophytosis, satin gene coat, chronic renal disease, amyloidosis, hypothyroidism, nutritional deficiency (low-protein [<16%] or all-seed diet), neoplasia (cutaneous lymphoma)
  - Infectious causes
    - Demodectic mange: lesions usually located over dorsum and abdomen
      - *D. aurati:* elongate mite found in hair follicles
      - *D. criceti*: short mite found in cutaneous pits
    - Sarcoptic mange: extreme pruritus; lesions typically are found around the head, limbs, and genitals
    - Satin gene carrier: thin or sparse hair, which may be normal or greasy in appearance
- Cutaneous masses: neoplasia, inflammation, abscess, HaPV
- Crusting, flaking of skin: dermatophytosis, mange, nutritional deficiencies
- Localized erythema, pododermatitis: contact allergy, contact irritation (cleaners), trauma from bedding/cage material
- Red mites on hamster: *O. bacoti*

INITIAL DATABASE

- Full dietary history
- Genetic history (for satin gene suspects)
- Full history for potential toxin exposure
- Dermatologic examination
  - Skin scraping (sedation or general anesthesia is recommended): demodectic and sarcoptic mites
  - Acetate tape preparation: *Malassezia,* ectoparasites, bacterial dermatitis
- Dental examination (sedation or anesthesia is required)
  - Dental disease may contribute to inappropriate nutrition, altered grooming.
    - Fine-needle aspirate and cytologic examination of cutaneous masses
    - Serum biochemistry if systemic disorder is suspected. Increase in ALP may be seen with hyperadrenocorticism.
    - Hamsters secrete both cortisol and corticosterone; cortisol levels alone may not be sufficient to diagnose hyperadrenocorticism. Limited blood volume often limits determination of blood corticosteroid levels.

ADVANCED OR CONFIRMATORY TESTING

- Dermatophyte culture
- Radiographs: to rule out underlying skeletal abnormalities (e.g., osteoarthritis; osteomyelitis) in cases of pododermatitis
- Biopsy and histopathologic examination of skin lesion

TREATMENT

THERAPEUTIC GOALS

- Infectious disease: eliminate the underlying organism on the animal and in the environment
- Noninfectious disease: eliminate discomfort associated with lesions; alleviate signs associated with cause

ACUTE GENERAL TREATMENT

Will vary depending on the cause:

- Nutritional deficiency: improve diet; provide access to commercial pelleted diet and appropriate vegetables and sources of animal protein
- Hamster polyomavirus: no effective treatment; consider euthanasia if risk of transmission to other hamsters exists
- Infectious
  - Sarcoptic mites and *O. bacoti*
    - Ivermectin 0.2-0.4 mg/kg SC, PO q 7-14 d; higher dose is recommended
    - Selamectin 15-30 mg/kg topically q 14-28 d
    - Regular bedding changes, cage cleaning
  - Demodectic mites: Ivermectin 0.2-0.3 mg/kg PO q 24 h until clinical signs resolve and skin scrapings are negative for parasites
  - Dermatophytosis
    - Systemic antifungal therapy
      - Terbinafine 10-30 mg/kg PO q 24 h
      - Itraconazole 5-10 mg/kg PO q 24 h
    - Topical antifungal therapy may be used in combination with systemic therapy:
      - Enilconazole 1:50 dilution, spray or moist wipe
      - Miconazole/chlorhexidine shampoos
      - Lime sulfur dips 1:40 dilution, q 7 d
    - Environmental decontamination: frequent damp mopping of hard surfaces rather than sweeping can reduce environmental spread of spores; 1:10 bleach solution can be used to clean environment; contact time: 10 minutes
    - Monitoring: once-weekly dermatophyte test medium (DTM) cultures; discontinue treatment once two consecutive negative cultures are obtained. Fungal cultures of the environment can also be obtained.
  - Skin abscesses
    - Lance, débride, and flush.
    - If abscess intact, may sometimes be surgically removed in toto
    - Systemic antibiotic therapy based on culture and sensitivity; start empirical treatment with trimethoprim-sulfa pending culture
      - Trimethoprim-sulfa 30 mg/kg PO q 12 h
      - Chloramphenicol 30-50 mg/kg PO q 8 h
      - Enrofloxacin 10-20 mg/kg PO q 12-24 h
- Pododermatitis
  - Débridement and wound care (application of colloidal or silver-impregnated bandages or gels may be beneficial)
  - Systemic antibiotics
  - Analgesia: meloxicam 0.3-0.5 mg/kg PO, SC q 24 h
- Neoplasia: mass removal; clean margins may not be obtained
- Hyperadrenocorticism
  - Medical management has been reported but is usually unrewarding.
    - Mitotane 5 mg PO q 24 h and metyrapone 8 mg PO q 24 h have been used.

CHRONIC TREATMENT

Dermatophytosis and demodectic mange will often require long-term therapy.

DRUG INTERACTIONS

Hamsters are particularly susceptible to antibiotic-induced dysbacteriosis; monitor hamsters on oral antibiotics carefully; consider concomitant probiotic therapy.

POSSIBLE COMPLICATIONS

Hamsters may ingest any topical medications as they groom. Therefore, avoid topical use of inappropriate antibiotics and corticosteroids.

RECOMMENDED MONITORING

Weekly DTM cultures for dermatophytosis cases

PROGNOSIS AND OUTCOME

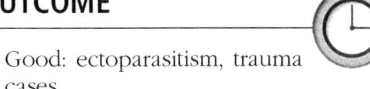

- Good: ectoparasitism, trauma cases
- Good to fair: dermatophytosis; pododermatitis (depending on severity of case, underlying cause)
- Fair to poor: neoplasia
- Poor: hamster polyomavirus; underlying systemic disease (renal failure, amyloidosis, hyperadrenocorticism)

PEARLS & CONSIDERATIONS

PREVENTION

- Provision of a commercial diet and a clean environment will go a long way toward reducing many skin conditions.
- Quarantine all new incoming animals for a minimum of 30 days before allowing contact with other animals.

CLIENT EDUCATION

- Dermatophytes are contagious; owners should be instructed that they should seek medical advice if lesions are found on humans in the household.
- Appropriate hamster bedding should be used. Woods containing volatile oils should be avoided.
- Care should be taken when cleaning the hamster's cage to remove all traces of any potentially toxic or caustic cleaners.
- The Syrian hamster satin gene is dominant; breeding of two satin hamsters will yield some offspring with the sparse satin coat.

SUGGESTED READINGS

Beco L, et al: Comparison of subcutaneous ivermectin and oral moxidectin for the treatment of notoedric acariasis in hamsters, Vet Rec 149:324–327, 2001.

Tani K, et al: Ivermectin treatment of demodicosis in 56 hamsters, J Vet Med Sci 63:1245–1247, 2001.

CROSS-REFERENCES TO OTHER SECTIONS

Hamster: Dental Disease
Guinea Pig: Skin Diseases

AUTHOR: **DOMINIQUE L. KELLER**

EDITOR: **CHRISTOPH MANS**

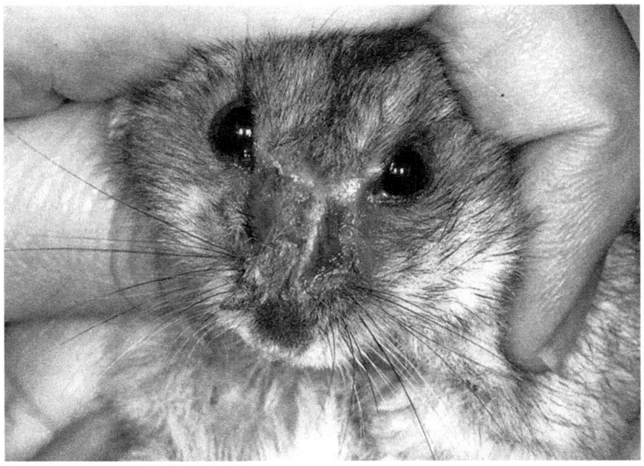

Skin Diseases Deep ulcerative bacterial dermatitis in a Russian dwarf hamster.

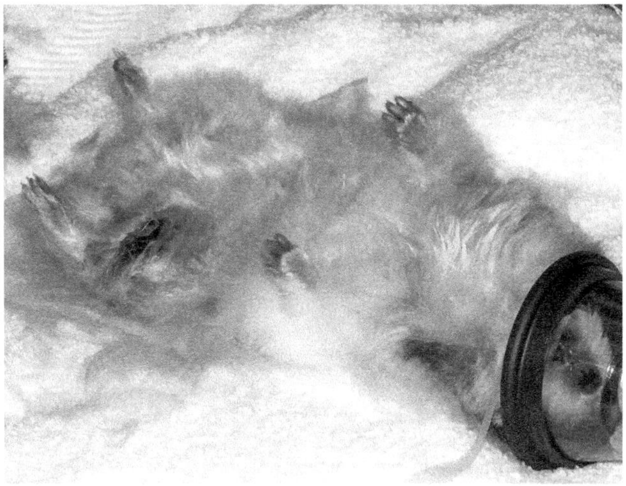

Skin Diseases Abscess secondary to a bite wound in the left inguinal region of a Syrian hamster.

SMALL MAMMALS: GERBILS

Ovarian Disease

BASIC INFORMATION

DEFINITION

Spontaneous pathologies of the ovaries

SYNONYMS

Cystic ovaries, ovarian cysts, ovarian tumors, ovarian neoplasia

EPIDEMIOLOGY

SPECIES, AGE, SEX Female Mongolian gerbils *(Meriones unguiculatus)* 2 years of age and older have a high incidence of ovarian disease.

GENETICS AND BREED PREDISPOSITION Other species of gerbils such as Sundevall's jird *(Meriones crassus)*, Libyan jird *(Meriones libycus)*, Shaw's jird *(Meriones shawi)*, and Tristram's jird *(Meriones tristrami)* show a tendency to develop granulosa cell ovarian tumors after 30 months of age.

RISK FACTORS

- Cystic ovaries increase significantly with age.
- Females between 12 and 20 months have a reported incidence of 47%.

ASSOCIATED CONDITIONS AND DISORDERS

- Ovulation and corpus luteum formation can continue to occur in gerbils with cystic ovaries if one ovary is affected.
- Reduction in fertility and litter size occurs when both ovaries are affected.

CLINICAL PRESENTATION

DISEASE FORMS/SUBTYPES

- Cystic ovarian disease
- Ovarian neoplasia

HISTORY, CHIEF COMPLAINT

- Abdominal distention
- Dyspnea
- Symmetric alopecia
- Weight loss
- Reduced food intake
- Decreased litter sizes and infertility

PHYSICAL EXAM FINDINGS

- Palpation of enlarged cysts/ovarian tissue
- Increased respiratory effort and respiratory rate due to abdominal compression from large cyst(s)
- Alopecia, bilateral, particularly affecting the flanks
- Hypotension and/or hypovolemia secondary to large ovarian cyst rupture

ETIOLOGY AND PATHOPHYSIOLOGY

- Ovarian cysts can be follicular (common), serous, or paraovarian (rare). Although histologic studies on the type of cyst have not been published, it appears that most are follicular cysts.
  - The incidence increases significantly with age: from 6-12 months, generally one ovary is affected in 5% of gerbils; from 20-30 months, one or both ovaries are affected in 73% of gerbils.
  - Cysts range in diameter from 1 mm to 5 cm; smaller cysts are common in younger animals; large cysts are more frequent in older animals and may contain up to 30 mL of fluid, accounting for 15% of the animal's weight.
  - Ovarian tissue becomes stretched to a thin film on the surface of the cyst, and the gerbil becomes infertile.
- Clinically symmetric alopecia and poor coat quality may be seen because of increased estrogen from ovarian cysts.
- Ovarian tumors, predominantly granulosa cell tumors, are the most common tumor of Mongolian gerbils. Studies have reported an incidence ranging from 13% in 2-year-old gerbils to 80% in 3-year-old gerbils. Other reported ovarian neoplasms are ovarian teratomas and dysgerminomas.
- With granulosa cell tumors:
  - >60% are bilateral.
  - In animals aged 1-2 years, a higher incidence is seen in virgin females than in parous females, but a greater incidence is noted in parous females >3 years of age than in virgin females.
  - Metastases occur in the abdomen; they are rarely found in the thorax.

DIAGNOSIS

DIFFERENTIAL DIAGNOSIS

- Abdominal distention
  - Dystocia
  - Hepatomegaly
  - Uterine disease
  - Renal disease
- Dyspnea/tachypnea
  - Lung metastasis
  - Primary respiratory disease
  - Pain
- Symmetric alopecia
  - Senile alopecia

INITIAL DATABASE

- Radiographs will rule out potential metastatic lung lesions.
- Abdominal ultrasound will confirm the presence of cysts and/or the presence of abnormal ovarian tissue.

ADVANCED OR CONFIRMATORY TESTING

- Percutaneous aspiration of ovarian cysts can be performed using ultrasonography.
- Fine-needle aspiration and cytologic examination may help to identify ovarian tumors histologically.
- Exploratory laparotomy is often needed to confirm the diagnosis.

TREATMENT

THERAPEUTIC GOALS

- Alleviation of dyspnea and tachypnea
- Alleviation of pain and discomfort
- Alleviation of excessive estrogen levels

ACUTE GENERAL TREATMENT

- Ovarian cysts can be percutaneously aspirated to reduce abdominal distention and secondary dyspnea. This will result in temporary alleviation of respiratory distress and abdominal distention. However, aspiration usually needs to be followed by surgical or medical treatment to prevent rapid reaccumulation of cyst fluid.
- Treatment of hormone-producing ovarian follicular cysts with human chorionic gonadotropin (hCG) (100 IU/kg SC, at least 3 injections q 10-14 d); however, hCG can cause local irritation, edema, and pain at site of injection. Alternative treatment consists of gonadotropin-releasing hormone (GnRH) (25 mcg/animal SC, 2 injections q 14 d).
- The treatment of choice for serous and paraovarian cysts and ovarian tumors is ovariohysterectomy. Metastatic spread of ovarian neoplasia should be ruled out before surgical treatment is provided.

POSSIBLE COMPLICATIONS

- Adhesions of the ovaries to other abdominal organs may complicate surgical removal.
- Large blood-filled cysts are frequently associated with granulosa cell tumors. Surgical removal of these cysts, together with the ovaries, or percutaneous aspiration carries the risk of inducing hypovolemic shock.

RECOMMENDED MONITORING

Submit surgically removed ovaries for histopathologic examination to rule out neoplasia. Ovaries with cysts may also have foci of neoplasia.

PROGNOSIS AND OUTCOME

- Ovarian cystic disease: percutaneous aspiration is a temporary therapeutic measure, as recurrence of cyst dilatation can recur in as little as 7 days. Ovariohysterectomy is curative.
- Ovarian neoplasm: ovariohysterectomy is curative if metastases have not occurred before surgical intervention

SUGGESTED READINGS

Guzman-Silva MA, et al: Incipient spontaneous granulosa cell tumour in the gerbil, *Meriones unguiculatus*. Lab Anim 40:96–101, 2006.

Norris ML, et al: Incidence of cystic ovaries and reproductive performance in the mongolian gerbil, *Meriones unguiculatus*. Lab Anim 6:337–342, 1972.

AUTHORS: **LA'TOYA LATNEY AND THOMAS M. DONNELLY**

EDITOR: **CHRISTOPH MANS**

Cardiac Disease

BASIC INFORMATION

DEFINITION

- *Cardiac disease* is an umbrella term for a variety of diseases affecting the heart.
- Heart murmurs are abnormal heart sounds that are produced as a result of turbulent blood flow that is sufficient to produce an audible sound. Heart murmurs can be pathologic or benign (innocent).

SYNONYMS

Heart disease, cardiopathy, cardiomyopathy

SPECIAL SPECIES CONSIDERATIONS

The prevalence of heart murmurs in chinchillas has been reported to be 23% in one study. Most heart murmurs are considered innocent, i.e., a murmur arising from a physiologic condition outside the heart, as opposed to a structural defect in the heart.

EPIDEMIOLOGY

SPECIES, AGE, SEX Older chinchillas are more likely to have a heart murmur and cardiac disease. No correlation with the sex has been demonstrated.

RISK FACTORS Heart murmur of grade 3 or greater is positively correlated with the presence of heart disease in chinchillas.

CLINICAL PRESENTATION

HISTORY, CHIEF COMPLAINT

- Heart murmurs are often incidental findings during physical examination in chinchillas that are otherwise healthy.
- Cardiac disease
  - Weakness
  - Reduced activity
  - Decrease in appetite
  - Labored breathing
  - Sudden death

PHYSICAL EXAM FINDINGS

- Innocent heart murmurs may be the only physical abnormality noticed in many chinchillas.
- Findings in chinchillas suffering from cardiac disease include the following:
  - Depression
  - Poor body condition
  - Heart murmur
  - Tachycardia (normal heart rate 100-150 bpm)
  - Dyspnea and tachypnea (normal respiratory rate 40-80 bpm)
  - Pale mucous membrane

ETIOLOGY AND PATHOPHYSIOLOGY

Different types of cardiopathies have been described in chinchillas, including hypertrophic cardiomyopathy, ventricular septal defect, and dynamic right ventricular tract outflow obstruction. The most common cardiac disease seems to be valvulopathy involving the mitral and less commonly the tricuspid valve.

DIAGNOSIS

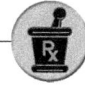

DIFFERENTIAL DIAGNOSIS

- Innocent heart murmur, which seems to be common in chinchillas
- Dyspnea: primary pulmonary disease, neoplasm, pleural effusion
- Depression: systemic bacterial infection, ketoacidosis, gastrointestinal disease
- Poor body condition: dental disease

INITIAL DATABASE

- Radiographs of the chest (lateral and dorsoventral views) may reveal an enlarged shadow of the heart but are often normal and may not be helpful for diagnosis.
- Echocardiography is the diagnostic modality of choice. It may reveal changes in the anatomy of ventricular walls, thickening of the valves, and atrial enlargement. Doppler studies are useful for assessing velocity, acceleration of flow in different parts of the heart, and mitral or tricuspid regurgitation.
- Electrocardiography

ADVANCED OR CONFIRMATORY TESTING

Most cases are diagnosed only at necropsy.

TREATMENT

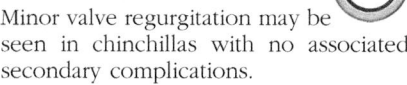

THERAPEUTIC GOALS

- Improve cardiac function.
- Decrease respiratory distress.

ACUTE GENERAL TREATMENT

- Treatment is needed only if significant abnormalities are found on echocardiography, or if the animal is showing clinical signs secondary to cardiac disease.
- At present, clinical management of cardiac disease in chinchillas is empirical, and treatment is extrapolated from other species.
- Severely dyspneic patients should be supplemented with oxygen; and handling and stress should be minimized.
- Pleural and/or abdominal tap if indicated (sedation or general anesthesia recommended)
- Diuretics: furosemide 2-10 mg/kg IM, SC, PO q 2-12 h for treatment of pulmonary edema and pleural effusion secondary to congestive heart failure

CHRONIC TREATMENT

- Enalapril 0.5 mg/kg PO q 24 h
- Furosemide 1-2 mg/kg PO q 8-12 h

DRUG INTERACTIONS

- The combination of angiotensin-converting enzyme (ACE) inhibitors and furosemide might result in azotemia, particularly in patients with concurrent renal dysfunction.

POSSIBLE COMPLICATIONS

- Sudden death
- Vascular thromboembolism
- Iatrogenic dehydration due to furosemide administration

RECOMMENDED MONITORING

- Behavior: monitor for weakness and reduced activity
- Body weight and appetite
- Respiratory rate
- Echocardiography recheck every 6 months

PROGNOSIS AND OUTCOME

Minor valve regurgitation may be seen in chinchillas with no associated secondary complications.

PEARLS & CONSIDERATIONS

COMMENTS

Currently, cardiac diseases in chinchillas are poorly understood and might be underdiagnosed. Echocardiography should be performed in chinchillas with a heart murmur of grade 3 or greater.

SUGGESTED READINGS

Heatley J: Cardiovascular anatomy, physiology and disease of rodents and small exotic mammals, Vet Clin Exot Anim 12:99–113, 2009.

Linde A, et al: Echocardiography in chinchilla, J Vet Intern Med 18:772–774, 2004.

Pignon C, et al: Evaluation of cardiac murmurs in chinchillas *(Chinchilla lanigera)*: a retrospective, multi-institutional study, Seattle, Proceedings of the AEMV Conference, August 6-7, 2011, p 149.

AUTHOR: **CHARLY PIGNON**

EDITOR: **CHRISTOPH MANS**

SMALL MAMMALS: CHINCHILLAS

Dental Disease

Additional Images Available on Website

BASIC INFORMATION

DEFINITION

Disorders affecting the dentition and associated structures

SYNONYMS

Dental malocclusion, periodontal disease, caries, tooth overgrowth

SPECIAL SPECIES CONSIDERATIONS

- Dental formula: 2(I1C0P1M3) = 20
- Incisor teeth and cheek teeth grow continuously throughout life (elodont).
- Incisor teeth and cheek teeth have a long crown (hypsodont) and no anatomic root (aradicular).
- Each tooth can be divided into a *clinical crown* (above the gingival sulcus) and the *reserve crown* (subgingival part).
- Incisor teeth in chinchillas are orange to yellow in color owing to pigmentation of the superficial layer of the labial enamel.
- Premolar and molar cheek teeth are morphologically identical in chinchillas and therefore can be termed *cheek teeth* (CT) 1-4.
- The occlusal planes of the cheek teeth are horizontal.
- Abnormalities related to subclinical dental disease can be detected in more than 30% of apparently healthy chinchillas presented for routine physical examination.

EPIDEMIOLOGY

SPECIES, AGE, SEX Acquired dental disease is common in chinchillas >5 years of age.

ASSOCIATED CONDITIONS AND DISORDERS Epiphora, poor coat condition, fur chewing, hepatic lipidosis, ketoacidosis, constipation, weight loss

CLINICAL PRESENTATION

DISEASE FORMS/SUBTYPES

- Incisor teeth disorders
- Cheek teeth disorders
- Periapical abscesses (rare)

HISTORY, CHIEF COMPLAINT

- Reduced food intake
- Change in food preferences toward more easily chewed feed items
- Reduced fecal output and small and irregular fecal pellets
- Weight loss
- Poor coat condition
- Fur-chewing (see Fur Disorders)
- Clear ocular discharge ("wet eye")
- Lethargy
- Wet fur around mouth and chin ("slobbers")

PHYSICAL EXAM FINDINGS

- General loss of condition
- Palpable bony swellings or irregularities on ventrolateral aspects of mandibles, which reflect apical elongation of the mandibular cheek teeth
- Salivation and soiled or wet fur around mouth, chin, and forefeet
- Poor coat condition
- Lethargy
- Small and irregular fecal pellets
- Constipation
- Epiphora
- Malocclusion of incisor teeth
- Fractured incisor teeth
- Facial abscesses (uncommon)
- Exophthalmia (uncommon)
- Intraoral examination
  - General anesthesia is mandatory for a complete intraoral examination; preferably the exam is performed under endoscopic guidance (stomatoscopy).
  - Gingival hyperplasia (mainly affecting the maxillary gingiva)
  - Buccal erosions and ulceration
  - Cheek teeth
    - Coronal elongation
    - Formation of sharp enamel points or spurs leading to buccal and lingual mucosal erosions and discomfort; most commonly, the maxillary cheek teeth are affected.
    - Change in occlusal surface plane
    - Periodontal disease
    - Mobility secondary to periodontal disease
    - Increased interproximal spaces, impacted with food or debris
    - Caries and resorptive lesions affecting the occlusal and interproximal surfaces (brown to black discoloration, tooth substance loss)
    - Missing teeth

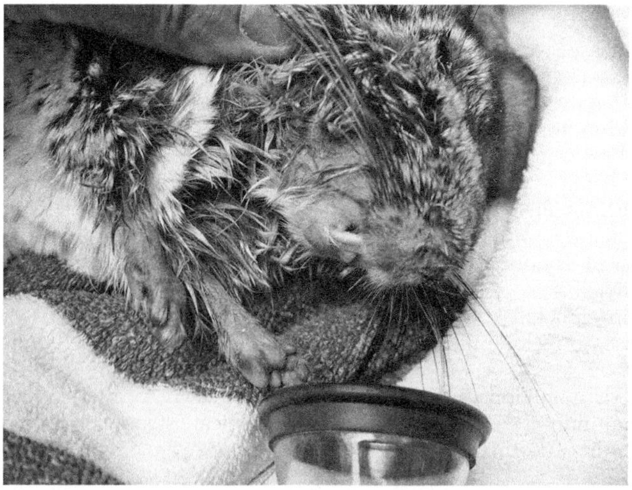

Dental Disease Wet fur around the mouth and chin (slobbers) in a chinchilla is caused by increased salivation secondary to dental disease. *(Photo courtesy Jörg Mayer, The University of Georgia, Athens.)*

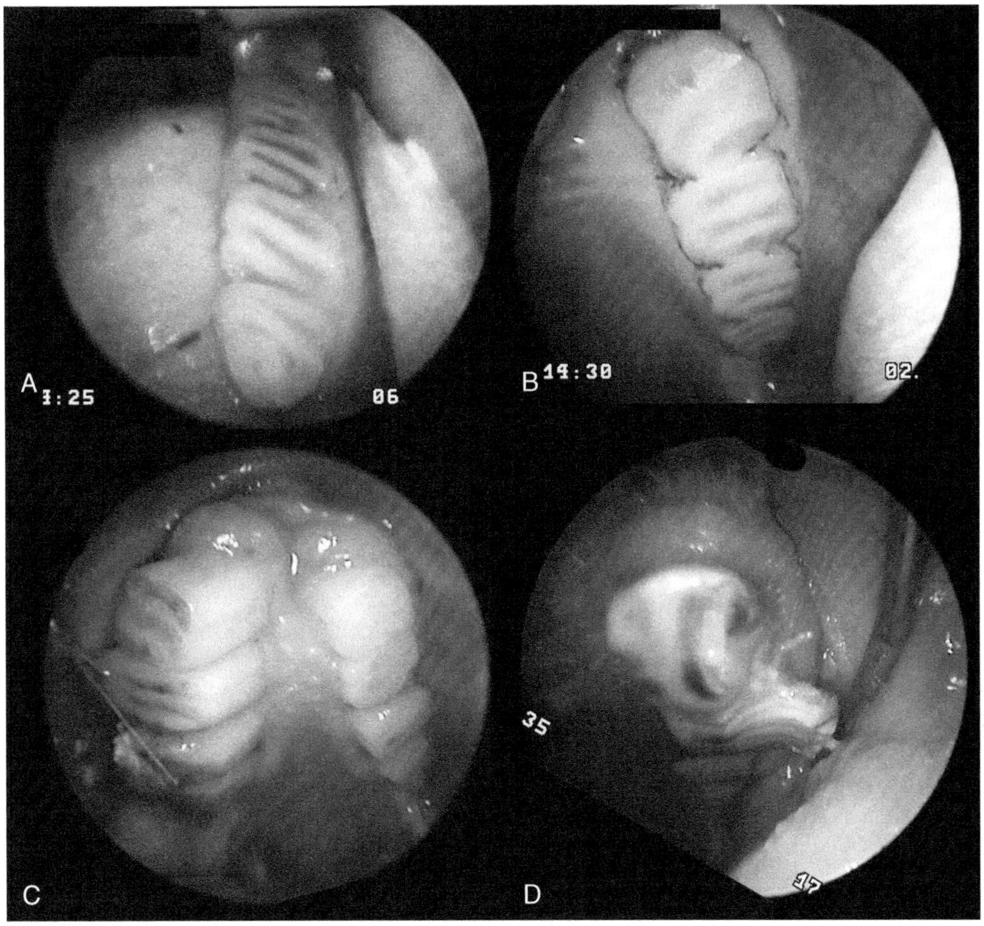

Dental Disease Endoscopy-guided intraoral examination in chinchillas. **A,** Normal left mandibulary cheek teeth. Note the short clinical crowns, the horizontal occlusal plane and the very narrow intercoronal spaces. **B,** Normal left maxillary cheek teeth. Note the normal gingiva and short clinical crowns. **C,** Severe elongation of the right maxillary cheek teeth. **D,** Left maxillary cheek teeth. Note the sharp enamel edge formation on the buccal aspect of 2nd cheek tooth (CT2). Also note the gingival hyperplasia if compared to **A** and the elongation of the clinical crowns of CT1.

ETIOLOGY AND PATHOPHYSIOLOGY

- Incisor teeth disorders
  - Incisor malocclusion occurs commonly secondary to cheek teeth malocclusion.
  - Trauma (e.g., excessive chewing on cage bars or cage furnishings, iatrogenic)
  - Depigmentation
- Cheek teeth disorders
  - Malocclusion and sharp enamel spur formation may be seen secondary to coronal elongation. Currently, it is believed that tooth elongation may be secondary to insufficient tooth wear because of feeding of inappropriate (low-fiber) diets.
  - In captivity, diets are often significantly lower in fiber compared with diets of wild chinchillas. Ingestion of less abrasive food requires less mastication, resulting in less dietary abrasion of the cheek teeth and consequently elongation of clinical and reserve crowns.
  - Other nutritional causes such as abnormal calcium and/or vitamin D metabolism and genetic predisposition have been suggested but have not been proven in chinchillas.
- Epiphora
  - Partial or complete obstruction of the nasolacrimal duct secondary to bone remodeling around the elongated apical reserve crowns of the maxillary cheek teeth

DIAGNOSIS

DIFFERENTIAL DIAGNOSIS

- Weight loss
  - Systemic disease (i.e., metabolic, infectious, organ failure)
  - Gastrointestinal disease (see Gastrointestinal Disorders)
- Constipation
  - Gastrointestinal disease
- Anorexia
  - Systemic disease (i.e., metabolic, infectious, organ failure)
  - Pain
- Poor coat condition
  - Lack of a sand bath
  - High humidity
  - Stress or pain leading to fur chewing
- Exophthalmia
  - Buphthalmia
  - Retrobulbar cyst or neoplasia
- Facial swelling
  - Neoplasia
  - Foreign body–induced abscess

INITIAL DATABASE

- Complete intraoral examination under general anesthesia
  - Endoscopically guided intraoral examination (stomatoscopy) is preferred for a complete intraoral examination.
  - Use magnification and focal illumination if stomatoscopy cannot be performed.
- Imaging

- Skull radiographs (five views: lateral, left and right oblique, ventrodorsal, rostrocaudal)
- CT scan of head: preferred over skull radiographs
- Urine analysis: ketonuria, low pH (normal urine pH 8-9), glucosuria
- Biochemistry profile: may be normal; hyperglycemia and azotemia may be evident. Rule out concurrent diseases that would affect the prognosis (e.g., hepatic lipidosis, ketoacidosis, renal insufficiency).
- Complete blood count: may be normal; hemoconcentration or anemia may be seen.

TREATMENT

THERAPEUTIC GOALS

- Resolve intraoral soft tissue trauma, which causes discomfort and pain.
- Reduce periodontal disease, which causes discomfort and pain.
- Restore normal occlusion if possible.
- Recover or maintain the animal's ability to eat unaided.

ACUTE GENERAL TREATMENT

- Provide supportive care as needed:
  - Fluid therapy: 60-100 mL/kg/d SC, PO, IV
  - Nutritional support: syringe-feed with high-fiber diet for herbivores (e.g., Oxbow Critical Care for Herbivores, 50-80 mL/kg PO q 24 h, divided into 4-5 feedings) or crushed and soaked pellets
  - Analgesia
    - Buprenorphine 0.03-0.05 mg/kg SC q 8-12 h
    - Meloxicam 0.3-0.5 mg/kg PO or SC q 12-24 h, once adequately hydrated
- Treatment of cheek teeth malocclusion
  - General anesthesia required
  - Specialized equipment required
    - Use low-speed dental drill, a diamond burr, cheek dilators, and a mouth gag.
    - Use appropriate magnification and illumination; preferably a rigid endoscope or otoscope is used.
  - Avoid iatrogenic damage to the soft tissue during dental procedures.
  - Remove sharp enamel spurs, which lead to soft tissue trauma buccally and lingually. Maxillary cheek teeth form spurs buccally; mandibular cheek teeth form spurs lingually.
  - Shorten elongated clinical crowns.
  - Restore the physiologically horizontal occlusal surfaces.
  - Do not attempt to extract cheek teeth unless severely diseased and mobile, secondary to periodontal infection or fracture. Cheek teeth extraction in chinchillas is technically challenging and complete extraction is often not achieved.
- Treatment of periodontal disease
  - Probe pathologic interproximal spaces and gingival and periodontal pockets.
  - Remove impacted debris.
  - Rinse cleaned gingival and periodontal pockets carefully with 2% hydrogen peroxide or diluted chlorhexidine solution. Use a 0.5-1 mL syringe and a 25- to 28-gauge needle. Avoid aspiration of rinse.
  - Consider placement of Doxirobe Gel (Pfizer Animal Health, New York, NY) in deep (>5 mm) gingival and periodontal pockets; this may help delay reimpaction with debris and may reduce periodontal inflammation.
  - If evidence of significant periodontal infection is found, consider long-term antibiotic therapy. Ensure appropriate coverage against anaerobic bacteria predominating in periodontal infections. Long-acting penicillin benzathine 40,000-60,000 IU/kg SC q 5 d is recommended.
- Treatment of caries
  - Remove diseased tooth substance with use of a low-speed or high-speed dental drill and appropriate burr.
- Treatment of incisor teeth malocclusion
  - Sedation or general anesthesia required
  - Specialized equipment required
    - Use a low-speed with diamond or carbon cutting blade dental drill or a high-speed dental drill.
    - Avoid iatrogenic damage to the soft tissue during incisor teeth trimming.
    - Use a tongue depressor or a spatula to protect the lips and tongue during trimming.
    - Do not use nail clippers or scissors to trim incisor teeth.
    - Avoid excessive shortening of clinical crowns; this will lead to temporary functional loss of the incisor teeth.
- Antibiotic therapy
  - Indicated if evidence of periodontal or periapical infection exists
  - Ensure appropriate coverage against anaerobic bacteria.
  - Penicillin G benzathine 40,000-60,000 IU/kg SC q 5 d
  - Trimethoprim-sulfa 30 mg/kg PO q 12 h. Combine with metronidazole for improved anaerobic coverage
  - Enrofloxacin 10-20 mg/kg PO q 12-24 h. Combine with metronidazole for anaerobic coverage
  - Metronidazole 20-30 mg/kg PO q 12 h. Combine with trimethoprim-sulfa or enrofloxacin for aerobic coverage. Dependent on the oral formulation of metronidazole used, chinchillas may become temporarily anorexic.
  - Chloramphenicol 30-50 mg/kg PO q 8 h
  - Azithromycin 30 mg/kg PO q 24 h
  - Epiphora (see Ocular Disorders)

CHRONIC TREATMENT

- Repeated treatments of cheek teeth and incisor teeth malocclusion, periodontal disease, and caries under general anesthesia. Recheck examination should be performed 2-8 weeks after the initial exam and treatment, depending on the severity of diagnosed intraoral disease.
- Analgesia: meloxicam 0.3-0.5 mg/kg PO q 12-24 h
- Long-term antibiotic therapy for cases suffering from severe periodontal disease: consider pulse therapy using penicillin G benzathine 40,000-60,000 IU/kg SC q 5 d
- Nutritional support: syringe-feed with high-fiber diet for herbivores (e.g., Oxbow Critical Care for Herbivores, 50-80 mL/kg PO q 24 h, divided into 4-5 feedings) or crushed and soaked chinchilla pellets until the animal is eating sufficient quantities unaided
- Periapical abscesses treatment (rarely indicated)
  - Several techniques have been reported in rabbits and are applicable to chinchillas.
  - Consider referral to a specialist if periapical abscess treatment is necessary.
- Tooth extraction (rarely indicated):
  - Technically challenging
  - Consider referral to a specialist for assessment and possible extractions.

DRUG INTERACTIONS

- Do not administer cephalosporins, penicillins, erythromycin, or clindamycin orally.
- Do not administer meloxicam to dehydrated animals.
- Dependent on the oral formulation of metronidazole used, chinchillas may become anorexic. Use penicillin G benzathine administered SC instead, if anorexia occurs. Discontinue metronidazole and provide nutritional support, until the animal regains a normal appetite.

POSSIBLE COMPLICATIONS

- Incomplete extraction of elodont teeth may result in regrowth if germinative tissue has not been completely removed during extraction.

- Iatrogenic damage to the teeth, tongue, or buccal mucosa

RECOMMENDED MONITORING

- Food intake
- Fecal output
- Body weight
- Urine ketones

PROGNOSIS AND OUTCOME

- Good to fair for animal with no secondary complications and if client is compliant with recommended treatment
- Guarded to poor if animal is in poor body condition or is suffering from systemic disease (i.e., severe and non-responsive ketoacidosis), or if client is not compliant with recommended treatments

CONTROVERSY

- A limited intraoral examination can be performed using a pediatric laryngoscope, an otoscope, or a vaginal speculum in a conscious animal, but up to 50% of intraoral lesions can be missed.
- Coronal reduction of elongated cheek teeth is often complicated and limited in chinchillas by the presence of gingival hyperplasia.

PEARLS & CONSIDERATIONS

Make sure to carefully evaluate the buccal aspects of the maxillary last cheek teeth (CT4) for spurs. Buccal spurs of CT4 are often missed during intraoral examination because they can be difficult to visualize and often are buried deep in the buccal tissue, causing soft tissue trauma and discomfort.

COMMENTS

- Despite sometimes dramatic elongation of reserve and clinical crowns of the cheek teeth, chinchillas often have no difficulty eating and maintain a good body condition until severe changes and complications, such as soft tissue trauma from sharp dental spurs or periodontal infection, have occurred.
- Congenital dental disease is rare in rodents; most dental disease is acquired.

PREVENTION

- Provision of an appropriate diet that is high in fiber allows for appropriate wear of cheek teeth.
- Sugary treats should be avoided.

CLIENT EDUCATION

- Educate owners about the appropriate dietary requirements of chinchillas.
- Owners must be informed that repeated and often lifelong treatment of dental malocclusion and periodontal disease under general anesthesia is required.

SUGGESTED READINGS

Crossley DA: Dental disease in chinchillas in the UK, J Small Anim Pract 42:12–19, 2001.
Jekl V, et al: Quantitative and qualitative assessments of intraoral lesions in 180 small herbivorous mammals, Vet Rec 162:442–449, 2008.
Mans C, et al: Disease problems of chinchillas. In Carpenter JW, et al, editors: Ferrets, rabbits and rodents: clinical medicine and surgery, ed 3, St Louis, 2012, WB Saunders, pp 311–325.

CROSS-REFERENCES TO OTHER SECTIONS

Fur Disorders
Gastrointestinal Disorders
Ocular Disorders

AUTHOR: **CHRISTOPH MANS**

EDITOR: **THOMAS M. DONNELLY**

SMALL MAMMALS: CHINCHILLAS

Fur Disorders

BASIC INFORMATION

DEFINITION

Fur disorders include normal physiologic response (e.g., fur-slip) and infectious, metabolic, nutritional, behavioral, and traumatic disorders of the pelage.

SYNONYMS

Fur-chewing, fur-slip, cotton fur syndrome

EPIDEMIOLOGY

SPECIES, AGE, SEX

- Chinchillas have an extremely dense hair coat (1000 follicles/cm^2). Chinchilla hair is tufted, but each filament actually grows from an independent root within a hair follicle. In chinchillas, as many as 60-90 hairs grow from each hair follicle.
- Provision of a special chinchilla sand or dust bath for 15 minutes daily is critical for a chinchilla to maintain a healthy coat.

GENETICS AND BREED PREDISPOSITION Anecdotally, the inheritability of fur-chewing has been reported.

RISK FACTORS

- Overcrowding and other stressors, such as chronic pain (e.g., from dental disease), are believed to be underlying causes of fur-chewing.
- Nutritional deficiencies
- Deprivation of sand bathing
- Contact with dermatophyte-infected animal

CONTAGION AND ZOONOSIS Dermatophytosis is a zoonotic disease.

GEOGRAPHY AND SEAONALITY Outdoor housing in geographic regions with high humidity (>80%) and high temperatures (>25°C [>77°F]), can lead to matted fur.

CLINICAL PRESENTATION

DISEASE FORMS/SUBTYPES

- Fur-slip
  - Chinchillas possess a predator avoidance mechanism known as fur-slip. When the animal is fighting or is roughly handled, it can release a large patch of fur, thus enabling it to escape. A clean smooth area of skin is left; hair may require several months to regrow.
  - Fur-slip should not be confused with fur-chewing.
- Fur-chewing
  - Fur-chewing occurs when a chinchilla bites off areas of its own fur or another animal's fur, resulting in a moth-eaten coat.
  - In chinchilla fur farms, an incidence of 15%-20% has been reported.

HISTORY, CHIEF COMPLAINT

- Dependent on underlying cause
- Fur loss (circumscribed, diffuse)
- Dry, flaky skin
- Patchy hair coat
- Darkening, discoloration of hair coat
- Fur-chewing/barbering
- Matted fur
- Sudden patchy fur loss after handling
- Wavy and weak hair

PHYSICAL EXAM FINDINGS

- Nutritional deficiency disorders: difficult to distinguish between different nutritional disorders
  - Fatty acid deficiency: mild skin flaking to alopecia due to fur loss and reduced hair regrowth; in severe cases, cutaneous ulcers, debilitation, and easy epilation of the fur
  - Pantothenic acid deficiency: patchy alopecia, fur epilates easily, skin may be thickened, roughened and scaly; fur can appear dull grey owing to depigmentation; possible hyperactivity, anorexia, and poor body condition; stunting in young animals
  - Zinc deficiency: alopecia and scaly skin
- Cotton fur syndrome: wavy, weak hair with cotton-like appearance
- Fur-chewing: focal areas of alopecia or short stubbly hair coat. Commonly affected areas include shoulders, flanks, and paws. In severe cases, only the head and neck remain furred ("lion's mane").
- Matted fur: hair is thickly matted
- Fur-slip: well-circumscribed focal alopecia; clean and smooth skin exposed
- Dermatophytosis: small scaly patches of alopecia on the nose, behind the ears, or on the forefeet. Lesions may appear on any part of the body; in advanced cases, a large circumscribed area of inflammation with scab formation is evident.

ETIOLOGY AND PATHOPHYSIOLOGY

- Nutritional deficiency disorders: rare in pet chinchillas fed a diet of appropriate quality
  - Fatty acid deficiency: diet deficient in unsaturated fatty acids due to poorly preserved food (incorrect storage) or lack of antioxidants in diet, causing rancidity of food
  - Pantothenic acid deficiency: water-soluble vitamin (B_5) essential for normal skin and hair formation
  - Zinc deficiency: important cofactor in many critical physiologic processes
- Cotton fur syndrome: high protein content in diet (crude protein >28%)
- Behavioral/environmental disorders
  - Fur-chewing: suspected to be due to overcrowding or other stressors, boredom, pain (e.g., from dental disease), or nutritional deficiency. Heritability of the condition is also suspected. However, no definitive evidence for any of these theories has been established.
  - Matted fur: chinchillas are adapted to an arid environment and exhibit increased productivity of the sebaceous glands. They are unsuited to an environment of high humidity (>80%) and high temperatures. When deprived of access to sand suitable for cleaning oil from the pelage, their coat becomes matted and greasy-looking.
  - Fur-slip: physiologic defense mechanism
- Infectious
  - Dermatophytosis: most commonly due to *Trichophyton mentagrophytes*, less commonly to *Microsporum gypseum* and *Microsporum canis*; direct and indirect transmission
    - Immune status of host is critical (high prevalence in very young, old, and immune suppressed animals).
    - Infection is usually self-resolving, and reinfection is prevented by the development of long-term immunity.
    - Chronic or recurrent infection is indicative of an inappropriate immune response.
    - Infected animals can be asymptomatic and are a constant source of infection.
    - *T. mentagrophytes* has been cultured from 5% of fur-ranched chinchillas with normal fur and 30% of animals with fur damage.

DIAGNOSIS

DIFFERENTIAL DIAGNOSIS

- Alopecia (circumscribed/diffuse): nutritional deficiencies, fur-slip, fur-chewing, dermatophytosis
- Thickened, flaky skin: nutritional deficiencies (fatty acid, pantothenic acid or zinc), dermatophytosis
- Circumscribed alopecia of nose, chin, and forefeet: dental disease (see Dental Disease) with excessive salivation, dermatophytosis

INITIAL DATABASE

- Thorough analysis of diet and husbandry
- Microscopic examination of hair and superficial skin scraping
- *T. mentagrophytes* will not fluoresce if fur is examined with an ultraviolet light (i.e., Wood's lamp).

ADVANCED OR CONFIRMATORY TESTING

- Dermatophyte (ringworm) culture
- Skin biopsy
- Intraoral exam (fur-chewing)

TREATMENT

THERAPEUTIC GOALS

- Dependent on cause of disease
- Dermatophytosis: eradication of infectious material from the affected animal, from in-contact animals, and from the environment

ACUTE GENERAL TREATMENT

- Dependent on cause of disease
- Nutritional deficiency disorders: correct diet; provide high-quality hay and commercial chinchilla pellets. Supplement diet with deficient nutrient until condition is resolved.
  - Fatty acid deficiency: correct diet and supplement feed with essential fatty acids. Veterinary preparations contain a combination of fish oil (eicosapentaenoic and docosahexaenoic acids) and vegetable oil (gamma linolenic acid). Because of the unique nature of each commercially available product, see actual label directions for specific dosage recommendations.
  - Pantothenic acid deficiency: give dexpanthenol (alcohol of D-pantothenic acid) 20 mg/kg IM for 2-3 days and correct diet
  - Zinc deficiency: dietary correction alone usually resolves deficiency, but supplementation with zinc sulfate 10 mg/kg PO daily for 2-3 weeks can expedite the process
- Cotton fur syndrome: reduce crude protein content of diet to 15%
- Behavioral/environmental disorders
  - Fur-chewing: multifaceted approach: reduce stressors, ensure appropriate environment, and offer high-quality diet. Remove dark undercoat to promote fur regrowth.
  - Matted fur: provision of sand bath for about 15 minutes daily and reduction of environmental humidity to <80%
  - Fur slip: no therapy necessary
- Infectious
  - Dermatophytosis
    - Sanitation of animals and disinfection of cages and environment (chlorine laundry bleach solution 1:10)
    - Trace carrier and in-contact animals.
    - Isolate affected and nonaffected animals.
    - Gently clip affected fur to discard and loosen infectious hair and scales.
    - Sanitation of animals and disinfection of cages and owner's environment
      - Environment: chlorine laundry bleach solution 1:10
      - Animal: topical therapy with 2% chlorhexidine/2% miconazole shampoo, 0.2% enilconazole rinse, or lime-sulfur dips (4-8 oz per gallon)

- Provide systemic antifungal therapy: first choice: terbinafine 10-30 mg/kg PO q 24 h; second choice: itraconazole 5-10 mg/kg PO q 24 h or griseofulvin in microsized form 50-100 mg/kg PO in 2-3 divided doses q 24 h
- Animal studies have shown that terbinafine is safer and more effective than commonly used antifungal drugs such as itraconazole or griseofulvin.
- Treatment is terminated after fungal cultures are negative twice, with a 4-week interval between cultures.
- If secondary bacterial infection occurs, start appropriate antibiotic therapy.

POSSIBLE COMPLICATIONS

Ingestion of topical medication

PROGNOSIS AND OUTCOME

Dependent on cause

PEARLS & CONSIDERATIONS

COMMENTS

- Controversy
  - A current popular theory suggests that fur-chewing is a behavioral disorder in which mothers transmit the vice to offspring. Chinchilla breeders also suggest that the higher incidence of fur-chewing in commercial herds is evidence of maladapted displacement behavior. Affected animals suffer from malnutrition; a third theory is that chinchillas chew their fur for dietary requirements. Multiple food factors are probably involved in this type of malnutrition, but the further dietary studies are needed to determine the cause.
  - Comparison of fungal cultures of skin and fur from fur-ranched chinchillas shows a 5% incidence of *T. mentagrophytes* in animals with normal skin and a 30% incidence in animals with fur damage. Fur ranchers often add fungicide to the sand bath to prevent damage to the pelt. However, topical treatment removes spores only from hair shafts, not from hair follicles. If clinical dermatophytosis occurs in a colony, topical treatment does not resolve it, and the infection becomes subclinical.
  - A previous theory for fur-chewing suggested that fur-chewing is due to abnormal endocrine activity because affected animals show increased thyroidal and adrenocortical activity. Thyroid hyperplasia has been shown to correlate with the size of chewed fur over the body and most likely is a reactive response of the thyroid to insulation loss following fur removal.
  - Other theories for fur-chewing include stress or overcrowding and dietary deficiencies, especially lack of fiber. None of these hypotheses has been proven.
- Never grasp a chinchilla by the skin at the back of its neck for restraint because this can cause fur-slip.
- Dermatophytes colonize keratin tissue (stratum corneum of skin, hair, nails); in the immune competent host, no living tissue is invaded. Dermatophytes have the ability to use keratin as a nutrient source. The presence of fungal organisms and their metabolic products is believed to induce allergic and inflammatory eczematous responses in the host. The type and severity of host response are related to the species and strain of dermatophyte.

PREVENTION

General: good hygiene (particularly in groups of young weanling chinchillas), good-quality high-fiber diet, and minimization of stress

CLIENT EDUCATION

- Dietary recommendations of high-quality hay and commercial chinchilla pellets should be given.
- A sand bath should be provided for about 15 minutes daily. Commercial chinchilla sand baths that are cement byproducts are recommended. Alternative sand baths consist of perfume-free talc powder and dietetic grade cornstarch. Recently, volcanic ash has been used.
- Excessive sand bathing may cause irritation of the eyes, resulting in mild conjunctivitis.
- Dermatophytosis is a zoonotic disease. Recommend thorough cleaning and disinfection of the household and handwashing after handling of affected animals. If clients experience dermatologic problems, encourage a consultation with their physician.

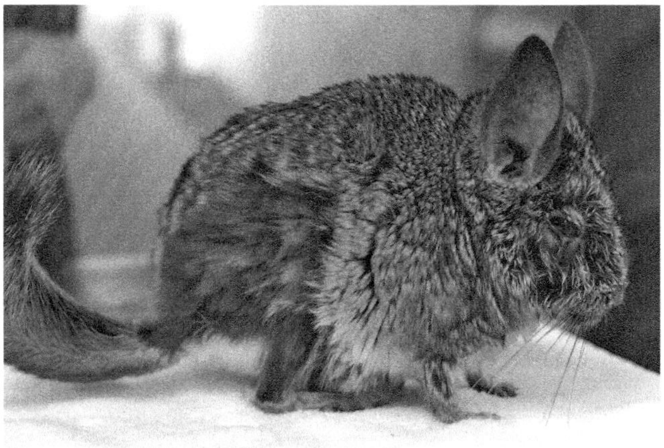

Fur Disorders Fur-chewing in a chinchilla.

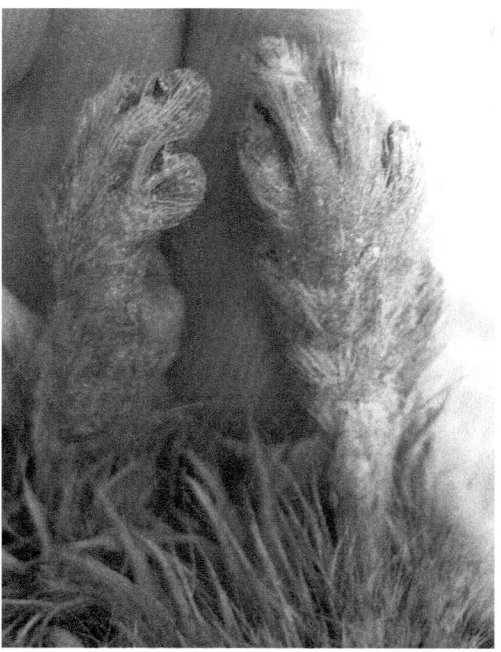

Fur Disorders Alopecia of the dorsal aspects of forelimbs in a chinchilla that presented for hypersalivation, secondary to dental disease.

SUGGESTED READINGS

Barber N, et al: Sandbathing reduces fur lipids of chinchillas, *Chinchilla laniger*, Anim Behav 39:403–405, 1990.
Donnelly TM, et al: Ringworm in small exotic pets, Semin Avian Exot Pet Med 9:82–93, 2000.

CROSS-REFERENCES TO OTHER SECTIONS

Dental Disease

AUTHOR: **CHRISTOPH MANS**

EDITOR: **THOMAS M. DONNELLY**

SMALL MAMMALS: CHINCHILLAS

Gastrointestinal Disorders

Additional Images Available on Website

BASIC INFORMATION

DEFINITION

Common disorders affecting the gastrointestinal tract of pet chinchillas can be classified as primary noninfectious and infectious disorders. Some primary noninfectious disorders can be complicated by secondary opportunistic infections.

SYNONYMS

Diarrhea, tympany, bloat, constipation, dysbacteriosis, enteritis, rectal tissue prolapse, intussusception

SPECIAL SPECIES CONSIDERATIONS

- The digestive tract of chinchillas allows digestion of a dry high-fiber diet. Digestion of fiber occurs in the voluminous cecum and in a highly sacculated ascending colon.
- The physiologic bacterial flora consists of predominantly Gram-positive aerobic and anaerobic bacteria (e.g., *Bacteroides, Bifidobacterium, Peptostreptococcus, Eubacterium, Lactobacillus*).
- Normal gastrointestinal transit time is 12 to 15 hours, similar to other rodents.
- Normal fecal pellets are rice grain shaped (8-12 × 3 mm), dark and firm.
- Chinchillas produce nitrogen-rich cecotrophs and nitrogen-poor normal fecal pellets.
- Because chinchillas are nocturnal, most food intake and defecation occurs overnight; cecotrophs may be passed during the daylight period.
- Chinchillas should be fed predominantly high-quality grass hay. Supplemental commercial chinchilla pellets should be offered. Treats such as dried or fresh fruits and vegetables should be offered only occasionally; preference should be given to items low in carbohydrates. Fresh water must be available at all times.

EPIDEMIOLOGY

SPECIES, AGE, SEX Although *Giardia duodenalis* and *Eimeria chinchillae* infections are often asymptomatic, they can cause significant morbidity and mortality, predominantly in young (<3 months) or immune compromised chinchillas.

RISK FACTORS
- Inappropriate diet
- Sudden diet changes
- Dental disease
- Systemic disease
- Stress
- Pain
- Inappropriate oral antibiotic therapy
- Poor sanitation

CONTAGION AND ZOONOSIS
- *G. duodenalis* and *E. chinchillae* are transmitted by the oral-fecal route.
- Excreted *G. duodenalis* cysts remain infectious for up to 3 weeks and sporulated *E. chinchillae* oocyts for several months.
- *Rodentolepis nana* ("mouse tapeworm") is zoonotic, does not require an intermediate host, and therefore can cause severe infection, particularly in immune compromised humans.

ASSOCIATED CONDITIONS AND DISORDERS
- Dental disease
- Ketoacidosis and hepatic lipidosis
- Poor coat condition

CLINICAL PRESENTATION

DISEASE FORMS/SUBTYPES
- Constipation
- Enteritis/Dysbacteriosis/Diarrhea
- Rectal tissue prolapse

HISTORY, CHIEF COMPLAINT
- Any systemic disease or painful or stressful condition may result in secondary gastrointestinal problems with nonspecific clinical signs such as anorexia, lack of fecal output, and lethargy.
- General complaints include the following:
  - Anorexia
  - Lethargy
  - Depression
  - Weight loss
  - Poor general condition
  - Poor coat condition
  - Teeth grinding
- Constipation
  - Small, firm, irregularly shaped fecal pellets
  - Reduced or no fecal output
- Dysbacteriosis/Enteritis/Diarrhea
  - Soft feces or diarrhea
  - Fecal staining of resting board
  - Fecal matting around anus
  - Distended abdomen
  - Rapid breathing
- Tympany
  - Distended abdomen
  - Hunched body posture
  - Rapid breathing
- Rectal tissue prolapse and intussusception
  - Prolapsed red tissue from anus
  - Increased preening around anus
  - Lack of fecal output
  - Straining

PHYSICAL EXAM FINDINGS
- Nonspecific findings can include the following:
  - Depression and lethargy
  - Dehydration
  - Cachexia
  - Poor coat condition
  - Perianal staining
  - Hunched body posture
- Constipation
  - Abdominal palpation reveals impaction of cecum and colon.
- Dysbacteriosis/Enteritis/Diarrhea
  - Perianal fecal soiling
  - Malodorous, soft fecal material
  - Tympanic intestine on abdominal palpation
  - In severe cases, animals can develop endotoxemia, septicemia and metabolic disturbances; therefore animals become more depressed and might progress into shock
- Tympany
  - Severity of clinical signs changes with progression and degree of tympany
  - Distended and tense abdomen
  - Hunched body posture or lateral recumbence in advanced cases
  - If animal is in shock, clinical findings can include hypothermia, tachypnea, tachycardia, severe

depression, and pale mucous membrane

- Rectal tissue prolapse
  - Prolapsed tissue from rectum, which can be edematous, hyperemic, or necrotic
  - Abdominal palpation might reveal a turgid cylindrical mass reflecting the intussuscepted portion of the intestine

ETIOLOGY AND PATHOPHYSIOLOGY

- Gastrointestinal disorders can be caused by a variety of infectious and noninfectious causes.
- Dysbacteriosis is defined as a disorder caused by an imbalance of the normal flora of the gastrointestinal tract. Dysbacteriosis is present in most cases of gastrointestinal disease in chinchillas.
- Constipation
  - Anorexia secondary to stress, or pain, for example due to dental disease, can lead to constipation. Insufficient food and water intake and possibly reduced gastrointestinal motility will lead to constipation and reduced output of smaller and irregular fecal pellets.
  - Systemic disease (i.e., systemic bacterial infection [e.g., *Pseudomonas aeruginosa*, organ failure, ketoacidosis) is an important factor leading to the development of constipation due to reduced food intake and gastrointestinal hypomotility.
  - Typhlitis and colitis can lead to constipation and abnormally shaped and smaller fecal pellets.
  - Thickened or impacted intestinal contents due to constipation are most commonly found in the cecum and the colonic flexure.
- Enteritis/Dysbacteriosis/Diarrhea
  - Dietary causes are considered more common in pet chinchillas: overfeeding of fresh green feed or items high in simple carbohydrates (treats, grains); sudden changes in diet, overfeeding, etc.
  - Iatrogenic: antibiotic-induced dysbacteriosis secondary to oral administration of inappropriate antibiotics or ingestion of topical antibiotics such as ointments used for topical wound management (e.g., triple antibiotic ointment)
- Infectious
  - Primary infectious causes are rare in pet chinchillas.
  - Primary bacterial enteritis caused by *Salmonella typhimurium, Salmonella enteritidis, Yersinia enterocolitica* is rare in pet chinchillas.
  - Secondary infections with opportunistic pathogens are common and develop after an initial disturbance of the normal intestinal flora, leading to dysbacteriosis and overgrowth of opportunistic pathogenic bacterial, parasitic, or fungal organisms.
    - *Escherichia coli,* a ubiquitous organism that is not considered part of the physiologic intestinal flora in chinchillas, can cause enteritis, septicemia, and endotoxemia.
    - *P. aeruginosa, Klebsiella* spp., *Proteus* spp., etc.
    - *Cyniclomyces guttulatus* (previously *Saccharomycopsis guttulata*)
      - Yeast; opportunistic fungal pathogen and physiologic part of the gastrointestinal flora
      - Overgrowth and diarrhea can be seen in cases of dysbacteriosis due to another (primary) cause such as sudden diet change.
      - Overgrowth is always considered a secondary problem; therefore, the primary cause should be identified.
    - *Giardia duodenalis*
      - Common parasite in chinchillas
      - Healthy chinchillas can harbor *G. duodenalis* organisms in low numbers in the small intestine; experimental infection of healthy chinchillas with *Giardia* cysts failed to induce clinical disease.
      - Predisposing factors such as stress and poor husbandry are believed to cause an increase in parasite numbers, resulting in diarrhea and potentially death.
      - Morbidity and mortality mainly in young (<3 months) or immune compromised animals
      - Subclinical carriers and chronic shedding without clinical signs are common. Disturbance of the normal intestinal microbial flora can lead to massive remultiplication of the organism and clinical giardiasis.
    - *Eimeria chinchillae*
      - Strict host-specific infection leads to damage of the intestinal mucosa, with subsequent disturbance of the physiologic flora and secondary intestinal fungal or bacterial enteritis.
      - Morbidity and mortality mainly in young (<3 months) or immune compromised chinchillas
    - *Rodentolepis nana*
      - Cestode do not require an intermediate host and therefore high numbers of parasites can be found in chinchillas, causing disease.
      - Infection can occur by direct transmission via the fecal-oral route.
      - Mild infections may be subclinical and are more common.
      - Heavy infection will result in anorexia, diarrhea, weight loss, poor fur condition, and possible death.
- Tympany
  - Secondary to gastroenteritis, dysbacteriosis, or ileus
  - In rare cases, tympany may be secondary to intestinal torsion or luminal obstruction.
  - Fiber-deficient diet, sudden diet changes, high-protein diet (fresh young grass), and foods rich in carbohydrates (e.g., grains, treats)
  - Inappropriate oral antibiotic treatment (cephalosporins, penicillins, erythromycin, clindamycin)
- Rectal tissue prolapse
  - Cause unknown; dysbacteriosis, enteritis, diarrhea, or tenesmus may be predisposing causes.
  - It is important to differentiate between prolapse of the rectum itself and prolapse of a more distal segment of the intestine, through the rectum, secondary to an intussusception.
  - The amount of small or large intestine involved in the intussusception can be extensive.

DIAGNOSIS

DIFFERENTIAL DIAGNOSIS

- Constipation: functional ileus, partial obstruction
- Lack of fecal output: intestinal intussusception
- Tympany: intestinal torsion, obstruction, gastroenteritis
- Anorexia: systemic disease (e.g., metabolic, infectious, organ failure), pain
- Tense or painful abdomen: parturition pain, urolithiasis, and nephrolithiasis

INITIAL DATABASE

- Identifying the underlying cause of gastroenteritis and dysbacteriosis is important to improve the therapeutic outcome and reduce the chance of recurrence.
- Full dietary history
- Full environmental history
- Consider the following tests based on clinical presentation:
  - Fecal flotation
  - Fecal wet mount
  - Fecal cytologic examination
  - Whole-body radiographs
  - Biochemistry profile: may be normal. Hyperglycemia, dehydration, and azotemia may be evident. Rule out concurrent diseases that would affect the prognosis (e.g., hepatic lipidosis, ketoacidosis, renal insufficiency).

- Complete blood count: Hemoconcentration, anemia, leukocytosis, or leukopenia
- Urine analysis: ketonuria, low/acidic pH (normal urine pH 8-9), glucosuria

• Specific tests for rectal tissue prolapse
  - Differentiate between a true rectal prolapse and an intestinal prolapse secondary to an intussusception. This is very important for establishing a correct diagnosis, prognosis, and therapy.
  - Passage of a lubricated probe at the mucocutaneous junction of the anus will be impossible in cases of true rectal prolapse. However, in cases of intestinal prolapse secondary to intussusception, passing a lubricated probe will be possible.

ADVANCED OR CONFIRMATORY TESTING

- Fecal culture for enteric opportunistic pathogens (e.g., *E. coli, P. aeruginosa*): interpretation may be difficult
- *Giardia* antigen testing: clinically healthy chinchillas can be positive
- Dental examination: rule out intraoral lesions (see Dental Disease)
- Abdominal ultrasound: identify intussuscepted intestinal segment
- Exploratory laparotomy: confirm intestinal intussusception and assess extent and viability of tissue

TREATMENT

THERAPEUTIC GOALS

- Rehydration and relief of discomfort
- Treatment of secondary infections and complications
- Treatment of primary underlying causes if possible

ACUTE GENERAL TREATMENT

- If animal is anorexic, dehydrated, or in discomfort, provide supportive care as needed:
  - Fluid therapy
    - Maintenance fluid rate: 60-100 mL/kg/d SC, PO, IV, IO
    - Replace fluid deficits and maintain normovolemia
    - For cases of constipation, use the enteral (oral) route to rehydrate intestinal contents
  - Nutritional support
    - Syringe-feed with high-fiber diet for herbivores (e.g., Oxbow Critical Care for Herbivores, 50-80 mL/kg PO q 24 h, divided into 4-5 feedings) or crushed and soaked pellets
  - Analgesia
    - Buprenorphine 0.03-0.05 mg/kg SC q 8-12 h
- Antibiotic therapy
  - Not necessary if chinchilla is in stable condition, bright, alert, and not anorexic.
  - Consider antibiotic treatment of predominantly Gram-negative opportunistic pathogens in chinchillas with severe dysbacteriosis, and when an infectious cause is suspected but unconfirmed and the animal is in a compromised general condition.
  - Give antibiotics by injection (SC, IM, IV); avoid the oral route in debilitated patients and in animals suspected to be septicemic.
    - Trimethoprim-sulfa 30 mg/kg PO q 12 h
    - Enrofloxacin 10-20 mg/kg SC, PO q 12-24 h
- Antiparasitic therapy
  - Treat in-contact animals
  - Clean and disinfect the environment to prevent reinfection: regular bedding changes and cage cleaning. Discard cage furnishings that cannot be disinfected (e.g., wood-based furnishings)
  - Metronidazole 20-30 mg/kg PO q 12-24 h for 5 days: for treatment of *Giardia*. Dependent on the oral formulation of metronidazole used, chinchillas may become anorexic.
  - Fenbendazole 20-50 mg/kg PO q 24 h for 5 days: for treatment of *Giardia*
  - Trimethoprim-sulfa 30 mg/kg PO q 12-24 h for 5-10 days: for treatment of *Eimeria*
  - Praziquantel 5-10 mg/kg SC, PO q 10 d: for treatment of cestodes
- Antifungal therapy
  - Nystatin 100,000 IU/kg PO q 8 h for 5 days, if *C. guttulatus* overgrowth is high or no response is noted following treatment of primary cause and dietary changes
- Constipation
  - After animal is rehydrated by parenteral fluid therapy, switch to enteral fluid therapy to rehydrate dehydrated and impacted ingesta. Give up to 100 mL/kg PO divided into 4-5 doses.
  - Syringe-feed high-fiber diet for herbivores (e.g., Oxbow Critical Care for Herbivores, 50-80 mL/kg PO q 24 h, divided into 4-5 feedings) or crushed and soaked pellets.
  - Increase fiber content of diet
- Tympany
  - Depends on degree of tympany. Mild cases should be treated with supportive care (see earlier). Severe cases require aggressive cardiovascular support: oxygen, intravenous/intraosseous fluid therapy, and parental antibiotic therapy. After patient has been stabilized, diagnose and treat the underlying cause.
  - Decompression via an orogastric tube placed under sedation or trocarization is controversial.
- Rectal tissue prolapse
  - Treatment of rectal prolapse, after an intussusception has been ruled out, consists of cleaning and soaking of edematous prolapsed rectal tissue in a concentrated sugar solution (50% dextrose). Replace the prolapsed tissue, and place a perianal purse-string suture.
  - Treatment of intussusception and intestinal prolapse should be considered only after an exploratory laparotomy has allowed assessment of the extent of intussusception and viability of affected tissue. Reduction of the intussusception during laparotomy is recommended. Chance of recurrence is high. Intestinal resection and anastomosis are required if viability of tissue is questionable.
  - Treatment of underlying cause to prevent recurrence

CHRONIC TREATMENT

Repeated and often lifelong treatment of dental malocclusion and periodontal disease under general anesthesia is required (see Dental Disease).

POSSIBLE COMPLICATIONS

In all cases of severe dysbacteriosis or impaired intestinal wall integrity, septicemia and endotoxemia have to be considered as secondary complications.

RECOMMENDED MONITORING

- Quality and quantity of fecal output
- Appetite
- Urine ketones

PROGNOSIS AND OUTCOME

- Prognosis is generally better if an underlying primary cause can be identified and successfully treated.
- Good: acute diarrhea or constipation, if animal is still eating
- Good to fair: constipation or diarrhea if animal has reduced appetite
- Fair: If animal is suffering from systemic disease such as ketoacidosis
- Fair: Rectal tissue prolapse without intussusception and prolapse of more proximal intestinal segment
- Fair to poor: severely depressed animal, severe ketoacidosis, dehydration
- Poor: rectal tissue prolapse secondary to an intussusception, severe tympany

CONTROVERSY

The use of prokinetic drugs in chinchillas is controversial, and clinical efficacy has not been demonstrated for any of the drugs recommended in the veterinary literature. Prokinetic drugs are contraindicated in cases in which an infectious process or an obstruction cannot be ruled out. Most chinchillas with gastrointestinal disease will respond to appropriate supportive care alone, including fluid therapy, analgesia, and nutritional support, making the use of prokinetic drugs unnecessary.

PEARLS & CONSIDERATIONS

COMMENTS

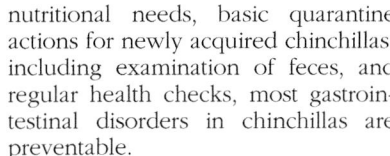

After stabilization of the patient and restoration of gastrointestinal motility, the goal should be to identify and treat the primary underlying cause to improve the case outcome and reduce the risk of recurrence of disease.

PREVENTION

- Most gastrointestinal disorders in pet chinchillas are directly or indirectly husbandry and diet related. Through adequate client education regarding nutritional needs, basic quarantine actions for newly acquired chinchillas, including examination of feces, and regular health checks, most gastrointestinal disorders in chinchillas are preventable.
- Do not administer antibiotics such as cephalosporins, penicillins, erythromycin, and clindamycin orally. Do not use topical ointments that contain bacitracin (e.g., triple antibiotic ointment) because of risk of ingestion by chinchillas. If these antibiotics are administered orally or are accidentally ingested, dysbacteriosis, endotoxemia, enterotoxemia, and death may result.

CLIENT EDUCATION

Chinchillas should be fed predominantly high-quality grass hay. Supplemental commercial chinchilla pellets should be offered. Treats such as dried or fresh fruits and vegetables should be offered only occasionally; preference should be given to items low in carbohydrates. Fresh water must be available at all times.

SUGGESTED READINGS

Mans C, et al: Disease problems of chinchillas. In Carpenter JW, et al, editors: Ferrets, rabbits, and rodents: clinical medicine and surgery, ed 3, St Louis, 2012, WB Saunders, pp 311–325.

Quesenberry KE, et al: Biology, husbandry, and clinical techniques of guinea pigs and chinchillas. In Carpenter JW, et al, editors: Ferrets, rabbits and rodents: clinical medicine and surgery, ed 3, St Louis, 2012, WB Saunders, pp 279–294.

Ward M: Rodents: digestive system disorders. In Keeble E, et al, editors: BSAVA manual of rodents and ferrets, Gloucester, UK, 2009, British Small Animal Veterinary Association, pp 123–141.

CROSS-REFERENCES TO OTHER SECTIONS

Dental Disease

AUTHOR: **CHRISTOPH MANS**

EDITOR: **THOMAS M. DONNELLY**

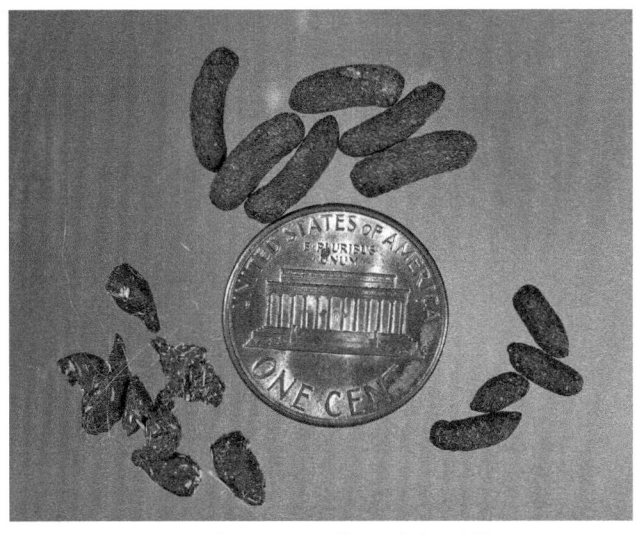

Gastrointestinal Disorders Fecal pellets of chinchillas. Top: Normal sized and regular shaped fecal pellets of a healthy chinchilla. Right: Fecal pellets from a chinchilla with constipation. Fecal pellets are smaller and irregular in size and shape. Left: Fecal pellets from a chinchilla with a mild *Eimeria chinchillae* infection. Fecal pellets are soft and misshapen.

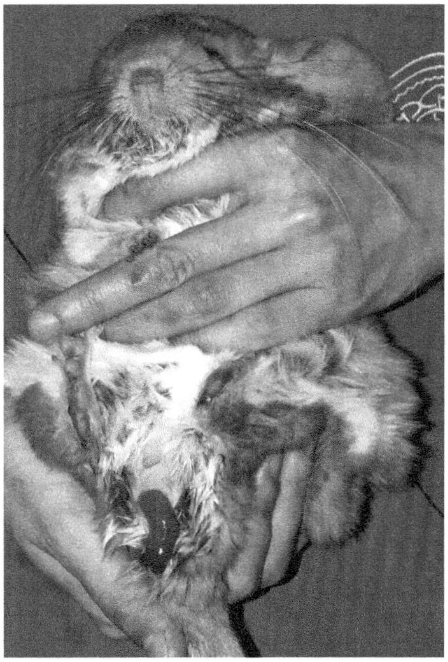

Gastrointestinal Disorders Rectal tissue prolapse in a young chinchilla.

SMALL MAMMALS: CHINCHILLAS

Ocular Disorders

BASIC INFORMATION

DEFINITION

Diseases of the eyes and surrounding structures

SYNONYMS

Epiphora, wet eye, conjunctivitis, corneal ulcer, ulcerative keratitis, keratitis

SPECIAL SPECIES CONSIDERATIONS

- Chinchillas have a large and exposed corneal segment, predisposing them to corneal trauma.

- Chinchillas have a vertical slit pupil.
- The third eyelid is only rudimentary developed as a small conjunctival fold at the medial canthus.
- The lacrimal drainage system consists of two lacrimal punctae at the medial canthus of the upper and lower eyelids. Both drain into a single lacrimal duct. The nasolacrimal duct runs in a similar course as in other rodents and lagomorphs and enters the nasal chamber just inside the nares.
- Catheterization of the lacrimal punctae for diagnostic and therapeutic purposes is not possible.
- Caruncular trichiasis occurs in chinchillas but is usually not associated with any secondary ocular disease (epiphora, conjunctivitis, corneal irritation), and therefore might be a normal variation.

EPIDEMIOLOGY

RISK FACTORS

- Inappropriate cage interior (sharp objects)
- Immune suppression
- Dental disease
- Excessive dust bathing
- Poor environmental hygiene

CONTAGION AND ZOONOSIS

- *Pseudomonas aeruginosa* infection can cause conjunctivitis and can occur sporadically or as epizootic outbreaks. Transmission between chinchillas is unlikely, but common sources of infection should be investigated (e.g., water bottles) to reduce chances of exposure and infection of other chinchillas.
- Human herpesvirus type 1 (HSV-1) can be transmitted from humans to chinchillas (anthroponosis), and rapidly develop into a rapid and fatal disease syndrome. Ulcerative keratitis and retinitis have been reported in chinchillas infected experimentally with HSV-1.

ASSOCIATED CONDITIONS AND DISORDERS

- Dental disease
- Systemic infection with *P. aeruginosa*
- HSV-1 infection (rare)

CLINICAL PRESENTATION

DISEASE FORMS/SUBTYPES

- Unilateral vs. bilateral disease
- Epiphora
- Conjunctivitis
- Corneal ulceration: simple, complex, or indolent (refractory) ulcer

HISTORY, CHIEF COMPLAINT

- Wet fur around eyes ("wet eye"), unilateral or bilateral
- Purulent eye discharge, unilateral or bilateral
- Painful red eye, squinting
- Cloudy eye
- Depression
- Anorexia

PHYSICAL EXAM FINDINGS

- Epiphora
  - Serous discharge
  - Unilateral or bilateral
  - Wetting or crusting of the periocular fur, and potentially periocular alopecia and dermatitis
  - Palpable apical elongation of the mandibular or maxillary cheek teeth, indicating underlying dental abnormalities
- Conjunctivitis
  - Unilateral: trauma, topical irritants, intraocular disease (e.g., uveitis)
  - Bilateral: primary infectious (e.g., *P. aeruginosa*)
  - Conjunctival hyperemia and edema
  - Mucopurulent ocular discharge
  - Periocular crusting
  - Blepharospasm
  - Depression and anorexia are common in cases of systemic *P. aeruginosa* infection
- Corneal ulceration
  - Retention of fluorescein dye in corneal stroma
    - No dye retention in case of complex ulcers, with stroma loss and exposure of Descemet's membrane
  - Corneal edema: focal (simple)—diffuse (complex corneal ulcer)
  - Blepharospasm (might be absent with indolent ulcers)
  - Conjunctivitis
  - Ocular discharge: serous (simple)—mucopurulent (complex corneal ulcer)
  - Loose corneal epithelial ulcer margins (indolent ulcer)

ETIOLOGY AND PATHOPHYSIOLOGY

- Epiphora
  - Secondary bone remodeling around the elongated apical reserve crowns of the maxillary cheek teeth can cause complete or partial compression and consequent obstruction of the nasolacrimal duct.
- Conjunctivitis
  - Irritation from excessive sand bathing, inadequate cage ventilation, or underlying nasolacrimal duct obstruction is often the cause.
  - Primary bacterial conjunctivitis caused by *P. aeruginosa* can occur as a localized infection or as part of a systemic infection.
- Corneal ulceration
  - The large and prominent corneal surface most likely predisposes chinchillas to corneal trauma.
  - Excessive sand bathing, providing inappropriate sand for bathing, and inappropriate housing conditions should be considered as possible underlying causes.
  - Corneal ulceration most frequently is primarily traumatic, followed by secondary colonization and infection by bacteria, and less commonly by fungi.
  - Tear film abnormalities, caused by insufficient tear production (i.e., keratoconjunctivitis sicca) have not been reported in chinchillas.

DIAGNOSIS

DIFFERENTIAL DIAGNOSIS

- Exophthalmos
- Eyelid deformities: trichiasis, distichiasis, entropion
- Facial nerve paralysis (typically secondary to otitis media)
- Corneal dystrophy or degeneration
- Anterior uveitis
- Glaucoma

INITIAL DATABASE

- Complete ophthalmologic examination
- Submit a conjunctival (or corneal) swab for aerobic bacterial culture and sensitivity. Collect samples before further diagnostics are performed.
- Assess cranial nerve reflexes: palpebral, corneal, and pupillary light reflexes
- Fluorescein dye application
  - Necessary to rule out damage to the corneal surface
  - Avoid direct contact between fluorescein-impregnated test strips and the corneal surface because this can result in false-positive fluorescein staining.

ADVANCED OR CONFIRMATORY TESTING

- Intraocular pressure (IOP) measurement
  - Reference ranges: 17.71 ± 4.17 mm Hg (by applanation tonometry); 2.9 ± 1.8 mm Hg (by rebound tonometry)
- Measurement of tear production
  - Schirmer tear test: reference range: 1.07 mm/min
  - Phenol red thread tear test: reference range: 14.0 mm/15 sec
- Corneal cytologic examination
- Conjunctival biopsy
- Ocular ultrasound or skull CT for evaluation of retrobulbar space in case of exophthalmos

TREATMENT

THERAPEUTIC GOALS

- Treat underlying cause
- Eliminate infection

- Eliminate ocular pain
- Prevent progressive loss of corneal stroma and corneal rupture
- Promote corneal reepithelialization

ACUTE GENERAL TREATMENT

- Epiphora
  - Topical nonsteroidal antiinflammatory drugs (NSAIDs)
    - Flurbiprofen 0.03% solution q 6-12 h for 10-14 d
    - Diclofenac 0.1% solution q 6-12 h for 10-14 d
  - Topical broad-spectrum antibiotics (e.g., tobramycin, gentamicin, oxytetracycline/polymyxin B combination) q 6-8 h for 7-10 d
  - Systemic NSAIDs
    - Meloxicam 0.3-0.5 mg/kg PO q 12-24 h for 10-14 d
- Conjunctivitis
  - Thoroughly lavage the conjunctival sac with physiologic saline.
  - Topical broad-spectrum antibiotics (e.g., tobramycin, gentamicin, oxytetracycline/polymyxin B combination) q 4-8 h for 7-10 d
  - Systemic antibiotic therapy for animals that present with depression and anorexia in addition to mucopurulent (usually bilateral) conjunctivitis, as these animals often suffer from systemic infection with *P. aeruginosa.* Empirical treatment should be initiated, pending aerobic bacterial culture results:
    - Enrofloxacin 10-20 mg/kg SC, IM, IV q 12-24 h
    - Ceftazidime 25 mg/kg SC, IM, IV q 8 h
- Corneal ulceration
  - Topical broad-spectrum antibiotics (e.g., tobramycin, gentamicin, oxytetracycline/polymyxin B combination, ciprofloxacin) q 4-6 h for 7-10 d
  - Consider atropine 1% solution or ointment topical q 12-48 h
  - Consider systemic administration of nonsteroidal antiinflammatory medication (e.g., meloxicam 0.3-0.5 mg/kg SC, PO q 12-24 h)
  - Anticollagenase therapy is indicated for melting or stromal corneal ulcers
    - Autogenous serum q 1-4 h
    - Oxytetracycline/polymyxin B ointment q 4-6 h
- Access to a sand bath should be restricted until the chinchilla has fully recovered.
- Supportive care is indicated for any chinchilla that is anorexic and depressed. Provide nutritional support, correct fluid deficits, and provide analgesia.
- Hospitalize animals with severe ocular disease or that are depressed and anorexic.

CHRONIC TREATMENT

- Indolent/refractory corneal ulcers
  - Perform corneal débridement and grid keratotomy after any potential infection is eradicated.
- For recurrent simple corneal ulcers in which no primary underlying cause can be identified, long-term treatment with lubricant eye drops might prevent recurrence.

POSSIBLE COMPLICATIONS

Do not use any topical formulations that contain bacitracin because ingestion can result in fatal dysbacteriosis.

PROGNOSIS AND OUTCOME

- Variable depending on cause
- Epiphora
  - Recurrence is common.
  - If underlying dental disease is responsible for the nasolacrimal duct obstruction, regaining permanent patency of the nasolacrimal duct is unlikely because no effective treatment is known for apical reserve crown elongation.
- Conjunctivitis
  - Good for unilateral disease
  - Good to guarded if normal Gram-positive bacterial flora is cultured
  - Guarded to poor if *P. aeruginosa* is cultured and the animal is showing signs of systemic disease (i.e., depression, reduced fecal output and anorexia)
- Corneal ulceration
  - Good for simple ulcers
  - Good to guarded if the underlying cause is identified
  - Guarded to poor for complex or melting ulcers, with significant bacterial infection

CONTROVERSY

- It is controversial whether *P. aeruginosa* is part of the normal conjunctival flora, which consists predominantly of Gram-positive organisms, including *Staphylococcus, Streptococcus,* and *Corynebacterium* species.
- Use of topical steroids in rodents is controversial because of possible systemic immune suppressive effects.

PEARLS & CONSIDERATIONS

COMMENTS

Because of the very small size of the lacrimal punctae, visualizing and catheterizing the lacrimal duct for flushing is very difficult and is not routinely performed.

CLIENT EDUCATION

Monitor for signs of recurrence.

SUGGESTED READINGS

Mans C, et al: Disease problems of chinchillas. In Quesenberry KE, et al, editors: Ferrets, rabbits and rodents, ed 3, St Louis, 2012, Saunders, pp 311–325.

Lima L, et al: The chinchilla eye: morphologic observations, echobiometric findings and reference values for selected ophthalmic diagnostic tests, Vet Ophthalmol 13:14–25, 2010.

Müller K, et al: Reference values for selected ophthalmic diagnostic tests and clinical characteristics of chinchilla eyes *(Chinchilla lanigera)*, Vet Ophthalmol 13:29–34, 2010.

AUTHOR: **CHRISTOPH MANS**

EDITOR: **THOMAS M. DONNELLY**

SMALL MAMMALS: CHINCHILLAS

Penile Disorders

BASIC INFORMATION

DEFINITION

- Penile disorders in chinchillas include a variety of conditions, which might be incidental findings during physical examination or may cause clinical disease.
- "Fur ring" is a descriptive term for the accumulation of hair around the base of the glans penis within the prepuce in chinchillas.
- Balanoposthitis is an inflammatory condition of the prepuce and glans penis that is usually secondary to infection.
- Paraphimosis is a condition in which the prepuce becomes trapped behind the glans penis and cannot be reduced.
- Phimosis is a condition in which the prepuce cannot be fully retracted from the glans penis.

SYNONYMS

Fur ring, paraphimosis, phimosis, balanoposthitis, preputial infection, preputial abscess

CLINICAL PRESENTATION

DISEASE FORMS/SUBTYPES

- Fur ring
- Balanoposthitis
- Preputial abscesses
- Paraphimosis
- Phimosis

HISTORY, CHIEF COMPLAINT

- Most fur rings and cases of phimosis are incidental findings during physical examination.
- Excessive grooming in preputial/perianal area
- Swelling in the area of the penis/prepuce
- Stranguria
- Dysuria
- Anuria
- Pollakiuria
- Anorexia
- Lethargy

PHYSICAL EXAM FINDINGS

- Accumulation of fur around the base of the glans penis within the prepuce
- Swelling of the prepuce
- Congested and edematous prolapsed glans penis and edema of the prepuce
- Dried and demarcated penile tissue if prolapse has been present for some time
- Inappetence and apathy due to pain or systemic infection
- Enlarged urinary bladder if urinary blockage due to urethral compression has occurred

ETIOLOGY AND PATHOPHYSIOLOGY

- Fur rings
    - Accumulation of hair ("fur ring"), smegma, or both around the base of the glans penis within the prepuce is common in chinchillas.
    - Fur rings can be found in single-housed as well as breeding males.
    - Fur rings are often incidental findings that cause no clinical signs, unless they lead to constriction and/or infection, and subsequently to balanoposthitis, preputial abscesses, or paraphimosis.
- Balanoposthitis
    - Infection of the prepuce and glans penis occurs secondary to the accumulation of fur and/or smegma.
    - Acute balanoposthitis can be seen as part of a systemic *Pseudomonas aeruginosa* infection, which usually leads to anorexia, constipation, and infection of other organs, such as conjunctivitis, pneumonia, or otitis.
    - Chronic balanoposthitis can present as a preputial abscess, which prevents the penis from extrusion from the prepuce.
- Paraphimosis
    - Is usually a complication of a fur ring or balanoposthitis
    - As a result of swelling and inflammation of the prepuce and/or glans penis, the glans penis is prolapsed from the prepuce, and manual reduction is not possible.
    - In reproductivally active males, a differential of paraphimosis is penile paralysis due to sexual exhaustion. This is seen in male chinchillas that are housed together with several females, or that were separated during copulation. However, swelling or edema is not present in cases of penile paralysis.
    - Bite injuries leading to inflammation and paraphimosis can occur if intact males are housed together.
- Phimosis
    - A poorly described condition in chinchillas and often an incidental finding during routine physical examination
    - Characterized by an inability to completely extrude the glans penis from the prepuce because of the formation of adhesions between the visceral layer of the prepuce and the glans penis, or because of stricture formation of the preputial opening
    - The cause of phimosis is unknown. In other species, phimosis can be congenital or acquired (i.e., secondary to chronic inflammation or trauma).
    - Phimosis may lead to the development of balanoposthitis as a result of the accumulation of smegma, which promotes secondary infection.

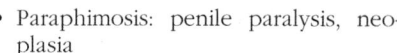

DIAGNOSIS

DIFFERENTIAL DIAGNOSIS

- Paraphimosis: penile paralysis, neoplasia
- Stranguria/dysuria: urolithiasis
- Penile abscess: neoplasia

INITIAL DATABASE

- Detailed examination of prepuce and glans penis
    - Closely examine for bite wounds or other injuries.
    - Completely extract glans penis from prepuce to examine for fur accumulation, fur rings, smegma, pustules, or necrotic tissue.
- Aspiration of edematous or inflamed tissue or preputial abscesses for cytologic examination and aerobic bacterial culture and sensitivity
- If the general condition of the animal is impaired, consider biochemistry profile, complete blood count, and urine analysis.
- Whole-body radiographs are taken to rule out urolithiasis if animal is dysuric, stranguric, or anuric.

TREATMENT

THERAPEUTIC GOALS

- Resolution of edema, inflammation, and infection
- Resolution of paraphimosis and phimosis
- Normal urination
- Prevent reoccurrence of penile disorder

ACUTE GENERAL TREATMENT

- Asymptomatic fur rings, accumulation of hair and smegma
    - Can be removed in conscious animals. Wear gloves, use lubrication, and carefully remove all fur and debris. Clean glans penis with diluted chlorhexidine solution, and replace into prepuce. No further treatment is necessary.
- Balanoposthitis
    - Treat primary underlying cause (e.g., fur ring, debris accumulation).
    - Consider systemic antibiotic therapy if severe infection and tissue damage are present.
- Preputial abscess
    - Aspirate abscess percutaneously to relieve pressure and allow for manual extrusion of the glans penis from the prepuce.
    - Treat primary underlying cause (e.g., fur ring, debris accumulation).
    - Consider systemic antibiotic therapy.
- Paraphimosis
    - Immediate treatment is necessary to prevent further tissue damage.
    - Initial assessment and treatments should be performed with the patient under sedation or general anesthesia.
    - Careful cleaning of the prepuce and prolapsed penis should be done with warm water.
    - Thoroughly examine the penis for a fur ring and for wounds.
    - If significant edema of the prepuce is present, apply 50% dextrose solution or crystalline sugar to reduce edema.
    - Apply lubricant gel or petroleum ointment (e.g., Vaseline) to facilitate repositioning of glans penis in the prepuce, if possible. Do not attempt to reposition the glans penis if significant preputial swelling is present and substantial force is necessary. Apply ointments or hydrogels to the

everted prepuce and glans penis to prevent drying of exposed tissue. Topical treatment should be performed 3 to 4 times daily. Wear gloves.
  - If self-mutilation or overgrooming occurs, an E-collar should be considered. Ensure that the animal can eat unaided, despite the E-collar.
  - Treat with systemic antibiotics.
  - Provide pain relief and antiinflammatory drugs
    - Buprenorphine 0.03-0.05 mg/kg SC q 8-12 h
    - Meloxicam 0.3-0.5 mg/kg PO or SC q 12-24 h, if adequately hydrated
  - Phimosis
    - Rule out concurrent balanoposthitis, and treat if present. Initiate systemic antibiotic therapy, pending surgical treatment, if indicated.
    - With the patient under general anesthesia, surgically remove adhesions between the visceral layer of the prepuce and the glans penis. Use surgical loops for improved magnification. Examine the glans penis carefully for the presence of fur rings or signs of infection, and clean with diluted chlorhexidine solution.
    - Following surgery, manually extrude the glans penis from the prepuce and apply ointment once daily for 7 days. Then reduce the frequency of treatment to once weekly, and monitor for the formation of new adhesions.
- Antibiotic therapy
  - Not necessary if chinchilla is in stable condition or if no evidence of infection can be found
  - Consider use of antibiotic treatment for predominantly Gram-negative opportunistic pathogens, particular *P. aeruginosa*, and when an infectious cause is suspected but unconfirmed and the animal is in a compromised general condition.
  - Give antibiotics by injection (SC, IM, IV) and avoid the oral route in debilitated patients, animals with impaired gastrointestinal function, and animals suspected to be septicemic.
    - Enrofloxacin 10-20 mg/kg SC, PO q 12-24 h
    - Trimethoprim-sulfa 30 mg/kg PO q 12 h
    - Chloramphenicol 30-50 mg/kg PO q 8 h
- If animal is anorexic and/or dehydrated, provide supportive care:
  - Fluid therapy
    - Maintenance fluid rate 60-100 mL/kg/d SC, PO, IV, IO
    - Replace fluid deficits and maintain normovolemia.
    - For cases of constipation, use the enteral (oral) route to rehydrate intestinal contents.
  - Nutritional support
    - Syringe-feed high-fiber diet for herbivores (e.g., Oxbow Critical Care for Herbivores, 50 to 80 mL/kg PO q 24 h, divided into 4 to 5 feedings) or crushed and soaked pellets.

CHRONIC TREATMENT

Paraphimosis might require long-term topical treatment, which usually can be provided by the owner.

POSSIBLE COMPLICATIONS

- Necrosis of prepuce and glans penis
- Recurrence of infection or inflammation
- Recurrence of fur or debris accumulation
- Recurrence of phimosis
- Post-renal azotemia
- Sepsis and death due to systemic *P. aeruginosa* infection
- Antibiotic-induced dysbacteriosis: do not use topical ointments that contain bacitracin (e.g., triple antibiotic ointment) because of the risk of ingestion by chinchillas. If ingestion occurs, dysbacteriosis, endotoxemia, and death may follow.

RECOMMENDED MONITORING

- Urination
- Appetite
- Fecal output

PROGNOSIS AND OUTCOME

- Excellent: fur rings and smegma accumulation, without secondary complications
- Good: simple balanoposthitis and preputial abscess if a primary cause can be identified and successfully treated
- Good: phimosis
- Guarded: paraphimosis
- Poor: penile and preputial necrosis, animals in poor general condition (i.e., severely ketoacidotic, cachexic), systemic *P. aeruginosa* infection

PEARLS & CONSIDERATIONS

COMMENTS

- In the literature, penile problems have been linked to reproductive activity. However, penile disorders are seen frequently in single-housed pet chinchillas.
- A complete physical examination in a male chinchilla includes complete extrusion of the glans penis from the prepuce and close examination for accumulation of fur or debris.
- Animals with diagnosed paraphimosis due to fur rings should be examined at least 4 times a year for recurrence.

PREVENTION

Regular examination of the glans penis for accumulation of fur or debris, by complete manual extraction from the prepuce

CLIENT EDUCATION

- Remove sand baths until complete recovery.
- Remove inappropriate bedding material, use of paper towels or newspaper.

SUGGESTED READINGS

Doerning BJ, et al: *Pseudomonas aeruginosa* infection in a *Chinchilla lanigera*, Lab Anim 27:131–133, 1993.

Ivey ES, et al: What's your diagnosis? Pollakiuria in a chinchilla, Lab Anim (NY) 27:21–22, 1998.

Mans C, et al: Disease problems of chinchillas. In Carpenter JW, et al, editors: Ferrets, rabbits and rodents, clinical medicine and surgery, ed 3, St Louis, 2012, WB Saunders, pp 311–325.

Quesenberry KE, et al: Biology, husbandry, and clinical techniques of guinea pigs and chinchillas. In Carpenter JW, et al, editors: Ferrets, rabbits and rodents: clinical medicine and surgery, ed 3, St Louis, 2012, WB Saunders, pp 279–294.

AUTHOR: **CHRISTOPH MANS**

EDITOR: **THOMAS M. DONNELLY**

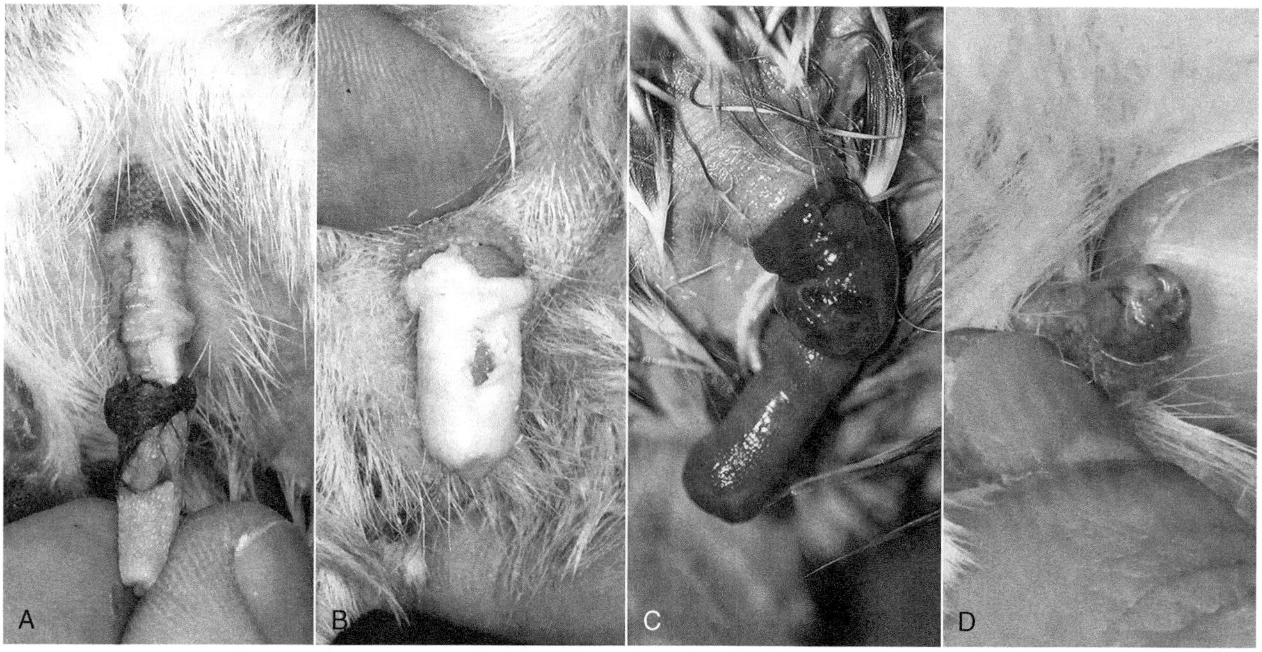

Penile Disorders Penile disorders in chinchillas: **A,** Hair accumulation ("fur ring") around the base of the glans penis. **B,** Excessive smegma accumulation. **C,** Paraphimosis, secondary to severe edema and infection of the prepuce. **D,** Phimosis.

SMALL MAMMALS: PRAIRIE DOGS

Odontoma

BASIC INFORMATION

DEFINITION

Odontomas are benign neoplasms of the teeth but are considered by many to be odontogenic hamartomas rather than true neoplasms. Hamartomas are benign tumor-like lesions composed of an overgrowth of mature tissue that normally occurs in the affected part of the body but with disorganization and often with one element predominating. In the case of odontomas, the tumor may consist of multiple, small, tooth-like structures (compound odontoma), or it may be a conglomerate mass of odontogenic hard and soft tissue (complex odontoma). The term *elodontoma* has been proposed to replace the term *odontoma* for hamartomatous jaw lesions in prairie dogs and similar species with elodont teeth. *Elodontoma* would then be defined as a hamartoma of continuously developing odontogenic tissue and alveolar bone at the periapical bud of elodont teeth.

SYNONYM

Elodontoma

SPECIAL SPECIES CONSIDERATIONS

- Prairie dogs are obligate nasal breathers. In prairie dogs, odontoma formation occurs at the apical aspect of the upper incisors, resulting in functional obstruction of the nasal passages and subsequent difficult breathing, which is a life-threatening condition.
- Prairie dogs have elodont incisors (i.e., continually growing teeth) with no anatomic root. Owing to the continuously developing nature of these teeth, all stages of odontogenesis occur from the apical end to the incisal edge. A permanently maintained apical bud is present at the apex of continuously growing teeth and contains self-renewing adult stem cells.

EPIDEMIOLOGY

RISK FACTORS Traumatic injury to the teeth

CONTAGION AND ZOONOSIS Clinical signs and presenting complaints may be similar to those of plague *(Yersinia pestis)*, which is rarely diagnosed in pet prairie dogs—plague is seen in wild prairie dogs.

ASSOCIATED CONDITIONS AND DISORDERS
- Weight loss
- Respiratory tract infection
- Cardiac disease

CLINICAL PRESENTATION

DISEASE FORMS/SUBTYPES
- Mild = Occasional sneezing and audible respiratory sounds
- Moderate = Sneezing, nasal discharge, audible respiratory sounds, decreased appetite, weight loss, mild dyspnea, and pawing at nose or mouth
- Severe = Sneezing, nasal discharge, audible respiratory sounds, complete anorexia, weight loss, and open-mouth breathing with profound dyspnea

HISTORY, CHIEF COMPLAINT Difficult breathing and/or respiratory distress are common presenting complaints. Weight loss and inappetence may occur. Signs of pain and discomfort, such as pawing at the mouth, and reluctance to maintain previously normal activity are often evident to owners.

PHYSICAL EXAM FINDINGS

- Purulent or serous nasal discharge
- Open-mouth breathing
- Weight loss
- Referred upper airway sounds
- Asymmetric air flow (e.g., demonstrated when a cotton wisp is placed in front of nares and asymmetric movement is seen)
- Poor body condition related to decreased food intake
- Unilateral or bilateral nodular hard palate lesions and malocclusion with erosion or notching of upper incisors

ETIOLOGY AND PATHOPHYSIOLOGY

- Odontomas appear to form in reaction to mechanical trauma of the upper incisors and bone around the incisors.
- Expansive growth of the tooth root occurs, creating a space-occupying mass.
- Eventually, the space-occupying mass extends deep into the sinus cavity, resulting in respiratory tract occlusion and distress.

DIAGNOSIS

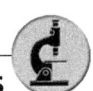

DIFFERENTIAL DIAGNOSIS

- Pneumonia
- Upper respiratory tract infection
- Heart failure resulting in respiratory signs
- Osteosarcoma of the maxillary bones
- Epiglottal fibrosarcoma

INITIAL DATABASE

- Skull (including oblique views) and thoracic radiographs
- Oral examination

ADVANCED OR CONFIRMATORY TESTING

- CT scan of the skull
- Skull radiographs are often sufficient to confirm a diagnosis.

TREATMENT

THERAPEUTIC GOALS

- Reestablish air passage through the nasal cavity.
- Provision of supportive care until surgery is considered or euthanasia is elected.

ACUTE GENERAL TREATMENT

- Rhinotomy via trephination into the nasal passages with stent placement. Use an 8-French polypropylene modified urinary catheter as the stent.
- Incisor extraction
  - Follow the same procedure as for a rabbit.
  - More challenging procedure owing to the hyperplasia surrounding both hard and soft tissues
  - Root deformation increases likelihood of incisor fracture during extraction procedure.
- Tracheostomy—not intended for long-term management of this condition
- Corticosteroids as palliative treatment with the goal of decreasing inflammation in the acute respiratory distress phase
  - Dexamethasone 4-5 mg/kg SC, IM, IP or IV once; prednisone 0.5-2.2 mg/kg PO, SC, or IM daily
- Supportive care can include the following:
  - Oxygen therapy
  - Fluid therapy with standard crystalloids at 60-100 mL/kg/d (adjusted accordingly for dehydration) given SC or IV to maintain hydration
  - Nutritional support in the form of assisted or syringe feeding a commercial diet (e.g., Oxbow Critical Care, Lafeber's Emeraid Herbivore)
  - Antibiotic therapy to treat secondary infection (e.g., ciprofloxacin at 5-20 mg/kg PO twice daily or enrofloxacin at 10-20 mg/kg PO, SC, or IM q 12-24 h)

CHRONIC TREATMENT

- Meloxicam 0.3-0.5 mg/kg PO q 12-24 h
- Antibiotic therapy
  - Enrofloxacin 10-20 mg/kg PO q 12-24 h or ciprofloxacin 10-20 mg/kg PO q 12-24 h
- Corticosteroids are used if desired effect is not achieved with nonsteroidal antiinflammatory drugs (NSAIDs) (do not use corticosteroids with NSAIDs).
- Prednisolone 0.5-1 mg/kg PO q 12-24 h
- Acetylcysteine (10% to 20% solution) diluted 1:1 with isotonic saline 0.1-0.25 mL twice daily is flushed into nasal stent to break down mucus and/or inspissated mucus plugs, to maintain a patent airway.
- In contrast to rats, prairie dogs do not tolerate nebulization well. They struggle to escape in a chamber and fight if a breathing mask is held over their muzzle.

DRUG INTERACTIONS

Do not combine the use of corticosteroids with NSAIDs.

POSSIBLE COMPLICATIONS

- Hypoxia and suffocation
- Hemorrhage and aspiration (including death) during rhinotomy or incisor extraction because a patent airway is difficult to obtain
- Endotracheal intubation is technically difficult in prairie dogs, owing to their anatomy. Endoscopy-guided endotracheal intubation is feasible, but requires specialized equipment.

RECOMMENDED MONITORING

- Serial radiographs or CT scans of the skull to monitor airway patency
- Pulse oximetry to monitor oxygen saturation and degree of respiratory compromise
- Monitor body weight because progressive weight loss is an indication of a worsening condition.

PROGNOSIS AND OUTCOME

- Prognosis in all cases is guarded to grave.
- The best chance for long-term survival is rhinotomy or incisor extraction, although these procedures are not without risk and may end in death of the patient.
- Chronic respiratory distress
  - Produces a chronic state of hypoxemia and fatigue
  - Results in animals with poor body condition and nutritional depletion because most of their efforts are spent breathing rather than eating
  - Results in debilitation, which correlates with poor postoperative survival

CONTROVERSY

Chronic mild trauma such as that caused by cage biting might distort the epithelial cords, causing minor anatomic abnormalities in the teeth (i.e., irregular enamel formation on the labial surfaces), but is unlikely to cause odontomas.

PEARLS & CONSIDERATIONS

COMMENTS

- The formation of large odontoma-like masses probably results from severe trauma that extensively damages odontogenic tissue and the surrounding follicle. For example, after trauma to the normally developing elodont tooth, bone regeneration may cause bone trabeculae to disrupt the epithelial cords, but they may also have been torn by bone trabeculae on impact, resulting in several odontogenic epithelial islands. Each daughter island of epithelium, because of its continuously proliferating nature in elodont teeth, continues to form its own hard

and soft tissue components, but in a haphazard manner, leading to the formation of odontomas.
- Odontomas have been reported in lemmings, voles, guinea pigs, degus, deer mice, and tree-squirrels.

PREVENTION

- Reduce risk of upper incisor trauma:
  - No wire cages, and remove all hard objects that the prairie dog may chew
  - Do not leave prairie dogs unattended on tables or objects from which they may fall.
- Good nutrition and husbandry
  - At present, no research has documented the "best" diet for captive prairie dogs.

CLIENT EDUCATION

Recommended reading for clients: Stoica K, et al: Bringing a prairie dog pup into your home, Canton, OH, 2001, K. Stoica.

SUGGESTED READINGS

Boy SC, et al: Odontoma-like tumours of squirrel elodont incisors—elodontomas, J Comp Pathol 135:56–61, 2006.

Capello V: Incisor extraction to resolve clinical signs of odontoma in a prairie dog, Exotic DVM 4:9, 2002.

Wagner RA, et al: Rhinotomy for treatment of odontoma in prairie dogs, Exotic DVM 3:29–34, 2001.

AUTHORS: **ANTHONY A. PILNY AND THOMAS M. DONNELLY**

EDITOR: **CHRISTOPH MANS**

SMALL MAMMALS: DEGUS

Behavioral Disorders

BASIC INFORMATION

DEFINITION

Any of various forms of abnormal behavior that have no underlying organic cause

SPECIAL SPECIES CONSIDERATIONS

- Degus are diurnal, ground-dwelling, curious, and very active animals.
- Degus are highly social animals; social contacts are crucial for their welfare.
- In the wild, degus live in groups of 10 to 15 animals of both sexes. Several groups form a colony.
- Separate hierarchies exist for males and females in each group.
- Degus exhibit considerable social tolerance in captivity. New animals are normally easy to introduce into established groups of animals.
- Mixed sex groups are usually nonproblematic in captivity.

EPIDEMIOLOGY

RISK FACTORS Single pet, inappropriate housing, inappropriate diet

ASSOCIATED CONDITIONS AND DISORDERS Secondary fungal and/or bacterial infection of skin lesions

CLINICAL PRESENTATION

HISTORY, CHIEF COMPLAINT

- Skin injuries
- Hair loss
- Fur chewing
- Biting
- Aggressiveness

PHYSICAL EXAM FINDINGS

- Skin wounds
- Fur damage
- Alopecia

ETIOLOGY AND PATHOPHYSIOLOGY

- Stereotypical behaviors, such as persistent gnawing of cage bars, extensive rubbing on cage bars, or continuous exaggerated self-grooming, are believed to be linked to stress.
- Stress factors: lack of social interaction, environmental stress (noises, light regime)
- Lack of environmental enrichment: diet, cage interior, no exercise, no sand bath
- Fur damage/alopecia
  - Localized over nose: results from constant rubbing/chewing on bars of cage—stereotypical behavior
  - Localized over back of nose: exaggerated grooming by cagemate-behavioral disorder
  - Fur chewing: may reflect stereotypical behavior or secondary to a severely fiber-deficient diet
- Mate aggressiveness (less common than in other rodent species)
  - Recent introduction to established group or solitary animal

DIAGNOSIS

DIFFERENTIAL DIAGNOSIS

- Skin injury
  - Traumatic injury by cage interior (sharp objects, etc.)
  - Bacterial dermatitis
  - Parasitic infection (uncommon)
  - Neoplasia
- Fur damage/alopecia
  - Fungal infection
  - Exaggerated social preening by cagemate
  - Fiber-deficient diet
  - Inappropriate sand bath (e.g., quartz sand)
  - Age-related in older animal

INITIAL DATABASE

- Fur damage/alopecia
  - Microscopic examination of skin scraping and hairs: rule out parasites (uncommon)
  - Fungal culture: rule out dermatophytosis
- Skin injuries
  - Bacterial/fungal culture if secondary infection suspected

ADVANCED OR CONFIRMATORY TESTING

- Skin injuries
  - Biopsy if suspicion of neoplasia or chronic nonhealing wound

TREATMENT

THERAPEUTIC GOALS

- Decrease abnormal behavior
- Resolve secondary complications (bacterial and/or fungal infections)

ACUTE GENERAL TREATMENT

- Stress-induced misbehavior
  - Remove excessive stimuli such as noises, activity around cage, and inappropriate circadian lighting (i.e., light during night).
  - Provide appropriate environment stimulation (space, sand bath, running wheel, branches).
  - Provide appropriate diet.
- Mate aggressiveness
  - Keep separate

- Reintroduce in steps: contact through wire first, animals in separate cages.
- Clean and rearrange the cage, then place new animal first; after 30 minutes, place long-standing animal.
- Skin injuries
  - Wound management
  - Surgical treatment if indicated
  - Pain management if indicated
  - Treatment of secondary fungal and/or bacterial infection

PROGNOSIS AND OUTCOME

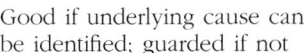

Good if underlying cause can be identified; guarded if not

PEARLS & CONSIDERATIONS

PREVENTION

Appropriate husbandry and diet

CLIENT EDUCATION

- Degus are social animals and enjoy human attention
- Never keep degus solitary; always house in groups.
- Provide sand bath, stimulating environment, enough space.
- Provide appropriate diet (minimum fiber content, 16% to 18%), high-quality hay, vegetables, branches, no fruits, and no molasses-containing rodent chow.

SUGGESTED READINGS

Jekl V, et al: Diseases in pet degus: a retrospective study in 300 animals, J Small Anim Pract 52:107–112, 2011.
Johnnson D: What veterinarians need to know about degus, Exotic DVM 4:39–42, 2002.
Najecki D, et al: Husbandry and management of the degu, Lab Anim (NY) 28:54–62, 1999.

AUTHOR: **CHRISTOPH MANS**

EDITOR: **THOMAS M. DONNELLY**

SMALL MAMMALS: DEGUS

Dental Disease

BASIC INFORMATION

DEFINITION

Disorders affecting the dentition and associated structures

SYNONYMS

Dental malocclusion, tooth overgrowth, periodontal disease, elodontoma

SPECIAL SPECIES CONSIDERATIONS

- Dental formula: 2(I1C0P1M3) = 20 teeth
- Incisor teeth and cheek teeth grow continuously throughout life (elodont).
- Incisor teeth and cheek teeth have a long crown (hypsodont) and no anatomic root (aradicular).
- Each tooth can be divided into a "clinical crown" (above the gingival sulcus) and the "reserve crown" (subgingival part).
- Incisor teeth in degus are orange to yellow in color owing to pigmentation of the superficial layer of the labial enamel.
- The figure-of-eight–shaped premolar and molar cheek teeth are morphologically indistinguishable in degus and therefore can be termed *cheek teeth (CT) 1-4*.
- The occlusal planes of the cheek teeth are nearly horizontal.

EPIDEMIOLOGY

SPECIES, AGE, SEX

- Acquired dental disease is common in captive degus.
- Acquired dental disease is significantly more common in older degus (>2 years).

RISK FACTORS

- High dietary intake of phosphorus (e.g., grains, treats) and inappropriate Ca : P ratio (<2 : 1)
- Low-fiber/less abrasive diet
- Trauma
- Age

ASSOCIATED CONDITIONS AND DISORDERS

- Weight loss
- Dyspnea
- Nasal discharge
- Epiphora

CLINICAL PRESENTATION

DISEASE FORMS/SUBTYPES

- Incisor teeth disorders
- Cheek teeth disorders
- Elodontomas

HISTORY, CHIEF COMPLAINT

- Reduced food intake
- Change in food preferences toward more easily chewed feed items
- Weight loss
- Soft feces-diarrhea
- Clear ocular discharge
- Lethargy
- Poor coat condition
- Sneezing
- Nasal discharge
- Dyspnea (elodontoma)
- Stridor (elodontoma)
- Open-mouth breathing (elodontoma)

PHYSICAL EXAM FINDINGS

- General loss of condition
- Palpable bony swellings or irregularities on ventrolateral aspects of mandibles reflect apical elongation of the mandibular cheek teeth.
- Depigmentation of the incisor teeth
- Malocclusion of the incisor teeth
- Tympany or reduced filling of gastrointestinal tract on abdominal palpation
- Soft feces-diarrhea
- Lethargy
- Epiphora
- Poor coat condition
- Facial abscesses
- Sneezing
- Nasal discharge
- Dyspnea, stridor, open mouth breathing (elodontoma)
- Cyanosis (elodontoma)
- Intraoral examination
  - General anesthesia is mandatory for a complete intraoral exam; it is preferred that the exam is performed under endoscopic guidance (stomatoscopy).
  - Cheek teeth
    - Coronal elongation
    - Formation of sharp enamel points or spurs leading to buccal and lingual mucosal erosions and discomfort. Most commonly, the maxillary cheek teeth are affected.
    - Change in occlusal surface plane
    - Periodontal disease
    - Mobility secondary to periodontal disease
    - Increased interproximal spaces, impacted with food or debris

- Caries affecting occlusal and interproximal surfaces (brown to black discoloration, tooth substance defects)
- Missing teeth

ETIOLOGY AND PATHOPHYSIOLOGY

- Cheek teeth disorders
  - The natural diet of degus consists mainly of foliage, bark, and grasses.
  - In captivity, degus will selectively ingest inappropriate food items, which are energy-dense, low in fiber, and high in phosphorus, such as grains, nuts, and seeds.
  - In degus, acquired dental disease can be induced by feeding of high-phosphorus diets or diets with a Ca:P ratio <2:1. This will result in coronal and apical cheek teeth elongation, leading to malocclusion and sharp enamel spur formation.
- Incisor teeth disorders
  - Incisor malocclusion occurs commonly secondary to cheek teeth malocclusion.
  - Depigmentation occurs secondary to a high-phosphorus diet or a diet with a Ca:P ratio <2:1.
  - Trauma (e.g., excessive chewing on cage bars or cage furnishings, iatrogenic)
- Elodontomas
  - An elodontoma is defined as a hamartoma of continuously developing odontogenic tissue and alveolar bone at the periapical bud of elodont teeth.
  - A hamartoma is a benign growth that resembles a neoplasm in the tissue of its origin. It is composed of tissue elements normally found at that site, but that are growing in a disorganized mass.
  - Elodontomas of the maxillary incisors appear to be common in captive degus.
  - The underlying cause for development of elodontomas is unknown. Repeated trauma (e.g., excessive chewing on cage bars or cage furnishings), age, and inflammation have been proposed as possible causes.
  - Stridor, dyspnea, and nasal discharge may occur secondary to partial to complete obstruction of the nasal cavities. In advanced stages, animals might present open-mouth breathing with cyanotic mucous membranes.

DIAGNOSIS

DIFFERENTIAL DIAGNOSIS

- Weight loss
  - Systemic disease (i.e., metabolic, infectious, organ failure)
  - Gastrointestinal disease
- Soft feces—diarrhea
  - Gastrointestinal disease (infectious, noninfectious)
  - Dietary
- Anorexia
  - Systemic disease (i.e., metabolic, infectious, organ failure)
  - Pain
- Dyspnea, nasal discharge, stridor
  - Upper respiratory disease (i.e., infection, foreign body, etc.)
  - Neoplasia
  - Lower respiratory tract disease
  - Congestive heart failure
- Poor coat condition
  - Barbering (behavioral)
  - Systemic disease (i.e., metabolic, infectious, organ failure)
  - Primary dermatologic problem
- Facial abscesses
  - Neoplasia

INITIAL DATABASE

- Complete intraoral examination under general anesthesia
  - Endoscopic intraoral guidance (stomatoscopy) is preferred for complete intraoral examination.
  - Use magnification and focal illumination if stomatoscopy cannot be performed.
- Imaging
  - Skull radiographs (five views: lateral, left and right oblique, ventrodorsal, rostrocaudal)
  - CT scan of head: preferred over skull radiographs
- Biochemistry profile: may be normal. Hyperglycemia and azotemia may be evident. Rule out concurrent diseases, which will affect the prognosis (i.e., diabetes mellitus [see Diabetes Mellitus], ketoacidosis, renal insufficiency).
- Complete blood count: may be normal; hemoconcentration or anemia may be seen
- Urine analysis: glucosuria, ketonuria, low pH (normal urine pH 8 to 9)

TREATMENT

THERAPEUTIC GOALS

- Resolve intraoral soft-tissue trauma, which causes discomfort and pain.
- Reduce periodontal disease, which causes discomfort and pain.
- Restore normal occlusion if possible.
- Recover or maintain the animal's ability to eat unaided.
- Reduce dyspnea caused by elodontoma formation.

ACUTE GENERAL TREATMENT

- Fluid therapy: 60-100 mL/kg/d SC, PO, IV
- Nutritional support: syringe-feed high-fiber diet for herbivores (e.g., Oxbow Critical Care for Herbivores, 50-80 mL/kg/d PO, divided into 4 to 5 feedings) or crushed and soaked pellets
- Analgesia
  - Buprenorphine 0.03-0.05 mg/kg SC q 8-12 h
  - Meloxicam 0.3-0.5 mg/kg PO or SC q 12-24 h once adequately hydrated
- Treatment of cheek teeth malocclusion
  - General anesthesia required
  - Specialized equipment required
  - Use a low-speed dental drill, a diamond burr, cheek dilators, and a mouth gag.
  - Use appropriate magnification and illumination. It is preferred that a rigid endoscope or video otoscope is used.
  - Avoid iatrogenic damage to the soft tissue during dental procedures.
  - Remove sharp enamel spurs, which lead to soft tissue trauma buccally and lingually. Maxillary cheek teeth form spurs buccally; mandibular cheek teeth form spurs lingually.
  - Shorten elongated clinical crowns.
  - Restore physiologically horizontal occlusal surfaces.
  - Do not attempt to extract cheek teeth unless severely diseased and severely mobile, secondary to periodontal infection or fracture. Cheek teeth extractions in degus are technically challenging, and complete extraction is often not possible.
  - Consider referral to a specialist for reassessment if extractions are deemed necessary.
- Treatment of periodontal disease
  - Probe pathologic interproximal spaces and gingival and periodontal pockets.
  - Remove impacted debris.
  - Rinse cleaned gingival and periodontal pockets carefully with 2% hydrogen peroxide or diluted chlorhexidine solution. Use a 0.5- to 1-mL syringe and a 25- to 28-gauge needle. Avoid aspiration of rinse.
  - Consider placement of Doxirobe Gel (Pfizer Animal Health, New York, NY) in deep (>5 mm) gingival and periodontal pockets; this may help delay re-impaction with debris and may reduce periodontal inflammation.
  - If evidence of significant periodontal infection is found, consider long-term antibiotic therapy. Ensure appropriate coverage against anaerobic bacteria predominating in periodontal infection. Long-acting penicillin G benzathine 40,000-60,000 IU/kg SC q 5 d is recommended.
- Treatment of caries

- Remove diseased tooth substance with a low-speed or high-speed dental drill and appropriate burr.
- Treatment of incisor teeth malocclusion
  - Sedation or general anesthesia is required.
  - Specialized equipment is required.
    - Use a low-speed with diamond or carbon cutting blade or a high-speed dental drill.
  - Avoid iatrogenic damage to the soft tissue during incisor teeth trimming.
    - Use a tongue depressor or spatula to protect the lips and tongue during trimming.
    - Do not use nail clippers or scissors to trim incisor teeth.
  - Avoid excessive shortening of the clinical crowns because this will lead to temporary functional loss of the incisor teeth.
- Antibiotic therapy
  - Indicated if evidence of periodontal or periapical infection is found
  - Ensure appropriate coverage against anaerobic bacteria.
  - Penicillin G benzathine 40,000-60,000 IU/kg SC q 5 d
  - Trimethoprim-sulfa 30 mg/kg PO q 12 h. *Combine with metronidazole for improved anaerobic coverage.*
  - Enrofloxacin 10-20 mg/kg PO q 12-24 h. *Combine with metronidazole for anaerobic coverage.*
  - Metronidazole 20-30 mg/kg PO q 12 h. *Combine with trimethoprim-sulfa or enrofloxacin for aerobic coverage.*
  - Chloramphenicol 30-50 mg/kg PO q 8 h
- Elodontoma treatment
  - No successful treatment has been reported for elodontoma in degus.
  - Rhinotomy to bypass the obstruction of the nasal cavity has been reported as a treatment option for elodontomas in prairie dogs.
  - Surgical extraction of diseased maxillary incisors might be an option in early stages of the disease. At advanced stages, complete extraction of the maxillary incisors and complete removal of all neoplastic tissue are not feasible.
  - Provide supportive care, including oxygen therapy if necessary, until surgery is considered or euthanasia is elected.
  - Any treatment attempts should be considered palliative.

CHRONIC TREATMENT

- Repeated treatment of cheek teeth and incisor teeth malocclusion, periodontal disease, and caries under general anesthesia. Recheck examination should be performed 2 to 8 weeks after initial examination and treatment, depending on the severity of diagnosed intraoral disease.
- Analgesia: meloxicam 0.3-0.5 mg/kg PO q 12-24 h
- Long-term antibiotic therapy for cases with severe periodontal disease. Consider pulse therapy using penicillin G benzathine 40,000-60,000 IU/kg SC q 5 d.
- Nutritional support: syringe-feed high-fiber diet for herbivores (e.g., Oxbow Critical Care for Herbivores, 50 to 80 mL/kg PO q 24 h, divided into 4 to 5 feedings) or crushed and soaked chinchilla pellets until the animal is eating sufficient amounts unaided
- Periapical abscess treatment
  - Several techniques have been reported in rabbits and are applicable to degus.
  - Consider referral to a specialist if periapical abscess treatment is necessary.
- Tooth extraction (rarely indicated)
  - Technically challenging
  - High risk of iatrogenic trauma
  - Consider referral to a specialist for assessment and possible extractions.

DRUG INTERACTIONS

- Do not administer cephalosporins, penicillins, erythromycin, or clindamycin orally.
- Do not administer meloxicam to dehydrated animals.

POSSIBLE COMPLICATIONS

- Incomplete extraction of elodont teeth may result in regrowth if germinative tissue has not been completely removed during extraction.
- Iatrogenic damage to the teeth, tongue, or buccal mucosa during dental procedures
- Elodontomas
  - Hypoxia and suffocation
  - Hemorrhage and aspiration (including death) during rhinotomy or incisor extraction because a patent airway is difficult to obtain

RECOMMENDED MONITORING

- Food intake
- Fecal output
- Body weight

PROGNOSIS AND OUTCOME

- Good to fair for animal with no secondary complications, and if client is compliant with recommended treatments
- Guarded to poor if animal is in poor body condition or is suffering from systemic disease, or if client is not compliant with recommended treatments
- Poor for animals diagnosed with elodontomas

CONTROVERSY

- A limited intraoral examination can be performed using a pediatric laryngoscope, otoscope, or vaginal speculum in a conscious animal, but up to 50% of intraoral lesions can be missed.
- Do not use nail trimmers to cut incisor teeth.

PEARLS & CONSIDERATIONS

COMMENTS

- Despite sometimes dramatic elongation of reserve and clinical crowns of the cheek teeth, degus often have no difficulty eating and maintain a good body condition until severe changes and complications, such as soft-tissue trauma from sharp dental spurs, or periodontal infection have occurred.
- Congenital dental disease is rare in rodents; most dental disease is acquired.

PREVENTION

- Provision of a diet containing >16% fiber with Ca:P ratio of 2:1. This can be achieved by feeding predominantly high-quality grass hay and hay-based commercial degu or chinchilla pellets. As supplementation, consider offering nontoxic tree branches, herbs, and restricted quantities of dark leafy greens or carrots.
- Do not feed grains, raisins, nuts, seeds, or other treats; they are high-energy and high-phosphorus food items. Feeding these inappropriate food items will contribute to development of acquired dental disease, diabetes mellitus, and gastrointestinal disease.

CLIENT EDUCATION

- Educate owners on the appropriate dietary requirements of degus.
- Owners must be informed that repeated and often lifelong treatment of dental malocclusion and periodontal disease under general anesthesia is required.
- Owners must be informed that treatment of acquired dental disease is usually only palliative.
- No successful treatment has been reported for degus suffering from elodontomas; therefore, the prognosis is poor.

SUGGESTED READINGS

Jekl V, et al: Diseases in pet degus: a retrospective study in 300 animals, J Small Anim Pract 52:107–112, 2011.

Jekl V, et al: Elodontoma in a degu *(Octodon degus)*, J Exot Pet Med 17:216–220, 2008.

Jekl V, et al: Impact of pelleted diets with different mineral composition on the crown size of mandibular cheek teeth and mandibular relative density in degus *(Octodon degus)*, Vet Rec 168:641–646, 2011.

CROSS-REFERENCES TO OTHER SECTIONS

Behavioral Disorders
Diabetes Mellitus
Odontomas (Prairie Dogs)

AUTHOR: **CHRISTOPH MANS**

EDITOR: **THOMAS M. DONNELLY**

SMALL MAMMALS: DEGUS

Diabetes Mellitus

BASIC INFORMATION

DEFINITION

Chronic metabolic disorder caused by hypoinsulinemia, secondary to pancreatic pathology, with consequences of hyperglycemia, glucosuria, and diabetic cataract formation in degus.

SPECIAL SPECIES CONSIDERATIONS

- The natural diet of degus is high in fiber and low in simple carbohydrates.
- Glucose metabolism differs from other mammalian species.
- Lens contains high activity of the enzyme aldose-reductase.

EPIDEMIOLOGY

SPECIES, AGE, SEX Most affected animals are between 6 months and 2.5 years of age by the time clinical signs are noticeable.

GENETICS AND BREED PREDISPOSITION Cataracts have also been reported in wild degus; therefore, a familial predisposition is likely.

RISK FACTORS

- Diet: high-sugar items (fruits, treats), rodent chow containing molasses
- Pregnancy: diabetic females in late gestation are at increased risk for pregnancy toxemia, similar to that described in the guinea-pig.

ASSOCIATED CONDITIONS AND DISORDERS

- Cataracts
- Ketoacidosis
- Secondary infection due to immune suppression
- Decreased wound healing
- Hepatic lipidosis

CLINICAL PRESENTATION

HISTORY, CHIEF COMPLAINT

- Polydipsia
- Polyuria
- Polyphagia
- Decreased body weight
- Lethargy
- Unilateral or bilateral "white eyes" (cataracts)
- Decreased fertility

PHYSICAL EXAM FINDINGS

- Cataract unilateral or bilateral
- Decreased body condition

ETIOLOGY AND PATHOPHYSIOLOGY

- Inappropriate diet containing large quantities of easily digestible carbohydrates is believed to cause hyperinsulinemia initially, subsequently progressing to failure of beta cells of the pancreas and hypoinsulinemia.
- Familial predisposition
- Other causes such as viral (cytomegalovirus) and pancreatic amyloidosis have been proposed but are most likely coincidental findings.
- Lens of degus contain high activity of the enzyme aldose-reductase, which catalyzes the reduction of glucose to sorbitol. Accumulation of sorbitol within the lens results in increased osmolarity in the lens and consequent influx of water, which leads to alteration of lens fibers and subsequent cataract formation.
- Diabetic cataracts in degus are classified as cortical.

DIAGNOSIS

DIFFERENTIAL DIAGNOSIS

- Polydipsia/polyuria: behavioral, excessive mineral salt intake, chronic renal insufficiency, other endocrine disorders
- Hyperglycemia: stress induced, other endocrine disorders
- Glucosuria: stress induced, other endocrine disorders
- Anorexia/weight loss: dental disease, gastrointestinal disease, any systemic disease, pain, stress, neoplasia
- Cataracts: congenital, senile

INITIAL DATABASE

- Blood biochemistry
  - Hyperglycemia (reference range, 128-176 mg/dL [7.1-9.8 mmol/L])
    - A single high blood glucose value is not diagnostic
    - Suspicious if blood glucose >200 mg/dL (>11 mmol/L)
    - Hyperglycemia may only be present in the acute phase of the disease. Some animals will become normoglycemic again
- Urinalysis
  - Glucosuria: may only be present in the acute stage of the disease. Some animals will become normoglycemic again.

TREATMENT

THERAPEUTIC GOALS

- Normoglycemia
- Elimination of clinical signs (cataracts are irreversible)

ACUTE GENERAL TREATMENT

Dependent on clinical signs

- Cataracts but no hyperglycemia and glucosuria: adjust diet
- Hyperglycemia/glucosuria (repeated measurements), no ketoacidosis: adjust diet
- Hyperglycemia/glucosuria (repeated measurements) + ketoacidosis: supportive care, insulin therapy should be considered
  - Insulin therapy
    - Owners should be thoroughly educated about lifelong treatment, costs, daily injections, increased

stress for animal, and questionable long-term success of therapy.
- Repeated blood collection for determination of blood glucose curve will be challenging.
- Initial dose insulin 1 IU/kg SC q 12-24 h may induce hypoglycemia.
- Adjustment of dosing regimen necessary dependent on response to treatment
- Owners should monitor response to treatment at home by testing the urine for glucose with test strips.

CHRONIC TREATMENT

- Dietary adjustments: diet low in simple carbohydrates
  - Hay *ad libitum*; dark leafy greens, vegetables (carrots, beet)
  - Do not offer fruits (high content of fructose).
  - Avoid rodent pellets, which contain molasses (check ingredient list), avoid minimum crude fiber (16%), and avoid low fat. Feed commercial degu or chinchilla pellets.
- If deemed appropriate: insulin therapy

POSSIBLE COMPLICATIONS

Insulin therapy: hypoglycemia

RECOMMENDED MONITORING

Glucose levels in blood and urine

PROGNOSIS AND OUTCOME

- If ketoacidosis: poor
- If no significant weight loss or secondary complications: good to guarded
- Animals with bilateral cataracts will handle blindness well in familiar environment.

PEARLS & CONSIDERATIONS

COMMENTS

- Insulin and glucagon have different molecular structures compared with most other mammals.
- Experimentally, cataracts developed within 4 weeks after degus became diabetic; treatment with Sorbinil (aldose-reductase inhibitor) prevented cataract formation for up to 6 months. Sorbinil currently is not available in most countries.

PREVENTION

- Appropriate diet
- Do not breed animals that have a medical history of diabetes mellitus (suspected inheritability).
- If animals tend to become obese with offered diet, do not feed ad libitum.

CLIENT EDUCATION

Appropriate diet is most important in prevention of diabetes mellitus in degus.

SUGGESTED READINGS

Brown C, et al: Cataracts and reduced fertility in degus *(Octodon degus)*, Lab Anim (NY) 30:25–26, 2000.
Jekl V, et al: Diseases in pet degus: a retrospective study in 300 animals, J Small Anim Pract 52:107–112, 2011.
Najecki D, et al: Husbandry and management of the degu, Lab Anim 28:54–62, 1999.

AUTHOR: **CHRISTOPH MANS**

EDITOR: **THOMAS M. DONNELLY**

SMALL MAMMALS: HEDGEHOGS

Cardiomyopathy

BASIC INFORMATION

DEFINITION

Dilated cardiomyopathy (DCM) is the term given to diseases in African pygmy hedgehogs in which myocardial failure is present for unknown reasons. This form of myocardial dysfunction is characterized by a primary increase in left ventricular end-systolic diameter and volume.

SYNONYMS

Idiopathic primary myocardial failure, congestive cardiomyopathy

SPECIAL SPECIES CONSIDERATIONS

African pygmy hedgehogs are nocturnal and spend much of the daytime sleeping.

EPIDEMIOLOGY

SPECIES, AGE, SEX

- African pygmy hedgehogs *(Atelerix albiventris)*
- Generally present at 3 years or older, although the disease may occur in animals as young as 1 year of age
- Males may be slightly more overrepresented.

GENETICS AND BREED PREDISPOSITION A genetic predisposition has been suggested.

ASSOCIATED CONDITIONS AND DISORDERS Other forms of cardiomyopathy can present with similar clinical signs.

CLINICAL PRESENTATION

HISTORY, CHIEF COMPLAINT

- Sudden death; in acute forms, the animal may die without premonitory signs
- Dyspnea
- Decreased activity
- Reduced food intake
- Weight loss

PHYSICAL EXAM FINDINGS

- Dyspnea/tachypnea (normal respiratory rate: 25-50 bpm)
- Tachycardia (normal heart rate: 180-280 bpm)
- Heart murmur
- Ascites

ETIOLOGY AND PATHOPHYSIOLOGY

- Cause unknown
- DCM is characterized by a primary increase in left ventricular end-systolic diameter and volume, leading to left ventricular dilatation.

DIAGNOSIS

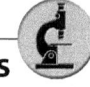

DIFFERENTIAL DIAGNOSIS

- Primary respiratory tract disease, such as pneumonia
- Neoplasia, particular lymphoma

INITIAL DATABASE

- Full-body radiographs (lateral and dorsoventral views); possible findings include the following:
  - Enlargement of the cardiac silhouette
  - Pulmonary edema
  - Pleural effusion
  - Hepatomegaly
  - Ascites
- Biochemistry: usually normal; in severe cases, might reveal prerenal azotemia, hyponatremia, and hypochloremia
- Complete blood count: usually normal

ADVANCED OR CONFIRMATORY TESTING

- Echocardiography is the diagnostic modality of choice for diagnosing DCM. Possible findings include the following:
  - Thin ventricular walls
  - Enlarged left ventricular end-systolic and end-diastolic dimensions
  - Left atrial enlargement
  - Reduced fractional shortening
- Unfortunately, many cases are diagnosed or confirmed only at necropsy.

TREATMENT

THERAPEUTIC GOALS

- Alleviate respiratory distress.
- Improve cardiac function (only short term).
- Minimize length of hospitalization.

ACUTE GENERAL TREATMENT

- Provide oxygen supplementation if dyspneic.
- Minimize handling and stress.
- Diuretics such as injectable furosemide are most useful initially in hospitalized patients. Oral furosemide should be considered for outpatients.
  - Furosemide 1-8 mg/kg PO, IM, SC q 8-12 h

CHRONIC TREATMENT

- Enalapril 0.5 mg/kg PO q 24 h
- Furosemide 1-2 mg/kg PO q 8-12 h for long-term therapy

DRUG INTERACTIONS

The combination of an angiotensin-converting enzyme (ACE) blocker (e.g., enalapril) and furosemide might result in azotemia, particularly in patients with concurrent renal dysfunction.

POSSIBLE COMPLICATIONS

- Vascular thromboembolism
- Renal tubular necrosis/ interstitial nephritis
- Hepatic lipidosis
- Iatrogenic dehydration from furosemide administration

RECOMMENDED MONITORING

- Body weight
- Respiratory rate and character
- Appetite

PROGNOSIS AND OUTCOME

Long-term prognosis is poor.

PEARLS & CONSIDERATIONS

COMMENTS

Hedgehogs, like many other exotic animals, will often hide signs of illness. Diligent monitoring of these animals is paramount for early detection of systemic disease.

SUGGESTED READING

Black PA, et al: Cardiac assessment of African hedgehogs *(Atelerix albiventris)*, J Zoo Wildl Med 42:49–53, 2011.

Raymond JT, et al: Cardiomyopathy in captive African hedgehogs *(Atelerix albiventris)*, J Vet Diagn Invest 12:468–472, 2000.

AUTHOR: **JAIME CHIN**

EDITOR: **CHRISTOPH MANS**

SMALL MAMMALS: HEDGEHOGS

Neoplasia

BASIC INFORMATION

DEFINITION

Transformation of normal body cells into malignant ones; can result in abnormal growths or infiltration of body organs, in which cell multiplication is uncontrolled and progressive.

SYNONYMS

Cancer, malignancy, tumors

SPECIAL SPECIES CONSIDERATIONS

Neoplasia is common in African pygmy hedgehogs; a wide variety of tumors and disseminated neoplastic processes affecting different body systems have been reported. Most tumors in African pygmy hedgehogs are malignant. Some hedgehogs present with more than one neoplasm.

EPIDEMIOLOGY

SPECIES, AGE, SEX African pygmy hedgehogs *(Atelerix albiventris)*. No gender predilection is known. One study showed that median age at the time of tumor diagnosis was 3.5 years (range, 2 to 5.5 years), although neoplasia has been reported in hedgehogs at 1 month of age. Retrospective studies in hedgehogs at necropsy have shown the prevalence of neoplasia to range from 29% to 52%.

RISK FACTORS Certain types of sarcomas and lymphoma in hedgehogs may be associated with retroviral infection.

ASSOCIATED CONDITIONS AND DISORDERS Hepatic lipidosis, renal infarction

CLINICAL PRESENTATION

DISEASE FORMS/SUBTYPES

- Integumentary
  - Cutaneous hemangiosarcoma, cutaneous histiocytic sarcoma, malignant cutaneous plasmacytoma, mast cell tumors
  - Mammary gland adenocarcinoma (common), mammary gland papillary carcinoma
- Hemolymphatic
  - Lymphosarcoma (common), myelogenous leukemia
- Digestive system
  - Oral squamous cell carcinoma (common), oral fibrosarcoma, gastric adenocarcinoma, pancreatic exocrine carcinoma, metastatic hepatocellular carcinoma
- Endocrine system
  - Adrenal cortical carcinoma, thyroid adenocarcinoma, islet cell tumor, pituitary adenoma, malignant neuroendocrine tumor
- Reproductive system
  - Uterine adenocarcinoma (common) and leiomyosarcoma
- Other reported neoplasms
  - Peripheral nerve sheath tumor, astrocytoma, neurofibroma, neurofibrosarcoma, schwannoma, osteosarcoma, fibrosarcoma, hemangioma

HISTORY, CHIEF COMPLAINT

- Chronic weight loss
- Anorexia
- Lethargy
- Diarrhea
- Dyspnea
- Distended abdomen
- Abnormal growths

PHYSICAL EXAM FINDINGS

- Presence of swellings and/or solitary or masses
- Emaciation
- Abdominal distention
- Loss of dentition and/or ptyalism (oral squamous cell carcinoma)
- Hind limb ataxia (adrenal cortical carcinoma)

ETIOLOGY AND PATHOPHYSIOLOGY

Possible causes include increased lifespan in captivity, genetic disorders, and retroviral infections.

DIAGNOSIS

DIFFERENTIAL DIAGNOSIS

- Wobbly hedgehog syndrome (see Wobbly Hedgehog Syndrome)
- Hepatic lipidosis
- Salivation/oral abnormalities: periodontitis, tooth abscesses, fractured teeth, oropharyngeal foreign body
- Abdominal distention/masses: intestinal foreign body/obstruction
- Diarrhea: gastroenteritis
- Dyspnea: pneumonia, congestive heart failure (see Cardiomyopathy)
- Congestive heart failure (in cases with dyspnea/ascites)

INITIAL DATABASE

- Fine-needle aspiration (including that of regional lymph nodes)
- Complete blood count: anemia, leukemia, cytologic abnormalities in leukocytes may be seen
- Serum biochemistry: changes depend on underlying neoplasm and secondary complications; hypercalcemia and hyperbilirubinemia are common findings
- Urinalysis
- Thoracic and abdominal radiography to assess for the following:
  - Metastatic disease
  - Heart and/or lung disease in cases presented for dyspnea

ADVANCED OR CONFIRMATORY TESTING

- Abdominal ultrasonography and ultrasound-guided fine-needle aspiration for intraabdominal masses, enlarged liver, and/or mesenteric lymph nodes
- Biopsy and histopathologic examination of masses and growths (incisional/excisional)
- Bone marrow aspiration should be performed for diagnosis of hematopoietic neoplasms and staging of other neoplasms.
- Advanced imaging: CT and MRI should be considered, but interpretation might be complicated because of the small size of the patient.
- Definitive diagnosis is often made only at necropsy.

TREATMENT

THERAPEUTIC GOALS

Palliative care in many cases

ACUTE GENERAL TREATMENT

- Surgical excision is considered the standard of care.
- Excision with wide margins combined with ovariohysterectomy is recommended in hedgehogs with mammary tumors.
- Analgesia if indicated
  - Buprenorphine 0.01-0.05 mg/kg SC, IM q 8-12 h
  - Butorphanol 0.2-0.4 mg/kg SC, IM q 6-8 h
  - Meloxicam 0.2 mg/kg SC, PO q 24 h
- Supportive care and nutritional support if indicated

CHRONIC TREATMENT

Currently, no effective chemotherapy protocols have been reported for African pygmy hedgehogs.

DRUG INTERACTIONS

Because renal disorders have a high prevalence in African pygmy hedgehogs, appropriate renal function and hydration should be confirmed before nonsteroidal antiinflammatory drugs are prescribed.

PROGNOSIS AND OUTCOME

- Prognosis depends on the type of tumor diagnosed.
- Oral squamous cell carcinomas and mammary carcinomas tend to be highly locally invasive and warrant a poor prognosis.
- In some cases, complete surgical excision of a tumor may result in remission.
- Up to 85% of hedgehog neoplasms are malignant—these carry a poor prognosis.

PEARLS & CONSIDERATIONS

COMMENTS

Neoplasia appears to be very common in the aged African pygmy hedgehog. Life span in captivity ranges from 3 to 8 years. Hedgehogs older than 2 years should be considered geriatric. Early detection of disease will enable optimal treatment, potentially improving the long-term prognosis in affected animals.

CLIENT EDUCATION

Annual wellness checks are recommended for hedgehogs beginning at 1 year of age. Semiannual physical examinations are recommended for hedgehogs over 2 years of age.

SUGGESTED READINGS

Heatley JJ, et al: A review of neoplasia in the captive African hedgehog *(Atelerix albiventris)*, Semin Avian Exot Pet Med 14:182–192, 2005.

Juan-Salles C, et al: Cytologic diagnosis of diseases of hedgehogs, Vet Clin North Am Exot Anim Pract 10:51–59, 2007.

Raymond JT, et al: Spontaneous tumors in captive African hedgehogs *(Atelerix albiventris)*: a retrospective study, J Comp Pathol 124:128–133, 2001.

CROSS-REFERENCES TO OTHER SECTIONS

Cardiomyopathy
Wobbly Hedgehog Syndrome

AUTHOR: **JAIME CHIN**

EDITOR: **CHRISTOPH MANS**

SMALL MAMMALS: HEDGEHOGS

Skin Diseases—Infectious

BASIC INFORMATION

DEFINITION

Any condition affecting the integument of African pygmy hedgehogs and resulting from infectious agents such as ectoparasites, fungi, or bacteria

EPIDEMIOLOGY

SPECIES, AGE, SEX African pygmy hedgehogs *(Atletrix albiventris)* of all species, both genders, and any age can be affected.

RISK FACTORS Overcrowding, poor hygiene, poor husbandry leading to malnutrition, inappropriate substrate, housing in close proximity to other species of animals

CONTAGION AND ZOONOSIS

- Dermatophytes are potentially zoonotic.

- One report of notoedric mange due to *Notoedres cati* in the African pygmy hedgehog

ASSOCIATED CONDITIONS AND DISORDERS Secondary bacterial dermatitis, allergic dermatitis

CLINICAL PRESENTATION

PHYSICAL EXAM FINDINGS

- Seborrhea
- Quill loss
- White or brownish crusts at the base of quills, around face and eyes
- Flaking of skin

ETIOLOGY AND PATHOPHYSIOLOGY

- Acariasis: Chorioptic and Notoedric mange have been reported.
- Fungal infection
  - Dermatophytosis is rare in African pygmy hedgehogs compared with infection of European hedgehogs *(Erinaceus europaeus)* by *Trichophyton mentagrophytes* var. *erinacei*. Infrequent cases are described in African pygmy hedgehogs in Japan with *T. mentagrophytes* var. *erinacei*.
  - Dermatomycosis caused by *Paecilomyces variotii* is described in one case in Korea.
- Fleas, ticks, and lice have been reported in wild caught African pygmy hedgehogs.

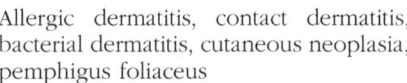

DIAGNOSIS

DIFFERENTIAL DIAGNOSIS

Allergic dermatitis, contact dermatitis, bacterial dermatitis, cutaneous neoplasia, pemphigus foliaceus

INITIAL DATABASE

- Obtain samples of loose quills and skin flakes for identification of mites under light microscopy
- Dermatophyte culture

ADVANCED OR CONFIRMATORY TESTING

- Skin scrapings (usually under sedation or general anesthesia, especially for obtaining samples from around the face)
- Aerobic bacterial culture
- Skin biopsy

TREATMENT

THERAPEUTIC GOALS

- Relieve pruritus and reduce environmental contamination.
- Resolution of parasitic, fungal, or bacterial infections.

ACUTE GENERAL TREATMENT

- Acariasis
  - Ivermectin 0.2-0.4 mg/kg SC, PO q 10-14 d
  - Selamectin 6-10 mg/kg topical q 21-28 d
  - Application of 1% permethrin may also be effective.
- Dermatophytosis
  - Terbinafine 10-30 mg/kg PO q 24 h
  - Itraconazole 5-10 mg/kg PO q 12-24 h
  - Shampoos and sprays containing enilconazole (0.2%) or miconazole may be used as adjunctive topical therapy.
  - Monitor response to antifungal treatment by weekly dermatophyte cultures. Discontinue treatment once two consecutive negative cultures are obtained.
- Dermatomycosis: Itraconazole 5-10 mg/kg PO q 12-24 h
- Fleas/Ticks
  - Fipronil spray, 1 pump/hedgehog
  - Selamectin 6-10 mg/kg topical
- Bacterial infection
  - Cephalexin 30 mg/kg PO q 12 h
  - Amoxicillin/clavulanic acid 15 mg/kg PO q 12 h
  - Trimethoprim-sulfa 30 mg/kg PO q 12 h
  - Enrofloxacin 5-10 mg/kg PO q 12-24 h

POSSIBLE COMPLICATIONS

Clinical signs may recur if concomitant environment decontamination is not achieved.

PROGNOSIS AND OUTCOME

Prognosis is usually very good with appropriate therapy and owner compliance.

PEARLS & CONSIDERATIONS

PREVENTION

- Regular application of topical products can be effective in preventing flea/tick infestations.
- Ensure regular changing of substrate/bedding and cleaning of cages.

CLIENT EDUCATION

Dermatophytes are potentially zoonotic.

SUGGESTED READINGS

Heatly JJ: Chapter 16, Hedgehogs. In Mitchell M, et al, editors: Manual of exotic pet practice, Philadelphia, 2008, Saunders, pp 433–455.

Ivy E, et al: African hedgehogs. In Carpenter JW, et al, editors: Ferrets, rabbits and rodents: clinical medicine and surgery, ed 3, St Louis, 2012, WB Saunders, pp 411–427.

AUTHOR: **JAIME CHIN**

EDITOR: **CHRISTOPH MANS**

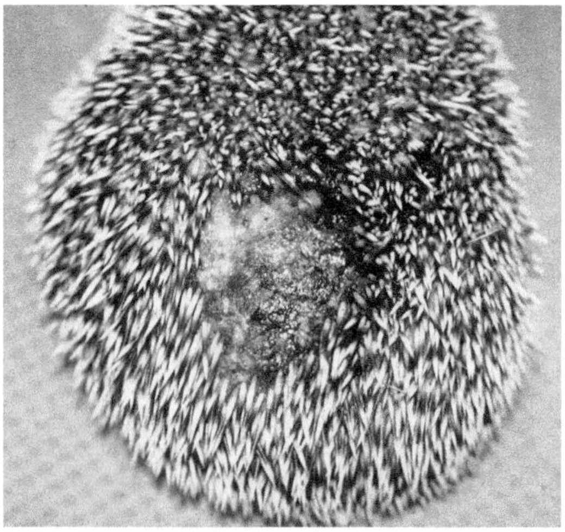

Skin Diseases Dorsal view of an African pygmy hedgehog with quill loss and severe erythematous and edematous skin. The primary differential diagnoses were fungal and/or bacterial infection. The actual diagnosis was cutaneous T-cell lymphoma (mycosis fungoides). Cutaneous neoplasms can mimic infectious skin diseases and neoplasia must always be considered a differential diagnosis until ruled out.

SMALL MAMMALS: HEDGEHOGS

Wobbly Hedgehog Syndrome

Client Education Sheet Available on Website

BASIC INFORMATION

DEFINITION

Wobbly hedgehog syndrome (WHS) is a fatal neurodegenerative disease affecting the brain and spinal cord, resulting in progressive paralysis and other neurologic deficits in African pygmy hedgehogs.

SYNONYMS

Degenerative myelopathy, spongiform leukoencephalopathy

SPECIAL SPECIES CONSIDERATIONS

WHS is predominantly reported in African pygmy hedgehogs (*Atelerix* spp.), but a similar syndrome has been reported in European hedgehogs (*Erinaceus europaeus*).

EPIDEMIOLOGY

SPECIES, AGE, SEX

- African hedgehogs (*Atelerix albiventris*) and Algerian hedgehogs (*Atelerix algirus*) are affected.
- Most animals that show clinical signs of WHS are younger than 2 years of age, but WHS can occur at any age.
- No gender bias is evident.

GENETICS AND BREED PREDISPOSITION Familial tendency toward the disease has been suggested in African hedgehogs.

RISK FACTORS Up to 10% of captive African hedgehogs in the United States appear to be affected by WHS.

CONTAGION AND ZOONOSIS Currently unknown

ASSOCIATED CONDITIONS AND DISORDERS

- Self-mutilation
- Abrasions on the dorsal aspect of the feet caused by paresis

CLINICAL PRESENTATION

HISTORY, CHIEF COMPLAINT

- Inability to close the hood (contraction of the circular orbicularis panniculi muscle, which extends along the sides and across the neck and rump, allows the formation of a muscular pouch into which the head, body, and legs can be brought)
- Incoordination, falling to one side, tripping, wobbling
- Seizures
- Weight loss
- Dysphagia

PHYSICAL EXAM FINDINGS

- Ataxia
- Ascending paralysis/paresis of the limbs that progresses to tetraparesis
- Generalized weakness
- Emaciation
- Muscle atrophy
- Seizures
- Scoliosis
- Unilateral exophthalmos

ETIOLOGY AND PATHOPHYSIOLOGY

- The cause of WHS remains unknown.
- WHS is a progressive neurodegenerative disease. Neurodegeneration results from spongiform changes in the white matter of the brain and spinal cord.
- Demyelination, axon degeneration, and occasional neuronal necrosis are also seen.

DIAGNOSIS

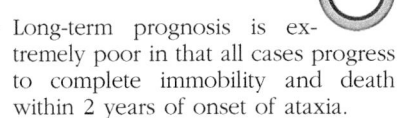

DIFFERENTIAL DIAGNOSIS

- Brain tumors
- Intervertebral disc disease
- Hepatic encephalopathy
- Infectious CNS disease (uncommon; e.g., canine distemper virus, *Baylisascaris procyonis*, rabies)

INITIAL DATABASE

- Antemortem diagnosis can only be presumptive based on appropriate clinical signs.
- Definitive diagnosis can be made only by postmortem examination.

ADVANCED OR CONFIRMATORY TESTING

The primary histologic lesion in hedgehogs with WHS is vacuolization of the white matter tracts of the cerebrum, cerebellum, and brainstem. The lesion also occurs in the white matter tracts throughout the spinal cord. Inflammation of the brain and spinal cord is NOT a feature of WHS.

TREATMENT

THERAPEUTIC GOALS

- Provide palliative care only.
- No treatment has been shown to stop the progression of neurologic deficits.

ACUTE GENERAL TREATMENT

- Supportive care (e.g., assisted feeding) is paramount.
- Antibiotics may be indicated to treat any concurrent infection (e.g., skin infection):
  - Cephalexin 30 mg/kg PO q 12 h
  - Amoxicillin/clavulanic acid 15 mg/kg PO q 12 h
- Removal of obstacles, exercise wheels from the enclosure to prevent injury

CHRONIC TREATMENT

Almost all hedgehogs in advanced stages of WHS require assisted feeding. A liquid diet (e.g., Oxbow Carnivore Care) is preferred and can be offered in bowls or by syringe.

POSSIBLE COMPLICATIONS

- Self-trauma
- Choking

RECOMMENDED MONITORING

- Progression of neurologic deficits
- Quality of life

PROGNOSIS AND OUTCOME

- Long-term prognosis is extremely poor in that all cases progress to complete immobility and death within 2 years of onset of ataxia.
- Many hedgehogs can maintain a reasonable quality of life with good supportive care in the initial stages of the disease.

PEARLS & CONSIDERATIONS

COMMENTS

- A variety of empirical treatments have been reported, including vitamin supplementation, antiinflammatory drugs, homeopathy, acupuncture, and physical therapy. None of the reported treatments is successful in stopping the progression of neurologic deficits.
- In early stages, the clinical signs of WHS can be remittent and relapsing, and the progression of WHS can be variable. Therefore, if empirical treatment is attempted, intermittent improvement in clinical signs should not be confused with a response to initiated treatment.

CLIENT EDUCATION

Because of a potential hereditary component, clients should avoid breeding from affected individuals or those from the same family lineage.

SUGGESTED READINGS

Graesser D, et al: Wobbly hedgehog syndrome in African pygmy hedgehogs, J Exot Pet Med 15:59–65, 2006.

Heatley JJ: Hedgehogs. In Tully T, et al, editors: Manual of exotic pet practice, St Louis, 2009, Saunders, pp 433–455.

AUTHOR: **JAIME CHIN**

EDITOR: **CHRISTOPH MANS**

SMALL MAMMALS: SUGAR GLIDERS

Behavioral Disorders

BASIC INFORMATION

DEFINITION

Any of a variety of behavioral abnormalities that manifest as a result of stress and/or improper husbandry

SYNONYM

Self mutilation syndrome

SPECIAL SPECIES CONSIDERATIONS

- Sugar gliders are highly gregarious, nocturnal, and arboreal animals.
- In the wild, sugar gliders typically live in colonies of 6 to 10 animals.
- Sugar gliders are territorial; aggression is common when new animals are introduced to established colonies.
- Sugar gliders are a laboratory model for serotonin deficiency depression, which is induced by housing animals alone.

EPIDEMIOLOGY

RISK FACTORS Solitary housing, inadequate socialization, improper husbandry

ASSOCIATED CONDITIONS AND DISORDERS Animals may also suffer from nutritional diseases owing to improper husbandry and diet.

CLINICAL PRESENTATION

DISEASE FORMS/SUBTYPES Animals may present with abnormalities ranging from aggression toward owners to self-mutilation and a variety of other aberrant behaviors.

HISTORY, CHIEF COMPLAINT

- History may include improper husbandry, poor socialization, and/or solitary housing.
- Animals may present with wounds or self-mutilation, hair loss, aggression toward owners.
- Coprophagy, polyphagia, polydipsia, and/or pacing might also be reported.

PHYSICAL EXAM FINDINGS

- Alopecia
- Wounds on the tail, limbs, scrotum, and/or penis

ETIOLOGY AND PATHOPHYSIOLOGY

- Increased adrenal activity or fur-pulling during stress may result in alopecia.
- Sexual frustration in pubescent males may play a role in self-mutilation of genitals.
- Aggression toward owners may be part of normal social behavior or a result of improper socialization.
- Housing animals alone or sudden changes in social structure may induce stress-related behaviors.

DIAGNOSIS

DIFFERENTIAL DIAGNOSIS

- Alopecia
    - Dermatitis (bacterial, fungal, parasitic)
- Skin wounds
    - Trauma from cagemates or environment
- Skin wounds caused by self-mutilation due to other underlying causes:
    - Pain from recent surgical procedure, traumatic injury, or urogenital disease
    - Neoplasia
    - Aberrant migration of a duodenal nematode (rare)

INITIAL DATABASE

- Thorough history, including husbandry practices, most important for diagnosis
- Complete physical examination
- Dermatologic evaluation
    - Skin cytologic examination and fungal and/or bacterial cultures if indicated for alopecia or skin wounds
- Consider radiographs, complete blood count, blood biochemistry, urinalysis, and fecal parasite analysis if suspicious for underlying disease process.

ADVANCED OR CONFIRMATORY TESTING

Biopsy and histopathologic examination if wounds are chronic or nonhealing, or if neoplasia is suspected

TREATMENT

THERAPEUTIC GOALS

- Decrease or end abnormal behavior.
- Resolve secondary wounds and/or alopecia.

ACUTE GENERAL TREATMENT

- Appropriate wound care, analgesics, and systemic antibiotics if indicated
    - Analgesics
        - Buprenorphine 0.01-0.03 mg/kg SC, IM, PO q 8-12 h
        - Butorphanol 0.1-0.5 mg/kg SC, PO q 6-8 h
        - Meloxicam 0.1-0.2 mg/kg SC, PO q 24 h
    - Antibiotics
        - Amoxicillin/clavulanic acid: 12.5 mg/kg PO q 12 h
        - Enrofloxacin 2.5-5 mg/kg PO, SC, IM q 12 h (dilute 1:1 with saline for parenteral injection; may cause tissue necrosis)
        - Trimethoprim/sulfamethoxazole 15 mg/kg PO q 12 h
        - Or other appropriate antibiotic based on culture and sensitivity
- Address underlying social stress and husbandry issues:
    - Provide socialization and environmental enrichment.
    - Correct dietary imbalances.
    - Provide foraging opportunities.
- Castration of intact males with scrotal injury
- E-collar may be necessary for cases of self-mutilation.
- Some animals may benefit from behavior-modifying drugs while husbandry issues are addressed. All doses are anecdotal.
    - Fluoxetine 1-5 mg/kg PO q 12 h
        - Start with lower dose and increase if needed.
    - Haloperidol 0.15 mg/kg PO q 24 h
        - Haloperidol may cause sedation and/or extrapyramidal effects (ataxia, weakness or rigidity, restlessness).

CHRONIC TREATMENT

- Husbandry changes must be maintained.
- Behavior-modifying drugs may have to be continued for months and be gradually tapered.

DRUG INTERACTIONS

Fluoxetine may increase extrapyramidal side effects of haloperidol. It is not recommended to use both drugs concurrently as initial treatment for self-mutilation.

POSSIBLE COMPLICATIONS

Wounds from self-mutilation can be extensive and potentially fatal.

PROGNOSIS AND OUTCOME

Good for some cases if husbandry changes are made, but guarded in cases of recurrent or prolonged self-mutilation

PEARLS & CONSIDERATIONS

COMMENTS

Sugar gliders are a communal species and should not be housed alone.

PREVENTION

- Do not keep sugar gliders housed alone.
- Reduce stress through appropriate husbandry and socialization.

CLIENT EDUCATION

- Housing in groups of at least 2 animals is recommended, although introduction of new animals into established groups may result in aggression.
- Cages should be of adequate size and height (minimum 36 × 24 × 36 inches, but larger preferred) and should contain areas for climbing and foraging.
- Animals should be socialized for at least 2 hours per day (especially if housed in smaller groups or singly), preferably at night when animals are typically active.

SUGGESTED READINGS

Association of Sugar Glider Veterinarians: Veterinarian Care Guide: Stress-related disorders and self-mutilation, 2011; Web-based care guide. http://www.asgv.org/interactive-care-guide/#diseases

Jones IH, et al: Towards a sociobiological model of depression. A marsupial model *(Petaurus breviceps),* Br J Psychiatry 166: 475–479, 1995.

Sobie JL: Sugar gliders. In Tynes VV, editor: Behavior of exotic pets, Ames, IA, 2010, Wiley-Blackwell, pp 181–189.

AUTHOR: **KIMBERLEE B. WOJCICK**

EDITOR: **CHRISTOPH MANS**

SMALL MAMMALS: SUGAR GLIDERS

Nutritional Disorders

BASIC INFORMATION

DEFINITION

Any of a variety of disorders caused by dietary imbalances and deficiencies

SYNONYMS

Nutritional osteodystrophy, metabolic bone disease, nutritional secondary hyperparathyroidism

SPECIAL SPECIES CONSIDERATIONS

- Sugar gliders are omnivorous with a natural diet consisting of plant exudates (sap, gum, nectar, manna, honeydew), pollen, and insects/arachnids.
- The natural diet will vary by season, with insect and arachnid prey forming a larger portion of the diet during spring and summer.
- Enlarged lower incisors aid in chewing bark, and modified fourth digits aid in extraction of insects.
- Sugar gliders have an enlarged cecum that is likely responsible for digestion of complex carbohydrates.

EPIDEMIOLOGY

RISK FACTORS Diets high in lean meat, insects, and fruit

ASSOCIATED CONDITIONS AND DISORDERS Cardiac, hepatic, and pancreatic disease may be associated with obesity. Anemia, hypoproteinemia, and renal and/or hepatic dysfunction may be seen in severely malnourished animals.

CLINICAL PRESENTATION

DISEASE FORMS/SUBTYPES Animals may present with abnormalities ranging from obesity and periodontal disease to severe malnutrition and signs of nutritional osteodystrophy.

HISTORY, CHIEF COMPLAINT

- Dietary deficiencies: increased quantities of fruit, lean meat, and insects, or feeding of inappropriate diet items such as processed human foods (cereals, items high in sugar)
- Weakness, lethargy, acute collapse, seizures, and/or hind limb paresis/paralysis
- Periodontal disease and obesity are often recognized during routine examination, but owners rarely present their pets for these disorders because they do not recognize them as problems.

PHYSICAL EXAM FINDINGS

- A range of findings may be noted depending on the severity of the dietary imbalance:
  - Obesity or thin body condition
  - Weakness/lethargy/debilitation
  - Seizures
  - Hind limb paresis or paralysis
  - Dehydration
  - Pale mucous membranes
  - Long bone fractures
  - Periodontal disease
  - Corneal opacities or cataracts

ETIOLOGY AND PATHOPHYSIOLOGY

- Obesity may result from a diet too high in fat or protein and can lead to cardiac, hepatic, and pancreatic disease.
- Hypoglycemia resulting from malnutrition and/or anorexia may present with seizures.
- Hypocalcemia resulting from dietary imbalances of calcium, phosphorus, and vitamin D may lead to osteoporosis and pathologic fractures, seizures, and/or hind limb paresis/paralysis.
- Inadequate intake of protein may result in anemia and hypoproteinemia, leading to weakness and general debilitation with poor body condition and pale mucous membranes.
- Corneal lipid deposits or cataracts may develop in juvenile animals if the mother was fed a diet too high in fat.
- Periodontal disease and dental calculus can form secondary to soft diets high in carbohydrates.

DIAGNOSIS

DIFFERENTIAL DIAGNOSIS

- Pathologic fracture
  - Traumatic fracture

- Hind limb paresis/paralysis
  - Spinal trauma
  - Hind limb or pelvic fracture (pathologic or traumatic)
  - Other spinal cord diseases (degenerative, neoplastic, vascular, inflammatory)
- Seizures
  - Cranial trauma (most common)
  - Parasitic CNS disease (toxoplasmosis, *Baylisascaris* larval migration)
  - Disseminated fungal disease (e.g., cryptococcosis)
  - Bacterial meningitis
  - Intoxication (e.g., lead)
  - Neoplasia
- Corneal opacities
  - Ulceration with edema
  - Scarring from previous trauma
- Cataracts
  - Vitamin A deficiency
  - Maternal pouch infection

INITIAL DATABASE

- Thorough history, including detailed diet composition, is important for diagnosis:
  - Blood biochemistry profile, including ionized calcium: hypoproteinemia, hypocalcemia, and hypoglycemia are commonly noted
  - Complete blood count: Anemia
  - Whole-body two-view radiographs: decreased density of long bones, pelvis, and vertebrae ± pathologic fracture may be noted

ADVANCED OR CONFIRMATORY TESTING

Advanced imaging (myelography, CT, or MRI) and/or CSF analysis may be helpful in cases with neurologic signs wherein a nutritional cause cannot be determined; however, such tests will be technically challenging and interpretation may be limited owing to patient size.

TREATMENT

THERAPEUTIC GOALS

- Correct underlying dietary deficiencies and restore normal calcium, phosphorus, and vitamin D homeostasis.
- Provide acute management of seizures and general debilitation while dietary causes are corrected.
- Allow healing of pathologic fractures and return of normal bone density.
- Promote weight loss for animals with obese body condition.
- Correct dental disease and prevent recurrence with dietary modifications.

ACUTE GENERAL TREATMENT

- Provide supportive care, including nutritional and fluid support:
  - Fluids may be administered subcutaneously; consider the intraosseous route in severely debilitated animals.
- Correct hypoglycemia if present.
- Correct hypocalcemia if present:
  - Calcium glubionate 150 mg/kg PO q 24 h
  - Calcium gluconate 100 mg/kg SC or IM q 12 h × 3-5 d (dilute in saline to 10 mg/mL). Initial doses may be administered IV or IO in animals with seizures or severe debilitation—administer slowly and monitor for bradycardia.
- Administer anticonvulsants if seizures are prolonged and/or are not controlled with correction of hypocalcemia and hypoglycemia.
  - Diazepam 0.5-2.0 mg/kg IV, IN, IM or midazolam 0.5-1 mg/kg IN, SC, IM
- Dental scaling and polishing ± extractions for animals with periodontal disease under general anesthesia. Extraction of mandibular incisors may result in fracture of the mandibular symphysis.
- Calcitonin 50-100 IU/kg SC has been recommended for animals severely affected by nutritional osteodystrophy. It decreases calcium resorption from bone. Use only when blood calcium level is within normal range and in conjunction with an oral calcium supplement, to avoid hypocalcemia.

CHRONIC TREATMENT

- Dietary changes must be maintained.
- Cage rest and oral calcium supplementation are continued until pathologic fractures heal and bone density is improved.

RECOMMENDED MONITORING

- Regular monitoring of body weight
- Serial blood biochemical analyses and radiographs are recommended to monitor resolution of clinical pathologic abnormalities, healing of fractures, and return of normal bone density.

PROGNOSIS AND OUTCOME

- Prognosis is good with supportive care and dietary correction if animals have not yet reached a stage of severe debilitation.
- Vertebral fractures may result in permanent neurologic deficits.

CONTROVERSY

The ideal diet for captive sugar gliders is unknown; many dietary variations can be adequate to maintain good health.

PEARLS & CONSIDERATIONS

COMMENTS

Diseases caused by inadequate or inappropriate nutrition are common in captive sugar gliders but can be easily prevented through client education.

PREVENTION

An appropriate diet with adequate amounts of protein and calcium is essential.

CLIENT EDUCATION

- Sugar gliders are omnivores that require a specialized diet. Several options are available to meet dietary requirements.
  - Diet example #1
    - 50% commercial insectivore or carnivore pelleted diet, 50% Leadbeater's mixture (150 mL water, 150 mL honey, one shelled hard-boiled egg, 25 g high-protein baby cereal, 1 teaspoon vitamin and calcium supplement). Use small quantities of lean meat, diced fruit, or gut-loaded insects as treat items (<5% of total diet).
  - Diet example #2
    - 5 g dry or 10 g semi-moist cat food, 5 g berries, 5 g citrus, 5 g other fruit, 5 g sweet potato, 1 g mealworm or other invertebrate prey
  - Diet example #3
    - 75% commercial sugar glider pelleted diet, 25% fresh fruits and vegetables, vitamin and calcium supplement, small quantities of treat items (<5% of total diet)
- Requirements for protein and calcium may be higher in growing or reproductively active animals. In these animals, the pelleted/commercial portion of the diet should be increased.

SUGGESTED READINGS

Association of Sugar Glider Veterinarians: www.asgv.org.

Dierenfeld ES: Feeding behavior and nutrition of the sugar glider *(Petaurus breviceps)*, Vet Clin Exot Anim 12:209–215, 2009.

Dierenfeld ES, et al: Comparison of commonly used diets on intake, digestion, growth, and health in captive sugar gliders *(Petaurus breviceps)*, J Exot Pet Med 15:218–224, 2006.

AUTHOR: **KIMBERLEE B. WOJICK**

EDITOR: **CHRISTOPH MANS**

RABBITS

Abscesses

Client Education Sheet Available on Website

BASIC INFORMATION

DEFINITION

Localized collections of pus in a cavity formed by tissue disintegration. Most abscesses in rabbits are formed after a bacterial insult.

SPECIAL SPECIES CONSIDERATIONS

In rabbits, abscesses are often encased in a fibrous capsule and contain thick caseous pus. They do not respond to traditional drainage methods used in cats and dogs.

EPIDEMIOLOGY

SPECIES, AGE, SEX Abscesses are diagnosed in all breeds, genders, and ages.

RISK FACTORS

- Dental disease (see Dental Disease)
- Multi-rabbit housing that leads to fight wounds (especially nonneutered hutch mates)
- Wire cages that lead to penetrating wounds and pododermatitis (see Pododermatitis)
- Skin wounds (see Dermatopathies)

ASSOCIATED CONDITIONS AND DISORDERS Some rabbit abscesses, especially those associated with the teeth, can result in inappetence and gastrointestinal stasis. In these cases, supportive treatment must be provided before the abscess is surgically treated.

CLINICAL PRESENTATION

DISEASE FORMS/SUBTYPES Abscesses in rabbits can present in many forms. The effect of the abscess(es) will depend on the location and the organs affected. Common presentations include the following:

- Dental disease–associated abscess, often presenting as a facial abscess
- Hepatic abscess (see Hepatic Disorders)
- Pulmonary abscess
- Reproductive tract abscess
- Subcutaneous abscess (see Cutaneous Masses)
- Retrobulbar abscess

HISTORY, CHIEF COMPLAINT

- Unlike in cats and dogs, pain, lethargy, and pyrexia are rarely associated with abscesses in the rabbit.
- Rabbits may present in apparent good health, particularly those with subcutaneous abscessation that may present as a slow-growing hard lump or soft swelling. These abscesses can be single or multiple.
- Internal or pulmonary abscesses may result in lethargy and inappetence or organ-specific disease.
- Dental abscesses may present with inappetence and drooling.
- Retrobulbar abscessation may present with exophthalmos and may be associated with dental disease.
- Occasionally, abscesses may burst and extrude caseous and/or odorous material.

PHYSICAL EXAM FINDINGS

- Subcutaneous abscesses can present as a firm or soft, slow-growing mass anywhere on the body. They can be single or multiple. Skin necrosis may be seen over the abscess.
- Facial abscesses are often the result of dental disease; an underlying bony mass can sometimes be palpated on the mandible or skull.
- Retrobulbar abscesses are often the result of a dental disease–associated abscessation in the maxillary premolars or molars.
- An internal abscess (hepatic, pulmonary, uterine [see Uterine Disorders]) can present as ill thrift, lethargy, respiratory distress, or gastrointestinal stasis.

ETIOLOGY AND PATHOPHYSIOLOGY

- Rabbit neutrophils possess little lysozyme activity. Lysozymes break down bacterial cell walls and liquefy necrotic tissue. With reduced lysozyme activity, rabbit pus remains caseated and does not drain well. The abscess often becomes encased in a fibrous capsule that minimizes antibiotic penetration.
- Bacterial content of rabbit abscesses is often a mixed infection, including both aerobic and anaerobic species (e.g., *Pasteurella multocida* [see Pasteurellosis], *Staphylococcus aureus* [see Staphylococcosis], *Pseudomonas* spp., *Bacteroides* spp., *Proteus* spp., and *Fusobacterium necrophorum*).

DIAGNOSIS

DIFFERENTIAL DIAGNOSIS

- Neoplasia
- Cyst
- Granuloma
- Hematoma
- Mucocele

INITIAL DATABASE

- Radiography of underlying structures (e.g., teeth/skull, limbs)
- Blood biochemistry and hematology, and urinalysis
- Ultrasonography (internal abscesses)
- Fine-needle aspiration of mass; not always diagnostic owing to the thick caseous nature of pus
- Gram stain of aspirate and/or bacterial culture and sensitivity

ADVANCED OR CONFIRMATORY TESTING

- Complete oral and dental examination under sedation or anesthesia
- CT scan to examine and determine the extent of internal abscesses and facial abscesses
- Bacterial culture and sensitivity of abscess capsule. Culture of pus is often unrewarding owing to low presence of bacteria; often culture of the capsule is more successful. This should include both aerobic and anaerobic culture.
- Thoracic radiographs

TREATMENT

THERAPEUTIC GOALS

- Identify and resolve the underlying cause of the abscess.
- Surgically remove the abscess(es) and any associated diseased tissue.

ACUTE GENERAL TREATMENT

- Abscesses can be associated with generalized disease (e.g., gastrointestinal stasis) that requires stabilization before anesthesia and surgery.
- Anorexia associated with dental disease requires supportive care via assisted feeding and hydration (see Anorexia).

CHRONIC TREATMENT

- Treatment options are many and varied. Often a multifactorial treatment plan is required.
- Antibiotic therapy alone is often unrewarding.
- Antibiotic therapy often requires a minimum duration of 4 to 6 weeks.
- Antibiotic choice should consider patient safety, spectrum of activity, and concentration in infected tissues.
- Suitable first-line antibiotics may include procaine penicillin 40,000-60,000 IU/kg q 24 h SC, IM, or azithromycin 15-30 mg/kg PO q 24 h
- Surgical débridement is essential because of the caseous nature of rabbit abscesses:
  - Lancing and drainage (e.g., Penrose drains) are generally unsuccessful.

- Surgical approach is similar to tumor removal with en bloc resection technique and wide margins.
- Removal of the abscess capsule is essential to ensure complete resolution.
- Infected tissue, including bone, teeth, and soft tissue, requires removal; otherwise, recurrence is likely (e.g., infected teeth and associated osteomyelitis).

- Surgical treatment and postoperative wound care may involve the following:
  - Marsupialization, which involves conversion of the abscess cavity into an open pouch by suturing the skin to the edges of the débrided abscess cavity. This promotes healing by second intention and allows treatment of the cavity as an open wound. The open wound can be flushed and irrigated daily with 0.05% chlorhexidine or 0.1% povidone-iodine solution. Postoperative management may be intensive, requiring 4 to 6 weeks of treatment.
  - Application of honey, glucose, or concentrated sugar solutions to the abscess cavity may be beneficial. These solutions have hygroscopic and bactericidal properties. Honey promotes wound healing; some types (e.g., Manuka honey from New Zealand) are thought to have additional antimicrobial properties.
  - Antibiotic-impregnated polymethylmethacrylate (AIPMMA) bead placement after débridement. Wounds are then closed. The beads slowly release antibiotic into the surrounding tissue for many months. Choice of antibiotics should be based on culture and sensitivity. Surgical removal of all infected tissue is essential for the success of this technique.
  - Calcium hydroxide has been used to treat dental condition–associated abscesses. It is used in cavities after surgical débridement of bony abscesses and is reputed to have antibacterial properties. The main disadvantage of calcium hydroxide is the severe collateral soft tissue damage.
- Palliative care with lifelong antibiotics and analgesia is often an option.

POSSIBLE COMPLICATIONS

Recurrence is common, especially if all infected tissue is not removed.

RECOMMENDED MONITORING

Depends on site of abscessation; monitor for abscess regrowth

PROGNOSIS AND OUTCOME

- Prognosis varies according to underlying cause of the infection and completeness of surgical resection.
- Multiple surgeries may be required.
- Dental abscesses have a varying prognosis depending on the extent of dental disease. Involvement of multiple teeth and/or multiple dental quadrants can greatly reduce the likelihood of resolution.
- Internal and pulmonary abscesses carry a poorer prognosis, even with complete surgical excision.

CONTROVERSY

Underlying metabolic bone disease may be associated with dental disease and subsequent infection and abscess formation.

PEARLS & CONSIDERATIONS

COMMENTS

- Radical surgery, medical treatment, and a diagnosis of the underlying cause are required for complete resolution of rabbit abscesses.
- Surgery may not completely control or be an option for multifocal abscessation. In these patients, treatments are palliative and should be aimed at maintaining quality of life.

PREVENTION

- Optimum dietary nutrition, including high-fiber content, to minimize dental disease
- Good sanitation
- Removal of "sharp" edges within cages and environment
- Neutering of rabbits housed together
- Prevention of skin wounds

CLIENT EDUCATION

Client education is essential before treatment is provided for any abscess. Often, multiple surgical procedures are required because many abscesses have a tendency to recur. Both intensive wound management and postoperative nursing require client participation and frequent rechecks. In some cases, resolution of an abscess is not possible. These rabbits can be offered a good quality of life with long-term antibiotic and analgesic therapy.

SUGGESTED READINGS

Harcourt Brown F: Abscesses. In textbook of rabbit medicine, Oxford, UK, 2002, Butterworth-Heinemann, pp 206–223.

Molan PC: The role of honey in the management of wounds, J Wound Care 8:415–418, 1999.

Tyrrell KL, et al: Periodontal bacteria in rabbit mandibular and maxillary abscesses, J Clin Microbiol 40:1044–1047, 2002.

CROSS-REFERENCES TO OTHER SECTIONS

Anorexia
Cutaneous Masses
Dental Disease
Dermatopathies
Hepatic Disorders
Lower Respiratory Tract Disorders
Mammary Gland Disorders
Myxomatosis
Otitis
Pasteurellosis
Pododermatitis
Staphylococcosis
Upper Respiratory Tract Disorders
Uterine Disorders

AUTHOR: **NARELLE WALTER**

EDITOR: **DAVID VELLA**

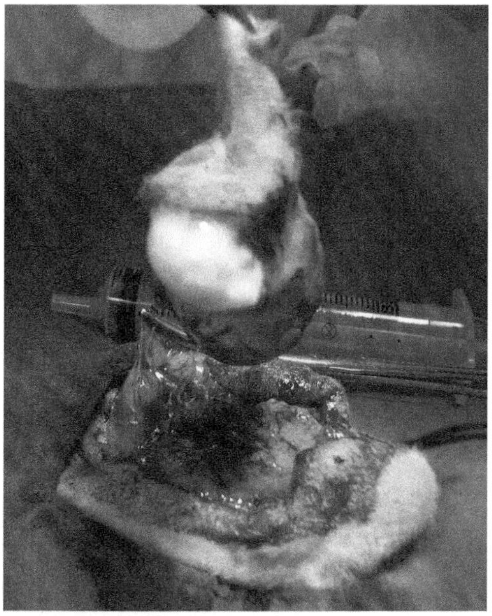

Abscesses Surgical removal of a dental-related encapsulated abscess from a rabbit's mandible. The thick white caseous pus is typical. Rabbit abscesses must be excised and are not amenable to lancing and draining. *(Photo courtesy Jörg Mayer, The University of Georgia, Athens.)*

Anorexia

BASIC INFORMATION

DEFINITION

Lack or loss of appetite for food; often accompanied by an aversion to food and/or an inability to eat

SYNONYM

Inappetence

SPECIAL SPECIES CONSIDERATIONS

Anorexia is a presenting complaint in rabbits. Many diseases and conditions affect the gastrointestinal tract, resulting in a decrease in or cessation of appetite. Urgent supportive treatment is necessary in most cases of anorexia to help reestablish hydration and control metabolic imbalances. Only then should investigation into the cause of anorexia be initiated.

EPIDEMIOLOGY

SPECIES, AGE, SEX Diagnosed across all breeds, genders, and age

RISK FACTORS

- Diets low in fiber and high in carbohydrates and proteins (pellets and grains)
- Dental disease (see Dental Disease)
- Stress
- Moulting (minimal brushing by owner or absence of companion rabbit) and subsequent ingestion of hair
- Concurrent underlying illness/disease

ASSOCIATED CONDITIONS AND DISORDERS Anorexia can quickly progress to hepatic lipidosis (see Hepatic Disorders) and metabolic acidosis if not treated promptly.

CLINICAL PRESENTATION

DISEASE FORMS/SUBTYPES Anorexia is a clinical sign with numerous underlying causes:

- Gastrointestinal hypomotility
- Dental disease
- Status post surgery/anesthetic
- Enteric disorders
- Pain
- Chronic renal failure (see Renal Disorders)
- Systemic disease
- Vestibular disease
- Metabolic disease
- Behavioral problem
- Stress

HISTORY, CHIEF COMPLAINT

- Loss of appetite for longer than 12 hours requires investigation and supportive treatment for the rabbit.
- Owners do not always notice a decrease in food intake or a change in feed preference, especially in rabbits that are group-housed or are not seen frequently (e.g., rabbits kept outside).
- In some chronic cases, weight loss may be the initial presenting sign.

PHYSICAL EXAM FINDINGS A complete clinical examination can help differentiate among the various causes of anorexia. Important areas to note in the rabbit are the following:

- Hydration stasis
- Presence or absence of feces, diarrhea, or uneaten cecotrophs (mistaken for diarrhea in rabbits)
- Upper respiratory disturbances
- Palpation of abdominal contents can indicate the following:
  - Solid fiber mat in stomach indicating dehydration (not blockage)
  - Fluid-filled stomach or intestinal loops indicating blockage
  - Gas-filled cecum indicating hypomotility
- Examination of dental arcade. Dental disease cannot be ruled out unless examination is performed in an anesthetized animal and skull radiographs are taken.
- Weight loss

ETIOLOGY AND PATHOPHYSIOLOGY

- Stress and/or other illness can have a dramatic effect on the gastrointestinal system. Sympathetic nerve stimulation inhibits gut motility. Slow gastric emptying can result in dehydration and solidification of intestinal contents, in particular the fiber mat always present in the rabbit's stomach.
- Slow gut motility results in gas accumulation in the stomach and cecum; this in turn results in pain.
- The physiologic effects of reduced gut motility can include gastric dilation/impaction, gastric ulceration, gastric trichobezoar formation, alterations in water/electrolyte secretion and absorption, hypovolemia, acid-base and electrolyte imbalances, and dehydration.
- Because glucose and lactate are produced in the cecum in response to fermentation, a decrease in their production and absorption (via cecotrophs) has deleterious effects.
- A decrease in gut motility decreases the production and absorption of fatty acids from the cecum (a product of bacterial fermentation). This decrease, along with a reduction in blood glucose, stimulates fatty acid mobilization from adipose stores.
- Hepatic inundation of fatty acids can cause hepatic lipidosis and liver failure. This occurs most readily in obese rabbits.
- Oxidation of these free fatty acids can result in ketoacidosis, leading to depression and further anorexia.

DIAGNOSIS

DIFFERENTIAL DIAGNOSIS

Anorexia can be caused by many and numerous conditions. Irrespective of the cause, anorexia can initiate a flow on effect that results in hepatic lipidosis and liver failure. Common causes of anorexia include the following:

- Dental disease
- Dietary insufficiencies
- Upper respiratory disease
- Toxicities
- Cecal impaction
- Metabolic disease
- Gastrointestinal hypomotility
- Neoplasia

INITIAL DATABASE

- Packed cell volume (or hematocrit) and total protein
- Blood glucose levels
- Complete blood count, serum biochemistry panel, and urinalysis

ADVANCED OR CONFIRMATORY TESTING

- Complete oral and dental examination under anesthesia
- Dental and skull radiographs
- Survey radiographs, including complete thoracic and abdominal radiographs. Skeletal radiographs can indicate the presence of arthritis.
- Abdominal ultrasound

TREATMENT

THERAPEUTIC GOALS

- Provide supportive treatment (hydration/supportive feeding).
- Identify the chief cause of inappetence.

ACUTE GENERAL TREATMENT

- Monitor vital signs closely, including heart rate, body temperature, and systolic blood pressure.
- Provide parenteral fluid therapy via intravenous or intraosseous route. Crystalloids may be used. Maintenance fluid rates are considered 100-120 mL/kg q 24 h.

- Provide assisted feeding through use of commercial formulas (e.g., Oxbow Critical Care or Lafeber Emeraid).
- Provide prokinetic drugs (only in non-obstructive cases) such as cisapride 0.5 mg/kg PO q 8 h or metoclopramide 0.2-1.0 mg/kg PO, SC q 6-8 h
- Provide anti-ulcer drugs (e.g., ranitidine 2-5 mg/kg PO, SC q 12 h) as gastric ulceration occurs with stress and gastrointestinal hypomotility.
- Provide analgesia if indicated by underlying condition. Ensure patient is adequately hydrated before using NSAIDs (e.g., carprofen 2-4 mg/kg PO, SC q 24 h; meloxicam 0.1- 0.5 mg/kg PO, SC q 24 h; ketoprofen 1-3 mg/kg PO q 12 h) and/or opioids (e.g., buprenorphine 0.03 mg/kg SC, IM q 8 h)
- Investigation into underlying condition is essential. If no cause is obvious, initial steps should include full blood profile, survey radiographs, and oral examination under anesthesia.

CHRONIC TREATMENT

- Dietary changes are required in rabbits on a low-fiber high-protein/carbohydrate diet (high-pellet diet). High fiber stimulates intestinal motility.
- Investigation into dental disease requires oral examination under anesthetic. This cannot be ruled out if mouth is viewed while awake/sedated. Spurs causing mucosal damage are a common cause of anorexia in rabbits. Dental radiographs are often required to outline the condition and rule out tooth root abscessation.
- Cecal impaction is an often insidious cause of anorexia in rabbits. Diagnosis is determined via abdominal radiographs. Treatment is required early in the course of disease and is often unsuccessful. Treatment includes hydration, increased dietary fiber, use of intestinal motility agents, supportive feeding, and paraffin liquid and progesterone treatment.

RECOMMENDED MONITORING

Dental disease may require regular dental examination and treatment.

PROGNOSIS AND OUTCOME

- Prognosis varies according to the underlying cause of anorexia.
- Dental disease may be an ongoing condition requiring long-term control of dietary change and regular molar examinations.

PEARLS & CONSIDERATIONS

COMMENTS

Anorexia is a common reason for owners to present pet rabbits for veterinary treatment. The list of potential causes is long. Clinicians should be aware that the anorexic rabbit often poses an enormous diagnostic challenge.

PREVENTION

- Optimum dietary nutrition, including high fiber content
- Regular dental examinations
- Regular grooming during moults
- Regular general health checks

SUGGESTED READINGS

Harcourt-Brown F: Anorexia in rabbits: 1. Causes and effects, In Pract 24:358–367, 2002.

Harcourt-Brown F: Anorexia in rabbits: 2. Diagnosis and treatment, In Pract 24:450–467, 2002.

CROSS-REFERENCES TO OTHER SECTIONS

Dental Disease
Gastric Disorders
Hepatic Disorders
Renal Disorders
Intestinal Disorders
Fluid Therapy in Rabbits and Rodents (Section II)

AUTHOR: **NARELLE WALTER**

EDITOR: **DAVID VELLA**

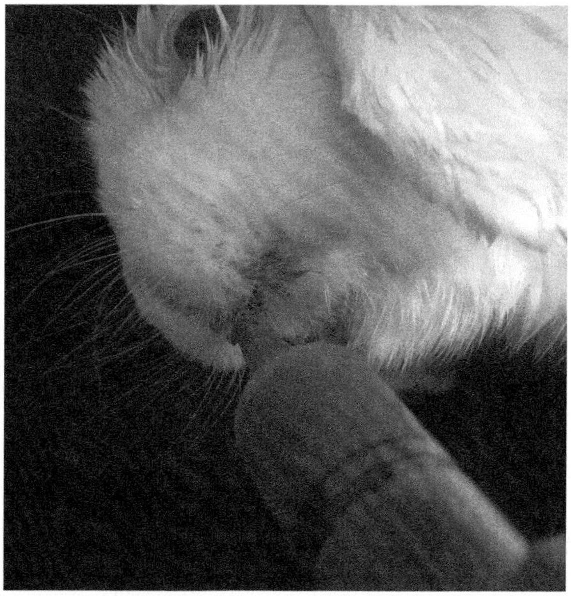

Anorexia Anorectic rabbit being fed with a syringe containing a commercial assisted-feeding formula. Anorectic rabbits must receive supportive care in the form of nutritional supplements. *(Photo courtesy Jörg Mayer, The University of Georgia, Athens.)*

RABBITS

Arthritis

BASIC INFORMATION

DEFINITION

- Describes inflammation of one (or more) joints; may be osteoarthritis or septic arthritis
- Progressive, inflammatory, irreversible deterioration of articular cartilage

SYNONYMS

Osteoarthritis, degenerative joint disease, osteoarthrosis, septic arthritis

SPECIAL SPECIES CONSIDERATIONS

Increasing prevalence with age

EPIDEMIOLOGY

SPECIES, AGE, SEX

- Osteoarthritis
  - No gender predilection. little breed predilection; however, giant breeds may be more prone to osteoarthritis of the stifles owing to increased weight loading and conformation

- Likely more common in older animals, although may be seen post trauma in animals of any age. May be secondary to developmental disorders in younger animals
- Septic arthritis
  - No gender, breed, or age predilection unless linked to specific cause (e.g., hock joint infection following progression of pododermatitis into flexor tendon sheaths may be more common in breeds more vulnerable to developing pododermatitis, such as Rex and giant breeds)

RISK FACTORS

- Osteoarthritis
  - More common following injury. In particular, poor handling technique may predispose to injury of the lumbar and lumbosacral joints.
  - Obesity
  - Hypervitaminosis A—induced polyarthropathy with hyperostosis and ankylosis of various joints has been described in a rabbit after chronic ingestion of a diet made up almost exclusively of carrots.
- Septic arthritis
  - Concurrent or previous infection/abscess allowing ascending spread to joint or, more commonly, hematogenous spread
  - Any factors that may predispose to pododermatitis risk further development into septic arthritis in joints of affected feet.

CONTAGION AND ZOONOSIS Not infectious, although septic arthritis may be seen in conjunction with infections with *Staphylococcus aureus* and *Pasteurella multocida*

ASSOCIATED CONDITIONS AND DISORDERS The main clinical consequence of arthritis is pain. Therefore, any rabbit showing pain-related signs, especially inactivity, urine stasis (including urolith formation and urine sludging), and gut hypomotility, should have arthritis considered as part of the underlying differential diagnosis.

CLINICAL PRESENTATION

DISEASE FORMS/SUBTYPES

- Osteoarthritis
- Septic arthritis
- Rheumatoid arthritis
- Secondary osteoarthritis: commonly results from trauma, joint instability, incongruity, and immobilization
- May affect any joint, in particular stifle, hocks, and elbows.

HISTORY, CHIEF COMPLAINT

- Reluctance to ambulate and move (often gradual decline)
- Hunched posture
- Lameness and stiffness after excessive exercise or prolonged rest
- Irritable behavior when approached or touched
- Reduced/restricted range of motion (e.g., lack of grooming, reduced cecotrophy, not using stairs, altered gait)
- Urine and fecal soiling of perineum
- Associated pain may lead to other problems (e.g., gut stasis, dysuria)

PHYSICAL EXAM FINDINGS

- Stiff or altered gait
- Lameness
- Abnormalities during joint manipulation (flexion and extension): joint pain, crepitus, instability, and/or decreased range of motion
- Joint effusion
- Joint thickening
- Muscle atrophy
- Other signs associated with secondary effects of pain (e.g., gut stasis)

ETIOLOGY AND PATHOPHYSIOLOGY

- Joint homeostasis is disrupted by abnormal cartilage and membrane cell functions, nutrition, or joint biomechanics.
- A catabolic imbalance results with chondrocytes unable to replace degraded extracellular matrix (degradation via cytokines and other inflammatory mediators).
- This cycle progresses irreversibly as the weakened biomechanical integrity of articular cartilage potentiates further dysfunction and disease.
- Periarticular fibrosis is a secondary process directed toward stabilizing the joint.
- Osteoarthritis
  - Excess "wear and tear." May be exacerbated by altered conformation and excessive weight. More common in aged rabbits
  - Secondary to joint trauma
- Septic arthritis
  - Ascending spread of bacteria from infection
  - Hematogenous spread (bacterial, spirochetal, mycoplasmal, rickettsial, viral, fungal, and protozoal)
  - Direct entry of bacteria into joint when damaged/injured
- Rheumatoid
  - Autoimmune
  - Chronic antigen-induced arthritis exacerbates vascular lesions in rabbits with atherosclerosis.

DIAGNOSIS

DIFFERENTIAL DIAGNOSIS

- Skeletal disease
  - Arthritis (osteoarthritis, septic, rheumatoid)
  - Osteomyelitis
  - Hypertrophy
  - Fracture
  - Neoplasia
  - Limb deformity
  - Spondylosis
  - Vertebral subluxation
- Pododermatitis
- Neurologic disease
  - Trauma (central or peripheral)
  - Infection (encephalitozoonosis, toxoplasmosis, neosporosis, cerebral nematodiasis, herpes, rabies)
  - Neoplasia
- Paresis
  - Metabolic disease (e.g., renal failure, hypokalemia, hepatic lipidosis, hypoglycemia)
  - Cardiovascular disease
  - Nutritional deficiency (e.g., vitamin E deficiency, hypovitaminosis A)
  - Toxins (e.g., woolly pod milkweed [*Asclepias eriocarpa*])
  - Generalized muscle weakness ("floppy rabbit syndrome")
- Other underlying disease causing general malaise (e.g., urogenital tract disease, gastrointestinal tract disease, dental disease)

INITIAL DATABASE

- Physical examination, including
  - Assessment of movement and gait: rabbits are often reluctant to move in the examination room. In some cases, it may be useful to ask the owners to film the rabbit at home.
  - Palpation and flexion/extension of joints to assess range of movement and to attempt to localize joint pain: should be done with great care owing to risk of causing further damage (especially when assessing the spine). The stifles should be assessed for draw if caudal cruciate (not cranial as in dogs) rupture with associated arthritis is likely. This should be done under anesthesia.
- Radiography: radiographic signs may be present only when changes are well advanced. Therefore, failure to see changes does not rule out arthritis. Typical radiographic lesions include subchondral sclerosis, joint space narrowing, osteophytosis, enthesiophytosis, joint capsule thickening, subchondral bone attrition, intraarticular calcified bodies, soft tissue calcification, and subchondral cysts.

ADVANCED OR CONFIRMATORY TESTING

- Arthrocentesis and synovial fluid analysis: especially useful in diagnosing septic arthritis. Often frank pus (hard to aspirate) is found. This may be submitted for culture and sensitivity, but failure to culture bacteria is common. Cytologic examination is far more sensitive and may reveal inflammatory cells ± microbes.
- Synovial biopsy and histopathologic examination

- Myelography: may be required with spinal problems
- Arthroscopy: in larger breeds, some joints may be amenable to this technique, allowing examination of synovium, cartilage, ligaments, and menisci
- CT may confirm joint incongruity.
- MRI may identify morphologic cartilage changes.
- Nuclear scintigraphy may help to localize osteoarthritis.

TREATMENT

THERAPEUTIC GOALS

- Pain alleviation
- Improved function
- Limited disease progression
- Facilitation of joint reparative process

ACUTE GENERAL TREATMENT

- General supportive care for any rabbit experiencing reduced or nil food intake (e.g., fluid therapy, assist feeding, analgesia, management of gut stasis)
- Provide parenteral fluid therapy (crystalloids may be used); maintenance fluid rate is considered to be 100-120 mL/kg q 24 h.
- Provide assist feeding by using commercial assist feeding formulas (e.g., Oxbow critical care feeding formula; Oxbow Pet Products, Murdock, NE).
- Analgesia
  - Nonsteroidal antiinflammatory drugs (NSAIDs; e.g., carprofen 2-4 mg/kg PO, SC q 24 h; meloxicam 0.3-0.5 mg/kg PO, SC q 24 h; ketoprofen 1-3 mg/kg PO q 12 h)
  - Opioids (e.g., buprenorphine 0.03 mg/kg SC, IM q 8 h)
- Septic arthritis
  - Antibiosis: pending culture and sensitivity results, select antibiotic that is likely to penetrate pus and be active against a range of organisms, including anaerobes (e.g., trimethoprim/sulfonamides 30 mg/kg PO q 12 h; azithromycin 30 mg/kg PO q 24 h). Antibiotics may be required for a period of 6 to 8 weeks.

CHRONIC TREATMENT

- Osteoarthritis
  - Surgical treatment for cause of joint degeneration (e.g., repair of an articular fracture, stabilization of cruciate deficient stifle, femoral head ostectomy, management of intervertebral disc disease): arthrodesis likely to be indicated only in cases of limited chronic joint instability of the forelimb. Amputation of affected limb may be performed in severe cases as a salvage procedure.
  - Analgesia: long-term treatment may be indicated, especially NSAIDs. Periodically monitor renal function in such cases. Tramadol 5-11mg/kg PO q 24 h may be indicated for renally compromised rabbits.
  - Chondroprotective agents (e.g., polysulfated glycosaminoglycans, pentosan polysulfate 3 mg/kg SC q 7 d × 4 doses)
  - Acupuncture may be useful.
  - Lifestyle changes: to obtain reduced loading on joints (weight control via dietary modification); reduced need to climb stairs, ramps, etc.; suitable substrate to avoid slipping and falls and to provide foot protection
  - Physical therapy: to improve joint motion and limb function
- Septic arthritis
  - Analgesia as for osteoarthritis
  - Long-term antibiosis may achieve control but is unlikely to solve the problem.
  - In mild cases, joint flushing (with saline) and instillation of antibiotic solutions may help; however, the nature of rabbit pus makes this approach much less effective than in other mammals.
  - Surgical intervention is often required. Arthrotomy with curettage and débridement may help. Alternatively, implantation of antibiotic-impregnated polymethylmethacrylate (AIPPMA) beads may be considered post débridement with closure of the joint space. Antibiotic type should be based on culture and sensitivity. The beads slowly release antibiotic into surrounding tissue for several weeks/months and should be removed after 6 to 12 weeks. Choice of antibiotics should be based on culture and sensitivity; choices typically include cephalosporins (e.g., cefazolin, ceftiofur) and aminoglycosides (e.g., gentamicin, tobramycin, amikacin).
  - Long-term management of subsequent osteoarthritis will be required. Repeat surgical débridement may be required, and in severe cases, joint amputation may be considered. However, care must be taken that the other limbs can cope with the subsequent increase in weight bearing.

DRUG INTERACTIONS

- Care must always be taken when using long-term antibiotics.
- NSAIDs: monitor renal function when using for long periods

POSSIBLE COMPLICATIONS

- Avoid use of oral preparations of lincomycin, clindamycin, erythromycin, and penicillins owing to risk of developing dysbiosis and enterotoxemia
- Renal dysfunction and/or gastric ulceration (NSAIDs)
- Gradual worsening of osteoarthritis will necessitate regular review of drugs and dosages; eventually may require euthanasia

RECOMMENDED MONITORING

- Body weight
- Full physical examination every 1 to 3 months; assess quality of life
- Renal function
- Repeat radiographic imaging of affected joints

PROGNOSIS AND OUTCOME

- Osteoarthritis: reasonable if pain can be controlled and owners are willing to make necessary lifestyle modifications
- Septic arthritis: good if seen early; if advanced, prognosis is poor for the joint but good for the rabbit if the limb can be amputated.

CONTROVERSY

Avoid using corticosteroids in rabbits because their use can precipitate clinical disease in a subclinically affected animal.

PEARLS & CONSIDERATIONS

COMMENTS

- Radiographic signs of osteoarthritis may not correlate with clinical signs. Treatment decisions cannot be made on the basis of radiographic findings alone.
- Efficacy of cartilage modifiers is not as well documented as that of NSAIDs.

PREVENTION

- General good care and appropriate housing and diet will reduce some of the "wear-and-tear" on joints. Good handling technique will reduce the chances of injury.
- Prompt recognition and early intervention may delay progression of disease.

SUGGESTED READINGS

Frater J: Hyperostotic polyarthropathy in a rabbit—a suspected case of chronic hypervitaminosis A from a diet of carrots, Aust Vet J 79:608–611, 2001.

Fu X, et al: Assessment of the efficacy of joint lavage in rabbits with osteoarthritis of the knee, J Orthop Res 27:91–96, 2009.

Keeble E: Common neurological and musculoskeletal problems in rabbits, In Pract 28: 212–218, 2006.

Lennox AM: Care of the geriatric rabbit, Vet Clin North Am Exot Anim Pract 13:123–133, 2010.

AUTHORS: **JOHN CHITTY AND DAVID VELLA**

EDITOR: **THOMAS M. DONNELLY**

Behavioral Disorders

Client Education Sheet Available on Website

BASIC INFORMATION

DEFINITION

- This can be seen at any age and in males or females. It is more prevalent in sexually entire rabbits. It may be due to learned behavior from an early age. Rabbits have different personalities that exhibit different levels of tolerance to handling and restraint.
- The natural defense of rabbits when danger is impending is to run away. When confined or caged and unable to run away, a rabbit is more likely to defend itself by lunging at a person to bite or by standing up on hind legs and attacking with its front limbs.

SYNONYMS

Biting behavior, food aggression

EPIDEMIOLOGY

RISK FACTORS

- "Adolescent behaviors"
- Hormonal changes with sexual maturity, pregnancy, or pseudopregnancy
- Pain or illness may elicit aggressive behaviors.
- Previous trauma may create aggressive behaviors.

ASSOCIATED CONDITIONS AND DISORDERS

- Chewing
- Digging
- Urine spraying
- Fecal marking
- Destruction

CLINICAL PRESENTATION

HISTORY, CHIEF COMPLAINT Clients complain that their rabbit is aggressive, irritable, and difficult to handle. Obtain a history of the behaviors and the context in which they occur.

PHYSICAL EXAM FINDINGS Usually unremarkable, although occasionally wounds caused by fighting with bonded mates when establishing social hierarchy may be evident on the rabbit.

ETIOLOGY AND PATHOPHYSIOLOGY

- Rabbit-to-rabbit aggression
  - Usually due to territorial defense, fear, and dominance. Aggression among young males at puberty precludes keeping entire males in groups. The space for one male to run away is not available, and serious injury can follow if the rabbits are not separated. In contrast, aggression is minimal among groups of female rabbits grouped at a young age.
- Rabbit-to-human aggression
  - Usually due to fear or distrust
  - May be due to learned dominance/aggression when aggressive behavior is unchallenged (e.g., a rabbit bites its owner, who stops handling it—the rabbit learns that biting keeps humans away)
  - Females with newborn kits and that are pseudopregnant tend to be more aggressive.
  - May be associated with territorial behaviors and food. Rabbit perceives human hand offering food as "taking" food away.
- Rabbits have a blind spot in front of their noses owing to lateral eye placement. They may bite inadvertently, mistaking a hand or fingers for food or for a threatening foreign object.
  - Avoid reaching beneath a rabbit's chin to pet it.
- Highly territorial rabbits in their enclosure may attack a caregiver over food competition or fear of feed removal.
  - Owners must assert dominance (e.g., say, "Move over," "Get out of the way," or "Stop what you are doing").

DIAGNOSIS

DIFFERENTIAL DIAGNOSIS

Aggression and other behavioral changes that may be related to a medical problem should be ruled out (e.g., pain-related problems such as gastrointestinal stasis and urinary tract disorders).

INITIAL DATABASE

- Complete blood count, serum biochemistry profile, and urinalysis are generally unremarkable.
- Fecal direct smear, flotation, and cytologic examination are generally unremarkable.
- Radiographs are generally unremarkable unless gastrointestinal stasis, gastrointestinal foreign body, neoplasia, abscess, urinary calculi, or calciuria is present.

TREATMENT

THERAPEUTIC GOALS

To rectify any abnormal behaviors.

ACUTE GENERAL TREATMENT

- To help alleviate food aggression, owners should relocate food bowls in different areas of the rabbit's territory. When taking food bowls into and out of the enclosure, owners should provide distraction with favored food items.
- Early socialization when the rabbit is young and gentle handling, are important. Socialization includes gentle handling of kit rabbits and patience to gain the rabbit's trust.
- Young children should not be allowed to pick up or carry a rabbit. Instruct children to interact with rabbits on the floor while allowing rabbits to approach them.
- Reaching down to pick up a rabbit through the top of the cage may seem less threatening to the confined rabbit than reaching in through the side door of a cage.
- If a rabbit bites hard, the handler should respond immediately with a high-pitched yelp (as a littermate might during rough play fighting) to deter the behavior.

CHRONIC TREATMENT

- Chronic treatment: behavior modification for biting
  - Owners should plan to spend several sessions over a few weeks or months, allowing the rabbit to relearn slowly to trust humans.
    - This should be done in a quiet place that is neutral territory to the rabbit.
    - Owners should wear gloves and protective clothing.
    - Owners should remain motionless even if the rabbit charges or bites.
    - An attacking rabbit will accept that a resting, calm owner will not respond to attempts to dominate, and that the owner will not attack the rabbit in return.
    - Progress may wax and wane as time goes on.
    - Owners should gradually offer food treats and eventually their hand.
    - Owners should end each session on a positive note and when possible begin to pet the rabbit and to pick it up.
- Chronic treatment: for rabbit-to-rabbit aggression

- A slow and patient bonding process (once the rabbits are neutered) is necessary.
  - Bonding takes time and patience.
  - Direct adult supervision is necessary to prevent injury.
- A social hierarchy must be established when rabbits are introduced; some fighting should be expected.
- Preparations should be made to separate fighting rabbits:
  - Owners can wear heavy leather gloves or put sneakers (canvas shoes) on their hands to allow separation of rabbits without injury to themselves.
- Initiate socialization by placing cages near each other, so the presence of a new rabbit is established; do not place cages too close because injuries can occur through wire caging.
- Allow one rabbit at a time to explore a rabbit-safe area. Then replace that rabbit in its cage and let the other rabbit into the same area. This allows each rabbit to familiarize with the others' scent.
- Introductions should be made in neutral territory such as a room into which neither rabbit has entered:
  - Decreases or avoids territorial defense
  - May make the rabbits interested in exploring the new environment
  - May make rabbits insecure and more likely to require the presence of another rabbit before exploring
- In neutral territory, put both rabbits in harnesses to allow each rabbit to see and smell the other without getting too close:
  - After several such situations, rabbits may appear less hostile to each other. Then allow each rabbit to approach the other rabbit, but be prepared to separate the rabbits if they fight.
  - If bite wounds occur, instruct owners to see their veterinarian—bite wounds can become infected and abscess.
- Continue introductions in neutral territory. Eventually, the rabbits can be left together in the neutral territory. Although some fighting may occur, they may tolerate each other and become bonded.
- Establish novel situations in which rabbits comfort each other:
  - Place rabbits in a clean, dry bathtub with some hay and greens as a distraction. Bathtubs are slippery, and rabbits find it difficult to move.
  - Place rabbits in a laundry basket on the floor of a car, and drive around in tight circles (in an empty parking lot).
- Some rabbits are not compatible with other rabbits:
  - Owners should be prepared for incompatibility by realizing that a new rabbit may need to have its own cage and space in the house if it does not bond to the rabbit(s) already present.

PEARLS & CONSIDERATIONS

COMMENTS

- Rabbits that are ready to attack will hold up their tail, adopt a strained stance, tense their body, and pull back their ears. Such a rabbit may be hunched to lunge and bite and may exhibit harsh snorts, grunts, hissing, or barking growls.
- Anger and aggression may also be exhibited by:
  - Shredding substrate with front paws and teeth
  - Head butting objects
  - Picking up objects and flinging them
- Thumping with rear feet is commonly seen to issue a warning, to announce danger, and to signal dislike of a situation.
- If a rabbit is nervous or scared, it will flatten against the ground with ears pinned against its head, eyes bulging, and muscles tight.

CLIENT EDUCATION

Demonstrate to clients the following:

- The proper way to handle rabbits
- What interaction is acceptable for children with pet rabbits
- How to appreciate and respect normal, instinctive behavior in rabbits

SUGGESTED READINGS

Bradley Bays T: Rabbit behavior. In Bradley Bays T, et al (eds): Exotic pet behavior, birds, reptiles, and small mammals, St Louis, 2006, Saunders-Elsevier, pp 1–49.

Harriman M: House rabbit handbook: how to live with an urban rabbit, ed 4, Alameda, CA, 2005, Drollery Press.

McBride A: Why does my rabbit...? London, 1998, Souvenir Press.

House Rabbit Society: Rabbit Behavior Resources Index. Information for clients. http://www.rabbit.org/behavior/index.html Accessed Aug 16, 2012.

CROSS-REFERENCES TO OTHER SECTIONS

- Dermatopathies
- Lower urinary tract disorders

AUTHORS: **TERESA BRADLEY BAYS AND THOMAS M. DONNELLY**

EDITOR: **DAVID VELLA**

RABBITS

Buphthalmia and Glaucoma

BASIC INFORMATION

DEFINITION

- Glaucoma is an increase in intraocular pressure (IOP) that is incompatible with normal visual function. Two types of glaucoma, hereditary and acquired, have been described in rabbits.
- The term *buphthalmia* (literally, "ox-eye") commonly refers to hereditary glaucoma seen especially in young rabbits. *Buphthalmia* or *buphthalmos* is a descriptive term for enlargement of an eye owing to increased IOP.
- In young animals, where scleral collagen is relatively soft, the globe expands readily, giving rise to buphthalmia. Clinically, pain does not appear obvious.
- Acquired glaucoma, as opposed to inherited glaucoma, usually occurs secondary to uveitis or intraocular neoplasia. Buphthalmia can also be seen as an extension of glaucoma in older rabbits.

SYNONYMS

- Ocular hypertension
- Megaglobus (antonym of *microphthalmos*): incorrect use of term for ocular lesion due to increased IOP
- Congenital glaucoma: inappropriate term for *buphthalmia* in young rabbits as condition is inherited
- Hydrophthalmos/hydrophthalmia

SPECIAL SPECIES CONSIDERATIONS

Buphthalmia is difficult to differentiate from exophthalmos and poses a potential problem in general practice. The third eyelid is often in a normal position with buphthalmos, and the third eyelid is often protruding in exophthalmos secondary to retrobulbar disease. Diagnosis of buphthalmos or exophthalmos requires an accurate method to measure IOP; ocular ultrasound is useful for measuring the diameter of the normal and abnormal globe. Although most practices have a Schiøtz tonometer, the rabbit must be on its side for a Schiøtz tonometer to be used correctly. Increased IOP occurs if the rabbit struggles or is held too tightly. Sedation of the rabbit slightly decreases IOP. Veterinary ophthalmologists use a pen-sized, handheld, digital applanation tonometer (TonoPen) that is reliable for measuring IOP.

EPIDEMIOLOGY

SPECIES, AGE, SEX

- Buphthalmia
  - IOP >30 mm Hg in rabbits >1 month of age is indicative of glaucoma. Normal IOP in rabbits >1 month is 15 to 23 mm Hg.
- Secondary glaucoma due to
  - Uveitis (see Uveitis): no age predilection
  - Intraocular neoplasia: usually seen in older animals (>7 years)
  - Lens luxation is rare and usually affects young to middle-aged rabbits (1 to 4 years)

GENETICS AND BREED PREDISPOSITION

- Buphthalmia is inherited as an autosomal recessive trait and is seen most frequently in New Zealand white rabbits.
- Glaucoma secondary to *Encephalitozoon cuniculi*–associated uveitis and cataract may be seen more frequently in dwarf rabbits; some authors claim these rabbits are more susceptible to *E. cuniculi* phacoclastic uveitis.

RISK FACTORS

- Anterior uveitis due to *E. cuniculi*–associated phacoclastic uveitis
- Intraocular neoplasia

ASSOCIATED CONDITIONS AND DISORDERS Glaucoma may occur

- With primary eye disease (i.e., abnormalities of the drainage/iridocorneal angle; primary glaucoma)
- Secondary to other eye diseases (secondary glaucoma)
- With miscellaneous developmental anomalies of the anterior segment of the eye

CLINICAL PRESENTATION

DISEASE FORMS/SUBTYPES Glaucoma may be classified on the basis of

- Cause: primary or secondary
- Duration: acute (vision potential) versus chronic (typically blind, buphthalmic eye)

HISTORY, CHIEF COMPLAINT

- Sometimes cloudy, red eye
- Variable ocular pain, evident as reluctance to be touched around the face or blepharospasm
- History of visual impairment or blindness (e.g., bumping into objects)
- Enlargement of the globe (buphthalmos)

PHYSICAL EXAM FINDINGS

- Unilateral or bilateral ocular changes
  - Corneal edema is a variable sign, often diffuse
  - Episcleral vascular congestion (tortuous, engorged, episcleral vessels)
  - Dilated pupil with slow to absent pupillary light reflexes
  - Optic disc cupping and variable retinal changes occur late in disease

ETIOLOGY AND PATHOPHYSIOLOGY

- Obstruction to aqueous humor outflow, causing elevated IOP
- Elevated IOP damages the optic nerve head and retina.
- Onset and severity of glaucomatous changes are influenced by the length and degree of IOP elevation.

DIAGNOSIS

DIFFERENTIAL DIAGNOSIS

- Exophthalmos secondary to orbital disease
- Other causes of red eyes (see Cherry Eye) (e.g., conjunctival [see Conjunctival Disorders] and/or episcleral hyperemia)

INITIAL DATABASE

Complete ophthalmic examination, including tonometry (measurement of IOP):

- Normal reported IOP values
  - 24.4 mm Hg ± 1.3 (in "rabbits")
  - 19.3 mm Hg ± 1.3 (in New Zealand Red rabbits)
- Applanation (e.g., TonoPen) or rebound tonometry (e.g., TonoVet) may be performed.
- IOP may return to normal as the eye stretches.

ADVANCED OR CONFIRMATORY TESTING

- Referral to veterinary ophthalmologist for
  - Confirmation of diagnosis
  - Additional or multiple tonometric measurements
  - Gonioscopy (direct observation of the iridocorneal angle)
  - Ophthalmoscopy of the ocular fundus (posterior segment of the eye, including retina and optic nerve)
  - Ocular ultrasonography
    - To measure eye size
    - To evaluate deep ocular structures if cornea, aqueous humor, or lens is opaque
    - To visualize concurrent ocular abnormalities (e.g., lens luxation, lens capsule rupture, retinal detachment, intraocular masses)

TREATMENT

THERAPEUTIC GOALS

- Treat immediately.
- Lower IOP of affected eye to maintain vision for as long as possible.
- Eliminate ocular pain.
- Depending on pathogenesis, treat contralateral eye prophylactically with IOP-lowering drugs to delay onset of glaucoma.
- Treat any underlying disease, e.g. uveitis.

ACUTE GENERAL TREATMENT

- In acute cases, it is critical that the IOP be lowered as soon as possible to maintain or restore vision (topical and oral medications). If tonometry is unavailable, glaucoma suspects should be referred to a veterinary ophthalmologist (as an emergency) for IOP measurement. Early surgical intervention may permit better and longer control of IOP. The clinician is urged to consider early referral, especially when vision in one eye has already been lost.
- Drugs: regardless of the type of glaucoma, the following may be administered initially and then over the long term if indicated:
  - Topical β-adrenergic adrenergic receptor antagonists or blockers (these drugs reduce aqueous formation) (0.5% timolol or 0.5% betaxolol, usually q 8-12 h)
  - Topical or systemic carbonic anhydrase inhibitors (CAIs; topical: 2% dorzolamide or 1% brinzolamide q 8-12 h)
    - Combined dorzolamide/timolol combination eye drops are available.
  - Mannitol 1-2 g/kg IV over 20 minutes to rapidly lower IOP (first effects in 1 to 2 hours; maximum effect in 4 to 6 hours; duration ≈8 to 10 hours) when there is a chance for return of vision (e.g., acute primary glaucoma)
  - Topical (1% q 6 h) and/or systemic (1-2 mg/kg PO q 24 h) prednisolone is indicated when anterior uveitis is

also present, unless an infectious cause for the uveitis is documented or is strongly suspected.

CHRONIC TREATMENT

- Long-term treatment of glaucoma can be a frustrating endeavor because the disease tends to progress despite medical therapy, particularly with primary glaucoma. Diligent monitoring, regular reassessment of therapeutic success, and client education are critical.
- Drugs
  - ±Topical and/or systemic prednisolone: when anterior uveitis is also present, taper to lowest effective dose
  - In all primary glaucomas, the disease continues to progress even though IOP may be controlled; often, combinations of several topical and systemic IOP-lowering drugs or surgery is eventually necessary.
- Surgery
  - Laser cyclophotocoagulation and cryoablation are procedures offered by most veterinary ophthalmologists to lower IOP and prevent ocular pain. Efficacy in nonpigmented rabbits would be doubtful.
  - End-stage blind and painful, enlarged globes may be treated by:
    - Enucleation
    - Evisceration and intrascleral prosthesis
    - Enucleation, evisceration, and implant surgeries should be followed by histopathologic examination of removed tissue to help determine the cause of glaucoma (i.e., primary vs. secondary) and the prognosis for the other eye. Ruling out neoplasia is also an important consideration.

DRUG INTERACTIONS

- Topical β-adrenergic blockers may lower heart rate and blood pressure and may cause bronchoconstriction.
- Systemic CAIs may cause metabolic acidosis and electrolyte imbalances as evidenced by depression (perhaps related to hypokalemia) that require drug cessation. Topical CAI preparations are not associated with these side effects.
- Mannitol, an osmotic diuretic, should be avoided in patients with heart disease (risk of fluid overload/iatrogenic pulmonary edema) or oliguric/anuric renal failure (rarely concurrent with acute glaucoma).

POSSIBLE COMPLICATIONS

With poor or inadequate control of IOP, any or all of the following may occur:

- Enlarged globe causing increased corneal exposure, recurrent corneal ulceration, corneal vascularization, and/or corneal pigmentation
- Optic nerve and retinal degeneration
- Blindness
- Ocular pain
- Lens luxation or subluxation

RECOMMENDED MONITORING

- Regular reexaminations with tonometry (e.g., monthly once IOP control is initially achieved) are necessary to control IOP (should be maintained at <20 mm Hg) and maintain vision for as long as possible.
- As glaucoma progresses, increased frequency and/or additional topical and systemic drugs to lower IOP are usually necessary. Surgical management is needed when response to medication is poor.

PROGNOSIS AND OUTCOME

- Prognosis is usually poor for the first eye presented with the primary glaucoma because the disease is often advanced and refractory to medical therapy.
- Topical prophylactic therapy can significantly delay the onset of glaucoma.

PEARLS & CONSIDERATIONS

COMMENTS

- Patients with dilated pupils, corneal edema, and conjunctival hyperemia require tonometry to estimate IOP.
- Clinical management of glaucoma is often difficult; therefore, referral of these patients to a veterinary ophthalmologist is advised.
- Medical therapy for glaucoma is expensive and is often required long term.
- In a permanently blind, persistently glaucomatous eye, treatment (e.g., evisceration and implant, enucleation) is generally indicated.
- Digital pressure (pressing on the eyes through closed eyelids) cannot be used for accurately assessing IOP.

PREVENTION

The benefits of screening for *E. cuniculi* should be considered. Anterior uveitis that is unrecognized or inadequately treated and controlled will predispose an eye to the development of secondary glaucoma. Cataractous eyes (see Cataracts) should be examined regularly for

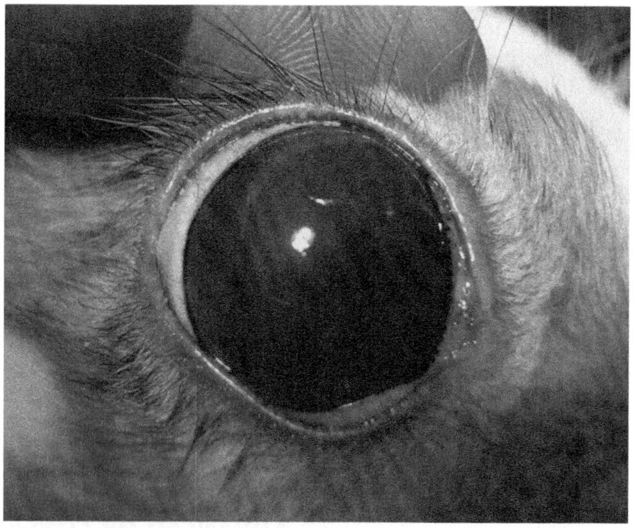

Buphthalmia and Glaucoma Buphthalmic eye in a 2-year-old male neutered dwarf rabbit. The enlargement of the eye is due to increased intraocular pressure. *(Photo courtesy Jörg Mayer, The University of Georgia, Athens.)*

evidence of lens-induced uveitis; treatment should be initiated when signs appear to prevent or delay the development of glaucoma.

CLIENT EDUCATION

- Glaucoma is a chronic disease that requires regular and diligent therapy. Missed medication will result in inadequate control of IOP, loss of sight, and pain.
- Rabbits with cataracts that are not surgical candidates require periodic eye examinations and tonometry indefinitely because they are at increased risk of developing glaucoma.

SUGGESTED READINGS

Bunt-Milam AH, et al: Hereditary glaucoma and buphthalmia in the rabbit, Prog Clin Biol Res 247:397–406, 1987.

Burrows AM, et al: Development of ocular hypertension in congenitally buphthalmic rabbits, Lab Anim Sci 45:443–449, 1995.

Hanna BL, et al: Recessive buphthalmos in the rabbit, Genetics 47:519–529, 1962.

Knepper PA, et al: Ultrastructural alterations in the aqueous outflow pathway of adult buphthalmic rabbits, Exp Eye Res 52:525–533, 1991.

Vareilles P, et al: Comparison of the effects of timolol and other adrenergic agents on intraocular pressure in the rabbit, Invest Ophthalmol Vis Sci 16:987–996, 1977.

CROSS-REFERENCES TO OTHER SECTIONS

Cataracts
Cherry Eye
Conjunctival Disorders
Dacryocystitis and Epiphora
Uveitis

AUTHORS: **THOMAS M. DONNELLY AND JEFFREY SMITH**

EDITOR: **DAVID VELLA**

RABBITS

Cardiovascular Disease

BASIC INFORMATION

DEFINITION

Cardiovascular disease refers to any disease process primarily involving the heart and/or blood vessels.

SYNONYMS

Cardiovascular disease is being diagnosed more commonly in rabbits. Congestive heart failure, both right- and left-sided, valvular disease, myocardial disease, congenital disease, vascular disease, arteriosclerosis, and atherosclerosis all have been described in the rabbit.

EPIDEMIOLOGY

SPECIES, AGE, SEX Incidence of acquired cardiovascular disease increases with age.

GENETICS AND BREED PREDISPOSITION

- Giant breeds are more prone to dilated cardiomyopathy.
- Arteriosclerosis has a higher incidence in New Zealand white rabbits and a lower incidence in Dutch rabbits.
- Some laboratory strains have been bred with a predisposition to develop atherosclerosis as research models (e.g., Watanabe heritable hyperlipidemic rabbit, St. Thomas's Hospital rabbit strain).

RISK FACTORS

- Genetics
- Dietary factors: cholesterol levels >0.5%, peanut oil in the diet, high levels of dietary saturated fat, vitamin E deficiency
- Chronic stress (e.g., from overcrowding)
- Hypertension
- Hypercalcemia secondary to hypervitaminosis D or chronic renal insufficiency
- Infection with pathogens that may cause cardiovascular disease (e.g., *Pasteurella multocida, Staphylococcus* spp., *Salmonella* spp., *Clostridium piriformis, Streptococcus viridans,* Coronavirus, and *Encephalitozoon cuniculi* [see Encephalitozoonosis])
- Doxorubicin has been shown experimentally to cause cardiac disease.
- Xylazine anesthesia can induce cardiomyopathy.

CONTAGION AND ZOONOSIS

- Very low risk of spread of infectious cardiac disease; cardiovascular lesions develop only occasionally after acute infection
- *Salmonella* spp. and *E. cuniculi* have some zoonotic risk.

ASSOCIATED CONDITIONS AND DISORDERS Rabbits recovering from *P. multocida, Salmonella* spp., and *C. piriformis* infections occasionally develop cardiomyopathy.

CLINICAL PRESENTATION

DISEASE FORMS/SUBTYPES Cardiovascular disease can be a life-threatening condition in some rabbits; in others, there may be few or no outward clinical signs.

HISTORY, CHIEF COMPLAINT

- Weakness
- Lethargy
- Weight loss (see Anorexia)
- Poor exercise tolerance
- Dyspnea
- Collapsing episodes
- Failure to grow
- Distended abdomen

PHYSICAL EXAM FINDINGS

- Mucosal color revealing cyanosis (assessment difficult in many breeds)
- Cold extremities (ear tips and toes)
- Increased capillary refill time
- Weak and irregular pulse
- Tachypnea
- Pulmonary crackles and wheezes
- Murmur
- Arrhythmia
- Exophthalmos
- Muffled heart sounds
- Ascites
- Peripheral edema

Not all findings will be present, and some signs such as ascites are rarely seen in rabbits.

ETIOLOGY AND PATHOPHYSIOLOGY

- Coronary arterial circulation is limited; this may predispose rabbits to myocardial ischemia.
- Hypercalcemia secondary to hypervitaminosis D or chronic renal insufficiency can lead to mineralization of the aortic arch.

DIAGNOSIS

DIFFERENTIAL DIAGNOSIS

- Respiratory disease (see Lower Respiratory Tract Disorders)
- Thoracic abscess

- Thymoma (see Thymoma)
- Other thoracic neoplasia

INITIAL DATABASE

- Radiography: cardiomegaly is the most common finding; pulmonary edema, plural effusion, and ascites are seen less frequently
- Echocardiography: most useful for the diagnosis of cardiac masses, pericardial effusions, and valvular disease, and for differentiation between different forms of cardiomyopathy
- Electrocardiography (see Electrocardiography, Sec. II): may be normal in the presence of cardiac disease; most useful for diagnosing arrhythmias; normal sinus rhythm seen in rabbits
- Blood pressure measurement: hypertension can occur secondary to noncardiac conditions such as chronic renal insufficiency
- Hematology: usually normal
- Biochemistry: sometimes normal. In cases of secondary hepatocellular swelling, alkaline phosphatase, aspartate transaminase, and alanine transaminase values may be moderately raised. Prerenal azotemia is seen when glomerular filtration rate is reduced.
- Pleural fluid cytologic examination and chemistry
- Abdominal fluid cytologic examination and chemistry

ADVANCED OR CONFIRMATORY TESTING

- Doppler echocardiography
- Magnetic resonance imaging
- Computed tomography

TREATMENT

THERAPEUTIC GOALS

- Remove underlying cause if possible.
- Provide supportive care to minimize clinical signs.
- Provide balanced therapeutic therapy to reduce rate of progression of the condition.
  - To extend and improve the patient's quality of life

ACUTE GENERAL TREATMENT

- Diuretics (e.g., furosemide 1-10 mg/kg q 8-12 h IM, IV to reduce pulmonary edema and/or reduce ventricular end-diastolic volume)
- Angiotensin-converting enzyme (ACE) inhibitors (e.g., benazepril 0.25-0.5 mg/kg q 24 h PO)
- Coronary vasodilators (e.g., nitroglycerin 2% ointment ≈1 mm/kg applied topically to the inner ear)
- Oxygen therapy (delivered via chamber, tent, face mask, or nasal catheter)
- Thoracocentesis to remove any significant effusions
- Restricted movement
- Monitoring of temperature for hypothermia and hyperthermia
- Supportive care and treatment of any secondary gastrointestinal hypomotility
- Midazolam 0.1-0.2 mg/kg IM to control stress

CHRONIC TREATMENT

- Benazepril 0.25-0.5 mg/kg q 24 h PO
- Furosemide 0.3-4 mg/kg q 8-12 h PO
- Pimobendan 0.1-0.3 mg/kg q 12 h PO for its inotropic and vasodilator effects
- Digoxin 0.003-0.030 mg/kg q 12-48 h PO (do not use with renal insufficiency)

DRUG INTERACTIONS

Benazepril, furosemide, and pimobendan combinations may have a clinically deleterious hypotensive effect.

POSSIBLE COMPLICATIONS

Hypotension with combination drug therapy. Occasionally, sole benazepril therapy can have a hypotensive effect.

RECOMMENDED MONITORING

- Monitor respiration rate and effort, body weight, and blood pressure monthly for the first 4 months. If on benazepril, monitor blood pressure after 3 days or when any deterioration in condition occurs.
- Repeat full workup if patient destabilizes.
- Perform electrocardiography if arrhythmias are present.
- Measure digoxin serum levels after 10 days of therapy. Significant individual variation has been noted. Use 0.5 to 2.0 ng/mL as a guide to therapeutic levels.

PROGNOSIS AND OUTCOME

Cardiac disease is rarely cured. It is most commonly managed through a balanced therapeutic approach.

PEARLS & CONSIDERATIONS

COMMENTS

Most often, treatment and management of cardiovascular disease in rabbits are extrapolated and modified from canine and feline medicine.

PREVENTION

- Minimize stress.
- Provide an appropriate diet.

SUGGESTED READING

Reusch B: Investigation and management of cardiovascular disease in rabbits, In Practice 27:418–425, 2005.

CROSS-REFERENCES TO OTHER SECTIONS

Anorexia
Encephalitozoonosis
Lower Respiratory Tract Disorders
Thymoma
Electrocardiography (Section II)

AUTHOR: **AIDAN RAFTERY**

EDITOR: **DAVID VELLA**

RABBITS

Cataracts

BASIC INFORMATION

DEFINITION

Any opacity, regardless of size, of the lens or its capsule is termed a *cataract.* A cataract results from a change in lens protein composition or lens fiber arrangement.

SYNONYM

Lens opacity

SPECIAL SPECIES CONSIDERATIONS

- Both congenital and acquired cataracts have been reported in rabbits.
- Cataracts can occur unilaterally or bilaterally.
- Many cataracts are idiopathic.
- An important cause of cataract in rabbits is infection with *Encephalitozoon cuniculi* (see Encephalitozoonosis).

EPIDEMIOLOGY

SPECIES, AGE, SEX

- The reported incidence of cataracts in laboratory rabbits is 4.0%. Males and females are equally affected.
- Older rabbits exhibit cataracts more often than young rabbits.
- Congenital cataracts (usually nuclear lenticular opacities) may be seen occasionally in a litter of rabbits. Based on research in laboratory rabbit fetuses, the prevalence of spontaneously occurring congenital cataracts is 3.6%.

GENETICS AND BREED PREDISPOSITION

- Based on toxicologic studies in laboratory rabbits, a significant difference in the incidence of cataracts exists between albino rabbits (e.g., New Zealand white; incidence 5.7%) and pigmented rabbits (e.g., New Zealand red; incidence 1.1%).
- The incidence of cataracts seen in toxicologic studies is consistent with an autosomal recessive mode of inheritance, but additional studies are needed to confirm the mode(s) of inheritance.

RISK FACTORS

- Major
  - Anterior uveitis associated with *E. cuniculi*
- Minor
  - Retinal disease
  - Lens luxation

CONTAGION AND ZOONOSIS *E. cuniculi* is considered a potential zoonotic disease.

ASSOCIATED CONDITIONS AND DISORDERS

- Ocular lesions develop after deposition of *E. cuniculi* spores in the lens. Sporulation leads to cataract formation, and subsequent disruption of the lens capsule evokes lens protein–induced phacoclastic uveitis.
- Intrauterine transmission of *E. cuniculi* is theorized to be the cause of intraocular development of the parasite because a mature lens capsule is considered too thick for microsporidia to penetrate, but during in utero development, the lens capsule is very thin or even absent.
- *Note:* Uveitis can occur with or without the presence of cataracts. The lesion typically is raised and off-white in the stroma of the iris.

CLINICAL PRESENTATION

HISTORY, CHIEF COMPLAINT Generally, owners describe a cloudy, white pupil. Occasionally, they may report vision disturbance.

PHYSICAL EXAM FINDINGS

- Opacity of the lens (unilateral or bilateral) with any or all of the following:
  - Anterior uveitis
  - Glaucoma
  - Lens subluxation or luxation (rare)
  - Retinal degeneration or detachment (rare)

ETIOLOGY AND PATHOPHYSIOLOGY

- Regardless of origin, all cataracts occur through a change in lens protein composition or lens fiber arrangement:
  - Inherited (rare)
  - Secondary to intraocular disease (common)
    - Uveitis (see Uveitis)
    - Glaucoma
  - Trauma to lens: blunt or penetrating (occasional)
  - Age-related (occasional)
  - Radiation therapy: injury when primary beam is near or on the globe
  - Electric shock
- Not all cataracts are progressive.

DIAGNOSIS

DIFFERENTIAL DIAGNOSIS

- Nuclear/lenticular sclerosis
  - Normal aging change
  - Usually seen in animals >6 years old
  - Does not cause vision loss
  - Center of lens becomes opalescent to hazy, but tapetal reflection in pupil is still visible, versus cataracts, which obstruct this reflection.
- Diseases causing diffuse corneal edema (bluish-white opacity on cornea, not in pupil; may obstruct ability to see the pupil), including
  - Glaucoma
  - Corneal endothelial degeneration or dystrophy
- Diseases causing secondary cataracts
  - Anterior uveitis
    - Cataracts are due to inflammation from trauma to lens
    - *E. cuniculi* anterior uveitis
    - Idiopathic uveitis
  - Lens luxation or subluxation
  - Retinal degeneration or detachment

INITIAL DATABASE

- Complete ophthalmic examination, including
  - Dazzle response
  - Evaluation of pupil size and symmetry and pupillary light reflexes
  - Intraocular pressure (IOP) measurement to rule out glaucoma
    - Normal intraocular pressure in rabbits is 15 to 23 mm Hg.
  - After IOP assessment (assuming normal result), dilate pupil with 1% tropicamide.
  - Use penlight or transilluminator to characterize the cataract and evaluate for concurrent uveitis.
  - Fundic (posterior segment) examination using indirect or direct ophthalmoscopy

ADVANCED OR CONFIRMATORY TESTING

- CBC, chemistry profile, and urinalysis to rule out systemic disease as either a cause of contributor of cataracts and/or to assess patient before considering referral for possible cataract surgery
- Electroretinogram (ERG) to assess retinal function (conducted by veterinary ophthalmologist before cataract surgery). Ocular ultrasound may be indicated at the same time.

TREATMENT

THERAPEUTIC GOALS

- Early immature cataracts do not require treatment.
- Progressive immature, mature, and hypermature cataracts should be surgically removed to
  - Restore vision (i.e., cataract surgery)
  - Prevent secondary uveitis and glaucoma

ACUTE GENERAL TREATMENT

- Treat associated uveitis with topical mydriatics (atropine 1% q 6-8 h until pupillary dilation is achieved and once daily thereafter) and topical antiinflammatories (nonsteroidal antiinflammatory drugs [NSAIDs]: flurbiprofen, diclofenac, or ketorolac q 6-8 h; corticosteroid: prednisolone acetate 1% or dexamethasone 0.1% q 6-8 h; frequency depends on severity of disease).
- Referral for cataract surgery if cataract is vision threatening and animal is systemically stable:
  - Cataract surgery requires preliminary posterior segment assessment.
  - Phacoemulsification (ultrasonic lens fragmentation) is performed to remove the cataract.
- If cataracts or uveitis is due to *E. cuniculi*, also treat with oral fenbendazole (20 mg/kg PO q 24 h × 28 d). This may not reverse ocular signs but may assist in the treatment of systemic infection.

CHRONIC TREATMENT

- After cataract surgery, treat as directed by the veterinary ophthalmologist:
  - Topical antibiotics and antiinflammatories (e.g., ofloxacin q 12 h × 7 d and dexamethasone 0.1% q 6-8 h × 4-5 d) (see Acute General Treatment above for drugs and doses)
  - Exercise restriction for 2 weeks

- Antiinflammatory therapy may be continued in a decreasing fashion for months or, in some cases, indefinitely.
- Frequent reevaluation of IOP, retinal examination, and inflammation control
- If cataract surgery is not an option:
  - Monitor cataracts for progression and treat associated uveitis with topical antiinflammatory drugs over the long term. If uveitis is due to *E. cuniculi*, also treat with fenbendazole (20 mg/kg PO q 24 h × 28 d).
  - Use IOP-lowering drugs in combination with antiinflammatories if secondary glaucoma develops.
  - Enucleation or evisceration of end-stage, blind, painful globes

DRUG INTERACTIONS

Use caution when applying any antiinflammatory agent to the cornea in the presence of corneal infection or ulceration.

POSSIBLE COMPLICATIONS

Without cataract surgery, the following can occur:

- Uveitis
- Glaucoma
- Blindness

After cataract surgery, the following can occur:

- Uveitis
- Glaucoma
- Corneal ulceration
- Surgical wound/incisional dehiscence
- Intraocular infection
- Retinal detachment
- Lens capsule proliferative fibrosis
- Corneal endothelial degeneration and secondary corneal edema

RECOMMENDED MONITORING

- Without cataract surgery, monitor for cataract progression and secondary complications every 2 to 4 months, or more or less frequently depending on the extent of cataract, the rate of cataract development, and the presence or absence of associated ocular complications.
- After cataract surgery, monitor according to recommendations of the veterinary ophthalmologist, which generally involve the following:
  - Reevaluations at postoperative weeks 2, 8, and 20
  - Long-term follow-up every 6 to 12 months for life
  - In addition to routine ophthalmic examinations, Schirmer tear test, IOP, menace response, and pupillary light reflexes should be evaluated each time the animal is presented to the veterinarian.

PROGNOSIS AND OUTCOME

- Rate of cataract progression is variable depending on cause and location of the cataract and age of the animal.
  - *E. cuniculi* cataracts and/or phacoclastic uveitis is an ocular emergency that must be treated immediately to save sight.
- Success of cataract surgery (i.e., phacoemulsification), as determined by a positive visual outcome, depends on concurrent disease. Without phacoclastic uveitis, 90% positive outcome; with phacoclastic uveitis, 50% positive outcome
- Success is increased with early referral (i.e., before animal is blind) and surgery, and with diligent postoperative monitoring and treatment.

CONTROVERSY

- Use of topical ophthalmic corticosteroids in rabbits is controversial owing to systemic absorption and potential side effects.
- Topical corticosteroids are more effective than NSAIDs in reducing inflammation associated with uveitis.

PEARLS & CONSIDERATIONS

COMMENTS

Evaluate any rabbit presenting with cataracts for *E. cuniculi* infection. In the author's experience, any rabbit presenting with *E. cuniculi* cataract/uveitis is at significant risk of developing encephalomeningitis and should be treated systemically for encephalitozoonosis (fenbendazole 20 mg/kg PO q 24 h × 28 d).

CLIENT EDUCATION

- It is essential that clients understand that not all cataracts are progressive.
- If a cataract is progressive, the client must make a decision with regard to surgery.
- Although surgery is associated with some risks, not opting for surgery is associated with risks of lens-induced uveitis, secondary glaucoma, retinal detachment, and ocular pain.

SUGGESTED READINGS

Felchle LM, et al: Phacoemulsification for the management of *Encephalitozoon cuniculi*–induced phacoclastic uveitis in a rabbit. Vet Ophthalmol 5:211–215, 2002.

Munger RJ, et al: Spontaneous cataracts in laboratory rabbits. Vet Ophthalmol 5:177–181, 2002.

Stiles J, et al: *Encephalitozoon cuniculi* in the lens of a rabbit with phacoclastic uveitis: confirmation and treatment. Vet Comp Ophthalmol 7:233–238, 1997.

CROSS-REFERENCES TO OTHER SECTIONS

Encephalitozoonosis
Uveitis

AUTHORS: **THOMAS M. DONNELLY AND CAMERON J.G. WHITTAKER**

EDITOR: **DAVID VELLA**

RABBITS

Cherry Eye

BASIC INFORMATION

DEFINITION

Cherry eye describes protrusion of a red tissue mass from the medial angle of the eye. This clinical condition is similar to cherry eye in dogs and is caused by prolapse of the deep gland of the third eyelid.

SYNONYMS

- Protrusion, prolapse, or eversion of the:
  - Deep lacrimal gland of the third eyelid
  - Deep gland of the nictitating membrane
  - Harderian gland

SPECIAL SPECIES CONSIDERATIONS

- The third eyelid (nictitating membrane) in rabbits is fairly prominent

and has a large, deep and a tiny superficial gland associated with it. The superficial gland of the third eyelid of the rabbit is a few millimeters long and lies against the convex surface of the slender, curved cartilage within the third eyelid.
- Other orbital glands include the lacrimal and accessory lacrimal glands, but these glands are not associated with the third eyelid and do not prolapse.
- The deep gland of the third eyelid prolapses commonly. Whereas the condition resembles cherry eye in the dog, a deep gland of the third eyelid is absent in dogs.
- The superficial gland of the third eyelid is often designated as the "nictitans gland." The deep gland of the third eyelid is also known as the *harderian gland.* It is:
  - A large, solid pyramidal gland that lies medially in the orbit
  - Composed of two definite units: a small dorsal white lobe and a more bulky ventral pink lobe. Despite differences in gross appearance, the histologic structure of the two lobes is similar. It is the pink lower lobe of the harderian gland that is seen in prolapse; that is why the protruding mass is typically red in color.

EPIDEMIOLOGY

SPECIES, AGE, SEX
- No known age or sex predisposition
- Reported cases are generally seen in rabbits younger than 2 years of age.

ASSOCIATED CONDITIONS AND DISORDERS
- Possible keratitis as a result of failure to blink well
- Exposure conjunctivitis
- Epiphora with facial wetting

CLINICAL PRESENTATION

HISTORY, CHIEF COMPLAINT Owners often describe the appearance of the prolapsed ocular gland as sudden.

PHYSICAL EXAM FINDINGS

- A 1- to 2-cm ovoid, pink to red mass covered with fine blood vessels is seen protruding from the medial angle of the eye.
- The mass does not appear to cause pain or distress.

ETIOLOGY AND PATHOPHYSIOLOGY

- The pathogenesis has not been determined but may be associated with fascial attachment abnormalities and/or inflammation of the gland.
- The protruding gland, which extends beyond the leading edge of the third eyelid, becomes abraded and dry, resulting in secondary inflammation and swelling.
- Protrusion is generally unilateral.
- Adenitis may be found on histologic examination.

DIAGNOSIS

DIFFERENTIAL DIAGNOSIS

- Pink or red masses
  - Neoplasia of the harderian gland or the superficial gland of the third eyelid presenting with third eyelid protrusion
- White masses
  - Retrobulbar fat prolapse: fat rabbits are also prone to protrusion of retrobulbar fat around the eye, including the area of the third eyelid.
  - Protrusion of the third eyelid secondary to retrobulbar neoplasia or inflammation
- Rare conditions
  - Third eyelid protrusion with Horner's syndrome
  - Hyperplasia of the lymphoid follicles of the third eyelid

INITIAL DATABASE

- Minimum database findings are nonspecific and generally normal.
- Cytology of the protruding gland may reveal nonspecific inflammation (adenitis).
- Imaging studies (ocular or orbital ultrasound, CT scan, MRI) are not necessary to diagnose this condition but may be indicated as part of the preoperative workup if the animal is older, or if concurrent disease is suspected.

ADVANCED OR CONFIRMATORY TESTING

In older rabbits, consider fine-needle aspiration (FNA) or biopsy to rule out neoplasia.

TREATMENT

THERAPEUTIC GOALS

- Replace the prolapsed gland.
- Topical treatment does not resolve the condition.

ACUTE GENERAL TREATMENT

- The condition generally is not painful and strong analgesia is not required.
- Provide lubrication and hydration to prolapsed gland (e.g., paraffin-based ophthalmic ointment or artificial tears applied frequently until surgery).
- Reduce inflammation and edema of the conjunctiva (e.g., topical antibiotics such as fusidic acid, chloramphenicol, or ciprofloxacin q 6 h) with or without topical corticosteroids (prednisolone acetate 1% q 6 h) or topical nonsteroidal antiinflammatory drugs (NSAIDs; flurbiprofen, diclofenac, or ketorolac q 4-6 h, depending on severity of inflammation).

CHRONIC TREATMENT

- Surgery
  - Return the prolapsed gland to a deeper position using the "pocket" technique described for cherry eye in dogs.
  - This procedure is difficult in the rabbit.
  - Repeat prolapse is common.
  - Refer to veterinary ophthalmologist.

DRUG INTERACTIONS

Use caution when applying any antiinflammatory agent to the cornea in the presence of corneal infection.

PROGNOSIS AND OUTCOME

- Prognosis is guarded.
- Warn owner that repeat prolapse can occur.
- Chronic protrusions are more difficult to replace.

CONTROVERSY

Use of topical ophthalmic corticosteroids in rabbits is controversial owing to systemic absorption and potential side effects.

PEARLS & CONSIDERATIONS

COMMENTS

- The harderian gland is wrapped behind the eyeball and is phylogenetically and anatomically associated with the third eyelid. It is generally horseshoe shaped and situated deep within the orbit. The single excretory duct opens at the base of the third eyelid, and the secretion provides lubrication for the edges of the eyelid.
- It is believed that the harderian gland has a significant function in social behavior. The secretion of the gland is a complex mixture of lipids, protein, and the pigment protoporphyrin.

SUGGESTED READINGS

Donnelly TM: Pink mass on the dorsomedial aspect of a rabbit's eye: cherry eye or prolapse of the deep gland of the nictitating membrane, Lab Anim (NY) 31:23–24, 2002.

Janssens G, et al: Bilateral prolapse of the deep gland of the third eyelid in a rabbit: diagnosis and treatment, Lab Anim Sci 49:105–109, 1999.

AUTHORS: **THOMAS M. DONNELLY AND JEFFREY SMITH**

EDITOR: **DAVID VELLA**

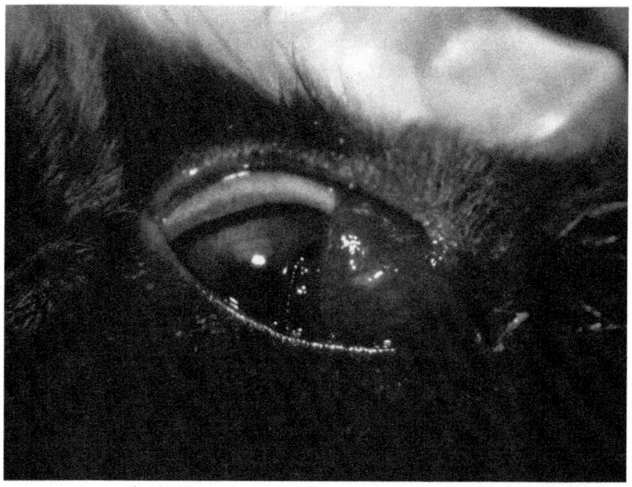

Cherry Eye Prolapse of the deep gland of the third eyelid (harderian gland) in a rabbit. The prolapsed gland is typically pink or red. Treatment requires returning the prolapsed gland to a deeper position using the "pocket" technique described for cherry eye in dogs. In severe cases, the gland needs to be surgically removed. *(Photo courtesy Jörg Mayer, The University of Georgia, Athens.)*

RABBITS

Coccidiosis

BASIC INFORMATION

DEFINITION

Coccidiosis is a hepatic or enteric disease caused by protozoan parasites of the subclass Coccidia, genus *Eimeria*. It is important to distinguish between infection by coccidia, which is common, and coccidiosis or overt disease, which is infrequent. Many rabbits are infected with coccidian parasites at least once during their life, and wild rabbits may be infected their entire lives with several species of coccidia that continually cycle through them, yet do not develop disease. Enhanced transmission of coccidia occurs when rabbits are brought together in large groups because of the rapid and direct life cycle of *Eimeria* species. Under these circumstances, coccidia cause disease. Consequently, coccidiosis is considered a major health problem in rabbits raised under intensive husbandry conditions.

SYNONYMS

- *Eimeria stiedai:* The spelling "stiedai" is used even though the original description used "stiedae." It was named for Ludwig Stieda, and according to the International Rules of Zoological Nomenclature, the genitive ending must be used. "-ae" would indicate that the species was named for a woman and "-ai" for a man.
- *Rabbit dysentery* is often used by rabbit breeders to describe intestinal coccidiosis.
- Intestinal coccidian:
  - *E. coecicola* (syn *E. oryctolagi*)
  - *E. irresidua* (syn *E. elongata*)
  - *E. media* (syn *E. flavescens*)
  - *E. intestinalis* (syn *E. piriformis, E. agnosta*)
  - *E. perforans* (syn *E. nana, E. lugdunumensis*)

SPECIAL SPECIES CONSIDERATIONS

- More than 12 *Eimeria* species are found in the rabbit:
  - *E. coecicola, E. exiqua, E. intestinalis, E. irresidua, E. magna, E. matsubayashii, E. media, E. nagpurensis, E. perforans, E. piriformis,* and *E. steidai* occur in domestic and wild rabbits.
  - *E. neoleporis* and *E. roobroucki* have been reported only in wild rabbits.

EPIDEMIOLOGY

SPECIES, AGE, SEX

- Intestinal coccidiosis
  - Suckling rabbits up to 16 days old are not susceptible to infection.
  - Young, recently weaned (e.g., 5- to 6-week-old) rabbits are most susceptible.
  - With increasing age, fecal oocyst output decreases progressively. It reaches a low level in animals older than 4 months but does not disappear completely without treatment.
  - Adults rarely develop clinical disease.

GENETICS AND BREED PREDISPOSITION No breed or gender susceptibility has been detected.

RISK FACTORS

- Most common in breeding colonies
- Poor hygiene results in large infective oocyst dose challenge.
- 1 to 4 months old: the overwhelming determinant of oocyst count is host age, with six species being most abundant in rabbits up to 4 months of age
- Immune suppressed rabbits of any age

CONTAGION AND ZOONOSIS

- Spores are infective 1 to 4 days after being passed in the feces and remain infective on soil or vegetation for several years.
- *Eimeria* species found in rabbits have not been shown to infect humans.

GEOGRAPHY AND SEASONALITY

- Geography
  - *E. irresidua, E. media,* and *E. perforans* occur throughout the world and are common.
  - *E. magna* occurs throughout the world but is uncommon.
  - *E. piriformis* is common in Australia.
- Seasonal differences are often detected in fecal oocyst counts of adults and young animals:
  - Peak intensity appears to occur from late spring to summer.

ASSOCIATED CONDITIONS AND DISORDERS

- Mixed infections of different *Eimeria* spp. are common.

- Eggs of the parasitic nematodes (see Endoparasites) (e.g., *Passalurus ambiguus*) are often seen in fecal samples of rabbits with heavy coccidial infections.

CLINICAL PRESENTATION

DISEASE FORMS/SUBTYPES

- Hepatic
  - Subclinical disease is common.
  - Acute mortality is associated with large infective oocyst dose.
  - When clinical disease is present, the signs are variable.
- Intestinal
  - Subclinical disease is common in adult rabbits. Pathogenicity varies with:
  - Species of *Eimeria*
    - All intestinal species of *Eimeria* appear to be pathogenic in young rabbits.
    - In adult rabbits, *E. coecicola, E. irresidua,* and *E. magna* are highly pathogenic; *E. piriformis* and *E. media* are moderately pathogenic; and *E. perforans* is mildly pathogenic.
  - Target organ
    - *E. perforans, E. irresidua,* and *E. intestinalis* may develop in the small intestine.
    - *E. magna* and *E. media* may develop in the small and the large intestine.
    - *E. coecicola* and *E. piriformis* may develop in the cecum.
  - Immune status of the rabbit
  - Infective oocyst dose

HISTORY, CHIEF COMPLAINT

- Hepatic
  - Weight loss
  - Stunting
  - Abdominal enlargement
  - Lethargy
  - Anorexia (see Anorexia)
  - Death
- Intestinal
  - Diarrhea sometimes with mucus and/or blood
  - Weight loss
  - Stunting
  - Lethargy
  - Anorexia (see Anorexia)
  - Death

PHYSICAL EXAM FINDINGS

- Hepatic
  - Ascites
  - Jaundice
  - Hepatomegaly
- Intestinal
  - Dehydration
  - Diarrhea
  - Occasionally intussusception and/or rectal prolapse

ETIOLOGY AND PATHOPHYSIOLOGY

- Hepatic coccidiosis
  - The liver is enlarged owing to papillary hyperplasia of the bile duct epithelium (and gallbladder occasionally) with different developmental stages of coccidia within bile ducts.
  - Acute cases may show numerous miliary hepatic abscesses.
  - Chronic cases develop a fibrotic response around affected ducts.
  - Other organs are not infected.
- Intestinal coccidiosis
  - In most cases, little or no reaction occurs.
  - When clinical disease occurs, a mixed inflammatory cell response is seen in the intestinal mucosa, with multifocal areas of intestinal necrosis, ulceration, edema, and hemorrhage.
  - Depending on the species of *Eimeria,* sporozoites may be found in the mesenteric lymph nodes and spleen (e.g., *E. coecicola* sporozoites present; *E. intestinalis* sporozoites absent).

DIAGNOSIS

DIFFERENTIAL DIAGNOSIS

- Hepatic
  - Adult rabbits
    - Toxin-induced hepatitis (e.g., drug, plant)
    - Chronic bacterial hepatitis (e.g., *Salmonella* spp.)
    - Chronic helminthic hepatitis (e.g., *Cysticercus pisiformis*)
  - Juvenile rabbits
    - Toxin-induced hepatitis (e.g., drug, plant)
    - Acute bacterial hepatitis (e.g., *Clostridium piliforme*)
- Intestinal
  - Mucoid enteropathy; however, it generally occurs in rabbits older than 10 weeks
  - Bacterial enteritis (e.g., clostridial enterotoxemia, colibacillosis, Tyzzer's disease, *C. piliforme*)
  - Viral enteritis (e.g., rotavirus, adenovirus, coronavirus and parvovirus have been isolated from young rabbits with diarrhea)

INITIAL DATABASE

- Detection of oocysts on examination of fecal smears or flotations. It is essential to distinguish between the different species of *Eimeria* because the oocysts look similar but their pathogenicity varies.
- Examination of sporulated oocysts is necessary to distinguish between certain intestinal *Eimeria* spp. Sporulation may take around three days.
- The prepatent period for intestinal *Eimeria* spp. is 14 to 18 days. In acute infection, oocysts may not be present.
- Blood biochemistry may demonstrate raised hepatic enzymes in hepatic coccidiosis.

ADVANCED OR CONFIRMATORY TESTING

- Demonstration of typical hepatic lesions (bile duct hyperplasia) on histopathologic examination is diagnostic for hepatic coccidiosis.
- Enzyme-linked immunosorbent assays (ELISAs) for detecting serum antibody in rabbits with coccidiosis have been developed experimentally but are not routinely available in diagnostic laboratories.

TREATMENT

THERAPEUTIC GOALS

- Eliminate the protozoa or slow their multiplication until immunity develops.
- Limit contamination of the environment with infective oocysts.
- Provide supportive care to optimize survival.

ACUTE GENERAL TREATMENT

- Anticoccidial drugs work best in the early stages of the disease:
  - Sulfonamides have the advantage that they are often also effective against secondary bacterial pathogens. Trimethoprim/sulfamethoxazole 30 mg/kg q 24 h PO; sulfadimethoxine 50 mg/kg first dose, then 25 mg/kg q 24 h PO
  - Toltrazuril (25 mg/kg daily for 2 days PO, then repeat after 5 days) is a highly effective anticoccidial treatment.
- Provide supportive care for dehydration:
  - Correct dehydration over 12 to 24 hours. Fluids (see Fluid Therapy in Rabbits and Rodents, Sec. II) can be given subcutaneously, intravenously, or intraosseously (see Intraosseous Catheters, Sec. II), depending on the patient. Crystalloids or colloid combinations are given depending on the condition of the patient.
  - In collapsed rabbits, track the response by monitoring blood pressure.
- Provide nutritional support by syringe feeding or via a nasogastric tube. Commercial products are available that provide effective nutritional support with a fiber content that helps promote normal gut function.
- Prokinetic drugs help normalize gut motility (e.g., metoclopramide 0.5-1 mg/kg q 6-8 h PO, SC; cisapride 0.5-1 mg/kg q 6-8 h PO)

- H2 histamine-receptor antagonists (e.g., ranitidine 2-5 mg/kg q 12 h PO) may stimulate gut motility but may also reduce the risk of gastric ulceration.

CHRONIC TREATMENT

- Vaccination of entire litters of rabbits by spraying a vaccine strain of oocysts into the nesting box has been shown effective in clinical trials of intensive production farm–reared rabbits.
- The vaccine strain is a precocious line (shortened life cycle) of oocysts derived from field isolates that display immunogenicity but are not pathogenic when administered at the correct oral dose.
- Immunization is quick and efficient because it does not require handling of rabbits.

POSSIBLE COMPLICATIONS

- Resistance to coccidiostats is seen increasingly in intensive production farm–reared rabbits.
- Intussusception subsequent to hyperperistalsis induced by coccidial infection of the intestines is reported in young rabbits.

RECOMMENDED MONITORING

- For breeding colonies with recurrent coccidiosis, investigate all cases of enteritis in young rabbits to ensure that preventive measures are working.
- Because the prepatent period for *E. stiedai* is 21 to 37 days, monitoring feces for oocysts is unlikely to be effective.

PROGNOSIS AND OUTCOME

Severe clinical signs carry a grave prognosis, especially for hepatic coccidiosis. Less severe clinical signs have a better prognosis. Subclinical infections will result in natural immunity.

PEARLS & CONSIDERATIONS

COMMENTS

- Parasitism with coccidia (and nematodes) does not appear to be an important cause of mortality in adult rabbit populations.
- Jaundice and abdominal effusion in a 4- to 16-week-old rabbit are virtually pathognomonic for hepatic coccidiosis.
- Intestinal coccidiosis is often difficult to confirm in a single patient because clinical disease is often aggravated by the proliferation of opportunistic pathogens (e.g., bacteria, viruses).
- Examination of sporulated oocysts is necessary to distinguish between some intestinal *Eimeria* spp.

PREVENTION

- Control is achieved by prevention of exposure to infective oocysts:
  - Frequent cleaning of rabbit accommodation, feeding, and water containers
  - Exposure to 140°F (60°C) for 60 minutes or to 176°F (80°C) for 15 minutes renders ≈80% of *Eimeria* species oocysts incapable of sporulation. *E. irresidua* oocysts tolerate exposure to 176°F (80°C) for 60 minutes.
  - Efficient removal of feces daily (before oocysts become infective)
    - Change bedding litter frequently, and keep it dry.
  - Control vermin and flies that could serve as mechanical vectors.
  - Avoid fecal contamination of food.
  - Keep rabbits younger than 4 months old out of contaminated areas.
  - Where there is a problem in spite of good husbandry, prophylactic anticoccidials may be needed.
  - Because coccidiosis primarily affects young rabbits just after weaning (5- to 6-week-old animals), disease prevention must be initiated before weaning.

CLIENT EDUCATION

- Warn clients of risks of mechanical transfer.
- Emphasize reason for good hygiene practices.
- Remove young rabbits from infected does as early as possible.
- Stop breeding with known infected does.

SUGGESTED READINGS

Barriga OO, et al: Pathophysiology of hepatic coccidiosis in rabbits, Vet Parasitol 8:201–210, 1981.
Levine ND, et al: Coccidia of the Leporidae, J Eukaryot Microbiol 19:572–581, 1972.
Pakandl M: Coccidia of rabbit: a review, Folia Parasitol (Praha) 56:153–166, 2009.

CROSS-REFERENCES TO OTHER SECTIONS

Anorexia
Endoparasites
Hepatic Disorders
Intestinal Disorders
Intraosseous Catheters (Section II)
Fluid Therapy in Rabbits and Rodents (Section II)

AUTHORS: **AIDAN RAFTERY AND THOMAS M. DONNELLY**

EDITOR: **DAVID VELLA**

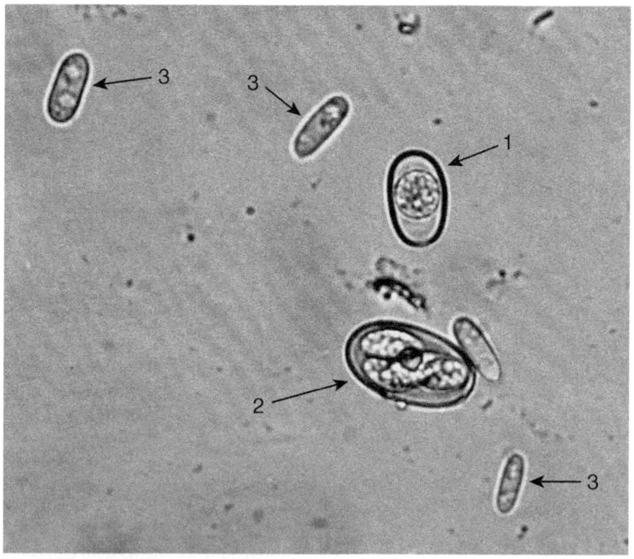

Coccidiosis Photomicrograph of a fecal floatation from a rabbit. *1,* Oocyst of intestinal *Eimeria* spp. Parasitologists identify Eimerian species by distinguishing morphologic features of the oocysts such as dimensions (length × width in μ), shape (e.g., ellipsoid, ovoid), wall (e.g., light yellow, colorless, light pink), micropyle (none, present, prominent), and residual body (none, variable, large). *2,* Egg of a parasitic nematode. *3,* The yeast *Cyniclomyces guttulatus* (previously *Saccharomycopsis guttulata*), which is a common and normal nonpathogenic inhabitant of the rabbit stomach and intestine. *(Photo courtesy Jörg Mayer, The University of Georgia, Athens.)*

Conjunctival Disorders

BASIC INFORMATION

DEFINITION

Conjunctivitis: inflammation of the conjunctiva, the vascular mucous membrane covering the anterior portion of the eye (bulbar portion), lining the eyelids and the nictitating membrane (palpebral portion)

Pseudopterygium: a rare acquired condition in which the conjunctiva grows across the cornea, usually leaving a very small opening in the center or fully covering the cornea

SYNONYMS

Conjunctivitis
- Red eye

Pseudopterygium
- Corneal occlusion syndrome
- Epicorneal, precorneal, or aberrant conjunctival membrane overgrowth
- Pseudosymblepharon

SPECIAL SPECIES CONSIDERATIONS

Conjunctivitis
- *Pasteurella multocida* is often considered the most common cause of conjunctivitis. However, in a survey of rabbits with conjunctivitis and dacryocystitis, when bacteria were isolated (in 78% of cases), *Staphylococcus* spp. were found in 48% of isolates and *Pasteurella* spp. were found in 12%.
- In healthy rabbits, bacteria have been recovered from 83% of animals. The most commonly recovered organisms are DNase-negative *Staphylococcus* spp. (57%), *Micrococcus* spp. (25%), and *Bacillus* spp. (19%).

Pseudopterygium
- Described only in rabbits
- A similar condition known as *pterygium* occurs in humans. However, in rabbits, the conjunctival overgrowth is not adherent to the corneal epithelium but lies on its surface, hence the name *pseudopterygium* (literally, "false pterygium").

EPIDEMIOLOGY

SPECIES, AGE, SEX

- Pseudopterygium is associated frequently with young (6 to 18 months) male rabbits.
- Most cases are reported in dwarf rabbits.

RISK FACTORS

Conjunctivitis
- Adnexal disease
- Trauma
- Hay dust
- Unsanitary conditions
  - Ammonia concentration >25 ppm is an ocular irritant that is often found in poorly ventilated rabbit farms.

Pseudopterygium
- No known risk factors.

CLINICAL PRESENTATION

HISTORY, CHIEF COMPLAINT

Conjunctivitis
- History of:
  - Previous treatment for dental disease
  - Nasal discharge
  - Previous upper respiratory tract infection
- Presenting complaint may include
  - No or mild clinical signs
  - Facial asymmetry, exophthalmos (usually in rabbits with tooth root abscesses)
  - Unilateral or bilateral alopecia, crusts, and/or matted fur in periocular area

Pseudopterygium
- Condition is conspicuous (overgrown conjunctiva covering the cornea).
- No pain is seen.

PHYSICAL EXAM FINDINGS

Conjunctivitis
- Conjunctival hyperemia
- Ocular discharge
- Chemosis (marked conjunctival edema)
- Facial pyoderma
- Dental disease

Pseudopterygium
- Fold of conjunctival tissue arising from the limbus
- Tissue is nonadherent to the cornea and may appear as a thin annulus or may cover a large portion of the ocular surface, even resulting in complete coverage of the corneal surface.
- Bilateral and symmetric

ETIOLOGY AND PATHOPHYSIOLOGY

Conjunctivitis
- Primary: infectious, environmental
- Secondary to an underlying ocular or systemic disease: tooth root disorders, glaucoma, uveitis (see Uveitis), neoplasia

Pseudopterygium
- Cause is not completely understood.

DIAGNOSIS

DIFFERENTIAL DIAGNOSIS

Conjunctivitis
- Attempt to distinguish primary conjunctivitis from inflammation secondary to ocular diseases:
  - Differentiate between conjunctival vessels and episcleral vessels; episcleral congestion indicates intraocular disease (e.g., glaucoma [see Buphthalmia and Glaucoma]), whereas conjunctival hyperemia may be a sign of primary conjunctivitis or intraocular disease.
- Unilateral condition with ocular pain and/or blepharospasm
  - Consider tooth root disorder, foreign body, or corneal injury/ulceration.
- Bilateral condition
  - Acute with severe eyelid edema: consider myxomatosis
  - Chronic; usually due to chronic upper respiratory tract infection or bilateral tooth root disorders (see Dental Disease)
- Epiphora (white discharge) confined to the medial canthus usually indicates dacryocystitis.

INITIAL DATABASE

Conjunctivitis
- History of exposure to chemical irritants
- Complete ophthalmic examination
- Schirmer tear test to rule out keratoconjunctivitis sicca (rare disease); reported normal values
  - 5.0 mm/min ± 2.5 in New Zealand White rabbits
  - 12.0 mm/min ± 2.5 in Netherlands Dwarf rabbits
- Test patency of nasolacrimal duct and rule out dacryocystitis:
  - Fluorescein dye solution applied to cornea: dye flows through the nasolacrimal system and reaches the external nares in approximately 10 seconds in normal rabbits
  - If no dye reaches external nares, perform nasolacrimal flush (see Dacryocystitis).
- Apply fluorescein stain to cornea to rule out ulcerative keratitis.
- Measure intraocular pressure to rule out glaucoma.
- Examine for signs of anterior uveitis (e.g., hypotony, aqueous flare, miosis).
- Perform thorough adnexal examination to rule out lid abnormalities (entropion, ectropion), lash abnormalities (distichiasis, trichiasis), and foreign bodies under nictitating membrane.
- Aerobic bacterial culture and sensitivity:
  - Consider with mucopurulent discharge.
  - Ideally take specimens before placing anything in the eye.

- Conjunctival cytologic examination may reveal a cause (e.g., eosinophilic keratitis) (rare).
- Conjunctival biopsy may be useful with mass lesions and immune-mediated disease and may help with chronic disease for which a definitive diagnosis has not been made.

ADVANCED OR CONFIRMATORY TESTING

Conjunctivitis

- Skull radiographs are obligatory to identify dental disease and nasal, sinus, or maxillary bone lesions, and, if present, to plan treatment strategies and monitor progression of treatment (see Dental Disease).
- To localize nasolacrimal duct obstruction and characterize associated lesions
  - CT or MRI is superior to radiography.
  - Dacryocystorhinography aids in localizing site of obstruction.
- Orbital ultrasonography aids in defining retrobulbar abscesses or neoplasia and the extent of the lesion.

TREATMENT

THERAPEUTIC GOAL

Treat any underlying disease that may be causing or exacerbating the condition (e.g., environment, dental disease, eyelid disorders).

ACUTE GENERAL TREATMENT

Conjunctivitis

- Usually treated as outpatient
  - If secondary to other disease, may require hospitalization while the underlying problem is diagnosed and treated
- Nasolacrimal duct flushing if obstruction is diagnosed or if inflamed (dacryocystitis)
  - Flushing of the duct often needs to be repeated, either daily for 2 to 3 consecutive days, or once every 3 to 4 days until irrigation produces a clear fluid.
  - Failure to keep ducts patent may result in scarring or permanent obstruction.
- Keep fur around face clean and dry.
- Initial treatment using broad-spectrum topical antibiotic or antibiotic based on results of Gram stain while awaiting culture results
  - Perform culture and sensitivity if patient is refractory to empirical treatment.
  - Apply triple antibiotic, chloramphenicol, gentamicin, or ciprofloxacin eye ointment q 6-12 h topically, depending on severity.
  - Systemic antibiotics are indicated in rabbits with tooth root abscess or upper respiratory infection as the cause of conjunctivitis.
- Topical nonsteroidal antiinflammatory agents (e.g., 0.03% flurbiprofen, 1% diclofenac) may help reduce inflammation and irritation.

Pseudopterygium

- Surgical correction is completed through a modified Arlt procedure. Introduced more than a century ago, the Arlt procedure (1903) is the classical enucleation method by which the conjunctiva is incised around the periphery of the cornea and dissected back. Conjunctival tissue is partially trimmed by sharp dissection into four quarters (divided in four along the horizontal and vertical axes), and the leading edge of each quadrant is sutured to the conjunctival fornix on the inside of the eyelids.
- If surgery is contemplated, the case should be referred to a veterinary ophthalmologist for treatment.

CHRONIC TREATMENT

Pseudopterygium

- Because of the likelihood that this disease is immune mediated, application of topical immune suppressants (e.g., cyclosporine, mitomycin C, steroid) appears effective in preventing recurrence. A limited number of cases have been reported.
  - Combination 0.1% topical dexamethasone and 0.2% cyclosporine ointments (3 cases) q 8 h × 7d, then q 12 h × 7d, then q 24 h × 14 d
  - Topical 0.4 mg/mL mitomycin C (3 cases) q 12 h × 28 d

DRUG INTERACTIONS

Conjunctivitis

- Never use topical corticosteroids if
  - Cornea retains fluorescein stain
  - Evidence of local or systemic bacterial infection

Pseudopterygium

- Topically administered immune suppressant drugs may result in systemic immune suppression and must be used with caution.

POSSIBLE COMPLICATIONS

Conjunctivitis

- Aggressive flushing of the nasolacrimal duct may cause temporary swelling of the periocular tissues. Swelling usually resolves within 12 to 48 hours.
- Topical aminoglycosides: may be irritating

RECOMMENDED MONITORING

Conjunctivitis: Recheck shortly after beginning of treatment (i.e., 5 to 7 days); then recheck as needed

PROGNOSIS AND OUTCOME

Conjunctivitis

- Prognosis is generally good with conjunctivitis not associated with rhinitis or dacryocystitis.
- Prognosis is good with mild conjunctivitis as part of upper respiratory tract infection (not pasteurellosis), although recurrence is common.
- Prognosis is poor with severe conjunctivitis associated with chronic pasteurellosis rhinitis ("snuffles"). Prolonged courses of antibiotics are often necessary, and recurrence is common (see Pasteurellosis).

Pseudopterygium

- Recurrence is common, and more than one surgery may be required.

PEARLS & CONSIDERATIONS

CLIENT EDUCATION

Conjunctivitis

- Warn clients that recurrence is common in patients with nasolacrimal obstruction (see Dacryocystitis and Epiphora). In many cases, acquisition of a second rabbit can be beneficial if the second rabbit grooms discharges from the affected rabbit's face.
- If ocular discharge is noted, instruct the client to clean the eyes and around the eyes before giving treatment.
  - Use sterile eyewash artificial tears in addition to hot compresses.
- If both solutions and ointments are prescribed, instruct the client to use the solution(s) before the ointment(s).
- If several solutions are prescribed, instruct the client to wait several minutes between treatments.
- Instruct the client to call for instructions if the condition worsens because this usually indicates that the condition may not be responsive or may be progressing, or that the animal may be having an adverse reaction to a prescribed medication.
- Inform client that an Elizabethan collar should be placed on the patient if self-trauma occurs.

SUGGESTED READINGS

Allgoewer I, et al: Aberrant conjunctival stricture and overgrowth in the rabbit, Vet Ophthalmol 11:18–22, 2008.
Cooper SC, et al: Conjunctival flora observed in 70 healthy domestic rabbits *(Oryctolagus cuniculus)*, Vet Rec 149:232–235, 2001.
Grinninger P, et al: Eosinophilic keratoconjunctivitis in two rabbits, Vet Ophthalmol 15:59–65, 2012.
Okuda H, et al: Conjunctival bacterial flora of the clinically normal New Zealand white rabbit, Lab Anim Sci 24:831–833, 1974.
Roze M, et al: Comparative morphology of epicorneal conjunctival membranes in rabbits and human pterygium, Vet Ophthalmol 4:171–174, 2001.

CROSS-REFERENCES TO OTHER SECTIONS

Buphthalmia and Glaucoma
Cataracts
Cherry Eye
Dacryocystitis and Epiphora
Dental Disease
Pasteurellosis
Uveitis

AUTHORS: **THOMAS M. DONNELLY AND JEFFREY SMITH**

EDITOR: **DAVID VELLA**

RABBITS

Cutaneous Masses

BASIC INFORMATION

DEFINITION

- Neoplasia arising from cells within the epidermis, dermis, subcutis, or skin adnexa. Cutaneous neoplasms may be benign or malignant. Malignant neoplasms may recur or metastasize. Tumorlike lesions are non-neoplastic masses that mimic a true neoplasm. Adenomas and carcinomas are epithelial in origin. Sarcomas are of connective tissue origin.
- In rabbits, malignant lymphoma frequently occurs in the cutis and subcutis without connection to the peripheral lymph nodes. (This neoplasm is discussed in Lymphosarcoma.)

SYNONYMS

- Trichoblastoma: basal cell tumor
- Collagenous hamartoma: collagenous nevus, fibroma
- Malignant peripheral nerve sheath tumor: neurofibrosarcoma

EPIDEMIOLOGY

RISK FACTORS

- In newborn, young juvenile, or immunosuppressed rabbits, viral-induced tumors may persist and metastasize, leading to the death of the animal.
- Biting arthropods (e.g., mosquitoes, fleas) transmit viral-induced tumors.

CONTAGION AND ZOONOSIS Lagomorph viruses that induce tumors are not transmissible to humans.

GEOGRAPHY AND SEASONALITY Viral-induced tumors most commonly occur during autumn.

CLINICAL PRESENTATION

DISEASE FORMS/SUBTYPES

- Benign tumors (in descending order of frequency)
  - Trichoblastoma: neoplasia arising from the outer root sheath of the hair follicle
  - Collagenous hamartoma: tumor-like lesion arising from dermal fibroblasts
  - Lipoma: neoplasia arising from adipocytes in the subcutis
  - Papilloma: viral or nonviral induced proliferation of the epidermis or outer root sheath epithelium
  - Trichoepithelioma: neoplasia arising from the hair follicle
  - Apocrine adenoma: neoplasia arising from sweat glands
  - Tricholemmoma: neoplasia arising from the hair follicle
- Malignant tumors (in descending order of frequency)
  - Myxosarcoma: neoplasia arising from fibroblast-like mesenchymal cells, embedded in a myxoid extracellular matrix
  - Malignant peripheral nerve sheath tumor: neoplasia arising from nerve sheaths
  - Fibrosarcoma: neoplasia arising from fibroblasts
  - Malignant melanoma: neoplasm arising from neuroectodermal melanocytes located in the epidermis, dermis, or hair follicles
  - Squamous cell carcinoma: neoplasia arising from epidermal keratinocytes
  - Leiomyosarcoma: neoplasia arising from smooth arrector pili muscles or vessel walls
  - Liposarcoma: neoplasia arising from pannicular adipose tissue
  - Osteosarcoma: neoplasia with bone formation
  - Hemangiosarcoma: neoplasia arising from blood vessels
  - Sebaceous gland carcinoma: neoplasia arising from sebaceous glands
  - Rhabdomyosarcoma: neoplasia arising from cross-striated muscle

PHYSICAL EXAM FINDINGS

- Most cutaneous neoplasms occur as solitary masses. However, viral papillomas, viral fibromas, malignant lymphoma, malignant melanoma, and collagenous hamartomas may occur as multinodular.
- Papillomas commonly occur on the ear or the eyelid.
- Lipomas commonly occur in the subcutis of the thorax or neck.
- Collagenous hamartomas commonly occur in the dermis of the abdomen or thorax.

ETIOLOGY AND PATHOPHYSIOLOGY

- Cutaneous neoplasms in rabbits can be divided into virus-induced and non–virus-induced tumors.
  - Viral papilloma is caused by a papillomavirus (family Papovaviridae, genus *Papillomavirus*) and is transmitted by biting arthropods and mosquitoes. Papillomas may undergo malignant transformation to squamous cell carcinoma. Papilloma virus strains are site specific. Strains causing cutaneous papillomas will not cause oral papillomas and vice versa.
  - Viral fibromas (e.g., Shope fibroma) are caused by different virus strains of the genus *Leporipoxvirus* that are endemic in the wild New World rabbit population (e.g., Eastern cottontail rabbit *[Sylvilagus floridanus]*) and are transmitted by biting arthropods and mosquitoes. Depending on the exact virus strain and rabbit breed or genetic background, viral strains that cause fibromas in wild New World rabbits may cause

myxomatosis in pet rabbits when transferred (see Lymphosarcoma and Myxomatosis).

DIAGNOSIS

DIFFERENTIAL DIAGNOSIS

- Abscesses, foreign body or fungal granulomas, mycobacteriosis, myxomatosis, cysts (see Abscesses and Myxomatosis)
- Inflammatory polyps frequently occur at the anorectal junction and mimic a true neoplasm.
- Differential diagnoses are ruled out by histopathologic examination of tissue biopsy or by fine-needle aspiration of the cutaneous mass.

INITIAL DATABASE

Cytologic examination (fine-needle aspirate) is a quick, fast, and inexpensive method used to diagnose skin tumors or to rule out differential diagnoses. Generally, fine-needle aspirates can be obtained from sedated rabbits. Enlarged lymph nodes should be aspirated for evaluation of possible metastasis. Cytologic examination will indicate only the malignancy (benign vs. malignant) of the neoplasm and a broad tumor category (epithelial vs. mesenchymal). Histopathologic examination (biopsy or excision) will lead to an exact diagnosis and generally is more reliable. However, anesthesia is necessary. Chest radiographs are indicated if metastasis of the tumor is likely.

ADVANCED OR CONFIRMATORY TESTING

The use of immunohistochemistry on rabbit tissue can be limited because many polyclonal antibodies used in the diagnosis of human, canine, feline, etc. tumors have been raised in rabbits.

TREATMENT

THERAPEUTIC GOALS

- Overall condition of the patient, age of the patient, and risk of anesthesia must be taken into account in the decision of whether or not a tumor is excised. In the absence of metastasis, malignant neoplasms should be fully excised. A benign neoplasm should be excised if the location or size of the mass jeopardizes the well-being of the patient. Some benign lesions may undergo malignant transformation (e.g., papilloma).
- Excision of malignant lymphoma is not indicated because it is a systemic or multicentric disease.

ACUTE GENERAL TREATMENT

- Complete excision is curative for benign neoplasms.
- Malignant neoplasms should be excised with wide margins; however, specific recommendations for the width of the margins have not been established for rabbits. To reach an accurate assessment of completeness of tumor excision, samples of the tumor periphery should be collected and submitted in a separate jar for histopathologic examination.

CHRONIC TREATMENT

Chemotherapy protocols or radiation protocols for the treatment of rabbit cancer patients have not been established. In an experimental setting, common chemotherapeutic drugs such as prednisone (0.5-2.0 mg/kg PO), doxorubicin (1 mg/kg IV q 14-21 d), mitoxantrone (5-6 mg/m^2 IV q 21 d), L-asparaginase (400 U/kg SC, IM), vincristine (0.5-0.7 mg/m^2 IV q 7-14 d), carboplatin (150-180 mg/m^2 IV q 21-28 d), cyclophosphamide (50 mg/m^2 PO q 24 h for 2-3 d q 7 d or 100-200 mg/m^2 IV q 7-21 d), and CCNU (50 mg/m^2 PO q 3-6 w) have been used.

POSSIBLE COMPLICATIONS

All neoplasms may recur when incompletely excised. Malignant neoplasms may recur even when margins are considered clean. Malignant neoplasms may metastasize to local lymph nodes, lung, or visceral organs. Sarcomas rarely metastasize but frequently recur at the original site. Carcinomas and malignant melanomas tend to recur and metastasize.

PROGNOSIS AND OUTCOME

- Benign tumors and tumorlike lesions carry a good prognosis unless the size of the mass or the tumor location is unfavorable.
- Sarcomas and carcinomas carry a guarded prognosis. Prognosis depends on overall health of the patient, surgery outcome, type of neoplasm, and status of tumor margins.
- Malignant melanoma, malignant lymphoma, hemangiosarcoma, and osteosarcoma carry a poor prognosis.

PEARLS & CONSIDERATIONS

COMMENTS

- In rabbits, osteosarcoma frequently occurs as soft-tissue osteosarcoma without bone involvement.
- Trichoblastoma can be pigmented and can clinically mimic a malignant melanoma.
- Cytologic examination is particularly useful in rabbits and should be attempted as a first line of diagnostics. In cases of insufficient results, a preoperative biopsy can be useful.

SUGGESTED READINGS

Heatley JJ, et al: Spontaneous neoplasms of lagomorphs, Vet Clin Exot Anim 7:561–577, 2004.

von Bomhard W, et al: Cutaneous neoplasms in pet rabbits: a retrospective study, Vet Pathol 44:579–588, 2007.

CROSS-REFERENCES TO OTHER SECTIONS

Abscesses
Dermatopathies
Ectoparasites
Lymphosarcoma
Mammary Gland Disorders
Myxomatosis

AUTHOR: **WOLF VON BOMHARD**

EDITOR: **DAVID VELLA**

RABBITS

Dacryocystitis and Epiphora

BASIC INFORMATION

DEFINITION

Inflammation of the nasolacrimal drainage system is one of the most common ocular problems seen in general practice. Epiphora is the presence of tear overflow from the eye onto the face.

SYNONYMS

- Nasolacrimal duct inflammation and/or blockage
- Dacryocystitis: inflammation of the lacrimal sac
- Dacryosolenitis: inflammation of the nasolacrimal duct
- Etymology: dacryo = a tear; solen = a duct; cyst = a sac or bladder

SPECIAL SPECIES CONSIDERATIONS

- The nasolacrimal drainage system provides a conduit for tears from the eye to the nares. Tears collect in the lacrimal lake, which is the triangular space at the medial angle of the eye. In the rabbit, a single lacrimal punctum (the opening of the nasolacrimal drainage system located 3 to 4 mm ventral to the lower eyelid margin at the medial canthus), canaliculus (lacrimal duct), lacrimal sac, nasolacrimal duct, and nasal meatus form this drainage system for each eye. The diameter of the nasolacrimal duct is small and variable throughout its length. The lumen narrows where it changes course in two places (the proximal maxillae and the base of the upper incisor). These two sites are important in the development of obstruction and for successful therapy.
- Epiphora in rabbits presents as a milky aqueous discharge that causes crusting of the facial fur near the medial canthus. It may be the result of excessive lacrimation or of nasolacrimal duct obstruction. The secretion of the Harderian gland (or the glands of the third eyelid—both superficial and deep) is white. Excessive lacrimation results from ocular irritation; a variety of external and intraocular disorders may be responsible (e.g., conjunctivitis). Inadequate tear drainage is caused by dacryocystitis and nasal duct obstruction.
- Epiphora should not be mistaken for an inflammatory discharge.

EPIDEMIOLOGY

SPECIES, AGE, SEX A retrospective study of 28 rabbits presenting with ocular discharge from the nasolacrimal duct opening showed the following:

- Mean age was 4.4 years.
- Dacryocystitis was a unilateral finding in 25 rabbits (89%).

RISK FACTORS Dacryocystitis and acquired nasal duct obstruction may arise from chronic rhinitis that travels up the nasolacrimal duct to the eye or from acquired dental disease such as tooth root inflammation or abscessation.

ASSOCIATED CONDITIONS AND DISORDERS

- Ocular discharge is a frequent finding in rabbits, ranging from epiphora with or without facial dermatitis that may include chronic scalding of the skin below the eye. The discharge can range from mucoid to mucopurulent to thick white purulent material.
- In severe cases, palpable distention of the lacrimal sac is evident and secondary conjunctivitis is often present. Close contact between the cornea and mucopurulent material in the lacrimal sac (the distended proximal end of the nasolacrimal duct) can lead to significant keratitis or even corneal ulceration.
- Establish whether the discharge signals a localized conjunctivitis or is the result of dacryocystitis (most common).

CLINICAL PRESENTATION

DISEASE FORMS/SUBTYPES

- Epiphora due to obstruction of the nasolacrimal duct
  - Acquired (most common cause)
  - Congenital causes (e.g., imperforate nasolacrimal punctum, nasolacrimal atresia) have not been described in rabbits.
- Epiphora due to overproduction of tears
  - Acquired (e.g., conjunctival foreign bodies, conjunctivitis): typically noninfectious and due to ocular irritants or allergens
  - Eyelid and eyelash abnormalities (e.g., distichiasis [eyelash in an abnormal location]): trichiasis (eyelash in a normal location but directed to the eye) or entropion

HISTORY, CHIEF COMPLAINT

- Ocular discharge, epiphora
- Conjunctivitis
- Constant sneezing, nasal discharge

PHYSICAL EXAM FINDINGS

- In early stages of dacryocystitis, affected rabbits present with epiphora and reddened eyelid margins.
- Later, white threads of mucus or pus appear at the medial canthus or in the ventral conjunctival cul-de-sac, with any or all of the following:
  - Conjunctivitis
  - Swelling in the medial canthal area

ETIOLOGY AND PATHOPHYSIOLOGY

- Dacryocystitis and acquired nasolacrimal duct obstruction may arise from chronic rhinitis that travels up the nasolacrimal duct to the eye or from acquired dental disease such as tooth root inflammation or abscessation.
- The tortuous nasolacrimal duct of the rabbit passes closely to the reserve crown ("root") apices of both the upper incisor and the first two cheek teeth. Any invasion or overgrowth of these tooth root apices into weakened maxillary bone may lead to narrowing of the nasolacrimal duct (dacryostenosis). Secondary dacryocystitis with infection often follows.
- Dacryocystorhinographic studies have shown that dacryostenosis occurs more commonly at incisor tooth apices than at cheek teeth apices in cases of acquired dental disease. Clinically, it is easier to visualize incisor teeth anomalies than cheek teeth disease (e.g., incisor tooth disease can sometimes be demonstrated by enamel dysplasia [the presence of horizontal ridging of the enamel seen on the labial side of the teeth], which is one of the first signs of acquired dental disease in rabbits).

DIAGNOSIS

DIFFERENTIAL DIAGNOSIS

- Epiphora
  - Ocular irritation and inflammation (including trichiasis and entropion)
  - Nasolacrimal duct obstruction due to trauma
  - Facial bone fractures (including iatrogenic causes)
  - Soft-tissue trauma involving the lower eyelid and medial canthus
- Conjunctivitis
  - Differentiate dacryocystitis from conjunctivitis by cannulation and irrigation of the nasolacrimal duct—if nasolacrimal duct is patent, consider conjunctivitis.

INITIAL DATABASE

- Perform thorough ocular examination.
- Examine both the lacrimal punctum and behind the third eyelid (use topical local anesthetics, e.g., proxymetacaine) because occasionally a foreign body may be found.
- Apply gentle digital pressure to the medial canthus of each eye. Check for the presence of abnormal exudate that may exude from the lacrimal sac.
- Inspect nose for the presence of nasal discharge.
- Examine incisor teeth and cheek teeth:
  - Ensure that any rabbit presenting with signs of ocular disease undergoes a thorough investigation for the presence of underlying dental disease.
  - Sedation or general anesthesia may be required to enhance inspection of the oral cavity and to perform skull/dental radiographic studies if dental disease is suspected.
- Check nasolacrimal duct patency using fluorescein dye.
- Flush the nasolacrimal duct of all rabbits presenting with epiphora:
  - Procedure is relatively easy: most rabbits tolerate cannulation of the lacrimal punctum after application of topical anesthesia, and generally do not require sedation. The lacrimal punctum is easy to find and cannulate because of its size. The procedure is more difficult to perform in dwarf rabbits.
  - Use a 22- to 25-gauge Teflon catheter (without the stylet) or stainless steel lacrimal or blunt cannulas to

cannulate the duct and insert catheter 10-15 mm. Preference for one type varies significantly between veterinarians. Avoid using rigid tomcat catheters because they can damage mucosa or rupture the nasolacrimal duct.
  - Irrigate with sterile saline and obtain a sample of the solution at the nasal meatus for bacteriologic studies.

ADVANCED OR CONFIRMATORY TESTING

- Bacterial culture and sensitivity of nasolacrimal flush solution and/or abnormal exudate from the lacrimal lake or punctum
- Dacryocystorhinography to assess for patency of nasolacrimal duct
  - Injection of contrast material into the lacrimal punctum will provide good radiographic detail of the nasolacrimal duct throughout its course and will show the site of obstruction. Use diluted Omnipaque (Iohexol 300 mg/mL; Amersham Health) or similar contrast media.
- Radiographic studies of skull/teeth with multiple views

TREATMENT

THERAPEUTIC GOAL

Diagnose and localize the cause of epiphora.

ACUTE GENERAL TREATMENT

- Treatment of epiphora
  - Rule out underlying predisposing disease.
  - Is usually frustrating if only topical antibiotics are used
  - Involves topical and systemic antibiotics and sometimes daily flushing with antibiotic-added saline
  - Suitable first-line ophthalmic antimicrobials include chloramphenicol, ciprofloxacin, ofloxacin, or fusidic acid.
  - Avoid aminoglycosides because their spectrum of activity is limited in the rabbit eye.

CHRONIC TREATMENT

- Continue administration of topical and systemic antibiotics and frequent flushing with antibiotic-added saline.
- Chronic cases of dacryocystitis are often obstructed. Attempts to flush the nasolacrimal duct usually result in:
  - Failure (common) or,
  - An opalescent, gritty material in the irrigation fluid at the nasal meatus
- Relieving the obstruction by frequent flushing is the ideal treatment but is not always successful:
  - Cannulation of an obstructed nasolacrimal duct with a monofilament nylon suture (0 to 2-0) is unrewarding and rarely succeeds because of abrupt changes and narrowing of the duct lumen in two locations.
- In long-standing cases of dacryocystitis, segments of the nasolacrimal duct may progressively narrow and be replaced with scar tissue until they are irreversibly obstructed. This results in permanent epiphora. Clip away matted hair and treat skin if affected by moist dermatitis. Owners should be advised accordingly.

DRUG INTERACTIONS

Topical aminoglycoside solutions are irritating to conjunctiva.

POSSIBLE COMPLICATIONS

Iatrogenic rupture of obstructed nasolacrimal duct from zealous attempts to flush

RECOMMENDED MONITORING

- Monitor patient for 7 days and evaluate for additional discharge if nasolacrimal flushing resolves the obstruction.
- Monitoring frequency and duration will depend on the underlying cause of the problem.

PROGNOSIS AND OUTCOME

- Early diagnosis and treatment improves the prognosis and outcome.
- Many animals require long-term treatment.
- A retrospective study of 28 rabbits diagnosed with dacryocystitis showed the following:
  - 12 rabbits (43%) had complete recovery.
  - 2 rabbits (7%) continued to display signs of dacryocystitis, and the owners continued to treat as clinical signs arose.
  - 14 rabbits (50%) were euthanized because of unrelated causes or were lost to follow-up.
- Most rabbits (96%) received topical antibiotic treatment. If necessary, additional topical (acetylcysteine, vitamin A ointment, nonsteroidal antiinflammatory drugs [NSAIDs]) or systemic treatment (antibiotics, NSAIDs, and glucocorticoids) was provided.
- Mean duration of therapy was 6 weeks.
- Nasolacrimal duct flushing was performed in 27 of 31 affected eyes (87%).
- Dentistry was performed in 80% of animals suffering from malocclusion.
- Determination of the cause of dacryocystitis indicated
  - No underlying cause in 10 rabbits (35%)
  - Dental malocclusion in 14 rabbits (50%)
  - Rhinitis in 2 rabbits (7%)
  - Panophthalmitis as presenting feature in 1 rabbit (4%)
- Some veterinary ophthalmologists consider that repeated flushing is indicated; others suggest that in cases unresponsive to topical medication, lifelong systemic antibiotic treatment is the only means of controlling the problem.

PEARLS & CONSIDERATIONS

COMMENTS

Every rabbit with corneal disease in the medioventral area of the eye should be examined for dacryocystitis.

CLIENT EDUCATION

In long-standing cases of dacryocystitis and conjunctivitis, the lacrimal punctum and segments of the nasolacrimal duct may progressively narrow and be replaced with scar tissue until they are irreversibly obstructed. This results in permanent epiphora, and owners should be advised accordingly.

SUGGESTED READINGS

Brown C: Nasolacrimal duct lavage in rabbits, Lab Anim (NY) 35:22–24, 2006.

Burling K, et al: Anatomy of the rabbit nasolacrimal duct and its clinical implications, Prog Vet Comp Ophthalmol 1:33–40, 1991.

Florin M, et al: Clinical presentation, treatment, and outcome of dacryocystitis in rabbits: a retrospective study of 28 cases (2003-2007), Vet Ophthalmol 12:350–356, 2009.

Marini RP, et al: Microbiologic, radiographic, and anatomic study of the nasolacrimal duct apparatus in the rabbit *(Oryctolagus cuniculus)*, Lab Anim Sci 46:656–662, 1996.

CROSS-REFERENCES TO OTHER SECTIONS

Bupthalmia and Glaucoma
Cataracts
Cherry Eye
Conjunctival Disorders
Dental Disease
Uveitis

AUTHORS: **THOMAS M. DONNELLY AND JEFFREY SMITH**

EDITOR: **DAVID VELLA**

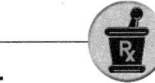

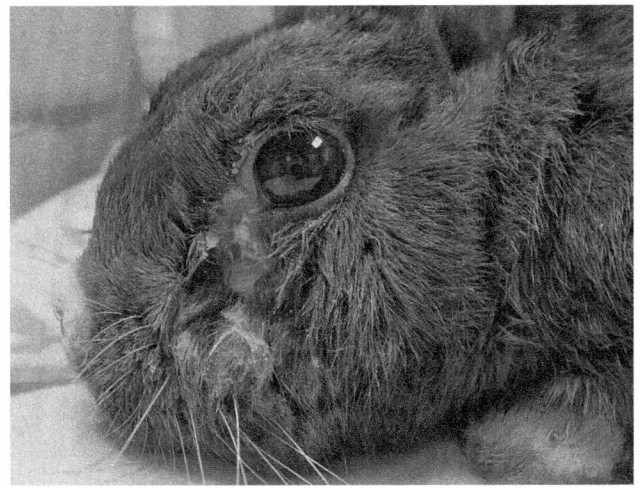

Dacryocystitis and Epiphora Tear overflow and periocular matting of hair are common signs of nasolacrimal duct blockage. *(Photo courtesy Jörg Mayer, The University of Georgia, Athens.)*

RABBITS

Dental Disease

Client Education Sheet Available on Website

BASIC INFORMATION

DEFINITION

Any disease, disorder, or malformation of the teeth and associated structures that results in dysphagia, masticatory malfunction, infection or malaise

SYNONYMS

Dental infection, dental malocclusion, dental associated disease, acquired dental disease (ADD), malocclusion, progressive syndrome of acquired dental disease (PSADD), tooth root abscess, apical abscessation, periapical abscessation, dental abscess

SPECIAL SPECIES CONSIDERATIONS

- The rabbit dental formula is I2/1 C0/0 PM3/2 M3/3 = 28.
- The incisors can be divided into maxillary and mandibular incisors. A second set of small maxillary incisors (peg teeth) are situated caudal to the larger main maxillary incisors.
- Premolars and molars can be collectively termed "cheek" teeth.
- Each tooth can be divided into the clinical crown (region of tooth exposed above the gingival margin) and the reserve crown (region of tooth buried below the gingival margin). The growing portion at the tip of the reserve crown is the apex, which is open in rabbit teeth.
- All teeth of rabbits are classified as elodont (continuously growing, with no anatomic "roots") and hypsodont (long-crowned). This leads to a dynamic state intrinsic to rabbit dentition, which can complicate dental disease.
- Dental disease is a very common presenting problem in pet rabbits.

EPIDEMIOLOGY

SPECIES, AGE, SEX Can affect rabbits of any age and gender

GENETICS AND BREED PREDISPOSITION

- Although breed dispositions have been suggested (especially in dwarf breeds), one study involving 1254 pet rabbits showed no significant relationship between breed and dental disease in rabbits. However, in the same study, significantly more males than females suffered from dental disease.
- Congenital malocclusions can occur.

RISK FACTORS

- Inappropriate diet (low fiber, poorly abrasive foods)
- Male gender
- Calcium and vitamin D imbalance
- Dental and jaw trauma

GEOGRAPHY AND SEASONALITY Occurs worldwide with no seasonality

ASSOCIATED CONDITIONS AND DISORDERS

- Dysphagia
- Anemia
- Abscessation
- Weight loss
- Ocular disease
- Nasal disease
- Dermatitis (see Dermatopathies)
- Obesity
- Myiasis

CLINICAL PRESENTATION

DISEASE FORMS/SUBTYPES

- Malocclusion may progress to further disease owing to improper masticatory ability, resulting in improper dental wear and attrition.
- Tooth elongation and dystrophy may result in malocclusion and/or dental spur formation.
- Dental associated infection can involve teeth, alveolar bone, surrounding bone, and soft tissue, leading to bony and soft-tissue abscessation.

HISTORY, CHIEF COMPLAINT

- The typical history of dental disease in rabbits can vary widely. Many of the signs associated with dental disease may go unnoticed for some time, in part because rabbits are a prey species and mask clinical signs of illness. Signs noted may include the following:
  - Anorexia (see Anorexia)
  - Dysphagia
  - Altered food preference
  - Weight loss
  - Halitosis
  - Chin wetness/drooling
  - Epiphora/ocular discharge (see Dacryocystitis and Epiphora)
  - Exophthalmos
  - Nasal discharge
  - Perineal soiling (urinary and/or fecal)
  - Unkempt coat

- o Wet/stained forelimbs
- o Facial/jaw swelling and/or abscessation

PHYSICAL EXAM FINDINGS

- Primary signs of dental disease may include malocclusion, dental asymmetry, tooth disfigurement/dystrophy, dental overgrowth, and dental spur formation. Enamel dysplasia (enamel ribbing of the incisors) may indicate underlying metabolic bone disease (MBD).
  - o When incisor teeth malocclude and overgrow, they usually follow a particular pattern of overgrowth. The lower incisors tend to protrude rostrally (unimpeded by lack of wear from the upper incisors). The main upper incisors tend to curl in a caudal direction. The peg teeth will often grow ventrolaterally. Maloccluded incisors may entrap hair as a result of attempted grooming.
  - o With cheek teeth, the array of misdirected growth is variable. However, production of dental spurs that impinge on the tongue or cheeks is more predictable. The upper cheek teeth tend to misdirect toward the cheek and produce spurs on their buccal sides. Hence buccal abrasions may be seen in this scenario. Conversely, the lower cheek teeth tend to misdirect toward and produce spurs on their lingual sides. Hence lingual abrasions may be seen. In severe cases, medial spurs of the lower cheek teeth may elongate sufficiently to cause laceration of the lingual artery, leading to a fatal hemorrhage.
  - o Diseased cheek teeth often exhibit "step-mouth" or "wave-mouth," which represents the pattern of unevenness of the occlusal plane of any one of the cheek teeth quadrants (i.e., upper or lower cheek teeth on right or left).
- Secondary signs that may alert to the presence of ADD include but are not limited to the following:
  - o Anorexia
  - o Dysphagia
  - o Loss of body condition
  - o Weight loss
  - o Change in dietary preference
  - o Halitosis
  - o Chin wetness/salivation
  - o Epiphora/ocular discharge
  - o Exophthalmos
  - o Nasal discharge
  - o Dyspnea
  - o Facial masses/swellings
  - o Altered mandibular movements
  - o Altered gape
  - o Perineal soiling (fecal and/or urinary)
  - o Uneaten cecotrophs
  - o Change in fecal consistency and quantity
  - o Unkempt coat/lack of grooming
  - o Wet/stained forearms

ETIOLOGY AND PATHOPHYSIOLOGY

- See Special Species Considerations above.
- Rabbits periodically "grind" their teeth to help shape the incisor tips to their characteristic chisel form. In normal resting occlusion, the mandibular incisor tips lay just caudal to the main maxillary incisors, in the space between the primary maxillary incisors and the peg teeth.
- The rabbit mouth features the following:
  - o Anisognathism, in which the mandibular cheek teeth are set narrower than the maxillary cheek teeth. This arrangement permits only one side of the mouth to be utilized for mastication at one time.
  - o A relatively long diastema: maximum open-mouth gape of a rabbit is 20° to 25°
  - o These two features make inspection of the oral cavity relatively difficult.
- Rabbits primarily use a vertical action to "cut" foliage with their incisors. Cut food is prehended into the mouth by the lips and then is masticated largely in a horizontal or lateral plane by the cheek teeth.
- Rabbits' teeth are shaped by continual processes of growth, dental attrition, and dietary abrasion. Rate of growth of the upper incisors is 2 mm/wk, and that of the lower incisors is 2.4 mm/wk. The rate of tooth growth may slow as dental disease advances.
- Many causes of dental disease in rabbits have been proposed. These can be grouped into congenital anomalies and acquired dental diseases. These events may occur individually or in combination; in any case, dental disease in rabbits tends to be progressive.
  - o Congenital causes include maxillary brachygnathia, mandibular prognathism, and jaw or teeth malformation.
  - o Acquired causes include trauma, inappropriate nutrition, MBD, trauma, and neoplasia.
  - o Effects of improper or insufficient wearing down of the teeth from an inappropriate diet are likely to have significant impact on the development of dental disease in rabbits.
  - o Strong evidence suggests that MBD (nutritional secondary hyperparathyroidism) also plays a major role in the formation of dental disease in rabbits.
- Incisors

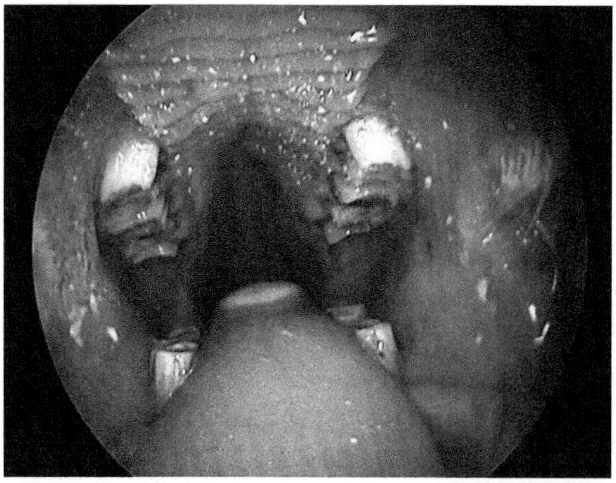

Dental Disease Evaluation of the cheek teeth is important in the stomatoscopy of dental status in the rabbit. Endoscopy-guided examination of the oral cavity while the rabbit is sedated or anesthetized allows a more detailed dental assessment. *(Photo courtesy Jörg Mayer, The University of Georgia, Athens.)*

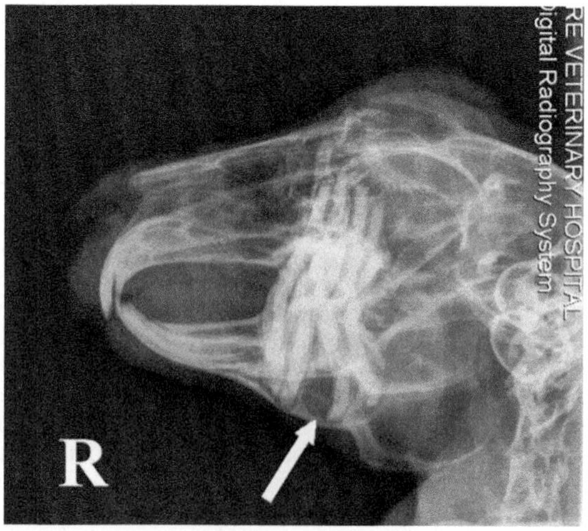

Dental Disease Left dorsal-right ventral oblique radiographic view of rabbit skull. There is a periapical infection associated with the right lower cheek tooth *(arrow)* demonstrated by osteolysis surrounding the apex. *(Courtesy David Vella.)*

- Malocclusion can be congenital. Acquired incisor malocclusion often results from disease of the cheek teeth. When incisor teeth malocclude and overgrow, they usually follow a particular pattern of overgrowth. The lower incisors tend to protrude rostrally (unimpeded by lack of wear from the upper incisors). The main upper incisors tend to curl in a caudal direction. The peg teeth will often grow ventrolaterally.

- Cheek teeth
  - Elongation can occur in both the clinical crown and reserve crown portions of the teeth. Increased length of the teeth or distortion of tooth shape secondary to weakness of the tooth and supportive structures leads to increased curvature of the teeth. This, coupled with loss of normal orientation of the teeth, leads to cheek teeth malocclusion.
  - Dental spurs (or spikes) can develop on overgrown cheek teeth, resulting in oral soft-tissue abrasions. Spurs tend to develop lingually on the lower cheek teeth and buccally on the upper cheek teeth.
- Regardless of the precise cause of dental disease, deviation of overgrown reserve crowns of cheek teeth results in predictable sites of their apical eruptions through associated cortical bone. In most instances, overgrown cheek teeth apices erupt through the cortical bone laterally, except for the first and last lower cheek teeth, which more often tend to erupt medially.
- Formation of infection and abscessation associated with dental disease in rabbits may have several causes, including endodontic infection, penetrating foreign bodies, trauma to teeth or jaw, and hematogenous spread.
  - One theory put forward on the development of tooth infection is the creation of periodontal pockets from loss of periodontal ligaments secondary to periodontitis. Although periodontitis is normally rare in rabbits, its incidence may increase as tooth growth is reduced. Once formed, these periodontal pockets may become inhabited by bacteria, initiate disease, and spread to the apex.
  - In another theory on formation of infection, accompanying alveolar bone demineralization may lead to widening of the periodontal spaces and subsequent loosening of the teeth. This phenomenon may allow bacteria and food particles to enter the periodontal space, generating periodontitis. Progression of this may lead to the development of periapical infection.
  - Infection involving the tooth apex and periapical tissue can progress to osteomyelitis of the supporting alveolar bone, soft tissue infection, and abscess formation.
  - Important features of dental associated abscesses in rabbits include the abscess capsule, necrotic tissue (dental, bony or soft tissue), and osteomyelitis. Thick caseous pus is nonamenable to simple lancing and drainage.
  - Dental abscesses in rabbits may harbor both mixed aerobic and anaerobic bacteria. *Fusobacterium nucleatum, Actinomyces* spp., *Streptococcus* spp., *Peptostreptococcus* spp., *Prevotella* spp., *Pasteurella* spp., *Staphylococcus* spp., *Pseudomonas aeruginosa, Enterococcus* spp., *Bacteroides* spp., and other microbes have been isolated from rabbit dental abscesses.
  - Even in severe cases, when infection or abscessation is present, typical signs presented in many other species affected by abscessation of any kind (malaise, pyrexia, pain, etc.) are not often seen in rabbits.

DIAGNOSIS

DIFFERENTIAL DIAGNOSIS

- Dental malocclusion
- Dental associated infection
- Facial/jaw trauma
- Other source of oral pain and discomfort
- Neoplasia of cutaneous, bony, or soft-tissue structures
- Unilateral exophthalmos (retrobulbar abscess, orbital abscess, neoplasia, hemorrhage, salivary mucocele, lacrimal apparatus disease, cellulitis, foreign body penetration, trauma, granuloma, cystic structures, including cysticercosis)

INITIAL DATABASE

- Thorough examination of face, jaw, and teeth
  - Facial palpation, especially in regions of ventral mandibles and lateral maxillae, for any unevenness, swellings, discomfort, or asymmetry. Any swelling of the face or jaw should raise the suspicion of dental disease and dental abscessation. Swellings associated with abscessation may be firm or soft but are usually nonpainful to touch. Often a ventral mandibular abscess may be hidden by the dewlap, hair growth, or normal head carriage of the rabbit. Occasionally, a ruptured abscess may be characterized by regional wetness and/or foul odor. The size of the facial abscess may not always give an indication of the severity or prognosis of the underlying dental disease problem.
  - Evaluation of degree of horizontal excursion of mandible
  - Inspection of incisors (occlusion, length, and quality). In normal resting occlusion, the mandibular incisor tips lay just caudal to the main maxillary incisors, in the space between the primary maxillary incisors and the peg teeth.
  - Inspection of cheek teeth (length, shape, arrangement, spurring). Use of otoscopes can aid examination of the first few cheek teeth. More specialized equipment such as the human bivalve nasal speculum (Model 26030, Welch Allyn, Skaneateles Falls, NY) can facilitate cheek teeth inspection by allowing retraction of the buccae and tongue away from the dental arcades.
- Examination of oral cavity under sedation or anesthesia: in sedated or anesthetized animals, inspection can be enhanced by the use of rabbit-specific instrumentation (e.g., mouth gags, cheek dilators, tabletop positioning stands). The use of stomatoscopy in anesthetized patients may offer a more detailed dental assessment.
- Hematology and blood biochemistry (many rabbits with chronic dental disease exhibit anemia)
- Skull radiography is considered essential for evaluating the extent of dental disease in rabbits. Four minimum views required are lateral, left and right lateral obliques, and dorsoventral. The rostrocaudal view can also be taken but may be less useful.
  - Lateral view
    - The overall impression of the shape of the skull is attained. Overall radiodensity of the skull bone can be assessed for evidence of osteopenia.
    - Incisor and cheek teeth occlusion can be assessed. The cheek teeth normally occlude in a zig-zag array.
    - The apex of the maxillary incisors may be assessed for their potential incursion into the incisive bone of the hard palate.
    - Nasal cavity assessment can also be made.
  - Lateral oblique views
    - Both left upper/right lower and right upper/left lower projections are necessary at an angle no greater than 30°. These projections reveal a mandible with associated cheek teeth set and its contralateral upper cheek teeth quadrant.
    - Evidence of deformities, curvatures, misalignments, dystrophic

calcification, resorptive lesions, and erosions in each tooth can be examined.
- The development of incisor abnormalities is believed to follow a course of elongation, closure of the pulp cavity, and dystrophic calcification of the reserve crown and surrounding bone.
- For cheek teeth, the interproximal spaces between teeth can be assessed. These spaces tend to widen with the presence of dental disease in rabbits. The apices of each cheek tooth can be closely examined for evidence of surrounding osteolysis, dystrophic calcification, elongation, and penetration into surrounding bone.
- In cheek teeth, elongation of the reserve crown appears to be the first change to take place in all rabbits with acquired dental disease. Subsequently, loss of the longitudinal radiodense enamel fold of the cheek teeth occurs.
- In dental diseased rabbits, the lower cheek teeth apical extremities often show penetration into the ventral mandibular cortex. Loss of the line of the lamina dura at the extremity of the dental socket occurs before this and is thus indicative of early dental disease.

- Dorsoventral view
  - In some cases may enable the detection of cheek teeth spurs despite superimposition of upper and lower cheek teeth sets
  - First upper premolars can be viewed without superimposition. Their associated surrounding lamina dura should be clearly visible bilaterally as a radiodense line in normal skulls.
  - Incisor reserve crowns can be viewed, as can part of the nasal cavity, which may be compared bilaterally.
  - Outlines of the mandible and the zygomatic arches can be partially inspected.

ADVANCED OR CONFIRMATORY TESTING

- CT imaging of skull: aids identification of dental associated infection, especially infections involving the nasal cavity and orbit
- Contrast dacryocystorhinography: may aid evaluation of patency of nasolacrimal ducts, especially in regions where teeth may impact on the duct (apices of main upper incisors and first two upper premolars). Cannulate the punctum lacrimale with a 22-to 24-gauge IV catheter, and insert a small amount of contrast agent (nonionic radiopaque contrast agent).
- Orbital ultrasound: may aid in evaluation of exophthalmos (for retrobulbar disease)
- If dental associated abscess is present, culture and sensitivity of abscess capsule: culture of pus is often unrewarding owing to low presence of bacteria; often culture of the capsule is more successful. This should include an anaerobic culture.

TREATMENT

THERAPEUTIC GOALS

- Restore normal eating ability.
- Correct dental anomalies.
- Resolve infection.
- Stop or slow progression of dental disease.
- Improve nutrition. Replace unsuitable diets with nutritionally balanced abrasive feed that encourages appropriate wearing down of teeth.

ACUTE GENERAL TREATMENT

- Provide general supportive care for any rabbit experiencing reduced or nil food intake (e.g., fluid therapy, assisted feeding, analgesia, management of gut stasis)
- Provide parenteral fluid therapy (crystalloids may be used). Maintenance fluid rates are considered 100 to 120 mL/kg/d.
- Provide assisted feeding with commercial assist feeding formulas (e.g., Oxbow Critical Care, Oxbow Pet Products, Murdock, NE; Emeraid Herbivore, Lafeber Vet, Cornell, IL; www.lafebervet.com).
- Analgesia
  - Nonsteroidal antiinflammatory drugs (NSAIDs; e.g., carprofen 2-4 mg/kg PO, SC q 24 h; meloxicam 0.3-0.5 mg/kg SC, PO q 12-24 h; ketoprofen 1-3 mg/kg PO q12 h)
  - Opioids (e.g., buprenorphine 0.03 mg/kg SC, IM q 8 h)
- Correct minor dental anomalies (e.g., corrective burring of dental spurs and overgrown teeth).
  - Incisors
    - Incisor trimming can be performed in sedated or anesthetized patients.
    - Use diamond discs or high-speed water-cooled dental burrs.
    - Avoid use of handheld clippers, nail cutters, etc. Longitudinal fractures may result in pain, pulpitis, and extension into periapical infection. Creation of a rough edge following this technique may lead to soft-tissue damage.
    - Avoid cutting to the level of the pulp. The pulp can be viewed as pink coloration within the tooth. Cutting into pulp may cause pain, pulpitis, necrosis, and infection. Accidental pulp exposure should be rectified via partial pulpectomy and pulp capping with calcium hydroxide.
    - Repeat incisor trimming may be required every 4 to 8 weeks.
    - Incisor malocclusions are often best treated via total incisor set extraction.
  - Cheek teeth
    - Cheek teeth procedures should always be performed with the patient anesthetized.
    - Provide adequate exposure of the oral cavity with cheek dilators and mouth gags and suitable light source. Commercial rodent/lagomorph table-top gags are available for this purpose.
    - Use soft tissue protection when burring cheek teeth.
    - Low-speed burrs on straight dental nose cones are available for use in rabbits.
    - Correctively burr away spurs and overgrown teeth. Do not reduce the height of the clinical crowns of all cheek teeth excessively (e.g., to the level of the gum line).
    - Regular water cooling during the burring process is advisable to minimize the potential for thermal injury.
    - Avoid the use of handheld rasps, files, or clippers in most situations.
    - Trimming of spurs may be required frequently (every 6 to 8 weeks).

CHRONIC TREATMENT

- Extraction of maloccluded or infected teeth
  - Incisors
    - In most instances, incisor malocclusions are best treated via total incisor set extraction. Rabbits can eat pellets and hay with incisors removed—they cannot graze pasture.
    - Use general anesthesia with local anesthetic nerve blocks (infraorbital and mental nerves) and adequate analgesia.
    - Rabbit incisor luxators can be inserted into the mesial and distal, and then onto the labial and lingual, aspects of the teeth before loosening and extraction.
    - Great care must be taken because teeth are fragile and can easily fracture.
  - Cheek teeth
    - Cheek teeth extraction in rabbits can be very difficult and laborious.

  - Use general anesthesia with local anesthetic nerve blocks where possible (e.g., mandibular, maxillary, and palatine nerves) and adequate analgesia.
  - Indicated for loosened, severely maloccluded, or infected cheek teeth. Cheek teeth that develop spurs are not generally routinely extracted.
  - Cheek teeth may require extraction via an extraoral approach because of their complex involvement in infection or fragmentation secondary to disease.
  - Intraoral approaches use rabbit cheek teeth luxators to free periodontal ligaments on the mesial, buccal, distal, and lingual aspects of the tooth. Gentle extraction of the tooth can be achieved with the use of rabbit cheek tooth extraction forceps.
- Dental infection
  - Medical therapy alone is largely considered a palliative measure only.
  - Resolution of dental infection and dental associated abscessation can be achieved in some cases with high-level care and dental procedures; can be a lengthy and difficult process with possible recurrence
  - Suitable first-line antibiotics may include azithromycin 30 mg/kg PO q 24 h or penicillin G 60,000 IU/kg SC, IM q 24 h. Avoid use of enrofloxacin alone. If used, enrofloxacin should be dosed at 10 mg/kg PO, SC q 12 h and combined with metronidazole 20 mg/kg PO q 12 h.
    - If dental associated abscess is present, perform culture and sensitivity of abscess capsule. Culture of pus is often unrewarding owing to low presence of bacteria; often culture of the capsule is more successful. This should include an anaerobic culture.
  - Analgesia as outlined previously
  - For minor dental infection restricted to the periapical space, tooth extraction orally and antibiosis may suffice. For more complicated infections involving bone and soft tissue, more extensive débridement is necessary.
  - Placement of wound drains does not produce suitable drainage in rabbit dental abscesses.
  - Many techniques describe surgical resection of the abscess capsule in conjunction with instillation of the surgical site with various compounds such as clindamycin powder, clindamycin capsules, antibiotic-impregnated polymethylmethacrylate beads (AIPMMA beads), calcium hydroxide, antibiotic preparations such as doxycycline-containing polymer gel, sugar and honey solutions, and bioactive ceramics. Each of these treatment modalities has reported varied success rates and should not be relied upon as a sole mode of therapy.
  - For complex infections, infected teeth need to be accurately diagnosed and targeted for extraction, along with infection of any associated tissue (bone, soft tissue, abscess, abscess capsule).
  - Surgical wounds are often marsupialized to allow healing by assisted secondary intention. This approach minimizes the recurrence of infection by attempting to eliminate infected tissue and avoiding closure of an infected wound.
    - Follow-up wound care (flushing, débriding, suture removal) is generally required for 2 to 4 weeks following surgery.
  - Alternatively, implantation of AIPMMA beads may be considered post débridement with closure of the wound. Antibiotic type should be based on culture and sensitivity. The beads slowly release antibiotic into surrounding tissue for several months. Choice of antibiotics should be based on culture and sensitivity; cephalosporins (e.g., cefazolin, ceftiofur) and aminoglycosides (e.g., gentamicin, tobramycin, amikacin) are typically used. Beads may be left within the wound or removed after several months.
  - In terms of surgical difficulty and prognosis for successful resolution, the tooth or teeth associated with the infection and the extent of the infection are important factors. Infection associated with the caudal cheek teeth (lower cheek teeth 4 and 5, and upper cheek teeth 3 to 6) is considered more difficult to access. Anatomic traits that affect access to the last two lower cheek teeth include the presence of the masseter muscle and the relative thinness of the mandible in this area. Anatomically, the last four upper cheek teeth apices and reserve crowns are located in the ventral bony orbit surrounded by the alveolar bulla of the maxilla. The alveolar bulla can act as a bony cavity to any periapical infection of the teeth it contains. If infection erupts through the thin bone of the alveolar bulla, retrobulbar infection of soft tissue results. Surgical access to this area is impeded by the eye, periorbital tissues, and zygomatic arch. Enucleation, although not ideal, may be required to access this area. Alternatively, partial resection of the zygomatic arch or lateral canthotomy procedures may be performed. Stomatoscopy may enhance visualization in oral dental procedures.
  - Palliative care may be the only option in cases where infection cannot be resolved.

DRUG INTERACTIONS

- Avoid the use of oral preparations of lincomycin, clindamycin, erythromycin, and penicillins.
- Avoid the use of NSAIDs in dehydrated and renally compromised patients.

POSSIBLE COMPLICATIONS

- Non-resolution of infection
- Jaw fracture at tooth extraction
- Ongoing dysphagia

RECOMMENDED MONITORING

- Body condition and feeding ability
- Serial radiography of teeth and skull

PROGNOSIS AND OUTCOME

- Dental disease tends to be progressive in rabbits. Intervention is aimed at correcting immediate problems and stopping or slowing progression of disease.
- Prognosis can be good if malocclusion (especially of incisors) is detected and rectified early.
- Prognosis is more guarded with the presence of dental infection and abscessation.

CONTROVERSY

- MBD as a cause of dental disease
- Corrective burring of all cheek teeth to level of gingival level versus reducing spurs and overgrown teeth only
- Antibiotic use: availability of different antibiotics and formulations (e.g., oral liquid) varies by country
- Use of combination short- and long-acting parenteral penicillins together (e.g., procaine penicillin G with benzathine penicillin G) may not offer any advantage over use of procaine penicillin G alone and may promote bacterial resistance.
- Reports of successful techniques describing the packing of dental abscesses in rabbits are likely to be limited to primary periapical infection without secondary involvement of teeth and bone. This form of dental infection in rabbits constitutes a small percentage of the total forms of dental infection diagnosed.

PEARLS & CONSIDERATIONS

COMMENTS

- Inappropriate diet is believed to play the most important role in the development of dental disease in rabbits, whether directly via lack of appropriate abrasion and attrition and/or indirectly via metabolic disease.
- Lack of regular access to unfiltered sunlight may play an important role in the development of MBD in rabbits.
- Fine-needle aspiration or biopsy of a facial mass that has any degree of suspect underlying dental infection generally is not recommended. Dental infection should be confirmed radiographically, not just on the basis of aspirated pus. Furthermore, a break in the integrity of the abscess capsule by fine-needle aspiration may result in loss of containment of infection and may compromise future surgical resection.

PREVENTION

- Feed rabbits natural high-fiber diets/
- Provide regular thorough dental examinations.

CLIENT EDUCATION

- Emphasize the importance of appropriate feeding. Pet rabbit diets should consist largely of grass or grass hays (at least 80% of diet) (e.g., timothy, oaten hays). A variety of fresh leafy green vegetables can be added to the diet. Pellets (if fed at all) should be of the highest quality, viewed as a supplement, and fed in very limited amounts. Seed mixes, cereals, etc., should not be fed or should be offered only in very small amounts intermittently as treats.
- Educate clients on secondary signs of dental disease, and instruct clients on methods of performing regular facial palpation of pet rabbits.

SUGGESTED READINGS

Capello V: Clinical technique: treatment of periapical infections in pet rabbits and rodents. J Exot Pet Med 17:124–131, 2008.

Crossley DA: Oral biology and disorders of lagomorphs. Vet Clin Exot Anim 6:629–659, 2003.

Harcourt-Brown FM: Metabolic bone disease as a possible cause of acquired dental disease in pet rabbits, Thesis, London, 2006, Royal College of Veterinary Surgeons.

Harcourt-Brown FM: The progressive syndrome of acquired dental disease in rabbits. J Exot Pet Med 16:146–157, 2007.

CROSS-REFERENCES TO OTHER SECTIONS

Abscesses

Anorexia

Dacryocystitis and Epiphora

Dermatopathies

Upper Respiratory Tract Disorders

AUTHOR: **DAVID VELLA**

EDITOR: **THOMAS M. DONNELLY**

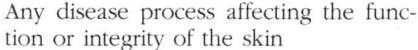

RABBITS

Dermatopathies

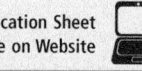

Client Education Sheet Available on Website

BASIC INFORMATION

DEFINITION

Any disease process affecting the function or integrity of the skin

SYNONYMS

- Alopecia (excessive moulting, hair loss)
- Dermatophytosis (ringworm)
- Necrobacillosis (Schmorl's disease)
- Pruritus (itch)

SPECIAL SPECIES CONSIDERATIONS

- Rabbit skin is very delicate compared with other exotic pet species, dogs, and cats.
- Rabbits are typically fastidious groomers. They spend about 16% of their daily activity on grooming.
- Rabbits moult biannually (spring and fall). Hair growth in rabbits occurs in periodic orderly waves, originating on the head and ventrum and spreading dorsally and caudally.
- Rabbits lack fleshy footpads. They rely on a normally thick covering of hair on the plantar and palmar surfaces of their feet. The underlying skin is thin, especially in the region of the metatarsus, increasing their vulnerability to developing pododermatitis.
- Female rabbits have a large fold of skin over the throat known as the *dewlap*. Breeding does pull fur from this area to line their nests before kindling.

EPIDEMIOLOGY

SPECIES, AGE, SEX

- Can affect rabbits of any age and gender
- In older breeding does, the dewlap can be large and easily mistaken for an abscess. Skin fold dermatitis and moist dermatitis often develop in this area.
- Dermatophytosis may be more common in young rabbits.
- Disseminated collagenous hamartomas are almost exclusively found in middle-aged male rabbits.

GENETICS AND BREED PREDISPOSITION

- Some breeds are more vulnerable to pododermatitis (e.g., short-coated breeds [Rex], large breeds).
- Long-haired breeds (e.g., Angora) are more vulnerable to hair matting.
- Some breeds (e.g., Angora) may moult in patchy fashion, leading to irregular coat length and the appearance of alopecia.
- Hereditary compulsive self-mutilation has been described in inbred Checkered Cross rabbits.
- Disseminated collagenous hamartomas are thought to have an X-linked recessive inheritance in male rabbits.
- A genetic defect is suspected with Ehlers-Danlos–like syndrome.

RISK FACTORS

- Moisture, any underlying problem leading to moisture/soiling of skin
- Unhygienic housing (especially damp bedding)
- Trauma, abrasions
- Large dewlap
- Infection (especially *Staphylococcus aureus* and *Pasteurella multocida*)

CONTAGION AND ZOONOSIS

- *S. aureus* and *P. multocida* may cause or complicate dermatitis, especially in moist conditions.
- Dermatophytes (*Trichophyton mentagrophytes, Microsporum gypseum, Microsporum canis*) may spread between rabbits and other mammalian species, including humans.
- *Fusobacterium necrophorum* can spread to humans via wound contamination and animal bite wounds (very rare).
- Cheyletiellosis is zoonotic and can cause popular dermatitis in humans.
- Some tick species that affect rabbits may carry zoonotic diseases.

GEOGRAPHY AND SEASONALITY

- Most conditions occur worldwide with no seasonality, apart from some that are associated with ectoparasites.
- Compulsive self-mutilation disorder in laboratory rabbits may be worse in late summer/fall.

ASSOCIATED CONDITIONS AND DISORDERS

- Abscesses (see Abscesses)
- Autoimmune disease
- Bacterial infection (necrobacillosis, staphylococcosis, pasteurellosis, treponematosis)
- Cutaneous neoplasms and nodules
- Dental disease
- Ectoparasite infestations (fleas, mites, lice, ticks, myiasis)
- Fungal infection (dermatophytosis)
- Hepatic disorders (see Hepatic Disorders)
- Mammary gland disorders
- Ocular disorders
- Otitis externa (see Otitis)
- Perineal soiling (urinary and/or fecal)
- Pododermatitis
- Upper respiratory tract disorders
- Viral infection (myxomatosis, Shope fibromatosis, Shope papillomavirus)

CLINICAL PRESENTATION

DISEASE FORMS/SUBTYPES

- Alopecia
- Moist dermatitis
- Pruritus
- Fungal infection (dermatophytosis)
- Bacterial infection (necrobacillosis, staphylococcosis, pasteurellosis, treponematosis)
- Viral infection (myxomatosis, Shope fibromatosis, Shope papillomavirus)
- Moulting
- Matting
- Scaling and crusting
- Sebaceous adenitis
- Self-mutilation
- Cellulitis
- Ehlers-Danlos–like syndrome
- Neoplasia (primary and secondary, benign and malignant tumors)
- Urine/fecal soiling
- Eosinophilic granuloma
- Ectoparasite infestations (fleas, mites, lice, ticks, myiasis)
- Pododermatitis

HISTORY, CHIEF COMPLAINT

- Pruritus, alopecia, scaling/crusting, mass effects, hair matting, hair discoloration, moist hair, odiferous coat, erythema and inflammation, self-mutilation
- In one survey, pruritus (40%) and alopecia (25%) were the most common presenting signs of a primary dermatologic condition for presentation to the vet.

PHYSICAL EXAM FINDINGS

- Pruritus
- Alopecia
- Scaling/crusting
- Mass effects
- Pain
- Hair matting
- Hair discoloration
- Moist hair
- Odiferous coat
- Erythema and inflammation
- Ectoparasite infestations
- Abscessation
- Dental disease
- Cutaneous nodules
- Soiled perineum (urinary and/or fecal)

ETIOLOGY AND PATHOPHYSIOLOGY

- Pruritus: rabbits may lick, bite, or chew rather than use their feet to scratch
- Parasites: ectoparasites such as fleas (*Spilopsyllus cuniculi, Ctenocephalides* spp.), mites (*Cheyletiella parasitovorax, Psoroptes cuniculi, Sarcoptes scabei, Notoedres cati, Leporacus gibbus, Demodex cuniculi*), lice (*Haemodipsus ventricosus*), ticks (*Haemaphysalis leporis-palustris, Amblyomma* spp., *Boophilus* spp., *Rhipicephalus* spp., *Dermacentor* spp., *Otobius* spp., *Ornithodoros* spp.), and myiasis may lead to pruritus, alopecia, and secondary infection. Many ectoparasites also serve as vectors for transmission of viral diseases such as myxomatosis and calicivirus (see Ectoparasites). The common rabbit intestinal worm *Passalurus ambiguus* may cause perianal pruritus and rectal prolapse (rare).
- Infection: bacterial infection and dermatophytosis may lead to pyoderma, cellulitis, and folliculitis
- Neoplasia: cutaneous lymphoma and other neoplastic diseases
- Self-mutilation: hereditary compulsive self-mutilation described in inbred Checkered Cross rabbits. Chemically-induced self-mutilation cases have been reported following hind leg intramuscular injections of ketamine and xylazine. Eosinophilic granuloma has been described in rabbits (rare).
- Allergic: verified cases of atopic dermatitis, food hypersensitivity, and contact hypersensitivity have not been confirmed in rabbits
- Injection site reactions may lead to alopecia, pruritus, and infection.
- Alopecia: loss of hair may be due to different processes, depending on the underlying cause:
  - New hair failing to grow when old hairs are lost (endocrine causes rare in rabbits)
  - Inflammation in hair follicles leading to hair loss (e.g., bacterial infection, dermatophytosis)
  - Breakage of hair due to trauma/pruritus (e.g., ectoparasitic infestation, self-mutilation)
  - Behavioral: pregnant and pseudopregnant does pull out hair from ventrum to line nest; barbering by dominant rabbit to submissive rabbit
  - Some breeds (e.g., Angora) may moult in patchy fashion, leading to irregular coat length and the appearance of alopecia.
  - Nutritional (rare): deficiencies in sulfur amino acids (e.g., lysine) and in Mg, Cu, and Zn can be associated with alopecia
  - Neoplasia, especially cutaneous lymphoma
  - Other causes include ischemia (e.g., postvaccinal vasculitis) and hair loss secondary to sebaceous adenitis, eosinophilic granuloma (rare).
- Moist dermatitis: can arise from excessive moisture on hair or coat, conformational and physical issues, or underlying disease. Affected areas may be moist, erythematous, edematous, painful, and odiferous. Hair discoloration may occur, especially with secondary *Pseudomonas* spp. infection (creating a blue-green color). Affected areas may also be vulnerable to myiasis.
  - Excessive moisture: wetting of hair or coat can lead to secondary infection if coat is not dried adequately. Dirty and damp conditions may predispose to dermatitis.
  - Conformational and physical issues
    - Dewlap: moist dermatitis may arise in skin folds associated with dewlap, especially in does with large dewlap
    - Long-haired breeds may experience difficulty in grooming effectively.
    - Matting of hair, especially in long-haired breeds, may evoke moist dermatitis.
    - Obesity and reduced flexibility and agility may hinder effective grooming.
    - Perineal skin folds may be excessive and vulnerable to moist dermatitis.
    - Reduced ability to adopt appropriate urination stance or ingestion of cecotrophs may evoke perineal dermatitis.
    - Trauma
  - Underlying disease
    - Dental disease may lead to drooling and excessive salivation and can result in chin wetness and moist dermatitis. Dental disease may also hinder effective grooming.
    - Ocular, nasolacrimal, and upper respiratory tract disease may lead to epiphora, mucopurulent ocular discharge, or nasal discharge, resulting in facial dermatitis.
    - Perineal dermatitis may follow soiling with urine or feces. Urinary and fecal soiling can result from genitourinary tract disease, gastrointestinal disease, musculoskeletal disease, any cause of polyuria, *Encephalitozoon cuniculi* (see Encephalitozoonosis) infection, inappropriate diet leading to

uneaten or excessive cecotrophs, and diarrhea.
- Mass effects, nodules, and swellings: various disease problems (infectious and noninfectious) can lead to cutaneous masses, nodules, and swellings
  - Noninfectious
    - Neoplasia: an array of primary and secondary, benign and malignant tumors have been reported in rabbits (see Cutaneous Masses)
    - Disseminated collagenous hamartomas: benign proliferations of connective tissue presenting as a solitary mass or disseminated; thought to have an X-linked recessive inheritance in male rabbits
    - Dermal fibrosis: thickening of skin of dorsum reported in two male rabbits; not associated with alopecia or pruritus
    - Eosinophilic granuloma (rare)
    - Hematoma
  - Infectious
    - Viral infection: myxomatosis, Shope fibromatosis, and Shope papilloma virus infection can lead to skin swelling, fibromas, and cutaneous masses. Shope fibroma virus and Shope papilloma virus are oncogenic. Atypical myxomatosis may result in scabby lesions on the face and body and is thought to occur from rabbits that have been previously vaccinated but did not receive the intradermal dose (see Cutaneous Masses and Myxomatosis).
    - Abscessation: resulting from skin wounds or bacteremia or secondary to otic, dental, or nasolacrimal duct disease
    - Bacterial infection: secondary bacterial infection of wounds may occur, especially with *S. aureus, P. multocida,* and *Pseudomonas aeruginosa,* leading to pyoderma and cellulitis. Primary infection with some bacterial organisms may also occur (e.g., *S. aureus, P. multocida, Treponema paraluiscuniculi* [rabbit syphilis]).
    - Necrobacillosis (Schmorl's disease): an uncommon disease associated with infection by *F. necrophorum,* which may be derived from rabbit feces. Wound contamination may lead to swelling, inflammation, abscessation, and ulceration, particularly on the face and neck. Caseous necrosis is a feature of infection.
    - Cellulitis: usually associated with bacterial infections *S. aureus* and *P. multocida*
    - Tapeworm cyst formation *(Coenurus serialis)* following ingestion of eggs and emergence of oncospheres from small intestine and later development of cysts in muscular and subcutaneous tissue
    - Warble fly *(Cuterebra cuniculi)* infestation: larvae enter host through a normal orifice and migrate to a subcutaneous site, resulting in a fistulated nodule
- Scaling and crusting
  - Dermatophytosis: infection with *T. mentagrophytes* and *M. canis.* Lesions usually appear as focal alopecia with variable scales and crusts and are more commonly found at the ear base, muzzle, paws, and nail beds. Lesions may be pruritic. Affected animals may be subclinical carriers.
  - Ectoparasites: *Cheyletiella parasitovorax* infestation may cause crusting scaling of skin, especially the dorsum with variable alopecia and pruritus
  - Treponematosis: *Treponema paraluiscuniculi* (rabbit syphilis) infection may result in crusty lesions on mucocutaneous junctions (nose, lips, eyelids, genitalia). Transmission is vertical and sexual.
  - Sebaceous adenitis: rare condition thought to be most likely due to an autoimmune disease directed at sebaceous glands and a defect in lipid metabolism. It features progressive exfoliative, nonpruritic dermatosis. Lesions usually begin at the face and neck. A case of exfoliative dermatitis with concurrent thymoma has been reported, as has a single case associated with autoimmune hepatitis.
- Other conditions
  - *Malassezia* dermatitis: considered rare in rabbits and most likely associated with other dermatologic conditions (e.g., sarcoptic mange)
  - Pododermatitis: has many possible causes; see Pododermatitis
  - Ehlers-Danlos–like syndrome featuring increased skin fragility and hypermobility secondary to collagen defect has been reported in two rabbits.

DIAGNOSIS

DIFFERENTIAL DIAGNOSIS

- Pruritus: may be associated with alopecia
  - Bacterial infection
  - Moist dermatitis
  - Dermatophytosis
  - Ectoparasite infestation
  - Self-mutilation
  - Vaccination site reaction
  - Eosinophilic granuloma (rare)
  - Allergy (rare)
- Alopecia: establishing pattern and association with inflammation/pruritus may aid in determining underlying cause
  - Symmetric with minimal inflammation
    - Behavioral
    - Barbering
    - Endocrinopathies (rare)
  - Symmetric with inflammation
    - Sebaceous adenitis
  - Localized or multifocal
    - Bacterial infection
    - Moist dermatitis
    - Dermatophytosis
    - Ectoparasite infestation
    - Self-mutilation
    - Moulting pattern
    - Ineffective grooming
    - Nutritional deficiency
    - Vaccination site reaction
    - Eosinophilic granuloma
    - Cutaneous lymphoma
- Moist dermatitis
  - Excessive moisture
    - Inadequate coat drying
    - Dirty or damp environment
  - Conformational and physical issues
    - Dewlap dermatitis
    - Inadequate grooming (long-haired breeds, matting of coat, obesity, reduced flexibility, dental disease)
    - Perineal skin fold excess
    - Improper urination stance
    - Trauma
  - Underlying disease
    - Dental disease
    - Ocular disease
    - Nasolacrimal and upper respiratory tract disease
    - Urinary or fecal soiling secondary to diseases of the genitourinary tract, gastrointestinal tract, musculoskeletal system; *E. cuniculi* infection; inappropriate diet and polyuria
- Mass effects, nodules, and swellings
  - Noninfectious
    - Neoplasia
    - Disseminated collagenous hamartoma
    - Dermal fibrosis
    - Eosinophilic granuloma
    - Hematoma
  - Infectious
    - Viral infection (myxomatosis, Shope fibromatosis, and Shope papilloma virus)
    - Abscessation
    - Necrobacillosis
    - Cellulitis
    - Tapeworm cyst formation
    - *C. cuniculi* infestation
- Scaling and crusting
  - Dermatophytosis
  - Ectoparasites
  - Treponematosis
  - Sebaceous adenitis
- Blue/green fur discoloration
  - *P. aeruginosa* infection

- Increased skin fragility and hypermobility
  - Ehlers-Danlos–like syndrome

INITIAL DATABASE

- Complete history and dermatologic examination, including thorough otoscopy
- Trichogram, acetate tape preparations, skin scraping, and skin impression cytologic examination
- Fine-needle aspirate of masses and swellings for cytologic and microbiological examination
- Wood's lamp examination (approximately 50% of strains of *M. canis* will fluoresce with an apple green color)
- Thorough dental examination (may require sedation or anesthesia)

ADVANCED OR CONFIRMATORY TESTING

- Dermatophyte culture
- Enzyme-linked immunosorbent assay (ELISA) available for *T. mentagrophytes* infection
- Blood biochemistry, hematologic analysis, and urinalysis to determine presence of underlying disease
- Skin biopsy and histopathologic examination, especially of masses
- Sampling of abscessation, deep pyoderma, or cellulitis for microbial culture and sensitivity
- Silver stains for *T. paraluiscuniculi* infection
- Darkfield microscopy for *T. paraluiscuniculi* infection
- Serologic examination for *T. paraluiscuniculi* infection
- Serologic examination for *E. cuniculi* infection
- Radiographic imaging of limbs and spine to assess for arthritis and spinal disorders (e.g., spondylosis)
- Radiographic imaging of skull to assess dental disease
- Radiographic imaging of abdo thorax to assess for neoplasia and genitourinary tract and gastrointestinal tract disease
- Abdominal ultrasonography may aid in assessment of gastrointestinal and genitourinary tract disease.
- Electron microscopy of skin: used to examine collagen structure to facilitate diagnosis of Ehlers-Danlos–like syndrome

TREATMENT

THERAPEUTIC GOAL

Alleviation of skin problem and any underlying condition

ACUTE GENERAL TREATMENT

- Depends on underlying cause(s)
- Moist dermatitis
  - Important to identify underlying cause
  - Gently clip and clean affected areas. Removal of hair facilitates drying of area; hair should be removed with careful use of clippers up to the area of unaffected skin. Remove all matted hair. Skin is very fragile and is prone to tearing.
  - Clipping may require light sedation. Consider midazolam 0.5-2 mg/kg IM, IV or diazepam 0.5-2 mg/kg IM.
  - Do not bathe skin until all hair is removed from affected areas. Use dilute chlorhexidine-based shampoos and ensure that area is dried thoroughly after bathing.
- Supportive care is vital, particularly nutritional and fluid support if rabbit has compromised status or is anorectic.
- For superficial infection, suitable first-line antibiotics may include procaine penicillin 40,000-60,000 IU/kg SC, IM q 24 h or enrofloxacin 10 mg/kg PO, SC q 12 h or trimethoprim/sulfonamides 30 mg/kg PO q 12 h.
- Topical antimicrobial therapy can also be employed but may be readily licked away by the rabbit, hence the choice of nontoxic compounds. Consider topical treatment with preparations containing fusidic acid, silver sulfadiazine/chlorhexidine, mupirocin calcium, or Manuka honey.
- Analgesia: some conditions may be associated with pain, especially perineal dermatitis
  - Nonsteroidal antiinflammatory drugs (NSAIDs) (e.g., carprofen 2-4 mg/kg PO, SC q 24 h; meloxicam 0.3-0.5 mg/kg PO, SC q 24 h; ketoprofen 1-3 mg/kg PO q 12 h)
  - Opioids (e.g., buprenorphine 0.03 mg/kg SC, IM q 8 h)
- Ectoparasite treatment (see Ectoparasites)
- Myxomatosis: consider euthanasia

CHRONIC TREATMENT

- Address underlying cause (e.g., dental disease, genitourinary tract disease)
- Dermatophytosis
  - May be difficult to eradicate in groups of rabbits because all in-contact rabbits require treatment
  - May require environmental decontamination: use diluted bleach (1:10)
  - Topical therapy options include applying or bathing with imidazoles (e.g., miconazole 2% twice weekly for 3 weeks, enilconazole 0.2% twice weekly for 3 weeks, clotrimazole 1% cream twice daily for 3 to 4 weeks) and lime sulfur dips. Bathing in rabbits should always be carried out carefully, ensuring adequate drying of coat afterward.
  - Systemic therapy may be employed for refractory cases (e.g., itraconazole 5 mg/kg PO q 24 h × 3-4 wk; griseofulvin 25 mg/kg PO q 24 h × 4-6 wk)
- Treponematosis: treat all exposed rabbits with penicillin G 42,000-84,000 IU/kg SC, IM q 7 d × 3 wk
- Surgery
  - Dermoplasty: surgical removal of excessive skin folds in the perineum and dewlap may aid in prevention of skin fold dermatitis
  - Abscessectomy: owing to the caseous nature of rabbit pus and the development of a thick abscess capsule, complete abscessectomy may be required to treat abscesses. Many abscesses may be refractory to medical therapy alone.
  - Cyst removal: subcutaneous cysts of *Coenurus serialis* may be surgically resected
  - Warble fly (*C. cuniculi*) larvae removal surgically: requires careful widening of fistula and retrieval without crushing larvae because this may otherwise evoke anaphylaxis. Further débridement and antibiosis may be required once larvae have been removed.
  - Ovariohysterectomy: for nonbreeding does that pull out hair
  - Shope papilloma virus: nodules may be resected
- Parasite treatment
  - Ectoparasite treatment (see Ectoparasites)
  - Myiasis: careful cleaning and clipping of affected areas. Treat as moist dermatitis. Remove maggots. Give ivermectin 0.4 mg/kg SC to treat larvae that hatch from unremoved eggs. Address underlying cause for attraction of flies to skin.
  - *Passalurus ambiguus*: treat all in-contact rabbits (fenbendazole 20 mg/kg PO × 5 d, repeated in 10-14 d)
- Address inappropriate diets: diets that lead to issues with cecotrophy should be addressed and nutritional deficiencies corrected
- Neoplasia: excision and/or chemotherapy depending on diagnosis
- Barbering: separation of rabbits
- Dermal fibrosis: no treatment necessary
- Disseminated collagenous hamartoma: none; resection of nodules if affecting rabbit
- Sebaceous adenitis: one report of successful treatment using cyclosporine A 5 mg/kg PO q 24 h combined with a medium-chain triglyceride solution (Miglyol 812, BUFA, Uitgeest, The Netherlands)
- Ehlers-Danlos–like syndrome: no specific treatment

DRUG INTERACTIONS

- Avoid use of oral preparations of lincomycin, clindamycin, erythromycin, and penicillins.
- Avoid the use of NSAIDs in dehydrated and renally compromised patients.

POSSIBLE COMPLICATIONS

- Worsening of lesions due to failure to address underlying cause(s)
- Antibiotic dysbiosis
- Nonimprovement of urinary and fecal soiling
- Myiasis

RECOMMENDED MONITORING

Lesion size and spread and response to therapy

PROGNOSIS AND OUTCOME

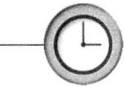

- Prognosis depends on underlying cause.
- Many dermatologic conditions in rabbits can be treated or managed.
- Myxomatosis carries a poor prognosis.
- Pododermatitis can be challenging and difficult to treat.

PEARLS & CONSIDERATIONS

COMMENTS

- Avoid using corticosteroids in rabbits because their use can precipitate clinical disease in a subclinically affected animal.
- Do not use fipronil in rabbits. Deaths following fipronil use have been reported in rabbits.
- Avoid use of organophosphates in rabbits.
- Pyrethrin-based products for use in dogs and cats may be toxic to rabbits.

PREVENTION

- Emphasize importance of appropriate feeding. Pet rabbit diets should consist largely of grass or grass hays (at least 80% of diet) (e.g., timothy, oaten hays). A variety of fresh leafy green vegetables can be added to the diet. Pellets (if fed at all) should be of the highest quality, viewed as a supplement, and fed in very limited amounts. Seed mixes, cereals, etc., should not be fed or should be offered only in very small amounts intermittently as treats.
- Encourage dry, clean, compliant bedding, and avoid moist conditions.
- Prevention of pododermatitis is enhanced by proper husbandry, diet, and client education.
- Avoid obesity (see Obesity).
- Vaccination against myxomatosis: vaccines are based on live attenuated Shope fibroma virus
- Ectoparasite prophylaxis in high-risk areas
- Neutering of female rabbits

CLIENT EDUCATION

- Measures to minimize development of pododermatitis such as suitable substrate provision and good diet are essential.
- Owners of breeds considered more vulnerable to pododermatitis (e.g., Rex, giant breeds) should have special emphasis placed on preventive measures and signs to be monitored.
- Emphasize importance of appropriate feeding. Pet rabbit diets should consist largely of grass or grass hays (at least 80% of diet) (e.g., timothy, oaten hays). A variety of fresh leafy green vegetables can be added to the diet. Pellets (if fed at all) should be of the highest quality, viewed as a supplement, and fed in very limited amounts. Seed mixes, cereals, etc., should not be fed or should be offered only in very small amounts intermittently as treats.
- Encourage regular grooming of rabbits, especially long-haired breeds.

SUGGESTED READINGS

Bomhard WV, et al: Disseminated collagenous hamartomas in rabbits—a new entity, Kleintierpraxis 53:224–230, 2008.

Florizoone K, et al: Symmetrical alopecia, scaling and hepatitis in a rabbit, Vet Dermatol 18:161–164, 2007.

Hill PB, et al: Survey of the prevalence, diagnosis and treatment of dermatological conditions in small animals in general practice, Vet Rec 158:533–539, 2006.

Jassies-van der Lee A, et al: Successful treatment of sebaceous adenitis in a rabbit with ciclosporin and triglycerides, Vet Dermatol 20:67–71, 2009.

White SD, et al: Dermatologic problems of rabbits, Comp Cont Ed Pract Vet 25:90–101, 2003.

White SD, et al: Lymphoma with cutaneous involvement in three domestic rabbits *(Oryctolagus cuniculus)*, Vet Dermatol 11: 61–67, 2000.

CROSS-REFERENCES TO OTHER SECTIONS

Abscesses
Cutaneous Masses
Dental Disease
Ectoparasites
Encephalitozoonosis
Endoparasites
Hepatic Disorders
Intestinal Disorders
Lower Urinary Tract Disorders
Myxomatosis
Obesity
Otitis
Pasteurellosis
Pododermatitis
Staphylococcosis
Treponematosis

AUTHOR: **DAVID VELLA**

EDITOR: **THOMAS M. DONNELLY**

RABBITS

Dysautonomia (Grass Sickness)

BASIC INFORMATION

DEFINITION

Clinical illness caused by dysfunction of the autonomic nervous system resulting from degenerative changes in neurons in the autonomic nervous system

SYNONYM

One form of constipative mucoid enteropathy

SPECIAL SPECIES CONSIDERATIONS

- Affects lagomorphs—rabbits and wild hares *(Lepus europaeus)*
- Has strong similarities to equine dysautonomia (grass sickness), feline and canine dysautonomia

EPIDEMIOLOGY

SPECIES, AGE, SEX Dysautonomia has been confirmed in domestic (show, pet, and laboratory) and wild rabbits. Weanling rabbits are particularly susceptible, but adults can also be affected. No sex predilection has been noted.

RISK FACTORS Weaning appears to be a risk factor, particularly if the change from a mainly milk to a low-fiber adult diet is abrupt. Other risk factors are not known.

CONTAGION AND ZOONOSIS
- A contagious nature is not confirmed, but multiple cases can occur at one site.
- No evidence suggests that it is a zoonosis.

GEOGRAPHY AND SEASONALITY Has been reported in domestic rabbits in Holland and seen in domestic and wild rabbits in England. Reports suggest that it occurs in France. (In wild hares, it has been confirmed in England and Scotland.)

ASSOCIATED CONDITIONS AND DISORDERS Clinical aspects of dysautonomia share features with the syndrome "constipative mucoid enteropathy." However, not all cases of mucoid enteropathy examined have had histologic evidence of neuronal degeneration in the ganglia.

CLINICAL PRESENTATION

HISTORY, CHIEF COMPLAINT Anorexia, obtundation, tooth grinding, palpable large bowel impaction, and the passage of mucus are characteristic clinical signs. Weight loss can be rapid.

PHYSICAL EXAM FINDINGS As well as diminished bowel function (distended stomach, impacted cecum) and bladder function (urinary retention and overflow incontinence), some show signs of swallowing difficulties (including debris in the mouth and perioral crusting with dry saliva and food) and inhalation pneumonia with crusting of the nostrils. Bradycardia, mydriasis, and dry mucosa have also been reported.

ETIOLOGY AND PATHOPHYSIOLOGY

- The causative agent is not known. A neurotoxin is postulated.
- In equine dysautonomia, evidence suggests that a toxico-infectious botulism caused by *Clostridium botulinum* type C toxin may be responsible for the neuronal degeneration.

DIAGNOSIS

DIFFERENTIAL DIAGNOSIS

- Other forms of "constipative mucoid enteropathy"
- Obstructive or inflammatory lesions involving the intestinal tract
- Severe coccidiosis

INITIAL DATABASE

- Diagnostic biochemical tests have not been identified.
- Radiographs can be helpful in evaluating abdominal contents.
- Fecal analysis to rule out coccidiosis

ADVANCED OR CONFIRMATORY TESTING

- No specific lab or imaging tests are available to validate an in vivo diagnosis.
- Confirmation of a suspected clinical diagnosis depends on careful postmortem dissection to retrieve ganglia (cranial mesenteric and cranial cervical are the easiest to locate, and the largest; stellate and caudal mesenteric can also provide a diagnosis). Diagnosis hinges on histopathologic confirmation of chromatolytic changes in various ganglionic neurons.
- Diagnostic chromatolytic changes are also present in autonomic preganglionic and somatic motor lower motor neurons in the brainstem, as well as in lower motor neurons in the spinal cord. The distribution of central changes is identical in horses, cats, dogs, and hares, with dysautonomia implying a shared origin.
- Systematic gross and histologic screening of the carcass for other lesions may provide an alternative explanation for the signs seen in vivo in suspect cases.

TREATMENT

THERAPEUTIC GOAL

In the absence of a specific premortem diagnosis, treatment of suspect cases is of necessity very nonspecific and involves supportive control of dehydration and hypoglycemia and provision of good hay bedding and fresh grass to try to restore an interest in eating and to promote bowel function.

ACUTE GENERAL TREATMENT

- Some have suggested that antibiotic treatment or prophylaxis at weaning may be helpful.
- Most rabbits require euthanasia on humane grounds after only a few days.
- Bowel motility stimulants may be appropriate.

CHRONIC TREATMENT

Very few cases will survive long enough to be considered chronic. However, it can only be helpful and can improve the chances of survival if efforts are made to control the secondary effects of bowel stasis.

POSSIBLE COMPLICATIONS

Oral administration of treatments is especially hazardous in cases with interference with the swallowing mechanism—and may lead to, or contribute to, inhalation pneumonia.

PROGNOSIS AND OUTCOME

Rabbit dysautonomia has a very poor prognosis. In a group of rabbits with suspected dysautonomia, it is advisable to have any early death(s) assessed by a postmortem examination with histopathologic examination when the carcass is still in fresh condition.

PEARLS & CONSIDERATIONS

COMMENTS

Because confirmation of suspect cases can be achieved only after histopathologic assessment of ganglia, the expense of a full necropsy examination is justified in an outbreak situation. Fresh tissues are essential, so close liaison with the lab is advisable.

PREVENTION

- Preventive measures are difficult to provide because the causes and trigger mechanisms for dysautonomia are not known.
- Avoidance of abrupt dietary changes, especially around the time of weaning

CLIENT EDUCATION

Clients should seek early veterinary advice with constipative conditions. Simple gentle abdominal palpation may provide early warning of trouble.

SUGGESTED READINGS

Hahn CN, et al: Neuropathological lesions resembling equine grass sickness in rabbits, Vet Rec 156:778–779, 2005.
Harcourt-Brown F: Dysautonomia. In Textbook of rabbit medicine, Oxfordshire, UK, 2002, Reed Educational and Professional Publishing Ltd, pp 278–280.
Harcourt-Brown F, et al: Rabbits and hares. In Mullineaux E, et al, editors: BSAVA manual of wildlife casualties, Quedgeley, UK, 2003, British Small Animal Veterinary Association, pp 109–122.
Van Der Hage MH, et al: Caecal impaction in the rabbit: relationships with dysautonomia, Toulouse, France, July 9–12, 1996, Proceedings 6th World Rabbit Congress, pp 77–80.
Whitwell K, et al: Mucoid enteropathy in UK rabbits: dysautonomia confirmed, Vet Rec 139:323–324, 1996.

CROSS-REFERENCES TO OTHER SECTIONS

Cardiovascular disease
Intestinal disorders
Lower respiratory tract disorders
Lower urinary tract disorders

AUTHORS: **KATHERINE E. WHITWELL AND CAROLINE HAHN**

EDITOR: **DAVID VELLA**

RABBITS

Ectoparasites

BASIC INFORMATION

DEFINITION

- Major ectoparasites of rabbit include *Cheyletiella parasitovorax,* fleas, *Notoedres cati, Psoroptes cuniculi,* and *Sarcoptes scabei.*
- Other ectoparasites include ticks, the fur mite *Leporacarus gibbus* (formerly *Listorphorus gibbus*), *Cuterebra cuniculi,* lice *(Haemodipsus ventricosus),* and fly larvae causing myiasis.

SYNONYMS

- *C. parasitovorax* = rabbit fur mite; "walking dandruff"
- Fleas = *Spilopsyllus cuniculi* (rabbit fleas), *Ctenocephalides felis* (cat flea), *Ctenocephalides canis* (dog flea)
- *Psoroptes cuniculi* = rabbit ear mites
- *Cuterebra cuniculi* = Warble flies
- *Haemodipsus ventricosus* = Pediculosis

SPECIAL SPECIES CONSIDERATIONS

- Parasites account for more than 80% of dermatologic diagnoses in exotic species; the most common diagnosis is unspecified mite infestation.
- In the United Kingdom and Europe, *P. cuniculi* are the most frequent cause of otitis in rabbits and may be the most frequent cause of dermatologic disease. However, the prevalence of ectoparasites and dermatologic conditions varies by region (tropic/temperate zone), country, and season (e.g., *S. scabei* is frequent in tropical countries/regions).

EPIDEMIOLOGY

SPECIES, AGE, SEX A survey of dermatologic conditions of small animals in general practice revealed that rabbits with parasitic disease ranged in age from 4 weeks to 10 years, with a median age of 2 years and a mode of <1 year. Any species, age, or sex of rabbit can be affected by ectoparasites.

RISK FACTORS

- Rabbits housed with other infected rabbits or with exposure to wild rabbits are at risk of infestation.
- Rabbits housed with dogs or cats may be exposed to *Ctenocephalides.*
- Pregnant does and kits may be more prone to severe rabbit flea infestation because ova of the flea mature only after the female feeds on a pregnant doe late in gestation.

CONTAGION AND ZOONOSIS

- Ectoparasites can be transmitted between rabbits.
- Cheyletiellosis is a zoonosis that causes papular dermatitis in humans and may be transmittable to other species, including dogs and cats.
- Rabbit fleas and lice are vectors for tularemia (see Tularemia, Sec. VI). They rarely bite humans but may bite dogs and cats.
- Ticks are important vectors of zoonotic disease (e.g., Rocky Mountain spotted fever, tularemia, Lyme disease). Most ticks that feed on rabbits rarely bite humans.

GEOGRAPHY AND SEASONALITY

- Some ectoparasites are more commonly seen in warmer months in temperate and cool climates (e.g., fleas).
- *Cuterebra cuniculi* are found in North America.
- Many tick species are specific to particular regions.

ASSOCIATED CONDITIONS AND DISORDERS

- The rabbit flea (*S. cuniculus*), rabbit louse (*H. ventricosus*) and the fur mite (*C. parasitovorax*) are vectors for myxomatosis (see Myxomatosis).
- Heavy infestations of fleas and lice may cause anemia.

CLINICAL PRESENTATION

HISTORY, CHIEF COMPLAINT Pruritus is the most common clinical sign.

PHYSICAL EXAM FINDINGS

- Physical examination findings include scales and crusts, and alopecia.
- *P. cuniculi* are associated with inflammation (hypersensitivity reaction to mite piercing skin to feed) and reddish-brown crusting of the external ear canal, head shaking, ear drooping, and pruritus; inflammation and crusting may be generalized in debilitated rabbits; severe infection can lead to eardrum perforation and neurologic signs.
- *C. parasitovorax* may be subclinical but more often causes a scaly, dry, sometimes pruritic dermatitis with patchy alopecia or broken hairs over the dorsal neck, trunk, hind end, and abdomen.
- *S. scabei* and *Notoedres cati* cause a crusty, pruritic dermatitis around the head, neck, and trunk.
- Flea infestations may manifest as a dull coat, easily epilated hair, and patchy alopecia with pruritus, skin erythema, and crusting, especially on the pinnae and face. Flea droppings may be seen in the coat.
- Lice infestations may cause weight loss, alopecia, pruritus and papule formation.

ETIOLOGY AND PATHOPHYSIOLOGY

- *P. cuniculi* are large, obligate, nonburrowing parasites with a 3-week life cycle and an ability to survive off the host for up to 21 days.
- The life cycle of the flea is controlled by the hormonal cycle of the host (this explains the sudden proliferation on pregnant does and young rabbits).
- *H. ventricosus* life cycle is 2 to 5 weeks
- *Cuterebra cuniculi* hatched larvae crawl into fur and enter host through a normal orifice and migrate to a subcutaneous site.

DIAGNOSIS

DIFFERENTIAL DIAGNOSIS

Other differentials for ectoparasites include dermatophytes, *Treponema paraluiscuniculi* and other bacterial infections, sebaceous adenitis, endocrine conditions, viral disease, dermal fibrosis, neoplasia, eosinophilic granuloma, Ehlers-Danlos syndrome, and dental disease (may cause moist dermatitis on chin or front legs from excessive drooling).

INITIAL DATABASE

- *Psoroptes* mites may be identified with the naked eye, an otoscope, or a microscope. Microscopic examination of crusts may reveal mites, mite feces, mite eggs, inflammatory cells, desquamated epithelial cells, and serum.
- *Cheyletiella* infection is diagnosed by clinical signs and microscopic examination of mites in skin scrapings, acetate tape preparations, or skin and hair debris that sticks to a flea comb.
- *S. scabei* and *Notoedres cati,* similar to *P. cuniculi,* are diagnosed by skin scraping.
- Fleas are diagnosed by identifying fleas and their droppings (flea dirt) on the rabbit.
- Lice (and their eggs) may be identified with the naked eye.
- *Cuterebra cuniculi* lesions may be diagnosed as a subcutaneous cyst with a central fistula (breathing hole).

TREATMENT

THERAPEUTIC GOAL

Ectoparasite eradication

ACUTE GENERAL TREATMENT

- *Psoroptes* can be treated with ivermectin (400 mcg/kg SC q 10-14 d for 3 treatments) or selamectin (6-18 mg/kg twice, 28 days apart). Less effective treatment methods include topical mineral oil, acaricides, and flea powder. Do not remove crusts from ears mechanically because this is painful (treatment should resolve).

- *Cheyletiella* can be treated with ivermectin (400 mcg/kg SC q 14 d for 3 treatments) or selamectin (6-18 mg/kg twice, 28 days apart). Other treatments include weekly lime sulfur dips for 3 to 6 weeks or application of carbaryl flea powder appropriate for cats twice weekly for 6 weeks.
- *S. scabei* and *N. cati* are treated similarly to *P. cuniculi.*
- Fleas can be treated with imidacloprid (Advantage; 10 mg/kg every month topically) and the insect growth regulator, lufenuron (Program; 30 mg/kg PO every month). Alternatively, carbaryl-based flea powder, safe for cats, can be used 1 to 2 times per week.
- Ticks can be treated topically with imidacloprid + permethrin (Advantix) at 10 + 50 mg/kg every month.
- Lice can be treated with imidacloprid 10 mg/kg topically
- *Cuterebra cuniculi* require surgical removal without damaging the larvae

CHRONIC TREATMENT

- Clean environment and treat contaminated areas with flea products.
- In flea infestations, treat the environment with insect growth regulator and insecticidal sprays (with rabbits removed from area until products have dried). Borate powder may be used on infected rugs.
- Ensure that all in-contact pet mammals are treated.

DRUG INTERACTIONS

- Fipronil (Frontline) is not recommended because adverse reactions (depression, anorexia, neurologic signs, and death), especially in small or young rabbits, have been reported.
- Organophosphates and flea collars are not appropriate for flea control because of their toxicity in rabbits.
- Over-the-counter permethrin or pyrethrin spray-on/spot-on are toxic to rabbits when applied in high concentrations.

POSSIBLE COMPLICATIONS

Permethrin- and pyrethrin-based environmental treatments may be ineffective because of flea resistance.

RECOMMENDED MONITORING

Monitor skin for signs of recurrence.

PROGNOSIS AND OUTCOME

Prognosis is good with appropriate therapy.

CONTROVERSY

- No evidence of the depot effect of selamectin has been noted in rabbits, although such evidence has been found in dogs and cats. Pharmacokinetic data indicate a short half-life after topical administration of 10 mg/kg in rabbits (0.93 d) compared with dogs (11.1 d) and cats (8.25 d). T_{max} (amount of time that drug is present at the maximum concentration in serum) is 0.5 days for 10 mg/kg and 20 mg/kg topical in rabbits.
- Rapid transdermal absorption may occur with other topical parasiticides in rabbits. Prolonged residual activity of topical parasiticides seen in dogs and cats may not occur in rabbits.
- Toxicity seen with fipronil may be due to rapid transdermal absorption.

PEARLS & CONSIDERATIONS

COMMENTS

Having environmental control of all ectoparasites is as important as treating the rabbit. This may involve regular changing of the bedding, treatment of in-contact animals, and chemical treatment of the environment.

PREVENTION

Minimize exposure to infected rabbits, dogs, and cats, as well as to wild rabbits.

CLIENT EDUCATION

Alert client to zoonotic potential of cheyletiellosis.

SUGGESTED READINGS

Hill PB, et al: Survey of the prevalence, diagnosis and treatment of dermatological conditions in small animals in general practice, Vet Rec 158:533–539, 2006.

White SD, et al: Dermatologic problems of rabbits, Compend Contin Educ Pract Vet 25:90–101, 2003.

CROSS-REFERENCES TO OTHER SECTIONS

Cutaneous Masses
Dermatopathies
Myxomatosis
Tularemia (Section VI)

AUTHOR: **JENNIFER GRAHAM**

EDITOR: **DAVID VELLA**

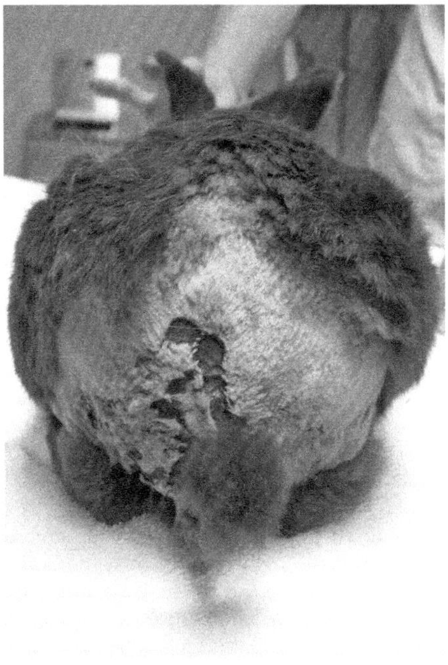

Ectoparasites Flystrike in a rabbit. The perianal area is often affected by flystrike; the area needs to be cleaned and wound management needs to be started after the maggots have been removed. *(Photo courtesy Jörg Mayer, The University of Georgia, Athens.)*

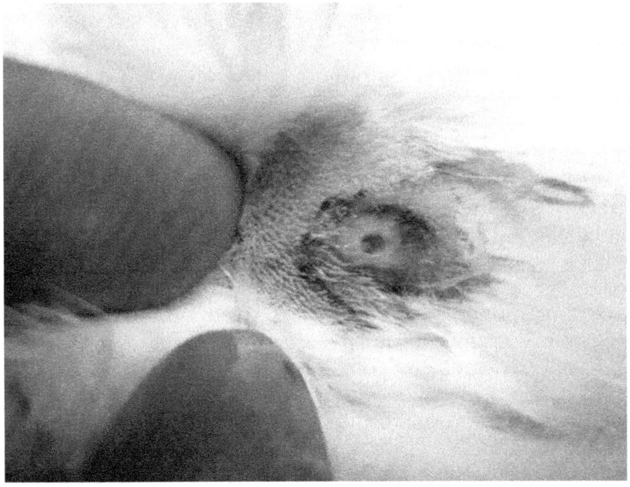

Ectoparasites Breathing hole of cuterebra larvae; the larvae are sitting just under the surface and move back and forth. Removal of the larvae requires local anesthesia. *(Photo courtesy Jörg Mayer, The University of Georgia, Athens.)*

RABBITS

Electrocution

BASIC INFORMATION

DEFINITION

Electrocution occurs when an animal becomes part of an electric circuit or is affected by the thermal effects of a nearby electrical arc. Passage of electricity through tissue results in electrophysiologic disruption of organs and burns. Classifications of electrical injuries generally focus on the power source (lightning or electrical), voltage (high or low voltage), and type of current (alternating [AC] or direct [DC]), each of which is associated with certain injury patterns. This topic reviews electrical injuries caused by manufactured electricity.

SYNONYMS

Electrical injury, electric shock

EPIDEMIOLOGY

SPECIES, AGE, SEX Any rabbit has the tendency to chew on cables and wires.
RISK FACTORS Environmental access to live cables and wires

CLINICAL PRESENTATION

- Anorexia due to oral burns
- Lethargy due to prolonged anorexia
- Dyspnea due to noncardiogenic pulmonary edema

DISEASE FORMS/SUBTYPES

- Electrical injuries are caused by
  - High-voltage AC (e.g., overhead high-voltage power line)
  - Low-voltage AC (this is the form always seen when animals bite into electrical cords in the home or an office setting)
  - DC (e.g., third energized rail of an electrical train system is contacted)

HISTORY, CHIEF COMPLAINT

- Sometimes witnessed; other times, the owner reports sudden onset of dyspnea, dysphagia, or collapse
  - Low-voltage AC injury without loss of consciousness and/or arrest; may result in significant injury with prolonged, tetanic muscle contraction
  - Low-voltage AC injury with loss of consciousness and/or arrest. In respiratory arrest or ventricular fibrillation that is not witnessed, electrical exposure may be difficult to diagnose.
- In mild cases, the only complaint is anorexia due to oral burns.

PHYSICAL EXAM FINDINGS

- Oral burns: to the tongue, palate, and commissures of the lips (sedation for the oral exam is often required)
- Singed hair around face, head, or body
- Respiratory problems: dyspnea, cyanosis, coughing
- Cardiac problems: arrhythmias
- Anorexia, lethargy

ETIOLOGY AND PATHOPHYSIOLOGY

- Electricity disrupts the electrophysiologic activity of tissue, causing muscle spasms, ventricular fibrillation, and vasomotor changes in the central nervous system, resulting in acute pulmonary edema
  - 60 Hz of alternating current or 120 volts is found in most households in the United States; in Europe and Australia, it is usually 50 Hz of alternating current or 220 volts.
- Electrical energy is also transformed into heat that causes coagulation of tissue proteins. Sudden death may result from these processes.
- Electrocution is almost always accidental, typically with an unconfined rabbit chewing on an electric cord.
- Electrocution experiments using rabbits resulted in complete arrest of respiration throughout the duration of shock with currents >50 mA; respiration restarted some seconds after the current was stopped.
  - When death occurred, the cause was asphyxia produced during the shock, arrest of circulation, or both.
  - With currents >1 ampere, significant tissue heating occurs with marked macroscopic and histologic changes at the sites of electrocution.

DIAGNOSIS

DIFFERENTIAL DIAGNOSIS

Chemical or thermal burns, exposure to fire, and smoke inhalation

INITIAL DATABASE

- Initial database is dependent on the severity of injury:
  - If the rabbit has no physical exam abnormalities, no testing is required.
  - If the rabbit is dyspneic or if pulmonary crackles are auscultated, chest radiographs are warranted.
  - In severely affected animals, complete blood count, serum biochemistry profile, coagulation profile, and urinalysis are warranted

ADVANCED OR CONFIRMATORY TESTING

- Arterial blood gas analysis may be useful in documenting hypoxemia.
  - In young or small animals, the stress of blood gas sample collection should be weighed against its potential benefits.

TREATMENT

THERAPEUTIC GOALS

- Treatment of pulmonary edema
- Treatment of burns
- Supportive care
  - Avoid development of hepatic lipidosis due to prolonged anorexia.

ACUTE GENERAL TREATMENT

- Noncardiogenic pulmonary edema is treated with rest and supplemental oxygen.
- Bronchodilators (e.g., albuterol 0.05 mg/kg PO q 8 h, or by aerosol; aminophylline 20 mg/kg PO q 12 h or 6-11 mg/kg PO, IM, or slow IV q 8 h) may help in clearing pulmonary edema.
- Intravenous fluid support may be required.
- Diuretics and glucocorticoids usually are not warranted.
- Positive-pressure ventilation with positive end-expiratory pressure in theory should help maximally distend the alveoli that are available and should keep the smaller airways open during the expiratory phase of respiration. However, if mechanical ventilation is deemed necessary, a poor outcome is likely.

CHRONIC TREATMENT

- Clean wounds.
- Treat burns with topical antibiotic (e.g., silver sulfadiazine).
- Provide soft food/feeding tube if burns are in the mouth.
- Surgical débridement and closure with extensive wounds
- Pain management (nonsteroidal anti-inflammatory drugs [NSAIDs] and opioids)
  - NSAIDs (e.g., carprofen 2-4 mg/kg PO, SC q 24 h; meloxicam 0.3-0.5 mg/kg PO, SC q 24 h; ketoprofen 1-3 mg/kg PO q 12 h)
  - Opioids (e.g., buprenorphine 0.03 mg/kg SC, IM q 8 h)

POSSIBLE COMPLICATIONS

- Infection of nonhealing burns
- Acute lung injury
- Acute respiratory distress syndrome
- Hepatic lipidosis due to prolonged (>24 hours) starvation

RECOMMENDED MONITORING

- Observation of food and water intake in immediate postinjury period is critical because supportive care (food/fluids) is often required.
- Monitor
  - Respiratory rate and effort
  - Healing of any burns

PROGNOSIS AND OUTCOME

- Depends on the degree of injury and severity of induced underlying disorders such as noncardiogenic pulmonary edema
- Critical period is the first 24 to 48 hours after electrical shock. If the animal survives this period and shows interest in food, prognosis is improved.

PEARLS & CONSIDERATIONS

COMMENTS

Noncardiogenic pulmonary edema can be the result of decreased alveolar pressure, increased vascular permeability, or neurological complications. Success of therapy will depend on the detection and treatment of the trigger factors. The basic approach to treatment includes oxygen and fluid therapy, and strict cage rest. To date there are no clear treatment recommendations. The prognosis is linked to the cause of edema and very often is guarded.

PREVENTION

- Remove access to wires that are plugged into outlets.
- Provide protective sheathing for all electrical cords and wires.

CLIENT EDUCATION

- Offer enough chew toys to rabbits, so there is less tendency or need to chew on inappropriate objects.
- Rabbit-proof any area in which the rabbit resides. Strictly supervise exercise outside of this area.

SUGGESTED READINGS

Lee WR, et al: Effects of electric shock on respiration in the rabbit, Br J Ind Med 21:135–144, 1964.

Spies C, et al: Narrative review: electrocution and life-threatening electrical injuries, Ann Intern Med 145:531–537, 2006.

CROSS-REFERENCES TO OTHER SECTIONS

Anorexia
Cardiovascular disease
Lower respiratory tract disorders

AUTHOR: **JÖRG MAYER AND THOMAS M. DONNELLY**

EDITOR: **DAVID VELLA**

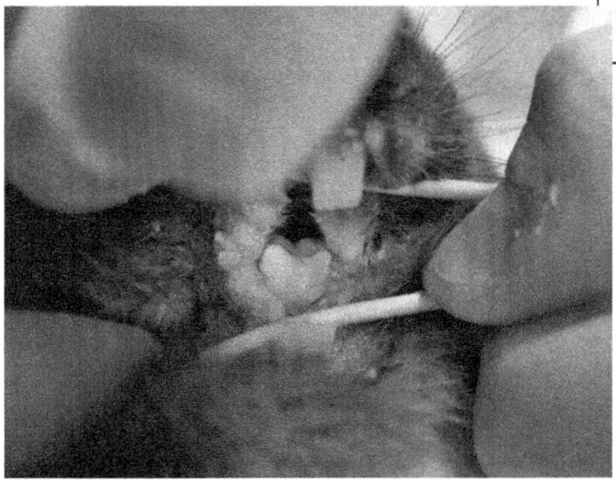

Electrocution Rabbit with lip, cheek, and tongue burns secondary to chewing an electrical cord. Note the pale avascular labial, lingual, and buccal necrotic tissue. The chief clinical sign was anorexia. *(Photo courtesy Jörg Mayer, The University of Georgia, Athens.)*

RABBITS

Encephalitis

BASIC INFORMATION

DEFINITION

Encephalitis is inflammation of the brain. Meningitis is inflammation of the membranes that cover the brain and spinal cord (meninges). Meningoencephalitis is concurrent inflammation of both the brain and the meninges.

SYNONYM

Encephalomeningitis

EPIDEMIOLOGY

GENETICS AND BREED PREDISPOSITION

- Lop-eared rabbits appear to be at increased risk for otitis externa, which may lead to meningitis in severe cases.
- Dwarf rabbits may have increased risk of exhibiting clinical signs due to *Encephalitozoon cuniculi* infection.

RISK FACTORS

- Otitis externa/media (see Otitis)
- Dental disease
- Positive *E. cuniculi* titer
- Exposure to toxins
- Exposure to raccoon feces
- Pasteurellosis (see Pasteurellosis)

CONTAGION AND ZOONOSIS

- *E. cuniculi* is a potential zoonosis, with immune suppressed individuals at particular risk.
- *Pasteurella multocida* contracted from a pet rabbit has resulted in fatal infection in one human.

GEOGRAPHY AND SEASONALITY

- Rabies is not present in the United Kingdom or Australia.
- *Baylisascaris procyonis* is found in North America.

ASSOCIATED CONDITIONS AND DISORDERS

- Otitis externa may be associated with increased risk of meningitis.
- *E. cuniculi* infection is positively associated with increased risk of seizure disorders and chronic renal disease (see Renal Disease).

CLINICAL PRESENTATION

DISEASE FORMS/SUBTYPES

- Meningitis may be further classified into:
  - Pachymeningitis (inflammation of the outer meningeal membrane)
  - Leptomeningitis (inflammation of the inner meningeal membrane)

HISTORY, CHIEF COMPLAINT

- Often an acute onset of clinical signs such as head tilt/rolling/urine scalding/falling/seizures
- Possible prior history of upper respiratory, dental, or aural disease
- Access to outdoors may be consistent with exposure to toxins (e.g., lead) and/or parasitic encephalitis (e.g., *B. procyonis*, toxoplasmosis, encephalitozoonosis).

PHYSICAL EXAM FINDINGS

- Neurologic signs will be the prominent findings:
  - Head tilt
  - Rolling
  - Ataxia
  - Nystagmus
  - Opisthotonus
  - Torticollis
  - Reduced mentation
- It is important to not ignore the non-neurologic signs (e.g., presence of urine scalding, otitis externa/media, dental disease, evidence of unexplained skin trauma/scuffing of nails).

ETIOLOGY AND PATHOPHYSIOLOGY

- Bacterial
  - Common
  - Related to dental, upper respiratory, or ear disease (pasteurellosis commonly implicated)
  - Listeriosis *(Listeria monocytogenes)* is a potential cause of meningoencephalitis in weanling rabbits.
- Protozoal
  - Exposure to *E. cuniculi* is common, but the incidence of disease caused by this organism is unknown.
  - Toxoplasmosis is seen sporadically.
- Viral
  - Rare
  - Rabies after a nonfatal bite is a potential differential diagnosis in endemic areas.
  - Herpes viral encephalitis after exposure to human herpes simplex virus has been reported.
- Parasitic
  - *B. procyonis* (raccoon roundworm) infestation is a possible cause in endemic areas, but occurrence is sporadic. A similar species, *B. columnaris,* is found in skunks but most reported cases of baylisascariasis are due to *B. procyonis.*
- Fungal
  - Not reported in rabbits currently, but in endemic areas should be considered
- Inflammatory
  - Heatstroke or granulomatous inflammation without evidence of causative organisms is a common postmortem finding. This has been suggested to be caused by *E. cuniculi.*
- Neoplastic
  - Potential differential diagnoses are pituitary adenomas and teratomas.
- Traumatic
- Toxic
  - Exposure to lead or organophosphate pesticides

DIAGNOSIS

DIFFERENTIAL DIAGNOSIS

- Seizures: epilepsy, uremia, hepatic encephalopathy, toxins, neoplasia, infection
- Urine scalding: urinary sludging, urolithiasis, cystitis, polyuria, spinal disease
- Head tilt/rolling: middle/inner ear disease
- Nystagmus: peripheral or central vestibular disease (see Vestibular Disease)
- Reduced mentation: sedation, uremia

INITIAL DATABASE

- Complete blood count and blood biochemistry
- Urinalysis, including trichrome stain to look for *E. cuniculi* spores
- Skull radiography
- Neurologic examination
- Fecal examination

ADVANCED OR CONFIRMATORY TESTING

- Aural examination under general anesthesia (using endoscope preferably) and cytologic and bacteriologic sampling from middle ear
- *E. cuniculi* serology
- *Toxoplasma* serology
- Rabies titer
- Serum lead evaluation
- Cerebrospinal fluid analysis
- Magnetic resonance imaging
- Computed tomography
- Necropsy, including histopathologic examination of the brain in cases where rabbit colonies are involved, or if rabies is suspected

TREATMENT

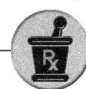

THERAPEUTIC GOALS

- To achieve sufficient neurologic function to allow good quality of life
- To control seizure activity
- To provide pain control as required

ACUTE GENERAL TREATMENT

- Provide safe, padded environment.
- Establish IV access and provide fluid and nutritional support as indicated.
- Control seizures with benzodiazepines (e.g., diazepam 1-5 mg/kg IV; midazolam 0.2-2 mg/kg IV IM).
- Cautious use of corticosteroids may be justified in severe cases (e.g., dexamethasone 1-2 mg/kg IM, IV once; prednisolone 0.05-2 mg/kg SC, IM once).
- Use of prochlorperazine (0.25-0.5 mg/kg q 8-12 h PO) may enhance stability.
- Broad-spectrum antibiotics with good central nervous system penetration (e.g., chloramphenicol 20-50 mg/kg q 8-12 h IM, IV, SC, PO; ceftazidime 50 mg/kg q 8 h IM, IV)

CHRONIC TREATMENT

- Benzimidazoles (e.g., fenbendazole 20 mg/kg q 24 h PO × 28 d for encephalitozoonosis; consider oxytetracycline 50 mg/kg q 12 h PO or enrofloxacin 5-10 mg/kg PO, SC, IM IV q 12 h in addition)
- *B. procyonis* infection: ivermectin 0.2-0.4 mg/kg q 7-10 d PO, SC; or oxibendazole 60 mg/kg q 24 h PO indefinitely
- Long-term antibiotics in response to culture and sensitivity results
- Long-term nonsteroidal antiinflammatory (NSAIDs) medication may prove beneficial (e.g., meloxicam 0.3-0.5 mg/kg q 12-24 h PO, SC).
- Supportive feeding as required
- Monitor for potential ongoing problems such as perineal cecotrophal soiling, urine scalding and associated dermal and urinary problems.
- Barbiturates to control chronic seizures (e.g., phenobarbital 2.5-5 mg/kg q 12 h PO; adjust accordingly)
- Lead toxicity: chelation therapy via NaCa-EDTA 27.5 mg/kg SC q 12 h × 5 d, repeated after 5 days. Repeat blood lead level 5 days after last treatment. Alternatively D-penicillamine 30 mg/kg q 12 h PO.

DRUG INTERACTIONS

NSAIDs and corticosteroids may interact, causing gastrointestinal ulceration.

POSSIBLE COMPLICATIONS

- Deterioration despite treatment
- Traumatic skeletal or ocular damage due to seizures or rolling
- Urine scalding
- Perineal cecotrophal soiling
- Gut stasis
- Status epilepticus

RECOMMENDED MONITORING

- Repeated neurologic examinations at intervals determined by rapidity of resolution of clinical signs
- Regular weighing and clinical examinations to ensure that the rabbit is adequately able to feed and clean itself
- Regular dental examinations
- Blood phenobarbital levels in rabbits receiving this drug

PROGNOSIS AND OUTCOME

- Dependent on causative agent/process and severity/duration of clinical signs at presentation
- Owners should be made aware of potentially prolonged recovery period and high risk of recurrence
- Part of the recovery process is learning to cope with clinical signs (rabbits and owners); failure of rabbit to cope may be triggered by other (unrelated) disease.

CONTROVERSY

- *E. cuniculi*: it is not yet known how many rabbits that are seropositive for encephalitozoonosis actually develop disease directly due to this organism
- Lufenuron is an oral chitin synthesis inhibitor. Although lufenuron probably does not kill *E. cuniculi,* it may hinder growth of microsporidia.

PEARLS & CONSIDERATIONS

COMMENTS

Many rabbits with seemingly insurmountable neurologic dysfunction are able to cope well within the home environment. It is better to assess this on "home ground" by looking at video footage or making a home visit, rather than on the basis of appearance in the examination room.

PREVENTION

- Avoid access to raccoon, skunk, and cat feces.
- Remove potential toxins from environment.
- Perform routine dental examinations to minimize the likelihood of untreated disease spreading into central nervous system.
- Use elevated food bowls and water bottles to reduce ingestion of *E. cuniculi* spores from urine-contaminated ground.
- Consider treating "in-contact" rabbits with fenbendazole prophylactically in cases where encephalitozoonosis is suspected.

CLIENT EDUCATION

To recognize early signs of disease and concurrent problems such as urine scalding

SUGGESTED READINGS

Carpenter JW: Diagnosing and treating common neurologic diseases in rabbits, Vet Med 101:728–736, 2006.

Gruber A, et al: A retrospective study of neurological disease in 118 rabbits, J Comp Pathol 140:31–37, 2009.

Keeble E: Common neurological and musculoskeletal problems in rabbits, In Pract 28: 212–218, 2006.

CROSS-REFERENCES TO OTHER SECTIONS

Abscesses
Encephalitozoonosis
Otitis
Pasteurellosis
Renal Disorders
Vestibular Disease

AUTHOR: **MOLLY VARGA**

EDITOR: **DAVID VELLA**

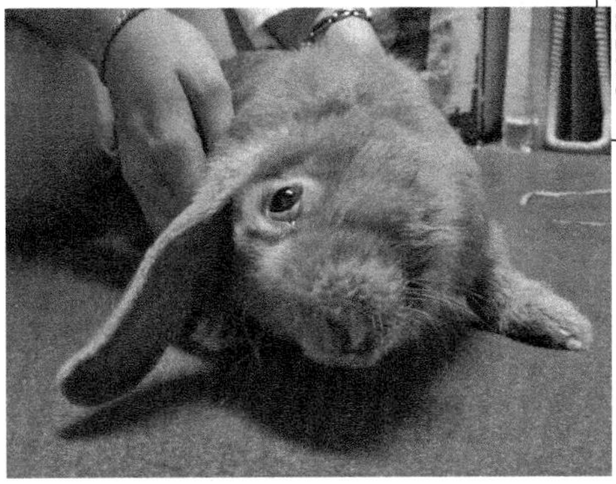

Encephalitis Torticollis is a common clinical sign of encephalitis in the rabbit. *(Photo courtesy Jörg Mayer, The University of Georgia, Athens.)*

RABBITS

Encephalitozoonosis

BASIC INFORMATION

DEFINITION

Encephalitozoonosis is a disease caused by a mammalian protozoal parasite belonging to the phylum Microsporidia. These obligate intracellular protozoa are spore-forming with a wide host distribution. Microsporidia are a diverse group of parasitic organisms, with more than 1200 recognized species in 143 genera.

SYNONYMS

- *Encephalitozoon cuniculi* is the most common microsporidian infection in mammals and has been reported in humans, rodents, guinea pigs, foxes, monkeys, cats, dogs, sheep, goats, pigs, and llamas.
- Three strains of *E. cuniculi:*
    - Strain I (rabbits and humans)
    - Strain II (rodents)
    - Strain III (dogs and humans)
- *Encephalitozoon intestinalis, Encephalitozoon hellem,* and *Enterocytozoon bieneusi* are reported commonly in humans as a cause of diarrhea. *E. bieneusi* has been described in wild and farmed rabbits in Spain. *E. hellem* can cause significant disease in immune compromised humans and psittacine birds. On further typing, previous reports of *E. cuniculi* in birds are now thought to be *E. hellem.*

SPECIAL SPECIES CONSIDERATIONS

Wide host distribution; clinical signs are most severe in rabbits, dogs, monkeys, and guinea pigs

EPIDEMIOLOGY

SPECIES, AGE, SEX Rabbits—any age and sex (no predilection to infection found in healthy rabbits). In the UK, 52% seroprevalence has been reported in healthy pet rabbits.

RISK FACTORS

- A study of healthy pet rabbits in the UK failed to identify any of the following as potential risk factors for infection: husbandry, diet, breed, age, sex, body weight, vaccination status, health status, contact with *E. cuniculi*–positive rabbits, and preventive medicine routine.
- Potential risk factors, however, include the following:
    - Contact with urine
    - Immune suppression
    - Juvenile animals and neonates with immature immune systems
    - Vertical transmission in utero

CONTAGION AND ZOONOSIS

- Transmission via oral ingestion of spores from infected urine or by contaminated food items and water
- Vertical transmission following transplacental infection reported
- Infection following inhalation also possible experimentally
- Environmental spore survival is, on average, 4 weeks.
- Spores are easily destroyed by disinfectants.
- Microsporidian infections are important in immune compromised humans and may cause severe life-threatening systemic disease. A direct link has never been identified between pet rabbits and human cases; however, *E. cuniculi* strains of human origin can infect rabbits and are immunologically and molecularly identical to those isolated from rabbits. It is likely that rabbits infected with *E. cuniculi* pose a zoonotic risk to immune compromised humans.

GEOGRAPHY AND SEASONALITY Microsporidial infections in humans have a worldwide distribution, except for Antarctica. Infection with *E. cuniculi* has been diagnosed in rabbits in Europe, Asia, Africa, America, and Australia. The parasite is frequently encountered in laboratory rabbits but is rare in wild rabbits in the UK. It is a newly emerging pathogen in pet rabbits.

ASSOCIATED CONDITIONS AND DISORDERS

- Clinical signs of encephalitozoonosis in rabbits can be indistinguishable from otitis media/interna and other causes of head tilt and neurologic disease in rabbits (differential diagnoses below).

- Rabbits:
  - Granulomatous interstitial pneumonitis
  - Focal interstitial granulomatous hepatitis
  - Granulomatous interstitial nephritis
  - Focal nonsuppurative granulomatous meningoencephalitis
  - Cataracts
  - Uveitis

CLINICAL PRESENTATION

DISEASE FORMS/SUBTYPES

- *E. cuniculi* infection in rabbits can cause severe life-threatening disease in some animals; others show no clinical signs.
- Carrier status with subclinical infection is common.

HISTORY, CHIEF COMPLAINT

- Urinary incontinence
- Head tilt
- Hind limb weakness
- Weight loss
- Anorexia
- Blepharospasm and ocular discharge

PHYSICAL EXAM FINDINGS

- Neurologic disease
  - Head tilt
  - Ataxia
  - Hind limb paresis
  - Torticollis
  - Paralysis
  - Retarded growth
  - Collapse
  - Tremors
  - Convulsions
  - Urinary incontinence
- Renal disease
  - Weight loss
  - Polyuria/polydipsia
  - Cystitis
- Ophthalmic disease
  - Cataract formation
  - Uveitis—primary or phacoclastic

ETIOLOGY AND PATHOPHYSIOLOGY

- Parasite is ingested and carried in macrophages via blood to target organs: liver, kidney, central nervous system, lungs, and heart.
- Serum immunoglobulin (Ig) G antibody titers rise 3 to 4 weeks post infection and peak at 6 to 9 weeks.
- Spores are excreted in the urine from 1 month post infection until 3 months post infection, when shedding stops.
- Host cell infected by injection of spore into cytoplasm using polar filament or phagocytosis
- Spore multiplies, causing cell rupture and spore release to extracellular spaces.
- Spores infect surrounding cells and are passed via circulation to other organs.
- Chronic diffuse cellular infiltration and granuloma formation occur with mononuclear cell infiltration.
- Ocular lesions due to spores deposited in developing lens post vertical transmission in utero. Spores later erupt to produce cataracts and lens-induced uveitis, secondary to lens rupture.

DIAGNOSIS

DIFFERENTIAL DIAGNOSIS

- Otitis media/otitis interna
- Spinal fracture secondary to trauma
- Bacterial central abscess (e.g., *Pasteurella* infection)
- Splay leg
- Lead toxicity
- Toxoplasmosis
- Listeriosis
- Heatstroke

INITIAL DATABASE

- Full neurologic examination
  - Central vestibular disease usually associated with multiple CNS signs
  - Not associated with facial nerve paralysis or Horner's syndrome
- Complete blood count
  - Anemia
  - Elevated total white cell count
- Serum biochemistry
  - Elevated blood urea nitrogen (BUN) and creatinine
  - Hyperkalemia
  - Hyponatremia
  - Elevated aspartate aminotransferase
  - Elevated glutamate dehydrogenase
- Urinalysis
  - Including cytologic examination and culture—to rule out other causes of urogenital tract disease
- Radiography
  - Routine skull radiography to rule out otitis media/interna
- Antibody assay tests
  - Serum antibody assay tests most widely used: immunofluorescent assays, ELISA assays, and carbon immunoassays
  - Serum ELISA tests commonly used to record IgG titers to *E. cuniculi*, with rising levels of antibodies at least 4 weeks apart indicating active infection
  - Antibody levels start to rise 2 weeks post infection, peaking at 10 weeks; spores present in the urine 3 to 4 weeks post infection
  - Wide variations in antibody response reported in rabbits, with some animals having persistently high levels of IgG for a long time, and others becoming negative after 8 weeks
  - Antibody levels can persist for years in rabbits with no clinical signs.
  - Severity of clinical signs not related to level of serum antibody titer
  - Single positive antibody test in a healthy rabbit
    - Indicates parasite exposure but does not indicate disease course. Three scenarios are possible: the rabbit could just have become infected (early infection) before the development of clinical signs; could be chronically infected, with no clinical signs; or could have been previously infected and then recovered.
  - Single positive antibody test in a rabbit showing clinical signs associated with *E. cuniculi* infection
    - If a single positive titer is recorded in a rabbit with CNS or renal disease, this suggests that active infection may be present, although rule out other differential diagnoses.
  - Single negative antibody response in a healthy animal
    - Does not rule out early infection in that seroconversion occurs 2 weeks post initial infection. If rabbit is healthy, repeat test 4 weeks later to rule out early infection, especially if the history indicates that the rabbit has already been in contact with another positive animal.
  - Single negative antibody test in a rabbit showing signs associated with *E. cuniculi* infection
    - In cases associated with clinical signs, however, a single negative result rules out *E. cuniculi* as a cause of clinical disease.
  - Seroconversion precedes renal shedding by 4 weeks, so antibody assay tests could be used in a multirabbit household to screen in-contact animals after a clinical case has occurred.
  - In the UK, serum IgM antibody titers may be measured with IgG, enabling potential distinction between acute active infection (elevation of both IgG and IgM) and chronic infection (IgG only elevated). Some chronic infections however may show elevation of both.
- PCR
  - Developed in humans for identification of *E. cuniculi* antigen in patient's urine or sputum
  - Available commercially in the UK for detection of *E. cuniculi* DNA in CSF and urine
  - In neurologic cases associated with known *E. cuniculi* infection, PCR on CSF samples detects 10% of cases, and PCR on urine detects 40% of cases.
  - Test depends on whether animal is excreting spores in urine at the time of sampling (excretion stopped by day 98 post infection).

  - Negative PCR result doesn't rule out disease and is more likely in chronic cases with neurological signs. In cases presenting with ocular clinical signs, PCR testing of aspirated lens material is highly diagnostic.
- Postmortem
  - Histopathologic demonstration of organism in rabbit kidney or brain is only definitive test.
  - Organism may not be found despite classic clinical signs and changes on histopathologic examination, making absolute diagnosis difficult.
- Other diagnostic tests (less commonly used):
  - Intradermal skin tests not sensitive and so no longer used
  - Culture of spores from urine or tissue samples on rabbit fibroblast monolayers
  - Urine samples centrifuged and examined for spores using modified trichrome stains or immunofluorescence
  - Urinary protein: creatinine ratio is not useful as no difference has been demonstrated between *E. cuniculi* serum IgG antibody positive and negative rabbits.

ADVANCED OR CONFIRMATORY TESTING

- Renal biopsy has been described for diagnosis of this disease in humans and rabbits by laparotomy or laparoscopy.
- CSF analysis: collect from cisterna magna or lumbosacral epidural space under general anesthesia. Mononuclear pleocytosis with elevated protein is a regular feature of rabbit encephalitozoonosis; however, these changes may be seen with other infections and are not on their own diagnostic for this disease.
- MRI and CT to rule out differential diagnoses (e.g., vestibular disease, CNS soft tissue masses)

TREATMENT

THERAPEUTIC GOALS

- Aim to reduce inflammation and inhibit spore formation.
- Response to treatment is variable, depending on how advanced the disease is.
- Chronic cases usually have neurologic signs associated with severe cell damage; successful treatment may not be possible.
- Acute cases with urinary incontinence may resolve with treatment.
- Ocular disease has a good prognosis, but in severe cases, phacoemulsification of the lens or enucleation may be indicated.

ACUTE GENERAL TREATMENT

- Oral fenbendazole 20 mg/kg PO q 24 h × 28 d. Inclusion of fenbendazole in a treatment protocol is associated with an increased survival rate.
- Covering broad-spectrum antibiosis, such as trimethoprim-sulfamethoxazole 30 mg/kg PO q 12 h, or enrofloxacin 10 mg/kg PO q 12 h × 10 d
- In acutely presenting cases, dexamethasone at 0.1-0.2 mg/kg SC q 48 h × 3 doses may be given.
- Glucocorticoids should be used with care in rabbits because they may lower white cell counts and affect cell-mediated immune response, thus limiting host defenses and increasing risk for other infections. Although one study showed 50% recovery rates in rabbits with neurologic signs treated with dexamethasone, a more recent study showed treatment with dexamethasone had no effect on neurological score or on short- or long-term survival.
- Severe neurologic signs may require sedation of the rabbit with diazepam or midazolam at 0.5 mg/kg SC, IM, or IV.
- Prochlorpherazine 0.2-0.5mg//kg PO q 8 h may be useful in rabbits with severe head tilt as it is used in humans with labyrinthitis
- Recent human research has found IFN-gamma useful in the treatment of *E. cuniculi.*

CHRONIC TREATMENT

A study in laboratory rabbits using fenbendazole showed it was safe and effective in reducing clinical signs in less advanced cases, and it prevented infection in exposed in-contact rabbits.

POSSIBLE COMPLICATIONS

Recent toxicity trials have indicated that fenbendazole is well tolerated by rabbits and has a wide safety margin (Winslet et al., 2007). Toxicities such as bone marrow suppression, which have been reported in other species associated with this drug, have not been recorded in rabbits at doses up to 85 mg/kg for 30 days.

RECOMMENDED MONITORING

- Repeat serologic screening for antibody titers post treatment is recommended after 28 days.
- In cases with altered hematologic and biochemical parameters, repeat blood samples should be taken during and after treatment.

PROGNOSIS AND OUTCOME

- Prognosis depends on clinical presentation. The prognosis is good for animals with ocular disease only following appropriate treatment.
- Subclinical infection appears to be common, with more than 50% of normal healthy pet rabbits having already been exposed and showing positive antibody titers.
- Rabbits with severe advanced neurologic disease may not respond to treatment; euthanasia should be considered in these cases.

PEARLS & CONSIDERATIONS

COMMENTS

- The rabbit–parasite relationship has yet to be fully understood.
- Establishment of infection and development of clinical signs are thought to be dependent on several factors: parasite species and strain, route of infection, age of the rabbit at the time of infection; and rabbit's immune status.
- If a balance between rate of infection and the rabbit's immunity is evident, clinical signs may not develop.
- Clinical signs may develop later on in association with concurrent infection, stress, or immune suppression.
- If the rabbit becomes immune suppressed following exposure, clinical disease is likely to develop.
- In immune deficient rabbits and in young and newborn animals with immature immune systems, disease is more likely.
- It is possible that clinical signs could develop at a later date in these cases as the result of concurrent infection, stress, or immune suppression. This is thought to be the case in the pet rabbit situation, where normal healthy seropositive animals can go on to develop clinical signs associated with infection at a later date.

PREVENTION

- Subclinical infection and carrier status make control of the disease difficult.
- Establishment of an *E. cuniculi*–free breeding colony is possible.
  - Healthy *E. cuniculi*–negative young rabbits are housed in complete isolation from other rabbits and in separate cages.
  - Serum antibody levels are tested every 2 weeks for 2 months; all positive animals, however weak the titer, are removed.
  - Testing continues until all animals are negative for 1 month.

- These animals set up the breeding colony, but testing should continue on a monthly basis to confirm disease-free status.
- In an outbreak, in-contact rabbits should be serologically screened to identify infected animals before the parasite is excreted in the urine.
  - These animals may be isolated, and treatment with fenbendazole commenced.
- Risk of infection can be reduced by using good hygiene practices such as regular disinfection of the cage, food bowls, and water containers, and by reducing urine contact between rabbits.

CLIENT EDUCATION

- Monitor closely for recurrence of clinical signs.
- Healthy positive rabbits may not require treatment with fenbendazole. These cases should be carefully monitored by serologic testing.
- Possible zoonotic infection may be found in immune compromised humans.
- Consider a prophylactic fenbendazole course for newly acquired rabbits at risk for previous infection.

SUGGESTED READINGS

Csokai J, et al: Encephalitozoonosis in pet rabbits *(Oryctolagus cuniculus)*: pathohistological findings in animals with latent infection versus clinical manifestation, Parasitol Res 104:629–635, 2009.
Jass A, et al: Analysis of cerebrospinal fluid in healthy rabbits and rabbits with clinically suspected encephalitozoonosis, Vet Rec 162:618–622, 2008.
Jeklova E, et al: Usefulness of detection of specific IgM and IgG antibodies for diagnosis of clinical encephalitozoonosis in pet rabbits, Vet Parasitol 170:143–148, 2010.
Keeble E: Encephalitozoonosis in rabbits—what we do and don't know, In Practice 33:426–435, 2011.
Sieg J, et al: Clinical evaluation of therapeutic success in rabbits with suspected encephalitozoonosis, Vet Parasitol 187:328–332, 2012.
Winslet V, et al: Evaluation of the safety of fenbendazole in rabbits. Birmingham, UK, 2007, BSAVA Congress 2007 Scientific Proceedings: Veterinary Programme, Section II: Clinical Research Abstracts, Exotics, pp 471.

CROSS-REFERENCES TO OTHER SECTIONS

Abscesses
Encephalitis
Endoparasites
Otitis
Pasteurellosis
Renal disorders
Upper respiratory tract disorders
Vestibular disease

AUTHOR: **EMMA KEEBLE**

EDITOR: **DAVID VELLA**

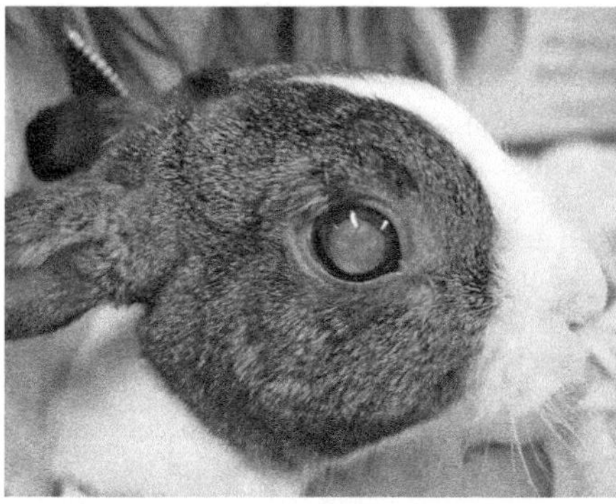

Encephalitozoonosis Severe cataract formation due to *Encephalitozoon cuniculi* infection; phacoemulsification or enucleation is treatment of choice. Histologic examination of the enucleated eye should always be performed to demonstrate causative agents. *(Photo courtesy Jörg Mayer, The University of Georgia, Athens.)*

RABBITS

Endoparasites

BASIC INFORMATION

DEFINITION

Any of various parasites that live in the internal organs and tissues of their host

SYNONYMS

- Parasite: most common use of the word refers to helminth (endoparasite) and arthropod (ectoparasite) parasites. Protozoa can also be endoparasites.
- Helminth: parasitic worm—nematode, cestode, or trematode
- Nematode: roundworm
- Pinworm: nematode worm. *Passalurus ambiguus* is the common pinworm of rabbits.
- Trichostrongylid: nematode worm. *Graphidium strigosum* and *Obeliscoides cuniculi* are stomach worms of rabbits; *Trichostrongylus retortaeformis* is found in the small intestine.
- Cestode: tapeworm. Numerous *Taenia* spp. are found in carnivores, and herbivores act as intermediate hosts throughout the world. Many species appear to have two scientific names because the larval (metacestode) stages in herbivores were often named as *Cysticercus, Strobilocercus,* or *Coenurus* spp., before it was realized that they were developmental stages of adult *Taenia* tapeworms found in carnivores. These terms are now considered to be invalid generic names.
- Cysticercosis: infection with metacestodes in the intermediate hosts of species-specific cestodes
- Trematode: a flatworm or fluke
- Protozoa: structurally and genetically diverse single-cell organisms. Major protozoal infections are discussed as separate topics (see Coccidiosis). Until recently, microsporidia *(Encephalitozoon cuniculi)* were classified as protozoa, but RNA analysis has resulted in reclassification of these pathogens to the fungi. See Encephalitozoonosis.

SPECIAL SPECIES CONSIDERATIONS

The most important endoparasitic diseases in pet rabbits are coccidiosis, encephalitozoonosis, and different helminthiases. Although numerous helminths have been described in wild rabbits, surveys of pet rabbits in Europe have shown an incidence of 5% *Passalurus ambiguus,* 1% trichostrongylids, and 0.5% trematodes.

Helminths

- Normal wild rabbits and many domestic rabbits have high numbers of pinworms in the cecum and colon.
- Trichostrongylid nematodes *(G. strigosum, O. cuniculi)* may be present in the stomach of wild rabbits. Infection rarely occurs in pet rabbits.
- Occasional reports describe cysticercosis in pet rabbits. Intermediate stages are found in wild rabbits and hares.
- *Taenia pisiformis* (formerly *Cysticercus pisiformis*) that forms cysts in visceral organs (especially liver)
- *Taenia serialis* (formerly *Coenurus serialis*) form cysts in intermuscular fascia or subcutis.
- More than 100 species, including rabbits, can be paratenic for the raccoon roundworm *Baylisascaris procyonis.* Infection of rabbits is reported infrequently in North America and Japan. Raccoons were introduced to Europe in the 1930s, but to date, no reports have described *B. procyonis* infection in rabbits in Europe.

- Rabbits are susceptible to infection with bovine liver fluke *Fasciola hepatica.* Infection is rare in pet rabbits.

Protozoa

- Rabbits are susceptible to infection with *Toxoplasma gondii.* Infection has been reported worldwide.

EPIDEMIOLOGY

SPECIES, AGE, SEX In wild rabbits, *G. strigosum* and *P. ambiguus* infections are greatest among older animals, whereas juvenile rabbits have the heaviest *T. retortaeformis* burdens.

RISK FACTORS

- Cysticercosis is rare in pet rabbits because most dogs are treated for tapeworms and are not fed raw intermediate herbivorous hosts. Risk of infection is higher when rabbits are allowed to graze on, or fed vegetables from, areas frequented by wild canids, including coyotes, wolves, and foxes.
- Contamination of feed by raccoon feces may result in larvae of the raccoon roundworm *B. procyonis* (and rarely larvae of *B. columnaris* from skunks), causing fatal cerebrospinal larva migrans.
- Nematodiasis is usually nonpathogenic in adult rabbits but may be associated with enteropathy in young rabbits. Endemic nematodes are rarely an important cause of mortality, except in rabbits that are overcrowded, food restricted, or exposed to severe weather.

CONTAGION AND ZOONOSIS Rabbits are intermediate hosts for a number of carnivore tapeworms; the most important of these are *Taenia serialis* and *Taenia pisiformis.* The life cycle is completed only when the rabbit is ingested by the definitive host—the rabbit does not shed eggs in the feces. Humans eating raw infected meat of rabbits with cysticercosis may be infected. Zoonotic risk is far greater from eating feed contaminated by feces of a definitive canid host.

GEOGRAPHY AND SEASONALITY Helminths described in this topic are found worldwide, except *T. retortaeformis* organisms, which are found in Europe and Australia but have not been reported in North America.

CLINICAL PRESENTATION

HISTORY, CHIEF COMPLAINT

- Some gastrointestinal parasites can cause diarrhea and weight loss.
- Heavy infestation with *P. ambiguus* may be associated with perineal dermatitis, anal irritation, and rectal prolapse.
- *E. cuniculi* and *T. gondii* infections are often subclinical but may cause clinical neurologic disease (e.g., convulsions, tremors, ataxia, paraplegia).
- Weanling rabbits are more susceptible to developing clinical disease from *Eimeria* spp., *Cryptosporidium* spp., and *T. retortaeformis* infections.

PHYSICAL EXAM FINDINGS

- Most rabbits with nematode infections are unremarkable on physical examination.
- Cysticercosis may be associated with subcutaneous, intramuscular, or abdominal masses. Cysts are often incidental findings found during ultrasonography, surgery, or postmortem examination.

ETIOLOGY AND PATHOPHYSIOLOGY

Protozoa

- *Coccidia:* see Coccidiosis
- *Encephalitozoon:* see Encephalitozoonosis
- *Cryptosporidium:* see Cryptosporidiosis, Sec. VI
- *Toxoplasma*
  - Rabbits are an intermediate host. Results of worldwide serologic surveys suggest that subclinical infections are prevalent, yet reports of clinical cases in rabbits are rare.
  - Type and severity of clinical illness depend on degree and localization of tissue injury. Tachyzoites are invasive asexual forms of the parasite that require intracellular existence for replication and survival. All cell types appear susceptible. Intracellular growth of *Toxoplasma* causes cell necrosis.

Helminths (disease related to location of parasite)

- Nematodes
  - Pinworms: *P. ambiguus*
    - Life cycle is direct: animals are infected through ingestion of eggs; cecotrophy provides continual reinfection with worms even in the presence of strict enclosure hygiene
    - Often found in high numbers within the cecum and the proximal colon without causing disease
  - Stomach worms: *G. strigosum* and *O. cuniculi*
    - Infection is often subclinical; severe infection is associated with gastritis and anemia.
  - *T. retortaeformis*
    - Found in the small intestine; infection is often subclinical; severe infection can induce atrophic enteritis
- Cestodes
  - *T. pisiformis*
    - Rabbits ingest tapeworm eggs that hatch in the small intestine and pass via the bloodstream to the liver. After 15 to 30 days, they penetrate the parenchyma and attach to the viscera as small cysts (size of a pea). Light infestations cause mild digestive disturbances; experimental heavy infestations cause severe liver damage and death.
  - *T. serialis*
    - Cysts develop in subcutaneous and intramuscular connective tissues and can have a diameter >4 cm.

DIAGNOSIS

DIFFERENTIAL DIAGNOSIS

- Nematodiasis
  - Other causes of diarrhea (e.g., dietary changes, neoplasia, bacterial and viral enteritis, toxicity)
  - Other causes of anal irritation (e.g., anal tumor, dermatitis, atopy, anal sacculitis)
  - Other causes of perineal dermatitis including urinary and fecal perineal soiling
- Cysticercosis
  - Other causes of fluid-filled cysts

INITIAL DATABASE

- Complete blood count and serum biochemistry: often, results are unremarkable
  - Eosinophilia is not a common accompaniment to intestinal helminth infection. Interleukin-5–mediated eosinophilia is induced by visceral migration of larval stages.
  - Eosinophilia is a not a manifestation of protozoal infection.
- Fecal endoparasite exam (flotation) and direct smear
- Aspiration of cyst fluid (fine-needle aspirate)
  - Cytologic examination of fluid: often observe clear, watery, sometimes flocculent fluid

ADVANCED OR CONFIRMATORY TESTING

- Toxoplasmosis
  - Serologic evidence of recent or active infection consisting of high immunoglobulin (Ig) M titers, or fourfold or greater, increasing or decreasing, IgG or other antibody titers
- Nematodiasis
  - Identification of nematode eggs based on characteristic appearance and size
- Cysticercosis
  - Microscopic appearance of formalin-fixed cyst
  - Immunohistochemical staining of fixed cyst
  - PCR analysis of aspirated cyst fluid for speciation of the cestode before surgical removal

TREATMENT

THERAPEUTIC GOAL

Eliminate parasitic infestation and eliminate clinical signs.

ACUTE GENERAL TREATMENT

- Toxoplasmosis
  - Available drugs usually suppress replication of *T. gondii* and are not completely effective in killing the parasite.
  - Clindamycin is used to treat humans, dogs, and cats but would likely kill rabbits from *Clostridium difficile*–induced enteritis.
  - Doxycycline is effective in experimental infections in mice and for cerebral toxoplasmosis in humans. No recommended dose has been put forth for rabbits. Try 4 mg/kg PO q 24 h for 4 weeks.
  - Currently, combination therapy with sulfadiazine (15 mg/kg PO q 24 h), pyrimethamine (1 mg/kg PO q 24 h), and folinic acid/leucovorin (1 mg/kg PO q 24 h) is considered effective. Doses listed are taken from dog/cat therapy. No recommended dose has been put forth for rabbits. Try combination therapy for 4 weeks.
- Nematodiasis
  - Nematodes can be treated with benzimidazoles (e.g., fenbendazole 20 mg/kg PO q 24 h × 5 d) or avermectins (e.g., selamectin 6-18 mg/kg topically).
  - Repeat treatment after 14 days.
- Cysticercosis
  - Surgical removal of cyst
  - When surgery presents unacceptable risk to patient, drainage of cyst fluid and use of praziquantel (6 mg/kg SC or intralesional, or 10 mg/kg PO; repeat in 10 d) are effective in killing mature cysts.

CHRONIC TREATMENT

Supportive care may be necessary in treating endoparasitic infestation because patients can range from poor condition to critical condition (typically with protozoan infestation).

DRUG INTERACTIONS

- Pyrimethamine is a folic acid antagonist that can cause bone marrow suppression. Addition of folinic acid (also known as *leucovorin*), the active metabolite of folic acid, to the diet minimizes bone marrow suppression.
- Use of the benzimidazole anthelmintics albendazole and fenbendazole is associated with idiosyncratic bone marrow suppression.

POSSIBLE COMPLICATIONS

Cysticercosis

- Treatment with praziquantel leads to a marked inflammatory reaction in the host. Corticosteroids have been advocated to reduce the inflammatory response in humans treated for neurocysticercosis with albendazole. However, doxycycline (4 mg/kg PO q 24 h 7-14 d) as a therapeutic agent for control of the inflammatory response offers an alternative treatment that is more suitable for rabbits because of sensitivity of this species to glucocorticoid-induced hepatic steatosis.

RECOMMENDED MONITORING

- Nematodiasis: repeated fecal analysis
- Cysticercosis: watch for evidence of inflammation at sites of killed tapeworm cysts

PROGNOSIS AND OUTCOME

- Overall prognosis varies from good to excellent when adult rabbits are treated.
- When immune compromised or young rabbits are treated, the prognosis varies from poor to good depending on how promptly the rabbit is diagnosed and treated.

PEARLS & CONSIDERATIONS

PREVENTION

Cysticercosis

- Prevent access to contaminated food materials
- Wash all vegetables thoroughly.
- Avoid access to grazing on vegetation contaminated by feces of foxes or of cats/dogs that are not regularly treated for cestodes, especially if they consume raw whole food items.

CLIENT EDUCATION

Always make clients aware of good husbandry and attention to hygiene within a colony or large group of rabbits.

SUGGESTED READINGS

Alvarez JI, et al: Doxycycline treatment decreases morbidity and mortality of murine neurocysticercosis: evidence for reduction of apoptosis and matrix metalloproteinase activity, Am J Pathol 175:685–695, 2009.

Deeb BJ, et al: Cerebral larva migrans caused by *Baylisascaris* sp in pet rabbits, J Am Vet Med Assoc 205:1744–1747, 1994.

Dubey JP, et al: Fatal toxoplasmosis in domestic rabbits in the USA, Vet Parasitol 44:305–309, 1992.

Elsheikha H, et al: Soft thoracic subcutaneous mass in a rabbit *(Oryctolagus cuniculus)*, Lab Anim (NY) 40:300–303, 2011.

O'Reilly A, et al: *Taenia serialis* causing exophthalmos in a pet rabbit, Vet Ophthalmol 5:227–230, 2002.

Schoeb TR, et al: Parasites of rabbits. In Baker DG, editor: Flynn's parasites of laboratory animals, Ames, IA, 2007, Blackwell Publications, pp 451–499.

Stassen T, et al: Fascioliasis in the rabbit [German], Tierarztl Prax Ausg K Kleintiere Heimtiere 32:355–362, 2004.

CROSS-REFERENCES TO OTHER SECTIONS

Coccidiosis
Cryptosporidiosis (Section VI)
Dermatopathies
Ectoparasites
Encephalitis
Encephalitozoonosis
Gastric Disorders
Intestinal Disorders

AUTHORS: **THOMAS M. DONNELLY AND VIVIANE SILVA RAYMUNDO**

EDITOR: **DAVID VELLA**

RABBITS

Floppy Rabbit Syndrome

BASIC INFORMATION

DEFINITION

Floppy rabbit syndrome (FRS) is a descriptive term for a condition with multiple possible origins. It is characterized by sudden onset of flaccid paresis or paralysis of all four limbs.

SYNONYMS

Generalized muscular weakness, flaccid paresis

EPIDEMIOLOGY

SPECIES, AGE, SEX

- The condition affects rabbits only.
- No age or sex predisposition is known.

RISK FACTORS Risk factors vary depending on the exact origin involved.

Trauma, dietary vitamin E deficiency, exposure to toxins, and generalized systemic disease leading to electrolyte disturbance are possible risk factors.

CONTAGION AND ZOONOSIS

- One differential diagnosis for FRS is botulism. This and other toxins may affect other animals, but only if the rabbit is subsequently consumed. Steps should be taken to avoid this possibility.

GEOGRAPHY AND SEASONALITY

- No seasonal incidence of this syndrome is known.
- FRS has been reported in Europe, North America, Asia, and Australia.

ASSOCIATED CONDITIONS AND DISORDERS FRS may be related to nutritional muscular dystrophy due to vitamin E deficiency. Lack of mobility and possible lack of appetite seen in FRS may cause or exacerbate gastrointestinal hypomotility.

CLINICAL PRESENTATION

DISEASE FORMS/SUBTYPES

- FRS has multiple possible causes.
- It resembles conditions such as spinal trauma and splayleg.
- It can be mistaken for sudden collapse due to general systemic disease.

HISTORY, CHIEF COMPLAINT Typically, rabbits with FRS present with sudden onset of generalized muscular weakness and a reduced but variable response to external stimuli.

PHYSICAL EXAM FINDINGS

- Flaccid paresis or paralysis
- Inability or reduction in ability to lift the head or move the limbs
- In nearly all cases, no other clinical abnormalities are noted.

ETIOLOGY AND PATHOPHYSIOLOGY

Many possible causes have been proposed, including hypokalemia, exposure or ingestion of plant or other toxins, nutritional muscular dystrophy, myasthenia gravis, cardiovascular disease, and unknown causes.

DIAGNOSIS

DIFFERENTIAL DIAGNOSIS

- Electrolyte disturbances
  - Hypokalemia
  - Hypomagnesemia
  - Hypercalcemia
- Infectious or parasitic events
  - *Encephalitozoon cuniculi*
  - Toxoplasmosis
  - Neosporosis
  - *Baylisascaris*
  - Rabies
- Toxic plants or other toxins
  - Heavy metals
  - Botulism
  - Milkweeds (*Asclepias* spp.) contain cardiac glycosides.
  - Lactucarium: desiccated juice from lettuce, *Lactuca* spp. The wild species *Lactuca virosa* is poisonous, but the common or garden lettuce, *Lactuca sativa,* is not toxic.
- Nutritional muscular dystrophy
  - Vitamin E/selenium deficiency
- Myasthenia gravis
- Cardiovascular disease (see Cardiovascular Disease)
- Severe systemic disease
- Splayleg (see Splayleg)

INITIAL DATABASE

- Blood biochemistry including electrolytes
- Hematologic examination including differential white blood cell count
- Serology for *Encephalitozoon cuniculi, Neospora caninum,* and *Toxoplasma gondii*
- Survey radiography to include the skull and the entire vertebral column

ADVANCED OR CONFIRMATORY TESTING

- Heavy metal analysis (e.g., lead and zinc)
- Myelography, CT or MRI scanning of skull and vertebral column
- Cerebrospinal fluid sample collection and analysis
- Electromyography
- Myasthenia gravis diagnostic tests
  - Pharmacologic testing with edrophonium chloride that elicits unequivocal improvement in strength
  - Serologic demonstration of acetylcholine receptor or muscle-specific tyrosine kinase antibodies

TREATMENT

THERAPEUTIC GOALS

- To treat any identified underlying cause
- If no identified cause, to provide nutritional support, fluid therapy (see Fluid Therapy in Rabbits and Rodents, Sec. II), and other supportive care as necessary until recovery

ACUTE GENERAL TREATMENT

- Treatment of any identified underlying cause
  - Chelation therapy for heavy metal toxicosis (calcium EDTA 13-27 mg/kg SC q 6-12 h)
  - Spinal trauma treatment including stabilization, antiinflammatory medication, and surgery
  - Selenium and/or vitamin E for nutritional muscular dystrophy (0.1 mg Se and 5 mg vitamin E/kg IM or SC every 14 days)
- Electrolyte replacement and/or correction of electrolyte and acid-base abnormalities
  - Administration of oral potassium supplementation may be useful (0.5-1.0 mEq PO q 12-24 h).
- If the rabbit is able to eat and drink, provide food and water in an accessible form. This may involve supporting the head or providing assisted feeding as necessary.
- If the animal is not able to prehend food, syringe or nasoesophageal administration of food and fluids and/or parenteral fluids may be necessary.
- Ensure that bladder emptying is occurring. Manually express the bladder or catheterize the urethra if necessary.

CHRONIC TREATMENT

- Provide continued nutritional and fluid support.
- Maintain good gastrointestinal function by feeding and if necessary using gastrointestinal prokinetic drugs (cisapride 0.5 mg/kg PO q 8-24 h).
- Avoid development of pressure sores on limbs.
- Monitor for fecal soiling.
- Monitor for urine scalding due to bladder overflow or inability to move while voiding urine.
- Monitor for ocular trauma if head is immobile.

POSSIBLE COMPLICATIONS

- Gastrointestinal stasis
- Pressure sores
- Fecal soiling
- Urine scalding
- Flystrike
- Ocular trauma

RECOMMENDED MONITORING

- Urine output
- Fecal output
- Appetite
- Body weight

PROGNOSIS AND OUTCOME

- Generally good
- Recovery typically occurs in 2 to 4 days.
- Prognosis worsens if complicating factors ensue.

PEARLS & CONSIDERATIONS

COMMENTS

- Controversy surrounds whether FRS is an actual syndrome or is simply a catch-all descriptive term for a number

of disparate entities. Although other problems can superficially resemble FRS (e.g., splayleg, severe systemic illness, encephalitozoonosis, spinal trauma, nutritional muscular dystrophy), true FRS appears to be a diagnosis arrived at by excluding other conditions with similar clinical signs. As yet, no indicator or diagnostic test can clearly identify the disorder. The exact cause is controversial, but hypokalemia appears to be implicated.
- When other serious diagnoses (e.g., spinal trauma) have been eliminated, the patient has a good to excellent prognosis for full recovery with supportive care in 2 to 4 days. However, the dramatic appearance of FRS, its similarity to spinal trauma, and lack of rapid recovery can lead owners to elect euthanasia if they are not counseled about the prognosis.

PREVENTION

- In most cases, no apparent precursors to FRS are noted. However, hypokalemia may contribute to development of the disease.
- Warn clients to avoid the following:
  - Diets containing 0.3% or less of potassium
  - Chronic gastrointestinal disease (because it may lead to hypokalemia)
  - Acute stress, fright, and hypothermia (because they may cause catecholamine-induced hypokalemia)

CLIENT EDUCATION

Clients should be advised to seek early veterinary attention for FRS rabbits. Once more serious causes have been ruled out, advise the client that supportive care and time will usually result in a favorable outcome, as long as complicating factors are avoided.

SUGGESTED READING

Generalised muscle weakness in rabbits. In Harcourt-Brown F, editor: Textbook of rabbit medicine, Oxford, 2002, Butterworth Heinemann, pp 315–318.

CROSS-REFERENCES TO OTHER SECTIONS

Cardiovascular Disease
Encephalitis
Encephalitozoonosis
Fluid Therapy in Rabbits and Rodents (Section II)
Gastric Stasis (Section III)
Splayleg

AUTHOR: **RICHARD A. SAUNDERS**

EDITOR: **DAVID VELLA**

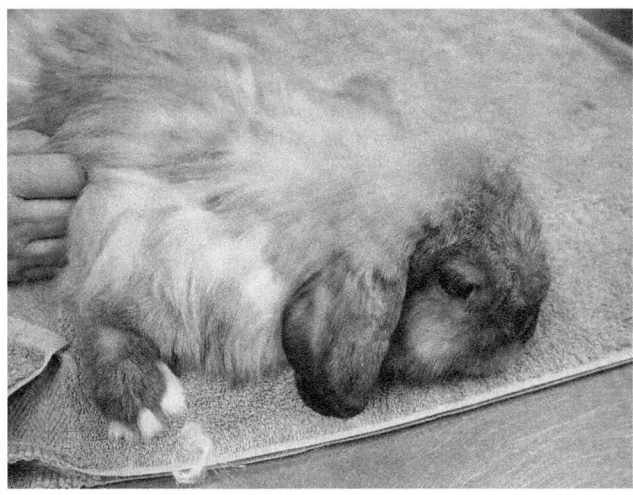

Floppy Rabbit Syndrome The floppy rabbit is usually unable to stand and often splays the legs. *(Photo courtesy Jörg Mayer, The University of Georgia, Athens.)*

RABBITS

Gastric Disorders

Client Education Sheet Available on Website

BASIC INFORMATION

DEFINITION

Disorders and diseases of the stomach

SYNONYMS

Gastritis, bloat, gastric tympany, gastric hypomotility/stasis, stasis, dilatation, obstruction, hairballs/trichobezoars, gastrointestinal hypomotility/stasis, rabbit gastrointestinal syndrome

SPECIAL SPECIES CONSIDERATIONS

- Rabbits have a relatively large, thin-walled stomach accounting for 15% of total gastrointestinal tract volume. Rabbits are unable to vomit owing in part to a well-developed cardiac sphincter.
- Rabbits are vulnerable to dietary imbalances that can result in cecal dysbiosis and alterations in proper gastrointestinal tract motility. Rabbits require regular ingestion of high-fiber diets consisting of grass and grass hays. Diets insufficient in fiber (such as seed mixes or pellet-only rations) can lead to gastrointestinal hypomotility and prolonged cecal retention times.
- Reduced food intake can rapidly result in hepatic lipidosis and ketoacidosis.

EPIDEMIOLOGY

SPECIES, AGE, SEX

- Adult rabbits have gastric contents that are highly acidic (pH 1 to 2). The acidity is slightly reduced during cecotroph ingestion (pH 3). Suckling rabbits have less acidic gastric contents (pH 5 to 6.5), which allow passage of some microbes to colonize the cecum and may also allow the passage of potentially pathogenic bacteria.
- Gastrointestinal hypomotility is seen most often in middle-aged to older rabbits.

GENETICS AND BREED PREDISPOSITION

- Gastric pyloric hypertrophy has been reported in the New Zealand White breed.
- Long-haired breeds may be more susceptible to the development of intestinal obstruction secondary to reingestion of compressed fecal hair pellets.

RISK FACTORS

- Low-fiber diets linked with gastrointestinal hypomotility
- Inappropriate diets containing grains, cereals, and fruits and lacking sufficient fiber may increase risks for hypomotility and cecal dysbiosis.

- Recent stressor or underlying disease: any underlying disease in rabbits can accompany gastrointestinal hypomotility; hence it is imperative to carry out a thorough physical examination
- Obesity may increase the risk of hepatic lipidosis in anorectic rabbits.

GEOGRAPHY AND SEASONALITY

Rabbits moult biannually (spring and fall). Moulting rabbits may ingest more hair during these times, which may predispose to the development of compressed fecal hair pellets and subsequent reingestion and gastrointestinal obstruction.

ASSOCIATED CONDITIONS AND DISORDERS

- Gastrointestinal hypomotility/stasis
- Mucoid enteropathy
- Dysautonomia

CLINICAL PRESENTATION

DISEASE FORMS/SUBTYPES

- Gastrointestinal hypomotility/stasis
- Gastric dilation
- Gastric obstruction
- Gastric trichobezoars

HISTORY, CHIEF COMPLAINT

- Anorexia (see Anorexia)
- Reduced appetite
- Weight loss
- Lethargy
- Weakness
- Small fecal pellets
- Reduced fecal output

PHYSICAL EXAM FINDINGS

- General: range from no abnormal findings to hunched posture/bruxism indicative of pain, shock, and dehydration
- Rabbits with gastrointestinal obstruction present acutely with pain, hypovolemic shock (bradycardia, weakness, pallor, hypothermia), and collapse and require immediate emergency care.
- Stomach palpation is important in distinguishing hypomotility, ingesta accumulation, and obstruction
  - Normally, the stomach is readily palpated as nonpainful, soft, and supple.
  - In hypomotile states, accumulated ingesta may result in a palpably enlarged stomach with doughy contents that can remain pitted when depressed and can progress to firm noncompressible contents in severe cases.
  - In acute gastrointestinal obstruction, gastric dilatation is noted (air, fluid), especially on the left side caudal to the ribs. Extreme distention and tympany of the stomach can result.
- Intestinal palpation can vary with the underlying disorder.
  - Normally, the intestines are readily palpated as nonpainful and devoid of large areas of gas or ingesta accumulation. Depending on the phase of digestion, hard fecal pellets may be palpated in the distal colon.
  - In gastrointestinal disease, no abnormal findings such as intestinal dilatation, intestinal fluid distention, intestinal impaction, intestinal "doughiness," and pain are reported. Large fluid and gas accumulation in the intestines is often indicative of a less acute condition.

ETIOLOGY AND PATHOPHYSIOLOGY

- Normal transit time for ingesta through the stomach is 3 to 6 hours.
- Rabbit stomach is vulnerable to dilatation (gaseous/fluid) in cases of outflow obstruction and hypomotility. With severe dilatation secondary to obstruction, compression of the caudal vena cava may impair venous return and cause significant pain.
- Foreign body obstruction most commonly occurs in the pylorus, the proximal duodenum, and the distal ileum.
- Gastric ulceration may occur secondarily with gastric disorders (most occur in the fundic region, although full-thickness ulcerations may be seen in the pyloric area).
- Many factors can affect gastrointestinal motility, including dietary fiber levels, pain and stressors, phase of fecal excretion, hormonal influences (e.g., catecholamines, prostaglandins, motilin), cecal volatile fatty acid fractions, underlying diseases, medications, and activity level.
- Physiologic effects of reduced gut motility can include gastric dilatation/impaction, gastric ulceration, gastric trichobezoar formation, alterations in water/electrolyte secretion and absorption, hypovolemia, acid-base and electrolyte imbalances, and dehydration.
- Reduced food intake can rapidly result in hepatic lipidosis and ketoacidosis in rabbits.
- Gastrointestinal obstruction: rapid accumulation of fluid proximal to the site of an intestinal obstruction due to the rabbit's inability to vomit, continual saliva production, water secretion into the stomach, and subsequent fermentation of contents can lead to severe gastric dilatation.
  - Obstruction secondary to re-ingestion of a compressed fecal hair pellet (most common) or ingestion of other foreign bodies and tumors
  - Compressed hair pellets from trichobezoars are different from hairballs. Compressed hair pellets are thought to form after compression of ingested hair into matted pellets in the large intestine, which are re-ingested during cecotrophy. This may occur more commonly in long-haired breeds or during moulting.
  - Obstruction secondary to ingestion of nonfood items such as fabric may also occur.
  - Obstruction secondary to strictures, adhesions, intussusception, neoplasia, and extraluminal compression (e.g., abscessation) is also possible.
- Gastric trichobezoars/hairballs generally develop as a result of reduced gastrointestinal motility rather than as the cause of it.
- Gastric dilatation secondary to aerophagia can occur in dyspneic rabbits with severe respiratory disease.
- Stomach worms (rare): trichostrongyloid nematodes
  - *Obeliscoides cuniculi* may produce gastric mucosal thickening and excessive production of mucus, leading to anorexia, lethargy, and weight loss
  - *Trichostrongylus retortaeformis*
  - *Graphidium strigosum*

DIAGNOSIS

DIFFERENTIAL DIAGNOSIS

- Gastrointestinal hypomotility/stasis
- Anorexia
- Gastrointestinal obstruction
- Gastric trichobezoar
- Mucoid enteropathy
- Gastric pyloric hypertrophy (New Zealand White breed)
- Gastric neoplasia (adenocarcinoma, leiomyoma reported)
- Dysautonomia
- Stomach worms
- Small and large intestinal disorders
- Accompanying underlying disease

INITIAL DATABASE

- Minimum database: blood biochemistry, hematology, and urinalysis (often unremarkable; however, may indicate dehydration, electrolyte imbalance, hepatopathy, and hyperglycemia)
- Abdominal radiography: gastric distention/impaction (gas, fluid, ingesta), intestinal distention/impaction, other organomegaly, free gas in abdominal cavity (gastrointestinal rupture), abdominal effusion
- Abdominal radiography: important diagnostic tool
  - Serial radiography can serve an important role in monitoring patient progress: monitor distention of gastrointestinal tract, gas patterns, and formation of feces
  - Normal gastrointestinal radiography
    - Stomach and cecum should nearly always contain ingesta.
    - Small amounts of gas may normally be present in the stomach and cecum (and very small amounts in the small intestine).

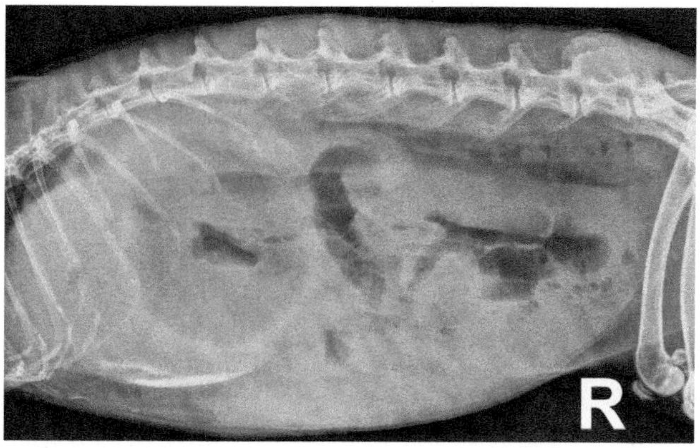

Gastric Disorders Right lateral abdominal radiograph image of a rabbit. Note the severe gastric distension. This was associated with a small intestinal obstruction. *(Photo courtesy Jörg Mayer, The University of Georgia, Athens.)*

  - Stomach is located caudal to the liver, usually within the confines of the rib cage. Gastric axis (the angle formed between the center of the fundus and the pylorus) in lateral view should be parallel with the ribs (lateral projection) and perpendicular to the spine (in ventrodorsal view).
  - Small intestines are typically located in the cranial abdomen dorsal to the cecum on the lateral projection, and in the left cranial abdomen on the ventrodorsal projection. The jejunum can extend into the midcaudal abdomen. The small intestines may be obscured by the large bowel.
  - Cecum typically occupies most of the right and ventral abdomen.
  - Distal colon and rectum can be more easily identified when spherical hard fecal balls are present.
  - Radiographic appearance of a rabbit's abdomen is largely affected by its current "phase" of digestion. During periods of cecotrophal ingestion, feeding tends to cease and the digestive tract is relatively emptier. When food is ingested, hard feces may be evident in the colon (rabbits often ingest food and pass hard feces simultaneously). Relative difference in radiographic appearance of an individual's abdomen can alter significantly during a 24-hour cycle.
- In hypomotile states, accumulated gastric ingesta may be crowned by a gas halo. The stomach normally contains small amounts of gas (gas cap), although a larger "crescenteric" gas cap may be more indicative of increased gas buildup. Gas accumulation may be evident in the intestines (especially the cecum).
- In acute gastrointestinal obstruction, severe gastric dilatation occurs (air, fluid), with the stomach extending well beyond the rib cage (Figure). Intestines may show little gas accumulation, although a small intestinal gas pattern suggestive of foreign body obstruction may be evident. Foreign bodies may not be discernible radiographically.
- Other organomegaly (e.g., hepatomegaly) may be evident.
- Free gas in abdominal cavity (gastrointestinal rupture) and abdominal effusions (e.g., peritonitis, cardiogenic) may be noted.
- Gastrointestinal contrast studies (e.g., pneumogastrogaphy, barium sulfate) are not usually diagnostically beneficial; these events carry procedural risks and are difficult to interpret.
- Abdominal ultrasound: may be hindered by the presence of large amounts of gastrointestinal gas

ADVANCED OR CONFIRMATORY TESTING

- Fecal flotation for trichostrongylid eggs of *O. cuniculi*
- Postmortem: histopathologic examination of intestinal ganglia for dysautonomia
- Exploratory laporotomy for suspected gastrointestinal obstruction

TREATMENT

THERAPEUTIC GOALS

- Return to normal appetite and gastrointestinal function.
- Provide supportive care during period of anorexia.
- Provide relief of obstruction, if present.

ACUTE GENERAL TREATMENT

- In cases of gastrointestinal hypomotility, it is essential to support hydration and nutritional needs.
  - Closely monitor vital signs, including heart rate, body temperature, and systolic blood pressure.
  - Provide parenteral fluid therapy via intravenous or intraosseous route. Crystalloids may be used. Maintenance fluid rates are considered 100 mL/kg/d.
  - Provide assist feeding by using commercial assist feeding formulas (e.g., Oxbow Critical Care Feeding Formula; Oxbow Pet Products, Murdock, NE).
  - Provide gut prokinetics (only in nonobstructive cases) via use of cisapride (0.5 mg/kg PO q 8 h), ranitidine 2-5 mg/kg PO, SC q 12 h.
  - Treat suspect gastric ulceration via ranitidine 2-5 mg/kg PO, SC q 12 h, omeprazole 0.5-1 mg/kg PO, IV q 24 h.
  - Offer analgesia (e.g., opioids, buprenorphine 0.03-0.05 mg/kg SC q 8-12 h; nonsteroidal antiinflammatory drugs [NSAIDs]: avoid use of NSAIDs in hypovolemic patients; meloxicam 0.3-0.5 mg/kg PO, SC q 12-24 h).
  - Provide regular movement/exercise and a quiet environment.
  - Surgical intervention for gastrointestinal hypomotility cases is rarely indicated and is likely to exacerbate hypomotile state.
- If gastric dilatation is present and gastrointestinal obstruction is suspected, treat as an emergency.
  - Institute supportive care measures for shock promptly while monitoring heart rate, body temperature, and systolic blood pressure.
    - Fluid therapy via IV or IO crystalloids is given at shock rates (60 mL/kg/h) for 1 hour. Alternatively, combine crystalloids (10-15 mL/kg) with colloids (5 mL/kg over 5-10 min q 15 min) to achieve systolic blood pressure >90 mm Hg.
    - Actively provide warmth using heat mats, hot water bottles, warmed fluids, or insulatory body wrapping. More advanced external heat sources such as forced air warmers can also be used.
  - Rapid decompression of stomach is necessary. Some patients may tolerate passage of orogastric or nasogastric tube, or sedation (e.g., midazolam 0.2-1 mg/kg IM, IV) may be necessary. Avoid percutaneous gastric trocarization because

thin-walled stomach may rupture severely.
  - Relieve obstruction via exploratory laparotomy (gastrotomy/enterotomy), although short period of patient stabilization may be required before surgery is performed.
  - Avoid per os medications and gut prokinetics until relief of obstruction is achieved.

CHRONIC TREATMENT

- Chronic intermittent gastrointestinal stasis occurs in some individuals. Underlying cause may be difficult to discern. Ensure that adequate dietary fiber is provided, and regularly groom long-haired rabbits.
- Trichostrongylosis can be treated via benzimidazoles (e.g., fenbendazole 20 mg/kg PO q 24 h × 5 d) or avermectins (e.g., selamectin 6-18 mg/kg topically).

DRUG INTERACTIONS

- Avoid use of oral preparations of lincomycin, clindamycin, erythromycin, and penicillins.
- Avoid use of NSAIDs in dehydrated and renally compromised patients.

POSSIBLE COMPLICATIONS

- Hypomotile states may be refractory to supportive care and treatment.
- Surgical intervention success rates are relatively low in obstructive disease, likely owing to rapid decompensation in rabbits with gastrointestinal obstruction.
- Untreated obstructive disease may result in gastric rupture and death.
- Postoperative adhesions and stricture formation may follow gastrointestinal surgery.

RECOMMENDED MONITORING

- Return of appetite and fecal production
- Regular vital sign measurement in compromised patients

PROGNOSIS AND OUTCOME

- Prognosis for gastrointestinal hypomotility is generally good in most cases, although this depends on underlying causes.
- Prognosis is guarded for gastrointestinal obstruction unless intervention is swift.

CONTROVERSY

- *Helicobacter* spp. have been isolated from rabbit stomachs, but significance of this is unknown.
- Metoclopramide may have little effectiveness in promoting gut motility but may provide some benefit in reducing nausea in rabbits.
- Routine use of antibiotics in gastrointestinal disease is not warranted. Limited cases (e.g., bacterial overgrowth, gastrointestinal surgery) may require antibiotics. Choose broad-spectrum antibiotics such as enrofloxacin or trimethoprim/sulfonamides.
- Use of products to enzymatically dissolve ingested hair (e.g., pineapple juice, papaya extract) is unlikely to achieve desired result.
- Use of orally medicated lubricants is unlikely to improve the passage of foreign bodies or trichobezoars.
- Simethicone (an oral antifoaming agent): may reduce size of gas bubbles (not reduce or prevent gas formation) within gastrointestinal tract, facilitating their passage

PEARLS & CONSIDERATIONS

COMMENTS

- Gastric trichobezoars are often the result of, rather than the cause of, gastrointestinal disease.
- Gastric ulceration is a common postmortem finding.

PREVENTION

- Ensure adequate dietary fiber.
- Avoid high-carbohydrate diets.
- Regularly groom pet rabbits.

CLIENT EDUCATION

- Emphasize importance of appropriate feeding. Pet rabbit diets should consist largely of grass or grass hays (at least 80% of diet; e.g., timothy, oaten hays). A variety of fresh leafy green vegetables can be added to the diet. Pellets (if fed at all) should be of the highest quality, viewed as a supplement, and fed in very limited amounts. Seed mixes, cereals, etc., should not be fed or should be offered only in very small amounts intermittently as treats.
- Educate clients on importance of monitoring food intake, fecal production, and activity level of rabbits.
- Encourage regular grooming of rabbits, especially long-haired breeds.
- Ensure that regular exercise and activity are provided to pet rabbits.

SUGGESTED READINGS

Harcourt-Brown FM: Gastric dilation and intestinal obstruction in 76 rabbits, Vet Rec 161:409–414, 2007.

Harcourt-Brown TH: Management of acute gastric dilation in rabbits, J Exot Pet Med 16:168–174, 2007.

CROSS-REFERENCES TO OTHER SECTIONS

Anorexia
Coccidiosis
Dental Disease
Dysautonomia (Grass Sickness)
Endoparasites
Hepatic Disorders
Intestinal Disorders

AUTHOR: **DAVID VELLA**

EDITOR: **THOMAS M. DONNELLY**

RABBITS

Hemorrhagic Disease

BASIC INFORMATION

DEFINITION

Rabbit hemorrhagic disease (RHD) is an acute, lethal disease of European rabbits *(Oryctolagus cuniculus)* caused by rabbit hemorrhagic disease virus (RHD virus), a calicivirus (genus, *Lagovirus*) that first emerged in China in 1984 in rabbits imported from Europe. The disease also emerged in Europe and was spread to many parts of the world, transported by rabbits or rabbit products.

SYNONYMS

- Rabbit calicivirus disease (RCD)
- Viral hemorrhagic disease (VHD) of rabbits
- Hemorrhagic pneumonia (China)
- Infectious necrotic hepatitis
- Malattia X (Italy before viral origin was understood)

EPIDEMIOLOGY

SPECIES, AGE, SEX

- RHD is seen only in European rabbits *(Oryctolagus cuniculus)*.

- Virus can infect rabbits of any age and sex, but very young rabbits (younger than 4 weeks of age) do not usually develop disease after infection. This age-related resistance wanes over subsequent weeks of life. It is present in the absence of maternal antibody, and despite resistance to disease, these rabbits still shed the virus and can infect in-contact rabbits.

GENETICS AND BREED PREDISPOSITION All breeds appear susceptible.

RISK FACTORS

- Contact with wild rabbits: virus can be spread mechanically by insects such as flies, mosquitoes, and fleas
- Introduction of virus on fomites such as cages and bedding
- Failure to quarantine introduced rabbits

CONTAGION AND ZOONOSIS

- Virus is highly infectious by oral, nasal, conjunctival, and parenteral routes.
- Insect vectors such as flies, fleas, and mosquitoes can spread the virus mechanically.
- Fomites are important in spread because the virus is resistant to environmental inactivation.
- The virus can persist in infected animal carcasses for long periods.
- No zoonotic potential is known.

GEOGRAPHY AND SEASONALITY

- The disease was originally reported in China in domestic rabbits imported from Europe.
- It is widespread in Europe and Britain and occurs in Cuba, Russia, the Middle East, and parts of Africa.
- RHD has occurred in farmed rabbits in the United States and Mexico but has been eradicated.
- The virus was accidentally released into the wild rabbit population in Australia, where subsequently it was deliberately spread as a biological control.
- It was illegally introduced into New Zealand, where it is now used similarly—as a biological control.
- In wild rabbit populations, strong seasonality is associated with epidemics because susceptible rabbit numbers build up in the population during the breeding season, but this differs between geographic regions, for example, spring in Spain and France and summer/early winter in Britain.

CLINICAL PRESENTATION

DISEASE FORMS/SUBTYPES

- Peracute infection: sudden death with no clinical signs
- Acute: rabbits may appear quiet and may have fever and an increased respiratory rate for up to 24 hours before death
- Subacute: jaundice and death over a period of several days to 2 weeks
- Subclinical: a small proportion of experimentally infected adult rabbits develop few or no clinical signs and clear the virus. Kits less than 4 to 8 weeks old are infected and shed virus but do not develop clinical signs other than fever.

HISTORY, CHIEF COMPLAINT

- Sudden death in adult or subadult rabbits, possibly preceded by a short period (24 hours or less) of malaise, increased respiratory rate, and fever. Death may be accompanied by a high-pitched squeal or by convulsions. Lateral recumbency, coma, and convulsions may occur in the hours before death.
- Typically, the disease may occur as an epidemic with high mortality among adult or sub-adult rabbits, but not in kits.

PHYSICAL EXAM FINDINGS

- Depressed demeanor
- Fever up to 42°C (108°F)
- Respiratory distress
- Jaundice may be present in subacute cases.
- Hematuria and bloody nasal discharge may be present in some cases.
- Convulsions, ataxia, posterior paresis, or CNS depression may occur.

ETIOLOGY AND PATHOPHYSIOLOGY

- Acute hepatic necrosis
- Nephrosis
- Disseminated intravascular coagulation (DIC)
- Hypoglycemia
- Hepatic encephalopathy (increased intracranial pressure; increased blood ammonia concentration)
- Leukopenia

DIAGNOSIS

DIFFERENTIAL DIAGNOSIS

- Sudden death
  - Enterotoxemia (*Clostridium perfringens* type E)
  - Peracute myxomatosis
  - Septicemia due to acute pasteurellosis, colibacillosis, or other bacteria that can cause disseminated intravascular coagulation
  - Poisoning such as sodium fluoroacetate (1080) or anticoagulants
  - Acute spinal trauma
  - Heatstroke
- Hepatic disorders
  - Acute necrotic hepatitis differentiates RHD from most other causes of sudden death.
- Bleeding disorders
- Neurologic disorders

INITIAL DATABASE

- Serum alanine aminotransferase (ALT), aspartate aminotransferase (AST), lactate dehydrogenase (LDH), alkaline phosphatase (ALP), and gamma glutamyltransferase (GGT) activities are dramatically elevated, particularly AST (from normal of 10 IU/L to 4000-14,000 IU/L).
- Increased serum bilirubin
- Leukopenia (dramatic decline in both lymphocytes and neutrophils)
- Increased prothrombin time (PT)

ADVANCED OR CONFIRMATORY TESTING

- Necropsy
  - Pale swollen liver (necrotizing hepatitis) with focal hemorrhages and pronounced lobular pattern
  - Dark kidneys
  - Enlarged dark spleen
  - Hemorrhagic, congested lungs
  - Hyperemic tracheal mucosa
  - Trachea may be filled with froth or fluid.
- Histopathologic examination: coagulative necrosis of hepatocytes at the periphery of lobules, nephrosis, disseminated intravascular coagulation (DIC) with thrombi, particularly in small renal and large pulmonary blood vessels. In rabbits that survive beyond acute infection, signs of liver regeneration may be present (e.g., connective tissue and bile duct proliferation; large, pale-staining binucleate hepatocytes).
- Reverse transcriptase-PCR (RT-PCR): this is the most common diagnostic assay. Virus can be detected in most tissues, including blood, but liver is the tissue with the highest concentration of virus. Virus RNA can be detected in the liver of some healthy rabbits.
- Electron microscopy: negative staining for virus particles concentrated from infected livers.
- Immunohistochemistry on liver impression smears or sections
- Virus cannot be grown in cell culture.
- Hemagglutination of human type O red blood cells or virus-capture ELISA can be used for diagnosis (not all strains hemagglutinate).
- Rabbit inoculation
- Serum antibody can be detected by hemagglutination-inhibition (HI) or with various ELISA-based assays in surviving animals. This could be useful in confirming outbreaks where young rabbits have not been clinically affected. If infected, seroconversion will occur, and a proportion of adult rabbits may survive subclinical infection and seroconvert. Low-level serologic cross-reaction with attenuated circulating caliciviruses has been noted.

- Care should be taken in interpreting positive reverse transcriptase (RT)-PCR and serology in the absence of liver pathology because of the prevalence of nonpathogenic strains of calicivirus that circulate in wild and some farmed rabbit populations.

TREATMENT

THERAPEUTIC GOAL

Therapy is purely supportive because no specific treatment has been identified.

ACUTE GENERAL TREATMENT

Supportive care only

PROGNOSIS AND OUTCOME

- All but a small proportion of patients with subacute disease will die.
  - Survival of individuals with subacute disease will depend on the degree of liver damage and the rate of hepatic regeneration, together with the degree of damage to other organs, particularly the kidneys. Chronic liver disease and cirrhosis may result.
- Rabbits that have been previously infected with an avirulent, naturally occurring field strain can have cross-protection yet may develop subacute disease. Some individuals may recover, and others may display prolonged disease course.

PEARLS & CONSIDERATIONS

COMMENTS

- RHD virus RNA has been detected in serum and liver from healthy rabbits many months after infection using nested RT-PCR. It is not clear whether this indicates chronic infection, or whether reactivation of viral replication and viral shedding can occur.
- Avirulent strains of a calicivirus closely related to RHD virus circulate in wild and farmed rabbit populations. It is assumed that RHD virus arose from these viruses. In some cases, previous infection with these viruses may provide cross-protection against virulent RHD virus.
- A related *Lagovirus* causes a disease similar to RHD in European brown hares and is termed *European brown hare syndrome virus (EBHSV)*. This disease emerged around the same time that RHD appeared. EBHSV does not infect rabbits, and RHD virus does not infect European brown hares. EBHSV may be less species-specific than RHD virus and has been recorded as infecting mountain hares *(Lepus timidus)* and Eastern cottontails *(Sylvilagus floridanus)*.
- In Australia and New Zealand, RHD virus is released as a biological control agent for wild European rabbit populations. Virus may spread from wild populations to pet rabbits.

PREVENTION

Vaccination with an adjuvanted killed vaccine derived from infected rabbit liver is regarded as effective. Manufacturer recommendations for vaccination should always be followed. A single shot is generally given at 10 to 12 weeks, along with an annual booster. Earlier vaccination may be necessary in some circumstances, but maternal immunity may interfere, and a second dose would be advisable. Antigenic variants of RHD virus can overcome vaccination.

CLIENT EDUCATION

- Vaccination
- Quarantine

SUGGESTED READINGS

Center for Food Security and Public Health, Iowa State University: http://www.cfsph.iastate.edu/Factsheets/pdfs/rabbit_hemorrhagic_disease.pdf. Accessed July 2008.

Cooke BD, et al: Rabbit haemorrhagic disease and the biological control of wild rabbits, *Oryctolagus cuniculus,* in Australia and New Zealand, Wildlife Res 29:689–706, 2002.

Ferreira PG, et al: Severe leukopenia and live biochemistry changes in adult rabbits after calicivirus infection, Res Vet Sci 80:218–225, 2006.

AUTHOR: **PETER KERR**

EDITOR: **DAVID VELLA**

RABBITS

Hepatic Disorders

BASIC INFORMATION

DEFINITION

Infectious and noninfectious diseases of the liver

SYNONYMS

Liver disease, hepatopathy

EPIDEMIOLOGY

SPECIES, AGE, SEX

- Dependent on the underlying cause
- Young animals are more susceptible to infections such as hepatic coccidiosis *(Eimeria stiedae)* and Tyzzer's disease *(Clostridium piliforme)*.

RISK FACTORS

- Anorexia can rapidly induce hepatic lipidosis in the rabbit.
- Obesity (see Obesity) is a risk factor for hepatic lipidosis.
- Pregnancy is a risk factor for hepatic lipidosis and pregnancy toxemia.

CONTAGION AND ZOONOSIS Salmonellosis, yersiniosis, and tularemia are causes of bacterial hepatitis in rabbits and of zoonotic diseases.

ASSOCIATED CONDITIONS AND DISORDERS Sebaceous adenitis and exfoliative dermatitis (1 case)

CLINICAL PRESENTATION

HISTORY, CHIEF COMPLAINT

- Lethargy, depression, weight loss, anorexia, and stunted growth
- Jaundice
  - Rare because the main product of heme breakdown in rabbits is biliverdin, not bilirubin
- Polydipsia and polyuria in some cases

PHYSICAL EXAM FINDINGS

- Abdominal distention
- Abdominal effusion
- Jaundice (rare)
- Hepatomegaly
- Diarrhea
- Dyspnea
- Bleeding (coagulopathies)
- Neurologic signs
- Seizures
- Collapse

ETIOLOGY AND PATHOPHYSIOLOGY

- Parasites
  - Hepatic coccidiosis *(Eimeria stiedai)* (see Rabbit Coccidiosis)
  - Hepatic cysts of *Taenia* spp. and hydatid cysts *(Echinococcus granulosus)*
  - Rare parasitic infection (e.g., liver fluke *[Fasciola hepatica]*, cryptosporidiosis, toxoplasmosis)

- Bacteria
  - Abscessation due to bacteremia or septicemia
  - Tyzzer's disease *(Clostridium piliformis)*
  - Ascending bacterial infection from gastrointestinal tract via portal vein (e.g., colibacillosis and salmonellosis; rarely, listeriosis, yersiniosis [pseudotuberculosis], tuberculosis, and tularemia)
- Viruses
  - Rabbit hemorrhagic disease (see Rabbit Hemorrhagic Disease) causes acute hepatic necrosis and disseminated intravascular coagulation (DIC).
- Toxins
  - Aflatoxicosis, lead, nonsteroidal antiinflammatory drugs (NSAIDs), and pine or cedar wood shavings
- Metabolic disorders
  - Hepatic lipidosis and pregnancy toxemia
- Neoplasms
  - Lymphoma, bile duct adenoma and carcinoma, metastatic disease
- Trauma
  - External abdominal trauma (e.g., road traffic accident, fall, predation, crush injury)
  - Torsion of caudate lobe of liver
- Autoimmune disease
  - One case of autoimmune hepatitis has been described in association with sebaceous adenitis and exfoliative dermatitis.

DIAGNOSIS

DIFFERENTIAL DIAGNOSIS

- Anorexia
  - Dental disease, any systemic disease (especially gastrointestinal), pain, stress
- Abdominal distention
  - Ileus and gaseous distention of gastrointestinal tract, abdominal mass, pregnancy, obesity
- Abdominal effusion
  - Abdominal neoplasia, cardiac disease
- Diarrhea
  - Bacterial or viral enteritis, clostridial enterotoxemia, gastric stasis/ileus, diet-related (low fiber/high carbohydrate)
- Dyspnea/collapse
  - Respiratory disease, cardiac disease, heatstroke, severe pain
- Jaundice
  - Prehepatic causes (e.g., hemolysis [hemolytic anemia], bacteremia, septicemia, DIC, excess kale, potato leaf, bracken ingestion)
- Neurologic signs
  - Encephalitozoonosis, heatstroke, trauma, brain abscess, toxoplasmosis, listeriosis, other bacterial encephalitis, viral encephalitis (e.g., herpesvirus), epilepsy (rare)
- Weight loss
  - Dental disease, any infectious or other metabolic disease, neoplasia, bullying

INITIAL DATABASE

- Serum liver enzymes (e.g., alanine aminotransferase [ALT], alkaline phosphatase [ALP], aspartate aminotransferase [AST], gamma glutamyltransferase [GGT], lactate dehydrogenase [LDH]) are elevated.
- Bilirubin is elevated.
- Bile acids are elevated.
- Serum protein is decreased.
- Clotting times may be increased.
- Packed cell volume may be decreased with liver lobe torsion.
- Abdominal radiography may show hepatomegaly and/or abdominal effusion.

ADVANCED OR CONFIRMATORY TESTING

- Selection of additional diagnostic tests is based on the history and clinical signs:
  - Abdominal ultrasonography and ultrasound-guided fine-needle aspiration (FNA) or Tru-Cut biopsy
  - Fecal analysis (hepatic coccidiosis, bacterial or viral enteritis)
  - Abdominocentesis if abdominal effusion is present
    - Measure specific gravity and protein content of effusion.
    - Perform cytologic examination and bacterial culture of effusion.
  - Laparoscopy or laparotomy and liver biopsy

TREATMENT

THERAPEUTIC GOAL

Dependent on cause of disease

ACUTE GENERAL TREATMENT

- Supportive treatment: fluid therapy, assisted feeding, vitamins, analgesia
- Milk thistle *(Silybum marianum)* has been suggested as an aid to hepatic regeneration.

CHRONIC TREATMENT

- Dependent on cause: specific treatments in addition to ongoing supportive care include the following:
  - Hepatic coccidiosis
    - Trimethoprim/sulfamethoxazole 30 mg/kg PO q 24 h; sulfadimethoxine 50 mg/kg first dose, then 25 mg/kg PO q 24 h; toltrazuril 25 mg/kg PO q 24 h for 2 d, then repeat after 5 days
    - Prevention of access to fresh feces, reduced stocking density
  - *Taenia* spp. hepatic cysts
    - Drainage and praziquantel 5-10 mg/kg SC, repeat in 10 d
  - *Echinococcus granulosus* cyst
    - Drainage and albendazole 1.7 mg/mL injected into each cyst
  - Liver fluke (*Fasciola* spp.)
    - Triclabendazole 45 mg/kg/d for 2 consecutive days
  - Bacterial hepatitis
    - Appropriate antibiotic therapy
    - Zoonotic considerations (salmonellosis, yersiniosis, tularemia) must be assessed.
  - Abscessation (see Abscesses)
    - Surgical removal
  - Lead toxicity
    - Calcium EDTA 27 mg/kg SC q 6-12 h as needed. Dilute to <10mg/mL with 0.45% NaCl/2.5% dextrose.
  - Metabolic disorders
    - Hepatic lipidosis: intravenous crystalloids and 5% dextrose
    - Pregnancy toxemia (see Pregnancy Toxemia): cesarean section
    - Treatment of dental disease, if this is cause of anorexia
  - Neoplasia
    - Surgical excision generally is not attempted.
    - Chemotherapy may be beneficial in cases of lymphoma.
  - Trauma
    - Surgical removal of twisted caudate liver lobe

RECOMMENDED MONITORING

- Serum liver enzymes and bilirubin
- Clotting times

PROGNOSIS AND OUTCOME

Dependent on cause

PEARLS & CONSIDERATIONS

COMMENTS

A specific diagnosis of hepatic disease is infrequently made in clinical practice because presenting signs are often vague and nonspecific, and diagnosis requires a wide range of diagnostic tests. Many conditions can cause liver impairment as a primary or a secondary condition, and it is likely that hepatic disease is underdiagnosed in rabbits.

PREVENTION

- General
  - Ensure good hygiene, particularly in groups of young weanling rabbits.
  - Provide quality high-fiber diet.
  - Prevent access to toxins.
- Vaccination

- Rabbit hemorrhagic disease in endemic countries
- Liver fluke
  - Avoid grazing of wet contaminated pasture.
- Hepatic coccidiosis (see Rabbit Coccidiosis)
  - Avoid fecal contamination of feed and water.
  - Keep stocking density low.
  - In-feed coccidiostats are indicated in some situations.

CLIENT EDUCATION

Anorexia should be treated as an emergency. Any rabbit not feeding for 24 hours must receive nutritional support to prevent development of hepatic lipidosis.

SUGGESTED READING

Meredith A, et al: Liver disease in rabbits, Semin Avian Exot Pet Med 9:146–152, 2000.
Stake NJ, et al: Successful outcome of hepatectomy as treatment for liver lobe torsion in four domestic rabbits, J Am Vet Med Assoc 238:1176–1183, 2011.
Stassen T, et al: Fascioliasis in the rabbit [German] Fasziolose beim Kaninchen, Tierarztl Prax Ausg K Kleintiere Heimtiere 32: 355–362, 2004.
Swartout MS, et al: Lead-induced toxicosis in two domestic rabbits, J Am Vet Med Assoc 191:717–719, 1987.

CROSS-REFERENCES TO OTHER SECTIONS

Abscesses
Anorexia
Coccidiosis
Endoparasites
Hemorrhagic Disease
Obesity
Pregnancy Toxemia

AUTHOR: **ANNA MEREDITH**

EDITOR: **DAVID VELLA**

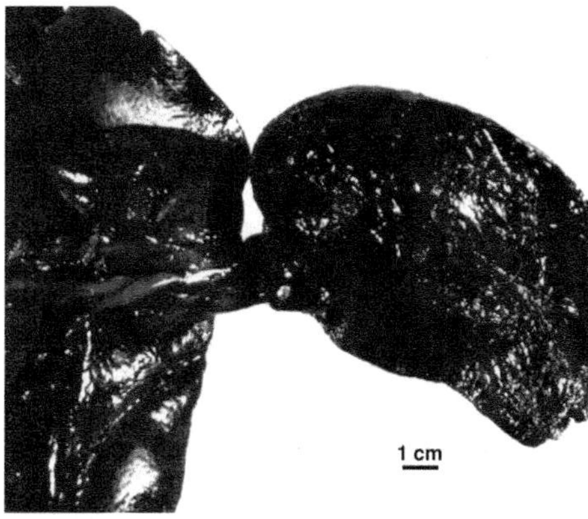

Hepatic Disorders Postmortem photograph of torsion of the caudate lobe in a 2-year-old female New Zealand white rabbit. Note the darkened (congested) state of the necrotic caudate lobe, and 360 degrees clockwise torsion at hilus. *(Photo courtesy Jörg Mayer, The University of Georgia, Athens.)*

RABBITS

Intestinal Disorders

BASIC INFORMATION

DEFINITION

Disorders and diseases of the intestine

SYNONYMS

Enteritis, foreign body, intestinal stasis, gut stasis, ileus, obstruction, gastrointestinal hypomotility/stasis, rabbit gastrointestinal syndrome, typhlitis, clostridial enteritis, clostridial enterotoxemia, enterotoxicosis, coccidiosis, proliferative enteritis/enteropathy/enterocolitis, histiocytic enteritis

SPECIAL SPECIES CONSIDERATIONS

- Rabbits are unable to vomit owing in part to a well-developed cardiac sphincter.
- Rabbits produce two types of feces: hard fecal pellets and cecotrophs. The latter are derived from the cecum and are re-ingested by the rabbit.
- As hindgut fermenters, rabbits host a wide variety of nonpathogenic microbes (bacteria, fungi, protozoa) in their cecum, many of which are vital to normal fermentative and digestive processes.
- Rabbits are vulnerable to dietary imbalances, which can result in cecal dysbiosis and alterations in proper gastrointestinal tract motility. Rabbits require regular ingestion of high-fiber diets consisting of grass and grass hays. Diets insufficient in fiber (such as seed mixes or pellet-only rations) can lead to gastrointestinal hypomotility and prolonged cecal retention times.
- Reduced food intake can rapidly result in hepatic lipidosis and ketoacidosis.

EPIDEMIOLOGY

SPECIES, AGE, SEX

- Infectious causes of enteritis are rare in adults. Adult rabbits have highly acidic gastric contents (pH 1 to 2), the acidity of which increases slightly during cecotroph ingestion (pH 3). Suckling rabbits have less acidic gastric contents (pH 5 to 6.5); this allows passage of some microbes to colonize the cecum and may also allow the passage of potentially pathogenic bacteria (e.g., susceptibility to pathogenic bacteria [*Escherichia coli, Clostridium* spp.] is greater in 3-week-old than in 6-week-old).
- Gastrointestinal hypomotility is seen most often in middle-aged to older rabbits.

GENETICS AND BREED PREDISPOSITION

- Gastric pyloric hypertrophy reported in New Zealand white breed
- Megacolon syndrome of homozygous spotted rabbits
- Long-haired breeds may be more susceptible to the development of intestinal obstruction secondary to re-ingestion of compressed fecal hair pellets.

RISK FACTORS

- Low-fiber diets linked with gastrointestinal hypomotility and increased cecal retention time
- Inappropriate diets containing grains, cereals, and fruits and lacking sufficient fiber may increase risks of hypomotility and cecal dysbiosis. High-carbohydrate diets are linked with increased risk of bacterial enteritis, especially clostridial enteritis, owing in part to their utilization of carbohydrates as fermentable substrate.
- Recent stressor or underlying disease: any underlying disease in rabbits can accompany gastrointestinal hypomotility, hence it is imperative to carry out a thorough physical examination
- Obesity may increase risk of hepatic lipidosis in anorectic rabbits.
- Inappropriate antibiotic use

- Contaminated environments and unsavory husbandry conditions
- Presence of multiple potential pathogens may induce a synergistic "co-pathogen" scenario in enteritis complex.

CONTAGION AND ZOONOSIS Salmonellosis presents potential zoonosis.

GEOGRAPHY AND SEASONALITY Rabbits moult biannually (spring and fall). Moulting rabbits may ingest more hair during these times, and this may predispose to the development of compressed fecal hair pellets and to subsequent re-ingestion and gastrointestinal obstruction.

ASSOCIATED CONDITIONS AND DISORDERS

- Gastrointestinal hypomotility/stasis
- Mucoid enteropathy
- Dysautonomia
- Coccidiosis
- Bacterial enteritis (e.g., *E. coli, Clostridium* spp.)
- Viral enteritis (e.g., rotavirus, coronavirus)
- Intestinal neoplasia
- Toxins (e.g., lead)

CLINICAL PRESENTATION

DISEASE FORMS/SUBTYPES Gastrointestinal hypomotility/stasis, enteritis, typhlitis

HISTORY, CHIEF COMPLAINT Anorexia, reduced appetite, weight loss, lethargy, weakness, small fecal pellets, reduced fecal output, perineal fecal soiling, diarrhea

PHYSICAL EXAM FINDINGS

- General: range from no abnormal findings to hunched posture/bruxism indicative of pain, shock, and dehydration
- Rabbits with gastrointestinal obstruction present acutely with pain, hypovolemic shock (bradycardia, weakness, pallor, hypothermia), and collapse and require immediate emergency care.
- Fecal staining of perineum or diarrhea: true diarrhea in rabbits accompanies lack of hard fecal pellets. The concurrent presence of hard fecal pellets and perineal fecal soiling indicates soft, poorly formed, or noningested cecotrophs rather than diarrhea. Cecotrophal soiling of the perineum is often mistaken for diarrhea.
- True diarrhea is more common in young rabbits and is uncommon in adults.
- Hematochezia and melena are rarely seen in rabbits.
- Stomach palpation is important in distinguishing hypomotility, ingesta accumulation, and obstruction.
  - Normally, the stomach is readily palpated as nonpainful, soft, and supple.
  - In hypomotile states, accumulated ingesta may result in a palpably enlarged stomach with doughy contents that can remain pitted when depressed, and that progress to firm noncompressible contents in more severe cases.
  - In acute gastrointestinal obstruction, gastric dilatation results (air, fluid), especially on the left side caudal to the ribs. Extreme distention and tympany of the stomach can occur.
- Intestinal palpation can vary with the underlying disorder.
  - Normally, the intestines are readily palpated as nonpainful and devoid of large areas of gas or ingesta accumulation. Depending on the phase of digestion, hard fecal pellets may be palpated in the distal colon.
  - In gastrointestinal disease, there may be no abnormal findings, intestinal dilatation, intestinal fluid distention, intestinal impaction, or intestinal "doughiness," and pain is possible. Large fluid and gas accumulation in the intestines is often indicative of less acute conditions.

ETIOLOGY AND PATHOPHYSIOLOGY

- Normal transit time for ingesta through small intestine is 10 to 60 minutes.
- Small intestine is relatively devoid of resident microbes.
- Much HCO_3^- is secreted into the duodenum to neutralize acidic digesta.
- Terminal portion of ileum (sacculus rotundus) contains an ileocecocolic valve that prevents backflow into the ileum.
- Colonic transit time for cecotrophs is 1.5 to 2.5 times faster than for hard feces.
- Rabbits produce on average 150 hard fecal pellets per day.
- The cecum, the largest organ in the abdominal cavity, holds about 40% of total ingesta. Fermentation of digestible fiber and production of volatile fatty acids occur within the cecum, with resulting cecotrophs passed and re-ingested by the rabbit. Cecotrophs serve as an important source of volatile fatty acids (energy), protein, and vitamins, and are important for cecal recolonization.
- Diet plays a key role in gastrointestinal well-being. A healthy cecal environment is governed by many factors and relies on a steady supply of fermentable fiber substrate. Cecal microflora is predominated by *Bacteroides* spp.; however, a mix of aerobic and anaerobic organisms is also present, including some potentially pathogenic bacteria in small numbers (e.g., *Clostridium* spp.). Alterations in the cecal environment (pH and floral population) can favor the proliferation of pathogenic bacteria.
- The fusus coli is a section of colon (separating proximal and distal portions) that is responsible for governing colonic motility. It is particularly sensitive to catecholamines, which can produce a reduction in gut motility.
- Rabbit stomachs are vulnerable to dilatation (gaseous/fluid) in cases of outflow obstruction and hypomotility. With severe dilatation secondary to obstruction, compression of the caudal vena cava may impair venous return and cause significant pain.
- Foreign body obstruction most commonly occurs in pylorus, proximal duodenum, and distal ileum.
- Many factors can affect gastrointestinal motility, including dietary fiber levels, pain and stressors, phase of fecal excretion, hormonal influences (e.g., catecholamines, prostaglandins, motilin), cecal volatile fatty acid fractions, underlying diseases, medications, and activity level.
- Physiologic effects of reduced gut motility can include gastric dilatation/impaction, gastric ulceration, gastric trichobezoar formation, alterations in water/electrolyte secretion and absorption, hypovolemia, acid-base and electrolyte imbalance, and dehydration.
- Reduced food intake can rapidly result in hepatic lipidosis and ketoacidosis in rabbits.
- Gastrointestinal obstruction: rapid accumulation of fluid proximal to the site of an intestinal obstruction due to rabbit's inability to vomit, continual production of saliva, water secretion into stomach, and subsequent fermentation of contents can lead to severe gastric dilatation
  - Obstruction secondary to re-ingestion of a compressed fecal hair pellet (most common) or to ingestion of other foreign bodies and tumors
  - Compressed hair pellets are different from trichobezoars and hairballs. Compressed hair pellets are thought to be formed after compression of ingested hair into matted pellets in the large intestine; these are then re-ingested during cecotrophy. This may occur more commonly in long-haired breeds or during moulting.
  - Obstructions also occur secondary to ingestion of nonfood item such as fabrics and clay-based cat litters.
  - Obstruction secondary to strictures, adhesions, intussusception, neoplasia, and extraluminal compression (e.g., abscessation, parasitic cysts, neoplasia, cystolith) is also possible.

- Cecotrophal soiling of perineum ("clagging," intermittent soft stools): often misinterpreted as diarrhea. Many factors influence cecotrophy. Diet especially plays an important role, with protein and fiber levels influencing this. Increased dietary fiber levels increase the level of cecotrophy, and increased dietary protein levels reduce cecotrophy. Other physical factors affecting cecotrophy include perineal pain (urine or fecal scalding), long-haired breeds, inflexibility, arthritis, spondylosis, obesity, dental disease, restrictive confinement, conformational anomalies, anorexia, neurologic disease, and cecotroph consistency.
- Infection: a host of bacterial, viral, and protozoal organisms can lead to gastrointestinal disease. Many may act synergistically as co-pathogens in the enteritis complex.
  - Protozoal
    - Coccidiosis: several *Eimeria* spp. are pathogenic to the intestinal tract. Infection may be dose-dependent, and the region of the intestines affected may be species-specific. Younger rabbits are more commonly affected. Diarrhea produced may be hemorrhagic but usually is green/brown and odiferous. Chronic infection may result in intussusception and rectal prolapse. Hepatic coccidiosis *(Eimeria stiedai)* may result in secondary diarrhea caused by severe hepatic dysfunction.
    - Cryptosporidiosis: *Cryptosporidium parvum* and *Cryptosporidium cuniculus* may affect young rabbits, resulting in transitory diarrhea and growth retardation; most likely acts as a co-pathogen
    - Flagellates: a host of nonpathogenic normal flora found in cecum and cecotrophs (e.g., *Entamoeba cuniculi, Giardia duodenalis, Monocercomonas cuniculi, Retortamonas cuniculi*)
  - Bacterial
    - Clostridial enterotoxemia: most commonly due to *C. spiroforme*, although *C. difficile, C. perfringens,* and *C. welchii* have also been implicated. Disruption of normal gut flora is considered to be an important predisposing factor (especially in adult rabbits). Low-fiber and high-carbohydrate diets and disruption of the normal cecal environment are more likely to influence disease, especially in younger (recently weaned) rabbits. Virtually all *C. spiroforme* isolates are toxigenic. Disease is usually severe and acute, with diarrhea, collapse, and death within 1 to 3 days. Antibiotic-associated dysbiosis of the cecum can lead to clostridial overgrowth. Avoid use of oral preparations of lincomycin, clindamycin, erythromycin, and penicillins.
    - Tyzzer's disease: caused by *Clostridium piliforme*; seen most often in weanling rabbits, leading to high morbidity and mortality. Transmitted by ingestion of spores. Organism colonizes cecum, resulting in typhlitis, and spread via portal circulation to liver leads to hepatitis. Further systemic spread can lead to myocarditis. Acute diarrhea and sudden death may be seen. Chronic forms of the disease may result in intestinal fibrosis, stenosis, hepatonecrosis, and myocarditis.
    - Coliform enteritis: *E. coli* is normally absent (or present in small numbers) in rabbit intestines. Suckling young and weaners are most susceptible (strain dependent). Enteropathogenic strains are most commonly seen in rabbits. Usually associated with concurrent disease or poor diet and act as co-pathogens. May produce yellowish diarrhea and death.
    - Proliferative enteritis/enterocolitis: *Lawsonia intracellularis* infection can result in proliferation and thickening of intestines (especially ileum). Mostly affects weanling and young rabbits, resulting in acute diarrhea. Rarely causes death unless coinfection occurs (e.g., *E. coli),* and can be difficult to eliminate.
    - Salmonellosis: *S. typhimurium* and *S. enteritidis* can cause diarrhea, septicemia, and rapid death
    - Other bacterial infections (rare): *Klebsiella pneumoniae, Pseudomonas* spp., *Campylobacter* spp., *Yersinia pseudotuberculosis, Mycobacterium paratuberculosis, Vibrio* spp.
  - Viral
    - Rotavirus: infection can result in enterocolitis and diarrhea. Severity of disease depends on viral strain and presence of co-pathogens (e.g., *E. coli, Eimeria* spp.). Mostly seen in weanlings because maternal immunity subsides at this time.
    - Coronavirus: coronaviral enteritis usually affects 3- to 10-week-old rabbits, resulting in diarrhea, lethargy, abdominal distention, and death
    - Other viral infections (rare): adenovirus, parvovirus
  - Yeasts
    - Cecotrophs and hard feces normally contain large numbers of yeasts (e.g., *Cyniclomyces guttulatus*). These are considered normal florae.
- Nematodiasis: *Passalurus ambiguus* (and *P. nonannulatus*) often found in large numbers in cecum and colon; usually nonpathogenic in adults but may be associated with enteritis complex in young rabbits
- Dysautonomia: suspected neurotoxin involved in producing constellation of signs associated with dysfunction of the autonomic nervous system. Anorexia, obtundation, tooth grinding, palpable cecal impaction, and passage of mucus are characteristic clinical signs. Prognosis is poor.
- Mucoid enteropathy: Unclear origin; may be associated with diet, co-pathogens, stressors, dysbiosis, toxins, and dysautonomia. Mostly affects weanlings and occasionally adults (usually after stressor). Diarrhea ± mucoid diarrhea features early and an impacted cecum. Stomach and small intestine may be distended with fluid and gas. Prognosis poor.
- Neoplasia: leiomyoma, leiomyosarcoma, papilloma, and polyps all reported as primary neoplasias of gastrointestinal tract; metastatic involvement of uterine adenocarcinoma also reported
- Toxicity: range of toxins potentially cause gastrointestinal signs (e.g., diarrhea, hypomotility) in rabbits, including lead, aflatoxins, some herbicides, and a variety of plants
- Neuromuscular disease: spinal disease or peripheral neuropathy can alter intestinal function and motility
- Inflammatory bowel disease and dietary intolerance are very rare in rabbits. An intestinal plasmacytosis has been reported in research rabbits.
- Megacolon syndrome of homozygous spotted rabbits: hereditary condition associated with impaired intestinal sodium absorption; increasing liquefaction of cecal and colonic contents leads to characteristic obstipation of cecum in end-stage disease

DIAGNOSIS

DIFFERENTIAL DIAGNOSIS

- Gastric hypomotility
- Anorexia
- Gastrointestinal obstruction
- Gastric trichobezoar
- Gastrointestinal infection (protozoal, bacterial, viral)
- Mucoid enteropathy
- Gastric pyloric hypertrophy (New Zealand white breed)

- Gastric neoplasia (adenocarcinoma, leiomyoma reported)
- Dysautonomia
- Stomach worms
- Accompanying underlying disease

INITIAL DATABASE

- Minimum database: blood biochemistry, hematologic examination, and urinalysis (often unremarkable; however, may indicate dehydration, electrolyte imbalance, hepatopathy, and hyperglycemia)
- Fecal analysis: especially for cases exhibiting diarrhea
  - Direct fecal smear exam ± fecal flotation: coccidiosis, nematodiasis; commensal yeast *C. guttulatus* often mistaken for coccidial oocysts or bacteria
  - Fecal Gram stain: may demonstrate *Clostridium* spp. or excessive Enterobacteriaceae
  - Fecal culture: more useful for suspect *Salmonella* infection because both *E. coli* and clostridial species may be present in small numbers in feces (culture of cecal contents may be more useful for isolation of latter two organisms in postmortem samples)
- Abdominal radiography: gastric distention/impaction (gas, fluid, ingesta), intestinal distention/impaction, other organomegaly, free gas in abdominal cavity (gastrointestinal rupture), abdominal effusion
- Abdominal radiography: important diagnostic tool
  - Serial radiography can serve an important role in monitoring patient progress: monitoring of distention of gastrointestinal tract, gas patterns, and formation of feces
  - Normal gastrointestinal radiography
    - Stomach and cecum should nearly always contain ingesta.
    - Small amounts of gas may normally be present in the stomach and cecum (and very small amounts in the small intestine).
    - Stomach is located caudal to the liver, usually within the confines of the rib cage. Gastric axis (angle formed between center of fundus and pyloris) in lateral view should be parallel with ribs (lateral projection) and perpendicular to spine (in ventrodorsal view).
    - Small intestines are typically located in the cranial abdomen dorsal to the cecum on the lateral projection and in the left cranial abdomen on the ventrodorsal projection. The jejunum can extend into the midcaudal abdomen. The small intestines may be obscured by the large bowel.
    - Cecum typically occupies most of the right and ventral abdomen.
    - Distal colon and rectum can be more easily identified when spherical hard fecal balls are present.
    - Radiographic appearance of a rabbit's abdomen is largely affected by its current "phase" of digestion. During periods of cecotrophal ingestion, feeding tends to cease, and the digestive tract is relatively emptier during this phase. When ingesting food, hard feces may be evident in the colon (rabbits often ingest food and pass hard feces simultaneously). The relative difference in radiographic appearance of an individual's abdomen can alter significantly during a 24-hour cycle.
  - In hypomotile states, accumulated gastric ingesta may be crowned by a gas halo. The stomach can normally contain small amounts of gas (gas cap), although a larger "crescenteric" gas cap may be indicative of increased gas buildup. Gas accumulation may also be evident in the intestines (especially the cecum).
  - In acute gastrointestinal obstruction, severe gastric dilatation results (air, fluid) with the stomach extending well beyond the rib cage. The intestines may have little gas accumulation, although a small intestinal gas pattern suggestive of foreign body obstruction may be evident. Foreign body may not be discernible radiographically.
  - Other organomegaly may be evident (e.g., hepatomegaly).
  - Free gas in abdominal cavity (gastrointestinal rupture) and abdominal effusions (e.g., peritonitis, cardiogenic) may be noted.
  - Gastrointestinal contrast studies (e.g., pneumogastrogaphy, barium sulfate) are not usually diagnostically beneficial, carry procedural risks, and are difficult to interpret.
- Abdominal ultrasound: may be hindered by the presence of large amounts of gastrointestinal gas, although may be useful to delineate gastrointestinal disease (obstructions, intussusception, neoplasia, extraluminal compression) and other structures of other organs
- Radiography of skull for investigation of dental disease
- Radiography of spine/pelvis for investigation of musculoskeletal and neurologic disease

ADVANCED OR CONFIRMATORY TESTING

- Postmortem
  - *C. spiroforme* infection: iota toxin isolation in cecal contents
  - Serotyping for suspect *E. coli* infection
  - Histopathologic examination of intestinal tract for *C. piliforme, E. coli, L. intracellularis,* salmonellosis, *K. pneumoniae, M. paratuberculosis,* rotavirus, *C. parvum*
  - Electron microscopy: identification of rotavirus and coronavirus
  - PCR: *L. intracellularis*
  - Histopathologic examination of intestinal ganglia for dysautonomia
  - Histopathologic examination of suspect neoplasia or area of intestinal strictures
  - Mucoid enteropathy: presence of much mucus in colon
- Advanced imaging
  - CT imaging of skull (further investigation of dental disease)
  - MRI/myelography of spine (further investigation of neurologic disease)
- Blood lead level determination: normal range considered 0.09 to 1.3 μmol/L (2 to 27 μg/dL)

TREATMENT

THERAPEUTIC GOALS

- Return to normal appetite and gastrointestinal function
- Treatment of underlying cause
- Relief of obstruction if present

ACUTE GENERAL TREATMENT

- In cases of gastrointestinal hypomotility, it is essential to support hydration and nutritional needs.
  - Monitor vital signs closely, including heart rate, body temperature, and systolic blood pressure.
  - Provide parenteral fluid therapy via intravenous or intraosseous route. Crystalloids may be used. Maintenance fluid rates are considered 100-120 mL/kg/d.
  - Provide assist feeding through use of commercial assist feeding formulas (e.g., Oxbow Critical Care Feeding Formula; Oxbow Pet Products, Murdock, NE).
  - Provide gut prokinetics (only in nonobstructive cases) via use of cisapride 0.5 mg/kg PO q 8 h; ranitidine 2-5 mg/kg PO, SC q 12 h.
  - Treat suspect gastric ulceration via ranitidine 2-5 mg/kg PO, SC q 12 h; omeprazole 0.5-1 mg/kg PO, IV q 24 h.
  - Offer analgesia (e.g., opioids; buprenorphine 0.03-0.05 mg/kg SC q 8-12 h), nonsteroidal antiinflammatory drugs (NSAIDs; avoid use of NSAIDs in hypovolemic patients); meloxicam 0.3-0.5 mg/kg PO, SC q 12-24 h.
  - Encourage regular movement/exercise and a quiet environment.

- Surgical intervention for gastrointestinal hypomotility cases is rarely indicated and is likely to exacerbate hypomotile state.
- If gastric dilatation is present and gastrointestinal obstruction is suspected, treat as emergency.
  - Promptly institute supportive care measures for shock while monitoring heart rate, body temperature, and systolic blood pressure.
    - Fluid therapy via IV or IO crystalloids at shock rates (60 mL/kg/h) for 1 hour; alternatively, combine crystalloids (10-15 mL/kg) with colloids (5 mL/kg over 5-10 min q 15 min) to achieve systolic blood pressure >90 mm Hg
    - Active warmth is provided via use of heat mats, hot water bottles, warmed fluids, insulatory body wrapping; more advanced external heat sources such as forced-air warmers can also be used.
  - Rapid decompression of stomach necessary: some patients may tolerate passage of orogastric or nasogastric tube, or sedation (e.g., midazolam 0.2-1 mg/kg IM, IV) may be necessary. Avoid percutaneous gastric trocarization because thin-walled stomach may rupture severely.
  - Relieve obstruction via exploratory laparotomy (gastrotomy/enterotomy), although short period of patient stabilization may be required before surgery.
  - Avoid per os medications and gut prokinetics until relief of obstruction is achieved.
- Coccidiosis: treatment via limiting access to hard feces (sporulation occurs in hard feces after about 3 days) and medicating with toltrazuril 25 mg/kg PO q 24 h × 2, repeated after 5 days
- Bacterial infections: based on results of culture and sensitivity testing. First-line choices include enrofloxacin 10 mg/kg PO, SC q 12 h; trimethoprim/sulfonamide 30 mg/kg PO q 12 h. For severe diarrhea, consider loperamide 0.1 mg/kg PO q 8 h.
  - *C. spiroforme* infection: try metronidazole 20 mg/kg PO q 12 h. Consider use of ion-exchange resin to aid in absorption of toxins (e.g., cholestyramine 0.5 g/kg PO q 12 h). Vitamin C 100 mg/kg PO, SC q 24 h may decrease toxin production/absorption.
  - *L. intracellularis* infection: try chloramphenicol 30-50 mg/kg PO q 8-12 h

CHRONIC TREATMENT

- Chronic intermittent gastrointestinal stasis occurs in some individuals. Underlying cause may be difficult to discern. Ensure that adequate dietary fiber is provided, and regularly groom long-haired rabbits.
- Nematodiasis can be treated via benzimidazoles (e.g., fenbendazole 20 mg/kg PO q 24 h × 5 d) or avermectins (e.g., selamectin 6-18 mg/kg topically).
- Lead toxicity: Calcium EDTA 27 mg/kg SC q 6-12 h as needed (usually 5 d minimum treatment). Dilute to <10 mg/mL with 0.45% NaCl/2.5% dextrose. Repeat blood lead level 5 days after last treatment. Repeat calcium EDTA therapy until blood levels return to normal (<40 μg/dL).

DRUG INTERACTIONS

- Avoid use of oral preparations of lincomycin, clindamycin, erythromycin, and penicillin.
- Avoid use of NSAIDs in dehydrated and renally compromised patients.

POSSIBLE COMPLICATIONS

Surgical intervention success rates relatively low; likely due to rapid decompensation in rabbits with gastrointestinal obstruction

RECOMMENDED MONITORING

Appetite, fecal production, and consistency

PROGNOSIS AND OUTCOME

- Prognosis for gastrointestinal hypomotility is generally good in most cases, although this depends on underlying causes.
- Prognosis is guarded for gastrointestinal obstruction unless intervention is swift.

CONTROVERSY

- *Helicobacter* spp. have been isolated from rabbit stomachs, but significance is unknown.
- Metoclopramide may have little effectiveness in promoting gut motility but may have some benefit in reducing nausea in rabbits.
- Routine use of antibiotics in gastrointestinal disease is not warranted. Limited cases may require antibiotics (bacterial overgrowth, gastrointestinal surgery). Choose broad-spectrum antibiotics such as enrofloxacin or trimethoprim/sulfonamides.
- Use of products to enzymatically dissolve ingested hair (e.g., pineapple juice, papaya extract) is unlikely to achieve desired result.
- Use of orally medicated lubricants is unlikely to improve the passage of foreign bodies or trichobezoars.
- Re-establishing cecal flora: commercial probiotics may not survive gastric transit owing to low pH. Process of "transfaunation" (collecting cecotrophs from healthy rabbit to feed to sick rabbit) may circumvent problem. However, cecotrophs need to be consumed whole by recipient without chewing to maintain protective mucous covering.
- Simethicone (an oral antifoaming agent): may reduce size of gas bubbles (not reduce or prevent gas formation) within gastrointestinal tract, facilitating their passage

PEARLS & CONSIDERATIONS

COMMENTS

- Gastric trichobezoars are often the result, rather than the cause, of gastrointestinal disease.
- Gastric ulceration is a common postmortem finding.

PREVENTION

- Ensure adequate dietary fiber.
- Avoid high-carbohydrate diets.
- Perform regular grooming of pet rabbits.
- An oral vaccine developed for coccidiosis (consists of nonpathogenic strains of *Eimeria magna*) is used mainly in commercial rabbitries.

CLIENT EDUCATION

- Emphasize importance of appropriate feeding. Pet rabbit diets should consist largely of grass or grass hays (at least 80% of diet) (e.g., timothy, oaten hays). A variety of fresh leafy green vegetables can be added to the diet. Pellets (if fed at all) should be of the highest quality, viewed as a supplement, and fed in very limited amounts. Seed mixes, cereals, etc., should not be fed or should be offered only in very small amounts intermittently as treats.
- Educate clients on importance of monitoring food intake, fecal production, and activity level of rabbits.
- Encourage regular grooming of rabbits, especially long-haired breeds.
- Ensure that regular exercise and activity are provided to pet rabbits.

SUGGESTED READINGS

Bödeker D, et al: Pathophysiological and functional aspects of the megacolon-syndrome of homozygous spotted rabbits, Zentralbl Veterinarmed A 42:549–559, 1995.

Harcourt-Brown FM: Gastric dilation and intestinal obstruction in 76 rabbits, Vet Rec 161:409–414, 2007.

Harcourt-Brown TH: Management of acute gastric dilation in rabbits, J Exot Pet Med 16:168–174, 2007.

Lipman NS, et al: Utilization of cholestyramine resin as a preventive treatment for antibiotic (clindamycin) induced enterotoxaemia in the rabbit, Lab Anim 26:1–8, 1992.

CROSS-REFERENCES TO OTHER SECTIONS

Anorexia
Coccidiosis
Dental Disease
Dysautonomia (Grass Sickness)
Endoparasites
Gastric Disorders
Hepatic Disorders

AUTHOR & EDITOR: **DAVID VELLA**

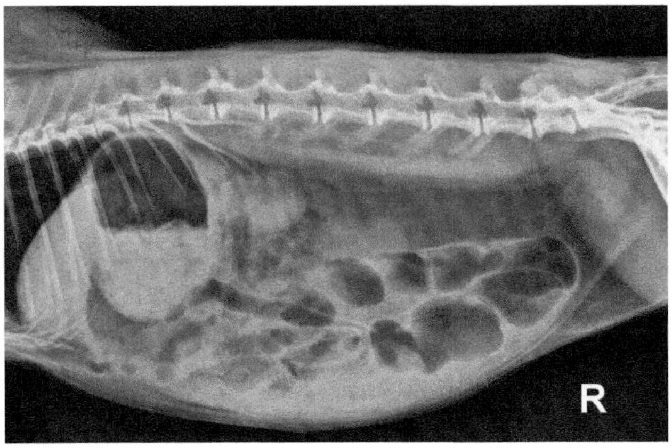

Intestinal Disorders Right lateral abdominal radiograph image of rabbit with gastrointestinal stasis. Note the gas accumulation in the cecum and gas cap in stomach. *(Photo courtesy Jörg Mayer, The University of Georgia, Athens.)*

RABBITS

Lower Respiratory Tract Disorders

BASIC INFORMATION

DEFINITION

Infectious and noninfectious diseases of the trachea, bronchi, lungs, and pleura

SYNONYMS

Lower airway disease, pneumonia, pleuritis, bronchitis, tracheitis, pulmonary disease, mediastinal disease

EPIDEMIOLOGY

RISK FACTORS

- Exposure to high levels of ammonia, dust, and other mucosal irritants can cause primary disease and can predispose to secondary bacterial infection (e.g., *Pasteurella multocida*).
- High stress levels and/or concurrent disease can lead to immune suppression and can predispose to development of bacterial lower respiratory tract disease (e.g., pasteurellosis).
- Sexually entire does are at higher risk of developing uterine neoplasia and metastatic lung disease.

ASSOCIATED CONDITIONS AND DISORDERS

- Cardiac disease
- Uterine neoplasia
- Hypertrophic osteodystrophy reported in association with pulmonary metastasis from uterine adenocarcinoma

CLINICAL PRESENTATION

HISTORY, CHIEF COMPLAINT Depression, lethargy, decreased appetite or anorexia (see Anorexia), weight loss

PHYSICAL EXAM FINDINGS

- Dyspnea (slow, deep breaths and mouth breathing)
- Cyanosis
- Auscultation of thorax
  - Rales (sometimes difficult to distinguish from upper airway sounds)
  - Muffled heart sounds and decreased or absent lung sounds (from pleural effusion, pneumothorax, consolidation, masses)
  - Friction rubs (pleuritis)
  - Fluid sounds (edema effusion)
- Percussion of thorax
  - Increased or decreased resonance
- Poor body condition
- Pyrexia or hypothermia
- Upper respiratory tract (URT) signs may also be present.
  - *Note:* Coughing is rare in the rabbit, even on tracheal manipulation.

ETIOLOGY AND PATHOPHYSIOLOGY

- Bacterial: *Pasteurella multocida, Bordetella bronchiseptica, Staphylococcus aureus, Pseudomonas aeruginosa, Escherichia coli, Mycobacterium* spp., *Moraxella catarrhalis, Moraxella bovis, Mycoplasma pulmonis, Chlamydophila* spp., CAR bacillus, *Francisella tularensis*
- Viral: amyxomatous myxoma virus (see Myxomatosis), rabbit hemorrhagic disease (RHD) (see Hemorrhagic Disease)
- Fungal: *Aspergillus* spp.
- Neoplastic: metastatic disease (uterine adenocarcinoma), lymphosarcoma (see Lymphosarcoma)
- Allergic/irritant: ammonia, smoke, allergens

- Trauma: lung lobe torsion, lung lobe rupture, tracheitis following endotracheal intubation
- Miscellaneous: foreign body aspiration, electrocution (see Electrocution), heatstroke, excessive fluid therapy
- Tracheal disease: obstructive (foreign body, granuloma), exudative
- Pulmonary disease
  - Alveolar: hemorrhage, edema, exudation, abscessation
  - Interstitial: metastatic neoplasia
- Pleural disease
  - Effusion: blood, pus, chyle, modified transudate, true transudate, air
  - Neoplasia
  - Abscess
  - Granuloma
- Mediastinal disease: thymoma (see Thymoma), lymphoma, abscess, granuloma, pneumomediastinum

DIAGNOSIS

DIFFERENTIAL DIAGNOSIS

Cardiovascular disease (see Cardiovascular Disease)

INITIAL DATABASE

- Thoracic radiography
  - Bronchial pattern (bronchopneumonia)
  - Fluid line (pleuritis, neoplasia, chylothorax)
  - Masses: pulmonary, mediastinal (neoplasia, abscess, granuloma)
  - Interstitial pattern (pneumonia)
  - Generalized pulmonary opacity (edema and effusion)
- Complete blood count (CBC)
  - Neutrophilia (acute infection/inflammation)
  - Leukopenia and/or reversed neutrophil/lymphocyte ratio (chronic infection/inflammation)
  - Anemia (chronic disease)

ADVANCED OR CONFIRMATORY TESTING

- Ultrasonography to identify masses and effusions
- Endoscopy (larynx, trachea, pleural space)
- Bronchoalveolar lavage: cytologic examination and culture
- Thoracocentesis: specific gravity, protein content, cytologic examination, culture
- Abdominal radiography (for primary neoplasm)
- Computed tomography
- Thoracoscopy, thoracotomy
- Biopsy and histopathologic examination (ultrasound-guided thoracoscopy or via thoracotomy: mediastinal or lung mass)
- Serologic examination: *P. multocida* (ELISA)

TREATMENT

THERAPEUTIC GOALS

- Dependent on the underlying cause
- Primary resolution where possible (e.g., surgical removal of neoplasm, abscess, foreign body, granuloma)
- Appropriate antibiotic or antifungal therapy for bacterial or fungus-associated disease
- Identification and removal of allergen or respiratory irritant
- For some conditions, palliative care may be all that is possible.

ACUTE GENERAL TREATMENT

- Oxygen therapy
- Supportive care: assisted feeding, fluid therapy, warmth
- Thoracocentesis (air, fluid)

CHRONIC TREATMENT

- Dependent on underlying cause; specific therapies include the following:
  - Antibiosis (tracheitis, bronchopneumonia, abscessation): systemic and via nebulization. A long course of treatment is often necessary (weeks to months). Antibiotics often used include fluoroquinolones (e.g., enrofloxacin 5-10 mg/kg PO q 12 h; marbofloxacin 5 mg/kg PO q 24 h), potentiated sulfonamides (e.g., trimethoprim/sulfa 30 mg/kg PO q 12 h), tetracyclines (e.g., doxycycline 2.5 mg/kg PO q 12 h) and penicillins (e.g., penicillin G procaine 60,000 IU/kg SC, IM q 24h).
  - Mucolytics have been suggested to help clear airways, e.g., N-acetylcysteine has a wide therapeutic range, with dosage usually 5-10 mg/kg and up to 100 mg/kg PO q 12 h; intranasal or aerosol delivery of 5%-20% solution has also been described. A drug that decreases mucous viscosity is bromhexine hydrochloride (not available in the US) at 0.7 mg/kg PO q 24 h or through aerosol delivery. However, conventional steam inhalation (e.g., placing the rabbit in a steamy room) or nebulizing hypertonic saline (7% sodium chloride) may also be useful.
  - Hyaluronidase may be of use in the treatment of pasteurellosis. The addition of hyaluronidase to a nebulization solution (100-150 U/100 ml) may render virulent strains with hyaluronic acid capsule susceptible to ingestion and killing by neutrophils.
  - Nonsteroidal antiinflammatory drugs (NSAIDs) (e.g., carprofen 2-4 mg/kg PO, SC q 24 h; meloxicam 0.3-0.5 mg/kg PO, SC q 12-24 h; ketoprofen 1-3 mg/kg PO q 12 h). Avoid use of NSAIDs in hypovolemic patients.
  - Diuretics (edema) (e.g., furosemide 1-4 mg/kg PO, SC, IM q 4-12 h; hydrochlorothiazide 0.5-2 mg/kg PO q 12 h; bendrofluazide 600 µg/kg PO q 24 h). Supplement patient with potassium and sodium if long-term treatment.
  - Surgical resection: lung lobe torsion, abscesses, neoplasia
  - Repeated thoracocentesis
  - Indwelling pleural drain and lavage

POSSIBLE COMPLICATIONS

- Anesthetic death (during radiography)
- Perioperative death
- Intrathoracic hemorrhage (from thoracocentesis)

RECOMMENDED MONITORING

Dependent on underlying cause:
- Radiography
- CBC

PROGNOSIS AND OUTCOME

- Dependent on underlying cause
- Very poor prognosis for neoplasia unless resectable
- Very poor prognosis for viral disease
- Moderate to good prognosis for alleviating clinical signs associated with bacterial bronchopneumonia, although complete elimination of the causative agent may not be possible

PEARLS & CONSIDERATIONS

COMMENTS

Although thoracotomy is the treatment of choice for several conditions of the lower respiratory tract, it is not commonly performed in the rabbit in general practice. Great attention must be paid to perioperative care and assessment of cardiovascular function.

SUGGESTED READINGS

Lennox AM: Respiratory disease and pasteurellosis. In Quesenberry KE, et al, editors: Ferrets, rabbit and rodents: clinical medicine and surgery, ed 3, St Louis, 2012, Elsevier, pp 205–216.

Marlier D, et al: Infectious agents associated with rabbit pneumonia: isolation of amyxomatous myxoma strains, Vet J 159:171–178, 2000.

Phaneuf LR, et al: Tracheal injury after endotracheal intubation and anesthesia in rabbits, J Am Assoc Lab Anim Sci 45:67–72, 2006.

CROSS-REFERENCES TO OTHER SECTIONS

Anorexia
Cardiovascular Disease
Electrocution
Hemorrhagic Disease
Lymphosarcoma
Myxomatosis
Pasteurellosis
Thymoma
Upper Respiratory Tract Disorders
Uterine Disorders

AUTHOR: **ANNA MEREDITH**

EDITOR: **DAVID VELLA**

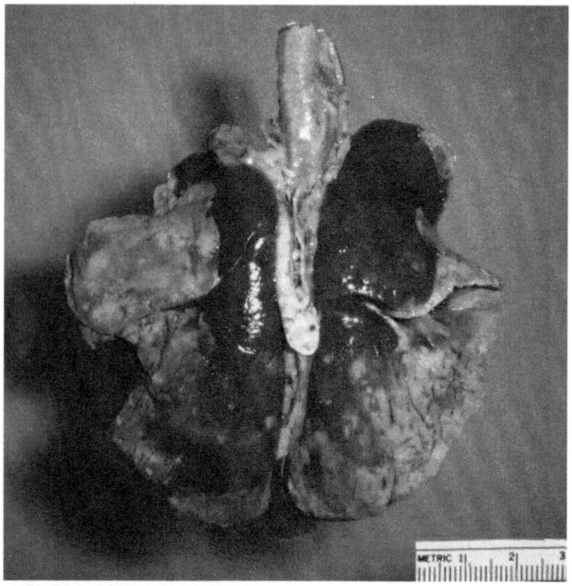

Lower Respiratory Tract Disorders Rabbit lung with a fibrinous pleuritis and pericarditis. *(Photo courtesy Jörg Mayer, The University of Georgia, Athens.)*

RABBITS

Lower Urinary Tract Disorders

Client Education Sheet Available on Website

BASIC INFORMATION

DEFINITION

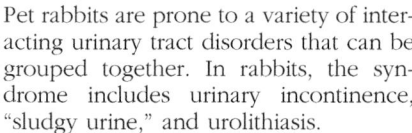

Pet rabbits are prone to a variety of interacting urinary tract disorders that can be grouped together. In rabbits, the syndrome includes urinary incontinence, "sludgy urine," and urolithiasis.

SYNONYMS

Lower urinary tract infection, sludgy urine, sludgy urine syndrome, urinary sludge syndrome, urolithiasis, dysuria, bladder atony, bladder overdistention, upper motor neuron (UMN) bladder, urine retention, urinary incontinence

SPECIAL SPECIES CONSIDERATIONS

- Little is published on normal rabbit urinalysis data.
- Normal urine output = 130 mL/kg/d.
- Urinary excretion of calcium is proportional to dietary calcium intake.

EPIDEMIOLOGY

GENETICS AND BREED PREDISPOSITION

- Lower urinary tract disease is commonly seen in older, overweight, physically inactive pet rabbits. The syndrome of rabbit lower urinary tract disorders is similar to feline lower urinary tract disease (FLUTD) in that these syndromes occur in "fat lazy cats" and "fat lazy pet rabbits."
- Consideration of the rabbit's mobility, husbandry, and general state of health is critical because there is an interrelationship between predisposing causes.

RISK FACTORS

- Urinary tract obstruction is most commonly caused by urolithiasis.
- Calciuria is normal in rabbits. Hypercalciuria results from excessive dietary calcium (e.g., feeding only alfalfa [also known as lucerne] hay).
- Urine retention leads to the development of sabulous calcium carbonate sediment ("sludge") in the bladder.
- Urine soiling and scalding of the perineum lead to urethritis and urinary incontinence. Common causes of urine scalding include the following:
  - Mobility problems caused by disease (e.g., hind limb paresis or paralysis, obesity, ulcerative pododermatitis, spondylosis) or husbandry (e.g., small, cramped cages) prevent a rabbit from adopting the correct stance for urinating.
  - Urinary incontinence due to loss of bladder control from neurologic disease (e.g., encephalitozoonosis) or spinal problems
  - Diseases causing polydipsia and polyuria: psychogenic polydipsia has been described in four female laboratory rabbits, and hormone-responsive incontinence has been described in two ovariohysterectomized does.
  - Anatomic and conformational conditions affecting the direction of the jet of urine (e.g., scarred preputial skin from bite wounds, obesity, or infection alters the direction of urination, so it lands on the skin)
- Perineal dermatitis may occur secondary to urinary scalding. It can also occur as a result of the following:
  - Ineffective grooming from pain or mobility problems
  - Matted fur soiled with uneaten cecotrophs from dental disease, obesity, and flexibility problems
  - Infection with *Treponema paraluis-cuniculi* (rabbit syphilis)
  - Neurologic disease
  - Upper and lower motor neuron disease, spinal cord injury/disease, peripheral nervous system disorders (including dysautonomia), urine retention, reflex dyssynergia, and dysautonomia
  - Urethral sphincter mechanism incontinence
  - Neoplasia of lower urinary tract, including bladder, is rare in rabbits.

CLINICAL PRESENTATION

HISTORY, CHIEF COMPLAINT Clinical signs can include inappropriate urination, depression, a hunched posture, teeth grinding, dysuria, pollakiuria, hematuria, stranguria, perineal urine soiling and scalding, urinary sludge, urinary incontinence, polyuria, and polydipsia.

PHYSICAL EXAM FINDINGS

- Abnormalities may not be detected
- Bladder palpation: may be normal or may reveal a large, distended, and firm bladder. Manual bladder expression may elicit thick, pastelike brownish urine. Cystoliths may be palpable. Pain may be present with underlying cystitis.
- Bladder expression may be easy or difficult (depending on sphincter tone, obstruction):
  - LMN (sacral lesion or peripheral nervous system): flaccid bladder, flaccid anus and tail
  - UMN (suprasacral lesion): turgid bladder, perineal tone intact
- Kidneys may palpate enlarged, irregular, or asymmetric
- Urethral calculi occasionally may be palpated in the penis.
- Urinary soiling and scalding of the perineal skin, inner thighs, tail, and rump

DIAGNOSIS

DIFFERENTIAL DIAGNOSIS

- Hematuria
  - Uterine disease (e.g., uterine adenocarcinoma), cystitis, urolithiasis, urethritis, coagulopathy
- Polyuria
  - Renal insufficiency/failure, severe hepatopathy, pyometra, hypercalcemia, hypokalemia, diabetes mellitus, endotoxemia, hyperproteinemia, pregnancy toxemia, postobstructive diuresis, polycythemia
- Polydipsia
  - Anorexia, pain/stress, psychogenic

INITIAL DATABASE

- Complete blood count/biochemistry
  - Usually unremarkable. Leukocytosis may be seen in rabbits with urinary tract infection. Red blood cell count and hematocrit may be depressed with chronic inflammation or causes of hematuria.
  - Blood calcium level measurement significance not determined. Rabbits have a relatively higher blood calcium level and range compared with other species. Their serum calcium concentration often reflects their dietary calcium intake.
  - Evidence for renal insufficiency (elevated blood urea nitrogen [BUN]/creatinine) may be seen. This should be checked with concurrent urine specific gravity measurement.
  - In cases of urinary outflow obstruction, postrenal azotemia (elevated BUN and creatinine) and hyperkalemia may be seen.
- Urinalysis
  - Affected animals may show hematuria. Proteinuria (30 mg/dL) is a common finding in both healthy and diseased animals. Urine sediment is normal in rabbits. Wet smear slides of urinary sediment frequently show carbonate and phosphate crystals even in healthy rabbits.
  - In cases of infection or inflammation, pyuria and hematuria may be evident. Bacteriuria may be seen occasionally. *Escherichia coli* is the most frequently isolated organism.

ADVANCED OR CONFIRMATORY TESTING

- Perform analysis of retrieved calculi for mineral composition.
- Perform microbiological examination and antimicrobial sensitivity on cystocentesis-collected urine samples.
- Diagnostic imaging
  - Abdominal radiography is nearly always indicated to evaluate kidneys, ureters, uterus, bladder, and urethra.
  - Diagnosis of urolithiasis is determined by abdominal and pelvic radiology because calcium-based calculi are radiopaque. When positioning the rabbit for abdominal radiographs, ensure that the entire caudal half of the body is captured on the radiograph (up to the distal tip of the urethra—the rabbit's penis is situated relatively caudal, ventral to the anus, and thus it is easy to miss the penile urethra with improper radiographic positioning). Pay attention to coccygeal area, and stretch hind limbs away from the body.
  - Uroliths often occur in more than one location simultaneously.
  - A small level of radiodense urine is common. Larger than normal deposits of urine sediment may result in an unusual level of bladder "sludge" that may indicate the problem. The presence of radiodense urine may hinder the identification of cystoliths.
- Ultrasonography
  - May be used to examine the bladder and the proximal urethra and to distinguish the presence of cystoliths within bladder sludge. Ultrasonography can also be useful in determining the presence of ureterolithiasis and secondary ureteral distention and hydronephrosis.
- Radiographic study of the spinal column is also indicated. Problems commonly found include spondylosis and vertebral subluxation.
- Other investigations:
  - Examine the oral cavity ± skull radiographs for the presence of dental disease.
  - Serologic testing for *Encephalitozoon cuniculi* may be required.
  - Evaluate renal function in rabbits with nephrolithiasis, hydronephrosis, or ureteral calculi.
  - Urethral catheterization can be both diagnostic and therapeutic in cases of urethral obstruction and bladder sludge removal; 3 to 3.5 Fr urinary catheters can be used.
  - To highlight the bladder wall lining, negative- and double-contrast radiographic techniques can be used, as in cats and dogs.
  - Cystoscopy and urethroscopy may be used to visualize urethral and bladder wall lining.

TREATMENT

THERAPEUTIC GOALS

- General considerations
  - Identify and treat underlying medical problems (e.g., spinal disorders, encephalitozoonosis, anatomic defects, ulcerative pododermatitis) and prevent husbandry from interfering with normal urination (e.g., provide clean dry bedding).
  - Gently clip and clean affected areas. Removal of hair facilitates drying of the area and clippers should be carefully used up to the area of unaffected skin. Remove all matted hair. Skin is very fragile and is prone to tearing.
  - Clipping may require light sedation. Consider midazolam 0.5-2 mg/kg IM, IV, or diazepam 0.5-2 mg/kg IM.
  - Do not bathe skin until all hair is removed from affected areas. Use dilute chlorhexidine-based shampoos, and ensure that the area is dried thoroughly after bathing.
  - Topical antimicrobial therapy can be employed but may be readily licked away by the rabbit, hence the choice of nontoxic compounds. Consider topical treatment with preparations containing fusidic acid, silver sulfadiazine/chlorhexidine, mupirocin calcium, or Manuka honey.
  - Provide analgesia.
  - Administer nonsteroidal antiinflammatory drugs (e.g., carprofen 2-4 mg/kg PO, SC q 24 h; meloxicam 0.3-0.5 mg/kg PO, SC q 24 h; ketoprofen 1-3 mg/kg PO q 12 h).

- Opioids (e.g., buprenorphine 0.03 mg/kg SC, IM q 8 h)
- Give antibiotics (e.g., enrofloxacin 10 mg/kg PO, SC q 12 h, or trimethoprim-sulfa 30 mg/kg PO q 12 h) to treat cystitis, urethritis, and secondary pyoderma.
  - Urine culture and sensitivity is always indicated.
  - Long courses of antibiotics may be necessary to treat cystitis.
- Provide the opportunity to exercise and urinate away from the bedding.

- Dealing with sabulous calcite sediment (sludge):
  - Sediment can be removed by manual expression of the bladder under sedation or general anesthesia. Sedation with a benzodiazepine may aid in relaxation of smooth muscle and may facilitate bladder expression (consider midazolam 0.5-2 mg/kg IM, IV, or diazepam 0.5-2 mg/kg IM). The process may require repeat attempts daily for several days. Provide analgesics post treatment.
  - Catheterize bladder to flush with sterile 0.9% saline. Provide analgesics post treatment.
  - Induce diuresis:
    - Intravenous fluid therapy
    - Subcutaneous fluid therapy
    - Increase voluntary water intake by sweetening the water with sucrose or fruit juice.
    - Provide leafy green vegetables. Some plants (e.g., dandelions, goose-grass, plantain, yarrow) may have diuretic properties.
    - Give a calcium-sparing thiazide diuretic such as hydrochlorothiazide 0.5-2 mg/kg PO q 12 h or bendrofluazide 600 μg/kg PO q 24 h, and supplement patient with potassium and sodium.
  - Provide an inhibitor of crystal formation such as potassium citrate.
  - Reduce the amount of calcium in the diet (e.g., avoid high-calcium foods such as alfalfa/lucerne hay).
  - Medical dissolution of uroliths in rabbits has not been reported.
  - Give the rabbit the opportunity to graze grass and the freedom to exercise.
- Surgical treatment: urolithiasis
  - Cystoliths and urethroliths require surgical removal.
  - Cystotomy closure: simple continuous appositional pattern closure is equal biomechanically and histologically to single-layer continuous Cushing closure.
  - Use synthetic absorbable monofilament sutures to close cystotomy (e.g., Monocryl, PDS II, Maxon).
- Surgical treatment: dermoplasty
  - Perform perineal dermoplasty on rabbits with deep perineal skin folds (e.g., obese female rabbits).
  - Perform corrective surgery on rabbits with scarred prepuces (e.g., to stop the jet of urine landing on the skin inside the thighs).

RECOMMENDED MONITORING

- Diet
  - A balanced diet with sufficient, but not excessive, quantities of calcium and phosphorus is required. Calcium deficiency can result in osteoporosis and dental problems. Phosphorus restriction increases urinary calcium excretion and exacerbates both hypercalciuria and bone loss.
  - Exclude all vitamin and mineral supplements and remove mineral blocks.
  - Feed rabbits fresh feed and low-calcium hay (e.g., timothy grass). Avoid pelleted diet.
  - Avoid high-calcium vegetables such as kale, broccoli, turnip, Chinese cabbage, and watercress.
  - Vegetables with moderate calcium content include cabbage, carrots, celery, and lettuce.
  - Encourage weight loss in overweight and obese rabbits.
  - Other
  - Urethral sphincter mechanism incontinence (USMI): consider diethylstilbestrol 0.5 mg per rabbit PO once to twice weekly. Phenylpropanolamine may also be used.
- Follow-up
  - Normal rabbit urine is alkaline, and owners or clinicians should try to estimate what the typical daily urine pH is for the animal. A rising urinary pH >8 (from ammonia production by urease-producing bacteria such as *E. coli*) is often a sign of bacterial cystitis.
- Patient monitoring
  - Obtain radiographs after surgery to verify complete removal of calculi.
  - Obtain abdominal radiographs of the bladder at 1 to 3 months postoperatively for early detection of calculus recurrence.
  - Collect urine samples via cystocentesis to perform urinalysis and examination of urinary sediment for crystals.
  - Ask the client how the rabbit is coping with the new low-calcium diet, and with receiving citrate and drinking water that includes sweetener to promote diuresis. Noncompliance reported when the rabbit will not eat the new diet or will not drink the sweetened water is a major reason for recurrence of calculi.
  - Act promptly to handle any episodes of perineal urinary soiling because scalding can result quickly, and affected skin is vulnerable to infection and myiasis.

PEARLS & CONSIDERATIONS

PREVENTION

- Reduce calcium in the diet (and if possible increase phosphorus in the diet).
- Give citrate daily in the diet, in the drinking water, or as an oral dose. Palatability may be an issue.
- Increase diuresis.
- Control bacterial cystitis.

CLIENT EDUCATION

- Avoid calcium-rich food items. Avoid alfalfa/lucerne–based pellets and hay.
- Increase water consumption. Provide multiple sources of fresh water. Consider flavoring water with small amounts of unsweetened fruit juice. Offer a variety of fresh leafy greens.

SUGGESTED READINGS

Donnelly TM: What's your diagnosis? Wet fur and dermatitis in a rabbit, Lab Anim (NY) 34:23–25, 2005.

Flatt RE, et al: Identification of crystalline material in urine of rabbits, Am J Vet Res 32:655–658, 1971.

Jens B, et al: Suture selection for lower urinary tract surgery in small animals, Comp Cont Educ Pract Vet 23:524–531, 2001.

Osborne CA, et al: Quantitative analysis of 4468 uroliths retrieved from farm animals, exotic species, and wildlife submitted to the Minnesota Urolith Center: 1981 to 2007, Vet Clin North Am Small Anim Pract 39:65–78, 2009.

Rogers KD, et al: Composition of uroliths in small domestic animals in the United Kingdom, Vet J 188:228–230, 2011.

CROSS-REFERENCES TO OTHER SECTIONS

Dysautonomia
Encephalitozoonosis
Obesity
Pododermatitis
Renal disorders
Treponematosis
Uterine disorders

AUTHOR: **THOMAS M. DONNELLY**

EDITOR: **DAVID VELLA**

Lymphosarcoma

BASIC INFORMATION

DEFINITION

Lymphoma is a neoplastic proliferation of lymphoreticular cells that arises most frequently from lymphoid tissues, but almost any tissue in the body can be involved.

SYNONYM

Malignant lymphoma, lymphoblastic lymphoma, lymphocytic lymphoma

EPIDEMIOLOGY

SPECIES, AGE, SEX Most lymphomas in rabbits occur in young adults, although the disease is reported in rabbits up to 10 years of age. Thymic lymphoma may occur more commonly in older rabbits. The true incidence of all forms of lymphosarcoma in rabbits is currently unknown.

GENETICS AND BREED PREDISPOSITION

- Not documented to have a breed predilection and seen in various rabbit breeds, including New Zealand white, Japanese white, Dutch, and Netherland dwarf rabbits
- Hereditary lymphosarcoma due to a recessive gene occurs in the inbred WH (wire-hair) strain of rabbit. Affected rabbits are generally less than 1 year of age. Lymphosarcoma is the cause of death in homozygotes and hemolytic anemia is the primary cause of death in heterozygotes with increasing lymphoproliferative disease, as rabbits grow older.

CONTAGION AND ZOONOSIS No infectious cause for lymphoma in rabbits has been identified. However, multiple research publications describe induction of lymphoma in laboratory rabbits with various viruses. These findings do not appear to have any bearing on spontaneous lymphoma in pet rabbits.

CLINICAL PRESENTATION

DISEASE FORMS/SUBTYPES

- Lymphoblastic (large cell) or lymphocytic (small cell) lymphoma
- Immunophenotype: B-cell, T-cell-rich-B-cell, and T-cell forms are described.
- Commonly multicentric (peripheral lymph nodes, abdominal organs, skin, blood [leukemic])
- Rare localized forms: cutaneous (usually associated with or progresses to multicentric form), thymic (usually T-cell), spinal, gastrointestinal, retro-orbital

HISTORY, CHIEF COMPLAINT

- Duration of illness before diagnosis varies from 1 week to 10 months.
- Clinical signs depend on location of disease but usually include one or more of: anorexia, lethargy, weakness, dyspnea, weight loss, cutaneous nodules (+/– ulceration, crusting, alopecia, erythema), blepharitis, diarrhea, peripheral lymphadenopathy.

PHYSICAL EXAM FINDINGS

- Thymic form: dyspnea, tachypnea, possibly bilateral exophthalmus and precaval syndrome due to the presence of a mediastinal mass
- Cutaneous form: multiple raised nonpainful nodules, ulcerated, crusty, erythematous lesions, alopecia
- Multicentric: enlarged peripheral nodes, emaciation, abdominal lymphadenopathy +/– cutaneous involvement

DIAGNOSIS

DIFFERENTIAL DIAGNOSIS

- Thymoma (see Thymoma) must be differentiated from thymic lymphoma by biopsy. Clinical signs and radiologic appearance of both diseases are similar.
- Cutaneous lymphoma: rule out infectious, allergic, traumatic (e.g. needle injections), parasitic, behavioral, and endocrine causes.

INITIAL DATABASE

- Clinical pathology
  - Complete blood count: normal or lymphocytosis (leukemic), mild anemia.
  - Chemistry profile: normal, or depending on organ involved: elevated AST, ALT, ALP, BUN, creatinine.
  - Hypercalcemia must be interpreted in light of the distinct calcium homeostasis in rabbits. Paraneoplastic hypercalcemia is extremely rare.
- Diagnostic imaging
  - Radiographs and computed tomography scan are useful in detecting thymic forms of lymphoma.
  - Ultrasonography is the imaging method of choice for most forms of lymphoma affecting the abdomen.
- Pathology.
  - Cytology: a fine-needle aspirate of enlarged lymph nodes, mediastinal mass, cutaneous nodules or other lesions should be performed and will often yield a diagnosis in cases of lymphoblastic (large cell) lymphoma.
  - Histopathology: to obtain a definitive diagnosis, especially in cases of lymphocytic (small cell) lymphoma, or to differentiate thymic lymphoma from thymoma.
  - Bone marrow aspirate: should be performed when a leukemic form is suspected.
  - Blood smear: may reveal circulating neoplastic lymphocytes.

ADVANCED OR CONFIRMATORY TESTING

- Immunohistochemistry can be performed on biopsy tissue to differentiate between T- and B-cell lymphoma.
- Immunohistochemical staining can be performed using CD3 antibody (a T-cell marker) and CD79a (a B-cell marker) antibodies. The most frequent subtype is B-cell lymphoma. The second most common subtype is T-cell–rich B-cell lymphoma—a lymphoma subtype that is rarely diagnosed in man, dogs, or cats, yet frequently occurs in horses.

TREATMENT

THERAPEUTIC GOALS

- Restoration of a good quality of life should be the primary therapeutic goal in case management. The owner should understand that the lymphoma most likely will be the animal's demise because cure is rarely if ever achieved.
- No well-established chemotherapy protocol is available for the rabbit, and each case must be managed individually. Ideally, an oncologist should be part of the treatment team.

ACUTE GENERAL TREATMENT

- Mediastinal form
  - Radiation has been used in rabbits with mediastinal lymphoma and appears mostly to be an efficacious and well-tolerated treatment. Recommended protocols usually involve several treatments a week, over a course of 2-4 weeks (definitive) or one treatment a week for 3-6 weeks (coarse fractionation/palliative). Cost can be limiting.
  - Systemic chemotherapy can be considered as adjuvant treatment in patients with thymic lymphoma (vs. thymoma). Oral prednisone therapy has been used successfully in a few

 - cases in which radiation or surgery were not an option.
 - Surgical excision of localized lesions after thorough staging should be considered (especially thymic, gastrointestinal forms). Perioperative mortality may be high.

CHRONIC TREATMENT

- The simplest form of chemotherapy for lymphoma is oral prednisolone at 1-2 mg/kg PO q 12-24 h. This treatment has been evaluated in a limited number of rabbits with variable results.
- Multiple-drug chemotherapy protocols are not published for rabbits, and treatment must be extrapolated from information available for other species, usually dog, cat, or ferret.
- Several chemotherapy agents have been used in rabbits, mostly in a laboratory setting, or anecdotally in pet rabbits. Doxorubicin (1 mg/kg IV q 14-21 d), mitoxantrone (5-6 mg/m^2 IV q 21 d), cyclophosphamide (5-6 mg/m^2 IV q 21 d), CCNU (50 mg/m^2 PO q 3-6 w), L-asparaginase (400 U/kg SC, IM), vincristine (0.5-0.7 mg/m^2 IV q 7-14 d), and carboplatin (150-180 mg/m^2 IV q 21-28 d) are reported.
- Chemotherapy can be administered intravenously, orally, or subcutaneously.
- The placement of an indwelling vascular access port has been described in rabbits in an experimental setting. It is used in other species receiving frequent chemotherapy administrations, and should be considered.
- The choice of the protocol should be based on the type of lymphoma, and owners should be well educated as to the effect of the drugs, expected outcome, and cost.

DRUG INTERACTIONS

- Chemotherapy side effects will be cumulative. Drugs should therefore be used following a defined protocol.

POSSIBLE COMPLICATIONS

- Chemotherapy can cause moderate to severe myelosuppression and gastrointestinal toxicity (mostly recognized as nausea and enteritis in rabbits). Rabbits may be more sensitive to the effects of chemotherapy agents. However there are currently no established doses of chemotherapy in rabbits
- Severe neutropenia can be encountered during the protocol because some rabbits appear to be extremely sensitive to myelosuppressive drugs. Secondary infection easily occurs if antibacterial therapy is not started.
- Doxorubicin can cause cardiotoxicity in other species. However, one author (JM) has used this drug aggressively without noting cardiotoxic effects in the rabbit.
  - In one study, doxorubicin was administered intravenously to male rabbits at doses of 3 mg/kg (50 mg/m^2) q 7 d for 10 wk without causing cardiac injury, suggesting that rabbits may be more tolerant than other species to doxorubicin.
- Administering high doses of corticosteroids to rabbits is controversial because of the immune suppressive effects of these drugs. However, the authors have not seen this side effect in rabbits with thymic lymphoma treated for several months with high doses of corticosteroids.

RECOMMENDED MONITORING

- Frequent complete blood counts are needed to monitor the degree of immune suppression in the patient.
- Doxorubicin cardiotoxicity has not yet been described in rabbits, but regular monitoring of cardiac function should be considered.
- Disease burden should be monitored for response to treatment, and the protocol adapted accordingly.

PROGNOSIS AND OUTCOME

- A cure for lymphoma is rarely achieved and the long-term prognosis is usually poor, independent of the treatment chosen, although survival data is lacking.

PEARLS & CONSIDERATIONS

CLIENT EDUCATION

Before starting any therapy, the client should understand that the treatment is aimed at improving the rabbit's quality of life for a certain time, and that a cure is rarely achievable.

SUGGESTED READINGS

Gomez L, et al: Lymphoma in a rabbit: histopathological and immunohistochemical findings, J Small Anim Pract 43:224–226, 2002.

Heatley JJ, et al: Spontaneous neoplasms of lagomorphs, Vet Clin Exot Anim 7:561–577, 2004.

Ishikawa M, et al: A case of lymphoma developing in the rabbit cecum, J Vet Med Sci 69:1183–1185, 2007.

Klimtová I, et al: Comparative study of chronic toxic effects of daunorubicin and doxorubicin in rabbits, Hum Exp Toxicol 21:649–657, 2002.

White SD, et al: Lymphoma with cutaneous involvement in three domestic rabbits *(Oryctolagus cuniculus)*, Vet Dermatol 11: 61–67, 2000.

Wolf B, et al: Morphological and immunohistochemical characterization of lymphoma in pet rabbits, J Comp Pathol 141:275, 2009.

CROSS-REFERENCES TO OTHER SECTIONS

Lymphoma, Ferrets
Thymoma

AUTHOR: **CECILIA ROBAT AND JÖRG MAYER**

EDITOR: **THOMAS M. DONNELLY**

Mammary Gland Disorders

Client Education Sheet Available on Website

BASIC INFORMATION

DEFINITION

Any disease process affecting the function or integrity of the mammary glands:
- Mastitis: inflammation of the mammary gland, often accompanied by sepsis
- Cystic: sterile mammary cysts derived from papillary ducts
- Neoplasia: benign mixed adenoma, mammary papilloma, mammary adenocarcinoma reported
- Dysplasia: hyperplasia of the mammary glands secondary to hormonal influence

SYNONYM

Cystic mastitis, mammary gland neoplasia, or dysplasia

SPECIAL SPECIES CONSIDERATIONS

Rabbit mammary tissue appears relatively sensitive to prolactin.

EPIDEMIOLOGY

SPECIES, AGE, SEX
- Mastitis: intact breeding does and does with pseudopregnancy
- Cystic mastitis usually occurs in nonbreeding entire does older than 3 years.
- Neoplasia: entire does older than 3 years of age
- Dysplasia: aged, primiparous, female, New Zealand white rabbits
- Mammary disease rarely occurs in male rabbits

GENETICS AND BREED PREDISPOSITION
- Mammary carcinoma has been reported frequently in laboratory rabbits, including Belgian and English Belgian, New Zealand white, and New Zealand white cross-breed does.
- Dysplasia reported only in New Zealand White rabbits

RISK FACTORS
- Mastitis: dirty environment, lactating does, pseudopregnancy, entire does, heavy lactation, abrasive bedding or caging, injury to a gland or teat
- Cystic mastitis: entire does
- Neoplasia: entire does
- Dysplasia: aged primiparous New Zealand White does

CONTAGION AND ZOONOSIS Mastitis: The bacteria responsible (e.g., *Staphylococcus aureus* [see Staphylococcosis], *Streptococcus* spp., and *Pasteurella* spp. [see Pasteurellosis]) may spread between does; can also be spread via kits that are fostered to another doe

ASSOCIATED CONDITIONS AND DISORDERS
- Does with cystic mastitis may show signs of pseudopregnancy.
- Cystic mastitis often occurs concurrently with endometrial hyperplasia or uterine adenocarcinoma.
- Cystic disease has been shown to progress to benign neoplasia followed by invasive adenocarcinoma.

CLINICAL PRESENTATION

DISEASE FORMS/SUBTYPES
- Mastitis: bacterial, cystic
- Neoplasia: benign mixed adenoma, mammary papilloma, mammary adenocarcinoma
- Dysplasia

HISTORY, CHIEF COMPLAINT
- Bacterial mastitis: inflamed mammary glands, anorexia, polydipsia, lethargy, and depression; death of the doe or kits
- Cystic mastitis: swollen glands, sometimes with blue coloration. Often accompanies uterine diseases (e.g., endometrial hyperplasia, uterine adenocarcinoma), hence other signs associated with these uterine diseases (e.g., hematuria) may be seen
- Neoplasia: mammary mass effects; signs of uterine disease may also be seen, as with cystic mastitis
- Dysplasia: one or more mammary glands swollen and firm with markedly enlarged teats; associated glandular tissue is usually discolored grey, blue, or greenish black

PHYSICAL EXAM FINDINGS
- Bacterial mastitis: hot, swollen, firm, painful glands; pyrexia; discoloration of overlying skin from red to dark blue; ulceration
- Cystic mastitis: variably sized subcutaneous nodules of variable duration that are usually fluctuant, are seldom painful, and may have discharge of milk or amber-colored liquid. Doe is not usually depressed. Swollen and firm glands with a clear to serosanguineous liquid expressed from the glands, with nipples distended
- Neoplasia: variably sized subcutaneous nodules of variable duration that are usually fluctuant, are seldom painful, and may have discharge of milk or amber-colored liquid
- Dysplasia: enlarged glands with discolored teats

ETIOLOGY AND PATHOPHYSIOLOGY

- Bacterial mastitis may arise from external contamination, abrasion, trauma, and hematogenous spread.
- Mastitis can occur concurrently with metritis.
- Milk retention from pseudopregnancy can lead to mastitis.
- Neoplasia may metastasize to regional lymph nodes or to distant organs (e.g., lungs).
- Cystic mammary glands may be associated with uterine hyperplasia and adenocarcinoma.
- Progression of cystic mammary gland disease may result in their coalescence and connective tissue formation around the cysts. This may evolve further to malignant changes and invasive mammary adenocarcinoma.
- Mammary dysplasia may be due to prolactin-producing pituitary adenomas.
- Mammary hyperplasia may be induced (in both genders) in New Zealand White rabbits after treatment with cyclosporin A.
- Mammary carcinoma can arise with no proceeding mammary abnormalities, or it can be a progressive disease starting with cystic disease, which progresses to benign neoplasia and then to invasive adenocarcinoma.
- A direct correlation has been noted between uterine tumors and mammary carcinomas.

DIAGNOSIS

DIFFERENTIAL DIAGNOSIS

Mammary mastitis, cystic mastitis, neoplasia, dysplasia, other cutaneous masses

INITIAL DATABASE

- Hematologic examination and biochemistry profile: usually unremarkable or may reflect inflammation; anemia may be present if underlying uterine disease is also present
- Mastitis: sampling of milk discharged or exudate from affected glands for microbial culture and sensitivity
- Mammary gland mass effects: fine-needle aspiration (FNA) and cytologic examination of swollen glands or biopsy and histopathologic examination to distinguish between cystic mastitis, neoplasia, and dysplasia

ADVANCED OR CONFIRMATORY TESTING

- Evaluate does for concurrent uterine disease (abdominal imaging via radiography and ultrasonography).
- Perform thoracic radiography to rule out metastasis if mammary or uterine neoplasia is suspected.

- For cystic mastitis, rule out bacterial mastitis via FNA and cytologic/microbiological examination.
- Histologic examination of affected mammary glands can differentiate between cystic mastitis, dysplasia, hyperplasia, and neoplasia.
- Advanced imaging: computed tomography or magnetic resonance imaging may be used to search for pituitary enlargement in cases of mammary hyperplasia
- Serum prolactin levels: normal ranges not fully established, although measurement may prove helpful in cases of suspected mammary dysplasia. Serum prolactin concentrations may be 10- to 1000-fold greater than those seen in nonpregnant rabbits.

TREATMENT

THERAPEUTIC GOALS

- Mastitis
  - Bacterial: resolve infection
  - Cystic: resolve cyst formation
- Neoplasia: remove affected tissue
- Dysplasia: provide potential management of pituitary adenoma

ACUTE GENERAL TREATMENT

- Bacterial mastitis: general supportive care for any rabbit experiencing reduced or nil food intake (e.g., fluid therapy, assist feeding, analgesia, management of gut stasis)
  - Provide parenteral fluid therapy (crystalloids may be used). Maintenance fluid rates are considered 100-120 mL/kg/d.
  - Provide assist feeding by using commercial assist feeding formulas (e.g., Oxbow Critical Care Feeding Formula; Oxbow Pet Products, Murdock, NE).
  - Analgesia
    - Nonsteroidal antiinflammatory drugs (NSAIDs; ensure that hydration is adequate and renal function is normal before use) (e.g., carprofen 2-4 mg/kg PO, SC q 24 h; meloxicam 0.3-0.5 mg/kg PO, SC q 24 h; ketoprofen 1-3 mg/kg PO q 12 h)
    - Opioids (e.g., buprenorphine 0.03 mg/kg SC, IM q 8 h)
  - Suitable first-line antibiotics may include procaine penicillin 40,000-60,000 IU/kg SC, IM q 24 h, or trimethoprim/sulfonamides 30 mg/kg PO q 12 h, or enrofloxacin 10 mg/kg PO, SC q 12 h in combination with metronidazole 20 mg/kg PO q 12 h.
  - Use warm compresses to affected glands, and attempt gentle drainage of glands several times a day.
  - Remove kits to prevent bacterial enteritis or starvation.
- Cystic mastitis: ovariohysterectomy without removal of mammae usually causes regression.
- Neoplasia: complete mastectomy and ovariohysterectomy

CHRONIC TREATMENT

- Bacterial mastitis: drainage of abscess, surgical removal in severe cases
- Cystic mastitis: surgical removal of mammae if not regressed 3 to 4 weeks after ovariohysterectomy
- Dysplasia: dopamine agonists (e.g., bromocriptine, quinagolide, cabergoline) carry potential for treatment of hyperprolactinemia, although little clinical use in rabbits has been reported

DRUG INTERACTIONS

- Avoid use of oral preparations of lincomycin, clindamycin, erythromycin, and penicillin.
- Avoid use of NSAIDs in dehydrated and renally compromised patients.

POSSIBLE COMPLICATIONS

- Cystic mastitis left untreated can progress to benign and malignant neoplasm.
- Neoplasia: metastasis to regional lymph nodes or distant organs (especially lungs) and associated complications
- Mastitis: kits may die from peracute septicemia or starvation

RECOMMENDED MONITORING

Repeat thoracic radiography if neoplasia is diagnosed.

PROGNOSIS AND OUTCOME

- Mastitis
  - Bacterial: good with early intervention
  - Cystic: excellent with ovariohysterectomy
- Neoplasia: good with treatment before metastasis
- Dysplasia: guarded if associated with pituitary neoplasia

PEARLS & CONSIDERATIONS

PREVENTION

Early neutering for females not intended for reproduction

CLIENT EDUCATION

Advise on neutering, and provide reasons and advantages associated with this procedure.

SUGGESTED READINGS

Adlam C, et al: Natural and experimental staphylococcal mastitis in rabbits, J Comp Pathol 86:581–593, 1976.

Atherton J, et al: Cystic mastitis disease in the female rabbit, Vet Rec 145:648, 1999.

Krimer PM, et al: Reversible fibroadenomatous mammary hyperplasia in male and female New Zealand white rabbits associated with cyclosporine A administration, Vet Pathol 46:1144–1148, 2009.

Sikoski P, et al: Cystic mammary adenocarcinoma associated with a prolactin-secreting pituitary adenoma in a New Zealand white rabbit *(Oryctolagus cuniculus)*, Comp Med 58:297–300, 2008.

CROSS-REFERENCES TO OTHER SECTIONS

Abscesses
Cutaneous Masses
Pasteurellosis
Staphylococcosis
Uterine Disorders

AUTHORS: **MICHELLE BINGLEY AND DAVID VELLA**

EDITOR: **THOMAS M. DONNELLY**

RABBITS

Myxomatosis

BASIC INFORMATION

DEFINITION

Myxomatosis is a generalized, fulminant, frequently lethal disease of domestic and wild European rabbits caused by Myxoma virus, a poxvirus in the genus *Leporipoxvirus*.

- Myxomatosis is not the same disease as rabbit pox, which is caused by strains of vaccinia virus.

SPECIAL SPECIES CONSIDERATIONS

Myxoma virus infects only lagomorphs—rabbits and hares. It causes generalized disease only in European rabbits and occasionally in European and mountain hares. It causes a cutaneous fibroma in some species of American lagomorphs: *Sylvilagus brasiliensis* (tapeti), *S. bachmani* (brush rabbit); and experimentally in *S. audubonni* (desert cottontail) and *S. nuttalli* (mountain cottontail).

EPIDEMIOLOGY

SPECIES, AGE, SEX

- Rabbits
- No age predisposition; however, kittens may be partially protected or the disease course modified by maternal antibody if born to immune does
- No sex predisposition

GENETICS AND BREED PREDISPOSITION All breeds of domestic rabbits appear to be susceptible. Wild European rabbits in Australia and Europe have undergone natural selection for resistance to myxomatosis since the release of the virus into wild populations in 1950 and 1952, respectively.

RISK FACTORS

- Exposure to biting arthropod vectors such as mosquitoes or fleas
- Close contact with wild European rabbits
- In western United States and Mexico, brush rabbits provide a natural host for Myxoma virus, and the virus can be transmitted to European rabbits by mosquitoes or other biting arthropod vectors.
- In South and central America, the tapeti (jungle rabbit) is the natural host.
- Introduction of new rabbits, including vaccinated rabbits, without adequate quarantine

CONTAGION AND ZOONOSIS

- Virus is normally spread from rabbit to rabbit on the mouthparts of blood-feeding arthropod vectors such as mosquitoes or fleas.
- Transmission is mechanical—the virus does not replicate in the vector.
- Virus is shed in oculonasal discharges from infected rabbits and may be transmitted from rabbit to rabbit by direct contact with mucosal surfaces or breaks in the skin (fighting, etc.) or by contaminated water bottles or feeders.
- Virus can readily be spread by handling infected rabbits and then susceptibles.
- There is no zoonotic potential because Myxoma virus does not replicate in humans.

GEOGRAPHY AND SEASONALITY

- Myxoma virus naturally occurs in the Americas. Two types are known: North American (Californian), which exists on the West coast of the United States and the Baja peninsula of Mexico in brush rabbits *(Sylvilagus bachmani);* and South American (Brazilian), which is found in tapeti *(S. brasiliensis).* The virus is able to spill over from cycles in its natural hosts to infect European rabbits, farmed or pets. In North America, this will occur in summer/autumn when mosquitoes are active, but in more tropical areas, mosquito activity will be less seasonal.
- Myxoma virus was introduced into wild European rabbits in France in 1952 and spread to the rest of Europe and Britain. Transmission depends on the predominant vector; in southern Europe, these are mosquitoes and fleas, whereas in Britain, the European rabbit flea is the main vector.
- Myxoma virus was introduced into wild European rabbits in Australia in 1950 as a biological control agent. The virus spills over from epidemics in the wild rabbit population to infect domestic European rabbits driven by mosquitoes or fleas. In temperate Australia, the risk is predominantly from spring to autumn, when epidemics are occurring in wild rabbit populations.
- Myxoma virus has been deliberately introduced into Chile and Argentina to control feral European rabbits and various islands.

ASSOCIATED CONDITIONS AND DISORDERS

- Secondary bacterial infections of the upper respiratory tract are common, and bacterial pneumonia may occur.
- Rabbits in North America can be infected by the closely related Shope fibroma virus, which causes a cutaneous fibroma (which is usually self-limiting) at the inoculation site but does not cause generalized disease in immunocompetent European rabbits. Its natural host is the Eastern cottontail *(Sylvilagus floridanus).*

CLINICAL PRESENTATION

DISEASE FORMS/SUBTYPES

- Peracute infection—also called *atypical myxomatosis.* Seen on the West coast of the United States in rabbits infected with Californian strains of Myxoma virus or hypervirulent field strains in Australia. There may be no clinical signs of myxomatosis, but neurologic signs such as convulsions have been described.
- Acute myxomatosis—classical form of the disease with mucocutaneous manifestations. A second "amyxomatous" form of the disease with few skin lesions is also described in Europe. Mortality rates are essentially 100%.
- Subacute infection—infection with attenuated strains of Myxoma virus produces more protracted disease course; up to 50% of rabbits may survive infection with some strains.

HISTORY, CHIEF COMPLAINT Classical myxomatosis is almost unmistakable. Rabbits present with swollen eyelids and mucopurulent conjunctivitis. The eyes may be partially or completely closed by swelling, depending on the stage of the disease. The face is typically swollen, and the ears may be swollen and drooping or just thickened, particularly at the base. Mucopurulent nasal discharge may be noted, along with acute congestion of the nasal passages, resulting in gasping or stertorous breathing. In severe cases, the head and neck are extended. Acute swelling of the anogenital region is common, and in males acute swelling of the scrotum and orchitis are common. Secondary lesions presenting as cutaneous lumps a few millimeters to several centimeters in diameter may be found on eyelids, face, nose, and ears, and also on the scrotum. Palpation of legs and body frequently reveals other secondary lesions. Depending on the timing of presentation, these lesions may be hemorrhagic, black, or scabbing.

PHYSICAL EXAM FINDINGS As above. Swollen lymph nodes can be readily palpated in prescapular and popliteal regions. Rectal temperature may be elevated to as high as 41°C (106°F), but in severe cases, rectal temperatures can be subnormal. Weight loss and dehydration are common. Variations in cutaneous lesions range from purple/blue "golf ball" swellings to flat, almost scablike lesions, depending on the strain of virus.

ETIOLOGY AND PATHOPHYSIOLOGY

- Virus is inoculated into the dermis by biting arthropods probing for a blood meal. Virus replicates locally initially in dendritic cells and then in epidermal cells, inducing the classical mucoid myxoma or primary lesion.
- From the skin, the virus moves to draining lymph nodes, where it replicates in T lymphocytes and macrophages and disseminates in lymphocytes and monocytes to distal tissues such as lungs, spleen, testes, skin, and particularly mucocutaneous sites such as eyelids. Replication at distal skin sites forms secondary lesions.
- Virus is shed in most discharges and reaches very high titers in skin lesions and lymph nodes.
- Replication in lymphoid tissues can lead to complete loss of T lymphocytes and destruction of B-cell follicles. T-lymphocyte responses are suppressed.
- Secondary bacterial infections are typical when the rabbit survives longer than a few days. In some farm environments, bacterial pneumonia is common; in other circumstances such as in laboratory rabbits, it is rarely seen.

- Low titers of serum antibody can be detected as early as 6 to 10 days after infection.
- In infection with attenuated strains, the virus is cleared by the immune response 10 to 20 days after infection. However, clinical signs, particularly due to secondary bacterial infection, may persist for many weeks or months.

DIAGNOSIS

DIFFERENTIAL DIAGNOSIS

- Bacterial upper respiratory tract infections (e.g., pasteurellosis)
- Bacterial conjunctivitis
- Bacterial pneumonia
- Keratoconjunctivitis of various causes
- Myxomatosis should be considered in cases of acute death.
- A herpesvirus infection of rabbits causing high morbidity and mortality has been reported in North America. It is associated with a swollen head, mucopurulent conjunctivitis, respiratory distress, and nodular, hemorrhagic skin lesions.

INITIAL DATABASE

- Initial diagnosis is almost exclusively based on clinical signs; differential diagnosis consists of primary bacterial infections such as pasteurellosis.
- Complete blood count: neutrophilia in acute cases for a couple of days before death, but otherwise unremarkable
- Necropsy: findings at postmortem are largely limited to external lesions, upper respiratory tract, testes, and lymphoid tissues. Lungs are typically clear in acute cases, but bronchopneumonia may be present in prolonged cases. In Europe, bacterial pneumonia is commonly described in farmed rabbits. In males, the scrotum may be acutely swollen, with up to 0.5 cm of edema on the cut surface. In hyperacute cases, pulmonary edema is common, with fluid dripping from the lungs and froth-filled trachea.

ADVANCED OR CONFIRMATORY TESTING

- Histopathologic examination of skin lesions or eyelids is distinctive and serves as the usual means of confirming the diagnosis. Epithelial proliferation with ballooning degeneration of epithelial cells is typical; neutrophilic infiltrates may occur in the deeper parts of the dermis and subdermis, but mononuclear cell infiltrates are uncommon in virulent infections. Large, stellate "myxoma cells," often appearing to bud out of small blood vessels, are a distinctive histologic feature. Lymph nodes are depleted of T cells, with destruction of B-cell follicles and proliferation of reticular cells. Spleens may show depletion of T cells with reticulum proliferation or may appear normal. Mild interstitial pneumonitis has been described in specific-pathogen–free rabbits infected with "amyxomatous" strains of Myxoma virus.
- Virus can be demonstrated by immunohistochemistry or electron microscopy.
- Specific antibody to Myxoma virus can be measured by ELISA, complement fixation, gel immunodiffusion, or virus neutralization assays. Antibody is useful for confirmatory testing on paired serum samples but is more likely to be used for epidemiologic studies. Very few laboratories will be set up to offer serologic diagnosis.
- Virus DNA detection by polymerase chain reaction on DNA extracted from conjunctival or nasal swabs, skin lesions, or tissues such as testes, lymph nodes, or lungs. This is straightforward, specific, and sensitive for rabbits with generalized disease. It may become negative in chronic cases in which the virus has been cleared.
- Virus isolation: during acute infection, Myxoma virus can be readily cultured in a variety of cell lines—both rabbit (RK13 cells, etc.) and primate (Buffalo green monkey kidney [BGMK], Vero, etc.)—from conjunctival swabs, skin lesions (needle biopsy), and tissues such as testes, lymph nodes, or lungs. Virus titers in the blood are low. Because the virus is associated with lymphocytes and monocytes, the buffy coat should be used if only blood is available for virus isolation. Depending on the inoculum titer, the virus may take 6 to 7 days to cause typical cytopathic effects in cell culture.

TREATMENT

THERAPEUTIC GOALS

- No specific treatment is available for myxomatosis. CMX001, an experimental derivative of cidofovir has activity against Myxoma virus in vitro and has been used in rabbits experimentally to treat poxvirus infections.
- The case fatality rate for virulent viruses is virtually 100%. Even attenuated strains of Myxoma virus may have case fatality rates of 50% to 90% in domestic rabbits.
- Treatment is aimed at providing nursing support (hydration/nutrition), controlling secondary bacterial infection, and minimizing distress.
- Keeping the rabbit warm is critical.
- If the decision is made to treat acute cases, consider the use of analgesics (e.g., buprenorphine 0.01-0.05 mg/kg SC q 6-12 h).

ACUTE GENERAL TREATMENT

No specific treatment is currently available. Consider broad-spectrum antibiotics to control secondary bacterial infection (e.g., fluoroquinolones, potentiated sulfonamides, tetracyclines).

RECOMMENDED MONITORING

- If the decision is made to attempt treatment, rabbits should be examined at least daily and an active decision made about euthanasia or continuing to monitor.
- Rectal temperature can provide a useful prognostic indicator. If this falls to subnormal, euthanasia should be actively considered.

PROGNOSIS AND OUTCOME

- Prognosis is extremely guarded for rabbits with acute myxomatosis. The disease course may be prolonged, but a very high proportion (50% to 100%) will die.
- Rabbits infected with strains of lower virulence that show mild clinical signs often recover with no treatment over a period of 3 to 5 weeks. Many of these rabbits will be left with a "moth-eaten" appearance around the ears and face from scars of secondary lesions. Chronic "snuffles" is not uncommon in rabbits that survive.

CONTROVERSY

- Myxomatosis was initially introduced to Australia, France, and Britain (illegally) as a biological control agent for wild European rabbits. The clinical appearance of infected rabbits has created controversy over this use. However, the disease is now firmly established in the wild rabbit populations of Europe and Australia. New Zealand has not permitted the introduction of Myxoma virus.
- Suggestions in the literature indicate that some rabbits become chronic carriers of the virus, and that recrudescent infection can be stimulated by immune suppression. Recovered rabbits treated with immune suppressant drugs apparently develop clinical signs that resemble myxomatosis, but virus cannot be isolated from nasal or conjunctival samples or from tissues other than the testes. The epidemiologic significance of this is unclear. Whether male rabbits can introduce myxomatosis into breeding units in this way has not been tested. However, semen from male rabbits with myxomatosis can transmit infection to does.

PEARLS & CONSIDERATIONS

COMMENTS

Myxomatosis appears to exist undiagnosed in rabbit farms in Europe, leading to its ready introduction into new units. This may be an issue in pet rabbits if such farms are supplying rabbits to the pet trade.

PREVENTION

- Vaccination using homologous live attenuated Myxoma virus or heterologous live attenuated virus (Shope fibroma virus):
  - In the United Kingdom, only one vaccine is available—an attenuated Shope fibroma virus (Nobivac Myxo, Intervet UK, Buckinghamshire, United Kingdom).
  - Myxomatosis vaccines are not readily available in North America.
  - The protection provided by the homologous vaccines appears to last longer (6 to 12 months) than that provided by Shope fibroma virus, which may wane after 3 months.
  - Some attenuated Myxoma virus vaccines have been associated with immune suppression in young rabbits.
  - Neither vaccine protects 100% of rabbits.
  - Vaccinated rabbits can become infected on challenge and can shed virus; this can occur within weeks of vaccination.
  - Regular booster vaccinations are necessary.
  - It is possible that maternal antibody may interfere with vaccination in the first 4 to 6 weeks of life.
  - Vaccination is not permitted in Australia.
- Prevention of flea and mosquito contact (e.g., housing indoors during summer, mosquito screens)
- Prevention of contact with wild rabbits
- Quarantine of introduced rabbits
- Isolation of clinical or suspect cases and in-contacts until diagnosis is confirmed

CLIENT EDUCATION

Emphasize prevention and vaccination where this is available.

SUGGESTED READINGS

Kerr PJ, Myxomatosis in Australia and Europe: a model for emerging infectious diseases, Antiviral Res 93:387–415, 2012.

Fenner F, et al: Biological control of vertebrate pests: the history of myxomatosis—an experiment in evolution, New York, 1999, CAB International.

Stanford MM, et al: Myxoma virus in the European rabbit: interactions between the virus and its susceptible host, Vet Res 38:299–318, 2007.

CROSS-REFERENCES TO OTHER SECTIONS

Conjunctival Disorders
Cutaneous Masses
Dermatopathies
Fluid Therapy in Rabbits and Rodents (Section II)
Lower Respiratory Tract Disorders
Pasteurellosis
Preventing Hypothermia During Anesthesia (Section II)
Testicular Tumors
Upper Respiratory Tract Disorders

AUTHOR: **PETER KERR**

EDITOR: **DAVID VELLA**

RABBITS

Obesity

BASIC INFORMATION

DEFINITION

An excessive accumulation of body fat, caused by greater caloric intake than expenditure

SYNONYMS

Overweight, fat, adiposity

EPIDEMIOLOGY

SPECIES, AGE, SEX Body weight standards vary with age, sex, and breed.

RISK FACTORS

- Inactivity
- Inadequate exercise
- Caged/sedentary rabbits
- Improper diet
- Geriatric rabbits
- Underlying chronic conditions (e.g., arthritis)
- Neutered rabbits

GEOGRAPHY AND SEASONALITY Obesity is more common in winter because of decreased activity due to limited outdoor access.

ASSOCIATED CONDITIONS AND DISORDERS

- Cardiovascular disease (see Cardiovascular Disease)
  - Atherosclerosis
  - Hemodynamic changes
  - High resting heart rate (resting tachycardia)
  - Hypertension
  - Cardiac hypertrophy
- Exercise intolerance
- Gastrointestinal disease
  - Gastrointestinal stasis
  - Fecal staining of perineum (inability to eat cecotrophs)
- Hepatic lipidosis
- Integument
  - Dermatitis (perineal urine soiling and scalding)
  - Poor hair coat due to inability to properly groom
  - Moist dermatitis (e.g., dewlap)
  - Increased susceptibility to ectoparasites (see Ectoparasites)
  - Myiasis
- Lower urinary tract disorders (see Lower Urinary Tract Disorders)
  - Sludgy urine
  - Cystitis
- Pregnancy toxemia (see Pregnancy Toxemia)
- Renal disease (see Renal Disorders)
  - Renal lipomatosis
- Musculoskeletal
  - Pododermatitis
  - Arthritis (see Arthritis)

CLINICAL PRESENTATION

HISTORY, CHIEF COMPLAINT

- Lethargy and/or inactivity
- Perineal soiling (urinary and/or fecal)
- Unkempt coat
- Skin fold dermatitis
- Gastrointestinal stasis
- Pododermatitis (see Pododermatitis)

PHYSICAL EXAM FINDINGS

- Overweight body condition
- Excessive subcutaneous body fat (e.g., axillary, inguinal, and dewlap regions)
  - Ribs difficult to palpate under thick fat
  - Excessive internal body fat; difficulty palpating internal organs as a result of excessive abdominal fat

- Excessive internal body fat: can result in difficulty palpating abdominal organs

ETIOLOGY AND PATHOPHYSIOLOGY

- Inappropriate diet
  - Obesity in rabbits is more likely due to feeding of nutrient-dense feed than to excessive intake of a nutritionally balanced diet.
- An accumulation of excess calories become transformed into fat.
- Excess fat gets deposited in various locations throughout the body.
- Obesity can lead to significant morbidity and mortality.
- Hypothyroidism is rare in rabbits.

DIAGNOSIS

DIFFERENTIAL DIAGNOSIS

- Pregnancy
- Abdominal enlargement
  - Organomegaly
  - Neoplasia
  - Effusion

INITIAL DATABASE

- Body weight and body condition assessment
- Radiography: may reveal excessive internal fat and joint abnormalities
- Blood biochemistry and hematology to assess for metabolic disease (e.g., diabetes mellitus [rare occurrence])

TREATMENT

THERAPEUTIC GOAL

Gradual weight loss and resolution of any associated conditions and disorders

ACUTE GENERAL TREATMENT

- Treat for any associated conditions and disorders (e.g., gastrointestinal stasis, hepatic lipidosis, pregnancy toxemia, arthritis).
- Clip and clean affected areas of coat (e.g., perineum, skin folds).

CHRONIC TREATMENT

- Clinicians should take an accurate diet history. It provides essential information about the rabbit's food intake and information about the food itself and the owner-pet bond.
- Measures to rectify or improve quality of diet (e.g., reduce nutrient-dense feed, increase fiber-rich feed):
  - If pelleted diet is offered, it should contain at least 18% to 20% fiber.
  - Dietary modifications should be conducted gradually.
- Promote gradual increase in rabbit's activity.

POSSIBLE COMPLICATIONS

- Hepatic lipidosis can occur rapidly if an obese rabbit is starved or becomes anorectic.
- Obese pregnant rabbits are predisposed to pregnancy toxemia. Do not fast a pregnant rabbit; allow ad libitum access to feed.

RECOMMENDED MONITORING

- Regular monitoring of weight and body condition
- Monitoring of serum liver enzymes for elevation (e.g., alanine aminotransferase [ALT], alkaline phosphatase [ALP], aspartate aminotransferase [AST], gamma glutamyltransferase [GGT], lactate dehydrogenase [LDH])
- Monitor fecal production to ensure that the rabbit is eating the new diet.

PROGNOSIS AND OUTCOME

- Dietary modification performed slowly and with close monitoring accompanied by increased activity has a good prognosis for a healthy weight loss.
- Diet and exercise changes must be long-term for the rabbit to maintain a healthy body condition.

PEARLS & CONSIDERATIONS

COMMENTS

- Obese rabbits are higher-risk anesthesia candidates.
- Obesity is seen commonly in pet rabbits because of inappropriate diet, excessive treats, and inadequate exercise.
- The mesometrium is a major fat storage site in female rabbits. Identification and ligation of broad ligament vessels during ovariohysterectomy may be challenging in obese rabbits.

PREVENTION

- Suggested food analysis for adult pet rabbits:
  - Crude fiber >18%
  - Indigestible fiber >12.5%
  - Crude protein 12%-16%
  - Fat 1%-4%
  - Calcium 0.6%-1.0%
  - Phosphorus 0.4%-0.8%
  - Vitamin A = 10,000-18,000 IU/kg
  - Vitamin D = 800-1200 IU/kg
  - Vitamin E = 40-70 mg/kg
  - Trace elements: magnesium 0.3%, zinc 0.5%, potassium 0.6%-0.7%
- Suitable exercise

CLIENT EDUCATION

- Encourage owners to feed a high-fiber diet (e.g., grass hays, green vegetables).
- Limit or avoid nutrient-dense feeds (e.g., commercial pelleted diets).
- Avoid mixed grain diets.
- Keep feed treats to a minimum.
- Make dietary changes gradually over a period of 2 to 3 weeks.
- Monitor fecal production closely to ensure that the rabbit is eating the new diet.
- Increase exercise by allowing free-range access, game playing, and sports (e.g., show jumping) and rabbit agility.

SUGGESTED READINGS

Cheeke PR: Rabbit feeding and nutrition, Orlando, 1987, Academic Press.

De Blas C, et al: The nutrition of the rabbit, Wallingford, UK, 1998, CAB International.

National Research Council, Subcommittee on Rabbit Nutrition: Nutrient requirements of rabbits, rev ed 2, Washington, DC, 1977, National Academy of Sciences.

CROSS-REFERENCES TO OTHER SECTIONS

Arthritis
Cardiovascular Disease
Dermatopathies
Ectoparasites
Hepatic Disorders
Intestinal Disorders
Lower Urinary Tract Disorders
Pregnancy Toxemia
Pododermatitis
Renal Disorders

AUTHOR: **ALANA SHRUBSOLE-COCKWILL**

EDITOR: **DAVID VELLA**

Otitis

Additional Images Available on Website

BASIC INFORMATION

DEFINITION

An acute or chronic inflammatory condition of the external, middle, or inner ear

SYNONYMS

- The terms *labyrinthitis* and *otitis labyrinthica* are synonymous with *otitis interna.*
- The terms *ear canker, ear mange, psoroptic mange, otoacariasis,* and *psoroptic scabies* are often used to describe cases of otitis externa.

EPIDEMIOLOGY

GENETICS AND BREED PREDISPOSITION Lop-eared breeds may be predisposed to otitis externa conformationally owing to ear canal stenosis.

RISK FACTORS

- Immune suppression (e.g., stress, corticosteroid use, concurrent disease)
- Exposure to rabbits (in pet stores, shelters, or multiple rabbit households) or fomites harboring *Psoroptes cuniculi* will increase the risk of developing otitis externa.
- Sharing of grooming equipment between rabbits may spread ectoparasites from one individual to another.
- Rabbits that are housed in or originate from establishments that suffer from outbreaks of respiratory disease are thought to be at higher risk of developing otitis media/interna.
- Overzealous cleaning of the ears and use of irritant topical medications may present risk.

CONTAGION AND ZOONOSIS

- Otitis may affect many rabbits within a group depending on the underlying cause. *P. cuniculi* mites, which often are associated with otitis externa, are transmitted by direct contact. *Pasteurella multocida* is frequently associated with otitis media/interna and respiratory disease. It is transmitted between rabbits by aerosol, by direct contact, via fomites, or venereally. Subclinical carriage of either organism is possible.
- Otitis is of limited zoonotic concern.

GEOGRAPHY AND SEASONALITY Worldwide

ASSOCIATED CONDITIONS AND DISORDERS

- Otitis externa: *P. cuniculi* infestation
- Otitis media/interna: pasteurellosis
- General debilitation may predispose rabbits to otitis.

CLINICAL PRESENTATION

DISEASE FORMS/SUBTYPES

- Otitis externa: usually associated with ectoparasite infestation; may cause intense pruritus with associated inflammation. Particularly severe cases may progress through the tympanic membrane to involve the middle ear, resulting in otitis media.
- Otitis media and otitis interna: frequently occur concurrently and are usually chronic problems by the time they are identified. Otitis media may extend through the tympanic membrane, resulting in a secondary otitis externa.

HISTORY, CHIEF COMPLAINT

- Otitis externa: may be subclinical, but head shaking, scratching of the ears, aural discomfort, and crusting of the medial pinnae are most common.
- Otitis media: may be subclinical, but moderate to severe cases may present with anorexia, inappetence, lethargy, aural discomfort, or pruritus associated with the base of the ear.
- Otitis interna: torticollis, falling, and/or ataxia

PHYSICAL EXAM FINDINGS

- Otitis externa: yellow-grey or brown crusting (up to 2 cm thick), erythema, and/or exudation (occasionally purulent) of the external ear canal; alopecia/excoriations of the pinnae; aural pain (sometimes with associated anorexia); occasionally dermatitis of the face/neck or generalized skin disease; stenotic or obstructed ear canals
- Otitis media: may be subclinical, or signs may include lethargy, para-aural swelling, unilateral or bilateral nasal discharge (if associated with upper respiratory tract infection), purulent material within the external ear canal (if tympanic membrane ruptured), facial asymmetry, abnormal cranial nerve reflexes, or corneal ulceration
- Otitis interna: mild to severe torticollis (head tilted toward the affected side), horizontal or rotatory nystagmus, strabismus, ataxia, falling or circling toward the affected side. Cases with bilateral disease may exhibit wide head excursions, a crouched stance, or an inability to stand.

ETIOLOGY AND PATHOPHYSIOLOGY

- Otitis externa: most frequently occurs because of infestation with the rabbit ear mite, *P. cuniculi.*
  - This nonburrowing mite feeds on loose epidermal debris, especially lipid material.
  - Antigenic material in the saliva and feces of the mite invokes an intense inflammatory reaction.
- Otitis externa may result from bacterial infection of the external ear canal (which may be secondary to *P. cuniculi* infestation), yeast infection, hypersensitivity, neoplasia, excessive cerumen production, and/or the presence of foreign material.
- Otitis media/interna
  - Most commonly due to bacterial infection (e.g., *P. multocida, Staphylococcus* spp., *Bordetella bronchiseptica, Pseudomonas aeruginosa, Listeria monocytogenes, Proteus mirabilis, Streptococcus epidermidis, Bacteroides* spp., and *Escherichia coli*)
  - Otitis media: bacteria gain access to the middle ear via the eustachian tube (from the upper respiratory tract) or less commonly via direct extension from the external ear canal
  - Otitis interna: infection usually results from an extension of otitis media
  - Hematogenous spread is also possible.

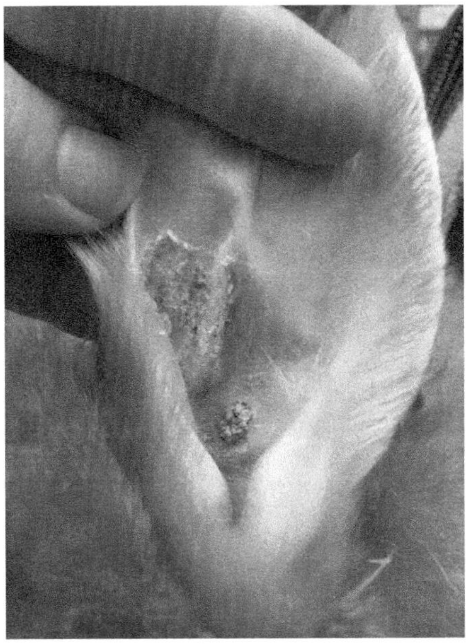

Otitis A mild case of otitis externa due to infestation with the rabbit ear mite, *Psoroptes cuniculus*. Crusting of the external ear canal and pruritus are the most common clinical signs. *(Photo courtesy Jörg Mayer, The University of Georgia, Athens.)*

- Otitis media may affect facial nerve function, but otitis interna usually involves the vestibulocochlear receptors.

DIAGNOSIS

DIFFERENTIAL DIAGNOSIS

- Otitis externa
  - Normal waxy exudate within the ear canal
- Otitis media/interna
  - Encephalitozoonosis
  - Cranial trauma
  - Cerebrovascular accident
  - Neoplasia of the central nervous system
  - Toxicosis
  - Ascarid migration
  - Cervical muscle contraction
  - Cervical scoliosis

INITIAL DATABASE

- Otitis externa
  - Otoscopic examination may reveal live ectoparasites, purulent material, and inflammation.
  - The ear canal features a tragus—a cartilaginous ridge that separates the main ear canal from a blind-ended diverticulum. Ensure that both sides of the tragus are examined, and where possible, aim to visualize the tympanic membrane.
  - Microscopy of crusts in mineral oil will readily detect ectoparasites; cytologic examination of other exudates may be similarly useful.
  - Bacterial culture (aerobic and anaerobic) of exudates
- Otitis media/interna
  - Neurologic examination: may reveal cranial nerve deficits
  - Otoscopic examination: under deep sedation or general anesthesia
  - Microscopy/culture of any exudate detected within the external auditory canal
  - Examination of the pharynx (under deep sedation or general anesthesia) to detect any purulent material or inflammation
  - Bacterial (aerobic and anaerobic) culture of deep nasal swabs if concurrent upper respiratory infection is present
  - Skull radiography may reveal increased opacity of the bullae or sclerosis, periosteal proliferation, or lysis of surrounding bone. However, in many cases, no demonstrable radiographic changes are noted.
  - Hematology may be a useful ancillary test, revealing leukopenia and an absolute or relative heterophilia if the condition is chronic. Total white blood cell count is often within normal limits.

ADVANCED OR CONFIRMATORY TESTING

- Otitis externa
  - Video-otoscopy to visualize the entire canal, including the tympanic membrane
  - Biopsy and histopathologic examination of any identified lesions
- Otitis media/interna
  - Skull CT (primarily to assess the integrity of the bullae): superior to radiography
  - Skull MRI (to detect presence of fluid in the middle ear and/or rule out differential diagnoses of central nervous system origin)
  - Positive-contrast canalography (for confirmation of tympanic membrane rupture)
  - Myringotomy (to obtain samples from the middle ear if the tympanic membrane is intact)
  - Ultrasonography (e.g., using saline in the ear canal as an acoustic window)
  - Bulla osteotomy and bacterial culture of samples collected during surgery
  - Biopsy and histopathologic examination of any abnormal tissue identified

TREATMENT

THERAPEUTIC GOALS

- Otitis externa: eradication of mite infestation and/or bacterial infection; removal of foreign material
- Otitis media/interna: eradication of infection and removal of exudates

ACUTE GENERAL TREATMENT

- Otitis externa
  - Antiparasitic or antibiotic treatment as indicated by initial database: this may be systemic and/or topical. Avoid products containing corticosteroids.
  - For bacterial infection, the use of an "ear wick" (i.e., a small piece of sponge impregnated with antibiotics implanted into the external ear canal for up to 1 week may provide an alternative to the frequent application of drops)
  - In cases of *P. cuniculi* infestation, treat with an avermectin (e.g., ivermectin 0.2-0.4 mg/kg SC or topically every 10-14 d for 2 or 3 treatments; or selamectin 6-18 mg/kg topically every 30 days), treat all in-contact rabbits, and replace bedding/disinfect/disinfect environment daily during treatment. Mites can survive in the environment for up to 21 days.
  - Do not manually remove crusts; doing so is extremely painful and will not hasten recovery.
  - Flushing the ear canal with sterile saline may be necessary to remove purulent material; sedation or anesthesia may be required.
  - Analgesia with nonsteroidal anti-inflammatory drugs (NSAIDs) and/or opioids
- Otitis media/interna
  - Systemic antibiotic therapy
  - Lavage of middle ear if tympanic membrane has ruptured
  - Analgesia with NSAIDs and/or opioids
  - Ocular lubrication if eyelid function is compromised
  - Supportive care, including assisted feeding, fluid therapy, and gut prokinetic medication when indicated

CHRONIC TREATMENT

- Prolonged course of antibiotics may be required for otitis media/interna.
- If medical therapy is unsuccessful, bulla osteotomy or total ear canal ablation may be considered for otitis media.
- Placement of antibiotic-impregnated polymethylmethacrylate beads in infected sites
- For severe protracted cases of otitis externa, lateral wall resection may be considered.

DRUG INTERACTIONS

Administration of corticosteroids is controversial and in most situations is inappropriate. Rabbits are highly sensitive to the immune suppressive and gastrointestinal effects of these drugs, and such treatment may in fact worsen the clinical outcome.

POSSIBLE COMPLICATIONS

- Failure to improve due to bacterial resistance to therapeutic agents, incomplete removal of typically caseous exudate, development of osteomyelitis, permanent destruction of neurologic tissue, poor client compliance, and/or progression of infection to involve central nervous tissue
- In cases with pronounced head tilt, aspiration secondary to abnormal body posture (especially if being syringe-fed)

RECOMMENDED MONITORING

- Repeated physical examination (including otoscopic and neurologic assessment)
- Monitoring of ability to ambulate, eat, drink, and groom unassisted
- Monitoring of eyelid function, tear production, and corneal integrity is important.

PROGNOSIS AND OUTCOME

- Otitis externa: good unless concurrent debilitating disease is present
- Otitis media/interna: dependent on the chronicity of the disease, the extent of bone involvement, and the reversibility of the neurologic damage; generally fair to poor

PEARLS & CONSIDERATIONS

COMMENTS

Rabbits use their hind limbs to clean their ears. As such, patients with hind limb dysfunction or hind limb amputees have increased susceptibility to the development of otitis externa in the ipsilateral ear. Owners of such rabbits should be encouraged to monitor and clean the rabbit's ears regularly.

PREVENTION

Prompt investigation, treatment, and isolation of rabbits with upper respiratory and/or external ear signs

CLIENT EDUCATION

- Ensure high standards of ventilation and sanitation.
- Disinfect grooming brushes and combs before reuse.
- Minimize stress.
- Long-term therapy required for otitis media/interna and residual deficits (head tilt/facial nerve paralysis) may persist following treatment, even if early improvement is noted.
- Recurrence of clinical signs following successful treatment is common.

SUGGESTED READINGS

Flatt RE, et al: Suppurative otitis media in the rabbit: prevalence, pathology and microbiology, Lab Anim Sci 27:343–347, 1977.

King AM, et al: Anatomy and ultrasonographic appearance of the tympanic bulla and associated structures in the rabbit, Vet J 173:512–521, 2007.

Kurtdede A, et al: Use of selamectin for the treatment of psoroptic and sarcoptic mite infestation in rabbits, Vet Dermatol 18:18–22, 2007.

CROSS-REFERENCES TO OTHER SECTIONS

Abscesses
Dermatopathies
Ectoparasites
Encephalitis
Encephalitozoonosis
Endoparasites
Pasteurellosis
Staphylococcosis
Upper Respiratory Tract Disorders
Vestibular Disease

AUTHOR: **MICHELLE L. CAMPBELL-WARD**

EDITOR: **DAVID VELLA**

RABBITS

Pasteurellosis

BASIC INFORMATION

DEFINITION

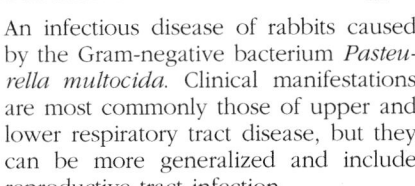

An infectious disease of rabbits caused by the Gram-negative bacterium *Pasteurella multocida.* Clinical manifestations are most commonly those of upper and lower respiratory tract disease, but they can be more generalized and include reproductive tract infection.

SYNONYM

Pasteurellosis is often referred to colloquially as "snuffles" when it affects the upper respiratory tract (see Upper Respiratory Tract Disease).

EPIDEMIOLOGY

GENETICS AND BREED PREDISPOSITION

- No known breed predisposition
- Common in meat breeds when kept commercially

RISK FACTORS

- Many rabbits are subclinical carriers. One or more stressors or anything that leads to immune suppression usually triggers development of overt clinical disease. Common examples are as follows:
  - High environmental ammonia levels
  - Overcrowding
  - Intercurrent disease
  - Transportation
  - Corticosteroid administration

CONTAGION AND ZOONOSIS

- Transmission is via aerosol, by direct contact, or via fomites.
- The main route of entry is via the nares.
- Entry of bacteria may occur through wounds.
- Venereal transmission to kits can occur if reproductive tract infection of the dam is present.
- Transmission via direct contact is more likely from rabbits with acute infection than from those with chronic infection
- Once the organism has entered the body and has colonized, infection can spread locally to contiguous tissues or hematogenously throughout the body.
- *P. multocida* can infect humans, but no reports have described direct transmission from rabbits to humans (see Pasteurellosis-Zoonosis, Sec. VI).

GEOGRAPHY AND SEASONALITY

- Worldwide incidence
- Ambient weather conditions may affect incidence, for example, very hot conditions are stressful to rabbits, and cold conditions may be associated with reduced ventilation in indoor situations.

ASSOCIATED CONDITIONS AND DISORDERS

- *P. multocida* may be present in association with other respiratory pathogens such as *Bordetella bronchiseptica,* and it is believed that their presence may enhance colonization by *P. multocida*.
- Clinical signs of pasteurellosis can be indistinguishable from those of other bacterial respiratory, otic, reproductive tract, and systemic infections.

CLINICAL PRESENTATION

DISEASE FORMS/SUBTYPES

- Rabbits challenged with *P. multocida* can:
  - Resist infection
  - Spontaneously eliminate infection
  - Become chronic carriers
  - Develop acute disease
  - Develop chronic disease

HISTORY, CHIEF COMPLAINT

- Depression
- Reduced appetite or anorexia (see Anorexia)
- Mucopurulent nasal and/or ocular discharge
- Head tilt
- Subcutaneous swellings (abscesses)

PHYSICAL EXAM FINDINGS

- Mucopurulent nasal discharge (rhinitis)

- Ocular discharge (dacryocystitis/conjunctivitis [see Conjunctival Disorders])
- Presence of discharge on medial aspect of forelimbs from grooming
- Sneezing
- Pyrexia (rare)
- Dyspnea
- Cyanosis
- Mouth breathing
- Head tilt (otitis interna/media)
- Other central neurologic signs (meningitis, brain abscessation)
- Subcutaneous swellings (abscesses)
- Abdominal masses (organ abscesses, pyometra)
- Orchitis
- Mastitis

ETIOLOGY AND PATHOPHYSIOLOGY

- Result of infection depends on strain virulence and host immune response.
- Most isolates from rabbits are capsular type A.

DIAGNOSIS

DIFFERENTIAL DIAGNOSIS

- Other bacterial respiratory tract infections
- Nasal foreign body
- Dental disease (see Dental Disease) (dacryocystitis, facial swellings)
- Vestibular disease (see Vestibular Disease)
- Other causes of head tilt or neurologic signs
- Cardiovascular disease (see Cardiovascular Disease)
- Neoplasia (e.g., lung, thymus, uterus)

INITIAL DATABASE

- Neutrophilia (acute infection only)
- Leukopenia (chronic disease): reversed neutrophil/lymphocyte ratio
- Anemia (chronic disease)
- Radiography: turbinate atrophy, bronchopneumonia, lung abscessation/consolidation

ADVANCED OR CONFIRMATORY TESTING

- Culture from deep nasal swab, abscess capsule
- Serologic testing: ELISA. High immunoglobulin (Ig) G levels correlate well with chronic infection. False negatives (acute disease, immune suppression) and false positives (cross-reaction with other related bacteria, especially in rabbits >1 year old) are possible.
- PCR on nasal swabs
- PCR in combination with serologic testing is currently the best method for diagnosis.

TREATMENT

THERAPEUTIC GOALS

- Elimination of the organism may not be possible, especially in cases of chronic disease.
- Treatment is aimed at alleviating clinical signs.

ACUTE GENERAL TREATMENT

- Antibiotic therapy, preferably based on culture and sensitivity testing
- Most strains of *P. multocida* are sensitive to fluoroquinolones (e.g., enrofloxacin 10 mg/kg PO q 12 h; marbofloxacin 7 mg/kg PO q 12 h), potentiated sulfonamides (e.g., trimethoprim/sulfamethoxazole 30 mg/kg PO q 12 h), and tetracyclines (e.g., doxycycline 4 mg/kg PO q 24 h; chloramphenicol 30 mg/kg PO q 12 h; penicillin G 42,000-84,000 IU/kg SC, IM, q 24 h). Tilmicosin, although reported to be successful in treating pasteurellosis in rabbits, has been associated with severe side effects, including anaphylaxis and death.
- Supplementary oxygen may be necessary if severe dyspnea or cyanosis is present.
- Supportive care is vital, particularly nutritional and fluid support where anorexia is present (see Fluid Therapy in Rabbits and Rodents, Sec II).

CHRONIC TREATMENT

- Prolonged courses of antibiotics are often necessary if chronic disease is present.
- Nebulization with antibiotics, mucolytics (e.g., bromhexine, acetylcysteine 50 mg as 2% solution with normal saline over 30-60 min), or hypertonic saline (7%)
- Steam therapy
- Nonsteroidal antiinflammatory drugs (e.g., carprofen 2-4 mg/kg PO, SC q 24 h; meloxicam 0.3-0.5 mg/kg PO q 24 h; ketoprofen 1-3 mg/kg PO q 12 h)
- Surgical removal of abscesses plus local antibiotic therapy if necessary
- Bulla osteotomy for chronic otitis media
- Nasolacrimal duct flushing for dacryocystitis
- Ovariohysterectomy or orchidectomy may be indicated in cases with reproductive tract involvement.
- Address any underlying husbandry issues or intercurrent disease.

RECOMMENDED MONITORING

- Improvement in clinical signs is most useful.
- Repeat radiography may be indicated in cases with lower respiratory tract involvement (see Lower Respiratory Tract Disease).

PROGNOSIS AND OUTCOME

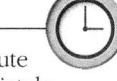

- Moderate prognosis in acute disease if treated appropriately
- More guarded prognosis in chronic disease, especially if turbinate atrophy and severe lung consolidation or abscessation is present
- Good prognosis for abscesses if completely removed
- Guarded prognosis for bulla osteotomy, although some cases may respond very well
- Severe chronic cases may require euthanasia.

PEARLS & CONSIDERATIONS

COMMENTS

- Nebulization with hyaluronidase (the capsule of *Pasteurella* contains hyaluronic acid) has been anecdotally reported to be of use.
- Take care when using corticosteroids in rabbits because their use can precipitate clinical disease in a subclinically affected animal.

PREVENTION

- No vaccine is commercially available; experimental vaccines have been shown to partially protect against severe disease but not infection.
- Prevention of stress
- Good husbandry (e.g., ventilation, low stocking density) and nutrition

CLIENT EDUCATION

Isolate any affected animals.

SUGGESTED READINGS

DiGiacomo RF, et al: Natural history of infection with *Pasteurella multocida*, J Am Vet Med Assoc 183:1172–1175, 1983.

DiGiacomo RF, et al: Transmission of *Pasteurella multocida* in rabbits, Lab Anim Sci 37:621–623, 1987.

Sanchez S, et al: Pasteurellosis in rabbits, Compend Contin Educ Pract Vet 22:344–351, 2000.

CROSS-REFERENCES TO OTHER SECTIONS

Abscesses
Anorexia
Cardiovascular Disease
Conjunctival Disorders
Cutaneous Masses
Dacryocystitis and Epiphora
Dental Disease

Encephalitis
Encephalitozoonosis
Fluid Therapy in Rabbits and Rodents (Section II)
Lower Respiratory Tract Disorders
Otitis
Pasteurellosis-Zoonosis (Section VI)
Upper Respiratory Tract Disorders
Uterine Disorders
Vestibular Disease

AUTHOR: **ANNA MEREDITH**

EDITOR: **DAVID VELLA**

RABBITS

Pododermatitis

BASIC INFORMATION

DEFINITION

Inflammation of the skin of the foot

SYNONYMS

Ulcerative pododermatitis, sore hocks, bumblefoot, avascular necrosis of the plantar aspect of the feet, pressure sores, suppurative pododermatitis

SPECIAL SPECIES CONSIDERATIONS

- Rabbits lack fleshy footpads. They rely on a normally thick covering of hair on the plantar and palmar surfaces of their feet. The underlying skin is thin, especially in the region of the metatarsus, increasing their vulnerability to developing pododermatitis.
- Thumping of hind feet displayed by some individuals may predispose to this condition.

EPIDEMIOLOGY

SPECIES, AGE, SEX Can affect rabbits of any age and gender

GENETICS AND BREED PREDISPOSITION

- Short-coated breeds (e.g., Rex) are predisposed owing to thin hair coverage on feet.
- Large breeds: giant rabbits may also be predisposed
- Hybrid meat rabbits and New Zealand white rabbits are more resistant to developing pododermatitis because of the dense hair coat on their footpads and metatarsus.

RISK FACTORS

- Moisture
- Unhygienic housing (especially damp bedding)
- Trauma
- Abrasions
- Iatrogenic (clipping of hair)
- Abrasive substrates (e.g., wire flooring, concrete, noncompliant substrates, some carpets)
- Poor conformation
- Obesity
- Emaciation
- Pregnancy
- Inactivity
- Excessive thumping
- Urinary/fecal soiling
- Lameness to any foot, leading to excessive weight bearing on other feet
- Infection (especially *Staphylococcus aureus* and *Pasteurella multocida*)

CONTAGION AND ZOONOSIS

- *S. aureus* and *P. multocida* may cause or complicate pododermatitis, especially in moist conditions.
- Specific high-virulence *S. aureus* strains do not seem to need these predisposing factors to cause disease.
- High-virulence *S. aureus* strains belonging to a specific bacterial clone have been isolated from meat rabbits within Europe and Australia.

GEOGRAPHY AND SEASONALITY Occurs worldwide with no seasonality

ASSOCIATED CONDITIONS AND DISORDERS

- Obesity, emaciation, pregnancy, and conditions that lead to inactivity, altered conformation, or soiling of the feet
- General immune suppression
- Limb deformities (congenital and acquired) and splayleg may predispose to development of pododermatitis.
- Any cause of paralysis, paresis, or altered gait

CLINICAL PRESENTATION

DISEASE FORMS/SUBTYPES Early forms may present with mild alopecia, erythema, and inflammation. Advanced cases can progress to severe ulceration and bone exposure. In advanced hindfoot cases, displacement of the superficial flexor tendon may occur.

HISTORY, CHIEF COMPLAINT Alopecia and inflammation (may be seen as redness in white or albino rabbits) of plantar and/or palmar aspects of the feet; lameness and swelling

PHYSICAL EXAM FINDINGS Alopecia, erythema, ulceration, pain, swelling, suppuration on plantar or palmar aspect of any foot, lameness

ETIOLOGY AND PATHOPHYSIOLOGY

- Rabbits lack footpads. The skin on their feet is very thin and adherent to underlying connective tissue.
- Hopping involves a digitigrade gait; while at rest, the hind feet are plantargrade, and weight is shared between the hind claws and the metatarsus.
- Noncompliant substrates (hard flooring) and wire floors prevent the hind feet from adopting normal plantargrade stance, causing most of the weight to be sustained by the metatarsus and hock, not by the claws.
- Some abrasive surfaces (e.g., carpet) may produce friction on the skin, thus exacerbating the problem.
- Ensuing abnormal weight bearing and loss of protective hair covering lead to development of pressure sores.
- Ischemia and necrosis of compressed soft tissue can develop and may lead to ulcerative and erosive lesions.
- Parts of the metatarsus most vulnerable include point of hock (calcaneus) and plantar prominence of central tarsal bone. The tip of each toe of any foot and the palmar carpal area can also be affected.
- Occasionally, ulcerative lesions can disrupt the integrity of the medial plantar vein or artery; this can result in significant hemorrhage and anemia.
- Advanced hindfoot cases can cause displacement of the superficial flexor tendon. This can cause permanent alteration of hindfoot conformation whereby toes are not able to flex appropriately, leading to extra weight bearing upon the point of the hock.
- Ulcerative pododermatitis is a vicious cycle whereby pain and disability reduce mobility, thus further exacerbating the condition.
- Moist and unhygienic conditions aggravate the condition, as can any condition that results in urinary and fecal soiling of the feet.

- Secondary infections that occur, primarily by *Staphylococcus aureus* and *Pasteurella multocida*, can lead to osteomyelitis and synovitis, predisposing to displacement of the superficial flexor tendon. Suppurative and exudative processes can lead to local hair matting and further contamination and abnormal pressure placement.
- Conditions that lead to lack of mobility (e.g., cramped housing, arthritis, spondylosis) can predispose to development of pododermatitis.
- Overweight, pregnant, and emaciated rabbits are more prone to developing the condition, as are large breed (>5 kg body weight) and Rex breed rabbits.
- Iatrogenic causes ensue if inadvertent removal of plantar or palmar hair occurs, or when hair is removed in preparation for surgery.
- Chronic infection may lead to anemia.
- Pain may result in aggression and gut stasis.

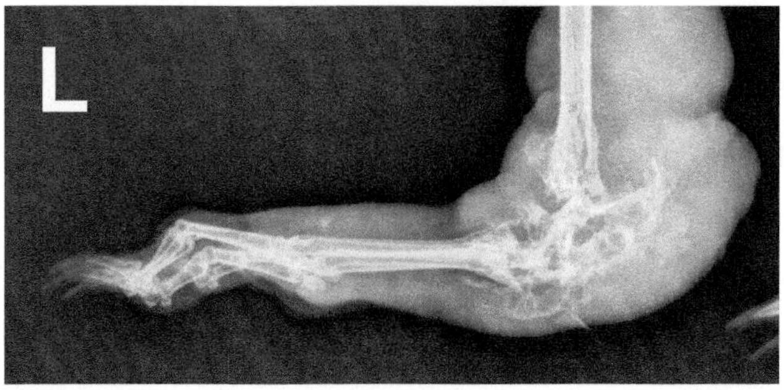

Pododermatitis Radiograph depicting severe septic arthritis secondary to pododermatitis in the left hock of a rabbit. *(Photo courtesy Jörg Mayer, The University of Georgia, Athens.)*

DIAGNOSIS

DIFFERENTIAL DIAGNOSIS

- Limb fracture
- Other causes of lameness (e.g., arthritis, trauma)
- Spondylosis
- Underlying chronic disease

INITIAL DATABASE

- Thorough palpation of limbs and digits
- Assessment of normal stance and gait on compliant surface (e.g., towel)
- Neurologic assessment of limbs
- Radiographic imaging of affected limb(s) to assess for underlying osteomyelitis in affected areas
- Radiographic imaging of full limb and spine to assess for arthritis and spinal disorders (e.g., spondylosis)
- Blood biochemistry and hematology to assess for underlying disease and anemic states

TREATMENT

THERAPEUTIC GOALS

- Alleviation of pain and infection
- Removal of inciting cause(s)
- Assessment for underlying disease
- Provision of compliant substrates
- Can be very difficult to treat and manage

ACUTE GENERAL TREATMENT

- Supportive care is vital, particularly nutritional and fluid support when anorexia is present
- Analgesia
  - Nonsteroidal antiinflammatory drugs (NSAIDs; e.g., carprofen 2-4 mg/kg PO, SC q 24 h; meloxicam 0.3-0.5 mg/kg PO, SC q 24 h; ketoprofen 1-3 mg/kg PO q 12 h)
  - Opioids (e.g., buprenorphine 0.03 mg/kg SC, IM q 8 h)
- Suitable first-line antibiotics may include procaine penicillin 40,000-60,000 IU/kg SC, IM q 24 h or enrofloxacin 10 mg/kg PO, SC q 12 h with metronidazole 20 mg/kg PO q 12 h.

CHRONIC TREATMENT

1. Address underlying cause(s):
   - Substrates: ensure that compliant substrates such as thick bedding of straw or hay are provided. Absorbent veterinary bedding or similar material can be used in areas where the rabbit spends most of its time. Eliminate course substrates such as wire flooring and concrete.
   - Body condition: address weight reduction in overweight individuals. Identify cause of poor body condition in underweight individuals.
   - Identify possible underlying disease: perform other diagnostics such as blood biochemistry and hematology and radiographic imaging of joints and spine.
2. Relieve pressure and minimize trauma to affected areas:
   - Mainly achieved by addressing substrate issues
   - Protective dressings may be employed but carry risk of secondary problems (e.g., overly tight, soiling, movement and intolerance).
   - Dressings can include a primary wound contact layer that is absorptive, as well as cushioning and protective material (e.g., Allevyn, Smith & Nephew, Andover, MA). Secondary dressings may include light gauze, and tertiary dressings such as Vetrap (3M, St Paul, MN) should be light. Close supervision of dressings is required.
   - Protective "boots" can also be employed. These may be developed by some creative caretakers.
3. Treat secondary infection (if present):
   - Given the potential seriousness of spread of infection in these areas, suitable first-line antibiotics should include systemic agents with both aerobic and anaerobic spectrum. Suitable first-line antibiotics were outlined previously.
   - Topical antimicrobial therapy can be employed but may be readily licked away by the rabbit, hence the choice of nontoxic compounds. Consider topical treatments with preparations containing fusidic acid, silver sulfadiazine/chlorhexidine, mupirocin calcium, or Manuka honey.
4. Offer analgesia:
   - Pododermatitis is potentially a very painful condition. Both short- and long-term analgesic strategies may need to be employed. NSAID therapy may be carried out as outlined earlier. For patients in which NSAID use may be contraindicated, consider the use of tramadol hydrochloride 5 mg/kg PO q 8-24 h.
5. Manage the lesions:
   - Apart from dressing the lesions, other measures can be taken in wound care. It is important to emphasize that minimal physical intervention should be provided. Further damage can readily occur following débridement. Trim hair only if it is affecting the lesions. Avoid clipping down to the level of the skin, remembering that hair provides a cushion for the foot. If débridement is necessary, carefully remove nonvital tissue and pus if present. This may require sedation or general anesthesia. In general, these wounds require open wound management and healing to occur by second intention.
6. Surgical intervention:
   - Débridement should be carried out only in a measured manner. Further damage can readily occur following débridement, as was outlined previously. In severely infected cases, implantation of

antibiotic-impregnated polymethylmethacrylate (AIPPMA) beads may be considered. Antibiotic type should be based on culture and sensitivity. The beads slowly release antibiotic into the surrounding tissue for several months. Choice of antibiotics should be based on culture and sensitivity, but options typically include cephalosporins (e.g., cefazolin, ceftiofur) and aminoglycosides (e.g., gentamicin, tobramycin, amikacin). Beads may be left within the wound or may be removed after several months.
- In severe cases (e.g., nonresponsive osteomyelitis, severe septic arthritis, displacement of the superficial digital flexor tendon), amputation of the affected limb may be considered. Conduct a midfemoral procedure for the hind limb or a midhumeral procedure for the forelimb. Although apparently radical in the first instance, this potentially leads to much relief in chronically affected individuals. Most rabbits appear to adapt well to a three-legged state, although the risk of pododermatitis developing in the remaining limbs is increased. It is imperative that steps are taken thereafter to minimize the development of pododermatitis in any other limb.

DRUG INTERACTIONS

Chronic or inappropriate antibiotic use may lead to dysbiosis.

POSSIBLE COMPLICATIONS

- Worsening of lesions due to failure to address underlying cause(s)
- Negative effects of inappropriate bandaging
- Antibiotic dysbiosis
- Urinary and fecal soiling due to reduced mobility
- Myiasis

RECOMMENDED MONITORING

- Patient comfort
- Lesion size and spread
- Serial radiography of osteomyelitic lesions

PROGNOSIS AND OUTCOME

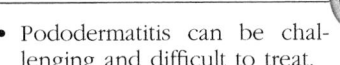

- Pododermatitis can be challenging and difficult to treat.
- Successful management is not always accomplished.
- In some animals with severe, chronic pododermatitis, euthanasia may be warranted. This is especially so if more than one limb is affected, or if other underlying complications are present.

PEARLS & CONSIDERATIONS

COMMENTS

- Avoid using corticosteroids in rabbits because their use can precipitate clinical disease in a subclinically affected animal.
- Rabbits use their hind limbs to clean their ears. As such, patients with hind limb dysfunction and hind limb amputees have increased susceptibility to the development of otitis externa in the ipsilateral ear. Owners of such rabbits should be encouraged to monitor and clean the rabbit's ears regularly.

PREVENTION

- Prevention of pododermatitis is enhanced by proper husbandry, diet, and client education.
- Avoid obesity.
- Encourage exercise and avoid cramped enclosures.

CLIENT EDUCATION

- Clients should be informed of potential risks of development of pododermatitis in each case.
- Measures to minimize the development of pododermatitis such as suitable substrate provision and good diet are essential.
- Owners of breeds considered more vulnerable (e.g., Rex, giant breeds) should have special emphasis placed on preventive measures and signs to monitor.

SUGGESTED READINGS

Harcourt-Brown F: Skin diseases. In Textbook of rabbit medicine, Oxford, 2002, Butterworth-Heinemann, pp 224–248.
Hermans K, et al: Rabbit staphylococcosis: difficult solutions for serious problems, Vet Microbiol 91:57–64, 2003.

CROSS-REFERENCES TO OTHER SECTIONS

Abscesses
Dermatopathies
Obesity
Pasteurellosis
Splayleg
Staphylococcosis
Vestibular Disease

AUTHOR: **DAVID VELLA**

EDITOR: **THOMAS M. DONNELLY**

RABBITS

Pregnancy Toxemia

BASIC INFORMATION

DEFINITION

Pregnancy toxemia is a metabolic disease primarily of pregnant does during late pregnancy (less frequently in postpartum, pseudopregnant, and nonpregnant does), characterized by low morbidity and high mortality. It occurs as the result of increased energy demand accompanied by insufficient nutrition.

SYNONYM

Ketosis

EPIDEMIOLOGY

SPECIES, AGE, SEX

- Rabbit
  - Most commonly in does in the last week of pregnancy
    - Primiparous vs. multiparous
  - Can also occur in postparturient, pseudopregnant, and nonpregnant does

GENETICS AND BREED PREDISPOSITION English, Polish, and Dutch breeds have a higher incidence.

RISK FACTORS

- Obesity
- Improper nutrition
  - Diet often too low in fiber
- Sudden stress
- Fasting during pregnancy
- Hereditary condition

ASSOCIATED CONDITIONS AND DISORDERS

- Anorexia and gastrointestinal (GI) stasis can accompany pregnancy toxemia.
- One report of a New Zealand white rabbit with pregnancy toxemia and concurrent pancreatitis

CLINICAL PRESENTATION

DISEASE FORMS/SUBTYPES Pregnancy toxemia can present as acute death or as progression of clinical signs over a period of 1 to 5 days.

HISTORY, CHIEF COMPLAINT

- Rabbits may be weak, depressed, and/or anorectic and usually are overweight.
- Owners may report that the rabbit is near the end of gestation, just recently has given birth, or may have just aborted.

PHYSICAL EXAM FINDINGS

- Dyspnea
- Ketonuria
- Acetone smell to the breathe
- Anorexia
- Incoordination
- Convulsions
- Coma

ETIOLOGY AND PATHOPHYSIOLOGY

- High-fat diets and obesity increase risk of hepatic lipidosis.
- Rabbits with fatty livers are more likely to develop pregnancy toxemia.
- Higher energy demands occur in late pregnancy and early lactation.
- Fat deposits become rapidly mobilized, resulting in hepatic lipidosis and ketosis.

DIAGNOSIS

DIFFERENTIAL DIAGNOSIS

- Ketosis
- Hepatic lipidosis
- Heatstroke

INITIAL DATABASE

- Complete blood count
  - Unremarkable
- Biochemistry panel
  - Hyperkalemia
  - Ketonemia
  - Hyperphosphatemia
  - Hypocalcemia
- Urinalysis
  - Acidic (pH 5 to 6)
  - Proteinuria
  - Ketonuria
- Clinicopathologic findings should not replace a high index of clinical suspicion because a low urine pH may be the only finding present in the initial database.

ADVANCED OR CONFIRMATORY TESTING

- On gross postmortem, rabbits often have abundant fat stores.
- On histologic examination, fatty infiltration of hepatocytes (hepatic lipidosis) and adrenal glands may be noted.

TREATMENT

THERAPEUTIC GOALS

- Treatment involves getting the rabbit stabilized and providing supportive care.
- Maintain a positive energy balance and good nutritional support.

ACUTE GENERAL TREATMENT

- Keep the animal warm.
- Fluid therapy containing 5% dextrose/glucose (intravenous or intraosseous)
- Calcium supplementation (parenteral or oral)
  - If hypocalcemic
- Nutritional support (syringe feeding, nasogastric or gastrostomy tube). Provide assisted feeding through use of commercial formulas (e.g., Oxbow Critical Care or Lafeber Emeraid).
- Provide prokinetic drugs (e.g., cisapride 0.5 mg/kg PO q 8 h or metoclopramide 0.2-1.0 mg/kg PO, SC q 6-8 h) and anti-ulcer drugs (e.g., ranitidine 2-5 mg/kg PO, SC q 12 h) if GI stasis is present.
- Cesarean section may be considered in stable patients.

RECOMMENDED MONITORING

- Monitor ketonuria.
- Monitor neurologic status.
- Monitor GI motility, food intake, and hydration status.

PROGNOSIS AND OUTCOME

- Most rabbits do not respond to treatment.
- Very poor prognosis
  - Prognosis improves if the rabbit has a spontaneous abortion.

PEARLS & CONSIDERATIONS

COMMENTS

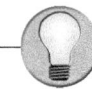

- Prevention plays a very important role because treatment often is not rewarding.
- Pregnancy toxemia is a multifactorial condition involving: anorexia, body condition, GI stasis, hepatic lipidosis, dietary status, and energy requirements.

PREVENTION

- Avoid obesity.
  - Rabbits should have a healthy body condition (3/5).
  - Provide late-term pregnant does with appropriate diets (with adequate fiber).
- Allow exercise during pregnancy.
- Avoid anorexia/starvation.
- Avoid stress.

CLIENT EDUCATION

- Pregnant does should be kept in good body condition and fed a high-fiber diet.
- Every effort should be made to reduce stress.
- A good-quality diet should be offered at all times.

SUGGESTED READINGS

Greene HSN: Toxemia of pregnancy in the rabbit: clinical manifestations and pathology, J Exp Med 65:809–832, 1937.

Harcourt-Brown F: Obesity, pregnancy toxaemia and hepatic lipidosis. In Harcourt-Brown F, editor: Textbook of rabbit medicine, London, 2002, Butterworth Heinemann.

Leland SE, et al: Pancreatitis and pregnancy toxemia in a New Zealand white rabbit, Contemp Top Lab Anim Sci 34:84–85, 1995.

CROSS-REFERENCES TO OTHER SECTIONS

Anorexia
Gastric Disorders
Hepatic Disorders
Obesity

AUTHOR: **ALANA SHRUBSOLE-COCKWILL**

EDITOR: **DAVID VELLA**

RABBITS

Pseudopregnancy

BASIC INFORMATION

DEFINITION

Pseudopregnancy is the development of signs of pregnancy without the presence of an implanted embryo or fetus. Characteristics and behaviors can vary, ranging from a mild change in behavior to nest building—the hallmark maternal sign of impending parturition. Duration of pseudopregnancy is estimated at between 15 and 18 days post ovulation and is related to the hormonal influence of persistent corpora lutea. Hallmark signs are seen at the end of a pseudopregnancy.

SYNONYMS

Pseudocyesis, false pregnancy, phantom pregnancy

EPIDEMIOLOGY

SPECIES, AGE, SEX

- Rabbits are induced ovulators and require the stimulation of coitus to ovulate.
- Ovulation in the absence of coitus and subsequent pseudopregnancy can result from:
  - Stimulation caused when one doe mounts another
  - A doe mounts the young in her own litter
  - Stressful situations (e.g., transportation in carrier to veterinarian, overnight hospitalization). A companion rabbit minimizes stress.

GENETICS AND BREED PREDISPOSITION

- Pseudopregnancy is rare in wild rabbits.
- Pseudopregnancy can occur in 20% of does group-housed compared with single-housed does.

RISK FACTORS

- Any intact female doe is at risk, even singly kept animals.
- Unfertilized ovulation resulting in pseudopregnancy can occur in 20% to 30% of artificially inseminated does injected with gonadotropin-releasing hormone (GnRH).

GEOGRAPHY AND SEASONALITY

Pseudopregnancy occurs during the breeding season. The wild European rabbit *(Oryctolagus cuniculus)* has a sharply defined main breeding season. In the northern hemisphere, the highest conception rate occurs in spring and the lowest in autumn, although sporadic breeding occurs during other months of the year. The breeding season of domestic European rabbits is less sharply defined, although mating occurs more often in spring and summer than in autumn and winter.

ASSOCIATED CONDITIONS AND DISORDERS

- Pseudopregnancy may lead to other uterine disorders (see Uterine Disorders) such as hydrometra.
- Pseudopregnancy may result in mammary gland development and milk production. Lactating rabbits may develop mastitis.
- Depending on the extent of behavioral changes during pseudopregnancy, rabbit-to-rabbit aggression can occur, resulting in bite wounds and abscesses.
- Mild alopecia or increased fur loss may result from maternal fur pulling and progesterone influences. Normally, the fur is tightly adhered to the skin, but during pregnancy and pseudopregnancy, it becomes loose.

CLINICAL PRESENTATION

HISTORY, CHIEF COMPLAINT

- Clients may describe:
  - History of recent introduction of male rabbit to group of rabbits
  - Observation of mounting on pseudopregnant rabbit by other females
- Pseudopregnant rabbits can present with:
  - Reproductive problems:
    - Breeding animals can present with failure to mate.
    - Rejection of buck during introduced mating sessions
    - Enlarged and well-developed mammary glands with milk production
  - Behavioral problems (see Dermatopathies):
    - Unexplained aggression or behavioral changes (e.g., biting, barbering, thumping of hindfeet) toward owners or toward other animals within the rabbit's social group
    - Territorial aggression
    - Fur pulling, which the owner may perceive as self-mutilation
    - Building of nests with fur and/or other material found in the environment
    - Excessive digging
  - Dermatologic problems (see Dermatopathies):
    - Some rabbits may present for patchy alopecia predominantly in the area of the dewlap and ventrum.
  - Gastrointestinal problems:
    - Pseudopregnant does can present with ileus.

PHYSICAL EXAM FINDINGS

- A nervous and aggressive rabbit during consultation
- Vital signs are often within normal limits
- Mammary development that may be accompanied by lactation
- Alopecia, usually around the area of the dewlap and ventrum
- Absence of palpable fetuses during abdominal palpation
  - Marble-shaped fetuses are distinguished between 12-14 days of pregnancy as they slip between thumb and fingers when gently moved back and forth with slight pressure. After 14-16 days of pregnancy distinguishing between fetuses and digestive organs is difficult.
  - Radiographic confirmation of fetuses is possible after 11-12 days of pregnancy.

ETIOLOGY AND PATHOPHYSIOLOGY

- The female rabbit is an induced ovulator:
  - An estrous cycle does not occur, although estrus behavior is observed.
  - Ovulation occurs after mating. Coitus provokes a reflex discharge of GnRH and hence LH from the pituitary, inducing ovulation.
  - Behavioral estrus in rabbits is characterized by lordosis and allowing other rabbits to mount.
- Ovulation can also be induced by:
  - Rabbit-to-rabbit interaction (even in the absence of a buck)
    - Mounting by other sexually active does or sterile bucks
    - Close proximity or scent of male rabbits
  - Transportation of female rabbits
    - This is a common cause of spontaneous ovulation.
- Normal gestation is 28-31 days. Hormones (primarily progesterone) secreted by the corpus luteum maintain pregnancy. After ovulation, even in the absence of fertilization and implantation, the uterus and mammary glands can still develop under the influence of the corpus luteum, which provides the hormonal influence for pseudopregnancy.
- In a nonpregnant rabbit, the corpus luteum regresses after 10 to 12 days.
- Pseudopregnancy lasts 15 to 18 days.

- After luteolysis, progesterone levels drop rapidly and maternal behaviors become apparent.
- Nest building and other maternal behaviors of the doe are controlled by a combination of hormones, including estrogen, progesterone, and prolactin.

DIAGNOSIS

DIFFERENTIAL DIAGNOSIS

- Late gestation
- Ovarian remnant after ovariectomy/ovariohysterectomy
- Adrenal tumors producing excessive sex hormones

INITIAL DATABASE

Signalment, history, and physical examination

ADVANCED OR CONFIRMATORY TESTING

- Abdominal radiography and ultrasound to rule out presence of fetuses
- Progesterone levels or hormonal panels can be measured:
  - Hormone measurements must be validated at the testing laboratory.
  - Hormone levels must be interpreted in relation to the behavior of the doe.
  - Pregnant and pseudopregnant rabbits cannot be differentiated accurately until day 19 of pregnancy/pseudopregnancy.

TREATMENT

THERAPEUTIC GOAL

Elimination of future occurrences of pseudopregnancy

ACUTE GENERAL TREATMENT

- Treatment is unnecessary in most cases because pseudopregnancy is self-limiting.
- One injection of prostaglandin $PGF_{2\alpha}$ (e.g., 200 µg alfaprostol SC) on the 10th or 11th day has been used in research laboratories and breeding farms to terminate pseudopregnancy. The doe can then be fertilized 14 days after an earlier infertile insemination. Without prostaglandin treatment, the doe cannot be fertilized again until 21 days after an infertile insemination. Use of prostaglandin $PGF_{2\alpha}$ is not recommended in pet rabbits. However, its use can be considered when extreme nesting behavior is refractory to treatment.

CHRONIC TREATMENT

The treatment of choice is neutering.

RECOMMENDED MONITORING

Because of the increasing incidence of uterine disorders with age, intact female rabbits should be assessed frequently.

PROGNOSIS AND OUTCOME

Prognosis is good because the condition is self-limiting.

PEARLS & CONSIDERATIONS

COMMENTS

- The core event in maternal behavior is construction of the maternal nest. Initially, the doe builds a nest of straw, hay, or other such material (described as the "straw nest"). At the end of pregnancy or pseudopregnancy, the female plucks fur from her body (chiefly from her dewlap and ventrum) and uses this to line the nest. This is called the *maternal nest*. This nest is built only under the condition of pregnancy or pseudopregnancy, or with appropriate experimental manipulations involving the hormones of pregnancy. Pregnant does generally keep a maternal nest free of feces and urine, whereas pseudopregnant does will fail to keep a maternal nest clean.
- Use of synthetic progesterone or androgens to terminate a pseudopregnancy is currently unproven and is restricted to research laboratory conditions.

PREVENTION

Pseudopregnancy is prevented by neutering.

CLIENT EDUCATION

- Pseudopregnancy often recurs and can be prevented by neutering.
- Potential uterine disorders can be prevented by neutering.

SUGGESTED READING

Gonzalez-Mariscal G, et al: Maternal care of rabbits in the lab and on the farm: endocrine regulation of behavior and productivity, Horm Behav 52:86–91, 2007.

CROSS-REFERENCES TO OTHER SECTIONS

Behavioral Disorders
Dermatopathies
Mammary Gland Disorders
Uterine Disorders

AUTHOR: **CATHY T.T. CHAN**

EDITOR: **DAVID VELLA**

RABBITS

Renal Disorders

BASIC INFORMATION

DEFINITION

- Infectious and noninfectious diseases of the kidney(s)
- Many different terms are used to describe renal function and its deterioration:
  - *Azotemia* refers to increased concentrations of urea nitrogen and creatinine and other nonproteinaceous nitrogenous waste products in the blood. *Renal azotemia* denotes azotemia caused by renal parenchymal changes.
  - *Uremia* is the presence of all urine constituents in the blood. Usually a toxic condition, it may occur secondary to renal failure or postrenal disorders, including urethral blockage.
  - *Renal reserve* may be thought of as the percentage of "extra" nephrons—those not necessary to maintain normal renal function. Although it probably varies from animal to animal, it is greater than 50% in most mammals.
  - *Renal insufficiency* begins when the renal reserve is lost. Animals with renal insufficiency outwardly appear normal but have a reduced capacity to compensate for stresses such as infection or dehydration and have lost urine-concentrating ability.
  - *Renal failure* is a state of decreased renal function that allows persistent abnormalities (azotemia and inability to concentrate urine) to exist; it refers to a level of organ function rather than to a specific disease entity. *Acute renal failure* generally refers to cases of sudden decline of glomerular filtration rate resulting in an accumulation of nitrogenous waste products and inability to

maintain normal fluid balance. *Chronic renal failure* generally refers to an insidious onset with slow progression (usually months to years) of azotemia and inadequately concentrated urine.
- It is important to realize that most of the renal diseases discussed can manifest as varying stages of compromise in renal reserve, renal insufficiency, or renal failure. If or when the disease process progresses depends on variables such as the specific disease in question, environmental factors, and the individual animal itself.

SYNONYMS

Renal disease, renal failure, kidney disease, kidney failure, nephropathy, renal insufficiency

SPECIAL SPECIES CONSIDERATIONS

- Kidney pathology is not uncommon in the rabbit; one review showed histologic lesions in 32.5% of 237 rabbits found dead or euthanized because of illness, and in 25% of 77 apparently healthy adult rabbits.
- Renal fibrosis with or without dystrophic calcification was the most common lesion observed in rabbits older than 10 months.
- Lesions associated with an infectious process such as renal abscesses, bacterial pyelitis, pyelonephritis, and nephritis were the primary finding in rabbits up to 5 months of age.
- Two cases of spontaneous amyloidosis—one associated with pyometritis and the other with renal calculi—were reported.
- Other causes of rabbit renal pathology include hypervitaminosis D, *Encephalitozoon cuniculi*, hydronephrosis, renal agenesis, renal cysts, and neoplasia.

EPIDEMIOLOGY

SPECIES, AGE, SEX Generally, kidney disease is associated with aging and loss of renal reserve over time.

RISK FACTORS
- Infection: *E. cuniculi*, pyelonephritis
- Acute obstructive disease secondary to urolithiasis
- Advanced age
- Nephrotoxins

CONTAGION AND ZOONOSIS *E. cuniculi*, one cause of rabbit renal disease, has shown zoonotic potential, especially in immune compromised humans such as transplant recipients and those infected with human immunodeficiency virus (HIV), as well as in children, and the elderly.

CLINICAL PRESENTATION

DISEASE FORMS/SUBTYPES
- *E. cuniculi*: kidney lesions do not always impair renal function, and latent infection can occur. Interstitial fibrosis is seen in later stages of the disease
- Pyelonephritis/suppurative nephritis: pyelonephritis in the rabbit may occur as the result of an ascending urinary tract infection or hematogenously during bacterial septicemia
- Obstructive disease: rabbits can have a combination of cystic, urethral, ureteral, and renal calculi. Neoplasia or adhesions related to surgery have been incriminated in obstructive disease.
- Hypervitaminosis D: rabbits are very sensitive to vitamin D toxicosis
- Nephrotoxicosis: aminoglycosides, dietary mycotoxins, tiletamine, inappropriate use of nonsteroidal antiinflammatory drugs (NSAIDs)
- Neoplasia
  - Lymphosarcoma is a common neoplastic condition in rabbits; higher incidence is noted in juvenile and young adult domestic rabbits younger than 8 months.
  - Embryonal nephromas are commonly found in domestic rabbits and usually are an incidental finding at necropsy.

HISTORY, CHIEF COMPLAINT
- Clinical signs and history vary with the severity of kidney pathology. Polydipsia and polyuria may be associated with loss of renal reserve in a rabbit that otherwise is doing well clinically. As progression to renal insufficiency or chronic renal failure progresses, rabbits will start to demonstrate a decreased appetite or total anorexia, weight loss, and lethargy.
- Perineal soiling resulting from polyuria or decreased grooming associated with lethargy and depression is not uncommon.
- Pollakiuria or hematuria may be present with urinary tract infection and subsequent ascending infection, resulting in suppurative nephritis or pyelonephritis.

PHYSICAL EXAM FINDINGS
- Depending on the progression of renal failure and uremia, the patient will present in varying states of lethargy, depression, decreased appetite or total anorexia, increased or decreased water intake, dehydration, and general malaise.
- Assess hydration status because azotemia may be caused by or worsened by dehydration.
- Secondary gastrointestinal (GI) stasis is not an uncommon finding because of lack of fiber ingestion, stress, or uremia-associated gastritis.
- Rabbits showing abdominal discomfort may grind their teeth or present in a tucked, hunched position.
- Rabbits with concurrent *Encephalitozoon* infection may show neurologic signs such as hind limb weakness or head tilt.
- Clinical signs of urolithiasis may include lethargy, decreased appetite, weight loss, anuria, stranguria, hematuria, and a hunched posture and bruxism, indicating abdominal pain. Perineal soiling and subsequent scald may occur because of pollakiuria and incontinence. A turgid bladder is evident if urethral obstruction is present, and nephromegaly may be palpable when hydronephrosis occurs secondary to ureteral obstruction.
- Clinical signs of pyelonephritis include pyrexia, lethargy, anorexia, and pain on palpation of the kidneys. Hematuria or pyuria may be present. Chronic, untreated pyelonephritis can result in renal failure manifested clinically as profound anorexia and lethargy with subsequent weight loss and declining condition.
- Clinical signs in rabbits suffering from vitamin D–related soft tissue mineralization are nonspecific and include anorexia, weight loss, dehydration, and infertility. Early clinical diagnosis is difficult because clinical signs are nebulous.
- Rabbits with renal lymphosarcoma may demonstrate organomegaly or nodular masses, which may be palpable on abdominal examination.

ETIOLOGY AND PATHOPHYSIOLOGY

- Chronic renal failure develops with aging and may be exacerbated by various renal insults, toxins, and bacterial infections.
- In spite of what is known about rabbit calcium metabolism, the causes of calculi formation are not understood and may relate to a combination of factors, including diet, genetics, anatomy, environment, and infection.
- Calculus-related urethral obstruction can result in acute post-renal failure. Ureteral stone obstruction can lead to hydroureter and hydronephrosis with loss of kidney function. Renal calculi cause varying degrees of pelvic obstruction. Many cases of renal calculi are bilateral or are present in conjunction with cystic calculi. Nephrolithiasis may be subclinical and found incidentally on abdominal radiographs. Over time, clinical signs of abdominal discomfort, hematuria, proteinuria, and isosthenuria may be seen. Eventually chronic renal failure may ensue.
- Pyelonephritis in the rabbit may occur as the result of an ascending urinary tract infection or hematogenously during bacterial septicemia.
- In rabbits with hypervitaminosis D, pathologic changes consist of mineral

deposition in a variety of tissues; kidneys and arteries (especially the aorta) are most sensitive.
- Initial target organs of *E. cuniculi* include those with high blood flow such as the kidney. Spores eventually develop, and over time, the pseudocyst becomes overcrowded and ruptures. Spores are spread to the urine via infected renal epithelial cells. Cell rupture is associated with a chronic inflammatory response and development of granulomatous lesions, primarily in the kidney.
- Systemic hypertension may be associated with chronic renal failure. Reduced perfusion of the kidneys results in hypertension via stimulation of the renin-angiotensin mechanism.

DIAGNOSIS

DIFFERENTIAL DIAGNOSIS

- *Encephalitozoon cuniculi*
- Pyelonephritis/suppurative nephritis
- Hypervitaminosis D
- Obstructive nephropathy
- Toxic nephropathy
- Neoplasia
- Renal agenesis

INITIAL DATABASE

- Clinical pathology
  - Glomerular function is evaluated by determination of blood urea nitrogen (BUN) and serum creatinine concentrations, both of which are freely filtered through the glomerular basement membrane.
  - Filtered urea, an end-product of protein catabolism, is reabsorbed through the renal tubules, and creatinine, an end-product of muscle metabolism, is released in the circulation at a constant rate and does not undergo tubular resorption.
    - When evaluating azotemia, establish whether it is prerenal, primary renal, or postrenal in origin.
    - Prerenal azotemia is not uncommon in rabbits and is found in association with stress, fright, water deprivation, severe dehydration, heatstroke, and toxic insults.
    - Primary or renal azotemia occurs with renal parenchymal disease and glomerular damage and is accompanied by variable increases in BUN and creatinine levels and isosthenuria.
    - Postrenal azotemia occurs with urinary tract obstruction, most commonly due to calculi. Urine specific gravity can vary in cases of postrenal azotemia.
  - The rabbit has a limited capacity to concentrate urea; therefore, dehydration may readily result in elevated (prerenal) values of BUN and creatinine that might otherwise be associated with renal disease in other species. In most cases of prerenal azotemia, elevations in BUN are less than 100 mg/dL (35.7 mmol/L) and are accompanied by an increase in urine specific gravity greater than 1.030.
  - Circulating levels of phosphorus are largely controlled by the kidneys, and consistent elevations in phosphorus in the face of isosthenuria and azotemia are not uncommon in animals with renal failure.
  - Vitamin D and parathyroid hormone influence intestinal absorption of phosphorus; parathyroid hormone stimulates renal excretion of phosphorus and conservation of calcium.
    - Hyperphosphatemia is seen in rabbits with kidney disease because of impaired renal phosphorus excretion.
    - In rabbits with chronic renal failure, hypercalcemia may occur because of impaired renal calcium excretion.
  - Anemia of chronic renal failure is a common entity that results from reduced erythropoietin production by damaged kidneys, uremic inhibition of red blood cell production, and increased red blood cell hemolysis.
  - Urinalysis serves as a tool for assessing urinary tract health, which should be assessed in any rabbit with suspected renal disease.
    - Urine specific gravity can help differentiate prerenal versus renal azotemia.
    - Urine protein can be elevated with urinary tract inflammation, hemorrhage, and infection, or can be an indication of renal damage. Protein levels in the urine must be interpreted along with urine specific gravity and sediment analysis. Glomerulonephritis and amyloidosis are the most common causes of renal-associated proteinuria.
    - Hematuria can result from upper or lower urinary tract disease or can be of uterine origin in intact females. Hematuria of renal origin is seen with pyelonephritis, neoplasia, nephroliths, or renal infarcts.
    - Urine sediment analysis can offer information on urinary tract hemorrhage, inflammation, bacteria, and renal tubular damage.
    - In cases of azotemic febrile rabbits with pyuria or bacteriuria, pyelonephritis must be ruled out.
  - Submit serology sample for *E. cuniculi* in any rabbit with azotemia of undetermined origin.
  - In rabbits with lymphosarcoma, anemia and azotemia may be seen clinically, and leukemia occasionally occurs.
- Imaging
  - Plain abdominal radiography can assess for increases or decreases in kidney size, radiopaque calculi within the urinary tract, abdominal masses associated with the urinary tract, and bladder distention.
  - Contrast cystography and urethrography can provide more specific information regarding the bladder and urethra. Intravenous pyelography, or excretory urography, is used to evaluate the size, shape, position, and internal structure of the kidneys, ureter, and urinary bladder, and is especially helpful at assessing the upper urinary tract (kidneys and ureters) for calculi, masses, or obstructive lesions.

ADVANCED OR CONFIRMATORY TESTING

- Advanced imaging
  - Renal ultrasonography plays a role in discerning size, contour, and texture of the kidneys, allowing for differentiation of focal versus diffuse disease and echodense versus echolucent lesions.
  - Ultrasonography of the entire urinary tract can help rule out obstructive nephropathy caused by urolithiasis or mass defects.
  - Ultrasonography and CT can help with the diagnosis of uroliths, pyelonephritis, hydronephrosis, or hydroureter, as well as renal cysts and abscesses.
- Blood pressure measurement
  - Indirect systolic blood pressure measurement can be determined using pneumatic cuffs and Doppler pulse detection units placed on limbs.

TREATMENT

THERAPEUTIC GOALS

- Treatment should be aimed at promoting diuresis and diminishing the consequences of uremia.
- Ultimate goal is to delay progression of renal disease and preserve overall patient well-being and quality of life.
- Determine severity of renal disease based on clinical signs, physical examination findings, and clinical pathology results to determine prognosis and tailor treatment.
- Look for underlying cause of renal disease to determine whether more definitively treatable.

ACUTE GENERAL TREATMENT

- Discontinue any potentially nephrotoxic drugs.
- Identify and treat any prerenal or postrenal abnormalities.
- Identify any treatable conditions such as urolithiasis or pyelonephritis.
- Initiate intravenous fluid therapy to induce diuresis and correct azotemia and electrolyte and acid-base imbalances. Replacement of dehydration deficits is done with the use of isotonic crystalloids. Maintenance fluids are given at 3-4 mL/kg/h in the rabbit.
- Potassium supplementation of fluids is based on blood potassium measurement.
- Monitor core body temperature; if hypothermic, warm patient with use of fluid warmers and warm air heating blankets.
- Assess for secondary GI stasis and treat accordingly. Consider nasogastric tube placement in cases of total anorexia and nutritional depletion.

CHRONIC TREATMENT

- Maintain long-term diuresis with subcutaneous fluid therapy (owners can be taught to do this at home). Normal water intake in rabbits is estimated to be 100 mL/kg/d.
- Dietary management: renal friendly dietary changes are difficult in rabbits because of specific dietary requirements. Avoid high-phosphorus and high-calcium feed. Offer low-protein grass hays and avoid legume hays.
  - Low-phosphorus Romaine, Boston, or bibb lettuces are healthy vegetable choices to add to the diet of a rabbit with renal disease.
  - Mature or second-cutting grass hays may contain less phosphorus (0.26% on a dry-matter [DM] basis) and are a good forage choice.
  - Maintaining adequate caloric intake to avoid weight loss takes precedence over nutrient composition of diet.
- If hyperphosphatemic, initiate enteric phosphate binders (e.g., aluminum hydroxide).
- Supplementation of water-soluble vitamins B and C may be considered because the excessive amount of urine production by failing kidneys commonly results in their loss.
- If anemia is present
  - Human recombinant (H-R) erythropoietin may be used to reverse the anemia associated with renal failure, although the patient may develop antibodies against the H-R erythropoietin.
  - Anabolic steroids (e.g., nandrolone 2 mg/kg SC) may be given.
- Consider use of omega-3 fatty acid supplements based on studies showing their beneficial effects in other species.
- Treat *E. cuniculi* if serology results are consistent with possible infection.
- Consider use of antihypertensives in hypertensive patients (e.g., angiotensin-converting enzyme [ACE] inhibitors, enalapril 0.25-0.5 mg/kg PO q 24-48 h).

DRUG INTERACTIONS

ACE inhibitors may potentially reduce glomerular filtration rate (GFR) and may exacerbate renal disease.

RECOMMENDED MONITORING

- Overall condition and clinical response to therapy should be assessed in all patients with renal disease. Frequency of follow-up assessments varies with initial diagnosis and severity of disease. Periodic assessments for azotemia, anemia, and phosphorus, potassium, and protein imbalances are recommended.
- Monitor body weight and condition, and adjust nutrition accordingly. Supplement with Critical Care for Herbivores (Oxbow Animal Health, Murdock, NE) as needed.
- Urinalysis and urine culture in patients being treated for pyelonephritis
- Regular monitoring of systemic blood pressure, especially in patients receiving ACE inhibitors

PROGNOSIS AND OUTCOME

- With any diagnosis of renal insufficiency or failure, prognosis varies with severity of clinical pathology findings, duration of disease, and severity of primary renal failure. If secondary to infection or obstructive disease, prognosis is determined by duration of disease process and success in treatment, medical or surgical, of the underlying condition and treatment of secondary renal insufficiency.
- Depending on initial diagnosis, disease severity, and response to therapy, quality of life issues and euthanasia should be discussed with the owner for any patient with renal failure.

CONTROVERSY

The use of ACE inhibitors for renal failure in rabbits has not been fully evaluated.

PEARLS & CONSIDERATIONS

COMMENTS

- For long-term administration of subcutaneous fluids, a subdermal SkinButton (Norfolk Vet Products, Skokie, IL; www.norfolkvetproducts.com) can be placed between the shoulder blades. Special accessing needles are used to administer subcutaneous fluids into the SkinButton.
- Peritoneal dialysis has been advocated in the management of some cases of acute renal failure.

CLIENT EDUCATION

Chronic renal failure requires continuous treatment and monitoring. Unless a specific underlying cause is diagnosed and treated successfully, treatment in many cases will be lifelong.

SUGGESTED READINGS

Fisher PG: Exotic mammal renal disease: causes and clinical presentation, Vet Clin North Am Exot Anim Pract 9:33–67, 2006.

Fisher PG: Exotic mammal renal disease: diagnosis and treatment, Vet Clin North Am Exot Anim Pract 9:69–96, 2006.

Harcourt-Brown F: Radiographic signs of renal disease in rabbits, Vet Rec 160:787–794, 2007.

Potter MP, et al: Apparent psychogenic polydipsia and secondary polyuria in laboratory-housed New Zealand white rabbits, Contemp Top Lab Anim Sci 37:87–89, 1998.

CROSS-REFERENCES TO OTHER SECTIONS

Encephalitozoonosis
Lower Urinary Tract Disorders
Lymphosarcoma
Uterine Disorders

AUTHOR: **PETER G. FISHER**

EDITOR: **DAVID VELLA**

RABBITS

Splayleg

BASIC INFORMATION

DEFINITION

A general descriptive term referring to any abnormality of rabbits that leads to an inability to adduct one or more limbs.

SYNONYMS

Congenital hip dislocation, congenital limb adduction, femoral neck anteversion, subluxation of hip, hip dysplasia

EPIDEMIOLOGY

GENETICS AND BREED PREDISPOSITION Certain types of splayleg have an autosomal recessive inheritance. Other types may be acquired. Larger breeds may be more susceptible.

RISK FACTORS

- Unsuitable flooring
- Inadequate diet in rapidly growing rabbits

CLINICAL PRESENTATION

HISTORY, CHIEF COMPLAINT

- Signs evident from early age: usually from several days to several months of age
- Inability to adduct one or more limbs resulting in lateral deviation of affected limb(s), hence the term *splayleg*
- Owners may report ataxia as the chief presenting sign.

PHYSICAL EXAM FINDINGS

- Inability to ambulate correctly or lift body off the ground. In some cases, complete paralysis is seen.
- Hind limbs most commonly affected
- May be present in all 4 limbs or just one limb
- Both affected and unaffected limbs may have pododermatitis.

ETIOLOGY AND PATHOPHYSIOLOGY

- Often a direct result of an autosomal recessive inherited condition
- Multifactorial origin suspected in many cases, with acquired factors such as inadequate substrate or diet implicated

DIAGNOSIS

DIFFERENTIAL DIAGNOSIS

Any condition resulting in ataxia or generalized muscular or skeletal weakness, including the following:

- Toxins
- Malnutrition
- Congenital abnormalities
- Floppy rabbit syndrome (see Floppy Rabbit Syndrome)
- Traumatic injury
- Hypokalemia
- Myasthenia gravis
- Vestibular disease
- *Encephalitozoon cuniculi*
- Toxoplasmosis
- Sarcocystis
- Spondylosis (usually in older animals)

INITIAL DATABASE

- Neurologic examination: inability to adduct one or more limbs
- Radiographs may reveal skeletal abnormalities such as:
  - Anteversion of the femoral neck
  - Subtrochanteric torsion of the femoral shaft
  - Subluxation of the hip
  - Lateral patellar luxation
  - Pelvic deformities
- Clinical pathology usually unremarkable unless related to disease from differential list

TREATMENT

THERAPEUTIC GOALS

- Correct underlying cause(s) where possible.
- Provide adequate quality of life.

ACUTE GENERAL TREATMENT

- Provide nutritional support if anorexia or gastrointestinal stasis is suspected.
- Provide pain relief where appropriate (e.g., meloxicam 0.3-0.5 mg/kg PO, SC q 12-24 h)

CHRONIC TREATMENT

- Correct underlying cause where possible (e.g., nonslip flooring).
- Amputation as a salvage procedure is an option if only one limb is affected.

POSSIBLE COMPLICATIONS

Mostly related to inability to ambulate:

- Pododermatitis (see Pododermatitis)
- Urine scald
- Perineal fecal/cecotrophal soiling
- Myiasis
- Gastrointestinal stasis

RECOMMENDED MONITORING

Regular reassessment to determine quality of life

PROGNOSIS AND OUTCOME

- Guarded prognosis in most cases
- Recovery unlikely
- Euthanasia is the outcome in many cases.
- Consider culling affected animals if inherited cause is determined.
- Some individuals cope with the long-term disability, especially if mild.
- Quality of life is the main consideration.

PEARLS & CONSIDERATIONS

COMMENTS

- *Splayleg* is a loose descriptive term; this condition results in adduction of one or more limbs.
- A variety of inherited or acquired causes may be involved.
- Inherited splayleg results in skeletal deformities in young growing rabbits.

PREVENTION

Correct underlying cause where possible.

CLIENT EDUCATION

- Quality of life must be constantly assessed.
- Do not breed from affected animals.

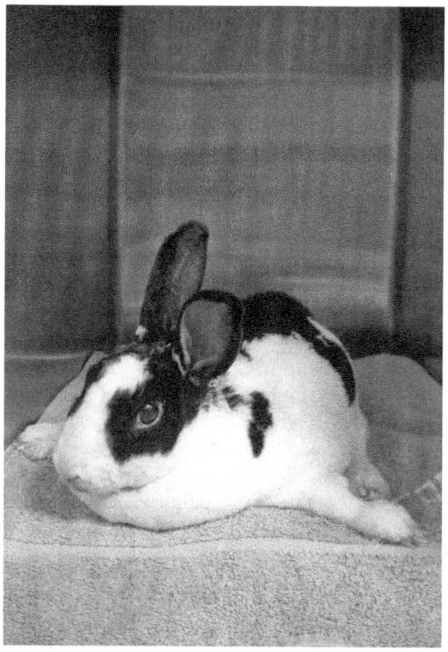

Splayleg Splayleg in a rabbit. Note the splayed position of the front legs. *(Photo courtesy Jörg Mayer, The University of Georgia, Athens.)*

SUGGESTED READINGS

Arendar GM, et al: Splay-leg: a recessively inherited form of femoral neck anteversion: femoral shaft torsion and subluxation of the hip in the laboratory lop rabbit, Clin Orthop Relat Res 44:221–229, 1966.

Jirmanova I: The splayleg disease: a form of congenital glucocorticoid myopathy? Vet Res Commun 6:91–101, 1983.

Joosten HF, et al: Splayleg: a spontaneous limb defect in rabbits. Genetics, gross anatomy and microscopy, Teratology 24:87–104, 1981.

CROSS-REFERENCES TO OTHER SECTIONS

Arthritis
Encephalitozoonosis
Floppy Rabbit Syndrome
Pododermatitis
Vestibular Disease

AUTHOR: **BRENDAN CARMEL**

EDITOR: **DAVID VELLA**

RABBITS

Staphylococcosis

BASIC INFORMATION

DEFINITION

Staphylococcosis in rabbits is an infection caused by the Gram-positive bacterium *Staphylococcus aureus.* The most common clinical signs are subcutaneous abscesses, pododermatitis, and mastitis.

SPECIAL SPECIES CONSIDERATIONS

- *Staphylococcus aureus* is a normal skin inhabitant in many animal species. It can cause wound infection in rabbits and in other species.
- Specific high-virulence strains, causing severe and disseminating infection in group-held animals, have been described only in rabbits.

EPIDEMIOLOGY

SPECIES, AGE, SEX

- Clinical signs vary depending on the age of the rabbit. All ages can be affected.
- No known sex predisposition; however, lactating does, especially primiparous does, are more prone to developing mastitis

GENETICS AND BREED PREDISPOSITION

- No known breed predisposition
- Hybrid meat rabbits and New Zealand White rabbits are more resistant to developing pododermatitis owing to the dense hair coat on their footpads and metatarsus.

RISK FACTORS

- Generally, *S. aureus* invades and causes disease when a skin wound is present. Sharp objects in the cage, moist bedding, an unsuitable wire mesh floor, and other abrasive substrates can cause skin lesions that predispose to the development of *S. aureus* infection.
- Specific high-virulence *S. aureus* strains do not appear to need these predisposing factors to cause disease.

CONTAGION AND ZOONOSIS

- Low-virulence *S. aureus* strains belong to the normal skin flora and usually cause problems through wound infection.
- Specific high-virulence *S. aureus* strains are highly contagious to other rabbits. Transmission can be direct or indirect and can occur through cages, hair, or feed.
  - Direct transmission of *S. aureus* may occur between does and suckling young, between littermates, and between cagemates.
  - Introduction of new breeding rabbits into a group is probably the most important source of infection.
  - Sperm (even after artificial insemination) also introduce potential risk of infection.
- No zoonotic potential has been described. Theoretically, *S. aureus* from rabbits can invade skin lesions in humans.

GEOGRAPHY AND SEASONALITY

- *S. aureus* infections occur worldwide with no seasonality.
- High-virulence *S. aureus* strains belonging to a specific bacterial clone have been isolated from meat rabbits within Europe and Australia. Their presence in other parts of the world has not been investigated.

ASSOCIATED CONDITIONS AND DISORDERS

- Pododermatitis
- Mastitis

CLINICAL PRESENTATION

DISEASE FORMS/SUBTYPES

- In farmed rabbits, two types of *S. aureus* infection can be distinguished at a group level:
  - Low-virulence strains
    - Most commonly seen
    - Usually remain limited to only one or a small number of animals
  - High-virulence strains
    - Less commonly seen
    - Consequences are severe owing to epizootic spread within the group.
- For individual pet rabbits, the distinction between low- and high-virulence strain infection is usually not made.
- With both types of infection, different clinical signs may be seen separately or concurrently.

HISTORY, CHIEF COMPLAINT

- Subcutaneous abscesses are most commonly seen.
- In lactating does, mastitis is often noticed. Consequently, the young may die owing to agalactia in the doe.
- Pododermatitis
- Newborn hairless rabbits may suffer from generalized pustular dermatitis.
- Less frequently seen problems include:
  - Septicemia
  - Bacteremia with localization primarily to liver, lungs, and uterus
  - Conjunctivitis
  - Purulent rhinitis
  - Arthritis
  - Head tilt due to otitis media
  - Vaginal discharge due to metritis

PHYSICAL EXAM FINDINGS

- The following findings may be present separately or concurrently:
  - Subcutaneous swellings (abscesses)
  - Swellings of the mammary gland(s), (mastitis)
  - Pododermatitis
  - Generalized pustular dermatitis in hairless young
  - Fever (septicemia)
  - Mucopurulent nasal discharge (rhinitis)
  - Ocular discharge (conjunctivitis)
  - Vaginal discharge (metritis)
  - Head tilt (otitis media)
  - Abdominal masses (abdominal/visceral abscesses)

ETIOLOGY AND PATHOPHYSIOLOGY

- The causative agent of staphylococcosis in rabbits is *Staphylococcus aureus.*

- Distinction between low- and high-virulence *S. aureus* strains can be made using a multiplex PCR test.
- In cases of pododermatitis, radiography may be used to detect the presence of osteomyelitis and arthritis.

DIAGNOSIS

DIFFERENTIAL DIAGNOSIS

- Subcutaneous abscesses due to other bacteria, e.g., *Pasteurella multocida*
- Facial abscesses due to dental associated disease
- Abdominal masses due to abscessation, granulomas, organomegaly, parasitic cysts, or neoplasia
- Bacterial rhinitis and conjunctivitis due to other bacterial infections, e.g., *P. multocida, Bordetella bronchiseptica,* and *Pseudomonas* spp.
- Head tilt due to bacterial otitis media or otitis interna, protozoal meningoencephalitis, and *Baylisascaris procyonis*
- Uterine disorders due to bacterial metritis, hydrometra/mucometra, and uterine neoplasia

INITIAL DATABASE

- Lancing of lesions usually reveals caseous pus.
- The most common differential diagnosis for *S. aureus* infections is *P. multocida*.
  - Microscopic evaluation of Diff-Quik–stained smears may reveal the presence of coccoid bacteria *(S. aureus)* or short rod–shaped bacteria *(P. multocida)*. Often bacteria are not seen, and only degenerating neutrophils are present on the smear.
- Imaging via radiography or ultrasonography may reveal affected internal organs.

ADVANCED OR CONFIRMATORY TESTING

- Bacterial culture and antimicrobial sensitivity testing
  - Swab samples should be taken from a recent skin lesion or from the interior wall of an opened abscess to minimize a false-negative culture result.
- Distinction between low- and high-virulence strains may be useful in epizootic outbreaks:
  - Previously, differentiation was performed by biotyping and then phage typing. The latter is a labor-intensive and time-consuming technique.
  - A quick multiplex PCR test has been developed that can be used to identify high-virulence strains after biotyping.
  - Confirmation is achieved with pulsed field gel electrophoresis (PFGE), which is expensive and is not readily available.

TREATMENT

THERAPEUTIC GOALS

- Low-virulence *S. aureus* strains:
  - Subclinical carriers should be considered normal and cannot be controlled.
  - Treatment is performed only on clinically affected animals.
- High-virulence *S. aureus* strains:
  - In group-housed rabbits, treatment of affected rabbits can be attempted. However, among farmed rabbits, eliminating high-virulence strains from all animals is virtually impossible; culling the entire group should be considered.
  - Among pet rabbits, treatment should be performed on all in-contact and clinically affected animals.

ACUTE GENERAL TREATMENT

- Supportive treatment is required in cases associated with anorexia and fever:
  - Assisted feeding (e.g., Oxbow Critical Care Feeding Formula; Oxbow Animal Health, Murdock, NE)
  - Fluid therapy: 120 mL/kg/d maintenance requirement + replacement fluid IV or SC
  - Nonsteroidal antiinflammatory drugs (NSAIDs; e.g., meloxicam 0.3-0.5 mg/kg PO, SC q 12-24 h)
- Surgical resection of abscesses
  - Débridement, cleaning, disinfection, and open wound drainage
  - Complete removal of the pus-containing abscess with its capsule
- Local and/or general antibiotic therapy
  - Ideally based on antimicrobial sensitivity testing
  - Oxytetracycline 100 mg/kg IM q 48 h, or enrofloxacin 10 mg/kg PO q12 h
  - Topical treatment of abscess cavities with either medical honey or antibiotic-impregnated polymethylmethacrylate (AIPMMA) beads.
- Pododermatitis (see Pododermatitis)

CHRONIC TREATMENT

- Abscesses, mastitis, and pododermatitis are difficult to cure and often require prolonged treatment and follow-up.
- Abscesses that have been treated surgically:
  - Wounds should remain open and abscess sites should be drained and cleaned daily until suppuration ceases.
- Pododermatitis
  - Affected animal should be kept on soft and dry bedding.

DRUG INTERACTIONS

Chronic or inappropriate antibiotic use may lead to intestinal dysbiosis.

PROGNOSIS AND OUTCOME

- Likelihood of abscess recurrence is high unless complete surgical resection is achieved.
- Guarded prognosis for severe pododermatitis: euthanasia should be considered
- Among group-housed rabbits, infection with high-virulence *S. aureus* strains carries a poor prognosis because clinical recurrence of disease is likely. Culling of entire group should be considered.

PEARLS & CONSIDERATIONS

COMMENTS

- High-virulence *S. aureus* strains
  - Have been described only in commercial meat–farmed rabbits throughout Europe and Australia.
  - Screening for *S. aureus* outside of these regions and in pet rabbits worldwide has not been performed.

PREVENTION

- A vaccine protecting against staphylococcosis does not exist.
- Some meat-rabbit owners claim to have fewer problems with high-virulence strains after administration of an autovaccine. Under experimental conditions, autovaccination gives limited protection.
- Materials used in enclosures should not give rise to wounds or foot lesions.

CLIENT EDUCATION

General husbandry on enclosure construction and maintenance

SUGGESTED READINGS

Hermans K, et al: Rabbit staphylococcosis: difficult solutions for serious problems, Vet Microbiol 91:57–64, 2003.

Vancraeynest D, et al: Multiplex PCR for the detection of high virulence *Staphylococcus aureus* strains from rabbits, Vet Microbiol 121:368–372, 2007.

CROSS-REFERENCES TO OTHER SECTIONS

Abscesses
Anorexia
Conjunctival Disorders
Cutaneous Masses
Dental Disease
Dermatopathies
Encephalitis
Encephalitozoonosis

Mammary Gland Disorders
Otitis
Pasteurellosis
Pododermatitis
Upper Respiratory Tract Disorders
Uterine Disorders
Vestibular Disease

AUTHOR: **KATLEEN HERMANS**

EDITOR: **DAVID VELLA**

RABBITS

Testicular Tumors

BASIC INFORMATION

DEFINITION

Testicular tumors are neoplasms arising within the testis. They can be functional (hormone secreting) or nonfunctional.

SYNONYMS

Testicular cancer, interstitial (Leydig) cell tumor, Sertoli cell tumor, seminoma, teratoma

SPECIAL SPECIES CONSIDERATIONS

Testicular tumors are infrequently reported in rabbits. The apparent low incidence in laboratory rabbits may be due to infrequent microscopic evaluation of testes and the fact that most laboratory rabbits do not live long enough to develop these neoplasms.

EPIDEMIOLOGY

SPECIES, AGE, SEX Older male rabbits (between 3 and 9 years of age) have a higher incidence.

RISK FACTORS Undescended testes present greater risk of neoplastic transformation.

ASSOCIATED CONDITIONS AND DISORDERS

- Orchitis and discomfort secondary to tumor growth
- Functional tumors can produce behavioral changes:
  - Increased incidence of collagenous hamartoma is seen with functional tumors.

CLINICAL PRESENTATION

DISEASE FORMS/SUBTYPES

- Unilateral or bilateral
- Neoplasms of different types can occur simultaneously in both testes (e.g., a Sertoli cell tumor in one, and a seminoma in the other). Interstitial cell tumors are the most commonly reported and are usually benign.

HISTORY, CHIEF COMPLAINT Enlargement or change of texture in one or both testes

PHYSICAL EXAM FINDINGS

- Testicular asymmetry
- Scrotal skin necrosis (rare)
- Gynecomastia (rare)

ETIOLOGY AND PATHOPHYSIOLOGY

- Causes of most forms in rabbits are not established.
- Most forms are benign and do not metastasize. However, malignant tumors (e.g., seminoma) may spread to local lymph nodes and lungs.
- Functional interstitial cell tumors are associated with increased serum testosterone levels:
  - May contribute to behavioral changes
  - May be associated with collagenous hamartomas

DIAGNOSIS

DIFFERENTIAL DIAGNOSIS

- Abscess (see Abscesses)
- Cysts
- Orchitis
- Testicular torsion
- Herniation of viscera

INITIAL DATABASE

Blood biochemistry and hematology

ADVANCED OR CONFIRMATORY TESTING

- Ultrasonography
  - Normal testes have regular echogenicity.
  - Testicular tumors may show mixed echotexture.
  - May be used to distinguish from herniated viscera, abscessation, and cysts
- Histopathologic examination to determine tumor type
  - Submit both testes for evaluation.
  - Include spermatic cord to evaluate for local invasion.
  - Multiple tumor types can occur in the same testes.
- Consider thoracic radiographs to check for lung metastases for malignant tumors.

TREATMENT

THERAPEUTIC GOAL

Surgical excision

ACUTE GENERAL TREATMENT

- Castration (closed technique)
  - Scrotal ablation may not be necessary unless tumor is excessively large.

CHRONIC TREATMENT

If castration is not an option, chronic treatment is palliative.

POSSIBLE COMPLICATIONS

Anesthetic risk associated with age of rabbit

PROGNOSIS AND OUTCOME

Excellent with complete excision

PEARLS & CONSIDERATIONS

COMMENTS

- Do not rely upon gross pathologic examination of excised testes to diagnose neoplasia because abscessation and cysts may appear similar.
- Submit both testes and spermatic cords for histopathologic examination.

PREVENTION

Castration is preventive.

CLIENT EDUCATION

Regular examination of testes in aged bucks

SUGGESTED READINGS

Hartmann M, et al: Testicular neoplasms in domestic rabbits [German], Tierarztliche Umschau 56:430–433, 2001.

Kojimoto A, et al: A scleroderma-like lesion in a rabbit with Leydig cell tumors, Jpn J Vet Anesth Surg 37:39–42, 2006.

Maratea KA, et al: Testicular interstitial cell tumor and gynecomastia in a rabbit, Vet Pathol 44:513–517, 2007.

CROSS-REFERENCES TO OTHER SECTIONS

Abscesses
Cutaneous masses
Pasteurellosis

AUTHORS: **WILL EASSON AND DAVID VELLA**

EDITOR: **THOMAS M. DONNELLY**

Thymoma

Client Education Sheet
Available on Website

BASIC INFORMATION

DEFINITION

Thymoma is a tumor of thymic epithelial origin, found in the cranial mediastinum.

EPIDEMIOLOGY

SPECIES, AGE, SEX More common in older rabbits (over 6 years of age)

ASSOCIATED CONDITIONS AND DISORDERS

- Paraneoplastic syndromes are less common in rabbits than in other species.
  - Hemolytic anemia (one report)
  - Exfoliative dermatitis (one report)
  - Immune disorders (e.g., myasthenia gravis) are associated with thymomas in cats, dogs, and man but have not been described in the rabbit.

CLINICAL PRESENTATION

DISEASE FORMS/SUBTYPES Thymomas generally are slow growing and are not metastatic. However, thymomas have the potential for local invasion and pleural dissemination.

HISTORY, CHIEF COMPLAINT

- Dyspnea, open-mouth breathing
- Lethargy, depression

PHYSICAL EXAM FINDINGS

- Clinical signs are those associated with a space-occupying lesion in the mediastinum.
- Dyspnea, open-mouth breathing
- Bilateral exophthalmos (due to partial occlusion of the cranial vena cava)
- Neck, head, and forelimb edema
- Reduced thoracic compliance, increased thoracic stiffness.

ETIOLOGY AND PATHOPHYSIOLOGY

- Neoplastic transformation of thymic epithelial cells
- Enlarging mediastinal mass causes dyspnea and venous occlusion.

DIAGNOSIS

DIFFERENTIAL DIAGNOSIS

- Thymic lymphoma
- Thymic carcinoma
- Mediastinal abscess (see Abscesses)
- Mediastinal hemorrhage
- Other neoplasia: thyroid carcinoma, mast cell tumor, metastatic tumor, chemodectoma (e.g., carotid body tumor)
- Thymic hyperplasia
- Thymic branchial cyst

INITIAL DATABASE

- Thoracic radiography (mediastinal mass)
  - Cranial masses can be difficult to distinguish from normal thoracic structures.
- Ultrasonography to characterize consistency of mass
  - Thymomas often show hypoechoic cystic areas.
- Complete blood count and biochemistry
  - Elevated white blood cell count and hemolytic anemia may be seen.

ADVANCED OR CONFIRMATORY TESTING

- CT plus intravenous contrast
- MRI
- Ultrasound-guided aspirate and cytology: may be nondiagnostic
- Histopathologic examination via:
  - Ultrasound-guided core needle biopsy
  - Thoracotomy and open incisional or excisional biopsy
  - Thoracoscopy and biopsy

TREATMENT

THERAPEUTIC GOALS

- Complete removal of the tumor
- If removal is not possible, significant reduction in size of the tumor to alleviate associated clinical signs and maintain quality of life

ACUTE GENERAL TREATMENT

- General supportive care, including oxygen therapy
- Surgical removal via a median sternotomy is the treatment of choice, although it does carry significant perioperative risk.

CHRONIC TREATMENT

- Few reports have described treatment for thymoma in the rabbit; more data are needed to assess the relative efficacy of different treatment options.
- Radiation therapy: after incomplete surgical removal or if rabbit is not a surgical candidate
- Corticosteroids may be used as adjuvant therapy in rabbits undergoing radiation therapy.
- Chemotherapy: efficacy not evaluated in rabbits; at present only suggested as an adjunct after surgery or radiation therapy

POSSIBLE COMPLICATIONS

- Surgery: acute perioperative death (due to pain, stress, ileus), inability to remove the tumor, pneumothorax, hemorrhage
- Radiation therapy: damage to adjacent normal critical tissues (heart, lung) (e.g., radiation pneumonitis and fibrosis, thrombosis of thoracic vessels). Cobalt 60 radiation units deliver radiation doses that may cause unacceptable toxicity for critical organs; a linear accelerator with electron capability is preferable.
- Anesthetic complications (repeated anesthetic episodes required for radiotherapy).
- Chemotherapy: complications depend on the drugs used but include bone marrow suppression, renal

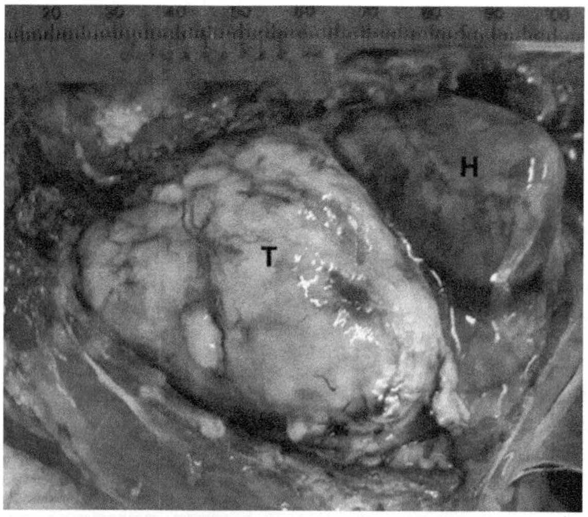

Thymoma Typical lesions of cutaneous lymphoma. Lesions normally are thick and raised but not painful. *(Photo courtesy Jörg Mayer, The University of Georgia, Athens.)*

toxicity, hepatic toxicity, and weight loss.

RECOMMENDED MONITORING

Follow-up radiography or, preferably, CT or MRI to monitor for recurrence

PROGNOSIS AND OUTCOME

- Prognosis should be good for surgical removal of a solitary tumor if perioperative complications are avoided.
- Reports have described survival time after radiation therapy ranging from 1 to 23 months.
- Survival time without treatment is reported as 4 months in only one case.

PEARLS & CONSIDERATIONS

COMMENTS

- Rabbits normally retain the thymus into adulthood.
- Thymomas are relatively rare tumors.
- Radiation therapy can provide benefit, but further development of a standardized protocol is required. Access to radiation treatment may be a significant factor.
- Treatment should be decided on a case-by-case basis, with particular emphasis on cardiopulmonary function and perioperative care, because a prolonged surgical period or repeated anesthetics (for radiation) may be required.
- Untreated thymomas may progress to metastatic thymic carcinoma, but death is likely to ensue as the result of a space-occupying mediastinal mass and dyspnea.

SUGGESTED READINGS

Andres KM, et al: The use of megavoltage radiation therapy in the treatment of thymomas in rabbits: 19 cases, Vet Comp Oncol 10:82–94, 2012.

Clippinger TL, et al: Removal of a thymoma via median sternotomy in a rabbit with recurrent appendicular neurofibrosarcoma, J Am Vet Med Assoc 213:1140–1143, 1998.

Künzel F, et al: Thymomas in rabbits: clinical evaluation, diagnosis, and treatment, J Am Anim Hosp Assoc 48:97–104, 2012.

Morrisey J, et al: Therapeutic options for thymoma in the rabbit, Semin Avian Exot Pet Med 14:175–181, 2005.

Sánchez-Migallón A, et al: Radiation therapy for the treatment of thymoma in rabbits *(Oryctolagus cuniculus)*, J Exotic Pet Med 15:138–144, 2006.

CROSS-REFERENCES TO OTHER SECTIONS

Abscesses

AUTHOR: **ANNA MEREDITH**

EDITOR: **DAVID VELLA**

RABBITS

Treponematosis

BASIC INFORMATION

DEFINITION

Treponematosis is a bacterial infection of rabbits caused by the spirochete *Treponema paraluiscuniculi* (previously *Treponema cuniculi*).

SYNONYMS

Rabbit syphilis, vent disease, venereal spirochetosis

SPECIAL SPECIES CONSIDERATIONS

- *T. paraluiscuniculi* infects only rabbits.
- A morphologically and serologically identical disease is found in European brown hares *(Lepus europaeus)* and is caused by *Treponema paraluisleporis*.

EPIDEMIOLOGY

SPECIES, AGE, SEX Young rabbits are resistant to infection.

RISK FACTORS Recent direct (especially sexual) contact with an infected rabbit. No evidence of vertical transmission in rabbits has been found. However, it is suspected that young rabbits can be infected during the kindling process, and seropositive rates usually increase with age.

CONTAGION AND ZOONOSIS

- Transmission is:
  - Sexual
  - Through direct contact
  - Although transplacental transmission has not been documented, cross-fostering experiments have shown that infection can occur at birth or during the nursing period.
- Subclinical carriers probably exist.
- *T. paraluiscuniculi* does not infect humans. However, *Treponema pallidum* (the causative organism of human syphilis) does infect rabbits.

GEOGRAPHY AND SEASONALITY

- Ubiquitous in distribution; however, the disease is virtually nonexistent in some wild rabbit populations in Australia
- No obvious seasonality, although more frequently seen during and just after breeding season

ASSOCIATED CONDITIONS AND DISORDERS Skin signs most common but will also cause abortion/neonatal death

CLINICAL PRESENTATION

DISEASE FORMS/SUBTYPES

- Skin disease
- Reproductive disease

HISTORY, CHIEF COMPLAINT

- The most frequent finding is crusting and erythema of the mucocutaneous junctions—nose, lips, eyelids, and especially external genitalia (known by rabbit breeders as the "vent").
- Skin lesions are initially hyperemic and edematous before progressing to erythematous papules and nodules that erode to form characteristic crusts.
- Localized lymphadenopathy may occur.
- Lesions may spread to eyelids and other parts of the skin with grooming.
- It is common to find genital lesions only. Occasionally, facial lesions only, probably caused by sniffing of infected genitalia, are found.
- Clinical signs can be slow to appear in infected animals.
- Signs usually appear 3 to 6 weeks after infection.

PHYSICAL EXAM FINDINGS Crusted skin lesions on genitalia and face

ETIOLOGY AND PATHOPHYSIOLOGY

- *T. paraluiscuniculi*, a spirochete bacterium
- Carried in the external genitalia (prepuce of males and vulva of females) or in open lesions on other parts of the body

- Infection is by sexual contact or direct contact (e.g., sniffing) with open lesions.
- Infection of the young can occur via the birth canal.
- Inflammatory lesions of the genitalia characterize the disease, although the face and regional lymph nodes are sometimes involved. In general, signs are related to the mucocutaneous junctions, although they are occasionally found on other parts of the skin. In some cases, abortion and neonatal death may occur.

DIAGNOSIS

DIFFERENTIAL DIAGNOSIS

- Early stages may resemble myxomatosis with swelling around mucocutaneous junctions.
- Typical skin lesions of treponematosis are unlikely to be confused with other diseases, especially if multiple rabbits are found with the same clinical signs.
- If an individual rabbit is found with genital lesions only, rule out trauma from fighting or injury.
- Obese females may have pyoderma around the vulval skin folds.

INITIAL DATABASE

- Physical examination
- Sampling of lesions
  - Perform cytologic examination or biopsy to rule out other causes and to attempt to identify the organism.

ADVANCED OR CONFIRMATORY TESTING

- Biopsy
  - Histologic examination of skin lesions will reveal hyperplasia of the epidermis, erosions and ulcerations, and an infiltrate composed of plasma cells, macrophages, and neutrophils. Standard stains can be inconclusive and will not stain the primary pathogen. Warthin-Starry silver staining is usually required to see spirochetal bacteria such as *Treponema*.
- Cytologic examination
  - Fresh, wet mounts of lesion scrapings provide a simpler method. Examined under a dark field microscopy, the organism can be readily identified by its characteristic spiral morphology and corkscrew motility.
  - Secondary bacterial infection is very common, and the primary organism may be hidden by subsequent inflammatory changes.
  - Do not overinterpret negative findings on cytologic examination or biopsy; do not rule out treponematosis.
- Serologic testing
  - Serological tests are commercially available.
  - The microhemagglutination test is more reliable than the rapid plasma reagin (RPR) test.
    - However, because both tests use *T. pallidum* as the antigen and antibodies are slow to rise, false-negatives can occur on antibody testing. Animals should be tested multiple times over several weeks to ensure a true-negative status.
    - False-negatives may occur where lesions are present before an antibody response occurs.
    - Infected rabbits may retain antibody titers (25% of serologically positive rabbits are subclinical). Antibody titers fall gradually with therapy.

TREATMENT

THERAPEUTIC GOAL

The treatment outlined is effective for individual rabbits and can be used to eradicate treponematosis from a colony if all animals are treated.

ACUTE GENERAL TREATMENT

- Penicillin is the treatment of choice. This is usually obtained in the form of three long-acting injections given subcutaneously 7 days apart.
- Parenteral benzathine penicillin G/ procaine penicillin G 25-50 mg/kg (42,000-84,000 IU/kg) SC q 7 d × three treatments
- 1 mg penicillin = 1667 IU penicillin

CHRONIC TREATMENT

Not applicable: complete resolution is normally seen within 10 days of therapy, and repeat treatments are generally unnecessary.

DRUG INTERACTIONS

Do not use corticosteroids (locally or systemically).

POSSIBLE COMPLICATIONS

When using penicillins in rabbits, risk of antibiotic-associated diarrhea is always present.

PROGNOSIS AND OUTCOME

Excellent with correct therapy

PEARLS & CONSIDERATIONS

COMMENTS

Use a high-fiber diet when using penicillins, and discuss the risks fully with owners before starting treatment.

PREVENTION

- In colonies that are free of infection, introduction of new breeding stock should be avoided.
- If it is necessary to bring in new animals, they should be examined for lesions and serologically tested before entering the colony.

CLIENT EDUCATION

- Education of rabbit breeders is vital.
- Many rabbit breeders believe that the condition "does not apply to them" if they have not seen signs. However, the presence of subclinical carriers means that disease prevention has to originate from the breeding colony.

SUGGESTED READINGS

Cunliffe-Beamer TL, et al: Venereal spirochetosis of rabbits. I, Description and diagnosis, Lab Anim Sci 31:366–371, 1981.

Cunliffe-Beamer TL, et al: Venereal spirochetosis of rabbits: II, Epizootiology, Lab Anim Sci 31:372–378, 1981.

Cunliffe-Beamer TL, et al: Venereal spirochetosis of rabbits: III, Eradication, Lab Anim Sci 31:379–381, 1981.

Saito K, et al: Chloramphenicol treatment for rabbit syphilis, J Vet Med Sci 66:1301–1304, 2004.

Saito K, et al: Clinical features of skin lesions in rabbit syphilis: a retrospective study of 63 cases (1999-2003), J Vet Med Sci 66:1247–1249, 2004.

Saito K, et al: Clinical features and rapid plasma reagin antibody titers in spontaneous and experimental rabbit syphilis, J Vet Med Sci 67:739–741, 2005.

CROSS-REFERENCES TO OTHER SECTIONS

Dermatopathies
Myxomatosis

AUTHOR: **JOHN CHITTY AND THOMAS M. DONNELLY**

EDITOR: **DAVID VELLA**

RABBITS

Upper Respiratory Tract Disorders

BASIC INFORMATION

DEFINITION

Infections and conditions affecting the nasal cavity and nasopharynx.

SYNONYMS

Snuffles, upper respiratory disease (URD), rhinitis, upper airway disease

SPECIAL SPECIES CONSIDERATIONS

- Rabbits are obligate nasal breathers; disease or infection of the upper respiratory tract can severely compromise respiration. This factor can make it difficult to differentiate between lower respiratory tract and upper respiratory tract disorders. Open-mouth breathing is a poor prognostic sign.
- Because of the rabbit's innate ability as a prey animal to mask signs of disease, many rabbits are not presented until late in the disease process.

EPIDEMIOLOGY

RISK FACTORS

- Concurrent disease
- Multirabbit housing
- High environmental ammonia levels (past and present)

ASSOCIATED CONDITIONS AND DISORDERS Upper respiratory disorders may result in dyspnea, hypovolemic shock, and/or inappetence. In these animals, supportive treatment is initiated concurrently with more specific therapy or investigation for the upper respiratory tract disorder.

CLINICAL PRESENTATION

DISEASE FORMS/SUBTYPES

- Chronic upper respiratory disorders: many chronic disorders can be due to past or present high levels of environmental ammonia levels, overcrowding/ fighting, malnutrition, intercurrent disease, or transportation and other stressors.
- Acute upper respiratory disorders: these can often be seen as an acute presentation of a chronic disorder

HISTORY, CHIEF COMPLAINT

- Sneezing
- Ocular discharge
- Unilateral or bilateral nasal discharge
- Dyspnea

PHYSICAL EXAM FINDINGS

- Mucopurulent to serous nasal discharge—unilateral or bilateral
- Rhinitis, sneezing
- Conjunctivitis
- Dacryocystitis
- Dyspnea, stridor, and/or open-mouth breathing
- Discharge matted on the medial aspect of the forepaws
- Otitis externa
- Inspiratory rales
- Audible harsh breathing
- Semi or non-patent nares (with respect to airflow)

ETIOLOGY AND PATHOPHYSIOLOGY

- Trauma, lysis, and infection of the nasoturbinates can cause mucosal irritation, rhinitis, and sneezing.
- Primary or secondary bacterial infection generates mucopurulent to serous nasal discharge.
- Extension of primary or secondary bacterial infection can irritate and infect the nasolacrimal duct.

DIAGNOSIS

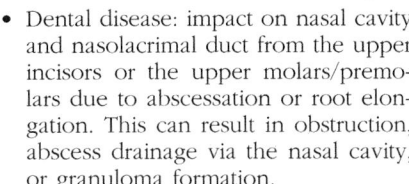

DIFFERENTIAL DIAGNOSIS

- Dental disease: impact on nasal cavity and nasolacrimal duct from the upper incisors or the upper molars/premolars due to abscessation or root elongation. This can result in obstruction, abscess drainage via the nasal cavity, or granuloma formation.
- Nasal foreign body (grass seed, etc.): often seen as sudden onset of unilateral mucopurulent discharge
- Mycotic disease (uncommon)
- Dacryocystitis
- Neoplasia (rare), e.g., lymphoma, nasopharyngeal carcinoma
- Allergic rhinitis (has been reported only anecdotally in rabbits)
- Primary bacterial rhinitis: attributing pathogenicity to any bacterial isolate can be challenging as bacterial rhinitis in rabbits is typically a mixed infection.
  - *Pasteurella multocida:* a common respiratory pathogen, although often thought to be a commensal organism; can often cause rhinitis and tracheitis
  - *Bordetella bronchiseptica:* Although a commensal of the upper respiratory tract in young or immune suppressed individuals, it may cause disease.
  - Other bacteria such as *Moraxella catarrhalis, Pseudomonas aeruginosa,* and *Staphylococcus aureus* may be present in upper respiratory tract disorders.

INITIAL DATABASE

- Complete auscultation of the upper and lower respiratory tract
- Extensive examination of the nares, using a light source and ensuring that both nares are patent
- Radiography of nasal turbinates and dental arcade: this may indicate erosion of nasal turbinates (chronic disease), sinus involvement or dental disease. Sensitivity of skull radiology is less than that of advanced imaging.
- Assessment of otitis
- Thoracic radiography to assess lower respiratory tract
- Complete blood count (lymphocyte-to-heterophil ratio may show changes)
  - Neutrophilia (acute infection/inflammation)
  - Leukopenia and/or reversed neutrophil/lymphocyte ratio (chronic infection/inflammation)
  - Anemia (chronic disease)
- Blood biochemistry
- Deep nasal culture using small-tipped swab in the medial aspect of each nare; this may require sedation and may not be diagnostic owing to the depth of the nasal cavity
- Gram stain of nasal discharge ± culture and sensitivity

ADVANCED OR CONFIRMATORY TESTING

- Complete nasal and sinus examination via endoscopy (rigid and flexible) under general anesthesia; size of patient may be inhibitory
- Biopsy and culture of tissue samples obtained via endoscopic evaluation
- CT/MRI to examine and determine dental involvement, nasal turbinate erosion, and tympanic bullae
- Culture and sensitivity of nasolacrimal duct flush, tracheal wash (caution should be undertaken), or nasal discharge: culture of nasal discharge alone can be unrewarding owing to low presence of bacteria. It should be noted that bacteria found in a culture may be secondary pathogens in the upper respiratory tract disorder.
- Serology *Pasteurella multocida* (ELISA): paired samples 3 weeks apart are ideal for assessing antibody response to active infection; controversial involvement in pet rabbits

TREATMENT

THERAPEUTIC GOALS

- Resolve dyspnea.

- Identifying and resolving the underlying cause.
- Halt the progression of chronic nasal turbinate destruction and control intermittent secondary infections.

ACUTE GENERAL TREATMENT

- Oxygen therapy may be required in dyspneic animals.
- Nebulizing can be an effective and, for some individuals, nonstressful treatment for acute upper respiratory tract disorder. Saline alone may be effective; additional medications such as antibiotics (fluoroquinolones [e.g., enrofloxacin 5-10 mg/kg PO q 12 h; marbofloxacin 5 mg/kg PO q 24 h], potentiated sulfonamides [e.g., trimethoprim/sulfa 30 mg/kg PO q 12 h], tetracyclines [e.g., doxycycline 2.5 mg/kg PO q 12 h] and penicillins [e.g., penicillin G procaine 60,000 IU/kg SC, IM q 24 h]), and mucolytics (e.g., N-acetylcysteine 5-10 mg/kg and up to 100 mg/kg PO q 12 h; intranasal or aerosol delivery of 5%-20% solution has also been described), may also be effective.
- Nonsteroidal therapy to reduce inflammation of the mucous membranes
- Antihistamines may be of little therapeutic use.
- Supportive care may be required for hypovolemic shock, hypothermia, and/or inappetence.

CHRONIC TREATMENT

- Is often nonspecific owing to difficulty in determining cause
- Antibacterial therapy should, without culture and sensitivity results, be broad spectrum. Antibiotics used with varying success include the quinolones, chloramphenicol, the aminoglycosides, parenteral penicillins, and trimethoprim-sulfa drugs.
- Topical ophthalmic medications and nasolacrimal duct flushing
- Antibiotic therapy should be received for a minimum of 14 days, and often for 2 to 3 months.
- Removal of environmental irritants such as dusty hay, mouldy hay, and exhaust fumes is advantageous.
- Regular removal of soiled litters will reduce urea contamination of the environment.
- Increase ventilation of housing
- Humidifier or vaporizer: this may provide a humid environment that may increase the bacterial load
- Stabilizing the environment: temporary indoor housing may assist some animals in recovery because they are less likely to be exposed to varying environmental temperatures
- Rhinostomy and rhinotomy surgical procedures may be considered in chronic cases unresponsive to medical therapy.

DRUG INTERACTIONS

Care should be undertaken with antibiotic therapy because of the predilection for intestinal dysbiosis, in particular with beta-lactams and macrolides.

POSSIBLE COMPLICATIONS

- Recurrence may be common owing to alterations in nasal turbinate architecture.
- Bacterial rhinitis can extend into the nasolacrimal duct, causing conjunctivitis. It can also result in otitis media and possibly vestibular disease via the eustachian tubes.
- Severe bacterial rhinitis may result in pneumonia.

PROGNOSIS AND OUTCOME

- Prognosis varies according to underlying causes of the disorder. Prognosis can vary widely and should be assessed on an individual basis.
- Elimination of bacterial rhinitis may not be possible owing to bacteria retained deep in the nasal passages.
- Primary and secondary bacterial infections can be lifelong, requiring continuing or intermittent treatment. This can provide individuals with good quality of life, although ongoing treatment requires owner dedication and early detection of recurrence.
- Chronic upper respiratory disease can result from damage to the nasal turbinates and subsequent secondary bacterial infection.
- Dyspnea (and especially open-mouth breathing) is a poor prognostic indicator.

CONTROVERSY

- *Pasteurella multocida:* prevalence of this pathogen in upper respiratory tract disease may be exaggerated. Full investigation into other causes of disease and awareness of secondary pathogens are required, although investigation often is not undertaken for various reasons. Antibody testing proves only exposure to the organism, not the cause of the disease.
- Corticosteroid treatment: corticosteroid treatment predisposing to an acute presentation of a chronic disorder is a controversial subject

PEARLS & CONSIDERATIONS

PREVENTION

- Good sanitation and low levels of environmental ammonia
- Stable environment to decrease stressors
- Low stocking rates

SUGGESTED READINGS

DiGiacomo RF, et al: Atrophic rhinitis in New Zealand white rabbits infected with *Pasteurella multocida*, Am J Vet Res 50:1460–1465, 1989.

Rougier S, et al: Epidemiology and susceptibility of pathogenic bacteria responsible for upper respiratory tract infections in pet rabbits, Vet Microbiol 115:192–198, 2006.

CROSS-REFERENCES TO OTHER SECTIONS

Conjunctival disorders
Dental disease
Lower respiratory tract disorders
Otitis
Pasteurellosis
Staphylococcosis
Vestibular disease

AUTHOR: **NARELLE WALTER**

EDITOR: **DAVID VELLA**

RABBITS

Uterine Disorders

BASIC INFORMATION

DEFINITION

Any disease process that affects the integrity or function of the uterus

SPECIAL SPECIES CONSIDERATIONS

Rabbits are induced ovulators (i.e., rabbits do not show an estrous cycle, and ovulation is dependent on coitus).

EPIDEMIOLOGY

SPECIES, AGE, SEX

- Intact female
- Uterine adenocarcinoma is rare in females younger than 2 years of age

but is present in approximately 60% of females after 4 years of age.

GENETICS AND BREED PREDISPOSITION Dutch, Tan, French Silver, Havana, Beveren, Chinchilla, Himalayan, and Polish rabbits are predisposed to uterine adenocarcinoma.

RISK FACTORS Previous breeding history appears to have no bearing on occurrence of neoplasia. Age is the strongest association with likelihood of uterine neoplasia.

CONTAGION AND ZOONOSIS *Pasteurella multocida* may cause transmural metritis; *Staphylococcus aureus* (see Staphylococcosis) is also a cause of infectious uterine disease. Spread may be venereal or hematogenous. *Chlamydophila* spp., *Listeria monocytogenes, Moraxella bovis, Actinomyces pyogenes, Brucella melitensis,* and *Salmonella* spp. all have been cultured from pyometra cases. Many of these bacteria can potentially infect humans.

ASSOCIATED CONDITIONS AND DISORDERS

Cystic mastitis is associated with uterine hyperplasia or neoplasia. Mammary neoplasia can be a consequence of untreated cystic mastitis.

CLINICAL PRESENTATION

DISEASE FORMS/SUBTYPES

- Benign endometrial hyperplasia
- Uterine adenoma
- Uterine adenocarcinoma
- Uterine leiomyoma
- Uterine leiomyosarcoma
- Uterine cysts
- Uterine polyps
- Hydrometra
- Mucometra
- Pyometra
- Endometrial venous aneurysms
- Endometriosis
- Many of these diseases show no obvious clinical signs.

HISTORY, CHIEF COMPLAINT

- Bloody urine
- Vulval discharge
- Infertility
- Swollen painful mammary glands
- Abdominal swelling
- Gastrointestinal stasis
- Dyspnea
- Loss of body condition

PHYSICAL EXAM FINDINGS

- Abdominal swelling with or without discomfort
- Multiple masses may be palpable cranial to the bladder if uterine enlargement is moderate. In severe cases, abdominal distention may be so great as to hinder palpation.
- Gut sounds may be reduced or absent.
- Bloody vulval discharge
- Pale mucous membranes due to anemia secondary to hemorrhage
- Fever
- Dyspnea due to lung metastases or excessive uterine enlargement may be seen in advanced disease.

ETIOLOGY AND PATHOPHYSIOLOGY

- Endometrial changes: venous aneurysms are considered a congenital defect. Previous trauma and bleeding disorders are not associated.
- Uterine adenocarcinoma is thought to be associated with the carcinogenic effects of estrogen; however, this hypothesis is controversial. Endometrial changes that may precede adenocarcinoma include endometritis, endometriosis, endometrial hyperplasia, endometrial polyps, and uterine adenoma.
- Endometriosis occurs owing to uterine contents flowing retrogradely into the peritoneal cavity through the space between the ovary and the infundibulum.
- Hydrometra: occurs as the result of accumulation of fluid within the uterus due to outflow obstruction (e.g., by endometrial hyperplasia). Increased secretion of fluids occurs when the uterus is under progesterone dominance (e.g., during pseudopregnancy [see Pseudopregnancy]).
- *Mucometra* refers to a form of hydrometra in which the fluid is mucinous.
- Pyometra: develops when the uterus is under the influence of progesterone, which initiates endometrial growth and secretions, providing a medium for bacterial colonization. It may be an endpoint of benign endometrial hyperplasia.

DIAGNOSIS

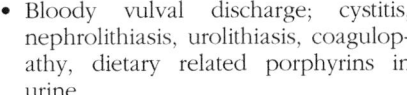

DIFFERENTIAL DIAGNOSIS

- Bloody vulval discharge; cystitis, nephrolithiasis, urolithiasis, coagulopathy, dietary related porphyrins in urine
- Gastrointestinal stasis: multiple causes
- Dyspnea: multiple causes
- Abdominal swellings: gastric tympany/bloat, pregnancy, ascites/abdominal effusions, organomegaly, mass lesions related to other structures, obesity

INITIAL DATABASE

- Complete blood count and blood biochemistry
- Urinalysis to rule out urinary system causes of clinical signs. In rabbits, urine fills the vaginal vault on voiding; therefore vulval discharges can appear as urinary problems.
- Abdominal ultrasonography
- Abdominal radiography
- Thoracic radiography (important to check for pulmonary metastases before anesthesia or sedation)
- Cytologic testing of vulval swab to determine characteristics of discharge

ADVANCED OR CONFIRMATORY TESTING

- Bacterial culture and sensitivity of any discharges, or aspirates from uterus
- Histopathologic examination of uterus
- Serologic testing for *Pasteurella multocida*

TREATMENT

THERAPEUTIC GOALS

- Depends on whether the rabbit is required for breeding
- Removal of cause of disease (e.g., ovariohysterectomy) and prevention of subsequent problems is the goal in pet rabbits.
- In breeding animals, a return to normal fertility may be the ultimate goal.

ACUTE GENERAL TREATMENT

- Provide fluid and nutritional support.
- Give blood transfusion if indicated.
- Initiate broad-spectrum antibiotics pending bacteriologic testing results (e.g., enrofloxacin 10 mg/kg PO q 12 h; metronidazole 20 mg/kg PO q 12 h; trimethoprim/sulfamethoxazole 30 mg/kg PO q 12 h).
- Ovariohysterectomy once patient is stable, if not intended for future breeding

CHRONIC TREATMENT

- Chemotherapeutic regimens for disseminated uterine adenocarcinoma; currently little information on chemotherapeutic protocols is available.
- Long-term NSAID treatment (e.g., meloxicam 0.3-0.5 mg/kg PO q 12-24 h)

POSSIBLE COMPLICATIONS

- Loss of subsequent fertility
- With uterine adenocarcinoma, metastatic spread to distant parts of body may occur (e.g., peritoneum, sublumbar lymph nodes, liver, lungs, bones).

RECOMMENDED MONITORING

Regular radiographic monitoring of thorax to screen for metastases in cases of uterine adenocarcinoma. Every 3 to 6 months is recommended.

PROGNOSIS AND OUTCOME

- Depends on cause of problem
- Good prognosis after ovariohysterectomy in cases of hydrometra,

mucometra, pyometra, uterine venous aneurysm, and uterine adenoma
- Guarded prognosis if uterine adenocarcinoma, particularly if dissemination has already occurred at time of diagnosis

CONTROVERSY

The role of estrogen in the development of uterine adenocarcinoma is uncertain.

PEARLS & CONSIDERATIONS

PREVENTION

Early neutering for females not intended for reproduction

CLIENT EDUCATION

Advise on neutering, and provide the reasons for and advantages associated with this procedure.

SUGGESTED READINGS

Elsinghorst TA, et al: Comparative pathology of endometrial carcinoma, Vet Q 6:200–208, 1984.

Johnson JH, et al: Ovarian abscesses and pyometra in a domestic rabbit, J Am Vet Med Assoc 203:667–669, 1993.

Saito K, et al: Uterine disorders diagnosed by ventrotomy in 47 rabbits, J Vet Med Sci 64:495–497, 2002.

Walter B, et al: Uterine disorders in 59 rabbits, Vet Rec 166:230–233, 2010.

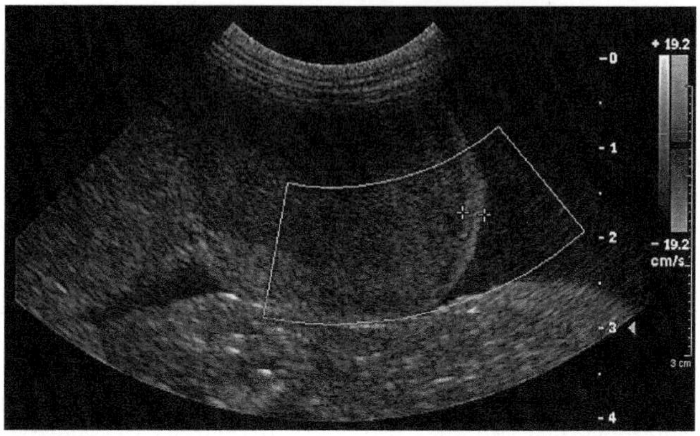

Uterine Disorders Ultrasound image of a uterine mass due to endometrial adenocarcinoma. Ultrasonography is the imaging modality of choice for visualization of the uterus. *(Photo courtesy Jörg Mayer, The University of Georgia, Athens.)*

CROSS-REFERENCES TO OTHER SECTIONS

Abscesses
Lower Urinary Tract Disorders
Mammary Gland Disorders
Pasteurellosis
Pregnancy Toxemia
Pseudopregnancy
Staphylococcosis

AUTHOR: **MOLLY VARGA**

EDITOR: **DAVID VELLA**

RABBITS

Uveitis

Client Education Sheet Available on Website

BASIC INFORMATION

DEFINITION

Inflammation of part of or the entire uveal tract, including iris, ciliary body, and choroid. May be associated with inflammation of adjacent structures such as retina, vitreous, lens, sclera, and cornea

SYNONYMS

- Anterior uveitis: iridocyclitis, cyclitis
- Panuveitis (inflammation of the entire uveal tract)
- Posterior uveitis: choroiditis, chorioretinitis, retinochoroiditis

SPECIAL SPECIES CONSIDERATIONS

- The primary cause of uveitis in rabbits is *Encephalitozoon cuniculi*–induced phacoclastic uveitis (*phaco* = lens-shaped; *clastic* = breaking up into pieces).
- Posterior uveitis is rarely seen in rabbits.

EPIDEMIOLOGY

SPECIES, AGE, SEX *E cuniculi* phacoclastic uveitis is seen more frequently in young rabbits (<2 years age).

CONTAGION AND ZOONOSIS *E cuniculi* is a potential zoonotic agent.

ASSOCIATED CONDITIONS AND DISORDERS
- Because uveitis has an immune complex basis, any antigen, endogenous or exogenous, is a potential initiator of uveal inflammation.
- Uveitis associated with *E. cuniculi* is likely to have associated systemic signs (e.g., central nervous system disorders).

CLINICAL PRESENTATION

HISTORY, CHIEF COMPLAINT Owner typically presents rabbit for change in appearance of the affected eye(s) and/or intraocular white mass.

PHYSICAL EXAM FINDINGS
- Conjunctiva and episclera
  - Red
- Cornea
  - Corneal edema of varying degrees, depending upon corneal endothelial cell damage. This occurs as a direct consequence of trauma or via interference by cellular aggregates from the inflamed iris (keratic precipitates [KPs]).
  - Corneal vascularization is also variable. Typically, vessels invading the corneal stroma are deep and straight rather than branching.
- Anterior chamber
  - Aqueous flare (cloudiness of the aqueous humor caused by increased protein levels)
  - Fibrin clots
  - Hyphema (blood in anterior chamber)
  - Hypopyon (pus in anterior chamber): may be confused easily with fibrin
- Iris
  - Color changes (e.g., blue iris becomes brown, brown iris becomes darker or depigmented)
  - Texture changes (e.g., thickened iris with visible neovascularization, as in rubeosis iridis)
  - Changes in contour (e.g., nodular appearance of the iris surface is often pink or white)
- Pupil
  - Often relatively constricted (miotic)
- Lens
  - Varying degrees of cataract
- Intraocular pressure (IOP) is low because of reduced aqueous

production by the inflamed ciliary body
  - Secondary glaucoma can occur. The pupil will dilate.

ETIOLOGY AND PATHOPHYSIOLOGY

- All types of uveitis involve tissue damage with potential vision loss (e.g., cataract formation).
- Clinical signs are attributed to disruption of the blood-ocular barrier (physiologic mechanism that prevents exchange of materials between blood and chambers of the eye) and release of numerous chemical mediators following tissue damage.
- Causes
  - Systemic illnesses
    - Endogenous source of immune complexes (e.g., bacterial infections)
  - Blunt and perforating trauma (e.g., ulcerative keratitis, surgical trauma [exogenous uveitis])
  - Lens-induced
    - Rapidly developing or hypermature cataracts leaking soluble lens proteins into the eye causing lens-induced uveitis (phacolytic or phacoclastic uveitis)
    - *E. cuniculi* causes phacoclastic uveitis by lens rupture.
  - Primary or secondary intraocular neoplasia (uncommon)

DIAGNOSIS

DIFFERENTIAL DIAGNOSIS

- Glaucoma
- Conjunctivitis
- Episcleritis or scleritis
- Keratitis
- Orbital disease

INITIAL DATABASE

- Complete ocular examination of both eyes
- IOP because glaucoma is a frequent complication of uveitis
  - Normal range in rabbits is 15 to 23 mm Hg.
  - A measurement of <10 mm Hg is consistent with uveitis; >30 mm Hg is consistent with glaucoma.
- Thorough general physical examination and history as systemic causes for uveitis are common.
- *E. cuniculi* titer
  - Positive titer indicates exposure to *E. cuniculi,* and lens-induced uveitis is a possible diagnosis.
  - Negative titer indicates no exposure to *E. cuniculi,* and lens-induced uveitis is highly unlikely.
- Ocular ultrasound is helpful in that opaque aqueous humor precludes thorough examination.
- Unless the cause is obvious, a systemic workup with complete blood count, serum biochemistry profile, and urinalysis is indicated.

ADVANCED OR CONFIRMATORY TESTING

Anterior chamber aqueous centesis in selective cases for culture, cytologic examination, and titers (refer to veterinary ophthalmologist)

TREATMENT

THERAPEUTIC GOALS

- Ameliorate the inflammation before inflammatory sequelae produce blindness.
- Whether rabbit is in pain is difficult to evaluate. If concomitant anorexia, treat for pain.
- Treat for *E. cuniculi* if infection suspected.

ACUTE GENERAL TREATMENT

In general, topical therapies are used for anterior uveitis.

- Reduce ocular inflammation with antiinflammatory drugs:
  - Corticosteroids
    - Topical and/or systemic depending on severity and location of uveitis.
    - Start with frequent dose, q 4-6 h, for topical (e.g., prednisolone acetate 1% or dexamethasone 0.1%) and antiinflammatory doses of systemic drug (e.g., prednisone 1 mg/kg per day).
  - Nonsteroidal antiinflammatory drugs (NSAIDs)
    - Topical and/or systemic depending on severity and location of uveitis
    - Topical (flurbiprofen, diclofenac, or ketorolac q 4-6 h, depending on severity of disease) and/or systemic (meloxicam 0.3 mg/kg PO q 24 h)
- Do not use systemic glucocorticoids and systemic NSAIDs concurrently because of their potential to cause gastrointestinal ulceration.
- Control ocular pain and prevent synechiae.
  - Topical atropine 1% q 12 h to dilate the pupil (i.e., mydriatic) in acute cases to minimize posterior synechiae and to prevent spasms of the ciliary body muscle (i.e., cycloplegic) that contribute to pain.
- Other therapies
  - If an infectious agent is the initiating cause, provide specific anti-infective therapy.
    - Focal abscesses in the iris can be treated with a combination of topical (e.g., ciprofloxacin q 6 h) and systemic antibiotics.
    - For *E. cuniculi,* treat with oral fenbendazole (20 mg/kg PO q 24 h × 28 d).
  - Tissue plasminogen activator 25 μg injected into the anterior chamber dissolves fibrin clots (refer to veterinary ophthalmologist).

CHRONIC TREATMENT

- After 7 to 10 days, antiinflammatory therapy is usually reduced in frequency if uveitis is controlled, and is continued for several weeks at a lower frequency and/or systemic dose.
- Lens removal by phacoemulsification may be essential if lens-induced uveitis is the cause.

DRUG INTERACTIONS

Use caution when applying any antiinflammatory agent to the cornea in the presence of corneal infection.

POSSIBLE COMPLICATIONS

- Blindness
- Glaucoma
- Cataracts
- Synechiae (adhesions) resulting in pupil immobility
- Retinal detachment
- Corneal opacity
- Prolonged ocular hypotony (low IOP) and eyeball shrinkage

RECOMMENDED MONITORING

- Animals with acute, severe forms of uveitis should be monitored frequently until inflammation begins to subside, and then weekly and biweekly.
- IOP should be monitored:
  - Because uveitis subsides and aqueous humor production usually normalizes, any outflow restrictions from adhesions/synechiae may become manifest as glaucoma and require therapy.

PROGNOSIS AND OUTCOME

- The prognosis is highly variable depending on severity of inflammation, stage at presentation, and underlying cause.
- Any significant inflammation of the interior of the eye should have a guarded prognosis for maintenance of ocular function.
- Atrophied (phthisis) eyeballs may require enucleation.

CONTROVERSY

- Use of topical ophthalmic corticosteroids in rabbits is controversial owing to systemic absorption and potential side effects.

- Topical corticosteroids are more effective than NSAIDs in reducing inflammation associated with uveitis.

PEARLS & CONSIDERATIONS

COMMENTS

- Phacoclastic uveitis in domestic animals and humans is usually caused by ocular trauma. In rabbits, it is primarily due to *E. cuniculi.*
- Not all cases of anterior uveitis in the rabbit are lens-induced.
  - *Pasteurella multocida*–associated cases may be encountered with a more classical uveitis characterized by episcleral congestion, miosis (pupil contraction), and hypopyon (pus in anterior chamber).
  - Some *P. multocida*–associated iridal inflammation is difficult to differentiate from lens-induced inflammatory disease, and anterior chamber paracentesis may be necessary.
  - Culture, cytologic examination, and titers

SUGGESTED READINGS

Felchle LM, et al: Phacoemulsification for the management of *Encephalitozoon cuniculi*-induced phacoclastic uveitis in a rabbit, Vet Ophthalmol 5:211–215, 2002.

Stiles J, et al: *Encephalitozoon cuniculi* in the lens of a rabbit with phacoclastic uveitis: confirmation and treatment, Vet Comp Ophthalmol 7:233–238, 1997.

CROSS-REFERENCES TO OTHER SECTIONS

Buphthalmia and Glaucoma
Cataracts
Conjunctival Disorders
Encephalitozoonosis
Pasteurellosis

AUTHORS: **THOMAS M. DONNELLY AND JEFFREY SMITH**

EDITOR: **DAVID VELLA**

RABBITS

Vestibular Disease

BASIC INFORMATION

DEFINITION

- The vestibular system is responsible for coordinating the position and movement of the head with those of the eyes, trunk, and limbs.
- Vestibular disease describes any disorder that disrupts this system.

SYNONYMS

Torticollis, wryneck, head tilt, labyrinthitis

EPIDEMIOLOGY

GENETICS AND BREED PREDISPOSITION Limited research suggests that vestibular disease in dwarf breeds is more likely to be due to granulomatous inflammation associated with *Encephalitozoon cuniculi* infection (central vestibular disease). Conversely, otitis media/interna with *Pasteurella multocida* infection may be a more likely cause in standard/laboratory breeds (peripheral vestibular disease).

RISK FACTORS

- Immune suppression
- Chronic upper respiratory infection
- Chronic ear disease
- Trauma
- Overzealous ear cleaning
- Exposure to feed contaminated with cat, raccoon, or skunk feces

CONTAGION AND ZOONOSIS

- The two primary differential diagnoses—*Encephalitozoon cuniculi* and *Pasteurella multocida*—are contagious. *E. cuniculi* is most often transmitted via ingestion of spores from the urine of infected rabbits. Transmission also occurs by inhalation and transplacentally. *P. multocida* is transmitted between rabbits by aerosol, direct contact, fomites, or venereally.
- Although transmission from rabbits to humans has not been documented, *E. cuniculi* does cause severe, life-threatening disease in humans with compromised immune function.
- Rabies is a less likely differential diagnosis but is a serious zoonosis.

GEOGRAPHY AND SEASONALITY Reported worldwide; no seasonality

ASSOCIATED CONDITIONS AND DISORDERS

- Rabbits with encephalitozoonosis may also have renal dysfunction and/or ocular lesions.
- Rabbits with pasteurellosis may also have upper and/or lower respiratory signs.
- Encephalitis or meningoencephalitis may accompany vestibular disorders, depending on the underlying cause.

CLINICAL PRESENTATION

HISTORY, CHIEF COMPLAINT

- Head tilt: usually acute onset
- Nystagmus
- Ataxia
- Circling
- Rolling
- Often described by owners as a "stroke"

PHYSICAL EXAM FINDINGS

- Head tilt: usually toward the lesion
- Spontaneous nystagmus
- Strabismus
- Ataxia
- Circling: usually toward the lesion
- Lateral recumbency and whole-body rolling: usually toward the lesion (central vestibular disease [CVD])

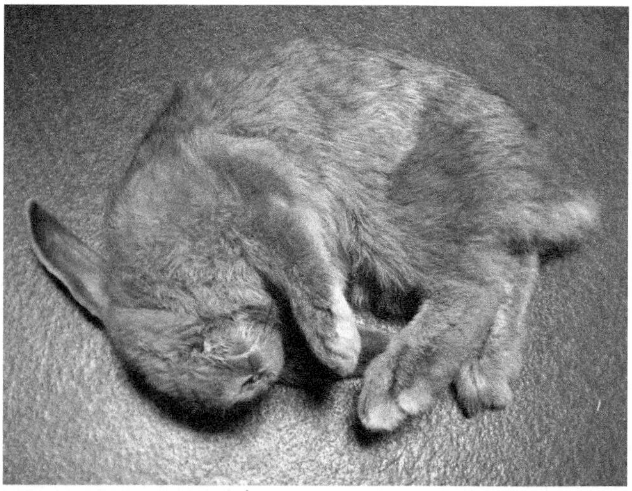

Vestibular Disease A rabbit with vestibular disease displaying severe head tilt and lateral recumbency. Regardless of whether the disease is central or peripheral, the head tilt is usually toward the direction of the lesion. *(Photo courtesy Jörg Mayer, The University of Georgia, Athens.)*

- Exudate within the external auditory canal in cases with otitis media
- Mental state:
  - CVD: likely to be altered (e.g., depression, stupor)
  - Peripheral vestibular disease (PVD): usually alert but may be disoriented
- Cranial nerve deficits (e.g., facial nerve paralysis) in cases of PVD
- Postural reaction deficits
- Wide head excursions, crouched stance, or an inability to stand may be observed with bilateral disease.
- Other neurologic signs (e.g., behavioral changes, seizures, hypermetria, intention tremors)

ETIOLOGY AND PATHOPHYSIOLOGY

- Etiology
  - PVD
    - Bacterial otitis interna (e.g., due to pasteurellosis [common], *Pseudomonas aeruginosa, Staphylococcus aureus*)
    - Toxins (e.g., aminoglycosides, lead)
    - Trauma (e.g., aggressive flushing, petrosal bone/tympanic bulla fracture)
    - Neoplasia (rare)
    - Idiopathic
  - CVD
    - Central nervous system parasitism (e.g., *E. cuniculi* [common], *Baylisascaris* spp., cerebral larval migrans [in endemic areas], toxoplasmosis)
    - Central nervous system infection (e.g., brain abscessation, brainstem meningoencephalitis with *Listeria monocytogenes*, herpesvirus encephalitis, rabies [in endemic areas], human herpes simplex 1 virus)
    - Immune-mediated encephalitis/meningoencephalitis
    - Trauma
    - Primary or metastatic neoplasia
    - Cerebrovascular disease
    - Degenerative disease
    - Hypovitaminosis A (rare)
    - Toxicity (e.g., lead, metronidazole [rare])
- Pathophysiology: damage to one or more of the following vestibular system components:
  - Peripheral vestibular system
    - Labyrinth within the inner ear and surrounding petrous temporal bone
    - Vestibular nerve that runs through the internal acoustic meatus
  - Central vestibular system
    - Vestibular nuclei within the medulla oblongata
    - Vestibular pathways of the brainstem and spinal cord
    - Components within the cerebellum or caudal cerebellar peduncle

DIAGNOSIS

DIFFERENTIAL DIAGNOSIS

- Otitis externa or media (causing temporary head tilt due to aural discomfort)
- Cervical muscle contraction
- Cervical scoliosis

INITIAL DATABASE

- Based on neurologic examination, aim to differentiate between central and peripheral vestibular disease.
- Complete blood count and serum biochemistry analysis: results may be normal
- Urinalysis: results may be normal. Gram stain of urine sediment may demonstrate protozoal spores that are excreted in the urine from 1 month postinfection until 3 months postinfection.
- Serologic assay to detect exposure to *E. cuniculi*
- PCR for *E. cuniculi* on urine or feces
- Otoscopic examination to rule out otitis externa and to assess integrity of tympanic membrane (when possible). The tympanic membrane may be discolored and bulging in cases of otitis media.
- Skull radiography may reveal increased opacity of the bullae or sclerosis, periosteal proliferation, or lysis of surrounding bone. However, in many cases, no demonstrable radiographic changes are noted.
- Examination of the pharynx (under deep sedation or general anesthesia) to detect purulent material or inflammation that may suggest otitis media due to bacteria of respiratory tract origin (e.g., *Pasteurella multocida*).

ADVANCED OR CONFIRMATORY TESTING

- Skull CT scan, especially if PVD is suspected
- Skull MRI provides excellent resolution of brain parenchyma; especially useful for investigating cases of suspected CVD
- Cerebrospinal fluid analysis to rule out encephalitis; sample from the cerebromedullary cistern
- Serologic testing for *Toxoplasma gondii*
- Bulla osteotomy to obtain material from the middle ear for culture
- Some cases may be definitively diagnosed only on postmortem examination, including histopathologic analysis of tissues.

TREATMENT

THERAPEUTIC GOALS

- Treatment should be based on the definitive diagnosis if it can be ascertained.
- Often empirical treatment will need to be started before results of the initial database are obtained.
- General supportive care should be provided.
- Rabbits with severe vestibular signs (e.g., uncontrollable rolling) and associated anorexia that fail to improve with initial treatment should be considered candidates for euthanasia.

ACUTE GENERAL TREATMENT

- Otitis media/interna
  - Systemic antibiotic therapy (e.g., oral or parenteral enrofloxacin 10 mg/kg q 12 h, trimethoprim/sulfa 30 mg/kg q 12 h, subcutaneous procaine benzylpenicillin 60,000 IU/kg q 2-7 d)
  - Lavage of middle ear with saline if tympanic membrane has ruptured
  - Analgesia with nonsteroidal anti-inflammatory drugs and/or opioids
  - Ocular lubrication if eyelid function is compromised
  - Supportive care, including assisted (hand or syringe) feeding, fluid therapy, and gut prokinetic medication, when indicated
- Encephalitozoonosis: oral benzimidazole therapy (e.g., fenbendazole 20 mg/kg q 24 h for 28 days; albendazole 20-30 mg/kg q 24 h for 30 days, then 15 mg/kg q 24 h for 30 days)
- Toxoplasmosis: trimethoprim-sulfa drugs, pyrimethamine, doxycycline
- Visceral larval migrans: oral oxibendazole 60 mg/kg q 24 h indefinitely and nonsteroidal antiinflammatory treatment (e.g., meloxicam 0.3-0.5 mg/kg PO q 24 h)
- General supportive care (all cases):
  - If signs are severe, ensure that cage is padded with deep bedding to prevent self-trauma.
  - Prochlorperazine, cyclizine, or meclizine to reduce disorientation
  - Short-term sedation with diazepam or midazolam (0.5 mg/kg SC) may be helpful in acute cases with severe neurologic signs.
  - Nutritional support (if unable to eat)
  - Fluid therapy (if unable to drink or dehydrated)
  - Metoclopramide to prevent nausea (which is known to accompany vestibular disorders in other species)

CHRONIC TREATMENT

- Prolonged course of antibiotics may be required for otitis media/interna (minimum, 4 to 6 weeks); ideally, drug selection is based on culture and sensitivity results.
- Daily gentle massaging of the neck muscles may help reduce spasms.
- If medical therapy is unsuccessful, bulla osteotomy or total ear canal

ablation may be considered for otitis media.
- Surgical resection of abscesses or tumors if accessible

POSSIBLE COMPLICATIONS

- A permanent, often mild, head tilt may persist after resolution of other clinical signs.
- Recurrence of head tilt following initial resolution is also possible, depending on the underlying cause.
- Other neurologic signs (e.g., urinary incontinence, development of perineal urine scald), seizures, hind limb paresis, deterioration of mental status
- Pressure sores from prolonged recumbency
- Aspiration secondary to abnormal body posture (especially if being syringe-fed)

RECOMMENDED MONITORING

- Regular monitoring of severity of head tilt and other neurologic signs
- Serial *E. cuniculi* titers

PROGNOSIS AND OUTCOME

- Dependent on the underlying cause and the severity of clinical signs
- Otitis media: dependent on the chronicity of the disease, the extent of bone involvement, and the reversibility of neurologic damage; generally fair to poor
- Encephalitozoonosis: fair to poor
- Encephalitis: guarded to poor
- Cerebral larval migrans: guarded to poor
- Neoplasia: poor

CONTROVERSY

- Administration of corticosteroids is controversial and in most situations is considered inappropriate. Although these drugs may reduce the inflammatory response to neurologic cell damage (e.g., in encephalitozoonosis), rabbits are highly sensitive to the immune suppressive and gastrointestinal effects of corticosteroids. Such treatment may in fact worsen the clinical outcome.
- If corticosteroids are used, a low dose of a short-acting formulation is preferred to reduce the risk of adverse effects. Providing some antibiotic cover concurrently is recommended.

PEARLS & CONSIDERATIONS

COMMENTS

- Some cases will spontaneously resolve or will improve over a period of weeks with or without treatment.
- Compensation for vestibular disorders will occur in many rabbits, regardless of lesion location. In such cases, clinical signs appear to wane somewhat with time despite the persistence of a head tilt.

PREVENTION

- Prompt investigation; treatment and isolation of rabbits with upper respiratory, neurologic, renal, and/or external ear signs
- Prophylactic fenbendazole has been shown to prevent experimental infection with *E. cuniculi* (20 mg/kg once daily for 9 days).
- Avoid access to skunk, raccoon, and cat feces.
- Select seronegative rabbits for breeding if possible.

CLIENT EDUCATION

- *E. cuniculi* is potentially zoonotic.
- Appropriate handling of this species can avoid unnecessary trauma.
- Encourage high standard of sanitation to minimize spread of infectious agents.
- Response to therapy may be unpredictable.
- Long-term nursing may be required.

SUGGESTED READINGS

Keeble E: Common neurological and musculoskeletal problems in rabbits, In Pract 28:212–218, 2006.

Rosenthal KR: Torticollis in rabbits, Proc North Am Vet Conf 2005:1378–1379, 2005.

CROSS-REFERENCES TO OTHER SECTIONS

Abscesses
Ectoparasites
Encephalitis
Encephalitozoonosis
Endoparasites
Otitis
Pasteurellosis
Renal Disorders
Staphylococcosis
Upper Respiratory Tract Disorders

AUTHOR: **MICHELLE L. CAMPBELL-WARD**

EDITOR: **DAVID VELLA**

FERRETS

Adrenal Disease

Client Education Sheet Available on Website

BASIC INFORMATION

DEFINITION

A condition in which a neoplastic change of the adrenal cortex results in increased androgens and/or estrogen in ferrets

SYNONYMS

Adrenal disease, adrenal gland disease, adrenal neoplasia, adrenal tumor, adrenocortical disease, adrenal endocrinopathy, hyperadrenocorticism

SPECIAL SPECIES CONSIDERATIONS

Ferrets are seasonal breeders. In the winter, when each day has less than 12 hours of light, plasma melatonin concentrations are high, resulting in a thick winter coat. High melatonin concentrations also suppress the release of gonadotropin-releasing hormone (GnRH) from the hypothalamus. With increasing day length, this suppression is lost and GnRH is released, resulting in the pulsatile release of luteinizing hormone (LH) and follicle-stimulating hormone (FSH) from the pituitary gland. These hormones in turn stimulate the release of estrogen and testosterone from the gonads, which in turn exert negative feedback on the hypothalamus and pituitary gland, resulting in suppression of release of GnRH, LH, and FSH. When ferrets are neutered, this negative feedback is lost, resulting in increased release of LH and FSH, which may promote steroidogenesis and induce nonneoplastic and neoplastic adrenocortical enlargement.

EPIDEMIOLOGY

SPECIES, AGE, SEX

- Ferrets 3 years of age and older are usually affected, but adrenal disease has been found in younger ferrets.
- There is no sex predilection.

GENETICS AND BREED PREDISPOSITION Although a genetic background has been suggested, a gene responsible for adrenal disease has not been detected.

RISK FACTORS Neutering most likely plays an important role in the origin of the disease.

GEOGRAPHY AND SEASONALITY Although the incidence of adrenal disease is considered prominent in the United States, it occurs as frequently in the Netherlands. In the United Kingdom, adrenal disease is being diagnosed more often, possibly because of a shift in neutering and indoor housing. These latter two factors are more probable risk factors for adrenal disease than geographic location.

ASSOCIATED CONDITIONS AND DISORDERS Ferrets commonly have multiple concurrent diseases. Frequently, a ferret with adrenal disease also has an insulinoma or a malignant lymphoma. Periprostatic cysts may be observed in males.

CLINICAL PRESENTATION

HISTORY, CHIEF COMPLAINT

- Clinical signs include
  - Symmetric alopecia, often starting at the base of the tail and then progressing cranially. The skin usually is not affected, although some excoriations may be seen.
  - Pruritus
  - Recurrence of sexual behavior after neutering
  - Vulvar swelling in neutered female ferrets
  - Occasional mammary gland enlargement in female ferrets
  - Urinary blockage in males due to periprostatic or periurethral cysts
- Different presentations of adrenal disease are possible depending on which clinical signs are most prominent. For example,
  - Alopecia is commonly seen, but many cases of adrenal disease have been diagnosed in ferrets without alopecia.
  - Pruritus or stranguria may be the only presenting clinical sign in some ferrets.

PHYSICAL EXAM FINDINGS

- Except for alopecia and vulvar swelling, no striking abnormalities are found during physical examination.
- During abdominal palpation, the left adrenal gland may be found, but abdominal fat may be a limiting factor.
- The right adrenal gland is more difficult to palpate because it is located more cranial and lays dorsal to the caudal vena cava and caudate lobe of the liver.

ETIOLOGY AND PATHOPHYSIOLOGY

- The most likely cause is neutering, which results in increased LH concentrations that activate LH receptors on adrenal cells. Continuous LH stimulation eventually leads to tumor formation in the adrenal cortex.
- A frequent suggestion is that neutering of very young ferrets causes adrenal disease. This is unlikely because ferrets are not neutered at an early age in the Netherlands, yet adrenal disease is just as common as it is in the United States.
- Increased light exposure, from ferrets being kept indoors, has also been suggested as a contributing factor for adrenal disease. This hypothesis is in agreement with increased LH levels. During increased light exposure, ferrets are under the influence of LH for a longer period compared with those kept under natural light conditions.
- Inbreeding (genetic background): although no specific genes have been identified, the genetic profile of ferrets may explain why this condition is seen in these animals, and not in other species routinely neutered.

DIAGNOSIS

DIFFERENTIAL DIAGNOSIS

- Functional ovarian remnant
- Seasonal alopecia: some clinicians speculate that seasonal alopecia is a very early sign of adrenal disease
- Food intolerance (allergy): clinical signs are identical to those of ferrets with adrenal disease

INITIAL DATABASE

- Clinical signs are the most useful tool in diagnosing adrenal disease.
- Clinical pathology
  - Obtain an "adrenal panel" consisting of estradiol, androstenedione, and 17α-hydroxyprogesterone measurements from a blood sample to see whether these hormones are elevated. However, the adrenal panel is of limited use in diagnosing adrenal disease because these hormones are also elevated in ferrets with a functional ovarian remnant. The adrenal panel will not allow differentiation between these two diseases.
  - Ovarian remnants are seen more commonly outside the United States, in countries where ferrets are kept for hunting.
  - The hormones within the adrenal panel have greater value in monitoring the effects of treatment.
  - For reference values, it is important to use those established by the laboratory that measures the adrenal panel, because results may vary significantly between the assays used.
- Urine
  - Urinary corticoid creatinine ratio (UCCR) is elevated in ferrets with adrenal disease. However, this test is unable to discriminate between a ferret with adrenal disease and a functional ovarian remnant.

ADVANCED OR CONFIRMATORY TESTING

- Abdominal ultrasound
  - Highly useful in locating affected adrenal gland(s); provides information on surgical possibilities
  - Potential remnant ovaries can also be located.
  - The prostate can be evaluated.
  - Concurrent disease, such as malignant lymphoma and insulinoma, may be found.

TREATMENT

THERAPEUTIC GOALS

- Alleviate clinical signs (e.g., relieve urinary blockage, address adrenal tumor, regrowth of fur).
- Surgically remove the tumor.
- Prevent recurrence of adrenal disease (e.g., hormone therapy with depot GnRH agonist).
- Depending on different circumstances (e.g., age of the ferret, adrenal gland involved, concurrent medical conditions of the ferret, financial restrictions of the owner), the owner may choose surgery, hormone therapy, or a combination.

ACUTE GENERAL TREATMENT

- For urinary blockage in males,
  - Insert a 3.5 Fr urinary catheter or a prepubic catheter to ensure proper bladder emptying.
  - Urinary tract catheterization is not always possible.
- The ideal treatment is a combination of unilateral adrenalectomy and hormone treatment with a depot GnRH agonist.
  - Leuprolide acetate 100 mcg per month SC for ferrets weighing <1 kg; 200 mcg per month SC in ferrets ≥1 kg
  - The implant Suprelorin (4.7 mg or 9.4 mg deslorelin) is given SC. It is registered for use in dogs in Australia and Europe as a contraceptive and remains active for approximately 2 and 4 years, respectively. In Europe the 9.4 mg deslorelin implant is now also registered as contraceptive in male ferrets.
- A close relationship exists between the right adrenal gland and the caudal vena cava; removal of the right adrenal gland is difficult and is not always recommended. Medical management is often the most appropriate treatment. Only experienced surgeons should perform a right adrenalectomy.

- When only the left adrenal gland is affected, an adrenalectomy immediately results in a decrease in adrenal hormones and has the quickest results in reducing pruritus and diminishing the size of the prostate.
- A GnRH agonist takes ≈14 days before an effect is seen; it initially causes a rise in circulating LH, resulting in brief stimulation of adrenal hormone production.

CHRONIC TREATMENT

- The author has managed many ferrets with adrenal disease for periods greater than 2 years in duration by using depot GnRH agonists such as leuprolide acetate or deslorelin. An SC implant of deslorelin eliminates clinical signs of adrenal disease and reduces steroid hormone concentrations; a 9.4-mg SC implant works for 12 months.
- In some cases, adrenal tumors become refractory to treatment, possibly owing to autonomous adrenal hormone production.
- The size of an adrenal tumor may increase dramatically in ≈5% of cases after a treatment period of 2 years or longer.

POSSIBLE COMPLICATIONS

- As with any surgery, there are risks. This is especially true when a right adrenalectomy is attempted because of the close association of the right adrenal gland with the caudal vena cava.
- When only a unilateral adrenalectomy is performed, continuous stimulation of the contralateral adrenal gland persists. Therefore, it is critical to treat with a GnRH agonist to prevent recurrence of adrenal disease.

RECOMMENDED MONITORING

Although adrenal tumors seldom continue to grow during GnRH agonist treatment, an annual abdominal ultrasound to monitor potential growth of the adrenal tumor is recommended.

PROGNOSIS AND OUTCOME

- Adrenal tumors seldom metastasize, regardless of the histologic diagnosis.
- Ferrets can be managed medically for many years.
- Most ferrets with adrenal disease will die from unrelated conditions.

CONTROVERSY

- Treatment with melatonin (0.5 mg PO daily or a subcutaneous implant containing 5.4 mg melatonin) has been suggested. Although recurrence of a beautiful pelage has been reported in these ferrets, their hormone concentrations, in general, increased while the adrenal tumors continued to grow.
- Because melatonin is available in drug stores in the United States, it is possible that home medication will delay initial presentation to veterinarians of ferrets with adrenal disease.
- Editors' note:
  - Surgical removal of the adrenal tumor is the only curative treatment.
  - Slow-release depot formulations of deslorelin are considered
    - A safe and minimally invasive alternative to adrenalectomy
    - Especially helpful in the treatment of old or medically compromised ferrets with adrenal disease that may not be able to undergo anesthesia and surgery
    - Helpful in ferrets with adrenal disease that have previously undergone unilateral adrenalectomy
  - Long-term effects of GnRH agonist implants on adrenal gland hyperplasia or adrenal tumor growth are unknown at present.

PEARLS & CONSIDERATIONS

COMMENTS

Because ferrets are usually neutered when presented to the pet market in the United States, it seems pivotal to convince the supplier not to neuter these ferrets in the future. Unwanted sexual behavior can be prevented by the use of depot GnRH agonists such as the deslorelin implant. However, the U.S. Food and Drug Administration's Center for Veterinary Medicine has currently not approved deslorelin for use in ferrets. Therefore, its use in ferrets is "off-label."

PREVENTION

Because adrenal disease is likely due to an increase in LH after neutering, an alternative to neutering is administering a depot GnRH agonist implant, such as deslorelin, to ferrets. These implants address all the reasons for which ferrets are neutered and cause decreased gonadotropin concentrations. Whether these implants decrease the incidence of adrenal disease remains to be elucidated.

SUGGESTED READINGS

Kuijten AM, et al: Ultrasonographic visualization of the adrenal glands of healthy and hyperadrenocorticoid ferrets, J Am Anim Hosp Assoc 43:78–84, 2007.

Schoemaker NJ: Hyperadrenocorticism in ferrets, PhD thesis, The Netherlands, 2003, Utrecht University. http://igitur-archive.library.uu.nl/dissertations/2003-1128-094343/inhoud.htm. Accessed July 12, 2012.

Schoemaker NJ, et al: Use of a gonadotropin releasing hormone agonist implant as an Alternative for surgical castration in male ferrets *(Mustela putorius furo)*, Theriogenology 70:161–167, 2008.

Swiderski, JK, et al: Long-term outcome of domestic ferrets treated surgically for hyperadrenocorticism: 130 cases (1995-2004), J Am Vet Med Assoc 232:1338–1343, 2008.

Wagner RA, et al: Clinical and endocrine responses to treatment with deslorelin acetate implants in ferrets with adrenocortical disease, Am J Vet Res 66:910–914, 2005.

CROSS-REFERENCES TO OTHER SECTIONS

Hyperestrogenism Anemia
Ovarian Remnant Syndrome
Prostatic Disease

AUTHOR: **NICO J. SCHOEMAKER**

EDITORS: **JAMES G. FOX AND ROBERT MARINI**

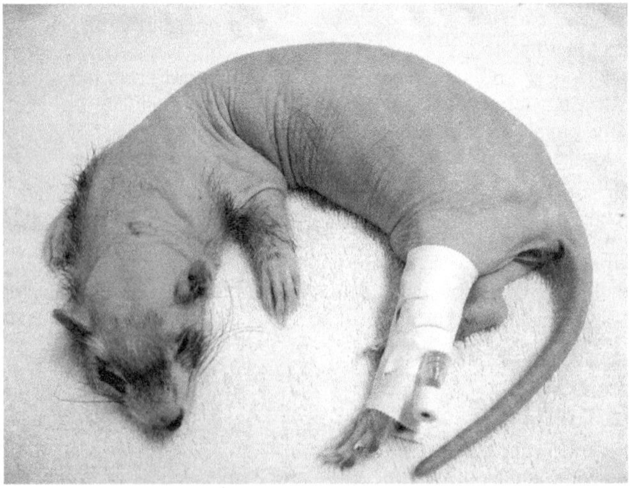

Adrenal Disease Generalized alopecia is a typical clinical sign of advanced adrenal disease in the ferret. *(Photo courtesy Jörg Mayer, The University of Georgia, Athens.)*

FERRETS

Aleutian Disease

Client Education Sheet Available on Website

BASIC INFORMATION

DEFINITION

Aleutian disease of ferrets is a disease complex with variable presentation caused by a parvovirus (Aleutian disease virus [ADV]). It was first described in mink, and much of the pertinent research on etiopathogenesis and viral characteristics was described in that species. Viruses causing Aleutian disease in ferrets are molecularly distinct from mink viruses, but cross-species infection can occur.

SPECIAL SPECIES CONSIDERATIONS

Mink of the Aleutian genotype, from which ADV derives its name, are predisposed to viral disease owing to reduced cell-mediated immune response. In adult mink, the disease is associated with immune complex glomerulonephritis, biliary hyperplasia, and arteritis; in kits, it is characterized by interstitial pneumonia. ADV-related glomerulonephritis and arteritis in ferrets may be less severe or nonexistent. In addition to mink and ferrets, antibodies to ADV have been found in raccoon, skunk, and fox. Disease associated with ADV has been reported only in ferret, mink, and skunk. Although ferret strains may infect mink, and vice versa, virulence is greater with their species-specific strain. The ferret strain of ADV is thought to have mutated from the original mink strain.

EPIDEMIOLOGY

SPECIES, AGE, SEX

- Both genders are affected.
- Most clinical cases occur in animals between 2 and 4 years old.
- Viral infections are more severe in young kits.

RISK FACTORS

- Immune suppressive conditions predispose to Aleutian disease.
- Ferret immune response plays a role in determining disease progression and outcome.

CONTAGION AND ZOONOSIS

- ADV may be transmitted by aerosol, fomite, and direct contact with ferret excreta or blood. Direct contact is considered the most important route of infection.
- Carrier ferrets may shed virus in urine and feces; viral DNA was detected in 2 of 4 urine and 2 of 2 fecal samples of a ferret without clinical signs.
- Vertical transmission has been documented in mink.
- Ease of transmission may be associated with strain virulence.
- ADV does not infect humans.

CLINICAL PRESENTATION

DISEASE FORMS/SUBTYPES

- In adult mink, three forms of the disease are described and are likely to exist in ferrets:
  - Progressive infection
  - Persistent nonprogressive infection
  - Nonpersistent, nonprogressive infection with clearance of the virus
- Most ferrets are without clinical signs.
- Disease presentation depends upon affected tissue.
- The most common disease presentations are chronic progressive wasting and ascending paresis or paralysis.

HISTORY, CHIEF COMPLAINT

- Weight loss, lethargy, inappetence
- Difficulty or inability in walking
- Seizures, muscle fasciculations
- Pallor

PHYSICAL EXAM FINDINGS Variable signs are associated with different forms of the disease.

- Chronic progressive wasting
  - Poor body condition
  - Pallor and melena if intestinal involvement or concomitant *Helicobacter mustelae* infection
  - Organomegaly (e.g., liver, spleen, mesenteric lymph node)
- Ascending neurologic disease
  - Atrophy of thigh muscles
  - Ataxia
  - Paresis to paralysis
  - Muscle fasciculation
  - Fecal and urinary staining from incontinence
  - Seizures

ETIOLOGY AND PATHOPHYSIOLOGY

- In neonates, ADV replication in type II pneumocytes culminates in interstitial pneumonia.
- In adults, the virus replicates and sequesters in macrophages and dendritic cells.
- Immune complex disease in various tissues, especially kidney, liver, and artery, is responsible for clinical signs.
- In ferrets, infiltration of multiple tissues with lymphocytes and plasma cells is the histopathologic hallmark of ADV infection.
- Lymphoplasmacytic proliferation may lead to hypergammaglobulinemia.
- Membranous glomerulopathy and vasculitis observed in mink may be less severe in ferrets.

DIAGNOSIS

DIFFERENTIAL DIAGNOSIS

- Chronic progressive wasting
  - Lymphoma
  - Eosinophilic gastroenteritis (see Eosinophilic Gastroenteritis)
  - *Helicobacter mustelae*–associated gastritis (see *Helicobacter mustelae*–Associated Gastritis and Ulcers)
  - Proliferative bowel disease (see Proliferative Bowel Disease)
  - Issues of food and water quality and access
- Posterior paresis or paralysis
  - Hypoglycemia (insulin-secreting pancreatic tumor)
  - Neoplasia (e.g., lymphoma)
  - Vertebral defect (e.g., hemivertebrae, vertebral fracture, intervertebral disk disease)
  - Hematomyelia associated with hyperestrogenism (see Hyperestrogenism Anemia)
  - Distemper (see Distemper)
  - Rabies
  - Fungal myelitis
  - *Mycobacterium* spp. infection
  - Thromboembolism

INITIAL DATABASE

- Complete blood count (animals may be anemic)
- Chemistry screen (azotemia, hypoalbuminemia, hyperglobulinemia, or elevated hepatic enzymes may be observed)
- Urinalysis (proteinuria, hematuria, casts may be seen)
- Radiography or ultrasound (to evaluate organomegaly or vertebral column integrity)

ADVANCED OR CONFIRMATORY TESTING

- If hyperglobulinemia exists, serum protein electrophoresis demonstrating that gamma globulins constitute 20% or more of total serum protein concentration is diagnostic.
- Counterimmunoelectrophoresis (CIEP)
  - This test, formerly produced by United Vaccines (Madison, WI), is a specific test for antibodies to ADV. Reportedly, it is insensitive to low titers, does not predict disease status, and does not report results in quantitative titers. It was the traditional ADV screening test but is no longer available.
- ELISA
  - A commercially available ELISA for ADV is marketed by Avecon

Diagnostics (Bath, PA) for in-house testing of blood or saliva. The test detects antibody to the NS1 protein and therefore detects only replicating virus.
 - An ELISA developed at The University of Georgia uses the entire virus and can detect chronic (persistent) disease as well as animals which have cleared the virus.
 - Use of both ELISAs is recommended.
- PCR and in situ hybridization are specific techniques available in academic settings (e.g., University of Georgia and Michigan State University).
- Histopathologic examination: submission of tissues collected by biopsy or whole organs in formalin fixative, with subsequent processing, staining, and evaluation, yields characteristic lesions.
 - Lymphoplasmacytic infiltrates in many organs
 - Renal tubular atrophy and degeneration, membranous glomerulopathy
 - Dilatation and proliferation of bile ducts
 - Vasculitis (in mink)
 - Perivascular lymphocytic cuffing in the brain and spinal cord
 - Lymphoplasmacytic meningitis
 - Hepatic periportal lymphoplasmacytic infiltrates that may have germinal centers
 - Lymphoid proliferation

TREATMENT

THERAPEUTIC GOALS

- No effective, specific antiviral therapy is available for ADV.
- Supportive care should be provided.
- No vaccine is available for ADV.

ACUTE GENERAL TREATMENT

- Supportive care directed by clinical signs and organ involvement may be palliative.
- In the short term, immune suppressive therapy (e.g., prednisone 2 mg/kg PO q 24 h) may be beneficial.

CHRONIC TREATMENT

- Immune modulatory agents (e.g., levamisole) used in mink have not been tested in ferrets and are of unknown efficacy.
- Cyclophosphamide was used to control ADV infection in mink for 16 weeks, but had no effect on viral titers.
- Melatonin may have some effect, presumably from immune modulation and antioxidant activity.

PROGNOSIS AND OUTCOME

Prognosis for ferrets with disease due to ADV is poor.

CONTROVERSY

- Culling ADV-positive ferrets that are free of clinical signs is not currently recommended.
- Breeding facilities may choose to eliminate ADV-positive jills and hobs when establishing ADV-negative colonies.

PEARLS & CONSIDERATIONS

COMMENTS

- A persistent carrier state exists.
- Hypergammaglobulinemia, pathognomonic for ADV-associated disease of mink, is not always observed in ferrets.
- A presumptive diagnosis may be made using history, clinical signs, and serology. A definitive diagnosis requires serology, PCR, in situ hybridization, and characteristic histopathologic lesions. Other diseases must be ruled out.
- Serology and PCR analysis may be used for an antemortem diagnosis of subclinical ADV infection.
- Antibodies to ADV generated by ferrets are nonprotective.

PREVENTION

- Separate housing with good sanitation probably suffices to minimize transmission in a colony or a multi-ferret household.
- Avoid handling ferrets at shows; handwashing and avoidance of potential fomites are important in preventing transmission.
- Sanitize using products with advertised efficacy against parvovirus (e.g., formalin, sodium hydroxide, phenolics, some quaternary ammonium disinfectants).

SUGGESTED READINGS

McCrackin Stevenson MA, et al: Aleutian mink disease parvovirus: implications for companion ferrets, Compend Cont Educ Pract Vet 23:178–187, 2001.

Palley LS, et al: Parvovirus-associated syndrome (Aleutian disease) in two ferrets, J Am Vet Med Assoc 201:100–106, 1992.

Pennick KE, et al: Persistent viral shedding during asymptomatic Aleutian mink disease parvoviral infection in a ferret, J Vet Diagn Invest 17:594–597, 2005.

CROSS-REFERENCES TO OTHER SECTIONS

Distemper
Eosinophilic Gastroenteritis
Helicobacter mustelae-Associated Gastritis and Ulcers
Hyperestrogenism Anemia
Insulinoma
Proliferative Bowel Disease

AUTHOR: **ROBERT P. MARINI**

EDITORS: **JAMES G. FOX**

FERRETS

Campylobacter spp. Infection

BASIC INFORMATION

DEFINITION

Campylobacter jejuni-associated diarrheal disease

SYNONYM

Campylobacteriosis

SPECIAL SPECIES CONSIDERATIONS

Similar to the disease seen in cats and dogs

EPIDEMIOLOGY

SPECIES, AGE, SEX Young weanling ferrets are most often affected; or can be diagnosed in adult ferrets

RISK FACTORS Weanling ferrets fed improperly cooked food—meat products, particularly poultry
CONTAGION AND ZOONOSIS Zoonotic risk due to fecal-oral spread of *C. jejuni*; can infect other susceptible pets in household
ASSOCIATED CONDITIONS AND DISORDERS Weanling animals with no prior acquired immunity to *C. jejuni* and loss of maternal immunity

CLINICAL PRESENTATION

DISEASE FORMS/SUBTYPES Mucus-laden, watery bile or blood-tinged diarrhea; asymptomatic infection can occur
HISTORY, CHIEF COMPLAINT Partial anorexia of several days' duration
PHYSICAL EXAM FINDINGS
- Fever
- Moderate weight loss
- Fecal staining of perineum

ETIOLOGY AND PATHOPHYSIOLOGY

- Campylobacteriosis is caused by different serotypes of *C. jejuni*.
- Inflammation of intestinal mucosa, often more pronounced in colon
- Experimentally, one can induce abortion, resorption of feti, and/or expulsion of dead feti.

DIAGNOSIS

DIFFERENTIAL DIAGNOSIS

- Proliferative colitis (see Proliferative Bowel Disease) caused by *Lawsonia* spp.
- Eosinophilic gastroenteritis
- Salmonellosis

INITIAL DATABASE

Growth of *C. jejuni* using selective media and microaerobic culture conditions

ADVANCED OR CONFIRMATORY TESTING

Organism is identified by specific biochemical tests that are readily available. Hippurate hydrolysis distinguishes *C. jejuni* from *C. coli*. PCR-based assays are available.

TREATMENT

THERAPEUTIC GOALS

- In general, efficacy of antibiotic therapy and treatment for *C. jejuni*–associated diarrhea in ferrets is unknown.
- Erythromycin, which is an effective treatment for campylobacteriosis in humans, is not effective in eradicating *C. jejuni* in ferrets. Erythromycin in feed (220 g/ton) controlled outbreak of *C. jejuni* colitis in mink kits.

ACUTE GENERAL TREATMENT

Provide parenteral fluid therapy if diarrhea is severe.

CHRONIC TREATMENT

Retreatment with other specific antibiotics such as enrofloxacin or tetracycline may be necessary.

DRUG INTERACTIONS

Monotherapy is recommended for treatment of *C. jejuni*.

POSSIBLE COMPLICATIONS

Chronic carriage of *C. jejuni* may pose continued zoonotic risk; may cause abortions

RECOMMENDED MONITORING

- Stress the importance of implementing appropriate hygienic measures.
- One may have to repeat fecal cultures to ensure absence of *C. jejuni* in feces.

PROGNOSIS AND OUTCOME

The diarrheal component of disease is usually self-limiting, even without antibiotic therapy.

CONTROVERSY

Potential for increased antibiotic-resistant *C. jejuni* in human and animal populations as a result of common use of antibiotics in feed and antibiotics sold over the counter.

PEARLS & CONSIDERATIONS

COMMENTS

Ferrets infected with *C. jejuni* pose a zoonotic risk, particularly in children.

PREVENTION

Eliminate raw or poorly cooked foods as a dietary source.

CLIENT EDUCATION

Practice sound hygienic practices when handling bedding and cages contaminated with feces, and sound handwashing using proper cleaning agents after handling ferrets.

SUGGESTED READING

Fox JG, editor: Biology and diseases of the ferret, ed 2, Baltimore, 1998, Williams & Wilkins.

CROSS-REFERENCES TO OTHER SECTIONS

Eosinophilic Gastroenteritis
Proliferative Bowel Disease

AUTHOR: **JAMES G. FOX**

EDITORS: **ROBERT P. MARINI**

FERRETS

Cataracts

BASIC INFORMATION

DEFINITION

A cataract is a complete or partial opacity of the lens or its capsule. The entire lens can be affected, or it can be localized. Cataracts result from a change in lens protein composition or lens fiber arrangement. Cataracts are the most common ferret ocular abnormality affecting vision.

SPECIAL SPECIES CONSIDERATIONS

- Progressive cataract formation has been reported in two studies of genetically unrelated populations of ferrets. In one population (n = 73), cataracts were observed in 47% of ferrets (11 to 12 months of age), and in another (n = 22), cataracts were seen in 44% of ferrets (>1 year old).
- Severity ranged from clinically insignificant, small punctate opacities in the posterior lens to blinding, complete cataracts in both anterior and posterior cortices of lens.
- In a large population (n = 3257) of juvenile ferrets (6 to 12 months age), 2.03% had bilateral cataracts and 0.15% had unilateral cataract.

EPIDEMIOLOGY

RISK FACTORS

- Anterior uveitis
- Age
- Nutritional imbalance
- Retinal degeneration
- Electrical shock

ASSOCIATED CONDITIONS AND DISORDERS

- Anterior uveitis
- Retinal degeneration
- Microphthalmia

CLINICAL PRESENTATION

DISEASE FORMS/SUBTYPES

- Cataracts are classified by age at onset, location, and severity, in addition to origin.
  - Age at onset: congenital, present at birth; juvenile, few months to 5 years; senile, >5 years
  - Location: capsule, anterior/posterior; cortex, anterior/posterior or equatorial; nucleus
  - Severity: incipient, <10% of retinal examination obstructed; immature (early, 10% to 50% of retinal examination obstructed; late, 50% to 99% of retinal examination obstructed); mature, 100% of retinal examination obstructed; hypermature, liquefaction/resorption with associated lens-induced uveitis
  - Morgagnian: nucleus falls ventrally in the capsule

HISTORY, CHIEF COMPLAINT

- Impaired vision
- Cloudy white pupil
- Anorexia/hyporexia (secondary to impaired vision)

PHYSICAL EXAM FINDINGS Ocular opacity: bilateral or unilateral

ETIOLOGY AND PATHOPHYSIOLOGY

- Regardless of origin, all cataracts occur through a change in lens protein composition or lens fiber arrangement:
  - Inherited: not documented in ferrets
  - Diabetes mellitus: cataracts not documented probably owing to rarity of this disease
  - Secondary to intraocular disease: uveitis, glaucoma, retinal degeneration
  - Trauma to lens: blunt or penetrating
  - Age-related
  - Nutritional: diet high in fat or deficient in vitamin E or protein may promote cataract formation
  - Electrical shock
- Not all cataracts are progressive.
- Cataracts can progress to become hypermature, resulting in lens-induced uveitis and increased risk of vitreal degeneration, retinal detachment, and secondary glaucoma.
- Congenital cataracts abolish binocularity if the ferret is deprived of patterned vision in one eye during postnatal development of the ocular cortex.

DIAGNOSIS

DIFFERENTIAL DIAGNOSIS

- Diagnosis of cataract is suspected based on observation of a cloudy pupil in an animal that may be visually compromised. It is confirmed by the finding of a lens opacity following complete dilatation of the pupil.
  - Nuclear/lenticular sclerosis: normal aging change usually seen in older animals; does not cause vision loss—center of lens becomes opalescent to hazy, but tapetal reflection in pupil is still visible, versus cataracts, which obstruct this reflection
  - Diseases causing diffuse corneal edema (bluish-white opacity on cornea, not in pupil; may obstruct ability to see the pupil), including glaucoma, anterior uveitis, and corneal endothelial degeneration or dystrophy
  - Diseases causing secondary cataracts
    - Retinal degeneration or detachment
    - Anterior uveitis (cataracts typically incomplete if due to inflammation; uveitis may occur secondary to cataracts)
    - Lens luxation
    - Diabetes mellitus (rare)

INITIAL DATABASE

- Complete ophthalmic examination, including
  - Menace response
  - Evaluation of pupil size and symmetry, pupillary light reflexes
  - Intraocular pressure (IOP): rule out glaucoma (upper limit of normal IOP reported as 25 to 30 mm Hg)
  - After IOP assessment (assuming normal result), dilate pupil with 1% tropicamide.
  - Penlight or transilluminator to characterize the cataract; evaluate for concurrent uveitis
  - Fundic (posterior segment) examination using indirect or direct ophthalmoscopy

ADVANCED OR CONFIRMATORY TESTING

- Complete blood count, serum biochemistry profile, and urinalysis primarily to assess patient before considering referral for possible cataract surgery, and secondarily to rule out systemic metabolic disease (e.g., diabetes mellitus) as cause of cataracts
- Ocular ultrasound if the cataract is immature or worse in severity and precludes accurate evaluation of the posterior segment of the eye

TREATMENT

THERAPEUTIC GOALS

- Incipient and nonprogressive early immature cataracts do not require treatment.
- Progressive immature, mature, and hypermature cataracts are treated to
  - Prevent secondary sequelae of cataracts: uveitis, glaucoma, and retinal detachment
- Referral to a veterinary ophthalmologist may help greatly in triage, diagnosis, and treatment of cataracts.

ACUTE GENERAL TREATMENT

- Treat associated uveitis with topical mydriatics and antiinflammatories.
- Treat secondary glaucoma accordingly.
- Referral for cataract surgery if cataract is causing secondary complications
  - Cataract surgery requires preliminary ocular ultrasound indicating that the posterior segment of the eye is normal.
  - Phacoemulsification (ultrasonic lens fragmentation) to remove the cataract
  - Artificial lenses are not available in a size suitable for ferrets. Without an intraocular lens implant, animals are hyperopic (far-sighted) and have little useful vision.

CHRONIC TREATMENT

- After cataract surgery, treat as directed by the veterinary ophthalmologist:
  - Topical antibiotics and antiinflammatories
  - Exercise restriction/Elizabethan collar for 1 to 2 weeks
  - Antiinflammatory therapy may be continued in a decreasing fashion for months or, in some cases, indefinitely.
  - Reevaluation of IOP, retinal examination, and inflammation control
- If cataract surgery is not an option,
  - Monitor cataracts for progression, and treat associated uveitis with topical antiinflammatories long term.
  - Use IOP-lowering drugs in combination with antiinflammatories if secondary glaucoma develops.
  - Enucleation or evisceration of end-stage, blind, painful globes

DRUG INTERACTIONS

Diazoxide (used in insulinoma treatment to prevent hypoglycemia) at a high dose causes reversible lenticular cataracts in dogs.

POSSIBLE COMPLICATIONS

- Without cataract surgery, the following can occur: uveitis, glaucoma, lens luxation, retinal detachment, and blindness.
- After cataract surgery, the following can occur: uveitis, glaucoma, corneal ulceration, surgical wound/incisional dehiscence, intraocular infection, retinal detachment, corneal endothelial degeneration, and secondary corneal edema.

RECOMMENDED MONITORING

- Without cataract surgery, monitor for cataract progression and secondary complications q 2-4 mo, or more or less frequently, depending on extent of cataract, rate of cataract development, and presence or absence of associated ocular complications.
- After cataract surgery, monitor according to recommendations of veterinary ophthalmologist; generally involve
  - Reevaluation at postoperative weeks 2, 8, and 20
  - Long-term follow-up q 6-12 mo for life
  - In addition to routine ophthalmic examinations, Schirmer tear test, IOP, menace response, and pupillary light reflexes should be evaluated each time the animal is presented for examination.

PROGNOSIS AND OUTCOME

- Rate of cataract progression is variable depending on the cause and location of the cataract and the age of the animal
- Success in preventing secondary complications is increased with early referral (before animal is blind) and surgery, and with diligent postoperative monitoring and treatment.
- Because artificial lenses are not available, cataract surgery does not lead to positive visual outcome—without an intraocular lens implant, animals have vision that, in human equivalence, is worse than 20/400 and corresponds to being "legally blind."

PEARLS & CONSIDERATIONS

PREVENTION

Prompt treatment of intraocular inflammation will decrease the likelihood of secondary cataracts.

CLIENT EDUCATION

- It is essential that clients understand that not all cataracts are progressive. Unilateral cataracts may not require surgery if vision is adequate in the unaffected eye, and if no underlying cause of the cataract would require additional treatment and/or monitoring.
- If a cataract is progressive, the client must make a decision with regard to surgery.
  - Although surgery is associated with some risks, not opting for surgery is associated with risks of lens-induced uveitis, secondary glaucoma, retinal detachment, and ocular pain.

SUGGESTED READINGS

Boyd K, et al: A closer look: secondary glaucoma more likely, Lab Anim (NY) 36:13–14, 2007.

Cutter-Schatzberg KV, et al: Juvenile ocular abnormalities in a ferret [Abstract 57], Vet Ophthalmol 6:361, 2003.

López Murcia MM, et al: Ocular findings in 22 adult ferrets *(Mustela putorius furo)* [Abstract 46], Vet Ophthalmol 7:433–434, 2004.

Miller PE, et al. Cataracts in a laboratory colony of ferrets, Lab Anim Sci 43:562–568, 1993.

Utroska B, et al: Bilateral cataracts in a ferret, Vet Med Small Anim Clin 74:1176–1177, 1979.

AUTHORS: **AMY J. FUNK AND THOMAS M. DONNELLY**

EDITORS: **JAMES G. FOX AND ROBERT MARINI**

FERRETS

Chordoma

BASIC INFORMATION

DEFINITION

Chordoma is a musculoskeletal tumor derived from notochord. It most commonly arises at the tail tip but may occur anywhere along the vertebral column. Cervical and thoracic vertebral chordomas have been described.

SPECIAL SPECIES CONSIDERATION

Chordoma is a rare neoplasm in animals; it occurs commonly only in ferrets.

EPIDEMIOLOGY

SPECIES, AGE, SEX

- Both genders are affected.
- Most affected ferrets are between 3 and 6 years of age.

RISK FACTORS

- Injury to the nucleus pulposus of intervertebral disks may predispose to development of chordoma.
- Wedge vertebra and other congenital vertebral abnormalities may create instability of the vertebral column, leading to disk injury.

CLINICAL PRESENTATION

DISEASE FORMS/SUBTYPES

- Tail tip
- Cervical or thoracic vertebral chordoma

HISTORY, CHIEF COMPLAINT

- Caudal vertebral chordoma
  - A mass is observed on the tail tip; potential for injury and ulceration of the mass
- Cervical or thoracic vertebral chordoma—signs may be sudden or slow in onset; distribution of signs depends on anatomic location of the mass
  - Motor dysfunction
  - Pain
  - Inability to urinate

PHYSICAL EXAM FINDINGS

- Caudal vertebral chordoma: a mass of variable size is observed at the tip of the tail; masses may be hard, round, or clublike
- Cervical or thoracic vertebral chordoma
  - Palpable mass involving the cervical or thoracic vertebral column
  - Paresis to paralysis
  - Hypoglycemia (insulin-secreting pancreatic tumor)
  - Tumor (e.g., lymphoma)
  - Vertebral defect (e.g., hemivertebrae, vertebral fracture, intervertebral disk disease)
  - Hematomyelia associated with hyperestrogenism
  - Distemper
  - Rabies
  - Fungal myelitis
  - *Mycobacterium* spp. infection
  - Thromboembolism

ETIOLOGY AND PATHOPHYSIOLOGY

- Derived from remnants of the notochord
- Local invasion and osteolysis
- Compression of the spinal cord

- Chordomas are slow growing and rarely metastasize.

DIAGNOSIS

DIFFERENTIAL DIAGNOSIS

- Caudal vertebral chordoma
  - Other neoplasms
  - Granuloma: fungal, bacterial, foreign body
- Cervical or thoracic vertebral chordoma
  - Vertebral mass
  - Other neoplasms
  - Granuloma: fungal, bacterial, foreign body
- Neurologic signs

INITIAL DATABASE

- Complete blood count
- Chemistry screen
- Radiography and myelography

ADVANCED OR CONFIRMATORY TESTING

- MRI
- Histopathologic examination: submission of tissues collected by tail tip amputation biopsy or debulking
  - Masses may be multilobulated.
  - Chordomas may have several histologic appearances. Three zones, which may be concentric, typically occur: a center of well-differentiated trabecular bone, an intermediate zone of cartilage, and a peripheral zone of physaliferous cells in a pale mucinous matrix.
    - Physaliferous cells are pathognomonic for chordomas. They are round to polygonal, have vacuolated cytoplasms, and may have nuclei that are central or peripheral. Physaliferous cells are also referred to as *bubble* or *bladder cells*.
    - Immunohistochemically, chordomas are cytokeratin and vimentin intermediate filament–positive and variably positive for S-100 protein and neuron-specific enolase. Chondrosarcomas, with which chordomas may be confused, are cytokeratin-negative.
    - Ataxia, loss of conscious proprioception
    - Loss of pain perception in limbs caudal to involved segment of spinal column

TREATMENT

THERAPEUTIC GOALS

- Removal of tumor; elimination of tumor burden
- Amelioration of neurologic signs

ACUTE GENERAL TREATMENT

- Caudal vertebral chordoma
  - Surgical amputation
  - Supportive perioperative and postoperative care
- Cervical or thoracic vertebral chordoma
  - Surgical removal or debulking
  - Laminectomy and spinal cord decompression
  - Steroid therapy: adapted from Cochrane reviews of clinical data in humans (e.g., methylprednisolone sodium succinate 15 mg/kg IV or IM initially, then 10 mg/kg IV or IM q 4 h for 24 h)
  - Cimetidine 5 mg/kg IM q 8-12 h

PROGNOSIS AND OUTCOME

- Prognosis for caudal vertebral chordoma is excellent.
- Prognosis for cervical or thoracic vertebral chordoma is poor to fair, depending on the amount of spinal cord injury and the success of tumor removal or debulking.

PEARLS & CONSIDERATIONS

COMMENTS

Chordomas are slow-growing and rarely metastasize.

SUGGESTED READINGS

Bracken MB: Steroids for acute spinal cord injury, Cochrane Database Syst Rev 1:CD001046, 2012.

Li X, et al: Neoplastic diseases in ferrets: 574 cases (1968-1977), J Am Vet Med Assoc 212:1402–1406, 1998.

Pye GW, et al: Thoracic vertebral chordoma in a domestic ferret *(Mustela putorius furo)*, J Zoo Wildl Med 31:107–111, 2000.

Williams BH, et al: Cervical chordoma in two ferrets *(Mustela putorius furo)*, Vet Pathol 30:204–206, 1993.

AUTHOR: **ROBERT P. MARINI**

EDITORS: **JAMES G. FOX**

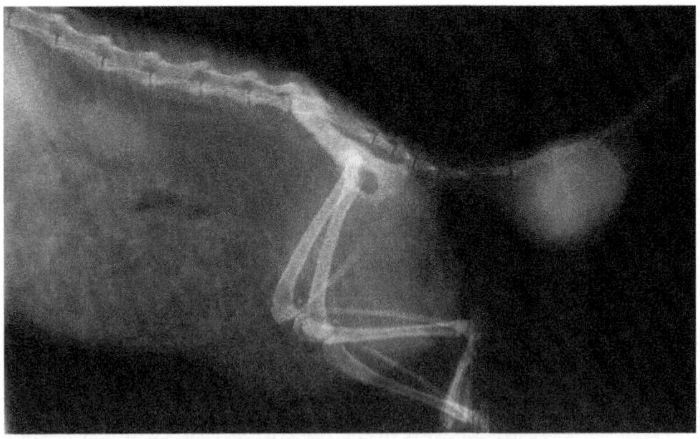

Chordoma Radiographic appearance of a tail chordoma; amputation is usually curative. *(Photo courtesy Jörg Mayer, The University of Georgia, Athens.)*

Cryptococcosis

BASIC INFORMATION

DEFINITION

- Systemic mycotic infection with the yeast form of *Cryptococcus gattii* or *Cryptococcus neoformans*
- *C. neoformans* is now divided into two varieties: *C. neoformans* var. *neoformans,* and *C. neoformans* var. *grubii*.
- *C. gattii* was formerly known as *C. neoformans* var. *gattii*.

SYNONYM

Cryptococcal infection

SPECIAL SPECIES CONSIDERATIONS

- Ferrets appear to display a varied spectrum of disease with cryptococcosis, including upper and lower respiratory tract, central nervous system, and skin disease.
- There has only been one report of ocular disease (bilateral chorioretinitis) in a ferret with generalized cryptococcosis.

EPIDEMIOLOGY

SPECIES, AGE, SEX Both genders and young/old ferrets can be affected.

RISK FACTORS

- *C. neoformans* is commonly associated with avian feces.
- *C. gattii* is associated with decaying plant matter in hollows of certain tree species (especially *Eucalyptus* spp.).

CONTAGION AND ZOONOSIS

- Cryptococcus can also affect other mammals, including humans, and birds.
- No reports have described animal-to-animal (including human) transfer of cryptococcal infection; it is not a contagious or anthropozoonotic disease. Infection appears to be the result of a common environmental source.
- *C. gattii* is considered an important emerging pathogen of immune competent humans in temperate regions of North America.

GEOGRAPHY AND SEASONALITY

- *C. neoformans* has a worldwide distribution, whereas *C. gattii* has a more tropical and subtropical distribution.
- Cryptococcal infections in ferrets have been documented in Australia, Canada, United States, Spain, and United Kingdom.
- No seasonality has been reported in ferrets.

CLINICAL PRESENTATION

DISEASE FORMS/SUBTYPES

- In ferrets, cryptococcosis can present as a varied spectrum of clinical disease, including
  - Upper respiratory tract disease (affecting nasal cavity and regional lymph nodes)
  - Lower respiratory tract disease (granulomatous pneumonia with or without pleurisy)
  - Lymphadenopathy
  - Abdominal cavity disease
  - Localized disease affecting limbs
  - Subcutaneous disease
  - Meningeal infection
  - Chorioretinitis

HISTORY, CHIEF COMPLAINT Depends on organ system affected

- Respiratory tract
  - Sneezing, nasal and ocular discharge
  - Coughing, dyspnea, and lethargy
- Localized disease affecting limbs and subcutaneous disease
  - Subcutaneous masses on nose, face, and limbs
- Meningeal infection
  - Seizures

PHYSICAL EXAM FINDINGS Depends on organ system affected

- Nasal and ocular discharge
- Tachypnea, dyspnea, harsh breathing sounds
- Lymphadenopathy
- Subcutaneous masses on nose, face, limbs
- Central neurologic deficits
- Chorioretinitis

ETIOLOGY AND PATHOPHYSIOLOGY

- *Cryptococcus* is a saprophytic, round, yeastlike dimorphic fungus with a large heteropolysaccharide capsule.
- Infection with *Cryptococcus* most likely occurs via aerosol of the nonencapsulated yeast form. Localized cutaneous infection may result from skin penetration.
- *Cryptococcus* appears to have a predilection for cooler parts of the body (e.g., respiratory tract, head, limbs).
- Hematogenous spread of *Cryptococcus* from a primary site of infection results in
  - Multifocal subcutaneous infection
  - Regional or generalized lymphadenomegaly
  - Central nervous system (CNS) infection. However, extension to the CNS

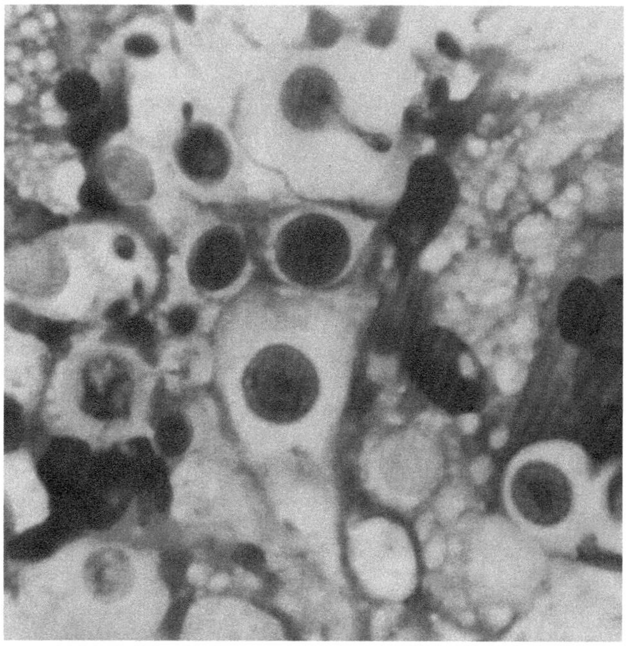

Cryptococcosis Cytologic examination reveals capsulate yeasts with narrow-neck budding and prominent unstained region surrounding each yeast (corresponding to capsule). Diff-Quik–stained smear. *(Image courtesy Richard Malik.)*

is more likely to occur from the nasal cavity (via cribriform plate and olfactory bulb).
- Pathogenicity is associated with polysaccharide capsule:
  - Aids resistance to host phagocytosis
  - Capsule thickens after infection
  - Has low stimulatory effect upon host proinflammatory cytokines
- *Cryptococcus neoformans* was previously defined by serotype. Cryptococcal strains worldwide are now divided into eight molecular types. Differences in epidemiology, pathogenicity, clinical traits, and drug susceptibility are associated with different cryptococcal species, varieties, and molecular types.

DIAGNOSIS

DIFFERENTIAL DIAGNOSIS

- Upper respiratory tract disorders, including inflammatory disease, viral infection (canine distemper virus, influenza, respiratory syncytial virus), bacterial infection, fungal infection, foreign body, and neoplasia
- Lower respiratory tract disorders, including inflammatory disease, viral infection (canine distemper virus, influenza, Aleutian disease), bacterial infection (including actinomycosis, *Streptococcus zooepidemicus, Streptococcus pneumoniae*, other *Streptococcus* spp., *Escherichia coli, Klebsiella pneumoniae, Pseudomonas aeruginosa, Bordetella bronchiseptica, Listeria monocytogenes*, mycobacteriosis), fungal infection (blastomycosis, coccidiomycosis, pneumocystosis), foreign body, heartworm disease *(Dirofilaria immitis)*, pulmonary edema, neoplasia (especially lymphoma), aspiration pneumonia, and pneumothorax
- Any other condition causing cough, including:
  - Pleural disorders: inflammation, infection, neoplasia
  - Esophageal disorders: inflammation, foreign body, neoplasia, esophageal duplication, cyst
  - Cardiac disease
- Subcutaneous swellings: infection, neoplasia, cyst
- Central neurologic disease: insulinoma, bacterial meningitis/encephalitis, CNS neoplasia

INITIAL DATABASE

- Blood biochemistry/hematology, urinalysis (all may be normal)
- Abdominal and thoracic radiographs
  - Especially to differentiate causes of lower respiratory tract disease
  - Early course of pneumonia may show interstitial pattern with progression to alveolar pattern as disease evolves. Radiographic changes indicative of late course of pneumonia may be patchy or generalized and/or may include lung lobe consolidation.

ADVANCED OR CONFIRMATORY TESTING

- Cytologic examination of needle aspirate from subcutaneous mass/lymph node or bronchoalveolar lavage/nasal wash
  - Assess sample by staining with modified Romanowsky, new methylene blue, or Gram stain; all are considered superior to India ink staining.
  - Characteristic capsulated round to oval yeast cells may be seen.
  - Failure to identify organisms after cytologic evaluation does not rule out infection because some yeasts are weakly capsulated and go unnoticed. Further diagnostics via culture and histopathologic examination are recommended in these cases.
- Microbiological examination of needle aspirate of subcutaneous mass, lymph node, bronchoalveolar lavage sample, exudates, CSF, and urine or tissue specimens
  - Both *C. neoformans* and *C. gattii* grow on most laboratory media; however, the preferred medium is Sabouraud's dextrose agar or bird seed agar.
  - Depending on sample site and chance of bacterial contamination, antibiotic additives can be included in Sabouraud's or bird seed agar to improve isolation of cryptococci.
  - Samples are cultured at 25°C (77°F) and 37°C (98.6°F), with growth expected between 2 and 10 days (usually between 2 and 3 days).
  - Colonies initially appear white/cream and then gradually yellow with age, displaying an increasing mucoid appearance relative to the level of capsular development.
  - Antifungal susceptibility testing is recommended because of the long duration of therapy required.
- Histopathologic examination of biopsy samples:
  - Histologic samples stained with hematoxylin-eosin (H&E) may reveal cryptococcal organisms.
  - Stains that more readily identify cryptococci include periodic acid-Schiff (PAS), methenamine silver, Fontana-Masson stain, and Mayer's mucicarmine, which is considered the most definitive by pathologists.
  - Immunohistochemistry can be used to distinguish *C. neoformans* strains in formalin-fixed tissue.
- Serologic testing
  - Assays are based on detection of cryptococcal capsular antigen by latex agglutination (latex cryptococcal antigen test [LCAT]). LCATs can be performed on serum or CSF and have established 90% to 100% sensitivity and 97% to 100% specificity in both human and animal studies. Other fluids such as pleural fluid or bronchoalveolar lavage fluid have been assessed with LCAT. Antigen titers as low as 1:2 are considered positive, and titer values are considered valuable in monitoring patient response to therapy.
  - Because titer values can differ between different test kits, it is critical to maintain test kit and test method consistency if response to treatment is being monitored.
  - In cryptococcosis treatment, a favorable response to therapy is indicated by a reduction in antigen titer. However, no correlation has been established between pretreatment titer value and prognosis.
- Molecular typing of cryptococcal species (e.g., PCR), in addition to serologic testing, is recommended for epidemiology.
- Diagnostic imaging (e.g., MRI) for ferrets exhibiting central neurologic signs

TREATMENT

THERAPEUTIC GOAL

Complete resolution of infection

ACUTE GENERAL TREATMENT

Supportive care if respiratory compromise (provide oxygen, hydration, nutrition), seizures, or inappetence

CHRONIC TREATMENT

- Antifungal agents (e.g., amphotericin B, flucytosine, azole antifungals [ketoconazole, fluconazole, itraconazole, voriconazole, pramiconazole, and posaconazole])
- Documented successful outcomes in ferrets treated with itraconazole at 10-20 mg/kg PO q 24 h × 10 months minimum
- Antifungal therapy should be maintained until LCAT titers are zero.
- Consider surgical debulking of nasal, subcutaneous, cutaneous, and lymph node lesions once medical therapy has commenced.

DRUG INTERACTIONS

- Amphotericin B use carries risk of nephrotoxicity.
- Flucytosine crosses the blood-brain barrier entering the CSF and may be

useful in CNS cases (no documented use in ferrets to date).
- Azole antifungals
  - Are fungistatic
  - Absorption is enhanced when given with food.
  - Itraconazole and ketoconazole should not be used with other hepatically metabolized drugs.

POSSIBLE COMPLICATIONS

- Azole antifungals may induce anorexia, vomiting, and hepatic disease.
  - Periodic monitoring of liver enzymes should be conducted.
- Amphotericin B may be nephrotoxic (lipid soluble forms may be less nephrotoxic).
  - Blood urea nitrogen (BUN) and creatinine levels should be assessed periodically.

RECOMMENDED MONITORING

- Hepatic function monitoring with azole antifungals
- Renal function monitoring with amphotericin B
- LCAT monitoring until antigen titer is zero

PROGNOSIS AND OUTCOME

- Prognosis is good.
- Early, aggressive, and prolonged treatment is usually necessary for success. Factors that may affect therapy include
  - Duration of infection
  - Extent of infection
  - Organ system involvement
  - Patient age and status
  - Renal and hepatic function
  - Patient temperament
  - Owner's financial and emotional commitment
- No correlation has been established between pretreatment LCAT titer values and prognosis.

PEARLS & CONSIDERATIONS

COMMENTS

Consider conducting diagnostic tests for cryptococcosis on ferrets that co-habitate with any positively diagnosed ferret.

PREVENTION

- No vaccine is available.
- Avoid avian feces and decaying plant matter.

SUGGESTED READINGS

Lester SJ, et al: Cryptococcosis: update and emergence of Cryptococcus gattii, Vet Clin Path 40:4–17, 2011.

Malik R, et al: Cryptococcosis. In Greene CE, editor: Infectious diseases of the dog and cat, ed 3, Philadelphia, 2006, Saunders Elsevier, pp 584–598.

Malik R, et al: Cryptococcosis in ferrets: a diverse spectrum of clinical disease, Aust Vet J 80:749–755, 2002.

Ropstad E-O, et al: Cryptococcus gattii chorioretinitis in a ferret, Vet Ophthalmol 14:262–266, 2011.

AUTHOR: **DAVID VELLA**

EDITORS: **JAMES G. FOX AND ROBERT P. MARINI**

FERRETS

Dental Disease

Client Education Sheet Available on Website

BASIC INFORMATION

DEFINITION

- Periodontal disease is infection of support structures of the teeth (gingiva, periodontal ligament, and periodontal alveolar bone).
- A fractured tooth consists of loss of tooth structure from trauma. It is problematic if the pulp canal is exposed.

EPIDEMIOLOGY

SPECIES, AGE, SEX No age or sex predilection

RISK FACTORS

- Periodontal disease
  - Soft food diet, previous periodontal disease (e.g., gingival recession)
- Fractured teeth
  - Ferrets have a normal curious, active nature.

CLINICAL PRESENTATION

HISTORY, CHIEF COMPLAINT

- Periodontal disease
  - Halitosis
  - Difficulty/reluctance to eat dry food in advanced disease
- Fractured teeth
  - Oral pain
  - Reluctance to eat/play

PHYSICAL EXAM FINDINGS

- Periodontal disease
  - Gingivitis
  - Gingival recession
  - Tooth mobility/loss in advanced disease
- Fractured teeth
  - Usually maxillary canine tooth
  - Loss of tooth crown
  - Discoloration (including translucency)
  - External nasal swelling or draining tract or fistula on buccal mucosa (root abscess)

ETIOLOGY AND PATHOPHYSIOLOGY

- Periodontal disease
  - Plaque buildup (especially buccal surfaces of maxillary canine and premolars)
  - Calculus formation (especially buccal surfaces of maxillary canine and premolars)
  - Gingival inflammation
  - Gingival recession
  - Periodontal ligament and bone loss
  - Tooth loss
- Fractured teeth
  - Head/oral trauma
  - Tooth fracture
  - Pulp canal exposure
  - Pulp canal infection
  - Tooth root abscess

DIAGNOSIS

DIFFERENTIAL DIAGNOSIS

- Periodontal disease
  - None, other than periodontal disease
- Fractured tooth
  - None, other than fractured tooth

INITIAL DATABASE

Oral examination

ADVANCED OR CONFIRMATORY TESTING

- Periodontal examination (requires general anesthesia)
- Dental radiography (requires general anesthesia)

TREATMENT

THERAPEUTIC GOALS

- Periodontal disease
  - Healthy gingiva
  - Clean tooth surfaces
- Fractured teeth
  - Removal and/or treatment of source of infection

ACUTE GENERAL TREATMENT

- Periodontal disease
  - Dental scaling and polishing
  - Tooth extractions (loose/abscessed teeth)
  - Antibiotics (e.g. Clavamox [amoxicillin/clavulanic acid] 12.5-25.0 mg/kg PO q 12 h; clindamycin 5.5-10.0 mg/kg PO q 12 h)
  - Pain management (if loose teeth or abscess) (e.g., buprenorphine 0.01-0.03 mg/kg SC, IM, IV q 8 h; carprofen 1 mg/kg PO q 12-24 h)
- Fractured teeth
  - Pain management
  - Antibiotics (if abscess)
  - Extraction
  - Endodontic treatment (root canal or vital pulpotomy)

CHRONIC TREATMENT

- Periodontal disease
  - Dental scaling and polishing
  - Tooth extractions (loose/abscessed teeth)
- Fractured teeth
  - Extraction
  - Endodontic (root canal or vital pulpotomy)

POSSIBLE COMPLICATIONS

- Tooth extractions
  - Incisional dehiscence
  - Root fracture
  - Jaw fracture
- Endodontic treatment
  - Failure (abscess development)

RECOMMENDED MONITORING

- Periodontal disease
  - Frequent oral examination
- Fractured teeth
  - Frequent oral examination
  - Dental radiographs (6 to 12 months after treatment)

PROGNOSIS AND OUTCOME

- Periodontal disease
  - Usually has an excellent prognosis
  - Gingivitis resolves with proper dental cleaning.
  - With proper closure, tooth extraction sites heal well (and remaining teeth will not shift).
- Fractured teeth
  - Usually have an excellent prognosis
  - With proper closure, tooth extraction sites heal well (and remaining teeth will not shift).

PEARLS & CONSIDERATIONS

COMMENTS

- Periodontal disease
  - Periodontal disease is common in ferrets.
  - Gingival recession is permanent, so early treatment and prevention are important.
  - Appreciation of normal gingiva and dentition is important to allow earlier treatment or preventive intervention.
- Fractured teeth
  - Oral pain is often subtle or overlooked.
  - Knowledge of normal dental anatomy and frequent oral examination will allow earlier diagnosis.

PREVENTION

- Periodontal disease
  - Start with a "clean slate" (young, healthy teeth and gums) of teeth and gums after proper dental cleaning.
  - Provide dry food and crunchy treats (more chewing causes more saliva to be released, which decreases plaque and calculus).
  - Daily tooth brushing (plaque builds up daily, mineralizes into calculus in less than 36 hours; plaque can be removed with brushing, calculus cannot)
  - Frequent dental examinations
  - Dental cleaning at appropriate intervals (prevents gingival recession)
- Fractured teeth
  - Difficult to prevent owing to ferrets' active nature
  - Early recognition of tooth fracture can prevent abscess.

CLIENT EDUCATION

- The oral cavity can be easily assessed by most owners.
- Halitosis is obvious, abnormal, and requires appropriate veterinary intervention.
- Educate owner about the combination of brushing or rubbing the tooth surfaces and the use of oral health care products.
  - Many pet ferrets do not mind tooth brushing as they like the taste of the toothpaste. Use cotton swabs for brushing and an enzymatic toothpaste (CET, Virbac, Fort Worth, TX) in either malt or poultry flavor.
- Whereas home oral hygiene is important to general health, emphasize that oral hygiene complements and does not replace professional dental care.

SUGGESTED READINGS

Church RR: The impact of diet on the dentition of the domesticated ferret, Exot DVM 9:30–39, 2007.

Fehr M, et al: Ferret dental disorders. Kleintierpraxis, 52:702–707, 2007.

Johnson-Delaney CA: Ferret dental disorders: pictorial of common clinical presentations, Exot DVM 9:40–43, 2007.

AUTHOR: **WILLIAM ROSENBLAD**

EDITORS: **JAMES G. FOX AND ROBERT MARINI**

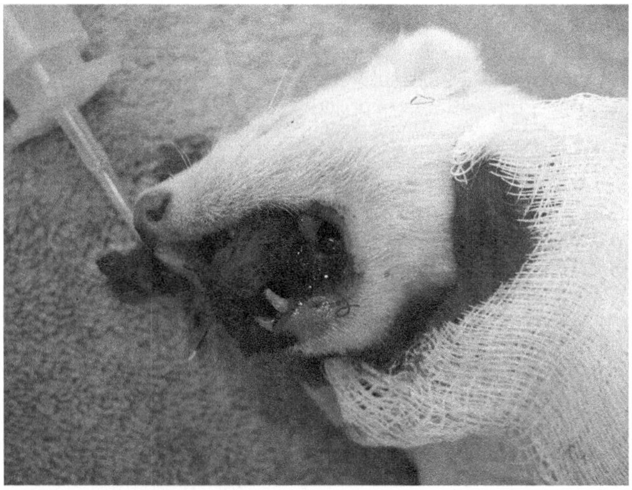

Dental Disease Dental calculus, gingivitis, and fractured teeth are very common in the ferret. When a dental procedure is performed, the animal must be intubated to avoid aspiration of fluids and blood. *(Photo courtesy Jörg Mayer, The University of Georgia, Athens.)*

Dirofilariasis

Client Education Sheet Available on Website

BASIC INFORMATION

DEFINITION

Heartworm disease is the clinicopathologic manifestation of infection with *Dirofilaria immitis*, an intravascular canid parasite that resides in the pulmonary arteries, the right side of the heart, and the venae cavae.

SYNONYMS

Heartworm disease, heartworm infection

SPECIAL SPECIES CONSIDERATIONS

- Studies have shown ferrets to be extremely susceptible to *D. immitis* infection, with recovery rates in experimental infections similar to those seen in dogs, and higher than those in cats.
- The ferret's small size can result in significant clinical disease and death, despite the presence of very few heartworms.

EPIDEMIOLOGY

SPECIES, AGE, SEX Ferrets are atypical hosts for this canine parasite.

RISK FACTORS

- Ferrets that have lived outdoors, or that spend time outdoors regularly in heartworm-endemic areas, are at greater risk.
- Varying seasonal individual risk is determined by season of the year and geographic location.

GEOGRAPHY AND SEASONALITY

- Reported worldwide and endemic throughout most parts of the United States, Australia, and Japan, and some Mediterranean countries
- Transmission is unlikely in regions or seasons where the ambient temperature does not average higher than 65°F (18°C) during a 30-day period.

ASSOCIATED CONDITIONS AND DISORDERS

- Aberrant larval migration (CNS): 1 case
- Caval syndrome resulting from retrograde migration of part of the worm burden into the right atrium and cavae: worm mass becomes entangled in tricuspid valve, causing intravascular hemolysis and signs of forward (hypoperfusion) and backward (congestive) heart failure (1 case)

CLINICAL PRESENTATION

DISEASE FORMS/SUBTYPES Classification of heartworm disease:

- Class 1: few or no overt clinical signs
- Class 2: moderate clinical signs
- Class 3: severe clinical signs
- Class 4: caval syndrome

HISTORY, CHIEF COMPLAINT

- Heartworm disease is not often diagnosed on routine wellness examinations owing to the fact that it causes severe clinical signs quickly.
- Infected ferrets are often presented in life-threatening respiratory distress.

PHYSICAL EXAM FINDINGS

- Owners usually notice a decrease in energy and anorexia that worsens over a period of days to weeks.
- Rapid and shallow breathing is a common presentation.
- Dyspnea, tachypnea, pale or cyanotic mucous membranes, and heart murmurs are often seen.

ETIOLOGY AND PATHOPHYSIOLOGY

- The disease mechanism is the same as in dogs:
  - Female mosquitoes serve as intermediate hosts after feeding on microfilaria-positive animals (usually dogs).
- Right-side heart failure: pronounced pulmonary hypertension leading to right-side heart enlargement with heart murmur
- Pleural effusion: large amount of serosanguineous thoracic fluid is often present
- Pulmonary parenchymal disease

DIAGNOSIS

DIFFERENTIAL DIAGNOSIS

- Thymic lymphoma
- Dilated cardiomyopathy
- Pyothorax

INITIAL DATABASE

- Complete blood count
  - Eosinophilia is not a common finding in ferret heartworm disease, but monocytosis may be seen
  - Mild nonregenerative anemia or eosinophilia
- Chemistry screen
  - Bilirubinuria and hypochloremia have been reported.
- Thoracic radiography: pneumonitis with interstitial lung pattern on radiographs

ADVANCED OR CONFIRMATORY TESTING

- ELISA-based antigen tests (e.g., IDEXX Snap Test; IDEXX Laboratories, Inc., Westbrook, ME)
  - Ferrets do not always show microfilaremia, so direct heartworm tests (e.g., filter and modified Knott's) are nondiagnostic.
  - IDEXX Snap Occult Heartworm test is effective 5 to 6 months after infection. This test detects only female heartworm protein; it may not be accurate in all cases.
- Echocardiography gives good assessment of the number of adult worms present:
  - Dilated pulmonary arteries
  - Parallel linear hyperechoic densities in pulmonary arteries, the right heart, and/or the venae cavae

TREATMENT

THERAPEUTIC GOALS

- Address complications:
  - Treat associated cardiac and pulmonary dysfunction.
- Prevent future infection.
- Elimination of adult heartworms with traditional treatments has been problematic:
  - Use of thiacetarsamide sodium 0.22 mL/kg IV q 12 h for 2 d as adulticide has 40% mortality.
  - Use of melarsomine 2.5 mg/kg at 1, 30, and 31 d IM as adulticide has 60% mortality.
  - Use of ivermectin ± corticosteroids has proved less than optimal, with most ferrets dying within 3 months.

ACUTE GENERAL TREATMENT

- Thoracocentesis is sometimes necessary for urgent treatment of severe pulmonary effusion. Up to 60 mL of serosanguineous fluid may be removed, allowing time for more conservative medical treatment.
- Symptomatic treatment of pulmonary congestion and cardiomyopathy should be instituted using furosemide 2 mg/kg IV, IM q 12-24 h and enalapril 0.5 mg/kg PO SID.
- Previous use of moxidectin (as ProHeart Injectable) at 0.17-2.0 mg SC had proved highly successful, with nearly 100% survival rate.
- Moxidectin is currently available in topical form as Advantage Multi (imidacloprid 10% + moxidectin 1%). It has not been tested as an adulticide, but empirically should prove effective and safe. It has proven efficacy as a chemoprophylactic at an approximate dose of 20 mg imidacloprid/2 mg moxidectin per kg

topically. (This is 0.4 mL of dose for cats up to 4 kg.)

CHRONIC TREATMENT

Long-term therapy for cardiac and pulmonary damage and complications may be necessary. Many ferrets require lifetime use of furosemide, enalapril, or corticosteroids.

PROGNOSIS AND OUTCOME

- Heartworm treatment and prevention have become more effective and safe in ferrets since the introduction of moxidectin.
- Number of adults in the heart is correlated with severity of disease:
  - A ferret in class 1 or 2 disease should be expected to survive treatment.
  - A ferret in class 3 disease has a significantly reduced chance of survival.

PEARLS & CONSIDERATIONS

COMMENTS

- Estimates of the pet ferret population in the United States range from 8 to 10 million, and most are not likely to receive heartworm chemoprophylaxis because of unfamiliarity with the problem on the part of both veterinarians and owners.
- Diagnosis may be difficult, requiring a high index of suspicion and multiple tests, including occult heartworm test, thoracic radiography, and echocardiography.
- As with cats, indoor living does not preclude infection. Although ferrets kept in outdoor cages are at higher risk, many ferrets kept on screened porches are also at risk, as are ferrets that go outside for walks with their owners.

PREVENTION

- All ferrets should be kept on heartworm chemoprophylaxis.
- Ivermectin 0.2 mg/kg PO, SC per month
- Moxidectin may be used topically at a dose of 2 mg/kg per month.

SUGGESTED READINGS

Bradbury C, et al: Transvenous heartworm extraction in a ferret with caval syndrome, J Am Anim Hosp Assoc 46:31–35, 2010.

Cottrell D: Use of moxidectin as a heartworm adulticide in four ferrets, Exot DVM 6:9–12, 2004.

McCall JW: Dirofilariasis in the domestic ferret, Clin Tech Small Anim Pract 13:109–112, 1998.

Schaper R, et al: Imidacloprid plus moxidectin to prevent heartworm infection *(Dirofilaria immitis)* in ferrets, Parasitol Res 101(Suppl 1):57–62, 2007.

CROSS-REFERENCES TO OTHER SECTIONS

Endoparasites

Heart Disease, Structural

AUTHOR: **DEBORAH COTTRELL**

EDITORS: **JAMES G. FOX AND ROBERT P. MARINI**

FERRETS

Distemper

Client Education Sheet Available on Website

BASIC INFORMATION

DEFINITION

Canine distemper virus (CDV) is an acute and often fatal febrile disease with respiratory and central nervous system signs most commonly seen in the ferret. Canine distemper is caused by a paramyxovirus of the genus *Morbillivirus.* Most terrestrial carnivores are susceptible to natural CDV infection. All animals in the Canidae family (e.g., dog, dingo, fox, coyote, wolf, jackal), the Mustelidae family (e.g., weasel, ferret, mink, skunk, badger, stoat, marten, otter), the Procyonidae family (e.g., kinkajou, coati, bassariscus, raccoon, red panda) may succumb to CDV infection. Large cats, marine mammals, and javelinas have also been found to be susceptible to CDV infection and disease.

SYNONYMS

Canine distemper, hard pad disease

SPECIAL SPECIES CONSIDERATIONS

Canine distemper is the most serious viral infection of ferrets, with mortality rates approaching 100%. Combination canine distemper vaccine or vaccines of ferret cell or low-passage canine cell origin should not be used in ferrets.

EPIDEMIOLOGY

RISK FACTORS Young animals are more susceptible than adults. Nonimmunized ferrets are at risk for disease if exposed to CDV-infected dogs or wild carnivores.

CONTAGION AND ZOONOSIS Viral transmission is most commonly by airborne and droplet exposure. Direct contact with exudates (conjunctival and nasal), urine, feces, and skin can also be a source of transmission. Fomites have been implicated in transmission. CDV is not a zoonotic disease.

ASSOCIATED CONDITIONS AND DISORDERS Clinical signs of CDV can appear similar to disseminated idiopathic myositis, influenza, and *Bordetella bronchiseptica.*

CLINICAL PRESENTATION

DISEASE FORMS/SUBTYPES CDV has a catarrhal phase (7 to 10 days post infection) and a CNS phase (may or may not be preceded by the catarrhal phase).

HISTORY, CHIEF COMPLAINT CDV should be considered based on clinical observation in any unvaccinated ferret with exposure.

PHYSICAL EXAM FINDINGS The catarrhal phase involves anorexia, pyrexia, photosensitivity, and serous nasal discharge. An erythematous pruritic rash may be seen spanning from the chin to the inguinal region. Footpad hyperkeratosis is an inconsistent feature. Mucopurulent ocular and nasal discharge with possible bacterial pneumonia may be seen with secondary bacterial infection. Ataxia, tremors, and paralysis may be seen in the CNS phase. Death from ferret strains of CDV occurs in 12 to 16 days.

ETIOLOGY AND PATHOPHYSIOLOGY

- CDV is transmitted by aerosol exposure.
- Ferrets shed virus in all body excretions; shedding begins about 7 days after exposure.
- The incubation period for CDV in ferrets is 7 to 10 days.
- Death can occur 12 to 16 days after exposure.
- One report of naturally occurring distemper calculated a minimum incubation period for six ferrets as 11 to 56 days, and in 13 ferrets the signs of disease lasted 14 to 34 days before death.

DIAGNOSIS

DIFFERENTIAL DIAGNOSIS

- Influenza
- *Bordetella bronchiseptica*
- Disseminated idiopathic myositis

INITIAL DATABASE

- Leukopenia
- Radiographic evidence of lung congestion/consolidation
- Positive antibody titer to CDV (vaccinated ferrets can have positive titer)

ADVANCED OR CONFIRMATORY TESTING

- Fluorescent antibody (FA) testing on conjunctival smears, mucous membranes, or blood smears
- Positive postmortem diagnosis based on histopathologic examination, immunofluorescence and/or immunocytochemistry, and virus isolation. Preferred tissues are lymph nodes, bladder epithelium, and cerebellum.

TREATMENT

THERAPEUTIC GOALS

- No specific treatment is available for CDV in ferrets; the mortality rate is almost 100%.
- Vaccination against CDV is the best prevention.

ACUTE GENERAL TREATMENT

- Isolate affected ferret.
- Provide supportive care and antibiotics to reduce secondary bacterial infections.
- Euthanasia may be the most humane option.

CHRONIC TREATMENT

- Vaccination is not helpful in the face of disease.
- Ferrets should be vaccinated against canine distemper virus. Currently, two vaccines for CDV have been approved for use in ferrets: Fervac-D (United Vaccines, Inc., Madison, WI) and PureVax (Merial, Athens, GA).

POSSIBLE COMPLICATIONS

Vaccine reaction (see Vaccine Reaction)

RECOMMENDED MONITORING

Assure routine vaccination.

PROGNOSIS AND OUTCOME

No specific treatment is known, and the mortality rate is almost 100%.

CONTROVERSY

Vaccine reaction

PEARLS & CONSIDERATIONS

COMMENTS

Combination canine distemper vaccine or vaccines of ferret cell or low-passage canine cell origin should not be used in ferrets.

PREVENTION

Use available ferret vaccines.

CLIENT EDUCATION

- Vaccination should begin at 6 to 8 weeks for kits, with booster vaccination provided every 3 to 4 weeks until 14 weeks old. Annual revaccination is recommended.

SUGGESTED READINGS

Bonami F, et al: Disease duration determines canine distemper virus neurovirulence, J Virol 81:12066–12070, 2007.

Deem SL, et al: Canine distemper in terrestrial carnivores: a review, J Zoo Wildl Med 31:441–451, 2000.

Perpinan D, et al: Outbreak of canine distemper in domestic ferrets *(Mustela putorius furo)*, Vet Rec 163:246–250, 2008.

Zehnder AM, et al: An unusual presentation of canine distemper virus infection in a domestic ferret *(Mustela putorius furo)*, Vet Dermatol 19:232–238, 2008.

CROSS-REFERENCES TO OTHER SECTIONS

Vaccine Reactions

AUTHOR: **JENNIFER GRAHAM**

EDITORS: **JAMES G. FOX AND ROBERT P. MARINI**

FERRETS

Ear Mites

BASIC INFORMATION

DEFINITION

Otodectes cynotis is an arthropod parasite of the class Arachnida that infests the ear canal of ferrets.

SPECIAL SPECIES CONSIDERATIONS

- This same mite species infests dogs and cats.
- Dark waxy debris in the ear canal is a normal finding in the ferret.
- The ferret ear canal is narrow and is flanked by long hairs. Administration of medications directly to the ear canal can be challenging.

EPIDEMIOLOGY

SPECIES, AGE, SEX Ferrets of any age and sex can be affected.

RISK FACTORS Ear mites are common in ferrets. Ferrets in contact with other animals that are infested with ear mites are at increased risk of becoming infested.

CONTAGION AND ZOONOSIS

- Transmission occurs by direct contact with infested animals such as dogs, cats, and other ferrets.
- The ferret ear mite is not transmissible to humans.

ASSOCIATED CONDITIONS AND DISORDERS Secondary otitis interna can occur with prolonged infestation. Signs include ataxia, circling, torticollis, and signs of Horner's syndrome.

CLINICAL PRESENTATION

HISTORY, CHIEF COMPLAINT

- Infestation is usually subclinical:
  - Clinical signs may include head shaking, scratching, or signs associated with otitis interna.

PHYSICAL EXAM FINDINGS On otoscopic examination, adult mites are often seen crawling within the ear canal.

ETIOLOGY AND PATHOPHYSIOLOGY

- *O. cynotis* has a direct, 3-week life cycle. The adult mite feeds on the host's blood from tissues in the ear canal. The adult lays its eggs that hatch in 3 weeks, thus completing the life cycle.
- *O. cynotis* can persist for up to 12 days off the host.

DIAGNOSIS

DIFFERENTIAL DIAGNOSIS

- Otitis externa, otitis media (e.g., *Malassezia*), otitis interna
- Horner's syndrome

INITIAL DATABASE

- Dark waxy debris in the ear canal is a normal finding in the ferret and should not be used as a diagnostic criterion for ear mites in this species.
- Microscopic examination is recommended for definitive diagnosis.
- Mite eggs, larvae, nymphs, and adults can be observed in ear canal debris; swab the ear canal gently and place debris on a slide with mineral oil.
- The slide should be examined shortly after collection before mites die or crawl off the slide.

TREATMENT

THERAPEUTIC GOAL

Eradication of ear mites

ACUTE GENERAL TREATMENT

- Affected and exposed ferrets should be treated simultaneously with an acaricide.
- Topical ivermectin is the preferred method:
  - 1% ivermectin diluted 1:10 in propylene glycol, administered at 400 mcg/kg twice, 2 weeks apart
  - Ear canals do not need to be cleaned before treatment; massage the ears after topical instillation.
  - Alternatively, ivermectin may be administered subcutaneously at 0.2-0.4 mg/kg repeated every 2 weeks for 3 or 4 treatments.
- For pregnant jills, in which ivermectin administered during the first 2-4 weeks of gestation at 0.2 mL of a 1% solution may cause congenital defects in offspring, topical thiabendazole compounds (such as Tresaderm) should be used instead of ivermectin. Administer once daily for 1 week followed by 1 week of rest followed by 1 additional week of therapy.
- More recently, selamectin (45 mg in the form of a complete 0.75-mL single-dose tube [Stronghold Cat/Revolution for Cats; Pfizer Animal Health, New York, NY], administered topically between the shoulder blades, without cleaning the external ear canal) has been effective in ferrets. A dose of 15 mg per ferret has also been reported to be efficacious.

CHRONIC TREATMENT

Chronic treatment is usually unnecessary.

DRUG INTERACTIONS

- Ivermectin administration to pregnant jills has been associated with congenital defects in kits and thus should be avoided; a topical thiabendazole compound should be used instead.
- Use of concurrent systemic and topical ivermectin should be avoided.

POSSIBLE COMPLICATIONS

- Recurrence of mites
  - Environmental decontamination (e.g., fipronil sprayed locally in the environment) and additional animal treatment may be required if reinfestation occurs.
  - Cleanse the ears.
  - Bathe the animal; wash the bedding in hot soapy water.
  - Disinfect the environment, ensuring that other animals in contact with the affected ferret have also been treated.
- Ivermectin toxicity
  - Ivermectin is a safe drug (therapeutic index = 33); toxicity is possible but has not been reported in ferrets.
  - Signs of toxicity include agitation, vocalization, anorexia, mydriasis, rear limb paresis, tremors, and disorientation; symptomatic and supportive care is recommended.
  - Congenital defects may occur in kits if pregnant jills are exposed.

RECOMMENDED MONITORING

Reexamine the ears and ear canal debris post therapy to ensure that all mites have been killed.

PROGNOSIS AND OUTCOME

- Topical ivermectin at the dose recommended previously has been found to be nearly 100% efficacious.
- Incomplete eradication is possible when thiabendazole is administered to pregnant jills; follow up with ivermectin postpartum if indicated.
- Recurrence is possible if the environment is infested or if ferrets are co-housed with other mite-infested animals.
- No significant long-term impairment is associated with uncomplicated ear mite infestation.

PEARLS & CONSIDERATIONS

COMMENTS

Topical ivermectin therapy is now considered the treatment of choice, as opposed to systemic therapy, which can result in incomplete eradication.

PREVENTION

Prevention may be accomplished by keeping the ferret isolated in an uncontaminated environment. However, this strategy may be undesirable for many pet owners and is unnecessary given the limited morbidity associated with ear mites.

CLIENT EDUCATION

Clients should be informed of the rationale for treatment at a 2-week interval because of the life cycle of the mite. In addition, knowledge of the mechanism of transmission and the need to keep the ferret's environment free of mites and eggs are important.

SUGGESTED READINGS

Fisher M, et al: Efficacy and safety of selamectin (Stronghold/RevolutionTM) used off-label in exotic pets, Int J Appl Res Vet Med 5:87–96, 2007.

Miller DS, et al: Efficacy and safety of selamectin in the treatment of *Otodectes cynotis* infestation in domestic ferrets, Vet Rec 159:748, 2006.

Patterson MM, et al: Comparison of three treatments for control of ear mites in ferrets, Lab Anim Sci 49:655–657, 1999.

CROSS-REFERENCES TO OTHER SECTIONS

Ectoparasites

AUTHOR: **SHARRON M. KIRCHAIN**

EDITORS: **JAMES G. FOX AND ROBERT P. MARINI**

FERRETS

Ectoparasites

BASIC INFORMATION

DEFINITION

Ferrets can be infested with fleas and mange mites (*Sarcoptes scabiei* and *Demodex* spp.). Ticks and fly larvae have been reported rarely in ferrets. (See Ear Mites.)

SYNONYMS

Scabies (sarcoptic mange), mange

EPIDEMIOLOGY

SPECIES, AGE, SEX No age or sex predisposition

RISK FACTORS

- Outdoor housing
- Possibly immune suppression for demodectic mange

CONTAGION AND ZOONOSIS Ferret fleas and sarcoptic mites can infest humans.

GEOGRAPHY AND SEASONALITY

- Worldwide
- More in warmer months

CLINICAL PRESENTATION

HISTORY, CHIEF COMPLAINT

- History of potential exposure
- Immune suppression associated with *Demodex* spp.
- Pruritus, dermatitis, alopecia

PHYSICAL EXAM FINDINGS

- Flea infestation can be clinically silent or can cause pruritus and signs of flea bite hypersensitivity.
- Sarcoptic mange manifests as:
  - A generalized condition with intense pruritus and focal or generalized alopecia, or
  - A pedal form whereby the feet become swollen and encrusted
- Ferrets with demodectic mange may present with mild pruritus, localized alopecia, and discolored skin.

ETIOLOGY AND PATHOPHYSIOLOGY

- Fleas are transmitted by direct contact:
  - *Ctenocephalides* spp. and *Pulex irritans* have been reported in ferrets.
- Direct contact, or fomites transmit *S. scabiei* to ferrets.
- Clinical demodicosis is rare. It has been reported in two ferrets that received an ear ointment containing triamcinolone acetonide and concurrently in a ferret with lymphoma:
  - *Demodex* spp. infects by direct contact.
  - Clinical demodicosis is commonly associated with concurrent immunosuppression (local or generalized).

DIAGNOSIS

DIFFERENTIAL DIAGNOSIS

Adrenal gland disease can cause pruritus and alopecia in ferrets.

INITIAL DATABASE

- Fleas or flea excreta ("flea dirt") can be identified on the animal, especially between the scapulae.
- Microscopic examination of skin scrapings or biopsies are used to identify mites:
  - For *S. scabiei,* repeated and deep scrapings may be required.

TREATMENT

THERAPEUTIC GOAL

Eradication of ectoparasite(s) from the ferret and its environment

ACUTE GENERAL TREATMENT

- Judicious use of products licensed for flea eradication in cats and dogs is effective in ferrets (e.g., topical imidacloprid by body weight from prepackaged cards q 4 wk; imidacloprid 10% + moxidectin 1% [Advantage Multi] 0.4 mL applied topically q 3-4 wk; lufenuron 30 mg/kg PO q 4 wk). Also treat the following:
  - Contact animals
  - The environment: pyrethrins are relatively safe, but the effect is short-lived and frequent treatments are often required. Organophosphates and dichlorvos-impregnated collars can be toxic to ferrets and are not recommended.
- Sarcoptic mange can be treated with ivermectin 200-400 mcg/kg SC q 2 wk until mites are eradicated.
- For demodicosis, ivermectin 200 to 400 mcg/kg SC q 2 wk or amitraz 0.0125%-0.0375 wash/dips q 5 d until negative has been used.

PROGNOSIS AND OUTCOME

Favorable with adequate and thorough treatment

PEARLS & CONSIDERATIONS

COMMENTS

- Extra-label use is involved when antiparasitic drugs are administered to ferrets.
- Ear mites are the most common parasite in ferrets.

PREVENTION

- Through examination of recently acquired animals
- Environmental control for fleas

SUGGESTED READINGS

Beaufrere H, et al: Demodectic mange associated with lymphoma in a ferret, J Exotic Pet Med 18:57–61, 2009.

Patterson M, et al: Parasites of ferrets. In Baker DG, editor: Flynn's parasites of laboratory animals, Ames, IA, 2007, Blackwell Publishing, pp 501–508.

Phillips PH, et al: Pedal Sarcoptes scabiei infestation in ferrets (Mustela putorius furo), Aust Vet J 64:289–290, 1987.

Powers LV: Bacterial and parasitic diseases of ferrets, Vet Clin North Am Exot Anim Pract 12:531–561, 2009.

Wenzel U, et al: Efficacy of imidacloprid 10%/moxidectin 1% (Advocate/Advantage multi) against fleas *(Ctenocephalides felis felis)* on ferrets *(Mustela putorius furo)*, Parasitol Res 103:231–234, 2008.

CROSS-REFERENCES TO OTHER SECTIONS

Ear Mites

AUTHOR: **MARY M. PATTERSON**

EDITORS: **JAMES G. FOX AND ROBERT P. MARINI**

FERRETS

Endoparasites

BASIC INFORMATION

DEFINITION

Internal parasites of the ferret are predominantly protozoal agents that affect the gastrointestinal tract (see Cryptococcosis, and Dirofilariasis).

SPECIAL SPECIES CONSIDERATIONS

- Wild mustelids and ranch mink may be infected with trematodes, nematodes, and cestodes. Such infections are rare in domestic ferrets.
- Coccidiosis and giardiasis are the most common endoparasitic conditions of ferrets.
  - Hepatic coccidiosis of mink *(Mustela vison)* caused by *Eimeria hiepei* has not been reported in the domestic ferret *(Mustela putorius furo)*.
  - Similarly, an outbreak of toxoplasmosis in black-footed ferrets *(Mustela nigripes)* presents both acute and chronic manifestations of disease, which have not been reported in toxoplasmosis of domestic ferrets.

EPIDEMIOLOGY

RISK FACTORS Younger animals under stress are at risk for coccidiosis.

CONTAGION AND ZOONOSIS

- Endoparasites are transmitted by the fecal-oral route, typically via contaminated food or water.
- Infection by *Toxoplasma gondii* is caused by ingestion of sporulated oocysts in cat feces or cyst-infected raw meat.
- *Giardia* spp. and *Cryptosporidium parvum* should be considered potentially zoonotic.
  - A zoonotic genotype of *G. intestinalis* has been described in ferrets.
  - *C. parvum* "ferret" genotype has been isolated from ferrets and American minks but not from humans. The reservoir status of the ferret for zoonotic genotypes of *C. parvum* is unknown (see Cryptosporidiosis-Zoonoses, Sec. VI).

ASSOCIATED CONDITIONS AND DISORDERS One report describes coinfection in ferrets by intestinal coccidia and *Lawsonia intracellularis*, the causative agent of proliferative bowel disease.

CLINICAL PRESENTATION

DISEASE FORMS/SUBTYPES

- Intestinal coccidiosis
- Giardiasis
- Toxoplasmosis
- Cryptosporidiosis

HISTORY, CHIEF COMPLAINT

- Most infections are subclinical and self-limiting.
- Coccidiosis may cause lethargy, diarrhea, and wasting.
- Unthriftiness in young animals may also be seen.
- Toxoplasmosis may cause death without premonitory signs.
- Cryptosporidiosis is usually subclinical.

PHYSICAL EXAM FINDINGS

- Coccidiosis may be characterized by:
  - No clinical signs or physical exam findings
  - Diarrhea (potentially severe) with dehydration and rectal prolapse, poor body condition, and fecal pasting
  - One case of hepatic coccidiosis in a ferret has been described (most likely caused by *Eimeria furonis*):
    - Emaciation
    - Mild icterus
- Toxoplasmosis may be characterized by:
  - No clinical signs or physical exam findings
  - Ataxia
  - Death without premonitory signs
- Giardiasis has not been associated with clinical signs or physical exam findings in the domestic ferret
- Cryptosporidiosis usually is not associated with physical exam findings in the domestic ferret.
  - Anorexia, depression, diarrhea, and death have been reported once.

ETIOLOGY AND PATHOPHYSIOLOGY

- Intestinal coccidiosis
  - Sporulated oocysts are ingested and release sporozoites.
  - Sporozoites invade enterocytes.
  - Asexual and sexual multiplication occurs; gametes (microgametes and macrogametes) fuse to become oocysts.
  - Absorptive enterocytes are destroyed as merozoites, and oocysts are released.
  - Inflammation further impacts absorption by remaining enterocytes.
  - Hyperplasia of enterocytes occurs during repair.
- Giardiasis
  - Cysts are ingested and become trophozoites in the small intestine.
  - Trophozoites adhere to enterocytes to cause malabsorption.
  - Putative "toxins" injure the metabolic machinery of absorptive cells.

DIAGNOSIS

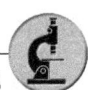

DIFFERENTIAL DIAGNOSIS

- Diarrhea
  - Rotavirus
  - Coronavirus
  - Coliform enteritis
  - Campylobacteriosis (see *Campylobacter* spp. Infections)
  - Salmonellosis
  - Proliferative bowel disease (see Proliferative Bowel Disease)
  - Eosinophilic gastroenteritis (see Eosinophilic Gastroenteritis)

INITIAL DATABASE

- Fecal flotation technique
- Direct smear of feces
- Rectal culture for agents of bacterial enteritis
- Serum chemistry and complete blood count for suspected cases of hepatic coccidiosis (elevations of hepatic enzyme concentration may be seen)
- Immunologic tests for *T. gondii* (Sabin-Feldman dye test, complement fixation, ELISA, latex agglutination test, modified agglutination test)

ADVANCED OR CONFIRMATORY TESTING

- Zinc sulfate centrifugation technique (*Giardia* spp.)
- ELISA for fecal antigen (*Giardia* spp.)
- Morphologic evaluation of oocysts
  - *Eimeria furonis* 12.8 × 12 μm: four sporocysts, each containing two sporozoites
  - *Eimeria ictidea* 23.6 × 17.5 μm: two sporocysts, each containing two sporozoites
  - *Isospora laidlawi* 34 × 29 μm: two sporocysts, each containing four sporozoites
  - *Cryptosporidium parvum* 5 μm (4 to 8 μm)
  - *Giardia* spp. 14 × 8 μm
- Acid-fast, auramine, or fluorescent antibody staining of concentrated fecal samples or acid-fast stain of direct smears *(C. parvum)*
- Histopathologic examination of tissue samples
  - Intestinal coccidiosis: jejunum and ileum demonstrate epithelial thickening with mild lymphoid and granulomatous enteritis with intraepithelial organisms
  - Hepatic coccidiosis: cholecystitis with cystic glandular proliferation and fibrosis; biliary duct proliferation with lymphoplasmacytic hepatitis and intralesional organisms

- *Cryptosporidia:* (in one report) mild eosinophilic enteritis in association with organisms (villous atrophy, blunting, and fusion in other species); (in another report) mixed inflammatory infiltrate with attachment of ovoid cryptosporidial bodies to the small intestinal and colonic brush border
  - *Toxoplasma:* multifocal necrosis of target organs associated with *Toxoplasma*-like organisms (lung, liver, and heart lesions documented in the ferret)
- Ultrastructural evaluation with electron microscopy may be used in academic settings.

TREATMENT

THERAPEUTIC GOALS

- Support ferrets that are wasting or that have diarrhea.
- Eliminate the parasite from the host and environment.
- Prevent reinfection.

ACUTE GENERAL TREATMENT

- Giardiasis
  - Metronidazole 50 mg/kg q 24 h PO for 5 d
  - Fenbendazole 50 mg/kg q 24 h PO for 3 d, repeated in 2 wk; used for dogs, unevaluated in ferrets
- Coccidiosis
  - Sulfadimethoxine 30 mg/kg q 24 h PO for 14 d
  - Sulfadiazine-trimethoprim 30 mg/kg q 24 h PO for 14 d
  - Amprolium 19 mg/kg q 24 h PO for 14 d
  - Decoquinate 0.5 mg/kg q 24 h PO for 14 d
- Toxoplasmosis
  - Sulfadiazine 60 mg/kg/d divided q 6 h PO, and pyrimethamine 0.5-1.0 mg/kg/24 h PO, may be used (used for cats, but not evaluated in ferrets). A 7- to 14-day course, to exceed improvement of clinical signs by several days, is recommended. Supplement with brewer's yeast ($^{1}/_{8}$-$^{1}/_{4}$ tsp PO q 24 h) to preclude folic acid deficiency.
- *Cryptosporidium*
  - No treatment is currently available.

RECOMMENDED MONITORING

- Periodic fecal monitoring for endoparasites is recommended.
  - One or two negative examinations after treatment
  - Screening at annual examinations

PROGNOSIS AND OUTCOME

Prognosis and outcome are good if ferrets are properly supported, parasites are eradicated, and reinfection is avoided by proper environmental management.

PEARLS & CONSIDERATIONS

COMMENTS

- Ferrets may be infected by several protozoa and helminths, although the latter are rare.
- Infection by *Toxascaris leonina, Toxocara cati, Ancylostoma* spp., and *Dipylidium caninum* is possible. One may use regimens developed in other species to treat these endoparasites in ferrets, but such use is considered extra-label, and treated animals should be monitored closely for adverse reactions.

PREVENTION

- Daily disposal of feces helps to prevent infection by eliminating oocysts before sporulation.
- Preventing ferrets from having access to dog and cat feces precludes fecal-oral transmission of parasites from those species.
- Food utensils should be kept species-specific.
- Sanitation or replacement of ferret housing, utensils, and other environmental items, which may be contaminated with oocysts or oocytes, should be carried out after initial treatment of infected ferrets.
- Environmental eradication may be attempted. Therapies reported to be efficacious include the following:
  - *Cryptosporidium* spp.: steam cleaning, prolonged exposure to 5% to 10% ammonia
  - *Giardia* spp.: 1% solution of sodium hypochlorite
  - Intestinal coccidia: heat sterilization of caging and utensils
- To prevent toxoplasmosis, avoid feeding ferrets uncooked meat or meat by-products, do not allow them to eat prey (mice, rats, rabbits), and keep cat

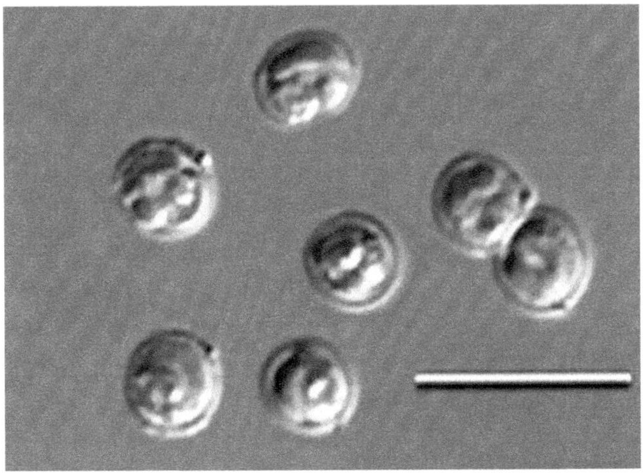

Endoparasites Photomicrograph of Cryptosporidium oocysts using differential interference contrast microscopy (Bar = 10 µm). Reports of cryptosporidiosis among ferrets have appeared for over 20 years. Recent molecular investigations have demonstrated that the ferret has unique genotype of Cryptosporidium. However, no human cases of cryptosporidiosis have been attributed to ferrets. *(Photo courtesy Jörg Mayer, The University of Georgia, Athens.)*

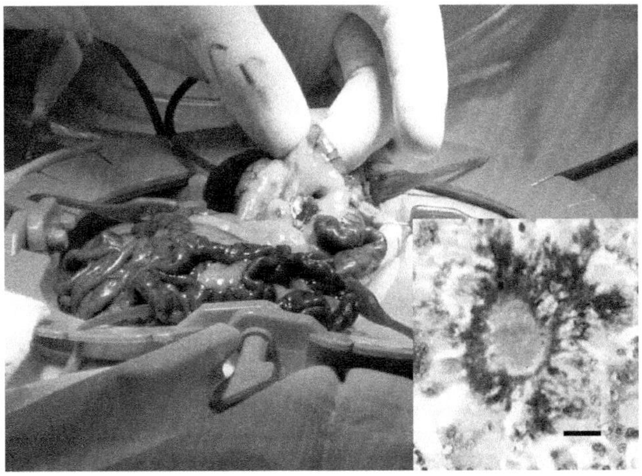

Endoparasites Ferret undergoing exploratory laparotomy. Enlarged mesenteric lymph nodes and a thickened intestine characterize eosinophilic gastroenteritis. Biopsy samples from ferrets with chronic diarrhea should include full-thickness intestinal and mesenteric lymph biopsies. Diagnosis of eosinophilic gastroenteritis requires microscopic demonstration of intestinal and/or mesenteric lymph node eosinophilic infiltration and presence of Splendore-Hoeppli bodies. *Inset,* Photomicrograph of mesenteric lymph node biopsy showing a Splendore-Hoeppli body characterized by radiating eosinophilic deposits from a central core surrounded by multinucleate giant cells and eosinophils. (H&E stain. Bar = 25 µm) *(Photo courtesy Jörg Mayer, The University of Georgia, Athens.)*

feces from contaminating ferret foods, litter boxes, and housing areas.

SUGGESTED READINGS

Blankenship-Paris TL, et al: Enteric coccidiosis in a ferret, Lab Anim Sci 43:361–363, 1993.
Patterson M, et al: Parasites of ferrets. In Baker DG, editor: Flynn's parasites of laboratory animals, ed 2, Ames, IA, 2007, Blackwell Publishing, pp 501–508.
Powers LV: Bacterial and parasitic diseases of ferrets, Vet Clin North Am Exot Anim Pract 12:531–561, 2009.

CROSS-REFERENCES TO OTHER SECTIONS

Campylobacter spp. Infections
Cryptococcosis
Dirofilariasis
Eosinophilic Gastroenteritis
Epizootic Catarrhal Enteritis
Proliferative Bowel Disease

AUTHOR: **ROBERT P. MARINI**

EDITORS: **JAMES G. FOX**

FERRETS

Eosinophilic Gastroenteritis

BASIC INFORMATION

DEFINITION

Disease characterized by eosinophilic infiltration of the gastrointestinal (GI) tract accompanied by GI signs. Affected ferrets frequently have eosinophilia.

SPECIAL SPECIES CONSIDERATIONS

Clinical and pathologic features are seen occasionally in cats.

EPIDEMIOLOGY

SPECIES, AGE, SEX

- No age or sex predilection
- Affected ferrets range in age from 6 months to 5 years

CLINICAL PRESENTATION

HISTORY, CHIEF COMPLAINT Chronic weight loss, anorexia, bloody mucus-laden diarrhea, episodic vomiting

PHYSICAL EXAM FINDINGS Enlarged mesenteric lymph nodes and thickened intestine on abdominal palpation

ETIOLOGY AND PATHOPHYSIOLOGY

- Cause unknown
- Infiltration of eosinophils into intestinal tissue
- Malabsorption
- Fluid loss
- Blood loss
- Electrolyte imbalance

DIAGNOSIS

DIFFERENTIAL DIAGNOSIS

- Inflammatory bowel disease (see Inflammatory Bowel Disease)
- Aleutian disease (see Aleutian Disease)
- Proliferative bowel disease (see Proliferative Bowel Disease)
- Lymphoma—intestinal (see Lymphoma)
- Campylobacteriosis (see *Campylobacter* spp. Infections)
- Salmonellosis
- *Helicobacter mustelae*–associated peptic ulcer disease (see *Helicobacter mustelae*–Associated Gastritis and Ulcers)
- GI foreign body (see Gastrointestinal Foreign Bodies)

INITIAL DATABASE

- Complete blood count (CBC)
  - Normal absolute blood count but relative eosinophilia that can be as high as 30% (in ferret heartworm disease, eosinophilia is often normal or mildly elevated)
- Chemistry profile
- Fecal flotation
- Aleutian virus serologic testing and/or PCR
- Radiographs
- Rectal bacterial cultures

ADVANCED OR CONFIRMATORY TESTING

- Intestinal biopsy—eosinophil infiltration
- Presence of eosinophilia
- Presence of Splendore-Hoeppli bodies (radiating club-shaped bodies of homogeneous eosinophilic material) in intestinal biopsy tissue.

TREATMENT

THERAPEUTIC GOAL

Supportive care: high-calorie dietary supplement (e.g., Nutrical)

ACUTE GENERAL TREATMENT

- If ferret is dehydrated, institute polyionic fluid therapy.
- Provide maintenance dose of 60 ml/kg over 24 hours.

CHRONIC TREATMENT

- Corticosteroid therapy
  - Prednisone 1.25-2.5 mg/kg SID PO until clinical signs abate
- An alternative therapy is ivermectin, which can be successful in individual cases:
  - 0.4 mg/kg SC q 2 wk for 2 doses

RECOMMENDED MONITORING

- Monitor hydration and weight during and after treatment.
- Monitor for peripheral eosinophil count by conducting CBCs.

PROGNOSIS AND OUTCOME

Guarded

CONTROVERSY

- Cause unknown
- Presence of Splendore-Hoeppli bodies is suggestive of an infectious origin (i.e., bacterial, fungal, or parasitic).

PEARLS & CONSIDERATIONS

COMMENTS

Peripheral eosinophilia is highly suggestive of the disease.

CLIENT EDUCATION

- Stress the need to monitor weight and appetite.
- Provide advice regarding complications arising from long-term corticosteroid therapy.

SUGGESTED READINGS

Carmel BC: Eosinophilic gastroenteritis in three ferrets, Vet Clin Exot Anim 9:707–712, 2006.
Fox JG, et al: Eosinophilic gastroenteritis with Splendore-Hoeppli material in the ferret *(Mustela putorius furo)*, Vet Pathol 29:21–26, 1992.
Palley LS, et al: Eosinophilic gastroenteritis in the ferret. In Kirk RW, et al, editors: Current veterinary therapy XI, Philadelphia, 1992, WB Saunders, pp 1182–1184.

CROSS-REFERENCES TO OTHER SECTIONS

Aleutian disease
Campylobacter spp. Infections
Gastrointestinal Foreign Bodies
Helicobacter mustelae–Associated Gastritis and Ulcers
Inflammatory Bowel Disease
Lymphoma
Proliferative Bowel Disease

AUTHOR: **JAMES G. FOX**

EDITORS: **ROBERT P. MARINI**

Epizootic Catarrhal Enteritis

BASIC INFORMATION

DEFINITION

Epizootic catarrhal enteritis (ECE) is an enteric viral disease of ferrets that is caused by a novel coronavirus, designated as ferret enteric coronavirus (FECV). In naïve ferrets, infection results in profuse greenish, mucoid diarrhea with high morbidity and low mortality.

SYNONYMS

Green diarrhea, greenies, green slime, ferret enteric coronavirus infection

SPECIAL SPECIES CONSIDERATIONS

FECV has been implicated anecdotally in diarrheal outbreaks in other Mustelid species.

EPIDEMIOLOGY

SPECIES, AGE, SEX

- Ferrets of all ages may be infected with FECV.
- Older animals may have more severe lesions caused by concomitant inflammatory bowel disease or other systemic illness.

RISK FACTORS

- Animals in facilities that routinely introduce new animals, such as shelters, are at risk.
- Older animals with concomitant disease, especially preexistent gastric *Helicobacter mustelae* infection, are at risk for more significant disease.

CONTAGION AND ZOONOSIS As with other group A coronaviruses, FECV is extremely contagious. The virus is spread easily in feces but may be spread mechanically by contaminated clothing, shoes, examination tables, and instruments.

GEOGRAPHY AND SEASONALITY

- Because of the immunity generated by previous infection, as well as production of maternal antibodies from jills on many breeding farms, true outbreaks of ECE are extremely rare in the United States.
- Most cases of ECE arise outside of the United States as a result of previously unexposed populations and importation of animals from North America for the pet trade.
- There is no seasonality.

ASSOCIATED CONDITIONS AND DISORDERS

- Acutely ill ferrets may develop gastric ulcers owing to the stress of illness and/or treatment.
- Affected animals may develop inflammatory bowel disease as a sequela of infection by FECV.

CLINICAL PRESENTATION

HISTORY, CHIEF COMPLAINT In most cases, the patient history will indicate recent introduction of a clinically normal ferret (often a kit from a pet store) into the house or facility within the last 48 to 72 hours. Naïve ferrets will subsequently develop profuse greenish diarrhea that quickly turns mucoid, ultimately exhibiting a "birdseed-like" consistency. Owners will report various degrees of anorexia in affected animals, with the suspect carrier showing no clinical signs.

PHYSICAL EXAM FINDINGS

- Clinical signs and physical findings are dependent on the duration of illness before presentation, as well as the age of the animal and the presence of concurrent illness.
- Young animals may exhibit no clinical signs besides mucoid diarrhea.
- Older animals may exhibit varying degrees of dehydration and anorexia.
- Clinical signs associated with gastric ulcers may be seen in animals that have been ill for several days.

ETIOLOGY AND PATHOPHYSIOLOGY

- A novel ferret group A coronavirus closely related to feline enteric coronavirus, canine coronavirus, and transmissible gastroenteritis of pigs causes ECE.
    - The virus infects mature enterocytes at villous tips, resulting in villous blunting and fusion.
    - Diarrhea results primarily from significant loss of absorptive surface in the gut, as well as from loss of digestive enzymes normally present in mature villous enteric epithelial cells.

DIAGNOSIS

DIFFERENTIAL DIAGNOSIS

- The differential diagnosis includes other infectious and noninfectious causes of diarrhea:
    - Coccidiosis
    - Campylobacteriosis
    - Rotavirus infection
    - Cryptosporidiosis
    - Salmonellosis
    - Lymphocytic and eosinophilic forms of inflammatory bowel disease

INITIAL DATABASE

- Clinicopathologic changes are not specific for ECE.
- Persistent lymphocytosis, hypoalbuminemia, and mild elevations in globulins suggest bowel inflammation but are not specific for this condition.
- Acutely ill animals may show an elevated alanine aminotransferase and rarely alkaline phosphatase as a result of inanition, starvation, and mobilization of fat stores to the liver.
- Rarely, acutely affected animals may exhibit hemoconcentration and mild electrolyte abnormalities, including hypernatremia, hypochloremia, and an increased anion gap.

ADVANCED OR CONFIRMATORY TESTING

- Definitive diagnosis requires biopsy of the intestine and evaluation for characteristic histopathologic lesions.
- Immunohistochemistry for coronaviral antigen in intestinal biopsy
- PCR on fecal samples or intestinal biopsy

TREATMENT

THERAPEUTIC GOALS

- The overall therapeutic goal is to combat dehydration and maldigestion/malabsorption, while preventing secondary bacterial infection.
- In chronic cases, amelioration of the effects of inflammatory bowel disease is required.

ACUTE GENERAL TREATMENT

- In dehydrated animals, volume replacement with up to 90 mL/kg/d of lactated Ringer's solution may be required.
- Broad-spectrum antibiotics (e.g., enrofloxacin 5 mg/kg bid PO or SC), although not helpful against coronaviral infection itself, are generally recommended to prevent secondary bacterial infection.
- Highly absorbable bland diets, such as Carnivore Care (Oxbow Foods, Inc., Murdock, NE) and Hill's products (Hill's Pet Nutrition, Inc., Topeka, KS), or meat-flavored baby foods, should be administered frequently in small amounts.
- If clinical signs of gastric ulcers are noted, palliative therapy is indicated:
    - Sucralfate 75 mg PO 10 min before meals

- Omeprazole 4 mg/kg PO q 24 h or
- Cimetidine 10 mg/kg PO q 8 h or
- Ranitidine bismuth citrate 24 mg/kg PO q 8 h
- Antibiotic therapy specific for *Helicobacter mustelae*

CHRONIC TREATMENT

- Animals that have recovered from epizootic catarrhal enteritis may develop "inflammatory bowel disease" after several months.
- These animals will often benefit from a bland diet and 0.5 mg/kg oral prednisone daily.
- Lifelong treatment may be required.

PROGNOSIS AND OUTCOME

- Most young, healthy animals will recover within 21 days.
- Older animals, especially those with other chronic illness, often experience more severe clinical signs and a longer disease course.

PEARLS & CONSIDERATIONS

COMMENTS

- Treatment success should be predicated on improvement of stool character over a period of weeks.
- Stools may vary significantly from day to day.

PREVENTION

Owing to prolonged shedding of the virus by carriers (up to 8 months), isolation of new arrivals is rarely beneficial in preventing epizootic catarrhal enteritis.

SUGGESTED READINGS

Williams BH, et al: Retrospective study: coronavirus-associated epizootic catarrhal enteritis (ECE) in ferrets *(Mustela putorius furo)*: 119 cases (1993-1998), J Am Vet Med Assoc 217:526–530, 2000.

Wise AG, et al: Molecular characterization of a novel coronavirus associated with epizootic catarrhal enteritis (ECE) in ferrets, Virology 349:164–174, 2006.

CROSS-REFERENCES TO OTHER SECTIONS

Campylobacter spp. Infection
Endoparasites
Helicobacter mustelae–Associated Gastritis and Ulcers
Inflammatory Bowel Disease

AUTHOR: **BRUCE H. WILLIAMS**

EDITORS: **JAMES G. FOX AND ROBERT P. MARINI**

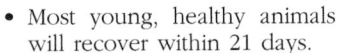

FERRETS

Ferret Systemic Coronaviral Disease (FSCD)

BASIC INFORMATION

DEFINITION

Ferret systemic coronaviral disease (FSCD) is a chronic, lethal disease of domestic ferrets. It is caused by a coronavirus initially designated as ferret systemic coronavirus (FSCV). Microscopic lesions in affected ferrets are identical to those seen in cats with the dry form of feline infectious peritonitis (FIP). The first cases of FSCD were seen in 2002.

SYNONYMS

- Granulomatous inflammatory syndrome (GIS) of ferrets
- Systemic coronavirus–associated disease
- Ferret systemic coronavirus infection
- FIP-like disease of ferrets

SPECIAL SPECIES CONSIDERATIONS

The disease is seen only in domestic ferrets.

EPIDEMIOLOGY

SPECIES, AGE, SEX

- FSCV can infect ferrets of any age and sex, but young ferrets (<1 year old) are more commonly affected. This age-related susceptibility may be due to immune suppression in ferrets that have been recently weaned, neutered, vaccinated, descented, and shipped to pet shops and private pet homes.
- The epidemiology of FSCD follows patterns similar to those of FIP, with outbreaks usually followed by a return to the endemic form of the disease.

RISK FACTORS

- Post-weaning stress and immune suppression due to surgeries, vaccination, overcrowding, and poor husbandry and shipment
- Failure to quarantine newly introduced young ferrets
- The role of fomites is unknown.

CONTAGION AND ZOONOSIS

- Transmission routes are unknown, but it is believed that the virus spreads by the same fecal-oral route as the FIP virus.
- No zoonotic potential is known.

GEOGRAPHY AND SEASONALITY

- The disease has been reported only in Europe and the United States.
- No seasonality is known.

ASSOCIATED CONDITIONS AND DISORDERS

- FSCV and ferret enteric coronavirus (FECV) are different but related viruses. However, it is unknown if there is a relationship between them as has been proposed in cats with FIP and feline enteric coronavirus.
- Many ferrets with FSCD have diarrhea days to months before the development of other signs.

CLINICAL PRESENTATION

DISEASE FORMS/SUBTYPES

- The disease is progressive, chronic, and lethal.
- Ferrets die or are euthanized days to months after the diagnosis. Average survival time after diagnosis is about 2 months.
- The disease is similar to the noneffusive (dry) form of FIP in cats. Lesions of FSCD resembling the effusive (wet) form of FIP have not been reported in ferrets.

HISTORY, CHIEF COMPLAINT

- Diarrhea may be the first clinical sign and can progress from brown-yellow to green-hemorrhagic.
- Weight loss, lethargy, anorexia, and hind limb weakness are common signs.
- Inability to gain weight is seen in growing animals.
- Less common clinical signs include vomiting, cough, sneezing, decreased consumption of water, and bruxism.
- Nasal discharge and rectal irritation have also been reported. Seizures may be observed before death.

PHYSICAL EXAM FINDINGS

- Common physical exam findings include palpable intraabdominal masses and splenomegaly. Intraabdominal irregular masses correspond more often with mesenteric lymphadenopathy, although the kidneys may also be enlarged.
- Fever greater than 40° C (104° F) can occur in some ferrets, but most animals show normal rectal temperature (39.3° C/102.7° F).
- Systolic murmurs, greenish urine, jaundice, and dehydration have rarely been reported.

ETIOLOGY AND PATHOPHYSIOLOGY

- FSCV infection
- Host response to FSCV infection is polyclonal hypergammaglobulinemia that results in systemic granulomatous inflammation.

DIAGNOSIS

DIFFERENTIAL DIAGNOSIS

- Aleutian disease (see Aleutian Disease)
  - Does not always cause mesenteric lymphadenopathy and hypergammaglobulinemia, and when present, these are less marked than in FSCD.
- Lymphoma (see Lymphoma)
  - Can produce gross lesions identical to FSCD, but lymphoma has not been linked to hypergammaglobulinemia in ferrets. Lymphocytosis and abnormal lymphocytes may be seen in some cases of lymphoma, but not in FSCD.
- Proliferative bowel disease
  - Produces diarrhea; mesenteric lymphadenopathy may be seen in rare cases as the result of extraintestinal translocation of colonic mucosa into regional lymph nodes. Hypergammaglobulinemia is not seen. Proliferative bowel disease is less commonly observed now than in the past. It generally affects ferrets younger than 16 weeks old, and the affected large bowel is usually thickened at palpation.
- Eosinophilic gastroenteritis
  - Produces diarrhea; in chronic cases, mesenteric lymphadenopathy occurs. Hypergammaglobulinemia has not been reported, but it might occur because of antigenic stimulation. Peripheral eosinophilia is commonly seen in cases of eosinophilic gastroenteritis.

INITIAL DATABASE

- Blood biochemistry
  - Total protein and protein electrophoresis: mild to moderate hyperproteinemia can be observed in about 50% of cases. Hypergammaglobulinemia is seen in most, if not all, cases. Globulins are usually higher than 4.2 g/dL, representing about 80% of total proteins. Gamma globulins are usually higher than 18 g/L, representing between 35% and 60% of total proteins. This gammopathy is polyclonal.
  - Remaining serum chemistry: nonspecific and dependent on the development of lesions in a particular organ
- Hematologic examination
  - Mild to moderate nonregenerative anemia is seen in about 50% of cases.
  - Mature neutrophilic leukocytosis, thrombocytopenia, and lymphopenia can be observed in some cases.
- Imaging
  - Loss of lumbar musculature, decreased peritoneal detail, presence of mid-abdominal soft-tissue masses and splenomegaly are the most significant radiographic signs.
  - Peritonitis, abdominal lymphadenopathy, splenomegaly, abdominal soft-tissue masses, nephromegaly, and changes in renal cortex echogenicity are potential ultrasonographic findings.
  - Ultrasound is superior to radiology when abdominal contrast is reduced, as frequently occurs in FSCV.

ADVANCED OR CONFIRMATORY TESTING

- Histopathologic examination
  - Multiple angiocentric granulomatous lesions can be observed in visceral organs and brain. These include diffuse granulomatous inflammation on serosal surfaces, and granulomas with or without neutrophils and necrosis. Observation of these microscopic lesions confirms FSCD.
  - If performing an exploratory laparotomy or laparoscopy, aim to biopsy abdominal organs (e.g., lymph nodes, spleen, liver, kidneys, small intestine, large intestine) that are nodular or that have pale, discolored foci on their surface.
- Immunohistochemistry on paraffin-embedded tissues is a confirmatory technique.
  - The monoclonal antibody FCV3-70 detects the presence of antigen in the cytoplasm of macrophages in different types of granulomatous lesions.
- Reverse-transcriptase PCR (RT-PCR)
  - Initially used for detection and characterization of the virus on some fresh-frozen tissues. Its usefulness for diagnostic purposes is unknown.
- Electron microscopy
  - Macrophages containing multiple intracytoplasmic virions, both within cytoplasmic membrane-bound vacuoles and free in the cytoplasm
- Virus isolation in cell culture has been unsuccessful.
- Necropsy
  - Multiple, white, irregular nodules or foci of white discoloration (0.5 to 3 cm) can be observed on the surface and within the parenchyma of different organs: lymph nodes, spleen, liver, kidneys, mesentery, lungs, and heart. Splenomegaly, renomegaly, hepatomegaly and lymph node enlargement can also be seen. Ascites/abdominal effusion has been observed only in a small number of cases.

TREATMENT

THERAPEUTIC GOALS

- Supportive therapy aimed at alleviating clinical signs is indicated.
- Specific treatment is directed at reducing the inflammation typical of the disease.
- Therapeutic protocols are based on those described to treat FIP in cats.
- Euthanasia should be considered.
- Progression to fatal FSCD may be the direct consequence of immune suppression.

CHRONIC TREATMENT

- Nonsteroidal antiinflammatory drugs (NSAIDs) reduce inflammation and do not cause marked immune suppression (e.g., carprofen 1 mg/kg PO q 12-24 h; meloxicam 0.2 mg/kg PO on first day, then 0.1 mg/kg SID PO).
- Antivirals such as ribavirin (50 mg/kg/d based on cat dose) may be effective, if combined with interferon (IFN). Whereas ribavirin is strongly inhibitory of FIP virus and SARS coronavirus in vitro, it is not effective against these viruses in vivo.
- The combination of a type I IFN (interferon alpha or beta) and a type II IFN (interferon gamma) may be helpful. Low doses should be used to avoid causing immune suppression.
- Corticosteroids are better used for a short period (e.g., prednisone 1 mg/kg PO q 24 h 7-14 d) once antiviral drugs have been administered to control viral replication.
- Antibiotics are indicated to control secondary infection.

DRUG INTERACTIONS

- Cytotoxic agents such as azathioprine, methotrexate, and cyclophosphamide could be used to control the immunopathologic consequences of viral infection, but they cause immune suppression.
- The most important side effect of these cytotoxic agents is marrow suppression. Owing to the high turnover of neutrophils, patients most frequently suffer neutropenia rather than thrombocytopenia or anemia. Neutropenia, as well as impaired humoral and cellular immune mechanisms, is responsible for increased susceptibility to bacterial, viral, or parasitic disease during immune suppressive therapy.

POSSIBLE COMPLICATIONS

Doses of ribavirin >100 mg/kg/d in ferrets are immune suppressive.

RECOMMENDED MONITORING

- Complete blood count should be monitored for nonregenerative anemia if the antiviral ribavirin is used.
- Protein electrophoresis is important to assess decrease of inflammation.

PROGNOSIS AND OUTCOME

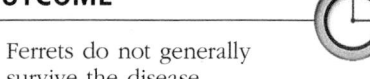

- Ferrets do not generally survive the disease.
- Affected ferrets usually die or are euthanized within 6 months of diagnosis.

CONTROVERSY

As in FIP, initial recoveries in ferrets treated for FSCD may be related not to effectiveness of treatment, but to the normal course of the disease.

PEARLS & CONSIDERATIONS

COMMENTS

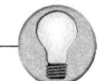

- FSCD is a recently described disease in ferrets, and information available on this condition is still scarce. Consequently, little is known about FSCV. However, partial sequencing of the coronavirus spike gene revealed that it is related to FECV. Hence, it has been proposed that a recent mutation in FECV could result in this disease, similar to the deletion mutation that occurs in feline coronavirus preceding the development of FIP.
- Extrapolation from FIP seems to be the most appropriate way to explain characteristics still unknown about FSCD.

PREVENTION

- Vaccination and noninvasive diagnostic testing are currently unavailable.
- Quarantine all animals, particularly young ferrets from an unknown origin.
- Avoid situations that combine poor hygiene, overcrowding, and stress in young ferrets (weaning, neutering, descenting, vaccination, and shipment in a short period). These situations favor infection and can be seen in shelters, farms, and pet shops.

CLIENT EDUCATION

- Quarantine
- Improved hygiene
- Avoid overcrowding.
- Reduce stress.

SUGGESTED READINGS

Dominguez ER, et al: Abdominal radiographic and ultrasonographic findings in ferrets *(Mustela putorius furo)* with systemic coronavirus infection, Vet Rec 169:231, 2011.

Garner MM, et al: Clinicopathologic features of a systemic coronavirus–associated disease resembling feline infectious peritonitis in the domestic ferret *(Mustela putorius)*, Vet Pathol 45:236–246, 2008.

Martínez J, et al: Identification of group 1 coronavirus antigen in multisystemic granulomatous lesions in ferrets *(Mustela putorius furo)*, J Comp Pathol 138:54–58, 2008.

Perpiñán D, et al: Clinical aspects of systemic granulomatous inflammatory syndrome in ferrets *(Mustela putorius furo)*, Vet Rec 162:180–184, 2008.

CROSS-REFERENCES TO OTHER SECTIONS

Aleutian Disease
Epizootic Catarrhal Enteritis
Lymphoma
Splenomegaly

AUTHORS: **DAVID PERPIÑÁN AND JORGE MARTÍNEZ**

EDITORS: **JAMES G. FOX AND ROBERT MARINI**

FERRETS

Gastrointestinal Foreign Bodies

Client Education Sheet Available on Website

BASIC INFORMATION

DEFINITION

The presence in the stomach and/or small intestine of an ingested object or material that is irritating and/or obstructive, or causes signs referable to partial or complete obstruction of the gastrointestinal (GI) tract

SYNONYM

GI foreign body (FB)

SPECIAL SPECIES CONSIDERATIONS

- The ferret has a short (2.5 to 4 hour) GI transit time, and so eats more frequently than most monogastrics.
- Ferrets allowed to roam can easily pick up foreign objects; ferrets are curious by nature.
- Ferrets are prone to trichobezoars from self-grooming.
- Ferrets are especially drawn to rubber, sponge, and foam materials that are easily ingested but poorly digested.
- No gross delineation can be made between the jejunum and the ileum, or between the ileum and the colon. Ferrets do not have a cecum.

EPIDEMIOLOGY

SPECIES, AGE, SEX

- No age or sex predisposition
- Trichobezoars tend to occur most often in older (>4 years) ferrets and in ferrets with pruritic skin (e.g., adrenal disease).
- Ingestion of foreign objects is more common in younger (<2- to 3-year-old) ferrets.

RISK FACTORS

- Excessive self-grooming
- Free-roaming ferrets
- Access to toys/objects made from foam, sponge, or rubber materials

ASSOCIATED CONDITIONS AND DISORDERS

- Conditions that cause delayed GI transit time, such as GI lymphosarcoma, gastric adenocarcinoma, inflammatory bowel disease (e.g., eosinophilic gastroenteritis), gastric ulcers, gastritis, *Helicobacter*, and ileus, may predispose to foreign body retention.
- Esophageal foreign bodies are rare but may occur with GI FB when multiple items are ingested.
- Pica due to liver disease or inflammatory bowel disease may predispose to GI FB ingestion.
- Hepatic lipidosis secondary to starvation may be seen with chronic FB.

CLINICAL PRESENTATION

DISEASE FORMS/SUBTYPES Partial or complete obstruction of the stomach and/or intestine

HISTORY, CHIEF COMPLAINT Lethargy, anorexia, decreased appetite, bruxism, ptyalism, pawing at mouth, vomiting, ± diarrhea, melena, weakness, weight loss, weakness, hematemesis

PHYSICAL EXAM FINDINGS May include the following:

- Dehydration, weakness, mucous membrane pallor
- Thin body condition

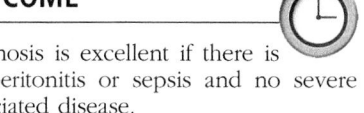

- Abdominal pain and/or distention
- Gas- and fluid-filled GI tract
- Palpable foreign object within the GI tract

ETIOLOGY AND PATHOPHYSIOLOGY

- Ingested foreign material (hair, foam, rubber, plastic, sponge) is too large to pass through the pylorus and/or small intestine, unaided.
- Ileus secondary to other causes does not permit the foreign object to pass.
- Primary ulceration of the mucosa may form, causing pain in the GI tract.
- Pressure necrosis, especially of the small intestine, may occur.

DIAGNOSIS

DIFFERENTIAL DIAGNOSIS

- Gastritis (possibly caused by *Helicobacter mustelae,* gastric mucosa–associated lymphoid tissue [MALT], lymphoma)
- Neoplasia (lymphosarcoma, adenocarcinoma, others)
- Gastric ulcer
- Inflammatory bowel disease (e.g., eosinophilic gastroenteritis)
- Intussusception
- Primary liver disease
- Primary renal disease (see Renal Disorders

INITIAL DATABASE

- Palpation of the abdomen
- Thoracoabdominal radiographs: look for obstructive pattern and effusion (peritonitis), as well as visible FB
- Complete blood count, biochemical profile (hypoglycemia, anemia, leukocytosis may be seen with GI FB)

ADVANCED OR CONFIRMATORY TESTING

- Positive-contrast radiography (barium, iodinated contrast media)
- Abdominal ultrasonography
- Endoscopy: limited to stomach because of small body size

TREATMENT

THERAPEUTIC GOALS

- Restore hydration and correct biochemical imbalances, if any.
- Remove FB(s).
- Treat any peritonitis.
- Reestablish normal GI motility and integrity.
- Return to oral alimentation.

ACUTE GENERAL TREATMENT

- Supportive care: IV catheter, fluids and electrolytes, glucose if hypoglycemic
- Endoscopic removal of FB, if possible
- Medical management in some cases (oral administration of a fluid lubricant) may induce passage of small, nonobstructing FBs.
- Surgical removal of FB
  - Preemptive analgesics, epidural
  - Abdominal exploratory
  - Liver biopsy for evaluation of hepatic lipidosis, other disease
  - Careful palpation of GI tract to look for multiple FBs
  - Gastric biopsy ± culture for *H. mustelae* if ulcers present, or if the gastric FB is chronic
  - Enterotomy or intestinal resection/anastomosis, as needed for intestinal FB (4-0 or 5-0 monofilament suture to close the bowel)
- Postoperative analgesics
  - Postop antacid ranitidine HCl 3.5 mg/kg IV or PO q 12 h
  - Famotidine 0.25-0.5 mg/kg PO, IV, SC q 12 h
  - Omeprazole 0.7 mg/kg PO q 24 h
- GI coating agents (sucralfate 2.5-5 mg/ferret q 12 h; do not give within 1 hour of other oral medications or food)
- Syringe-feed if needed to induce appetite in postoperative ferrets that are anorexic without discernible cause.

CHRONIC TREATMENT

- Cage rest 7 to 10 days before resuming normal activity or interacting with other ferrets
- Do not allow ferrets to roam freely without direct supervision.
- Remove all suspect FB material from the ferret's environment.
- Treat dermatologic problems promptly to prevent excessive self-grooming and hairball formation.

POSSIBLE COMPLICATIONS

- Incisional infection of subcutaneous fat, if proper sterile technique is not observed (change gloves and instruments, lavage abdomen and subcutaneous tissue, during surgery)
- Dehiscence of enterotomy and peritonitis
- Long-term stricture of enterotomy site (rarely a problem unless ferret ingests another FB[s]: it may lodge at stricture site that previously would have been large enough to allow FB to pass through the bowel)
- Morbidity from concurrent disease (hepatic lipidosis, GI neoplasia, inflammatory bowel disease, *Helicobacter* infection)

RECOMMENDED MONITORING

- Routine postop care:
  - Nothing by mouth (NPO) for 12 hours
  - Reintroduce food and water.
  - Watch for vomiting/diarrhea.
  - Treat coexisting medical problems.
- Observe for signs of obstruction in the future, especially if an enterotomy is done.
- Monitor access to foreign materials.

PROGNOSIS AND OUTCOME

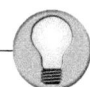

Prognosis is excellent if there is no peritonitis or sepsis and no severe associated disease.

CONTROVERSY

- Endoscopy: many ferret FB would be amenable to endoscopic removal with the proper equipment (small insertion tube ≈5 mm)
- When to do surgery?
  - If a FB is in the intestine, stabilize as much as possible and do surgery the same day.
  - If gastric nonobstructive FB: can stabilize over longer period, but still should do surgery within 24 hours of diagnosis

PEARLS & CONSIDERATIONS

COMMENTS

- Hairballs may be prevented by using a cat laxative at ¼ the recommended cat dose, 2 to 3 times weekly, if itching or excessive grooming is noted.
- Small FBs may be flushed through the GI tract by orally administering a lubricant, or during surgery by injecting a small bolus of saline solution into the small intestine with a 25-gauge needle, orad (in direction toward mouth) to the FB, then "milking" the FB out through the colon with the fluid.

PREVENTION

- Confine ferrets to a safe enclosure unless properly supervised.
- Do not provide materials that may be chewed up and ingested.
- Treat all skin diseases promptly.

CLIENT EDUCATION

Clients should be educated about ferret-proofing the environment and about signs to look for with FB ingestion.

SUGGESTED READINGS

Bixler H, et al: Ferret care and husbandry, Vet Clin North Am Exot Anim Pract 7:227–255, 2004.

Mullen HS, et al: Gastrointestinal foreign body in ferrets: 25 cases (1986-1990), J Am Anim Hosp Assoc 28:13–19, 1992.

Schwarz LA, et al: The normal upper gastrointestinal examination in the ferret, Vet Radiol Ultrasound 44:165–172, 2003.

Wagner R, et al: Diagnosing gastric hairballs in ferrets, Exot DVM 10:19–23, 2008.

CROSS-REFERENCES TO OTHER SECTIONS

Adrenal Disease
Eosinophilic Gastroenteritis
Helicobacter mustelae–Associated Gastritis and Ulcers
Hepatobiliary Disease
Renal Disorders

AUTHOR: **HOLLY S. MULLEN**

EDITORS: **JAMES G. FOX AND ROBERT MARINI**

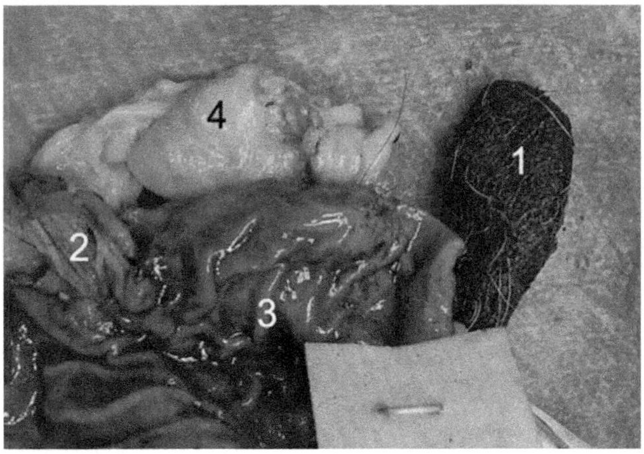

Gastrointestinal Foreign Bodies Necropsy examination of a ferret showing dissected stomach. Examination of the stomach revealed a gastric trichobezoar *(1)* and ulcerations of the gastric mucosa *(3)*. The esophagus *(2)* and mesenteric fat *(4)* are identified. Trichobezoars occur most frequently in older (>4 y) ferrets and in ferrets with pruritus (e.g. adrenal disease). *(Photo courtesy Jörg Mayer, The University of Georgia Athens.)*

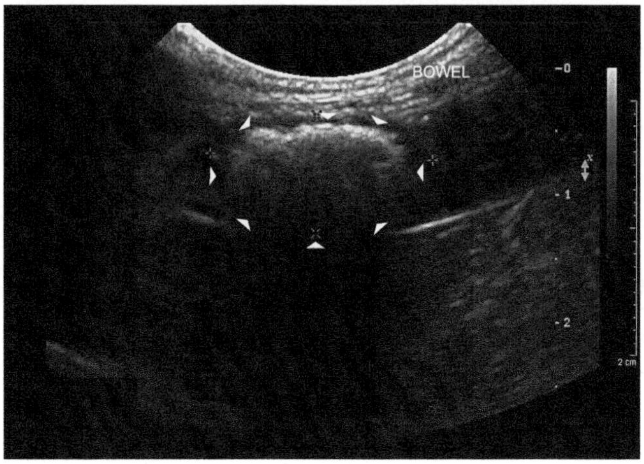

Gastrointestinal Foreign Bodies Ultrasonograph of young ferret with intestinal obstruction. Note the appearance of the foreign body (outlined by white arrowheads) in a distended loop of bowel. Ultrasonography is a useful imaging modality in aiding diagnosis of intestinal foreign bodies as the material comprising foreign bodies is often radiolucent and is not apparent on plain radiographs. *(Photo courtesy Jörg Mayer, The University of Georgia Athens.)*

FERRETS

Heart Disease, AV Block

BASIC INFORMATION

DEFINITION

Atrioventricular (AV) block refers to delayed or terminated conduction of the electrical impulse through the AV node, preventing normal transmission of the signal from the atria to the ventricles.

SYNONYM

Complete heart block is a synonym for third-degree AV block.

SPECIAL SPECIES CONSIDERATIONS

In a recent retrospective study of electrocardiographic diagnoses in ferrets, AV block was the most common electrocardiogram (ECG) abnormality diagnosed.

EPIDEMIOLOGY

SPECIES, AGE, SEX In general, heart disease in ferrets is most commonly diagnosed in middle-aged to older pets.

ASSOCIATED CONDITIONS AND DISORDERS Third-degree AV block may be associated with structural heart disease.

CLINICAL PRESENTATION

DISEASE FORMS/SUBTYPES

- First-degree AV block: slowing of conduction through the AV node, represented by a prolonged PR interval on the ECG (the expected PR interval in a ferret is 0.03 to 0.06 second)
- Second-degree AV block: occasional or regular nonconduction through the AV node represented by P waves not followed by a QRS (ventricular) complex on the ECG. Second-degree AV block may be further subcategorized as follows:
  - Mobitz type I (Wenckebach phenomenon): the PR interval becomes progressively prolonged, culminating in a nonconducted P wave (uncommon in ferrets)
  - Mobitz type II: the PR interval is constant, but some P waves are not conducted to the ventricles (not followed by a QRS complex). If nonconducted P waves occur in regular repetitions, this pattern can be described by using a ratio of P waves to QRS complexes (e.g., 3 : 1). This type of AV block may be further described as "high grade" if it occurs with three or more consecutive nonconducted P waves.
- Third-degree AV block: complete failure of the AV node to convey the atrial electrical impulse to the ventricles, leading to complete dissociation of P waves and QRS complexes on an ECG. With this bradyarrhythmia, P waves occur regularly and at a rate faster than the ventricular escape rate (rate of QRS complexes). QRS complexes are typically wide and bizarre in appearance owing to their ventricular origin, although they may appear

narrow if originating high in the ventricle or at the AV junction.

HISTORY, CHIEF COMPLAINT

- First- and second-degree AV blocks are most commonly diagnosed as an incidental finding in ferrets examined for another problem, or during a routine exam.
- Ferrets with third-degree AV block or high-grade second-degree AV block commonly present for collapse, weakness, or lethargy, or with signs of dyspnea due to congestive heart failure.

PHYSICAL EXAM FINDINGS

- First-degree AV block is not detectable on physical exam (the diagnosis is made on the basis of ECG findings).
- Second-degree AV block may be suspected on the basis of auscultation of pauses in heart rhythm. Overall heart rate may be decreased with higher grades of second-degree AV block.
- Third-degree AV block is suspected when the heart rate is significantly lower than normal for this species (180 to 250 bpm). If congestive heart failure (CHF) is present, ferrets may have an increased respiratory rate and effort, harsh lung sounds or crackles due to pulmonary edema, dull lung and heart sounds due to pleural effusion, and cyanotic mucous membranes.

ETIOLOGY AND PATHOPHYSIOLOGY

- First-degree AV block and low-grade second-degree AV block may occur as normal variants in ferrets, often concurrent with respiratory sinus arrhythmia.
- Many drugs can cause iatrogenic AV block, including beta-adrenergic blockers, calcium channel blockers, digoxin, and opioids.
- Pathologic disorders that increase vagal tone (i.e., gastrointestinal disorders) may lead to AV block.
- AV block may occur as the result of idiopathic fibrosis of the AV node, or after damage/infiltration associated with structural heart disease (e.g., dilated cardiomyopathy, hypertrophic cardiomyopathy).
- Severe hyperkalemia (as can occur with urethral obstruction) may lead to third-degree AV block.

DIAGNOSIS

DIFFERENTIAL DIAGNOSIS

- Ferrets that present with weakness, lethargy, or collapse: differential diagnoses include systemic diseases such as hypoglycemia, anemia, and neoplasia
- Ferrets who present with dyspnea:
  - Differential diagnoses include (CHF) secondary to structural heart disease (without AV block).
  - Primary respiratory disease such as pneumonia
  - Pneumothorax (usually secondary to trauma)
  - Pleural effusion secondary to heartworm disease or neoplasia such as lymphoma

INITIAL DATABASE

- Electrocardiogram (ECG): essential for definitively diagnosing AV block. An ECG may be obtained by placing the ferret in lateral recumbency, or by restraining the ferret using a scruff and hanging the ferret vertically if lateral positioning is resisted. Moistened gauze squares may be used to cushion the clamps, and the teeth on the alligator clips should be filed smooth before they are used. Alternatively, alligator clips may be used in conjunction with adhesive ECG electrodes used for infants (e.g., Tende-Trode, Vermed, Bellows Falls, VT).
- Complete blood count and serum biochemistry (including blood glucose) may be useful for differentiating metabolic or other systemic causes of weakness or collapse.

ADVANCED OR CONFIRMATORY TESTING

- Echocardiogram: useful in checking for structural heart disease. Most ferrets with first- or second-degree AV block have normal echocardiographic findings. Ferrets with third-degree AV block may have severe underlying structural disease, or evidence of chronic volume loading (chamber dilation), secondary to long-standing bradycardia.
- Thoracic radiographs should be obtained if dyspnea is present.

TREATMENT

THERAPEUTIC GOALS

- First-degree and low-grade second-degree AV block: no hemodynamic consequence; treatment not required
- Third-degree and high-grade second-degree AV block: if significant bradycardia and clinical signs attributable to this are present, the goal of therapy would be to increase the ventricular response rate (thereby improving cardiac output) via a pacemaker.
- CHF may accompany third degree AV block, and in these cases, diuretics are used to relieve congestion.

ACUTE GENERAL TREATMENT

- First- and low-grade second-degree AV block: treatment not required
- Third-degree and high-grade second-degree AV block causing clinical signs: IV isoproterenol (0.04-0.08 mcg/kg/min continuous-rate infusion) may be administered to severely symptomatic ferrets, but results in canine and feline species are often variable and unrewarding. For very unstable ferrets, transcutaneous emergency pacing (before plans are made for more permanent pacing) may be considered.

CHRONIC TREATMENT

- First- and low-grade second-degree AV block: treatment not usually required
- Third-degree AV block and high-grade second-degree AV block causing clinical signs: a pacemaker is the treatment of choice for these arrhythmias in canines, and may be considered for symptomatic ferrets. One case report describes an epicardial pacemaker used to treat third-degree AV block in a ferret.

POSSIBLE COMPLICATIONS

Epicardial pacemaker implantation is major surgery and is not routinely performed in this species. Potential complications include intraoperative mortality, infection, and equipment malfunction.

RECOMMENDED MONITORING

- Periodic auscultation ± ECG is prudent for ferrets with first- and second-degree AV block (although these milder forms of AV block uncommonly degenerate to third-degree AV block).
- For ferrets living with high-grade second-degree or third-degree AV block, periodic monitoring of ECGs, echocardiograms, and thoracic radiographs is advised.

PROGNOSIS AND OUTCOME

- Prognosis for first- and low-grade second-degree AV block in ferrets is excellent.
- Prognosis for ferrets with symptomatic third-degree and high-grade second-degree AV block is guarded to poor (without pacemaker implantation).

PEARLS & CONSIDERATIONS

COMMENTS

- First- and low-grade second-degree AV block is commonly diagnosed in ferrets without structural heart disease and typically is not a matter of clinical concern.
- In the author's experience, some ferrets with pauses in heart rhythm on auscultation can have a normal sinus rhythm recorded on a subsequent ECG. Presumably, increased sympathetic tone from the stress of the ECG recording is eliminating the AV block in these cases.
- Ventricular antiarrhythmic medications should not be administered to ferrets

with high-grade second-degree or third-degree AV block (without artificial pacing) because of risk of suppression of the ventricular escape rhythm.

SUGGESTED READINGS

Bublot I, et al: The surface electrocardiogram in domestic ferrets, J Vet Cardiol 8:87–93, 2006.

Malakoff RL, et al: Echocardiographic and electrocardiographic findings in ferrets: 95 cases (1994-2009), JAVMA 2012; accepted for publication.

Sanchez-Migallon Guzman D, et al: Pacemaker implantation in a ferret *(Mustela putorius furo)* with third-degree AV block, Vet Clin North Am Exot Anim Pract 9:677–687, 2006.

CROSS-REFERENCES TO OTHER SECTIONS

Hepatobiliary Disease
Renal Disorders

AUTHOR: **REBECCA L. MALAKOFF**

EDITORS: **JAMES G. FOX AND ROBERT P. MARINI**

FERRETS

Heart Disease, Structural

Client Education Sheet Available on Website

BASIC INFORMATION

DEFINITION

- Dilated cardiomyopathy (DCM): heart muscle disease characterized by a dilated, often spherical, left ventricular chamber with thin walls and depressed wall motion, and variable degrees of left atrial enlargement. The right atrium and ventricle may be affected as well.
- Hypertrophic cardiomyopathy (HCM): heart muscle disease characterized by thickening of the left ventricular walls, with small or normal left ventricular chamber size, and normal or hyperdynamic left ventricular wall motion
- Restrictive cardiomyopathy: heart muscle disease characterized by significant left or biatrial enlargement with relatively normal left ventricular wall thicknesses and motion
- Degenerative valvular heart disease: cardiac disease characterized by thickening and regurgitation of one or more valves

SYNONYM

Endocardiosis is a synonym for degenerative valvular heart disease.

SPECIAL SPECIES CONSIDERATION

The ferret has a long thoracic cavity bordered by 14 ribs (as opposed to 13 ribs in canine and feline species). The ferret heart is located farther caudally in the thorax than that of dogs and cats, lying roughly between the 6th and 8th ribs.

EPIDEMIOLOGY

SPECIES, AGE, SEX Heart disease is most commonly diagnosed in middle-aged to older ferrets.

ASSOCIATED CONDITIONS AND DISORDERS Systemic hypertension and hyperthyroidism have been associated with left ventricular hypertrophy in feline and canine species, but this has not been reported in ferrets.

CLINICAL PRESENTATION

DISEASE FORMS/SUBTYPES

- See the Definition section for the forms of cardiac disease most commonly seen in ferrets (DCM, HCM, etc.)
- Degenerative valvular disease is the most common echocardiographic diagnosis made in ferrets.
  - The aortic valve is most commonly affected, followed by the mitral valve.
  - Trivial aortic insufficiency is a common incidental echocardiographic finding in ferrets; it is usually of no clinical significance. More severe aortic regurgitation, especially in conjunction with mitral regurgitation, may be associated with congestive heart failure (CHF).
- CHF: may occur with any of the forms of structural heart disease described
  - Left-sided CHF is manifested as pulmonary edema and pulmonary vascular congestion. Right-sided CHF may be manifested as pleural effusion, pericardial effusion, hepatomegaly, and/or ascites.
  - DCM is often associated with CHF in ferrets.

HISTORY, CHIEF COMPLAINT Ferrets with heart disease may present for lethargy, dyspnea, decreased appetite, weight loss, weakness, collapse/syncope, or exercise intolerance.

PHYSICAL EXAM FINDINGS May include the following:

- Auscultation abnormalities: heart murmur, arrhythmia, gallop sounds, muffled heart or lung sounds (with pleural or pericardial effusion), harsh lung sounds or crackles (with pulmonary edema)
- Cyanotic mucous membranes
- Prolonged capillary refill time
- Jugular venous distention
- Pulse deficits
- Ascites and/or hepatomegaly

ETIOLOGY AND PATHOPHYSIOLOGY

- Although taurine deficiency has been found as a cause of dilated cardiomyopathy in feline and canine species, this has not been reported in ferrets.
- Nonbacterial thrombotic endocarditis affecting the aortic valve has been reported in a ferret treated for a bite wound. Histopathologic examination revealed both myxomatous degeneration of the valve (a typical finding in dogs with endocardiosis) and inflammatory changes (likely representing two distinct pathologic processes).

DIAGNOSIS

DIFFERENTIAL DIAGNOSIS

- Differential diagnoses for dyspnea/collapse include pneumonia, primary or metastatic neoplasia, pneumothorax (usually secondary to trauma), diaphragmatic hernia, hypoglycemia, metabolic acidosis, and anemia.
- Differential diagnoses for pleural effusion include neoplasia (e.g., lymphoma), heartworm disease, hemothorax, and chylothorax.
- Differential diagnoses for abdominal distention/ascites include neoplasia, hemoabdomen, uroabdomen, hypoalbuminemia (from GI or liver disease), and polycystic disease (renal, liver).

INITIAL DATABASE

- Thoracic radiographs: useful for detecting cardiomegaly, pulmonary vascular changes, pulmonary edema, or pleural effusion
- Complete blood count, chemistry screen (including blood glucose), and potentially blood gas may be useful in differentiating metabolic from other systemic causes of dyspnea and weakness.
- Occult heartworm ELISA (e.g., IDEXX SNAP Heartworm Test, IDEXX Laboratories, Westbrook, ME)

ADVANCED OR CONFIRMATORY TESTING

- Electrocardiogram (ECG): provides a diagnosis of underlying heart rhythm

(arrhythmias may be seen with structural heart disease)
  - An ECG may be obtained by placing the ferret in lateral recumbency or by restraining the ferret using a vertical scruff if lateral positioning is resisted.
  - Moistened gauze squares may be used to cushion the clamps, and the teeth should be filed smooth. Alternatively, adhesive pediatric electrodes may be applied to shaved skin and the clamps attached to the metal stud.
- Echocardiogram: provides detailed information about the size of cardiac chambers, wall thicknesses, systolic wall function, and valvular competency, in most cases allowing a definitive diagnosis of structural heart disease if one exists.

TREATMENT

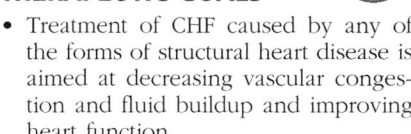

THERAPEUTIC GOALS

- Treatment of CHF caused by any of the forms of structural heart disease is aimed at decreasing vascular congestion and fluid buildup and improving heart function.
- Treatment of structural heart disease in ferrets in the preclinical (asymptomatic) phase is controversial but may be attempted, depending on the underlying cause and degree of secondary cardiac changes.

ACUTE GENERAL TREATMENT

- Acute CHF should be treated with parenteral furosemide (IV or IM, typically at doses of 1 to 4 mg/kg q 8-12 h) and supplemental oxygen in the emergency setting.
- If significant pleural effusion is present, thoracocentesis should be performed. Ideally, radiographic or ultrasound guidance should be used to determine the optimal location for thoracocentesis (may be cranial to the heart).
- Nitroglycerin paste may be used for acute CHF, but caution should be used to avoid hypotensive effects to which ferrets may be particularly prone.

CHRONIC TREATMENT

- Long-term oral therapy with furosemide or other diuretics is required for chronic management of CHF:
  - Furosemide is typically administered at doses of 1-4 mg/kg PO q 8-12 h (start low and titrate upward).
  - If CHF is refractory to standard treatment with furosemide, addition of thiazide diuretics and/or potassium-sparing diuretics may be considered (typically used at published feline dosages).
- Angiotensin-converting enzyme (ACE) inhibitors, such as enalapril, are commonly used with CHF to blunt activation of the renin-angiotensin-aldosterone system and decrease salt and water retention, to reduce afterload by vasodilatation, and to attempt to slow disease progression:
  - Ferrets can be sensitive to the hypotensive effects of ACE inhibitors, so caution should be used with dosing.
  - Enalapril doses starting at 0.25–0.5 mg/kg PO q 48 h may be given and titrated up to 0.5 mg/kg PO q 24 h if tolerated.
- Digoxin may be considered for ferrets with DCM and for those with supraventricular tachyarrhythmias. No data are available regarding the pharmacokinetics of this drug in ferrets; cautious dosing should be used, along with close monitoring for signs of toxicity (anorexia, vomiting, diarrhea):
  - Digoxin elixir is recommended for more accurate dosing in ferrets, typically starting at 0.01 mg/kg PO q 24 h, based on lean body weight (usually ≈75% of body weight).
  - Serum digoxin levels may be measured 6 to 8 hours after drug administration, although reference values for this species are not available (extrapolated reference values for dogs are often used for evaluation).
  - Use of digoxin is contraindicated in ferrets with significant azotemia, hypokalemia, severe bradyarrhythmias, or severe ventricular arrhythmias.
- Beta-adrenergic blockers (e.g., atenolol) may be used for ferrets with tachyarrhythmias and/or HCM. The recommended dosage of atenolol is 3.125 to 6.25 mg per ferret PO q 24 h.
- Calcium channel blockers (e.g., diltiazem) may be used for ferrets with tachyarrhythmias and/or HCM at a dosage of 3.75 to 7.5 mg per ferret PO q 12 h.
- Pimobendan is a phosphodiesterase-inhibiting, calcium-sensitizing inodilator that has recently become available for treatment of CHF caused by DCM or degenerative valvular disease in dogs. This drug provides inotropic support and vasodilatation. Extra-label use in ferrets with DCM has met with some anecdotal success. Dosages of pimobendan used in ferrets have included 0.25 mg/kg PO q 24 h, or ½ of a 1.25-mg tablet PO q 12 h.

DRUG INTERACTIONS

- Aggressive diuresis in conjunction with ACE inhibitors may predispose to hypotension.
- Avoid combining drugs with negative chronotropic and inotropic effects (i.e., beta-adrenergic blockers and calcium channel blockers).

POSSIBLE COMPLICATIONS

- Electrolyte abnormalities caused by diuretics and/or ACE inhibitors
- Dehydration (from diuretics)
- Azotemia (from decreased renal function related to ACE inhibitors, digoxin
- Pneumothorax secondary to thoracocentesis

RECOMMENDED MONITORING

- In the acute setting, monitoring of respiratory rate and effort is essential.
- Monitor for signs of hypotension (lethargy, anorexia).
- Monitor renal values and electrolytes closely.

PROGNOSIS AND OUTCOME

Prognosis is highly variable depending on the underlying heart disease and response to therapy.

CONTROVERSY

DCM has previously been described as the most commonly reported form of heart disease in ferrets. However, a recent retrospective study of echocardiographic diagnoses in ferrets demonstrates that chronic valvular disease is much more commonly diagnosed. Although DCM is infrequently diagnosed, it is often associated with CHF, and therefore remains a clinically important disease for this species.

PEARLS & CONSIDERATIONS

COMMENTS

Primary cardiac disease is a relatively common finding in pet ferrets. It is important for practitioners who work with this species to be able to recognize pertinent historical clues and physical exam findings, and to understand diagnostic and therapeutic options.

PREVENTION

To date, no methods are known for preventing structural cardiac disease in ferrets.

CLIENT EDUCATION

Clients should be educated to watch for signs of cardiac disease in their ferrets (dyspnea, weakness, etc.) and to be aware that diagnostic and treatment options are available if heart disease is present.

SUGGESTED READINGS

Gaztanaga R, et al: Clinical case: dilated cardiomyopathy in a ferret, Madrid, October 26-29, 2006, Proceedings of 41th AVEPA Congress.

Kottwitz JJ, et al: Nonbacterial thrombotic endocarditis in a ferret (*Mustela putorius furo*), J Zoo Wildl Med 37:197–201, 2006.

Malakoff RL, et al: Echocardiographic and electrocardiographic findings in ferrets: 95

cases (1994-2009), JAVMA 2012; accepted for publication.
Stepien RL, et al: M-mode and doppler echocardiographic findings in normal ferrets sedated with ketamine hydrochloride and midazolam, Vet Radiol Ultrasound 41:452–456, 2000.
Wyre NR, et al: Clinical technique: ferret thoracocentesis, Semin Avian Exot Pet Med 14:22–25, 2005.

CROSS-REFERENCES TO OTHER SECTIONS

Heart Disease, AV Block
Dirofilariasis

AUTHOR: **REBECCA L. MALAKOFF**

EDITORS: **JAMES G. FOX AND ROBERT P. MARINI**

FERRETS

Helicobacter mustelae-Associated Gastritis and Ulcers

Client Education Sheet Available on Website

BASIC INFORMATION

DEFINITION

Helicobacter mustelae chronic infection resulting in chronic gastritis, duodenitis, and ulcer formation

SYNONYM

Helicobacter-associated gastric disease

EPIDEMIOLOGY

SPECIES, AGE, SEX
- Acquired at young age
- Persistent infections
- No gender bias

GENETICS AND BREED PREDISPOSITION
- Virtually 100% prevalence in ferrets from selected commercial breeders in the United States
- Prevalence in other countries unknown

RISK FACTORS Fecal/oral spread of *H. mustelae* infection acquired by kits from older ferrets

ASSOCIATED CONDITIONS AND DISORDERS Chronic *H. mustelae* may result in development of gastric adenocarcinoma or gastric mucosa-associated lymphoid tissue (MALT) lymphoma.

CLINICAL PRESENTATION

DISEASE FORMS/SUBTYPES
- Chronic gastritis
- Gastric or duodenal ulcers
- Gastric cancer

HISTORY, CHIEF COMPLAINT
- Weight loss
- Vomiting
- Lethargy
- Bruxism (teeth grinding)
- Inappetence

PHYSICAL EXAM FINDINGS
- Black tarry stool (melena)
- Enlarged gastric lymph nodes
- Anemia

ETIOLOGY AND PATHOPHYSIOLOGY

- Chronic gastric inflammation with or without gastric or duodenal ulcers
- Recent stress (e.g., surgery) may precipitate ulcer formation.
- Diagnose by gastric biopsy and histologic examination, culture of the organism from stomach with subsequent identification. Identify with special silver stain on histologic examination.
- Diagnosis by endoscopy

DIAGNOSIS

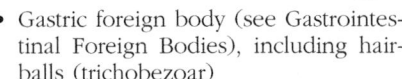

DIFFERENTIAL DIAGNOSIS

- Gastric foreign body (see Gastrointestinal Foreign Bodies), including hairballs (trichobezoar)
- Gastric tumor

INITIAL DATABASE

Complete blood count to determine degree of anemia, particularly if ferret has melena

ADVANCED OR CONFIRMATORY TESTING

- Use contrast barium radiography to depict ulcers.
- Diagnose by gastric biopsy and histologic examination.

TREATMENT

THERAPEUTIC GOALS

- Eradicate *H. mustelae* with antimicrobial therapy.
- Original triple therapy
  - Amoxicillin 10 mg/kg PO q 12 h; metronidazole 20 mg/kg PO q 12 h; bismuth subsalicylate 17 mg/kg (1 mL/kg) PO q 12 h
- Alternative therapies
  - Clarithromycin 12.5 mg/kg PO q 8 h; ranitidine bismuth citrate 24 mg/kg PO q 8 h, or
  - Clarithromycin 50 mg/kg PO q 24 h; omeprazole 4 mg/kg PO q 24 h; metronidazole 75 mg/kg PO q 24 h. 14 days of therapy are required for eradication.

ACUTE GENERAL TREATMENT

If ulcer is bleeding, perform endoscopy and cauterize or topically treat ulcer with epinephrine.

CHRONIC TREATMENT

- Treat ulcers using either
  - H2 blockers (e.g., cimetidine 10 mg/kg PO, SC, IM, IV q 8 h; ranitidine bismuth citrate 24 mg/kg PO q 8 h) or
  - Proton pump inhibitors (e.g., omeprazole 4 mg/kg PO q 24 h)
- Provide antacid and prostaglandin inhibitor:
  - Bismuth subsalicylate 17 mg/kg (1 mL/kg) PO q 8 h
- Protect against proteolytic enzymes in gastric tissue:
  - Sucralfate, a cytoprotective agent, 75 mg PO 10 min before meals

PROGNOSIS AND OUTCOME

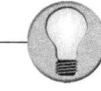

- If acute ulcers develop with bleeding: poor prognosis
- If *H. mustelae* is eradicated with antimicrobials: excellent prognosis

CONTROVERSY

- *H. mustelae* has been associated with splenomegaly.
- Use of silver stains to identify *H. mustelae* in gastric biopsies is an insensitive diagnostic test; quantification of *H. mustelae* using this method is not possible.

PEARLS & CONSIDERATIONS

COMMENTS

If chronic gastritis is present: highly probable that the ferret is infected with *H. mustelae*

PREVENTION

- Highly prevalent acquired infection in kits when co-housed with *H. mustelae*–infected adult ferrets
- Can successfully eradicate *H. mustelae* with antimicrobial therapy in pregnant jill in third trimester, and kits can be raised without becoming infected with *H. mustelae*

CLIENT EDUCATION

Highly likely that pets acquired from pet stores are infected with *H. mustelae*

SUGGESTED READINGS

Erdman SE, et al: *Helicobacter mustelae*–associated gastric MALT lymphoma in ferrets, Am J Pathol 151:273–280, 1997.

Fox JG, et al: *Helicobacter mustelae*-associated gastric adenocarcinoma in ferrets *(Mustela putorius furo)*, Vet Pathol 34:225–229, 1997.

Fox JG, et al: *Helicobacter mustelae*-associated gastritis in ferrets: an animal model of *Helicobacter pylori* gastritis in humans, Gastroenterology 99:352–361, 1990.

Marini RP, et al: Ranitidine bismuth citrate and clarithromycin alone or in combination, for eradication of *Helicobacter mustelae* infection in ferrets, Am J Vet Res 60:1280–1286, 1999.

CROSS-REFERENCES TO OTHER SECTIONS

Gastrointestinal Foreign Bodies

AUTHOR: **JAMES G. FOX**

EDITORS: **ROBERT P. MARINI**

FERRETS

Hepatobiliary Disease

BASIC INFORMATION

DEFINITION

Chronic cholangiohepatitis coupled with cellular proliferation ranging from hyperplasia to neoplasia

EPIDEMIOLOGY

SPECIES, AGE, SEX

- Ferrets, *Mustela putorius furo*, 5 to 8 years of age, castrated males and spayed females (not described in intact males and females)
- Risk factors
  - Not described
  - Preliminary evidence suggests that this condition may have an infectious origin.

CLINICAL PRESENTATION

HISTORY, CHIEF COMPLAINT

- Weight loss (most common)
- Anorexia
- Lethargy
- Diarrhea

PHYSICAL EXAM FINDINGS

- Poor body condition
- Enlarged liver

ETIOLOGY AND PATHOPHYSIOLOGY

- Presumptive etiopathogenesis
  - Chronic infection with a variety of potential pathogens causes hepatobiliary inflammation
  - Inflammation leads to oval cell hyperplasia, with the latter directed toward biliary hyperplasia.
  - Hepatobiliary inflammation and/or chronic infection leads to neoplastic transformation through alteration of cell population homeostasis.

DIAGNOSIS

DIFFERENTIAL DIAGNOSIS

- Infectious (*Helicobacter* spp., *Campylobacter* spp., [see *Campylobacter* spp. Infection] Aleutian disease virus [see Aleutian Disease])
- Metabolic (diabetes mellitus, pregnancy toxemia, anorexia)
- Neoplastic (primary carcinoma, lymphoma, hemangiosarcoma, or metastatic)
- Biliary obstruction
- Toxic (copper toxicosis)

INITIAL DATABASE

- Complete blood count
- Biochemical panel (high alanine aminotransferase is common; alkaline phosphatase may be elevated)
- Urinalysis
- Fecal examination horacic and abdominal radiographs
- Tests for Aleutian disease virus (see Aleutian Disease)

ADVANCED OR CONFIRMATORY TESTING

- Confirmatory tests include ultrasound for confirmation of liver involvement and excisional biopsy via laparotomy with subsequent histopathologic examination (including hematoxylin and eosin–stained and silver-stained sections) and microaerobic culture for *Helicobacter* spp., including antibiotic susceptibility testing. Liver biopsy samples need to be placed in special freeze media (brucella broth and 20% glycerol) and frozen at −80° C (−112° F) before microaerobic culture.
- *Note:* Ultrasound-guided liver biopsy may cause seeding of neoplastic hepatic tissue along the biopsy needle track.

TREATMENT

THERAPEUTIC GOALS

- Treat dehydration with isotonic fluids.
- Provide nutritional support to prevent further weight loss.

ACUTE GENERAL TREATMENT

- Surgical excision of circumscribed liver tumors may be performed.
- Antibiotics may be indicated if liver cultures are positive for *Helicobacter* spp.
  - Antibiotics: broad spectrum (e.g., enrofloxacin 5 mg/kg twice daily); clarithromycin for *Helicobacter* (12.5 mg/kg PO q 8 h)
- Fluid therapy administered according to criteria used in cats; B vitamin or dextrose may be added
- Nutritional support using gruel-feeding by syringe, 5-10 mL q 6-8 h. Foods include blended ferret chow, meat-containing baby foods, and meat-containing prescription diet. Nutrical (CSI Chemical Corporation, Bondurant, IA) is well liked by most ferrets and can be used to administer oral medications.

PROGNOSIS AND OUTCOME

Guarded to poor depending on clinical presentation and histopathologic diagnosis

PEARLS & CONSIDERATIONS

COMMENTS

General supportive care, including attention to nutrition, is recommended.

SUGGESTED READING

García A, et al: Hepatobiliary inflammation, neoplasia, and argyrophilic bacteria in a ferret colony, Vet Pathol 39:173–179, 2002.

Hauptman K, et al: Extrahepatic biliary tract obstuction in two ferrets (Mustela putorius furo), J Small Anim Pract 52:371–375, 2011.

CROSS-REFERENCES TO OTHER SECTIONS

Aleutian Disease
Campylobacter spp. Infection
Eosinophilic Gastroenteritis
Helicobacter mustelae–Associated Gastritis and Ulcers
Proliferative Bowel Disease

AUTHOR: **ALEXIS GARCÍA**

EDITORS: **JAMES G. FOX AND ROBERT P. MARINI**

FERRETS

Hyperestrogenism-Associated Anemia

BASIC INFORMATION

DEFINITION

In female ferrets, prolonged estrus results in estrogen-induced aplastic anemia, in which the bone marrow fails to produce adequate numbers of erythrocytes, leukocytes, and platelets.

SYNONYMS

Aplastic anemia, bone marrow hypoplasia, estrogen-induced bone marrow depression, estrogen toxicosis, estrus-associated anemia, hyperestrogenism, post-estrus anemia

SPECIAL SPECIES CONSIDERATIONS

- Female ferrets (jills) are induced ovulators and require the stimulation of coitus to ovulate. If the jill does not ovulate, she will remain in estrus, resulting in high levels of circulating estrogen that eventually cause bone marrow suppression.
- Jills have a defined breeding season influenced by photoperiod. In the Northern hemisphere, jills exhibit a constant estrus between late March and early August if they are not bred; and between August and January in the Southern hemisphere.
- Jills have both a pregnancy and a pseudopregnancy of 42 days' duration. During the breeding season, jills may return to estrus after pregnancy or pseudopregnancy.
- Exogenous hormonal induction of ovulation will induce pseudopregnancy.

EPIDEMIOLOGY

SPECIES, AGE, SEX Hyperestrogenism occurs in sexually mature jills.

RISK FACTORS Unmated intact jill

GEOGRAPHY AND SEASONALITY Hyperestrogenism is related to the breeding season of ferrets.

ASSOCIATED CONDITIONS AND DISORDERS

- Intact jills with hyperestrogenism may have concurrent hydrometra or pyometra.
- Neutropenia may result in pneumonia, pyometra, and other infections.
- Neutered jills with an ovarian remnant can develop hyperestrogenism.

CLINICAL PRESENTATION

DISEASE FORMS/SUBTYPES

- Mild anemia
  - Frequently associated with early stages of hyperestrogenism
- Severe anemia
  - Occurs with untreated hyperestrogenism

HISTORY, CHIEF COMPLAINT

- Vulval swelling and discharge
- Alopecia
- Lethargy and anorexia in early stage of disease
- Weakness, tachypnea, melena, and collapse in later stage of disease

PHYSICAL EXAM FINDINGS

- Alopecia
- Vulval swelling, discharge, and/or trauma
- Anemia
  - Mild anemia: anorexia, lethargy, pale mucous membranes
  - Severe anemia: as above, weakness, tachypnea, collapse, heart murmur (anemia-related), hemorrhage (petechiae, ecchymoses), hind limb paresis

ETIOLOGY AND PATHOPHYSIOLOGY

Elevated estrogen levels cause myeloid hyperplasia in the bone marrow followed by hypoplasia affecting all cell lines in the peripheral blood. After a brief initial leukocytosis, thrombocytopenia, anemia, and leukopenia occur. Death is usually associated with hemorrhage.

DIAGNOSIS

DIFFERENTIAL DIAGNOSIS

- Adrenal disease (see Adrenal disease)
- Seasonal alopecia
- Ovarian remnant
- Functional ovarian neoplasia
- Anemia
  - Mild anemia is often associated with chronic disease in older ferrets.
  - Mild to severe anemia may be associated with endocrinopathies or hematopoietic neoplasia.
  - Severe anemia occurs in gastric ulcerative disease with chronic hemorrhage (e.g., *Helicobacter mustelae* infection [see Helicobacter mustelae–Associated Gastritis and Ulcers]).
  - Severe anemia occurs with severe acute hemorrhage (e.g., trauma).

INITIAL DATABASE

- Hematology and blood biochemistry
- Anemia due to hyperestrogenism is characterized by
  - Nonregenerative normocytic anemia
  - Thrombocytopenia
  - Leukopenia
  - Hypoproteinemia

ADVANCED OR CONFIRMATORY TESTING

- Bone marrow aspiration
  - Hypocellular bone marrow contains 10% to 20% hematopoietic cells; the other 80% to 90% of cells are adipocytes, lymphocytes, erythrocytes, and hemosiderin-containing macrophages.
- Necropsy
  - Death is usually due to hemorrhage associated with ongoing thrombocytopenia. However, concurrent metritis/vaginitis can develop, leading to pyometra, collapse, and death.
  - Weight loss (normal weights: jills, 0.5 to 1.2 kg; hobs, 1.0 to 2.0 kg)
  - External
    - Pale tissues, cutaneous ecchymosis, and petechial hemorrhages
    - Vulval discharges indicate vaginitis/pyometra, often with culture of *Escherichia coli* and *Corynebacteria* spp.
  - Internal
    - Extensive blood pooling in stomach, small and large intestines
    - Hemorrhages in omentum, urinary bladder, uterus, and periovarian fat

- Cranial subdural hematoma
- Hematomyelia in thoracic and sacral vertebrae, associated with clinical ataxia and paraplegia

TREATMENT

THERAPEUTIC GOAL

To prevent a hemorrhagic death

ACUTE GENERAL TREATMENT

- Remove source of endogenous estrogens:
  - Ovariohysterectomy is indicated when the jill is no longer severely anemic, i.e., >25% packed cell volume (PCV).
  - Alternatively, when PCV is >25%, use ovariohysterectomy or hormonal therapy to induce ovulation (e.g., gonadotropin-releasing hormone [GnRH] agonists 20 mcg IM, or human chorionic gonadotropin [hCG] 100 mcg IM)
- If hormonal therapy is not an option (e.g., rapid removal of estrogen source/ovaries is deemed essential; inability to obtain hormones) then ovariohysterectomy may be necessary. However, it is not without risk of death to the patient and the following measures should be taken.
  - When PCV is 15%–25% perform blood transfusion before surgery.
  - When PCV is <15%, patient stabilization (including blood transfusion) must be performed before ovariohysterectomy (see Chronic Treatment).
- Blood transfusions
  - Required when PCV <15% to 25%
  - Ferrets have no discernible blood groups, and transfusion poses little clinical risk, even without cross-matching.
  - Transfusions involving fresh whole blood are preferable.
  - Multiple blood transfusions may be required.

CHRONIC TREATMENT

- Supportive care in the form of corticosteroids and anabolic steroids
- Antibiotics prophylactically for secondary bacterial infection
- Iron dextran (10 mg IM once) may be indicated for severe hemorrhage.
- Bone marrow transplant: intramedullary bone marrow transplantation can be attempted for severely anemic cases when bone marrow suppression has been prolonged

DRUG INTERACTIONS

Megestrol acetate has been used to delay estrus, but its use is discouraged in intact jills because of the risk of pyometra.

POSSIBLE COMPLICATIONS

- Irreversible bone marrow suppression may occur.
- Hematomyelia in thoracic and sacral vertebrae may result in spinal cord compression, ataxia, and paraplegia. Neurologic deficits may be irreversible.

RECOMMENDED MONITORING

- PCV
- Total plasma protein (TPP)

PROGNOSIS AND OUTCOME

- Good if early detection, and estrus has been <1 month
- Undetected estrus >2 months typically results in sudden death due to hemorrhage.
- PCV <10% is usually fatal.

PEARLS & CONSIDERATIONS

COMMENTS

- Subdural hemorrhage and hematoma formation may result in central nervous system signs.
- Hematomyelia in thoracic and sacral vertebrae may result in spinal cord compression, ataxia, and paraplegia.
- Older breeding jills may produce smaller litters, become sterile, and show alopecia without other signs of hyperestrogenism. This is probably the result of an ovarian tumor. Removal results in a healthy ferret with full coat regrowth.

PREVENTION

- Neutering of jills
- Breeding jills not being bred: consider use of sham mating (vasectomized male) or hormonal therapy to induce ovulation and luteinization (e.g., hCG 100 mcg IM)
  - Hormonal therapy is given after at least 10 days of estrus.
  - Vulval swelling usually diminishes within 1 week.
  - Repeat therapy may be required if jill remains in estrus.
  - Pseudopregnancy typically lasts 40 to 50 days, whereafter jills may or may not return to estrus.
- Alternatively, subcutaneous implants of slow-release formulations of GnRH agonists, such as implants containing deslorelin acetate (4.7 mg), suppresses ovarian follicular development. This is suitable treatment for nonbreeding jills because the average duration of treatment-induced ovarian quiescence with deslorelin is 698 ± 122 days (i.e., the first posttreatment estrus will not occur for at least 2 years).
- With sham mating or hCG treatment, normal post-treatment estrus will occur, and the jill will be able to conceive if mated and to carry pregnancy to term. In contrast, ferrets treated with deslorelin will show a delay in expression of the first post-treatment estrus and if mated will not conceive but will become pseudopregnant. However, second deslorelin post-treatment estrus should be normal, and if jills are mated, they should become pregnant and carry to term.

CLIENT EDUCATION

- Inform owners of the importance of neutering or inducing pseudopregnancy with sham mating or hCG if the jill is intended for breeding.
- Clients considering buying a female ferret should ensure that the ferret has been sterilized at a suitable age before purchase, and should obtain certification of neutering.

SUGGESTED READINGS

Lewington JH, et al: Ferret husbandry, medicine and surgery, ed 2, Philadelphia, 2007, Saunders Elsevier, pp 258–262.
McKay J: Ferret breeding, London, 2006, Swan Hill Press, pp 189–190.
Prohaczik A, et al: Comparison of four treatments to suppress ovarian activity in ferrets (*Mustela putorius furo*), Vet Rec 166:74–78, 2010.
Prohaczik A, et al: Deslorelin treatment of hyperoestrogenism in neutered ferrets (*Mustela putorius furo*): a case report, Vet Med (Praha) 54:89–95, 2009.
Sherrill A, et al: Bone marrow hypoplasia associated with estrus in ferrets, Lab Anim Sci 35:280–286, 1985.

CROSS-REFERENCES TO OTHER SECTIONS

Adrenal Disease
Heart Disease, AV Block
Heart Disease, Structural
Helicobacter mustelae-Associated Gastritis and Ulcers
Lymphoma
Ovarian Remnant Syndrome

AUTHOR: **JOHN HENRY LEWINGTON**

EDITORS: **JAMES G. FOX AND ROBERT P. MARINI**

FERRETS

Ibuprofen and Acetaminophen Toxicity

Client Education Sheet Available on Website

BASIC INFORMATION

DEFINITION

- Ibuprofen toxicosis results in prostaglandin inhibition and altered renal blood flow, gastrointestinal tract ulceration, and platelet dysfunction. Severe overdose of ibuprofen can cause renal failure.
- Acetaminophen toxicity causes depletion of red blood cell glutathione concentration, which results in methemoglobinemia. Hepatic necrosis may be associated with acetaminophen toxicity.

SYNONYMS

- For ibuprofen, common brand names are Motrin, Advil, and Midol.
- For acetaminophen, common brand names are Tylenol and Paracetamol.

EPIDEMIOLOGY

SPECIES, AGE, SEX A gender difference of acetaminophen-UDP-glucuronosyltransferase is apparent in ferrets, with intrinsic clearance values significantly higher in male than in female ferret livers. There is no specific breed predilection.

GENETICS AND BREED PREDISPOSITION In ferrets, glucuronidation of acetaminophen is relatively slow in the liver compared with all other species, except the cat. As in cats, this makes ferrets more vulnerable to acetaminophen toxicity than other species.

RISK FACTORS

- Over-the-counter medications are the fourth most common cause of poisoning in small animals.
- Acetaminophen and ibuprofen toxicities are relatively common because of increasing use of these drugs in human beings.

ASSOCIATED CONDITIONS AND DISORDERS Other toxicities

CLINICAL PRESENTATION

HISTORY, CHIEF COMPLAINT Owners may dose their pets, or animals may gain access to and ingest ibuprofen or acetaminophen.

PHYSICAL EXAM FINDINGS

- Clinical signs of the following:
  - Ibuprofen toxicosis can include vomiting, diarrhea, CNS depression, anorexia, and melena. Severe overdose can cause azotemia and oliguria or anuria from renal failure. Gastrointestinal signs can be seen within 2 to 6 hours after ingestion; renal signs can develop within 12 hours to 5 days after ingestion. Seizures may be observed with severe overdosage.
  - Acetaminophen toxicosis may present with progressive depression, salivation, vomiting, abdominal pain, tachypnea, and cyanosis. Chocolate-colored urine may be seen with hematuria or hemoglobinuria.

ETIOLOGY AND PATHOPHYSIOLOGY

- Ibuprofen toxicosis results in prostaglandin inhibition and altered renal blood flow, gastrointestinal tract ulceration, and platelet dysfunction. Severe overdose of ibuprofen can cause renal failure.
- Acetaminophen toxicity causes depletion of red blood cell glutathione concentration, which results in methemoglobinemia. Hepatic necrosis may be associated with acetaminophen toxicity.

DIAGNOSIS

DIFFERENTIAL DIAGNOSIS

Differentials for

- Ibuprofen include toxicities with other nonsteroidal antiinflammatories (NSAIDs) or disease, causing renal failure
- Acetaminophen include other drug toxicities that can cause methemoglobinemia (e.g., nitrites, phenacetin, nitrobenzene, phenol and cresol compounds, sulfites)

INITIAL DATABASE

- Ibuprofen toxicosis
  - Progressive rise of blood urea nitrogen (BUN), creatinine, and phosphate; metabolic acidosis; inability to concentrate urine. Liver enzymes may be elevated.
- Acetaminophen toxicosis
  - Methemoglobinemia with progressive rise of liver enzymes, hematuria, or hemoglobinuria

ADVANCED OR CONFIRMATORY TESTING

- Ibuprofen
  - Ibuprofen analysis can be performed in the ferret on serum, urine, or hepatic tissues. Renal papillary necrosis is seen in severe cases.
- Acetaminophen
  - Acetaminophen serum concentration is maximally elevated 1 to 3 hours after ingestion; blood glutathione is markedly depressed. Pulmonary edema and liver and kidney congestion may be seen.

TREATMENT

THERAPEUTIC GOALS

- Ibuprofen
  - The primary goal of treatment is to prevent or treat gastric ulceration, renal failure, CNS effects, and possible hepatic effects; however, stabilizing the ferret is the first priority.
- Acetaminophen
  - Patients with methemoglobinemia must be evaluated and treated promptly in an attempt to avoid a hemolytic crisis.

ACUTE GENERAL TREATMENT

- Ibuprofen: emesis and gastric lavage useful within 1 to 2 hours of ingestion; ± activated charcoal 1-3 g/kg PO and a cathartic unless animal is dehydrated; diuresis for 24 to 36 hours to prevent acute renal failure; gastrointestinal protectants; metoclopramide 0.5 mg/kg PO, SC, or IM q 6-8 h to control vomiting; antiseizure medications are indicated if patient is seizuring
- Acetaminophen: emesis and gastric lavage useful within 1 to 2 hours of ingestion; ± activated charcoal immediately after completion of emesis or gastric lavage; *N*-acetylcysteine; whole-blood transfusion may be needed if anemia, hematuria, or hemoglobinuria is severe; fluids and electrolytes (IV) to maintain hydration and electrolyte balance

CHRONIC TREATMENT

- Ibuprofen: gastrointestinal protectants should be used for 5 to 7 days post exposure to prevent gastric ulceration. Nutritional support is important for anorectic patients.
- Acetaminophen: clinical signs may be expected for 12 to 48 hours after ingestion; care should be continued while signs present. Continual monitoring of methemoglobinemia is vital for effective management. Nutritional support is important for anorectic patients.

DRUG INTERACTIONS

- Ibuprofen: substances that could cause an interaction with ibuprofen include coumarin-type anticoagulants, which could increase the risk of gastrointestinal bleeding. Glucocorticoids may

also increase the likelihood of GI ulcerations. Other NSAIDs, such as salicylates, phenylbutazone, and indomethacin, could potentiate the gastrointestinal effects of ibuprofen.
- Acetaminophen: drugs requiring activation or metabolism by the liver may be reduced in effectiveness.

POSSIBLE COMPLICATIONS

- Ibuprofen: renal failure is a potential complication, and papillary necrosis is considered irreversible
- Acetaminophen: liver necrosis and resulting fibrosis may compromise long-term liver function

RECOMMENDED MONITORING

- Ibuprofen: BUN, creatinine, urine specific gravity, and hepatic enzymes should be monitored closely (serum creatinine level alone may not accurately reflect the presence of renal failure in ferrets). Baseline values and then repeated values checked at 36, 48, and 72 hours post exposure are recommended. Urine output should be evaluated, and the ferret should be monitored for acidosis and electrolyte shifts. Hyperphosphatemia, hypocalcemia and reduced total carbon dioxide can be seen in ferrets with renal disease. The animal should be monitored for clinical signs suggestive of gastritis, which may include weight loss, vomiting, hypersalivation, and bruxism.
- Acetaminophen: continual monitoring of methemoglobinemia is vital for patient management; laboratory measurement of methemoglobin percentage ideally performed every 2 to 3 hours. Liver enzyme activities in serum should be determined q 12 h; measurement of blood glutathione provides evidence of effectiveness of treatment.

PROGNOSIS AND OUTCOME

- Ibuprofen: prognosis is good if the ferret is treated promptly and appropriately; delay in treatment can decrease survival potential. Papillary necrosis is generally considered an irreversible condition.
- Acetaminophen: progressively high serum liver enzymes 12 to 24 hours after ingestion warrant serious concern. Methemoglobin concentration in excess of 50% warrants a grave prognosis.

CONTROVERSY

Use of cimetidine with ibuprofen toxicosis appears to be controversial. Cimetidine decreases hepatic blood flow and inhibits hepatic microsomal enzymes. Pretreatment with cimetidine was found to increase both the rate and the extent of absorption of ibuprofen in rats; however, the extent of decreased clearance with single-dose ibuprofen ingestion in humans is considered insignificant.

PEARLS & CONSIDERATIONS

COMMENTS

- Ferrets: as in cats, glucuronidation of acetaminophen is relatively slow in the liver. However, unlike in cats, in which UGT1A6 is encoded by a pseudogene and is dysfunctional, there are no defects in the ferret *UGT1A6* gene that could account for the low level of activity.
- Over a 6-year period (2001-2007), the ASPCA (American Society for Prevention of Cruelty to Animals) Animal Poison Control handled 618 cases of ferrets suspected or observed to have exposure to various toxicants. Most of these exposures (more than 50% of reported cases) occurred to various medications. Ibuprofen, acetaminophen, and the antidepressant venlafaxine were the medications most frequently associated with toxicity.

PREVENTION

Acetaminophen and ibuprofen should be used cautiously (or avoided altogether) in ferrets.

CLIENT EDUCATION

Treatment may be prolonged and expensive in some cases. Prolonged management may be required in patients with significant renal or hepatic disease.

SUGGESTED READINGS

Court M: Acetaminophen UDP-glucuronosyltransferase in ferrets: species and gender differences, and sequence analysis of ferret UGT1A6, J Vet Pharmacol Ther 24:415–422, 2001.

Dunayer E: Toxicology of ferrets, Vet Clin North Am Exot Anim Pract 11:301–314, 2008.

Richardson J, et al: Ibuprofen ingestion in ferrets: 43 cases (January 1995-March 2000), J Vet Emerg Crit Care 11:53–59, 2001.

AUTHOR: **JENNIFER GRAHAM**

EDITORS: **JAMES G. FOX AND ROBERT P. MARINI**

FERRETS

Inflammatory Bowel Disease

Client Education Sheet Available on Website

BASIC INFORMATION

DEFINITION

Inflammatory bowel disease (IBD) is a poorly defined and often incorrectly used term in ferrets and other small animals for a systemic inflammatory disease primarily involving the gastrointestinal tract. Clinical disease results from dysregulation of the mucosal immune response. The umbrella term *IBD* used in ferrets and other small animals for a variety of gastrointestinal diseases is not the same disease that is seen in humans. Clinical signs, origin, endoscopic features, and histopathologic features are very different from those seen in humans. Continued use of the term *IBD* for these diseases in small animals is a source of frustration and confusion to clinicians and pathologists alike.

SYNONYMS

- Crohn's disease, ulcerative colitis
- Incorrectly used synonyms: antibiotic responsive enteritis, eosinophilic enteritis or eosinophilic gastroenteritis, epizootic catarrhal enteritis, food allergy, gluten hypersensitivity, lymphoplasmacytic enteritis, proliferative bowel disease or colitis

SPECIAL SPECIES CONSIDERATIONS

- Ferrets have been reported incorrectly to be susceptible to IBD.
- True IBD is rare in small animals.
- Cotton-top tamarins are natural animal models of human IBD.

EPIDEMIOLOGY

SPECIES, AGE, SEX

- Ferrets are susceptible to several gastrointestinal inflammatory conditions that have erroneously been placed under the umbrella term of IBD.

- The true incidence of IBD (Crohn's disease and ulcerative colitis) in ferrets is unknown.

GENETICS AND BREED PREDISPOSITION

- In contrast to human and canine IBD, no genetic predisposition to IBD in ferrets is known.
- Recent research on Crohn's disease in humans and mouse models of IBD has led to the idea that genetically susceptible individuals develop a dysregulated response of the mucosal immune system to commensal enteric flora. Many genetically susceptible humans, mice, and dogs have defects in intracellular pattern-recognition receptors (PRRs) (e.g., toll-like receptors [TLRs] and nuclear organization domain receptors [NODs]) that are responsible for clearing virulent and commensal bacteria. It is thought that this inability to clear commensal bacteria leads to chronic immune stimulation and harmful cytokine release, resulting in disease.

ASSOCIATED CONDITIONS AND DISORDERS

- IBD often results in extraintestinal disease.
  - Uveitis, cholangitis, and autoimmune liver, pancreatic, and joint disease is commonly seen in humans with IBD.
  - Soft-coated wheaten terriers with IBD often have concurrent protein-losing nephropathy.
  - IBD in cats is frequently associated with cholangiohepatitis and pancreatitis.
- IBD in ferrets may be seen in association with splenomegaly and/or cholangiohepatitis.

CLINICAL PRESENTATION

DISEASE FORMS/SUBTYPES

- Ferret IBD, by the more permissive use of the term, likely consists of a variety of many different diseases that have similar clinical signs and similar histopathologic changes.
- Clinical signs will result depending on which segment of the intestine (and/or abdominal organs) is involved, and the degree (e.g., mild, moderate, severe) of inflammation.
- Specific disease entities in ferrets include the following:
  - Eosinophilic gastroenteritis (see Eosinophilic Gastroenteritis)
  - Epizootic catarrhal enteritis (enteric coronavirus infection) (see Epizootic Catarrhal Enteritis)
  - *Helicobacter mustelae*–associated gastritis (see *Helicobacter mustelae*–Associated Gastritis and Ulcers
  - Proliferative bowel disease *(Lawsonia intracellularis)* (see Proliferative Bowel Disease)
  - Hepatobiliary disease (chronic cholangiohepatitis) (see Hepatobiliary Disease)
- Major forms of IBD in humans are Crohn's disease and ulcerative colitis. The primary difference between them lies in the location and nature of the inflammatory changes.
- Crohn's disease: affects the terminal ileum and colon, occasionally the small intestine, stomach, and esophagus, and rarely the rectum. On endoscopy, skip lesions (patchy areas of inflammation) are seen grossly.
- Ulcerative colitis: continuous colonic involvement beginning in the rectum. The ileum and the small intestine are rarely involved.

HISTORY, CHIEF COMPLAINT Diseases referred to as *IBD* in ferrets typically cause similar clinical signs, including anorexia, decreased appetite, ptyalism, bruxism, pawing at the mouth, weight loss, diarrhea, mucoid or "birdseed" stools, melena, abdominal pain, vomiting, poor hair coat, and ill-thrift.

PHYSICAL EXAM FINDINGS

- Weight loss
- Diarrhea and/or melena
- Abdominal pain
- Thickened rope–like intestines
- Enlarged mesenteric lymph nodes
- Splenomegaly

ETIOLOGY AND PATHOPHYSIOLOGY

- Various origins: usually infectious—*Helicobacter mustelae*, ferret enteric coronavirus, Aleutian disease parvovirus, *Giardia* spp., *Lawsonia intracellularis, Salmonella enterica,* (see Salmonellosis, Sec. VI) *Campylobacter jejuni, Cryptosporidium* spp (see Cryptosporidiosis, Sec. VI).
- Increased mucosal inflammation
- Dysregulated cytokine production
- Enterocyte destruction

DIAGNOSIS

DIFFERENTIAL DIAGNOSIS

- The spectrum of diseases termed in ferrets includes the following:
  - Food protein intolerance, as to cow's milk, peanuts, eggs, etc.
  - Gluten hypersensitivity
  - Autoimmune disorders
  - *H. mustelae*–associated chronic active gastritis
  - Eosinophilic gastroenteritis
  - Giardiasis
  - Microsporidiosis
  - Campylobacteriosis
  - Coccidiosis
  - Enteric coronavirus infection
  - Proliferative bowel disease
  - Salmonellosis
  - Chronic cholangiohepatitis
  - Mycobacteriosis
  - Enteropathy-associated T-cell lymphoma
  - Drug-induced enteropathies

INITIAL DATABASE

- Clinical examination
- Complete boold count (CBC) serum biochemistry: often results are unremarkable
  - In Crohn's disease and ulcerative colitis, iron deficiency anemia is seen.
- Fecal endoparasite exam (flotation) and direct smear

ADVANCED OR CONFIRMATORY TESTING

- Gastroscopic and colonoscopic biopsy and/or surgical biopsy
- Regardless of the portion of the gastrointestinal tract under consideration, histologic abnormalities of IBD are grouped under three broad headings:
  - Changes in mucosal architecture reflecting active or recent epithelial abnormality
  - Increased numbers of leukocytes in the lamina propria
  - Fibrosis within the lamina propria
- Epithelial changes are the most reliable, yet the least prevalent. Subjective impressions of increased numbers of leukocytes within the lamina propria represent the least reliable but the most widely used criterion for a diagnosis, simply because most biopsy samples do not have any other mucosal abnormalities.
- Histopathologic features that are wrongly interpreted as IBD include increased numbers of lamina propria lymphocytes, plasma cells, and eosinophils; increased numbers of goblet cells; villous blunting; and increased intraepithelial lymphocytes. These findings are nonspecific and can be seen in normal ferrets, older animals, and animals with numerous and different gastrointestinal diseases.
- Histopathologic features of Crohn's disease involve the deeper layers of the bowel wall with fissures, sinus tracts, fistulas, and fibrosis, all of which may produce radiographically or endoscopically evident areas of mural thickening and/or luminal stenosis. Most of these features cannot be evaluated in mucosal biopsy specimens and require full-thickness biopsies. Often seen are the following: a mixed inflammatory infiltrate; cryptitis and microabscesses; lymphoid aggregates; branching atrophic crypts; and Paneth cell metaplasia. Crohn's disease will also exhibit granulomas in the ileum or the colon that are unassociated with crypt rupture; disproportionate

submucosal inflammation; transmural lymphoid infiltrates; and serositis.

- Ulcerative colitis involves the mucosa in a diffuse and continuous fashion and always affects the rectum.
- Colonoscopy reveals erythema, edema, obscured normal vascular pattern, multiple ulcers and/or strictures, and stenosis.
- Other causes of diarrhea should be ruled out by using the appropriate tests (fecal flotation, fecal culture, food trials, serology, and endoscopy).
- Refer to appropriate section/topic for specific diseases.

TREATMENT

THERAPEUTIC GOALS

- Identifying the cause of the ferret IBD will determine the appropriate treatment.
- In Crohn's disease and ulcerative colitis, immune suppression is the mainstay of treatment.

ACUTE GENERAL TREATMENT

- Immunosuppressive agents that non-specifically reduce inflammation and immunity have been the mainstay of conventional therapies for IBD.
- Novel protein diets for 2 weeks or more to eliminate food intolerance or allergy (also try hydrolyzed peptide based diet); antibiotics (metronidazole 10-15 mg/kg PO q 12-24 h; tylosin 25 mg/kg PO q 12-24 h; tetracycline 20-25 mg q 8-12 h) to modify intestinal microflora; steroidal antiinflammatories (prednisone 2 mg/kg PO q 24 h initially for 1-2 weeks, then taper dose by half every 2 weeks), or immune suppressives (azathioprine 0.9 mg/kg PO q 24-72 h) are often used when a cause of IBD in ferrets cannot be determined.
- Responses to such treatments are unpredictable and all drug doses are strictly empirical. Adverse drug reactions may occur, especially with azathioprine. Regular monitoring of CBC is advised.
  - Mild to moderate disease (mild clinical signs). Try dietary change, antibiotics.
  - Moderate to severe disease (no response to dietary change/antibiotics or pronounced clinical signs). Try above plus corticosteroids (taper dose over 8-12 weeks).
  - Persistent clinical signs (>3 months) despite corticosteroid therapy or cachexia, persistent diarrhea and/or vomiting, abdominal pain. Try azathioprine.
- In Crohn's disease and ulcerative colitis, the most widely used treatment is mesalazine (5-aminosalicylic acid), an antiinflammatory drug that acts locally in the gastrointestinal tract.

CHRONIC TREATMENT

- Chronic treatment of IBD in ferrets is determined by the underlying cause. treatment is determined by the underlying cause.
- In Crohn's disease and ulcerative colitis, various antidiarrheals, elemental diets, antibiotics (metronidazole), antiinflammatories (corticosteroids), and immune suppressives (azathioprine, 6-mercaptopurine, methotrexate, cyclosporine) are used. Since 1998, anti–tumor necrosis factor α monoclonal antibodies—murine-chimeric (infliximab) or human (adalimumab)–have been used to induce and maintain remission of Crohn's disease. Surgery to remove affected bowel is sometimes required.
- Data using biological agents targeted against cytokines for treatment of IBD is lacking in dogs, cats, and ferrets.

POSSIBLE COMPLICATIONS

Care should be taken to differentiate chronic IBD in ferrets from early intestinal lymphoma.

PROGNOSIS AND OUTCOME

- The prognosis varies depending on the cause of the ferret IBD.
- Crohn's disease and ulcerative colitis are lifelong systemic diseases with recurrent flare-ups.

PEARLS & CONSIDERATIONS

COMMENTS

- IBD is a clinical syndrome for which it is difficult to develop a valid, objective histologic counterpart, and it should be a diagnosis of last resort, made by the clinician after alternatives such as food intolerance, motility disorders, and infectious disease have been ruled out.
- The pathophysiology resulting in IBD, the basis for phenotypic variation and the mechanism for unpredictable response to treatment are not known.
- The thoroughness of the clinical and laboratory investigation before endoscopic biopsy is used is influenced by the amount of time and money available to evaluate what are often elusive functional entities. Endoscopic biopsies are often done early, after symptomatic medical therapy (see Acute General Treatment) has failed to control clinical signs.
- It is not appropriate for a pathologist to issue a diagnosis of "inflammatory bowel disease." It is more appropriate to list the histologic findings, and to indicate that the changes could be "compatible with" a clinical diagnosis of that syndrome.

CLIENT EDUCATION

- Chronic gastrointestinal inflammatory disease in ferrets is not always cured.
- Emphasize that treatment is aimed at controlling clinical signs.

SUGGESTED READINGS

Allenspach K: Clinical immunology and immunopathology of the canine and feline intestine, Vet Clin North Am Small Anim Pract 41:345–360, 2011.

Brown CC, et al: Alimentary and peritoneum. In Maxie MG, et al, editors: Jubb, Kennedy, and Palmer's pathology of domestic animals, ed 5, New York, 2007, Elsevier Saunders, pp 105.

Dryden GW Jr: Overview of biologic therapy for Crohn's disease, Expert Opin Biol Ther 9:967–974, 2009.

Hecht GA: Inflammatory bowel disease—live transmission, N Engl J Med 358:528–530, 2008.

Jergens AE, et al: Inflammatory bowel disease in veterinary medicine, Front Biosci (Elite Ed) 4:1404–1419, 2012.

Malewska K, et al: Treatment of inflammatory bowel disease (IBD) in dogs and cats, Pol J Vet Sci 14:165–171, 2011.

CROSS-REFERENCES TO OTHER SECTIONS

Cryptosporidiosis (Section VI)
Eosinophilic Gastroenteritis
Epizootic Catarrhal Enteritis
Helicobacter mustelae-Associated Gastritis and Ulcers
Hepatobiliary Disease
Proliferative Bowel Disease
Salmonellosis (Section VI)

AUTHOR: **THOMAS M. DONNELLY**

EDITORS: **JAMES G. FOX AND ROBERT P. MARINI**

FERRETS

Influenza

BASIC INFORMATION

DEFINITION

Several strains of human influenza virus, family Orthomyxoviridae, can cause disease in ferrets. Severity of clinical signs in ferrets is dependent on virulence of the strain of virus.

SYNONYMS

Flu, Orthomyxoviridae

SPECIAL SPECIES CONSIDERATIONS

As in people, influenza in ferrets primarily causes upper respiratory signs. Influenza virus is transmitted via aerosol droplets from human to ferret or from ferret to human.

EPIDEMIOLOGY

SPECIES, AGE, SEX All ferrets are susceptible to influenza, but disease may be more severe in neonates as opposed to older ferrets. Death may occur in neonates from lower airway obstruction resulting from bronchiolitis, pneumonia, and lower respiratory tract infection.

RISK FACTORS Ferrets become infected after being exposed to humans infected with influenza virus or to other infected ferrets.

CONTAGION AND ZOONOSIS Influenza virus can be transmitted between humans and ferrets.

GEOGRAPHY AND SEASONALITY The incidence of disease is likely to be higher in ferrets during influenza season in humans.

ASSOCIATED CONDITIONS AND DISORDERS Hearing loss has been associated with influenza infection in ferrets. Limited enteritis can result because influenza virus can infect the cells of the intestinal mucosa. Hepatic dysfunction has been reported in ferrets experimentally infected with influenza.

CLINICAL PRESENTATION

HISTORY, CHIEF COMPLAINT Ferrets are infected following exposure to infected humans or ferrets. Owners may notice upper respiratory signs, including sneezing, eye watering, and nasal discharge. Ferrets may be lethargic or anorectic.

PHYSICAL EXAM FINDINGS Mucoid or mucopurulent nasal discharge is common, along with bouts of sneezing and serous ocular discharge. Photophobia and conjunctivitis may be observed, as well as otitis. Clinical signs are more commonly seen associated with the upper respiratory tract than with the lower respiratory tract. After a short incubation, ferrets may be initially febrile, with body temperature decreasing 48 hours later.

ETIOLOGY AND PATHOPHYSIOLOGY

- Influenza is caused by an orthomyxovirus. Human influenza viruses A and B are pathogenic to ferrets. Ferrets are also susceptible to avian, phocine, equine, and swine influenza, although only porcine influenza causes clinical signs.
- Transmission is via aerosol droplets and direct contact with virus transmitted at the height of pyrexia and continuing for the next 3 to 4 days.
- Upper respiratory signs are more common than lower respiratory signs because influenza virus generally remains localized in nasal epithelium in ferrets. Infection of the lower respiratory tract is usually confined to the bronchial epithelium and is the result of secondary bacterial infection. Death can occur from secondary pulmonary infection with Lancefield group C hemolytic streptococci. Neonates are likely to die from lower respiratory tract infection.

DIAGNOSIS

DIFFERENTIAL DIAGNOSIS

- Pneumonia
- Canine distemper virus
- Aleutian disease virus
- Respiratory syncytial virus

INITIAL DATABASE

- Diagnosis is based on clinical signs typical of infection, history of exposure, virus isolation from nasal secretions, and a high antibody titer.
- Transient leukopenia can be seen. Plasma biochemical values are usually within reference range, but increased values of blood urea nitrogen, creatinine, alanine aminotransferase, potassium, and albumin have been reported in infected ferrets.

ADVANCED OR CONFIRMATORY TESTING

- Virus isolation
- ELISA can detect antibodies against influenza A. Antibodies are detected 3 days after infection.

TREATMENT

THERAPEUTIC GOAL

Influenza has a 7- to 14-day course in adult ferrets and usually is associated with low mortality. Most ferrets can be treated at home via general supportive care measures.

ACUTE GENERAL TREATMENT

- Force-feed and give water via syringe if needed.
- A pediatric cough suppressant (without alcohol) and/or an antihistamine (such as diphenhydramine) can be given for symptomatic therapy.
- Intranasal delivery of phenylephrine can be given to relieve nasal congestion.
- Antiviral medications (amantadine, zanamivir, etc.) can be used but may not be necessary.
- Antibiotics can be used to control secondary infection of the respiratory tract (antibiotic therapy may reduce neonate mortality).
- Antipyretics generally are not recommended because fever may help restrict the severity of infection.

POSSIBLE COMPLICATIONS

Death in neonates from secondary bacterial infection

RECOMMENDED MONITORING

Monitor at home and hospitalize if nonresponsive to supportive care measures.

PROGNOSIS AND OUTCOME

- Most cases are self-limiting and associated with low mortality.
- Prognosis may be more guarded in neonates.

PEARLS & CONSIDERATIONS

COMMENTS

- Newborn ferrets are protected from disease by milk-derived antibodies from immunized dams.
- In experimental models, ferrets are resistant to infection from the same influenza strain for 5 weeks after primary infection.

PREVENTION

- Prevent exposure of ferrets to infected humans or ferrets.
- Vaccination is not generally recommended because disease is relatively benign in ferrets, and wide antigenic variation of virus makes vaccination difficult. Vaccination seems to provide only short-term immunity. If vaccines are used, live vaccine is recommended over inactivated because live vaccine induces greater protective effect and is more likely to stimulate local antibody production.

CLIENT EDUCATION

- Zoonotic potential of influenza virus between ferrets and humans
- Prevent exposure of ferrets to infected humans or ferrets. Wear mask and gloves if handling ferret while infected with influenza.

SUGGESTED READINGS

Kim YH, et al: Influenza B virus causes milder pathogenesis and weaker inflammatory responses in ferrets than influenza A virus, Viral Immunol 22:423–430, 2009.

McCullers JA, et al: Influenza enhances susceptibility to natural acquisition of and disease due to Streptococcus pneumoniae in ferrets, J Infect Dis 202:1287–1295, 2010.

Patterson AR, et al: Naturally occurring influenza infection in a ferret (*Mustela putorius furo*) colony, J Vet Diagn Invest 21:527–530, 2009.

Swenson SL, et al: Natural cases of 2009 pandemic H1N1 Influenza A virus in pet ferrets, J Vet Diagn Invest 22:784–788, 2010.

AUTHOR: **JENNIFER GRAHAM**

EDITORS: **JAMES G. FOX AND ROBERT P. MARINI**

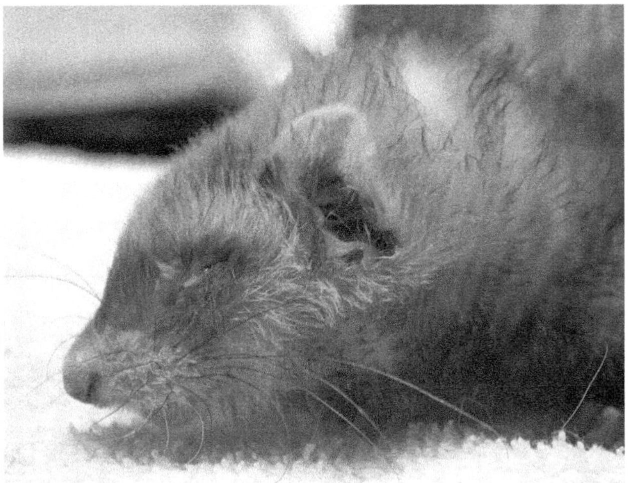

Influenza Upper respiratory disease can be a common problem in the ferret. The ferret is susceptible to human influenza virus. In the early stage, this often resembles distemper. *(Photo courtesy Jörg Mayer, The University of Georgia Athens.)*

FERRETS

Insulinoma

Client Education Sheet Available on Website

BASIC INFORMATION

DEFINITION

- A common functional tumor of the beta cells (β-cells) of the endocrine portion of the pancreas.
- Increased secretion of insulin leads to clinical signs associated with hypoglycemia.

SYNONYMS

β-Cell tumor, hyperinsulinism, insulin-secreting tumor, islet cell carcinoma, functional islet cell tumor

EPIDEMIOLOGY

SPECIES, AGE, SEX

- Occurs frequently in middle-aged to older ferrets
- No sex predilection

GENETICS AND BREED PREDISPOSITION Genetic predisposition is suspected but not proven.

RISK FACTORS High-carbohydrate diets may be a risk factor.

ASSOCIATED CONDITIONS AND DISORDERS Adrenal disease (hyperadrenocorticism) is a common concurrent disease (see Adrenal Disease).

CLINICAL PRESENTATION

DISEASE FORMS/SUBTYPES

- Acute or chronic
- Episodic or persistent

HISTORY, CHIEF COMPLAINT

- Lethargy
- Ataxia
- Weakness
- Abnormal behavior ("star-gazing," disorientation)
- Hypersalivation, pawing at mouth
- Weight loss
- In cases of severe hypoglycemia:
  - Seizures
  - Collapse
  - Coma
- A hypoglycemic episode may be precipitated by exercise, fasting, eating.

PHYSICAL EXAM FINDINGS

- None unless examined during a hypoglycemic event
- Acute: see History/Chief Complaint
- Chronic: Emaciation, muscle wasting
- Insulinomas are not usually palpable
- Other signs attributable to concurrent disease may be present (e.g., alopecia, vulvar swelling with adrenal disease)

ETIOLOGY AND PATHOPHYSIOLOGY

- Pancreatic β-cell tumors (adenoma or carcinoma) result in overproduction of insulin.
- In normal ferrets, when blood glucose concentrations decrease below ≈60 mg/dL (<3.2 mmol/L), insulin secretion stops, and catecholamines and glucagon are released to help return the blood glucose concentration to normal.
- In ferrets with insulinoma, neoplastic β-cells do not respond appropriately to inhibitory stimuli such as hypoglycemia or hyperinsulinemia, and continue to secrete insulin. When blood glucose levels increase rapidly, even when blood glucose concentration is low, excessive insulin release from these tumors can occur and will cause a marked rebound hypoglycemia.
- Clinical signs of insulinoma are classified as:
  - Neuroglycopenic: secondary to hypoglycemia at the level of the central nervous system. Includes weakness, ataxia, abnormal behavior, and seizures.

- Sympathoadrenergic: secondary to decreased blood glucose at the level of the hypothalamus leads to release of cathecolamines by the sympathetic nervous system. Includes agitation, muscle tremors/fasciculations, vocalization, and tachycardia.
- In ferrets, insulinoma develops within the right and left pancreatic lobes with equal frequency. Multiple nodules are present in up to 75% cases.
- Local tumor recurrence is common. Metastatic rate is low (regional lymph nodes, liver, spleen).

DIAGNOSIS

DIFFERENTIAL DIAGNOSIS

- Hypoglycemia
  - Fasting, severe hepatic disease, hypoadrenocorticism, sepsis, laboratory error
- Weakness
  - Cardiovascular (egg arrhythmias), metabolic (e.g. electrolyte imbalances, anemia), neurological, gastrointestinal
- Seizures
  - Cardiovascular (e.g., syncope), neurologic (e.g. epilepsy), toxins

INITIAL DATABASE

- Baseline glucose: ideally after a 3-hour fast; a value less than 60 mg/dL is highly suggestive of insulinoma when it occurs with typical signs
- Complete blood count and chemistry profile are usually unremarkable.
  - Normoglycemia may be present if counter-regulatory mechanisms are activated.

ADVANCED OR CONFIRMATORY TESTING

- Insulin levels: normal insulin levels have been reported to be between 5-40 μU/mL (35-278 pmol/L)
- Elevated insulin levels with concurrent hypoglycemia is highly suggestive of an insulinoma. A definitive diagnosis can be obtained on histopathology.
- Insulin-to-glucose ratios are not commonly used.
- Insulinoma should be suspected if insulin levels are normal in the face of hypoglycemia.

TREATMENT

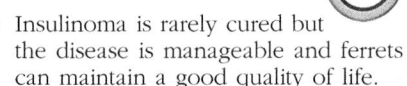

THERAPEUTIC GOAL

Correct clinical signs and maintain blood glucose above 60 mg/dL.

ACUTE GENERAL TREATMENT

- Seizures and emergency therapy
  - If signs are present but the patient is able to eat, feed a small meal.
  - If seizure or severe collapse/weakness is present, administer the following:
    - Glucose (e.g., corn syrup) gingival or sublingual, and/or
    - Intravenous slow bolus 0.25-2 mL/kg of 50% dextrose solution to effect
  - The goal is to abolish clinical signs. Blood glucose levels may remain below normal; acute treatment should not aim to normalize blood glucose levels because doing so may elicit greater insulin secretion from the tumor.

CHRONIC TREATMENT

- Diet:
  - Feed regularly and frequently. Feed 4 to 6 or more small meals per day of a diet high in protein, fat, and complex carbohydrates. Simple sugars should be avoided.
- Surgery:
  - Surgery is rarely curative but can improve disease free interval (DFI) and survival times (SI).
  - Multiple nodules are often present, nodulectomy or partial pancreatectomy can be performed.
  - Surgical complications are rare. Persistent hypoglycemia was present in 53% ferrets postsurgery in one study. Transient hyperglycemia has also been reported.
- Medical management: corticosteroids
  - Corticosteroids increase blood glucose levels by stimulating hepatic glycogenolysis and gluconeogenesis.
  - Initial dose of prednisolone or prednisone 0.25-0.5 mg/kg PO q 12 h. If clinical signs or hypoglycemia persist, the dose can be increased as needed up to 2.2 mg/kg PO q 12 h.
  - After initiation of glucocorticoid therapy, blood glucose should be rechecked monthly.
  - Owners should be advised to monitor clinical signs closely, as the goal of therapy is primarily to control signs of hypoglycemia rather than normalize blood glucose levels.
- Medical management: other drugs
  - Can be added if diet and corticosteroid therapy do not adequately control clinical signs
  - Diazoxide: (benzothiadiazine) inhibits insulin secretion, stimulates hepatic gluconeogenesis and glycogenolysis, and inhibits tissue use of glucose. Dose: 5-10 (up to 30) mg/kg/day divided q 8-12 h. Side effects include vomiting, diarrhea, hypertension, lethargy.
  - Octreotide: (somatostatin analog) inhibits insulin secretion and synthesis. Questionable efficacy. Requires subcutaneous injections q12h.
- Chemotherapy
  - Doxorubicin has been used in one study (1 mg/kg IV q3 weeks). It appears to be well tolerated and may be beneficial in the treatment of insulinoma. Further studies are needed.

DRUG INTERACTIONS

None

POSSIBLE COMPLICATIONS

Hyperglycemia (iatrogenic diabetes mellitus) from pancreatectomy: typically transient and resolves within 2-3 weeks, but may be persistent and will resolve as disease progresses. It can be controlled with insulin injections (empirical dose, 0.1-1 U/ferret SC q 12 q 12-24 h).

RECOMMENDED MONITORING

- Blood glucose
- At the start of medical therapy and 7 d later, then q 4-8 weeks
- Postsurgery: once to twice daily during hospitalization
- At home: if clinical signs of hypoglycemia recur

PROGNOSIS AND OUTCOME

- Insulinoma is rarely cured but the disease is manageable and ferrets can maintain a good quality of life.
- Survival times (ST) are difficult to predict as they are currently based on low numbers of reported cases
- Surgery appears to prolong disease free interval (DFI) and ST.
- Even after recurrence/progression of hypoglycemia, ferrets can still be adequately managed for several months (ST>DFI).
- With medical management alone, STs range from 5-504 days (DFI 0-262 d).
- With surgical+/− medical therapy, STs range from 93-1002 days (DFI 0-690 d).

CONTROVERSY

Insulinoma may be a consequence of a genetic disorder that also predisposes the ferret to hyperadrenocorticism and dilated cardiomyopathy. In humans, a similar genetic disorder called *multiple endocrine neoplasia (MEN)* occurs.

PEARLS & CONSIDERATIONS

COMMENTS

- Adding an annual blood glucose level as a general health recommendation can start at the age of 3 years.
- Many ferrets are concurrently diagnosed with adrenal gland disease and insulinoma.
- Alpha cell islet tumors (e.g., glucagonoma) can occur at the same time as beta cell tumors. Glucagonomas

result in hyperglycemia that is poorly responsive to insulin therapy.
- Prednisone oral solution 5 mg/mL contains 5% alcohol, which makes it difficult to administer to a ferret. Use pediatric prednisone solutions (e.g., Pediapred) that do not contain alcohol, or have a pharmacy compounded prednisone solution if pediatric solution is not concentrated enough for easy administration.

PREVENTION

Feeding a "carnivore" diet (lower carbohydrate levels, higher protein levels) may lower the risk of developing an insulinoma.

CLIENT EDUCATION

- Inform owners of clinical signs associated with the presence of an insulinoma
- Instruct clients to treat a hypoglycemic animal at home by applying sugar syrup (honey, cane syrup) onto oral mucous membranes, and seek veterinary advice rapidly.
- Inform owners that insulinoma is rarely curable but can be readily managed while maintaining a good quality of life for the patient.
- Instruct owners not to feed commercial treats that are often rich in simple sugars.

SUGGESTED READINGS

Caplan ER, et al: Diagnosis and treatment of insulin-secreting pancreatic islet cell tumors in ferrets: 57 cases (1986-1994), J Am Vet Med Assoc 209:1741–1745, 1996.

Chen S: Vet Clin North Am Exot Anim Pract 13:439–452, 2010.

Dutton MA: Case report: histopathologic changes in an islet cell tumor after doxorubicin chemotherapy in a ferret, Exot Mammal Med Surg 2:5–7, 2004.

Dutton MA: Case studies on doxorubicin for the treatment of ferret insulinoma (12 cases), Exot Mammal Med Surg 2:1–5, 2004.

Ehrhart N, et al: Pancreatic beta cell tumor in ferrets: 20 cases (1986-1994), J Am Vet Med Assoc 209:1737-1740, 1996.

Fox JG, et al: C-cell carcinoma (medullary thyroid carcinoma) associated with multiple endocrine neoplasms in a ferret *(Mustela putorius)*, Vet Pathol 37:278–282, 2000.

Weiss CA, et al: Insulinoma in the ferret: clinical findings and treatment comparison of 66 cases, J Am Anim Hosp Assoc 34:471–475, 1998.

CROSS-REFERENCES TO OTHER SECTIONS

Adrenal Disease
Heart Disease, AV Block
Heart Disease, Structural
Helicobacter mustelae–Associated Gastritis and Ulcers

AUTHORS: **CECILIA ROBAT AND MICHAEL DUTTON**

EDITORS: **JAMES G. FOX AND ROBERT P. MARINI**

FERRETS

Lymphoma

Client Education Sheet Available on Website

BASIC INFORMATION

DEFINITION

Lymphoma is a proliferation of lymphoreticular cells that arises most frequently from lymphoid tissues, but almost any tissue in the body can be involved.

SYNONYMS

- Lymphosarcoma
- Malignant lymphoma
- Lymphoblastic lymphoma or lymphocytic lymphoma
- High, medium, or low-grade lymphoma
- Mycosis fungoides (epitheliotropic T-cell lymphoma, cutaneous lymphoma)
- Gastric mucosa-associated lymphoid tissue (MALT) lymphoma

EPIDEMIOLOGY

SPECIES, AGE, SEX

- Lymphoma is seen at all ages; however, in the juvenile ferret (younger than 2 years of age), an aggressive form of lymphoma is often found (lymphoblastic lymphoma). Often a mediastinal mass is part of the initial finding.
- Older ferrets (older than 2 years of age) are more likely to develop a more indolent form of lymphoma (lymphocytic lymphoma). Common forms are multicentric or gastrointestinal lymphoma.

GENETICS AND BREED PREDISPOSITION Not documented

RISK FACTORS

- Some ferrets with lymphoma have tested positive for feline leukemia virus (FeLV).
- Ferrets should not be in contact with cats in which FeLV status is unknown or with cats that are positive.

CONTAGION AND ZOONOSIS An infectious origin has been suspected based on multiple outbreaks of lymphoma in a group of ferrets. Therefore isolation of the group should be recommended to avoid possible contamination of new arrivals.

CLINICAL PRESENTATION

DISEASE FORMS

- Lymphoma can be classified according to location/affected organs:
  - Multicentric
  - Mediastinal
  - Gastrointestinal
  - Cutaneous
  - Leukemic
  - Extranodal
  - Other
- In the young ferret, the mediastinal form is most common.
- In the adult ferret, the multicentric and gastrointestinal forms are most common.
- Another classification (used in domestic animals) for lymphoma is derived from the World Health Organization (WHO) scheme. The WHO system of disease classification is based on diagnosis of diseases rather than on cell types and requires complete patient data plus immunophenotyping:
  - Stage 1: involvement limited to a single node or lymphoid tissue in a single organ
  - Stage 2: involvement of many lymph nodes in a regional area
  - Stage 3: generalized lymph node involvement
  - Stage 4: liver and/or spleen involvement (with or without stage 3 disease)
  - Stage 5: manifestation in the blood and involvement of bone marrow and/or other organ systems (with or without stages 1-4 disease)
  - Substage a: without systemic signs
  - Substage b: with systemic signs
- T cell immunophenotype appears to be more common (especially mediastinal, cutaneous forms) in ferrets.

HISTORY, CHIEF COMPLAINT

- The history and clinical findings can vary significantly with different forms of lymphoma. Depending on the age of the animal and the site of the primary location, clinical signs can appear peracute (e.g., mediastinal T-cell lymphoma in a young ferret) to chronic.
- Owners may report inappetence, weight loss, increased respiratory effort, diarrhea or lethargy; or a ferret

may present for evaluation of a non-painful mass (most commonly in the mandibular area).
- The diagnosis of lymphoma should always involve biopsy with histopathologic examination. Fine-needle aspirates are often inconclusive owing to lack of the tissue architecture needed to diagnose and classify the lymphoma type. Diagnosis should be made on the basis of the combination of clinical history, clinical examination, and histopathologic examination. Hematologic examination is often unrewarding in diagnosing lymphoma.

PHYSICAL EXAM FINDINGS

- Mediastinal form
  - Young ferrets usually present peracute with severe respiratory distress and/or exercise intolerance.
- Gastrointestinal form
  - Diarrhea to melena, tenesmus, regurgitation/vomiting, emaciation, abdominal mass
- Multicentric form
  - Large palpable lymph nodes, splenomegaly, hepatomegaly, enlarged intra-abdominal lymph nodes
- Extranodal or solitary form. Depending on location of primary lesion, ferrets may present with
  - Lameness to paralysis (spinal form)
  - Single or multiple skin lesions, erythema, erosions or ulcers, crusts or plaques, may or may not be pruritic. Reported sites are the feet, face, or diffuse (cutaneous form).
  - Large spleen (splenic form)
  - Renal failure, renomegaly (renal form)
  - Exophthalmos, unilateral or bilateral (orbital form)

ETIOLOGY AND PATHOPHYSIOLOGY

Multiple viral agents (Aleutian disease parvovirus, FeLV, ferret retrovirus), as well as bacterial agents *(Helicobacter mustelae)*, have been suspected.

DIAGNOSIS

DIFFERENTIAL DIAGNOSIS

- Multicentric: fat depositions around lymph nodes in obese animals can mimic lymphadenopathy.
- Mediastinal: other neoplasms (e.g., thymoma) can cause a mediastinal mass.
- Gastrointestinal: chronic non-neoplastic inflammatory/infectious disease will cause enlargement of abdominal lymph nodes; other neoplasms (e.g., intestinal adenocarcinoma), gastric/intestinal foreign body.
- Splenic: extramedullary hematopoeisis causing splenomegaly is very common in ferrets.
- Cutaneous: other cutaneous neoplasms (e.g., mast cell tumor, sebaceous tumor), infectious disease (egg Sarcoptes scabei).

INITIAL DATABASE

- Clinical pathology
  - Blood work should not be used as a primary diagnostic tool but it should be performed in every patient with lymphoma, to evaluate overall health.
  - Anemia is common and is usually mild and non-regenerative.
  - Lymphocytosis should not be immediately interpreted as leukemia. Ferrets with chronic inflammatory/infectious disease will often present with persistent lymphocytosis.
  - A blood smear evaluation can be helpful in diagnosing lymphoblastic leukemia.
  - Hypercalcemia can be observed in ferrets with T-cell lymphoma.
  - Serum chemistry findings are usually non-pathognomonic. Ferrets with liver involvement may have elevated liver values; patients with renal lymphoma will often present with azotemia.
- Diagnostic imaging
  - Radiographs are useful in detecting mediastinal forms of lymphoma; ultrasonography is the imaging modality of choice for abdominal forms of lymphoma.
- Pathology
  - Cytology: in cases of lymphoblastic lymphoma, a diagnosis can readily be made on cytology (a homogeneous population of lymphoblasts will be present).
  - Histopathology: in cases of lymphocytic lymphoma, small neoplastic lymphocytes cannot be differentiated from normal non-neoplastic lymphocytes. A biopsy sample is necessary for diagnosis of lymphoma. e.g. surgical biopsy of enlarged mesenteric lymph nodes. Histopathologic evaluation is also recommended if cytology is non-diagnostic.
  - Bone marrow aspirate/biopsy: should be performed when stage 5 or leukemic disease are suspected.
    - Mandibular, superficial cervical (prescapular), superficial inguinal, and popliteal lymph nodes are easy to access to obtain a fine-needle aspirate/biopsy specimen.

ADVANCED OR CONFIRMATORY TESTING

Immunohistochemistry can be performed on the biopsy specimen to differentiate between T- and B-cell lymphoma.

- CD3 positive and CD79a negative: T cell lymphoma
- CD3 negative and CD79a positive: B cell lymphoma

TREATMENT

THERAPEUTIC GOALS

- Restoration of a good quality of life should be the primary therapeutic goal in case management. The owner should understand that lymphoma most likely will be the cause of the animal's demise because cure is rarely if ever achieved. Adult-onset lymphoma in aged ferrets can be slowly progressive, and ferrets "die with" rather than "die from" the disease.
- If the diagnosis of lymphoma was an incidental finding during a routine examination, and if the quality of life of the animal is generally considered good, aggressive chemotherapy might not be indicated because some cases have been described as representing a longitudinal subclinical form. Treatment can be initiated when clinical signs suggest progression of the disease.
- In cases where the animal appears to suffer from the disease, aggressive treatment such as chemotherapy, surgery, radiation, or a combination of these modalities should be considered.
- Different chemotherapeutic options are available, ranging from oral prednisolone as a sole agent to multimodal drug protocols. The different protocols are listed below.
- Topical retinoids have been used with some success in a ferret with cutaneous lymphoma.

ACUTE GENERAL TREATMENT

- Mediastinal form: radiation offers fast relief because the mass will often shrink significantly within hours after treatment. Because of the often-aggressive form of this disease, systemic chemotherapy should be used as adjuvant treatment.
- Multicentric form: in cases of severe splenomegaly, a splenectomy should be performed in animals at risk of splenic rupture, or when the presence of the enlarged spleen results in clinical signs. Often this occurs when the spleen occupies more than 50% of the abdomen. If large masses are present, they can be surgically removed before the start of chemotherapy.
- Gastrointestinal form: if the ultrasound examination reveals significant thickening of the bowel or a mass causing obstruction, abdominal surgery for intestinal resection and anastomosis may be indicated before the start of chemotherapy.
- Extranodal form: surgery is often indicated to remove the mass or the affected organ (if possible), or to provide relief. In cases of suspected spinal lymphoma, radiation therapy is indicated to provide fast relief.

PROTOCOL 1*			
Week	Day	Agent	Dosage
1	1	Prednisone	1-2 mg/kg PO q 12 h and continued throughout therapy
	1	Vincristine	0.025 mg/kg IV
	3	Cyclophosphamide	10 mg/kg PO, SC
2	8	Vincristine	0.025 mg/kg IV
3	15	Vincristine	0.025 mg/kg IV
4	22	Vincristine	0.025 mg/kg IV
	24	Cyclophosphamide	10 mg/kg PO, SC
7	46	Cyclophosphamide	10 mg/kg PO, SC
9	63	Prednisone	Gradually decrease dose to 0 over the next 4 wk

PROTOCOL 2[†]*		
Week	Agent	Dosage
1	Vincristine	0.025 mg/kg IV
	L-asparaginase	400 IU/kg IP
	Prednisone	1 mg/kg PO q 24 h and continued throughout therapy
2	Cyclophosphamide	10 mg/kg SC
3	Doxorubicin	1 mg/kg IV
4-6	As wk 1-3 above, but discontinue L-asparaginase	
8	Vincristine	0.025 mg/kg IV
10	Cyclophosphamide	10 mg/kg SC
12	Vincristine	0.025 mg/kg IV
14	Methotrexate	0.5 mg/kg IV

Source: From chemotherapy protocols for lymphoma in ferrets. In Carpenter JW, editor: Exotic animal formulary, ed 3, Philadelphia, 2005, WB Saunders, 2005, p 472.

*CBC should be checked weekly during therapy; after therapy is discontinued, continue to monitor CBC and do physical examination at 3-month intervals.

†Protocol is continued in sequence biweekly after week 14, making the therapy protocol less intensive.

CHRONIC TREATMENT

- Chemotherapy can be considered chronic treatment because the treatment usually lasts for weeks to months.
- The different chemotherapeutic regimens vary in terms of length, numbers of drugs used, invasiveness, and effectiveness.
- The simplest form of chemotherapy for lymphoma is oral prednisolone given at 1-2 mg/kg PO q 12-24 h. This treatment will achieve partial or complete, short-lived remission.
- Chemotherapy may be less effective in ferrets receiving chronic immunosuppressive doses of prednisolone at the start of therapy.
- Several multidrug chemotherapy protocols have been described, using L-asparaginase, vincristine, cyclophosphamide, doxorubicin, methotrexate, and prednisone.
- Unfortunately the paucity of information regarding remission durations and survival make comparison between the different protocols impossible. Most protocols and dosages are extrapolated from data available in dogs and cats. Multidrug protocols appear more efficacious than single agent therapies.
- The more rapidly progressive disease encountered in young animals should likely be treated more aggressively than the indolent form commonly seen in adult animals.
- IV drugs should be administered with great caution through a perfectly placed catheter. Doxorubicin, and to a lesser extent vincristine, extravasation injury can result in severe tissue sloughing
- Oral drugs can be compounded for accurate dosing.
- Chemotherapy administration should always be performed respecting rules of maximum safety (e.g., gloves, mask, gown, goggles, dedicated area, closed administration systems, surface decontamination with bleach etc.).
- To avoid the risk of extravasation and the need for repeated placement of intravenous catheters, use of a subcutaneous vascular access port (VAP) has been described. However, a surgical procedure is needed for placement of the VAP.
- In cases where repeated intravenous access is not feasible, and surgery to place a VAP is not an option, an oral and subcutaneous chemotherapy protocol has been used with success.
  - Advantages include that chemotherapeutic drugs are given orally or are injected under the skin or intramuscularly, the animal does not need to

Ferrets Meters Squares			
Kg	BSA	Kg	BSA
0.2	**0.034**	1.7	0.142
0.3	0.045	**1.8**	**0.148**
0.4	**0.054**	1.9	0.153
0.5	0.063	**2**	**0.159**
0.6	**0.071**	2.1	0.164
0.7	0.079	**2.2**	**0.169**
0.8	**0.086**	2.3	0.174
0.9	0.093	**2.4**	**0.179**
1	**0.100**	2.5	0.184
1.1	0.107	**2.6**	**0.189**
1.2	**0.113**	2.7	0.194
1.3	0.119	**2.8**	**0.199**
1.4	**0.125**	2.9	0.203
1.5	0.131	**3**	**0.208**
1.6	**0.137**		

be hospitalized, and the patient can be treated as an outpatient.

DRUG INTERACTIONS

Chemotherapy drugs should be used with caution, following a protocol, after consultation with a veterinary oncologist. Precise timing between treatment administrations should be respected as overlapping severe bone marrow or gastrointestinal toxicities will be seen if drugs are used inadequately.

POSSIBLE COMPLICATIONS

- Myelosuppression is the most common side-effect of chemotherapy drugs. A complete blood count should be performed prior to and 1 week post each treatment. Treatment should be delayed if the neutrophil count is less than 1500-2000/ul, or if the patient is unwell. Antibiotics should be administered if the neutrophil count at nadir (usually 1 week post treatment) is less than 1000/ul. If the patient is febrile and neutropenic, aggressive in-hospital treatment should be initiated, as death can occur rapidly in a septic patient. A 20% dose reduction should then be applied for subsequent doses.
- Gastrointestinal toxicity should be treated with supportive anti-emetic or anti-diarrheal therapy.
- Minimal hair loss and whisker loss may occur
- Specific drug complications:
  - Doxorubicin may cause cumulative cardiac or renal toxicity.
  - Cyclophosphamide may cause sterile cystitis.

RECOMMENDED MONITORING

- Tumor burden should be closely evaluated during treatment. If disease is stable, or if a remission (partial or complete) is noted, treatment should be continued. If disease progresses, the patient should be reevaluated and a different therapy should be considered.

- Quality of life remains the main goal of oncologic therapy. If a patient does not tolerate a treatment, dose adjustments or drug modifications should be applied.
- Appetite and weight should be monitored closely.

PROGNOSIS AND OUTCOME

- Lymphoma is rarely cured.
- Adult ferrets with lymphocytic lymphoma may enjoy remissions of 1-2 years with therapy.
- In young ferrets with lymphoblastic lymphoma, prognosis is poor despite treatment.

PEARLS & CONSIDERATIONS

PREVENTION

- It has been speculated that chronic long-standing forms of inflammatory bowel disease can lead to gastrointestinal lymphoma. Early detection of any gastrointestinal pathology is important to avoid potential progression toward lymphoma.
- In cases of a cluster appearance of lymphoma, a "closed herd" policy is best used to avoid transmitting any potentially infectious agent.

CLIENT EDUCATION

Before the start of any therapy, the client needs to understand that treatment is aimed toward improving the ferret's quality of life for a particular length of time, because cure is rarely achieved.

Tufts Chemotherapy Protocol for Lymphoma in Ferrets (No-IV Protocol)

			Weight				Weight
Week 1	L-ASP	____			both drugs *x 2 days*		
	CTX	____	____	Week 12	CBC*	____	____
	PRED	____		Week 13	CTX	____	____
Week 2	L-ASP	____		Week 15	PCB	____	____
	CBC*	____	____	Week 16	CBC*	____	____
Week 3	L-ASP	____		Week 17	CBC	____	____
	CYTOSAR	____	____	Week 18	CTX	____	____
	Cytosar x 2 days			Week 20	CYTOSAR	____	____
Week 4	CBC*	____	____		LEUK	____	
Week 5	CTX	____	____		both drugs *x 2 days*		
Week 7	MTX	____	____	Week 23	CTX	____	____
	CBC	____		Week 26	PCB	____	____
Week 8	CBC*	____	____	Week 27	CBC*	____	____
Week 9	CTX	____	____		CHEM	____	
Week 11	CYTOSAR	____	____				
	LEUK	____					

If not in remission, continue Weeks 20-26 for 3 cycles. If disease is progressive, discontinue protocol and consider alternative protocol.

Key:

PRED = Prednisone (non)	2 mg/kg PO daily X 1 week then q 48 h
L-ASP = L-asparaginase (non)	10,000 IU/m^2 SC
CTX = Cytoxan (mod)	250 mg/m^2 PO. At same time administer 50 mL/kg lactated Ringer's solution SC.
CYTOSAR = Cytosar (mod)	300 mg/m^2 SC X 2 days (dilute 100 mg with 1 mL H_2O)
MTX = Methotrexate (mild)	0.8 mg/kg IM
LEUK = Leukeran (mild)	1 tab/ferret PO (or ½ tablet daily for 2 days)
PCB = Procarbazine (mild)	50 mg/m^2 PO daily for 14 days

*Dose Reductions: If CBC indicates severe myelosuppression, reduce dosage by 25% for next treatment.

mod = moderately myelo-suppressive; **mild** = mildly myelo-suppressive, **non** = non-myelo-suppressive

Staging Protocol for Ferret Lymphoma

- ☐ CBC + Platelet Count
- ☐ Chemistry Profile
- ☐ Urinalysis (Culture if indicated)
- ☐ Thoracic Radiographs
- ☐ Abdominal Ultrasound
- ☐ Bone Marrow Aspirate
- ☐ Freeze Serum
- ☐ Histopathology

INSTRUCTIONS AND REMARKS FOR THE NON-INVASIVE CHEMOTHERAPY PROTOCOL FOR LYMPHOMA IN FERRETS

CONTACT DR. JÖRG MAYER (MAYERJ@UGA.EDU)

1. Adhere strictly to the protocol and make a note of any side effects which are observed during the treatment.
2. The myelosuppression is the most important factor in monitoring. Other side effects might include vomiting, diarrhea, or nausea. Systemic antibiotic therapy might be indicated very early in the protocol. L-ASP has the potential to cause anaphylaxis (I have not seen it, yet). In case any reaction is noticed after the first dose, premedicate with dexamethasone (1 mg/kg SC) 10 min before the subsequent treatments.

3. As indicated in the protocol, a 25% reduction of the myelosuppressive drugs should be initiated if the CBC shows a severe drop (segmented neutrophil count < 1000/μL). The myelosuppressive drugs are CTX, CYTOSAR, MTX, LEUK, and PCB. Start antibiotic therapy to prevent secondary infection.
4. When toxic side effects occur use the scale below in order to grade the toxicity.
5. The Cytoxan elixir (injectable drug prepared as oral medication) is usually prepared by a compounding pharmacy. Lactated Ringer's solution is given to avoid sterile cystitis.
6. Eventually we want to publish results and kindly ask you to share your findings (toxicity, blood work results, and outcome) with us.
7. If an animal should die during the therapy, try to get a necropsy, as any information available is vital.

Toxic Effect and Grade	Signs
Neutropenia	
0	None
1	1500-3000 neutrophils
2	1000-1500 neutrophils
3	500-1000 neutrophils
4	<500 neutrophils
Thrombocytopenia	
0	None
1	100,000-200,000
2	50,000-100,000
3	15,000-50,000
4	<15,000
Vomiting/Diarrhea	
0	None
1	Nausea, inappetence, soft stool
2	Sporadic vomiting, anorexia <2 days, 1-4 watery stools/day for <2 days
3	1-5 vomiting episodes/day <2 days, anorexia >3 but <5 days, 4-7 watery stools/day for >2 days
4	Hospitalization for vomiting/diarrhea, anorexia >5 days with 10% weight loss

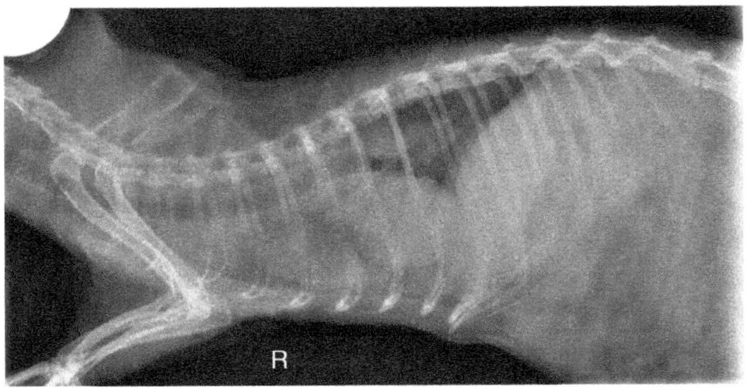

Lymphoma Mediastinal lymphoma (mass cranial to the heart) and pleural effusion in a ferret. *(Photo courtesy of Jörg Mayer, The University of Georgia, Athens.)*

SUGGESTED READINGS

Ammersbach M, et al: Laboratory findings, histopathology, and immunophenotype of lymphoma in domestic ferrets, Vet Pathol 45:663–673, 2008.

Coleman LA, et al: Immunophenotypic characterization of lymphomas from the mediastinum of young ferrets, Am J Vet Res 59:1281–1286, 1998.

Erdman SE, et al: Clinical and pathologic findings in ferrets with lymphoma: 60 cases (1982-1994), J Am Vet Med Assoc 208:1285–1289, 1996.

Erdman SE, et al: *Helicobacter mustelae*–associated gastric malt lymphoma in ferrets, Am J Pathol 151:273–280, 1997.

Rassnick KM, et al: Use of a vascular access system for administration of chemotherapeutic agents to a ferret with lymphoma, J Am Vet Med Assoc 206:500–504, 1995.

CROSS-REFERENCES TO OTHER SECTIONS

Ectoparasites
Eosinophilic Gastroenteritis
Epizootic Catarrhal Enteritis
Helicobacter mustelae–Associated Gastritis and Ulcers
Inflammatory Bowel Disease
Proliferative Bowel Disease
Splenomegaly

AUTHORS: **JÖRG MAYER AND CECILIA ROBAT**

EDITORS: **JAMES G. FOX AND ROBERT P. MARINI**

FERRETS

Mastitis

BASIC INFORMATION

DEFINITION

Inflammation of the mammary gland of ferrets is seen in lactating jills and is most commonly caused by hemolytic *Escherichia coli* and *Staphylococcus* spp.

SYNONYM

Gangrenous mastitis

EPIDEMIOLOGY

SPECIES, AGE, SEX Postpartum jills of breeding age are affected. Two peaks of disease incidence occur: one at early lactation, the other at 3 weeks postpartum, when peak lactation and teat trauma combine to predispose to infection.

RISK FACTORS
- No risk factors have been definitively established.
- Both normal and clinically affected ferrets may harbor hemolytic *E. coli* in their feces.
- In other species, bedding and sanitation may be contributory.

CONTAGION AND ZOONOSIS

- β-Hemolytic *E. coli* may be cultured from the feces of clinically normal ferrets, as well as ferrets with diarrhea and jills with mastitis. It may also be cultured from the mouths of suckling kits; the latter may transmit the organism from one gland to another, or to jills to which kits are fostered. Precautions should be used to avoid spreading causative organisms to other ferrets in the household.
- No case of zoonotic transmission has been reported.

GEOGRAPHY AND SEASONALITY

- The natural breeding season of jills extends from March through August. Seasonality of occurrence therefore depends upon the date of parturition. Kits are typically weaned at 6 weeks of age.
- The seasonality of mastitis incidence may be changed by altering the breeding season through photoperiod.

ASSOCIATED CONDITIONS AND DISORDERS

- Diarrhea of jills and suckling kits may occur.
- Sepsis of jills may occur.

CLINICAL PRESENTATION

DISEASE FORMS/SUBTYPES

- Acute, necrotizing (gangrenous) mastitis
- Chronic mastitis may be a sequela of acute mastitis or may occur independently at peak milk production as kits reach 3 weeks of age.

HISTORY, CHIEF COMPLAINT

- Acute
  - Lethargy, decreased appetite, lactational failure
  - Crying, restless kits
- Chronic
  - Decreased milk production
  - Failure of weight gain in kits

PHYSICAL EXAM FINDINGS

- Acute
  - Signs of mammary inflammation: heat, swelling, pain on palpation, erythema with subsequent discoloration of surrounding tissue
  - Ulceration, purulent discharge of skin and mammary tissue
  - Teat necrosis
  - Fever, depression, lethargy
- Chronic
  - Firm glands that are not discolored

ETIOLOGY AND PATHOPHYSIOLOGY

- Acute (β-hemolytic *E. coli*)
  - Ascending infection of the teat canal with β-hemolytic *E. coli* organisms
  - Exotoxin production (α-hemolysin, cytotoxic necrotizing factor 1 [CNF1], and P pili)
  - Release of endotoxin to create systemic manifestations of disease
  - Inflammation with subsequent or consequent necrosis; swelling of the teat canal may preclude natural drainage of milk
- Chronic *(S. intermedius)*
  - A common commensal of skin; this organism is commonly implicated

DIAGNOSIS

DIFFERENTIAL DIAGNOSIS

- Coliform mastitis
- Staphylococcal mastitis
- Other causes of necrosis and inflammation (e.g., heat pad–induced injury post cesarean section)

INITIAL DATABASE

- Complete blood count
- Microbiological culture of milk or purulent discharge; antibiotic sensitivity testing of *E. coli* isolates

ADVANCED OR CONFIRMATORY TESTING

- Histopathologic examination of biopsy material
  - Coagulative and liquefactive necrosis of glandular and adjacent tissues is a hallmark of acute coliform mastitis. Edema, congestion, hemorrhage, polymorphonuclear leukocytes bordering necrotic tissue, large numbers of bacteria, and thrombosis are additional features.
- Advanced proteomic, genomic, and serotypical evaluation of isolates
  - Necrotoxigenic *E. coli* have been isolated from cases of gangrenous mastitis. These organisms are characterized by the presence of a protein toxin, CNF1, which causes constitutive activation of Rho-GTPases, altering cellular signaling and precipitating a range of cellular changes.

TREATMENT

THERAPEUTIC GOALS

- Eliminate causative microorganisms.
- Administer supportive care.
- Maintain lactation.
- Salvage mammary tissue for future lactations.

ACUTE GENERAL TREATMENT

- Antibiotics should be administered immediately. Amoxicillin with clavulanate drops (18.75 mg PO q 12 h), chloramphenicol (50 mg/kg IM, SC q 12 h), or enrofloxacin (5 mg/kg SC, IM q 12 h, followed by the same dose in Nutri-Cal PO after 24-48 h of parenteral therapy) may be used pending bacterial culture and sensitivity results.
- Flunixin meglumine (1–2 mg/kg IM, SC, or IV q 12 h for 1–2 d only) or meloxicam (0.2 mg/kg initial dose, then 0.1 mg/kg q 24 h PO, SC; reduce to 0.025 mg/kg q 24-48 h for long-term use) may be used as an analgesic, antiinflammatory, and in the case of flunixin meglumine, an anti-endotoxic agent.
- Subcutaneous polyionic replacement fluids should be used in dehydrated jills.
- Lesion care (e.g., flushing with warm saline or dilute chlorhexidine) is beneficial.
- Débridement of necrotic tissue is beneficial.
- Nutritional support may be achieved by adding a gruel of warmed, blended ferret chow, meat-containing baby food, or meat-containing kitten chow to the jill's regular chow. Nutrical is liked by most ferrets and can be used to administer oral medications.
- Early and aggressive therapy may preserve lactation; kits should remain with the jill if possible. Kits may require supplementation during early stages of a jill's treatment. Kits maintained on jills with chronic mastitis will require thrice-daily supplementation to satiety with milk replacer.

CHRONIC TREATMENT

Antibiotic therapy should be attempted but may not be effective.

POSSIBLE COMPLICATIONS

- Gentamicin should be avoided as treatment because of potential nephrotoxicity.
- In acute mastitis, teats or entire glands may be lost:
  - Carpal carriage of kits nursing enrofloxacin-medicated jills is a theoretical, but undocumented possibility.

PROGNOSIS AND OUTCOME

- In acute mastitis, the prognosis for jill survival is good if early and aggressive therapy is used. The prognosis for successful future lactation is good if most glands were spared.
- In chronic mastitis, the prognosis for future lactation is poor.

CONTROVERSY

The author has found that use of enrofloxacin, flunixin meglumine, and early débridement and lesion care precludes the need for surgical resection of mammary glands.

PEARLS & CONSIDERATIONS

COMMENTS

- General supportive care, including attention to nutrition, is recommended.
- Kits may spread infectious microorganisms to foster jills. Jills to which kits are fostered should be monitored closely for signs of mastitis.
- Kits that develop diarrhea while nursing a jill with mastitis should receive oral antibiotics of the same types that are being used to treat the jill.

PREVENTION

Microorganisms responsible for mastitis are part of the commensal flora of ferrets. In a multi-ferret household or breeding establishment, enzootics may be avoided by segregating affected animals and their bedding, feeding, and confinement items. Containment practices should be employed.

SUGGESTED READINGS

Liberson AJ, et al: Mastitis caused by hemolytic *Escherichia coli* in the ferret, J Am Vet Med Assoc 183:1179–1181, 1983.

Marini RP, et al: Characterization of haemolytic *Escherichia coli* strains in ferrets: recognition of candidate virulence factor CNF1, J Clin Microb 42:5904–5908, 2004.

Pollock CG: Disorders of the urinary and reproductive systems. In Quesenberry KE, et al, editors: Ferrets, rabbits, and rodents: clinical medicine and surgery, ed 3, St Louis, 2012, Elsevier, pp 44–61.

AUTHOR: **ROBERT P. MARINI**

EDITOR: **JAMES G. FOX**

FERRETS

Megaesophagus

BASIC INFORMATION

DEFINITION

Megaesophagus is a descriptive term for an esophagus that lacks normal motility and appears dilated radiographically.

SYNONYM

Esophageal achalasia, which describes a specific condition of spasm of the lower esophageal sphincter, is sometimes used as a synonym for this condition in human literature. The term is sometimes incorrectly used in discussions of megaesophagus in the veterinary literature.

SPECIAL SPECIES CONSIDERATION

Megaesophagus in the ferret is infrequently diagnosed, and its origin is poorly characterized. In the dog and cat, the condition may be idiopathic, or it may be secondary to one of many primary diseases. The same may be assumed to be true in the ferret.

EPIDEMIOLOGY

SPECIES, AGE, SEX All reported cases of megaesophagus in the ferret have occurred as an acquired condition in adult animals. Both sexes are affected.

CLINICAL PRESENTATION

HISTORY, CHIEF COMPLAINT Owners may describe exaggerated swallowing efforts, coughing or choking motions, and regurgitation.

PHYSICAL EXAM FINDINGS

- Clinical signs include lethargy, dysphagia, inappetence or anorexia, and weight loss.
- Some ferrets have labored breathing.

ETIOLOGY AND PATHOPHYSIOLOGY

- The cause of megaesophagus in the ferret is unknown.
- The muscular anatomy of the ferret is similar to that of the dog.
- Consider the potential causes of the condition in dogs, and pursue the diagnostic workup accordingly.

DIAGNOSIS

DIFFERENTIAL DIAGNOSIS

- Esophageal or Gastrointestinal foreign body (see Gastrointestinal Foreign Bodies)
- Gastritis
- Influenza or other respiratory disease (see Influenza)
- Autoimmune myasthenia gravis

INITIAL DATABASE

- Diagnosis is based on clinical signs and radiographic imaging of both thorax and abdomen.
- Radiographically, cervical and thoracic portions of the esophagus may be dilated, and food may be visualized in the lumen.
- The thoracic trachea is displaced ventrally by the enlarged esophagus.
- Aspiration pneumonia and gastric gas may be seen.

ADVANCED OR CONFIRMATORY TESTING

- Confirm the esophageal dilatation by doing a contrast esophagogram to delineate the esophagus and to detect strictures or obstructions.
- Given the potential for aspiration, some practitioners avoid the use of barium and use iodine-based contrast media instead. Administer 5-10 mL/kg PO of liquid iodine–based contrast medium while holding the ferret vertically, then expose lateral and ventrodorsal radiographic views.
- Endoscopy may be used to visualize the esophageal mucosa for lesions and to detect strictures or foreign bodies.
- Contrast fluoroscopy may be used to determine esophageal motility.

TREATMENT

THERAPEUTIC GOAL

Management of ferrets with megaesophagus is patterned on the treatment of dogs with the condition.

ACUTE GENERAL TREATMENT

- Maintain hydration using parenteral fluids.
- Aggressive antibiotic therapy is indicated for aspiration pneumonia (e.g., enrofloxacin 10 mg/kg SC, IM, q12 h).
- It may be useful to place a pharyngogastric feeding tube so that the dysfunctional esophagus is "bypassed" until the animal is stabilized.

CHRONIC TREATMENT

- Feed the ferret a liquid or semifluid diet while maintaining the animal in an upright posture.
- The diet should be energy dense and of sufficient nutrient content to meet metabolic needs and prevent fat mobilization and hepatic lipidosis.
- Frequent small feedings 4 to 6 times daily may be necessary.
- Liquid formulations are easiest for pet owners to administer and will descend more readily into the lower GI tract for absorption.
- Maintain the animal in a vertical position for 10 to 15 minutes after feeding.
- If gastritis or gastric reflux esophagitis is suspected, H2 blockers such as

ranitidine (1-2 mg/kg PO q 8 h), famotidine (0.25-0.5 mg/kg SC q 24 h), or cimetidine (10 mg/kg SC, IM q 8 h) may be indicated.
- Metoclopramide (0.2-1 mg/kg PO, SC q 6-8 h) may be helpful for stimulating peristalsis of the esophagus.
- If a primary cause of the megaesophagus can be identified, treat accordingly (e.g., pyridostigmine bromide 1 mg/kg PO q 8 h in myasthenia gravis).

POSSIBLE COMPLICATIONS

- Most ferrets that present with megaesophagus have secondary aspiration pneumonia.
- Malnutrition and hepatic lipidosis due to mobilization of fat stores are common.

PROGNOSIS AND OUTCOME

- Prognosis is poor.
- Most ferrets die or are euthanized within days of diagnosis.

CONTROVERSY

Early anecdotal reports on myofascitis (see Myofascitis) or disseminated idiopathic myositis (DIM) of ferrets implicated it as a possible cause of megaesophagus.

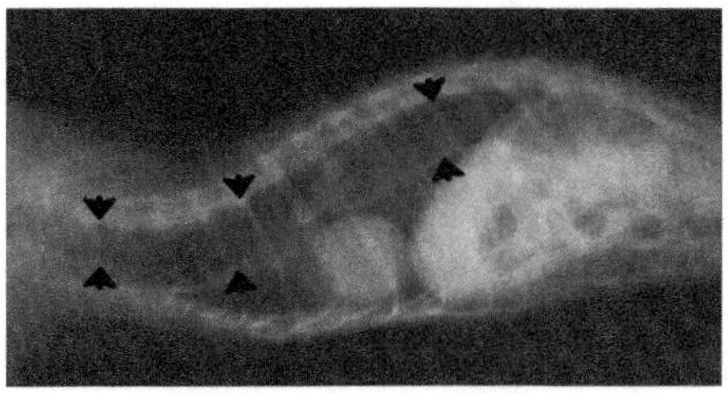

Megaesophagus Lateral thoracic radiographic view of a ferret with megaesophagus. The entire esophagus is dilated *(arrows)*. The trachea is deviated ventrally at the thoracic inlet. *(Photo courfesy Jörg Mayer, The University of Georgia Athens.)*

Subsequent studies demonstrated that DIM of ferrets causes suppurative inflammation of the muscle and fascia of the entire esophagus, with thickening of the organ wall, but does not cause dilatation of the esophageal lumen.

PEARLS & CONSIDERATIONS

COMMENTS

- Early detection and intensive dietary management and supportive care efforts probably yield the most successful outcomes.
- Pet owners should understand that lifelong nutritional and supportive care will be required, and that complications, especially aspiration pneumonia, are likely to occur.
- Until primary causes of this condition are identified, long-term maintenance of affected animals will be extremely challenging.

SUGGESTED READINGS

Blanco MC, et al: Megaesophagus in nine ferrets, J Am Vet Med Assoc 205:444–447, 1994.
Couturier J, et al: Autoimmune myasthenia gravis in a ferret, J Am Vet Med Assoc 235:1462–1466, 2009.
Garner MM, et al: Myofasciitis in the domestic ferret, Vet Pathol 44:25–38, 2007.

CROSS-REFERENCES TO OTHER SECTIONS

Cryptococcosis
Gastrointestinal Foreign Bodies
Helicobacter mustelae–Associated Gastritis and Ulcers
Influenza
Myofascitis

AUTHOR: **MICHAEL C. BLANCO**

EDITORS: **JAMES G. FOX AND ROBERT P. MARINI**

FERRETS

Myofascitis

BASIC INFORMATION

DEFINITION

Myofascitis (MF) is a sporadic fatal inflammatory disease affecting skeletal and cardiac muscle in young ferrets. The cause of this condition is currently unknown, but the disease has a mortality rate of 100%.

SYNONYMS

Because the condition is disseminated, and muscle is the predominant target tissue of the inflammatory process, the terms *polymyositis* and *disseminated idiopathic myositis* have also been used for this condition. However, inflammation may be seen in the fascia around muscle bundles and in adjacent adipose tissue of some animals, so MF seems a more appropriate morphologic term.

EPIDEMIOLOGY

SPECIES, AGE, SEX MF generally affects animals younger than 2 years of age. There is no sex predilection.

CONTAGION AND ZOONOSIS The disease is sporadic and is not believed to be contagious. There is no apparent zoonotic potential.

CLINICAL PRESENTATION

HISTORY, CHIEF COMPLAINT

- Affected animals are usually between 3 and 21 months of age with an acute history of anorexia, lethargy, weakness, and occasionally hyperesthesia, especially over the hind limbs.
- All ferrets reported to date with MF had received at least one vaccination for canine distemper.

PHYSICAL EXAM FINDINGS

- Weakness
- High fever (up to 106°F [41°C])
- Mild dehydration
- Painful, swollen lymph nodes
- Hyperesthesia of limbs, primarily hind limbs
- Muscle wasting
- Splenomegaly

ETIOLOGY AND PATHOPHYSIOLOGY

- The cause of this condition is currently unknown.
- Profound infiltration of neutrophils is seen in target organs—esophagus, heart, skeletal muscle, and occasionally lymph nodes.
- Based on histologic findings, bacterial and immune-mediated causes have been proposed but not proven.

DIAGNOSIS

DIFFERENTIAL DIAGNOSIS

- Ferret systemic coronaviral disease (see Ferret Systemic Coronaviral Disease)
- Megaesophagus (see Megaesophagus)
- Canine distemper infection (see Distemper)

INITIAL DATABASE

- Affected animals may exhibit
  - Profound leukocytosis (occasionally in excess of 50,000/cm^3) with a mature neutrophilia
  - Mild to moderate, usually nonregenerative anemia
  - Elevated liver enzymes (alanine aminotransferase [ALT], alkaline phosphatase) due to inanition
  - Mild hypoalbuminemia

- Creatine phosphokinase and aspartate aminotransferase (AST) are usually within normal limits.

ADVANCED OR CONFIRMATORY TESTING

- Biopsy of swollen painful lymph nodes and surrounding skeletal muscle with presence of suppurative to pyogranulomatous inflammation within biopsy samples
- Ultrasound may show slight thickening of esophageal musculature due to a profound cellular infiltrate in advanced cases.

TREATMENT

THERAPEUTIC GOALS

- Treatment is palliative in the vast majority of cases.
- A wide range of antibacterial, antiviral, antifungal, antiinflammatory, and immune-suppressive medications have been tried singly and in combination for the treatment of affected animals; however, all affected animals have died or been euthanized.
- A single case of temporary remission has been seen with interferon-α at a dosage of 600 IU/d for 2 months, but the animal's condition eventually relapsed, recurred, and it died.

ACUTE GENERAL TREATMENT

Palliative care

PROGNOSIS AND OUTCOME

The prognosis for myofascitis is grave, and all affected animals have died or been euthanized.

CONTROVERSY

Currently, two schools of thought have been reported on the origin of this condition: bacterial infection or an immune-mediated process. These are based upon the unique histologic finding of suppurative to pyogranulomatous inflammation in numerous organs. Although consistent histologically with a bacterial origin, no infectious agents have been isolated in any case. The histologic presentation is not consistent with any known immune-mediated condition of humans or animals.

PEARLS & CONSIDERATIONS

COMMENTS

This disease is currently considered uniformly fatal in ferrets.

SUGGESTED READING

Garner MM, et al: Myofasciitis in the domestic ferret, Vet Pathol 44:25–38, 2007.

CROSS-REFERENCES TO OTHER SECTIONS

Distemper
Ferret Systemic Coronaviral Disease
Megaesophagus

AUTHOR: **BRUCE H. WILLIAMS**

EDITORS: **JAMES G. FOX AND ROBERT P. MARINI**

FERRETS

Neonatal Disease

BASIC INFORMATION

DEFINITION

Conditions specific to animals before weaning: ophthalmia neonatorum, umbilical cord prolapse, infection and entanglement, congenital anomalies, and intercurrent bacterial or viral diseases. Kit health is also affected by maternal factors such as jill temperament and parity, general condition, maternal rejection or cannibalism, and lactational failure from mastitis, postparturient disease, or poor nutrition. Kits are typically weaned no earlier than 6 weeks of age.

SYNONYMS

- Diseases of kits
- Ophthalmia neonatorum = Neonatal conjunctivitis

SPECIAL SPECIES CONSIDERATIONS

- Ophthalmia neonatorum
  - The eyes of ferret kits open at 32 to 34 days; this postnatal delayed opening may be a factor in the development of subpalpebral infection.
- Umbilical-placental entanglement
  - The speed of parturition may prohibit adequate placental ingestion by the jill. This predisposes to entanglement of kits in placentae or placental remnants, umbilical cords, and bedding that creates an interwoven mass which binds the kits together.

EPIDEMIOLOGY

SPECIES, AGE, SEX Age: before weaning (≈6 weeks)

RISK FACTORS

- Umbilical entanglement
  - In the author's experience, fibrous, dry, or sharp-edged nesting material (e.g., aspen shavings) seems to predispose to umbilical entanglement.
- Neonatal infection and sepsis
  - Poor environmental conditions with excessive cold or heat, inadequate or excessive ventilation, and poor sanitation will predispose to neonatal infection and sepsis.
- General
  - Primiparous jills are more likely to reject or neglect their kits than multiparous jills
  - Noise, temperature >70°F (>21°C), and excessive human attention are all factors that may contribute to maternal neglect.
  - Food and water should be available just a short distance from the nest box; placing food and water in the nest box may help ambivalent jills accept their litters.

GEOGRAPHY AND SEASONALITY

- The natural ferret breeding season runs from March to August in the Northern hemisphere; diseases of kits will occur within this period and shortly beyond.
- In production facilities, where seasonality may be ablated by photoperiod, diseases of kits may occur throughout the year.

ASSOCIATED CONDITIONS AND DISORDERS

- Any disease affecting jills may influence neonatal health.
- Mastitis (see Mastitis) and metritis are particular conditions that impact neonatal health and may require supplemental feeding, early weaning, and other interventions in kits.

CLINICAL PRESENTATION

DISEASE FORMS/SUBTYPES

- Ophthalmia neonatorum
- Umbilical-placental entanglement
- Neonatal infection, intercurrent bacterial or viral disease, sepsis

HISTORY, CHIEF COMPLAINT

- Ophthalmia neonatorum
  - Unilateral or bilateral subpalpebral swelling of eyes is seen.
- Umbilical-placental entanglement
  - Masses of kits of varying numbers are found bound by their umbilical cords, placentae, and bedding.
- Neonatal infection, intercurrent bacterial or viral disease, sepsis
  - Depending on the nature of an infection, kits may be anorectic, poorly motile, or crying; if they have diarrhea, they may be "sticky" or may appear wet from maternal grooming.

PHYSICAL EXAM FINDINGS

- Ophthalmia neonatorum
  - Subpalpebral swelling in kits
- Umbilical-placental entanglement
  - Kits may be dehydrated, poorly motile, and hypothermic from failure to nurse.
  - Entanglement may be so severe that limbs are strangulated, leading to edema and eventual necrosis.
  - Umbilical prolapse, hematoma, or erythema may also be seen.
- Neonatal infection, intercurrent bacterial or viral disease, sepsis
  - Kits may be hypothermic, poorly motile, and dehydrated from infection and/or sepsis and subsequent failure to nurse.
  - Abdominal distention may be noted.
  - Perineal staining may be observed in kits with diarrhea.

ETIOLOGY AND PATHOPHYSIOLOGY

- Ophthalmia neonatorum
  - Accumulation of purulent debris within the conjunctival sac is responsible for this condition.
  - Skin microflora may be cultured:
    - How bacteria access the conjunctival sac is unknown.
    - Specific virulence factors have not been identified.
- Umbilical-placental entanglement
  - Speed of parturition, failure of the jill to ingest placentae, and desiccation of umbilical cords create this condition.
- Neonatal infection, intercurrent bacterial or viral disease, sepsis
  - Sepsis from umbilical infection with *Escherichia coli* or other organisms leads to shock, organ failure, and death.
  - Diarrhea from rotavirus infection may occur in kits from 1 to 42 days of age (most commonly observed in the first week of life).
    - As in other species, rotaviral diarrhea is due to small intestinal malabsorption secondary to villous blunting and vacuolization of villous epithelial cells.
    - Failure of passive immunity may predispose to disease.

DIAGNOSIS

DIFFERENTIAL DIAGNOSIS

- Neonatal infection, intercurrent bacterial or viral disease, sepsis
  - *Escherichia coli*
  - *Campylobacter jejuni* (see *Campylobacter* spp. Infection)
  - Rotavirus

INITIAL DATABASE

- Ophthalmia neonatorum
  - Physical examination suffices for diagnosis.
  - Culture and antibiotic sensitivity of the discharge
- Umbilical-placental entanglement
  - Physical examination suffices.
- Neonatal infection, intercurrent bacterial or viral disease, sepsis
  - Physical examination, complete blood count, serum chemistry

ADVANCED OR CONFIRMATORY TESTING

- Neonatal infection, intercurrent bacterial or viral disease, sepsis
  - Histopathologic examination of freshly dead or dying kits to demonstrate microorganisms in various organ systems (e.g., brain, liver, heart)
- Rotavirus
  - Intracytoplasmic inclusion bodies in villous epithelium
  - Electron microscopic evaluation of centrifuged fecal suspensions
  - The ferret rotavirus does not react with commercial immunoenzymes (e.g., Rotazyme).

TREATMENT

THERAPEUTIC GOALS

- Ophthalmia neonatorum
  - Drainage and eventual normal opening of the palpebral fissure
  - Restoration of euglycemia and body condition through resumption of nursing
- Umbilical-placental entanglement
  - Kit separation with preservation of limb function and normal umbilical anatomy
- Neonatal infection, intercurrent bacterial or viral disease, sepsis
  - Elimination of pathogens
  - Restoration of normal appetite, euglycemia, and euhydration

ACUTE GENERAL TREATMENT

- Ophthalmia neonatorum
  - Separation of the palpebrae along the fissure using a 25-gauge needle or a #11 scalpel blade
  - Lavage of the eye and flushing of the exudate with physiologic saline or eyewash
  - Application of topical ophthalmic antibiotic ointment (q 6-12 h) for as long as the eye remains open (with the healing palpebral fissure will reclose and eye[s] will reopen normally at 32 to 34 days)
- Umbilical-placental entanglement
  - Disentanglement achieved using microscissors
    - If the nexus of debris is inspissated, bathing it in warm moist fluid is helpful. As soon as one kit is unfettered from the mass, the others are separated with increasing ease.
- Neonatal infection, intercurrent bacterial or viral disease, sepsis
  - Administration of polyionic replacement fluid (e.g., lactated Ringer's solution 0.5-1.0 mL SC q 6-12 h, or as calculated to replace estimated deficits and insensible and ongoing losses and to provide maintenance)
  - Administration of glucose PO
  - Provision of supplemental heat (e.g., circulating hot water blanket, heat lamp, hot water bottle)
  - Administration of a broad-spectrum antibiotic (e.g., trimethoprim-sulfadiazine 30 mg/kg divided SC, PO; amoxicillin 20 mg/kg q 12 h SC, PO)
  - Supplemental feeding may be beneficial.
    - Provide puppy or kitten milk replacer with supplemental cream PO using eye dropper until kits are satiated.

CHRONIC TREATMENT

Kits should be kept with the jill as much as possible during and after veterinary intervention. Supplemental feeding and heat may be used as needed.

DRUG INTERACTIONS

- The commonly used fluoroquinolone antibiotic enrofloxacin has been shown to cause "carpal carriage" and chondrodystrophy in puppies, as well as retinal degeneration in cats. Neither of these effects has been described in ferrets.
- Retinal degeneration in cats is seen when enrofloxacin is used at doses greater than 5 mg/kg daily. Intravenous administration, prolonged course of treatment, and advanced age may predispose to this effect.

POSSIBLE COMPLICATIONS

- Ophthalmia neonatorum
  - Recurrence is possible because palpebrae close after drainage of purulent material.
- Umbilical-placental entanglement
  - Amputation of neonatal extremities is sometimes required.

RECOMMENDED MONITORING

- Ophthalmia neonatorum
  - Kits should be monitored for normal eye opening at 32 to 34 days of age.
- Umbilical-placental entanglement and neonatal infection
  - Kits should be monitored for body weight and condition.

PROGNOSIS AND OUTCOME

Prognosis is good for all conditions if recognized and treated early.

PEARLS & CONSIDERATIONS

COMMENTS

- Neonatal loss in mink is exacerbated by concurrent infection with Aleutian disease virus.
- Jill nutrition is essential to robust lactation and, consequently, to kit survival. Lactating jills require a meat-based diet containing 35% to 40% protein and 20% to 30% fat. Warming a jill's food may promote consumption.
- Maternal cannibalism is made more likely by noise, lack of privacy, and primiparous state (in a study of mortality in 107 black-footed ferrets, the most common cause of mortality was cannibalism at ≈40%). Some authors recommend not disturbing the jill and kits for several days.
- Thin, restless, vocalizing kits suggest that the jill is ill or has rejected the kits.
- Ferret kits may be fostered to another lactating jill if available.
- Kits older than 3 weeks can be fed supplemental milk replacer alone; those younger than 3 weeks should have replacer diluted at a 1 : 1 ratio with ferret milk.
- Kits may be "creep fed" moistened ferret chow at 3 weeks of age.

SUGGESTED READINGS

Bell JA: Periparturient and neonatal diseases. In Quesenberry KE, et al, editors: Ferrets, rabbits, and rodents: clinical medicine and surgery, ed 2, Philadelphia, 2004, Saunders, pp 50–57.

Bronson E, et al: Mortality of captive black-footed ferrets *(Mustela nigripes)* at Smithsonian's National Zoological Park, 1989-2004. J Zoo Wildl Med 38:169–176, 2007.

Manning DD, et al: Derivation of gnotobiotic ferrets; perinatal diet and hand-rearing requirements. Lab Anim Sci 40:51–55, 1990.

Pollock CG: Disorders of the urinary and reproductive systems. In Carpenter JW, Quesenberry KE, editors: Ferrets, rabbits, and rodents: clinical medicine and surgery, ed 3, Philadelphia, 2012, Elsevier, pp 46–61.

CROSS-REFERENCES TO OTHER SECTIONS

Campylobacter spp. Infection
Mastitis

AUTHOR: **ROBERT P. MARINI**

EDITOR: **JAMES G. FOX**

FERRETS

Osteoma

BASIC INFORMATION

DEFINITION

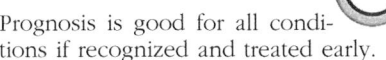

Slow-growing and well-circumscribed benign neoplasm of the bone

EPIDEMIOLOGY

SPECIES, AGE, SEX Any age (occurrence in ferrets 2 to 7 years old has been reported)

CLINICAL PRESENTATION

HISTORY, CHIEF COMPLAINT Firm, bony swelling most commonly arising from intramembranous bone of the skull and mandible, and rarely from the appendicular skeleton

PHYSICAL EXAM FINDINGS

- Irregularly contoured firm protuberance arising from the surface of bone
- Typically nonpainful
- Depending on location, may be a physical impediment
  - An osteoma at the base of the occipital bone compressed the larynx and trachea causing respiratory distress. One report described laryngeal compression and dyspnea.
  - A thoracic vertebral (T6-T9) osteoma causing spinal cord compression resulted in difficulty urinating and defecating for several weeks followed by acute onset of hind limb paralysis.

ETIOLOGY AND PATHOPHYSIOLOGY

Benign bone neoplasm composed of well-differentiated, densely sclerotic, compact (lamellar) bone

DIAGNOSIS

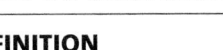

DIFFERENTIAL DIAGNOSIS

- Osseous metaplasia
- Connective tissue neoplasia or inflammation
- Multilobular osteoma (also known as *osteochondroma* or *osteochondrosarcoma)*
- Osteomyelitis
- Ameloblastoma (rare)
- Osteosarcoma

INITIAL DATABASE

- Clinical examination
- Radiography
  - Radiographs show a mineralized mass originating from adjacent bone.

ADVANCED OR CONFIRMATORY TESTING

- Computed tomography
  - In some ferrets, the extent of the mass may be adequately delineated by radiography. CT should be performed to adequately define an obscure bony mass and to assess the effects of the mass on surrounding structures.
- Histopathologic examination
  - Fine-needle aspirates are not diagnostic because tissue hardness severely limits amount of aspirate.

   - Biopsy may be difficult without surgical removal of the mass because of the extreme density of the tumor.
   - Histologically, osteomas appear identical to reactive bone or osseous metaplasia. For this reason, it is difficult, if not impossible, to distinguish the two entities by microscopic examination alone. The pathologist should always be sent associated radiographs.

TREATMENT

THERAPEUTIC GOAL

Surgical reduction to maintain function of affected area

CHRONIC TREATMENT

Typically, osteoma is a cosmetic issue, and many owners elect to monitor only.

POSSIBLE COMPLICATIONS

- Regrowth at original site is possible if complete excision of osteoma is incomplete.
- Right or left total mandibulectomy (previously referred to as *hemimandibulectomy*) and maxillectomy surgeries have the potential for profuse bleeding.

RECOMMENDED MONITORING

Periodic examinations for regrowth, if the tumor is surgically removed

PROGNOSIS AND OUTCOME

- Morbidity associated with osteomas is usually the result of a compressive effect of the tumor because the growth either impinges on the nasal cavity, pharynx, or spinal cord, and/or restricts range of motion of the mandible.
- Osteomas are usually progressive, slow growing, and do not metastasize. They can grow steadily, and then enter a quiescent period of a few to several years.
- If function is not impaired, prognosis is excellent.

PEARLS & CONSIDERATIONS

COMMENTS

- Osteomas generally are not locally invasive. When located on the maxilla or mandible they cause disfigurement.
- Treatment is often considered a cosmetic issue, and most owners elect to monitor.
- Osteomas in ferrets are uncommon.

CLIENT EDUCATION

- Discuss with owners the benign neoplastic nature of an osteoma and the need to monitor for:
   - Loss of function in affected area, or
   - Increased growth of the mass
- Animals adapt remarkably well after radical resection of oral tumors. The altered facial configuration is usually well accepted by owners if enough function can be restored to allow for independent eating and drinking. Clients should be shown before-and-after pictures of similar surgical cases to ensure their understanding of cosmetic changes.

SUGGESTED READINGS

de Voe RS, et al: Radiographic and CT imaging of a skull associated osteoma in a ferret, Vet Radiol Ultrasound 43:346–348, 2002.

Jensen WA, et al: Osteoma in a ferret, J Am Vet Med Assoc 187:1375–1376, 1985.

Perpiñán D, et al: Thoracic vertebral osteoma in a domestic ferret *(Mustela putorius furo)*, J Exot Pet Med 17:144–147, 2008.

Ryland LM: What is your diagnosis? Focal, ovoid, smooth-bordered, osseous proliferation compatible with an osteoma of the parietal bone, J Am Vet Med Assoc 197:1065–1066, 1990.

AUTHORS: **MICHAEL DUTTON AND THOMAS M. DONNELLY**

EDITORS: **JAMES G. FOX AND ROBERT P. MARINI**

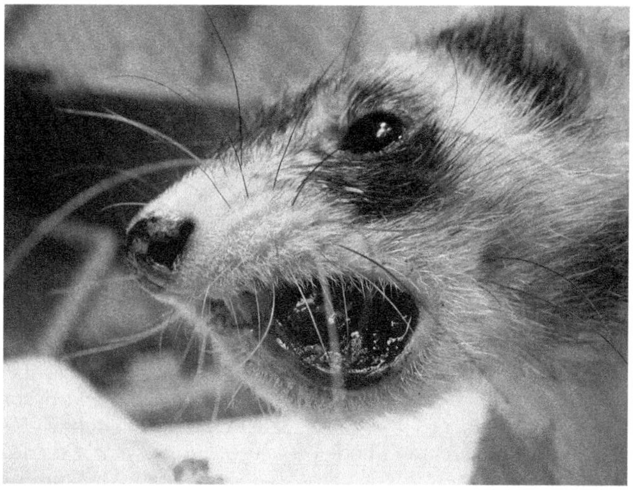

Osteoma Osteoma of the mandible in a ferret. *(Photo courtesy Jörg Mayer, The University of Georgia, Athens.)*

FERRETS

Ovarian Neoplasia

BASIC INFORMATION

DEFINITION

Tumors or cancers of the ovary are neoplasms that can be benign or malignant. They are classified according to the tissue of origin, such as surface epithelium, stromal endocrine cells, and totipotent germ cells. In intact female ferrets, ovarian neoplasia is a frequently-seen tumor. Ovarian neoplasia can also occur in spayed female ferrets that have an ovarian remnant after incomplete surgical sterilization (see Ovarian Remnant Syndnome).

SYNONYMS

Ovarian cancer, ovarian tumor, gonadal tumor

SPECIAL SPECIES CONSIDERATION

Reproductive system neoplasms, including ovarian neoplasia, are rarely reported in ferrets because most are acquired as gonadectomized pets.

EPIDEMIOLOGY

SPECIES, AGE, SEX Intact older female ferrets usually >2 years of age

RISK FACTORS Repeated treatment of unsterilized female ferrets in season with estrus-suppressing hormones such as megestrol acetate (Ovarid) or proligestone (Covinan), to avoid post-estrus anemia, may contribute to development of neoplastic changes in the ovaries.

GEOGRAPHY AND SEASONALITY

- Ovarian tumors are rarely seen in pet ferrets in the United States owing to the widespread practice of neutering ferrets at a young age (often at 6 weeks of age).
- Occasionally seen in Australia, the United Kingdom, and European countries where female ferrets may be kept for breeding purposes, or sterilized later in life

ASSOCIATED CONDITIONS AND DISORDERS

- Estrogen-induced bone marrow suppression with consequent anemia and thrombocytopenia may develop if the ovarian remnant secretes excess estradiol for a prolonged period.
- Adrenal-associated endocrinopathy-like disease (see Adrenal Disease) from elevated androstenedione and 17-hydroxyprogesterone, but not estradiol, has been associated with sex cord stromal tumors at the site of an ovarian pedicle in two neutered female ferrets. Both ferrets had alopecia. After surgical resection of abnormal tissue, the high hormone values decreased quickly, and hair regrowth ensued. Both ferrets had adrenal glands that were grossly normal in appearance.

CLINICAL PRESENTATION

DISEASE FORMS/SUBTYPES

- Most tumors (e.g., leiomyoma, leiomyosarcoma, fibromyoma) are of smooth muscle origin. Leiomyoma is the most commonly reported ovarian tumor.
- Primary gonadal tumors (sex cord or germ cell tumors) are less common:
  - Sex cord tumors: granulosa cell tumor, Leydig cell tumor, Sertoli-Leydig cell tumor (arrhenoblastoma)
  - Germ cell tumors: teratoma, teratocarcinoma
- More than 70% of ovarian tumors are malignant on histologic appearance, but metastasis has not been reported.

HISTORY, CHIEF COMPLAINT

- Infertility is often reported.
- Often incidental finding during ovariohysterectomy in older females or noted at necropsy.

PHYSICAL EXAM FINDINGS

- Often unremarkable
- Older female ferrets may have a palpable mass in the region of one of the ovaries.
- Persistent estrus with vulvar swelling
- Lethargy, anorexia, weakness, tachypnea, melena, pallor, and cardiac murmurs secondary to estrogen-induced aplastic anemia
- Alopecia that is more generalized compared with spreading lower dorsal distribution of alopecia in ferrets with adrenal disease

ETIOLOGY AND PATHOPHYSIOLOGY

- Clinical signs can be related to hormone production by sex cord tumors.
- Organ impingement due to space-occupying mass from tumor has not been reported.
- Abdominal effusion secondary to carcinomatosis has not been reported.

DIAGNOSIS

DIFFERENTIAL DIAGNOSIS

In intact females showing infertility, consider other causes of infertility such as metritis and hydrometra.

INITIAL DATABASE

- Clinical signs and history are the most useful diagnostic tools; older ferrets are more likely to be affected.
- Physical examination may detect a swollen vulva.
- Abdominal palpation is generally unrewarding because ovarian tumors are rarely large enough to be palpated.
- Complete blood count (CBC) is of benefit if the ferret has been showing signs of estrus for >3 weeks to screen for anemia and/or thrombocytopenia.
- Blood biochemistry is generally unremarkable

ADVANCED OR CONFIRMATORY TESTING

- Imaging
  - Diagnosis of ovarian neoplasia cysts by radiography is difficult because of frequent small size of the tumor and similar opacity to surrounding abdominal tissue.
  - Ultrasonography using B-mode ultrasound allows imaging of the inner structure of cystic tumors >2 cm in diameter.
- Exploratory laparotomy or laparoscopy

TREATMENT

THERAPEUTIC GOALS

- Alleviation of clinical signs, especially estrogen-induced bone marrow suppression, if present
- Surgical exploration and excision of neoplastic tissue

ACUTE GENERAL TREATMENT

- Surgical removal of the neoplastic ovary. This is usually curative because metastatic disease, even if ovarian tissue is malignant, is extremely rare.
  - In intact females, remove both ovaries and uterine horns. Explore the abdomen to detect other concomitant disease.
- In spayed ferrets, explore the whole abdomen and remove all abnormal tissue.
  - Check for any remaining uterine tissue, and surgically resect it as well. The remaining uterine stump is often cystic because of the influence of hormones secreted from neoplastic tissue.

POSSIBLE COMPLICATIONS

If any part of a functional ovarian neoplasm is missed and is not surgically removed, recurrence of clinical signs will ensue.

RECOMMENDED MONITORING

- Check that clinical signs have abated post surgery. Vulval swelling should diminish within 2 weeks of surgery.
- In ferrets that have an abnormal CBC or serum hormone elevations before surgery, repeat these tests 1 to 2 months after surgery to ensure that values are within normal range.

PROGNOSIS AND OUTCOME

Despite the common malignant histologic appearance of most ovarian tumors, metastasis has not been reported, and surgical excision is curative.

PEARLS & CONSIDERATIONS

COMMENTS

- Ovarian tumors may be unilateral or bilateral.
- Uterine tumors appear relatively uncommon in intact female ferrets.

PREVENTION

The permanent solution for avoiding ovarian neoplasia is complete surgical sterilization of female ferrets at 6 to 8 months of age. Locating and completely removing the ovaries (and uterus) at this age may be less difficult surgically than in ferrets <6 months of age, particularly for inexperienced surgeons.

CLIENT EDUCATION

Ovariohysterectomy will eliminate risks of ovarian tumors and hyperestrogenism-associated anemia (see Hyperestrogenism-Associated Anemia).

SUGGESTED READINGS

Beach JE, et al: Spontaneous neoplasia in the ferret *(Mustela putorius furo)*, J Comp Pathol 108:133–147, 1993.

Dillberger JE, et al: Neoplasia in ferrets: eleven cases with a review, J Comp Pathol 100:161–176, 1989.

Hauptman K, et al: Comparison of estradiol and progesterone serum levels in ferrets suffering from hyperoestrogenism and ovarian neoplasia, Vet Med (Praha) 54:532–536, 2009.

Martínez A, et al: Spontaneous thecoma in a spayed pet ferret *(Mustela putorius furo)* with alopecia and swollen vulva, J Exot Pet Med 20:308–312, 2011.

Patterson MM, et al: Alopecia attributed to neoplastic ovarian tissue in two ferrets, Comp Med 53:213–217, 2003.

CROSS-REFERENCES TO OTHER SECTIONS

Adrenal Disease
Hyperestrogenism-Associated Anemia
Ovarian Remnant Syndrome

AUTHORS: **BEVERLEY ANN ALDERTON AND THOMAS M. DONNELLY**

EDITORS: **JAMES G. FOX AND ROBERT P. MARINI**

FERRETS

Ovarian Remnant Syndrome

BASIC INFORMATION

DEFINITION

Ovarian remnant syndrome (ORS) refers to clinical signs indicating the presence of functional ovarian tissue in a previously ovariohysterectomized jill.

SYNONYM

Persistent estrus

EPIDEMIOLOGY

SPECIES, AGE, SEX Spayed female ferrets with an ovarian remnant after incomplete ovariohysterectomy are usually <2 years of age.

RISK FACTORS Inappropriate surgical technique that may predispose the patient to ORS includes inadequate exposure of the ovarian pedicles, resulting in poor visualization and inaccurate placement of clamps or ligatures.

GEOGRAPHY AND SEASONALITY Clinical signs may be more obvious during the ferret's breeding season, when the ovary is active and is secreting sex steroids. In the Northern hemisphere, this occurs from March/April through August/September; in the southern hemisphere, from August/September through March/April.

ASSOCIATED CONDITIONS AND DISORDERS Estrogen-induced bone marrow suppression with consequent anemia and thrombocytopenia may develop if the ovarian remnant secretes excess estradiol for a prolonged period.

CLINICAL PRESENTATION

DISEASE FORMS/SUBTYPES ORS results when functional normal or neoplastic ovarian tissue remains after ovariohysterectomy.

HISTORY, CHIEF COMPLAINT Neutered female ferrets will show signs of being in estrus, depending on the time of year. The vulva will swell, and the ferret's odor will increase owing to sex steroid production from the ovarian remnant.

PHYSICAL EXAM FINDINGS Young female ferrets usually show no obvious physical abnormalities apart from a swollen vulva and increased odor.

ETIOLOGY AND PATHOPHYSIOLOGY

Retention of ovarian tissue (may be microscopic in size) that remains functional and secretes sex steroids. The ovarian remnant may undergo hyperplasia and/or neoplasia with time.

DIAGNOSIS

DIFFERENTIAL DIAGNOSIS

- The primary differential diagnosis is adrenal disease. Similar clinical signs of estrus, vulvar swelling, and alopecia are noted.
- A plasma androgen and estrogen hormonal panel ("adrenal" panel) analysis, abdominal ultrasonography, and exploratory laparotomy can aid in diagnosis. However, the "adrenal panel" will not allow differentiation between these two diseases.
- Hormones within the "adrenal panel" have greater value in monitoring the effects of treatment. Upon removal of remnant ovarian tissue, clinical signs should resolve within days.

INITIAL DATABASE

- Clinical signs and history are the most useful diagnostic assessments.
- Physical examination will detect a swollen vulva.
- Abdominal palpation is generally unrewarding because ovarian remnants are rarely large enough to be felt.
- Complete blood count (CBC) is of benefit to check for anemia and/or thrombocytopenia if the ferret has been showing signs of estrus for >3 weeks.
- Blood biochemistry is usually unremarkable.

ADVANCED OR CONFIRMATORY TESTING

- Imaging
  - Diagnosis of ovarian remnant by plain radiography is difficult because of small size of the remnant and opacity of ovarian tissue similar to that of surrounding abdominal tissue.
  - Ultrasonography using B-mode ultrasound may allow imaging of the inner structure of a cystic ovarian remnant >2 cm in diameter.
- Response to estrus suppression treatment
  - Perform after the ferret has been showing estrus for at least 10 days
    - Proligestone (a progestogen) at 50 mg SC; if no response in 7 days, give another 25 mg SC
    - Human chorionic gonadotropin (hCG) at 100 IU/ferret IM; repeat in 14 days if no response
    - Gonadotropin-releasing hormone (GnRH) (e.g., Cystorelin) 20 mcg/ferret SC or IM
    - Buserelin (synthetic GnRH) at 0.25 mL IM; repeat in 14 days if no response
  - Ferrets with ovarian remnants will usually respond to these drugs by reduction of estrus signs within 1 to 2 weeks owing to negative pituitary

hormone feedback. A ferret with adrenal disease may show no or little response to these treatments, particularly proligestone.
- o Ferrets that have been in estrus for a prolonged period (>4 weeks) may not respond to hCG or GnRH, and differentiation between adrenal disease and the ovarian remnant is not possible.
- Exploratory laparotomy or laparoscopy
  - o Perform histopathologic examination to confirm that the tissue is ovarian, and whether it is normal or neoplastic.

TREATMENT

THERAPEUTIC GOALS

- Surgical exploration and excision of remnant ovarian tissue
- Alleviation of clinical signs, especially those related to estrogen-induced bone marrow suppression, if present

ACUTE GENERAL TREATMENT

- Surgical removal of ovarian remnant
  - o Explore the entire abdomen and remove all abnormal tissue.
  - o Do not assume that ovarian remnant is unilateral—remnant ovarian tissue may be bilateral.
  - o Check for any remaining uterine tissue, and surgically resect it as well. The remaining uterine stump can often become cystic under the influence of persistent sex steroid stimulation.

CHRONIC TREATMENT

- If surgery is declined by the owner or is complicated by the presence of other concurrent diseases, clinical signs in the jill may be managed by giving an estrus suppression drugs (see Advanced or Confirmatory Testing, above). This treatment is not ideal over the long term, and surgery should always be strongly recommended.
- Use of GnRH agonists, such as the deslorelin implant (Suprelorin) or leuprolide (Lupron), may be an alternative medical treatment for older entire female ferrets with functionally active neoplastic ovarian remnants.
- In ferrets with severe hormonally-induced alopecia, regular use of skin emollients will be required.

POSSIBLE COMPLICATIONS

Failure to remove any part of an ovarian remnant will result in recurrence of clinical signs. A second or third laparotomy may be required, especially if ovarian remnant is minuscule.

RECOMMENDED MONITORING

- Check that clinical signs have abated post surgery. Vulval swelling should diminish within 2 weeks of surgery.
- In ferrets that show abnormal CBC or hormone elevations before surgery, repeat these tests 1 to 2 months after surgery to ensure that values are within normal range.

PROGNOSIS AND OUTCOME

Because complete surgical removal of ovarian remnant(s) is usually curative, the prognosis and long-term outcome are good.

CONTROVERSY

- Continued use of progestogen injections to take jills out of estrus and to avoid estrogen-induced bone marrow suppression may predispose the uterus to development of endometritis and/ or pyometra. Unless the jill is used for breeding, sterilization or alternatives to sterilization are recommended (see Adrenal Disease).
- Repeated use of hCG to alleviate signs of estrus may stimulate antibody formation, making further doses less effective and potentially stimulating an allergic reaction following subsequent injections.
- Repeated use of any estrus suppression drugs may contribute to ovarian tumor development.

PEARLS & CONSIDERATIONS

COMMENTS

- Timing of exploratory surgery to remove ovarian remnants is important: surgery should be performed when the animal is under an estrogenic influence (i.e., breeding season) so ovarian tissue is enlarged and is easier to identify.
- In ferrets <5 months of age, the reproductive tract is small and friable.
- During ovariohysterectomy in very young ferrets (<8 weeks), the risk of inadvertent loss of the extirpated ovary into the abdominal cavity is increased, especially if it is not excised cleanly.
- Always examine the entire abdomen when looking for an ovarian remnant because torn ovarian tissue can implant anywhere in the abdominal cavity.

CLIENT EDUCATION

- Train owners to recognize signs of estrus in the jill.
- Clinicians and owners should discuss benefits and disadvantages of spaying nonbreeding jills while young.

SUGGESTED READINGS

de Wit M, et al: Signs of estrus in an ovariectomized ferret [Dutch], Tijdschr Diergeneeskd 126:526–528, 2001.

Eshar D, et al: Ovariohysterectomy in ferrets, Lab Anim (NY) 39:140–141, 2010.

Hauptman K, et al: Comparison of estradiol and progesterone serum levels in ferrets suffering from hyperoestrogenism and ovarian neoplasia, Vet Med (Praha) 54:532–536, 2009.

Martínez A, et al: Spontaneous thecoma in a spayed pet ferret *(Mustela putorius furo)* with alopecia and swollen vulva, J Exot Pet Med 20:308–312, 2011.

Patterson MM, et al: Alopecia attributed to neoplastic ovarian tissue in two ferrets, Comp Med 53:213–217, 2003.

Prohaczik A, et al: Deslorelin treatment of hyperoestrogenism in neutered ferrets *(Mustela putorius furo)*: a case report, Vet Med (Praha) 54:89–95, 2009.

CROSS-REFERENCES TO OTHER SECTIONS

Adrenal Disease
Hyperestrogenism-Associated Anemia
Ovarian Neoplasia

AUTHORS: **BEVERLEY ANN ALDERTON AND THOMAS M. DONNELLY**

EDITORS: **JAMES G. FOX AND ROBERT P. MARINI**

FERRETS

Pregnancy Toxemia

BASIC INFORMATION

DEFINITION

A serious, life-threatening disease seen in late pregnancy due to energy imbalance from high metabolic demand, inadequate nutrition, or both

SYNONYM

Eclampsia

SPECIAL SPECIES CONSIDERATIONS

- Pregnancy is 41 to 43 days.
- Sexual maturity occurs at 6 to 12 months and is dependent on season (see Hyperestrogenism-Associated Anemia).
- Litter size ranges from 1 to 18 kits, with average of 8 kits.

EPIDEMIOLOGY

SPECIES, AGE, SEX Ferret, female, more common in young jills

RISK FACTORS

- First litter
- Younger age of jill
- Large litter size
- Inadequate nutritional plane
- Obesity

ASSOCIATED CONDITIONS AND DISORDERS

- Hepatic lipidosis
- Gastric ulceration

CLINICAL PRESENTATION

HISTORY, CHIEF COMPLAINT

- Advanced pregnancy
- Acute onset of lethargy and/or anorexia
- Sudden death may occur.

PHYSICAL EXAM FINDINGS

- Large fetal load may be evident.
- One or more of the following may be seen:
  - Weight loss
  - Anorexia
  - Dehydration
  - Shedding
  - Diarrhea and/or tarry stool
  - Dyspnea
  - Pale or hyperemic or icteric mucous membranes
  - Doughy abdomen on palpation

ETIOLOGY AND PATHOPHYSIOLOGY

- Energy imbalance is due to high metabolic demand, inadequate nutritional plane, or both.
- Young jills with first litters are more susceptible owing to metabolic demands of their own growth as well as fetal growth.
- Larger litters (>10 kits) cause large metabolic demand, particularly in the last week of gestation (day 34 onward of pregnancy).
- Inadequate nutrition causes negative energy balance.
- This condition may be precipitated by stress, dietary change, or inadvertent restricted access to food or water.
- Negative energy balance leads to excessive fatty acid mobilization, especially in animals that were initially obese.
- Hypoglycemia may lead to ketosis.
- Hepatic lipidosis is a common finding.

DIAGNOSIS

DIFFERENTIAL DIAGNOSIS

- Dystocia
- Hypoglycemia due to pancreatic neoplasia
- Other systemic disease

INITIAL DATABASE

- Complete blood count: anemia common but nonspecific
- Chemistry screen: azotemia, hypoproteinemia, elevated aspartate aminotransferase (AST)/alanine aminotransferase (ALT)/lactate dehydrogenase.
  - Blood glucose may be low, normal, or elevated.
  - Electrolyte abnormalities may be present (e.g., hypocalcemia).
- Urinalysis: ketonuria, bilirubinuria
- Abdominal radiography: estimate stage of fetal development and number of kits (fetal load)

ADVANCED OR CONFIRMATORY TESTING

Hepatic lipidosis may be noted visually during cesarean section or histologically.

TREATMENT

THERAPEUTIC GOALS

- Restore energy balance by increasing energy supply and/or reducing energy demand.
- Correct associated clinical abnormalities.

ACUTE GENERAL TREATMENT

- Treatment must be prompt and aggressive.
- Parenteral fluids, including electrolytes and glucose
- Frequent meals of high-energy, high-protein diet (hand-feeding or force-feeding if necessary). Food made into slurry and warmed may be more palatable. Commercial high-energy nutritional supplements may also be used.
- Once the jill is stabilized, cesarean section is indicated in most cases. This procedure may be lifesaving for the jill, even if the kits do not survive.
- Gas anesthesia is indicated owing to decreased liver metabolism of injectable anesthetics.
- Surviving kits may be fostered or may be left with the jill once she has recovered from anesthesia. They may be fed canine or feline milk replacer 6 times daily as a supplement until the jill starts to lactate.

POSSIBLE COMPLICATIONS

- Kits will likely not survive at less than 40 days' gestation and may not survive even if full term.
- Death of the jill is possible, regardless of interventions.
- Agalactia is common, especially after cesarean section.
- Kits should be fostered if the jill dies or fails to lactate within 24 hours. Hand rearing is labor-intensive and is unlikely to be rewarding.

RECOMMENDED MONITORING

- Monitor food intake.
- Ensure that the jill is lactating.

PROGNOSIS AND OUTCOME

Prognosis for both the jill and the kits is poor.

PEARLS & CONSIDERATIONS

COMMENTS

Jills that survive and recover do not appear to have long-term effects, and do not appear to be predisposed to recurrence.

PREVENTION

- Pregnant jills should be monitored closely during the last half of gestation to ensure adequate food intake.
- Maintain a high plane of nutrition throughout pregnancy and lactation (at least 20% fat and 35% protein).
- Avoid changes in diet and other stresses during pregnancy.

- Ensure that water is freely available at all times, preferably from multiple sources (e.g., water bottle and open dish).
- Accidental withholding of food or water, even overnight, may precipitate toxemia.

CLIENT EDUCATION

- Clients who have the potential to breed ferrets should be made aware of the importance of maintaining good nutrition, access to food and water, and close monitoring.
- Prevention is far superior to treatment.

SUGGESTED READING

Batchelder MA, et al: Pregnancy toxemia in the European ferret *(Mustela putorius furo)*, Lab Anim Sci 49:372–379, 1999.
Prohaczik A, et al: Metabolic and endocrine characteristics of pregnancy toxemia in the ferret, Vet Med (Praha) 54:75–80, 2009.

CROSS-REFERENCES TO OTHER SECTIONS

Hyperestrogenism-Associated Anemia
Insulinoma

AUTHOR: **MARGARET BATCHELDER**

EDITORS: **JAMES G. FOX AND ROBERT P. MARINI**

FERRETS

Proliferative Bowel Disease

BASIC INFORMATION

DEFINITION

Proliferative lesions of the lower bowel (most frequently the colon) due to infection by the intracellular bacterium, *Lawsonia intracellularis*, which consists of epithelial hyperplasia and inflammation of colonic mucosa, and causes protracted bloody mucoid diarrhea

SYNONYMS

Proliferative colitis, *Lawsonia*-associated diarrhea

SPECIAL SPECIES CONSIDERATIONS

A similar disease syndrome also caused by *Lawsonia intracellularis* is seen in pigs, hamsters, rabbits, and macaques.

EPIDEMIOLOGY

SPECIES, AGE, SEX

- Young weanling ferrets
- Can occasionally be diagnosed in older ferrets

RISK FACTORS

- Rapidly growing ferrets are more susceptible to infectious diseases, particularly if diet is not adequate nutritionally.
- Stress of shipping

CONTAGION AND ZOONOSIS

- No known zoonotic risk
- It is not known whether *L. intracellularis*, which infects pigs and hamsters as well as other susceptible species (monkeys, rabbits), can infect ferrets, under natural conditions or experimentally.

ASSOCIATED CONDITIONS AND DISORDERS Often diagnosed in young, rapidly growing ferrets

CLINICAL PRESENTATION

HISTORY, CHIEF COMPLAINT

- Intermittent, chronic, mucohemorrhagic or bile-tinged diarrhea
- Weight loss, duration of illness less than 3 weeks to 18 weeks

PHYSICAL EXAM FINDINGS

- Partial prolapse of rectum
- Palpable segmented lower bowel
- Greater than 100-g weight loss during the first 2 to 4 weeks of illness.

ETIOLOGY AND PATHOPHYSIOLOGY

- Caused by intracellular bacterium, *L. intracellularis*
- Proliferative colonic epithelium
- Malabsorption
- Fluid loss
- Blood loss
- Proliferative epithelium can extend through serosa into regional lymph nodes and liver.

DIAGNOSIS

DIFFERENTIAL DIAGNOSIS

- Systemic granulomatous disease
- *Helicobacter mustelae*–associated diarrhea and peptic ulcers
- Inflammatory bowel disease
- Idiopathic eosinophilic gastroenteritis
- Gastrointestinal foreign body
- *Campylobacter jejuni*–associated diarrheal disease

INITIAL DATABASE

Specific *L. intracellularis* PCR–based assay performed on feces

ADVANCED OR CONFIRMATORY TESTING

- Colonic biopsy, followed by fluorescent antibody test specific for *Lawsonia* intracellular bacteria
- Curved intracytoplasmic bacteria noted histologically in formalin-fixed tissue by using silver stains

TREATMENT

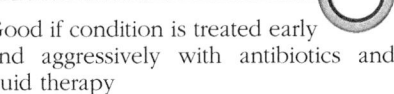

THERAPEUTIC GOALS

- Maintain fluid balance.
- Oral caloric and amino acid supplements
  - Nutrical (EVSCO Pharmaceuticals, Buena, NJ) is essential.
- Pharmacy-compounded oral chloramphenicol palmitate 50 mg/kg q 12 h for 10-14 d
- IM or SC chloramphenicol sodium succinate injectable 50 mg/kg q 12 h
- Alternatively, metronidazole PO 20 mg/kg q 12 h for 10-14 d

CHRONIC TREATMENT

- Provide supportive fluid therapy.
- Maintain high-nutritive diet.

POSSIBLE COMPLICATIONS

- Extraintestinal translocation of colonic mucosa into regional lymph nodes and liver
- Metastatic bone formation has been noted in affected translocated intestinal tissue.

RECOMMENDED MONITORING

Monitor weight during and after treatment.

PROGNOSIS AND OUTCOME

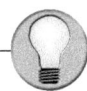

Good if condition is treated early and aggressively with antibiotics and fluid therapy

PEARLS & CONSIDERATIONS

COMMENTS

- Rectal prolapse, palpable thickened colon, and protracted diarrhea are highly suggestive of this disease in young weanling ferrets. *Campylobacter*-associated gastrointestinal disease does not cause thickening of the colon.

- *L. intracellularis* was previously referred to as an intracellular *Campylobacter*-like organism because the curved intracytoplasmic bacteria resemble *Campylobacter* species.
- Confusion over descriptions and treatments of *Campylobacter*-associated gastrointestinal disease and proliferative bowel disease may arise if publications before 1993 are reviewed, because both conditions were often written about as one disease.

PREVENTION

- Preventive measures are poorly understood, but fecal-oral spread is suspected.
- Maintain a high nutritional plane in rapidly growing ferrets.

CLIENT EDUCATION

- Emphasize the need for adequate diet and free access to potable water.
- Avoid overcrowding.
- Reduce stress and maintain adequate hygiene of ferret enclosures.
- Chloramphenicol must be handled with gloves to avoid absorption and idiosyncratic reactions.

SUGGESTED READINGS

Fox JG, et al: *Campylobacter*-like omega intracellular antigen in proliferative colitis in ferrets, Lab Anim Sci 38:34–36, 1988.
Fox JG, et al: Proliferative colitis in ferrets: epithelial dysplasia and translocation, Vet Pathol 26:515–517, 1989.
Fox JG, et al: Proliferative colitis in the ferret, Am J Vet Res 43:858–864, 1981.
Krueger KL, et al: Treatment of proliferative colitis in ferrets, J Am Vet Med Assoc 194:1435–1436, 1989.

CROSS-REFERENCES TO OTHER SECTIONS

Campylobacter spp. Infection
Metastatic Bone Formation
Osteoma

AUTHOR: **JAMES G. FOX**

EDITOR: **ROBERT P. MARINI**

FERRETS

Prostatic Disease

BASIC INFORMATION

DEFINITION

- Prostatic cysts: fluid-filled epithelial structures within the prostate that compress the urethra
- Prostatitis, prostatic abscess: infection or profound inflammation of the prostate gland
- Periurethral cyst: rare lesion that probably arises from embryonic remnants of urogenital ducts, müllerian structures, or mesonephric duct

SYNONYMS

Prostatomegaly, prostatic cysts, periprostatic cysts, periurethral cysts, prostatitis, prostatic abscess

SPECIAL SPECIES CONSIDERATIONS

Prostatic tissue surrounds the neck of the ferret bladder, and the urethra passes through the prostate.

EPIDEMIOLOGY

SPECIES, AGE, SEX Although prostatic disease may be seen at any age, disease is most common in middle-aged (3 to 4 years of age) to older, neutered male ferrets. Periurethral cysts may be seen in male and female ferrets.

RISK FACTORS Prepubertal gonadectomy and adrenocortical disease

CONTAGION AND ZOONOSIS Prostatic cysts associated with adrenal disease are often sterile. Heavy growth of *Staphylococcus* spp., nonhemolytic *Streptococcus* spp., *Escherichia coli, Proteus* spp., and *Pseudomonas* has been reported in prostatitis and prostatic abscesses. Reports have also described clostridial infection in paraprostatic cysts in dogs.

GEOGRAPHY AND SEASONALITY Prostatomegaly secondary to adrenocortical disease is much more common in ferrets from the United States. Adrenal disease has been correlated with early spay/neuter programs prevalent on American ferret breeding farms. In Europe, most ferrets are gonadectomized when several months of age, and adrenal disease is relatively uncommon.

ASSOCIATED CONDITIONS AND DISORDERS

- Adrenocortical disease is the most common cause of prostatomegaly in ferrets.
- Prostatomegaly may be associated with signs of cystitis, urinary incontinence, and preputial dermatitis, or with urethral obstruction.
- Prostatic lesions may also be caused by neoplasia.

CLINICAL PRESENTATION

DISEASE FORMS/SUBTYPES

- Urethral compression: enlarged prostate compresses the urethra, promoting urine stasis
- Urethral obstruction: prostatomegaly is extensive enough to obstruct urine outflow
- Prostatic disease in ferrets is generally sterile but sometimes can become infectious (prostatitis, prostatic abscesses).

HISTORY, CHIEF COMPLAINT

- Ferrets frequently present with signs of lower urinary tract disease: pollakiuria, hematuria, stranguria, dysuria, or anuria. Owners may misinterpret the straining observed as "constipation," or the tenesmus may lead to diarrhea or, in rare instances, rectal or vaginal prolapse. Owners may observe excessive licking at the prepuce.
- A previous history of adrenal surgery may be noted. Signs of adrenal disease, such as alopecia, pruritus, or behavioral changes (e.g., aggression, increased sexual activity), may be observed but are frequently absent.
- Severely affected ferrets (those with urethral obstruction, advanced cystitis, or prostatitis) may present with a history of anorexia, lethargy, depression, or even collapse. In some instances, nonspecific signs of illness may be observed without noticeable signs of dysuria.

PHYSICAL EXAM FINDINGS

- An enlarged prostate may be palpable as a mass lesion or as variably sized, fluctuant cysts near the base of the urinary bladder. The prostate may be larger than the bladder in some instances.
- Additional signs of adrenocortical disease such as alopecia or evidence

of pruritus may be seen but are frequently absent.
- Thick, white to yellow, opaque discharge may be observed at the distal urethra or may be associated with urination if the prostate is abscessed.
- The abdomen may be tense and painful with prostatitis, prostatic abscesses, or urethral obstruction.
- With urethral obstruction, the ferret is often depressed and weak, and the urinary bladder is distended and painful. The overly full bladder may dribble urine, creating a wet, urine-stained ventral abdomen.
- The prepuce may be red from frequent licking.

ETIOLOGY AND PATHOPHYSIOLOGY

- Adrenocortical disease is associated with elevated circulating sex steroid hormones, which may stimulate squamous metaplasia of prostatic ductular epithelium. The prostate then expands with multiple cysts of various sizes filled with keratin, neutrophils, and proteinaceous debris.
- Prostatic disease unrelated to adrenal disease is rare in the ferret. Prostatic tumors such as prostatic seminoma and carcinoma have been reported.
- The pathogenesis of prostatitis or prostatic abscesses is poorly understood in the ferret. Urine stasis secondary to prostatomegaly may promote bacteriuria and regional migration of bacteria into prostatic tissue. Bacteria may also enter the prostate hematogenously.
- Rare reports have described prostatic abscess associated with transitional cell tumors of the bladder.

DIAGNOSIS

DIFFERENTIAL DIAGNOSIS

- Cystitis
- Urolithiasis (see Urolithiasis)
- Neoplasia of the lower urinary tract (e.g., transitional cell carcinoma)

INITIAL DATABASE

- Complete blood count/serum biochemistry results may be unremarkable:
  - Inflammatory leukogram may be observed with prostatitis.
  - Mild to moderate normocytic, normochromic anemia is consistent with adrenocortical disease.
  - Urethral obstruction is associated with azotemia, hyperphosphatemia, metabolic acidosis, and hyperkalemia.
  - Compared with cats and dogs, the mean creatinine level in ferrets is lower (0.4 to 0.6 mg/dL) and the range for creatinine is narrower (0.2 to 0.9 mg/dL). Significant increases in creatinine are relatively moderate (generally <2 mg/dL).
  - Hypoglycemia may be seen with concurrent insulinoma (see Insulinoma).
- Urinalysis: inflammatory sediment may be present
- Survey radiographs
  - Evaluate the entire length of the urinary tract.
  - Prostatomegaly may appear as a mass lesion caudodorsal to the urinary bladder, displacing the bladder cranioventrally.

ADVANCED OR CONFIRMATORY TESTING

- Use abdominal ultrasound to evaluate adrenal glands, kidneys, bladder, and prostate.
  - Prostatic cysts contain hypoechoic to anechoic fluid.
  - Hyperechoic sediment may be seen within cysts with prostatitis or prostatic abscesses.
  - Fluid-filled periurethral cysts may be found caudal to the bladder encompassing the urethra.
- If ultrasonography is unavailable:
  - Contrast cystography may illustrate an irregular blockage around the bladder neck.
  - Use the adrenal hormone panel available through the University of Tennessee to confirm the presence of adrenocortical disease. The adrenal panel may also prove helpful if ultrasonographic assessment of the adrenal gland is equivocal.
- Perform fine-needle aspiration of prostatic fluid if the sonographic appearance of cysts suggests infection, or if the cysts are overly large. (Ideally, cyst aspiration should be ultrasound-guided and the patient should be sedated.)
  - Cytology: suppurative exudate
  - Aerobic and anaerobic bacterial culture/sensitivity
- Urine bacterial culture/sensitivity

TREATMENT

THERAPEUTIC GOALS

- Relieve urethral obstruction.
- Support renal perfusion.
- Alleviate urethral compression.
- Manage infection in ferrets with prostatitis or prostatic abscesses.

ACUTE GENERAL TREATMENT

Relieve urethral obstruction

- If the ferret is a good anesthetic risk at the time of presentation, place a urinary catheter under general anesthesia immediately.
  - Provide appropriate analgesia (e.g., buprenorphine 0.01-0.03 mg/kg q 8-12 h SC, IM, IV).
  - Carefully monitor the electrocardiogram (ECG) for evidence of hyperkalemia: loss of P wave, widening of QRS complex, peaked T waves, and short QT interval
  - Relief of obstruction and forced diuresis are usually sufficient in the management of hyperkalemia; however, medial treatment of hyperkalemia is indicated if an arrhythmia is present, in addition to poor perfusion or altered mentation. Give calcium gluconate 50-100 mg/kg slow bolus IV.
  - A 24-gauge catheter may be used to identify and dilate the small urethral opening near the tip of the J-shaped os penis.
  - Place a 3 Fr urinary catheter designed for use in ferrets. Alternatively, a 22- to 20-gauge jugular catheter may serve as a makeshift urinary catheter, or a 3.5 Fr red rubber catheter may be placed in a large male.
- If the ferret requires stabilization before anesthetic induction, perform cystocentesis using a 23- to 25-gauge needle to provide temporary relief. Provide fluid therapy and supportive care.
- If a urinary catheter cannot be placed, empty the bladder via cystocentesis, provide supportive care, then:
  - Perform an emergency cystotomy with anterograde flushing of the urethra.
  - Alternatively, tube cystostomy has been described in the ferret. A 5 or 8 Fr Foley catheter is passed through a ventral paramedian incision and into the bladder lumen, where it is secured with a purse-string suture.
  - In rare instances, an emergency perineal urethrostomy is required.

Support renal perfusion

- First, administer fluids to correct perfusion abnormalities, then rehydrate the patient. Maintenance fluid requirements in ferrets are estimated at 75 mL/kg/d.
- Discontinue any potentially nephrotoxic drugs.

Alleviate urethral compression

- Adrenalectomy is the treatment of choice for adrenocortical disease and associated prostatic cysts.
  - Unless emergency surgery must be performed (see earlier), perform adrenalectomy after hydration and urine production are restored and laboratory values are normal. Preoperative stabilization usually requires at least 24 to 36 hours.
  - Small to medium-sized, sterile prostatic cysts usually begin to resolve

within days after removal of the diseased adrenal gland.
- Administer leuprolide acetate monthly depot formulation at high doses (e.g., 250 mcg/kg IM) to ferrets with severe urethral compression.
  - This synthetic gonadotropin-releasing hormone (GnRH) analog can promote reduction of prostatic tissue within 12 to 48 hours of drug administration, allowing better urine flow through, and even voluntary micturition around, the urinary catheter.
  - Ancillary use of leuprolide may help to stabilize the patient preoperatively. Leuprolide may also be indicated in ferrets that are poor surgical candidates, or when owners decline surgery (see Chronic Treatment, below).
- Patient with profound urethral compression may also benefit from the smooth muscle relaxant, diazepam 0.5 mg/kg q 6-8 h IM, IV, PO.

Manage infection in ferrets with prostatitis or prostatic abscesses
- Select a lipid-soluble antibiotic that is known to penetrate the prostatic capsule, such as potentiated sulfas or fluoroquinolones.
- Exploratory laparotomy is indicated.
  - Some surgeons recommend marsupializing the prostatic abscess to the abdominal wall. Marsupialization allows repeated and prolonged abscess drainage and lavage. The stoma is then allowed to close by secondary intention.
  - Omentalization is currently the surgical technique of choice in the management of prostatic abscess in dogs. Aspirate the prostate to reduce contents, open and flush prostatic abscess, then suture omentum to the remaining prostate wall.

CHRONIC TREATMENT

- Antibiotics: use bacterial culture/sensitivity results to adjust antibiotic therapy for prostatitis or prostatic abscess. Administer antibiotics for at least 4 to 6 weeks.
- Medical management of adrenal disease: drug therapy may serve as an adjunct to surgery or an alternative to surgery in patients that are a poor surgical risk, or when there are financial constraints.
  - Therapies are extrapolated from drug use in other species, and considerable individual variation in clinical response has been noted. Medical management does not alter adrenal tumor growth.
  - Leuprolide acetate depot is most commonly used; however, other GnRH agonists such as deslorelin acetate implants and goserelin acetate have also been used, particularly in countries where leuprolide is not easily accessible.
  - Antiandrogen agents may be used as an adjunct to leuprolide or surgery:
    - Flutamide 10 mg/kg PO q 12-24 h as with leuprolide, effects may be seen within days in some ferrets, and some veterinarians advocate the use of flutamide instead of leuprolide. Use caution in patients with liver disease.
    - Bicalutimide 5 mg/kg PO q 24 h: sometimes recommended for ferrets with severe prostatic disease. Because bicalutimide increases testosterone and estradiol levels when used alone, it must be used in conjunction with an antigonadotropic agent like leuprolide to be effective.
    - Finasteride 5 mg/kg PO q 24 h
  - The antiestrogen agent anastrozole, 0.1 mg/kg PO q 24 h, may be useful as an adjunct to leuprolide for prostatic disease related to excess estradiol.
  - Melatonin has been advocated as adjunctive treatment for adrenal disease, but its effects are probably too delayed to be of any use in ferrets with urethral compression or obstruction.
- In rare instances of profound urethral compression, the alpha-adrenergic antagonists prazosin 0.05-0.10 mg/kg PO q 8 h and phenoxybenzamine 3.75-7.50 mg PO q 24-72 h may also be used. Use caution with these medications because of the potential for adverse gastrointestinal and cardiovascular effects.

DRUG INTERACTIONS

Remember that concurrent administration of a fluoroquinolone with any multivalent cation-containing product such as a magnesium/aluminum antacid (e.g., the phosphate binder, aluminum hydroxide) will substantially decrease quinolone absorption.

POSSIBLE COMPLICATIONS

- Recurrent cystitis
- Peritonitis
- Prostatic cysts may extend into bladder or urethral tissue. Therefore it is possible for severe prostatic disease or surgical repair to be associated with urinary incontinence, uroabdomen, or urethrocutaneous fistula formation.

RECOMMENDED MONITORING

- Monitor urine production in catheterized ferrets using a closed system attached to a small (100 to 250 mL) IV bag. (Normal urine production is up to 140 mL/d.)
- Culture prostatic fluid and urine 2 to 4 weeks after completion of antibiotic therapy in ferrets with prostatitis or prostatic abscess.
- Use serial abdominal ultrasonography to follow the progress of prostatic cysts, particularly prostatic abscesses.
- Monitor sex steroid hormone levels when selecting adjunctive medical therapy and to monitor patient progress.
- Exacerbation of *Helicobacter mustelae* (see *Helicobacter mustelae*–Associated Gastritis and Ulcers) is not uncommon in ferrets with concurrent illness causing gastritis and possible gastric erosions and ulcers. Monitor ferret for signs of gastrointestinal discomfort such as bruxism (tooth grinding), ptyalism (excessive drooling), pawing at the mouth, anorexia, and diarrhea, including melena. Consider prophylactic administration of gastroprotectants to critically ill ferrets (e.g., famotidine 0.5 mg/kg PO, IV, SC q 24 h and/or sucralfate 100 mg/kg PO q 8-12 h).

PROGNOSIS AND OUTCOME

- If left untreated, prostatic disease can lead to urethral blockage, acute renal failure, and death.
- Prognosis is generally good in ferrets that undergo aggressive therapy for underlying adrenocortical disease.
- Prognosis is fair for prostatitis or prostatic abscesses if managed aggressively, and poor for prostatic neoplasia.

CONTROVERSY

- Although leuprolide acetate depot injections are by far the most popular medical therapy for ferrets with prostatomegaly caused by adrenal disease, a host of other medications may be tried. However, few clinical trials and even fewer empirical data are available to help clinicians make informed choices.
- The prevalence of infectious prostatitis associated with adrenal disease in the ferret is unknown but appears to be relatively low.
- Debate continues about the best way to manage prostatitis and prostatic abscesses in the ferret. Some surgeons have advocated marsupialization; others recommend omentalization.

PEARLS & CONSIDERATIONS

COMMENTS

- Prostatomegaly secondary to adrenocortical disease is the leading cause of urinary tract disease in neutered male ferrets.

- Antibiotic therapy alone usually fails to resolve prostatic abscesses, and surgical management is indicated.
- Use ferret adrenal hormone panel results to guide selection of adjunctive medical therapy.

PREVENTION

- Early recognition of adrenal disease may reduce the risk of urethral compression secondary to prostatic disease. Twice-yearly physical examinations are strongly recommended for middle-aged (3 to 4 years of age) to older ferrets.
- Ensure that sterile prostatic cysts associated with adrenal disease resolve post adrenalectomy by following their sonographic appearance. Long-term persistence of cysts may promote the development of prostatitis and abscesses.
- Because a strong correlation has been established between early spay/neuter and adrenal disease in the ferret, gonadectomy at several months of age might reduce the incidence of disease in American ferrets. Of course, this practice would likely increase the incidence of other health problems (e.g., estrogen toxicity).

CLIENT EDUCATION

- Educate ferret owners on the prevalence of adrenal disease and on signs of the disease.
- Teach owners to recognize signs of cystitis and urethral compression.

SUGGESTED READINGS

Fisher PG: Exotic mammal renal disease: diagnosis and treatment, Vet Clin North Am Exot Anim Pract 9:69–96, 2006.

Johnson-Delaney CA: Medical therapies for ferret adrenal disease, J Exot Pet Med 13: 3–8, 2004.

Nolte DM, et al: Temporary tube cystostomy as treatment for urinary obstruction secondary to adrenal disease in four ferrets, J Am Anim Hosp Assoc 38:527–529, 2003.

Pollock CG: Disorders of the urinary and reproductive systems. In Quesenberry KE, et al, editors: Ferrets, rabbits, and rodents: clinical medicine and surgery, St Louis, 2012, Elsevier, pp 44–61.

Powers LV, et al: Omentalization of prostatic abscesses and large cysts in ferrets *(Mustela putorius furo)*, J Exot Pet Med 16:186–189, 2007.

CROSS-REFERENCES TO OTHER SECTIONS

Adrenal Disease

Helicobacter mustelae–Associated Gastritis and Ulcers

Hyperestrogenism Anemia

Ibuprofen and Acetaminophen Toxicity (Client Handout)

Insulinoma

Renal Disorders

Urolithiasis

AUTHOR: **CHRISTAL POLLOCK**

EDITORS: **JAMES G. FOX AND ROBERT P. MARINI**

FERRETS

Renal Disorders

Client Education Sheet Available on Website

BASIC INFORMATION

DEFINITION

- Infectious and noninfectious diseases of the kidney(s)
- Many different terms are used to describe renal function and its deterioration:
  - *Azotemia* refers to increased concentrations of urea nitrogen and creatinine and other nonproteinaceous nitrogenous waste products in the blood. *Renal azotemia* denotes azotemia caused by renal parenchymal changes.
  - *Uremia* is the presence of all urine constituents in the blood. Usually a toxic condition, it may occur secondary to renal failure or postrenal disorders, including urethral blockage.
  - *Renal reserve* may be thought of as the percentage of "extra" nephrons: those not necessary to maintain normal renal function. Although it probably varies from animal to animal, it is greater than 50% in most mammals.
  - *Renal insufficiency* begins when renal reserve is lost. Animals with renal insufficiency outwardly appear normal but have a reduced capacity to compensate for stresses such as infection or dehydration and have lost urine-concentrating ability.
  - *Renal failure* is a state of decreased renal function that allows persistent abnormalities (azotemia and inability to concentrate urine) to exist; it refers to a level of organ function rather than to a specific disease entity. *Acute renal failure* generally refers to cases of sudden decline of glomerular filtration rate resulting in accumulation of nitrogenous waste products and inability to maintain normal fluid balance. *Chronic renal failure* generally refers to an insidious onset with slow progression (usually months to years) of azotemia and inadequately concentrated urine.
- It is important to realize that most of the renal diseases discussed can manifest as varying stages of compromise in renal reserve, renal insufficiency, or renal failure. If or when the disease process progresses depends on variables such as the specific disease in question, environmental factors, and the individual animal itself.

SYNONYMS

Renal disease, renal failure, kidney disease, kidney failure, chronic renal failure, chronic renal disease, acute renal disease, acute renal failure, nephropathy

SPECIAL SPECIES CONSIDERATIONS

- Renal pathology is not uncommon in the ferret; many ferrets older than 4 years have varying degrees of chronic interstitial nephritis.
- A 1994 review of 61 cases showed that the most prevalent causes of ferret renal pathology included acute nephritis (22%), renal cysts (15%), glomerulonephritis (14%), pyelonephritis (6%), glomerulosclerosis (4%), congestion (4%), and tubular atrophy (4%).
- Other causes of ferret renal pathology include Aleutian disease, toxic nephropathies, and renal disease associated with urinary tract calculi and neoplasia.

EPIDEMIOLOGY

SPECIES, AGE, SEX

- Many ferrets older than 4 years of age have varying degrees of age-related chronic interstitial nephritis.
- Cystic renal diseases are common findings in domestic ferrets. A 2008 retrospective from 54 ferrets showed 69% of cases with documented renal cysts, 26% with primary polycystic disease consisting of polycystic kidney disease

(PKD) affecting renal tubules or, more commonly, glomerulocystic kidney disease (GCKD).
- The anatomy of the penis predisposes to urethral obstruction that may result in postrenal azotemia and acute renal failure.

GENETICS AND BREED PREDISPOSITION No genetic influence has been established for ferret cystic renal disease.

RISK FACTORS
- Nephrotoxins: vitamin D, ethylene glycol, heavy metals, nephrotoxic drugs (e.g., nonsteroidal antiinflammatory drugs [NSAIDs])
- Infection
  - Pyelonephritis
  - Aleutian disease
- Acute obstructive disease secondary to urolithiasis or adrenal disease–associated prostatic disease

ASSOCIATED CONDITIONS AND DISORDERS Cystic prostatic disease, prostatomegaly, and prostatic abscess secondary to adrenal disease may result in urethral obstruction, postrenal azotemia, and acute renal failure.

CLINICAL PRESENTATION

DISEASE FORMS/SUBTYPES
- Aleutian disease: parvoviral infection can lead to glomerular deposition of immune complexes and renal failure
- Chronic interstitial nephritis: varying degrees of chronic interstitial nephritis are commonly found on necropsy of geriatric ferrets. Chronic interstitial nephritis is a progressive disease, with lesions seen as early as 2 years and advanced cases resulting in renal failure as early as 4.5 years. Clinical signs vary with severity of kidney pathology.
- Renal cystic disease: in a 2008 retrospective,
  - PKD was found in one ferret, and GCKD accounted for 92% of cases with primary polycystic lesions.
  - Secondary renal cysts associated with developmental or chronic end-stage renal disease were identified in 20% of cases.
- Toxic nephropathy: ferrets often access potential toxic compounds in their environment. Iatrogenic drug toxicities are also common.
- Hydronephrosis is uncommon and has been associated with inadvertent ureteral ligation during ovariohysterectomy, ureterolithiasis, and renal pelvic neoplasia.
- Pyelonephritis is uncommon and is usually associated with an ascending bacterial urinary tract infection or septicemia. Cystitis and adrenal-associated prostatic disease are the most common causes of urinary tract infection, with *Escherichia coli* and *Staphylococcus aureus* being the most common causative agents.
- Neoplasia: urinary tract neoplasms are generally considered rare. Transitional cell carcinomas are the most commonly reported primary tumor of the ferret kidney (renal pelvis).

HISTORY, CHIEF COMPLAINT Clinical signs vary with severity of kidney pathology. Polydipsia and polyuria may be associated with early kidney failure, with progression to anorexia, weight loss, and lethargy as renal reserve is lost and renal insufficiency or chronic renal failure progresses.

PHYSICAL EXAM FINDINGS
- Depending on the progression of renal failure and uremia, the patient will present in varying states of lethargy, decreased appetite or total anorexia, increased or decreased water intake, dehydration, and general malaise.
- Assess hydration status because azotemia may be caused by or worsened by dehydration.
- Melena is not an uncommon finding because of stress- or uremia-associated gastritis and gastric ulceration.
- Teeth grinding or presentation in a tucked, hunched position may indicate pain.
- Clinical signs of urethral obstruction include stranguria, dysuria, pollakiuria and hematuria with anorexia, lethargy, and abdominal pain. Abdominal palpation reveals an enlarged turgid bladder.
- Ferrets with hydronephrosis will have a palpably enlarged kidney.
- Clinical signs of pyelonephritis include pyrexia, lethargy, anorexia, and pain on palpation of the kidneys. Chronic, untreated pyelonephritis can result in renal failure manifested clinically as profound anorexia and lethargy with subsequent weight loss and declining condition.

ETIOLOGY AND PATHOPHYSIOLOGY
- Aleutian disease: although the parvovirus itself causes little or no harm to the ferret, the marked inflammatory response generated by the host results in production of a large number of antigen-antibody complexes. These circulate in the body and over time cause systemic vasculitis, most notably in the glomerular capillaries. As the disease progresses, marked membranous glomerulonephritis and tubular interstitial nephritis may result in eventual renal failure and death.
- Chronic interstitial nephritis is usually a progressive disease associated with aging. Varying degrees of chronic interstitial nephritis are seen at necropsy of geriatric ferrets that have died from other causes.
- Renal cystic disease: renal cysts may be hereditary or acquired. The precise cause of cystic renal disease in the ferret is unknown. Theories suggest congenital causes or occurrence secondary to chronic urinary tract infection (UTI) and low-grade nephritis that predispose the kidneys to cysts. Ferrets with secondary renal cysts associated with developmental anomalies, membranous glomerulonephritis, or end-stage kidney disease will show hyperphosphatemia and elevated blood urea nitrogen (BUN) in comparison with those with primary cystic disease.
- Obstructive disease may occur as the result of renal, ureteral, or urethral cystic calculi; compression from prostatic cysts or abscesses associated with primary adrenal disease; or compression of the ureter or renal pelvis secondary to neoplasia; or it may occur iatrogenically as inadvertent ligation of a ureter during routine ovariohysterectomy. Acute renal failure secondary to urethral obstruction can be diagnosed by abnormalities in the biochemical profile, including elevated BUN and creatinine levels, hyperphosphatemia, and hyperkalemia.

DIAGNOSIS

DIFFERENTIAL DIAGNOSIS
- Aleutian disease
- Acute renal failure secondary to obstructive disease
- Renal calculi
- Hydronephrosis
- Chronic interstitial nephrosis
- Toxic nephropathy: NSAIDs, zinc, copper, nephrotoxic drugs
- Pyelonephritis
- Neoplasia

INITIAL DATABASE
- Clinical pathology
  - Glomerular function is evaluated by determination of BUN and serum creatinine concentrations that are freely filtered through the glomerular basement membrane.
  - Filtered urea, an end-product of protein catabolism, is reabsorbed through the renal tubules, while creatinine, an end-product of muscle metabolism, is released in the circulation at a constant rate and does not undergo tubular resorption. BUN of 10 to 45 mg/dL is considered normal in the ferret.
  - Ferrets are unique in that normal creatinine levels (0.2 to 0.6 mg/dL) are considerably lower than in other mammals and have a narrower range (0.2 to 0.9 mg/dL).

- When evaluating azotemia, it is important to establish whether it is prerenal, primary renal, or postrenal in origin.
- Primary or renal azotemia occurs with renal parenchymal disease and glomerular damage and is accompanied by variable increases in BUN and creatinine levels and an isosthenuric urine.
- Postrenal azotemia occurs with urinary tract obstruction, most commonly due to calculi. Urine specific gravity can vary in cases of postrenal azotemia.
  - Circulating levels of phosphorus are largely controlled by the kidneys, and consistent elevations in phosphorus in the face of isosthenuria and azotemia are not uncommon in animals with renal failure. A phosphorus level of 4.0 to 9.1 mg/dL is considered normal in the ferret.
  - Hyperphosphatemia that occurs in chronic renal failure is closely related to dietary protein intake inasmuch as protein-rich diets are also high in phosphorus.
- Anemia of chronic renal failure is a common entity that results from reduced erythropoietin production by damaged kidneys, uremic inhibition of red blood cell (RBC) production, increased red blood cell hemolysis, and blood loss associated with gastrointestinal (GI) ulceration.
- Urinalysis offers a tool for assessing urinary tract health, which should be assessed in any ferret with suspected renal disease.
- Specific gravity can help differentiate prerenal from renal azotemia.
- Urine protein can be elevated with urinary tract inflammation, hemorrhage, and infection or can be an indication of renal damage. Protein levels in the urine must be interpreted, along with urine specific gravity and sediment analysis. Glomerulonephritis and amyloidosis are the most common causes of renal-associated proteinuria.
- Hematuria of renal origin is seen with pyelonephritis, neoplasia, renoliths, or renal infarcts.
- Urine sediment analysis can offer information on urinary tract hemorrhage, inflammation, bacteria, and renal tubular damage.
- In cases of azotemic, febrile ferrets with pyuria or bacteriuria, pyelonephritis needs to be ruled out.

• Imaging
- Plain abdominal radiography can assess for increases or decreases in kidney size, radiopaque calculi within the urinary tract, abdominal masses associated with the urinary tract, and bladder distention.
- Contrast cystography and urethrography can provide more specific information about the bladder and urethra.
- Intravenous pyelography, or excretory urography, is used to evaluate the size, shape, position, and internal structure of the kidneys, ureter, and urinary bladder, and is especially helpful in assessing the upper urinary tract (kidneys and ureters) for calculi, masses, or obstructive lesions.
  - Iohexol (240 mg iodine/mL) at a dose of 720 mg iodine/kg and injected into a cephalic catheter is one iodinated contrast material used in ferrets for excretory urography.

ADVANCED OR CONFIRMATORY TESTING

• Advanced imaging
- Renal ultrasonography plays a role in discerning size, contour, and texture of the kidneys, allowing for differentiation of focal versus diffuse disease and echodense versus echolucent lesions.
- Ultrasonography of the entire urinary tract can help rule out obstructive nephropathy due to urolithiasis or mass defects.
- Ultrasonography and CT can help with the diagnosis of pyelonephritis, hydronephrosis, or hydroureter, as well as renal cysts and abscesses.

• Serology
- Diagnosis of Aleutian disease is confirmed antemortem with a positive serum titer coupled with hypergammaglobulinemia or lymphoplasmacytic inflammation in tissue biopsy samples.

TREATMENT

THERAPEUTIC GOALS

- Ultimate goal is to delay progression of renal disease to preserve overall patient well-being and quality of life.
- Determine severity of renal disease based on clinical signs, physical examination findings, and clinical pathologic examination results, to determine prognosis and tailor treatment.
- Treatment should be aimed at promoting diuresis and diminishing the consequences of uremia.
- Look for underlying cause of renal disease to determine if more definitively treatable.

ACUTE GENERAL TREATMENT

- Discontinue any potentially nephrotoxic drugs.
- Identify and treat any prerenal or postrenal abnormalities.
- Identify any treatable conditions such as urolithiasis or pyelonephritis.
- Initiate intravenous fluid therapy to induce diuresis and correct azotemia and electrolyte and acid-base imbalances. Replacement of dehydration deficits is done with the use of isotonic crystalloids. Maintenance fluids are 3 to 4 mL/kg/h in the ferret.
- Potassium supplementation of fluids is based on blood potassium measurement.
- Monitor core body temperature, and if hypothermic, warm patient with use of fluid warmers and warm air heating blankets.
- Once stable, consider esophagostomy tube placement in cases of total anorexia and nutritional depletion.
- Treatment for pyelonephritis includes fluid therapy and diuresis, nutritional support, and antibiotics based on sensitivity results. Parenteral antibiotics are recommended during initial treatment, followed by 4 to 6 weeks of oral antibiotic therapy. Posttreatment culture of a sterilely collected urine specimen is recommended to ensure that the bacterial infection is eliminated, and biochemical parameters are monitored for resolution of any preexisting azotemia.

CHRONIC TREATMENT

- Maintain long-term diuresis with subcutaneous fluid therapy (owners can be taught to do this at home). Volumes given vary with patient size; 50 to 60 mL per injection site in the ferret is routine.
- Dietary management: Recommended dietary protein levels vary; however, studies have shown that cats that consume a prescription kidney failure diet have increased survival compared with cats that do not (or will not) eat this type of diet. Many food manufacturers offer feline prescription renal-failure diets, but benefits of their long-term use in ferrets have not been published. Renal friendly dietary changes may be difficult to enforce in the ferret because of species-specific high protein requirements and/or olfactory imprinting, which determines dietary preference at an early age.
  - Maintaining adequate caloric intake to avoid weight loss takes precedence over nutrient composition of diet.
- If hyperphosphatemic, initiate enteric phosphate binders.
- Treat increased gastric acidity with H2 blockers (famotidine: 0.25-0.5 mg/kg PO, IV, SC q 24 h) and intestinal protectants (sucralfate: 1/8 of 1 gram tablet/animal PO q 6 h). Treat

associated gastroenteritis and nausea with metoclopramide (0.2-1.0 mg/kg PO, SC, IM q 6-8 h) or maropitant citrate (Cerenia, Pfizer Animal Health).
- Consider use of omega-3 fatty acid supplements based on studies showing their beneficial effects in other species.
- Multivitamin supplementation is recommended because the excessive urine production by failing kidneys commonly results in loss of water-soluble vitamins.
- Human recombinant erythropoietin may be used to reverse anemia associated with renal failure; however, no published studies of its use in ferrets.

POSSIBLE COMPLICATIONS

- Anorexia
- GI ulceration
- Hyperphosphatemia
- Acidosis
- Anemia

RECOMMENDED MONITORING

- Overall condition and clinical response to therapy should be assessed in all patients with renal disease. Frequency of follow-up assessments varies with initial diagnosis and severity of disease. Periodic assessments for azotemia, anemia, and phosphorus, potassium, and protein imbalances are recommended.
- Monitor stool for evidence of melena.
- Monitor body weight and condition, and adjust nutrition accordingly.
- Urinalysis and urine culture are performed for patients being treated for pyelonephritis.

PROGNOSIS AND OUTCOME

- With any diagnosis of renal insufficiency or failure, prognosis varies with severity of clinical pathology findings, duration of disease, and severity of primary renal failure. If secondary to infection or obstructive disease, prognosis is determined by duration of disease process and success of treatment—medical or surgical—for the underlying condition of secondary renal insufficiency.
- Depending on initial diagnosis, disease severity, and esponse to therapy, quality of life issues and euthanasia should be discussed with the owner for any patient with renal failure.

PEARLS & CONSIDERATIONS

COMMENTS

- Ferrets are unique in that creatinine levels (0.2 to 0.6 mg/dL) are considerably lower than in other mammals and have a narrower range (0.2 to 0.9 mg/dL). As a result, serum creatinine levels that can be considered high in the ferret could still be within the normal range for other species. Alternate mechanisms of creatinine excretion other than free glomerular filtration, such as renal tubular secretion or greater enteric degradation, may have a larger role in the excretion of creatinine in this species. Consequently, elevations in the concentration of BUN associated with renal failure are not always accompanied by increases in the concentration of serum creatinine above the normal range. Any increase in serum creatinine above normal should be considered significant in the ferret. BUN measurements greater than 100 mg/dL with concurrent creatinine of 2.0 mg/dL would be consistent with significant renal disease in the ferret. Creatinine and inulin clearance, although impractical in private practice because of the requirement for metabolic cages or placement of an indwelling catheter, can be used to adequately measure glomerular filtration rate and detect early renal insufficiency in ferrets. Creatinine and inulin clearance values in the ferret have been reported at 3.32 and 3.02 mL/min/kg, respectively.
- The pattern of microscopic histopathologic changes associated with chronic interstitial nephritis in the ferret is unique. At low magnification, linear bands of fibrosis are seen to extend from the capsule inward. Periglomerular and glomerular fibrosis results in glomerulosclerosis. The interstitium is expanded by fibrous connective tissue throughout; this consists of scattered moderate numbers of lymphocytes and plasma cells. Tubules within these radiating streaks of fibrosis exhibit variable degrees of atrophy. Pathologists with little ferret tissue experience may be tempted to diagnose chronic infarction. As the disease progresses, diffuse glomerulosclerosis is noted throughout the cortex, and fibrosis may progress so that large areas are devoid of functional glomeruli and tubules.
- For long-term administration of subcutaneous fluids, a subdermal SkinButton (Norfolk Vet Products, Skokie, IL; www.norfolkvetproducts.com) can be placed between the shoulder blades. Special accessing needles are used to administer subcutaneous fluids into the SkinButton.
- Peritoneal dialysis has been advocated in the management of some cases of acute renal failure.

CLIENT EDUCATION

Chronic renal failure requires continuous treatment and monitoring. Unless a specific underlying cause is diagnosed and treated successfully, treatment in many cases will be lifelong.

SUGGESTED READINGS

Fisher PG: Exotic mammal renal disease: causes and clinical presentation, Vet Clin North Am Exot Anim Pract 9:33–67, 2006.

Fisher PG: Exotic mammal renal disease: diagnosis and treatment, Vet Clin North Am Exot Anim Pract 9:69–96, 2006.

Jackson CN, et al: Cystic renal disease in the domestic ferret, Comp Med 58:161–167, 2008.

Kawasaki TA: Normal parameters and laboratory interpretation of disease states in the domestic ferret, Semin Avian Exot Pet Pract 3:40–47, 1994.

Orcutt CJ: Ferret urogenital diseases, Vet Clin North Am Exot Anim Pract 6:113–138, 2003.

Richardson JA, et al: Managing ferret toxicosis, Exot DVM 2:23–26, 2000.

Wojick K, et al: Clinical technique: peritoneal dialysis and percutaneous peritoneal dialysis catheter placement in small mammals, J Exot Pet Med 17:181–188, 2008.

CROSS-REFERENCES TO OTHER SECTIONS

Adrenal Disease
Aleutian Disease
Ibuprofen and Acetaminophen Toxicity
Prostatic Disease
Urolithiasis

AUTHOR: **PETER G. FISHER**

EDITORS: **JAMES G. FOX AND ROBERT P. MARINI**

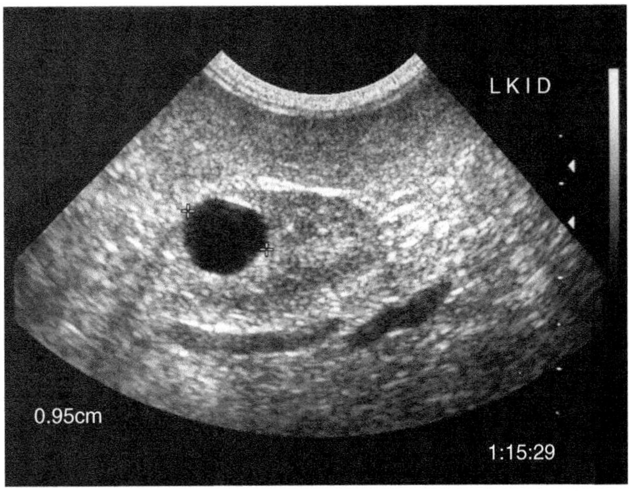

Renal Disorders Ultrasonograph of a ferret kidney highlighting a renal cyst. These are common incidental findings in ferrets and usually only require monitoring for growth. *(Photo courtesy Jörg Mayer, The University of Georgia, Athens.)*

FERRETS

Skin Tumors

Client Education Sheet Available on Website

BASIC INFORMATION

DEFINITION

Tumors affecting skin and adnexa

SYNONYMS

Skin cancer, skin neoplasia, integumentary or cutaneous tumor

SPECIAL SPECIES CONSIDERATIONS

- In two large surveys, tumors affecting skin and adnexa represent 13% and 18% of tumors, respectively.
- In contrast to other species, mast cell tumors of ferrets are benign.

EPIDEMIOLOGY

SPECIES, AGE, SEX

- *Mustela putorius furo*
- Both genders are affected. In one study, castrated males (gibs) had a significantly higher prevalence of cutaneous squamous cell carcinoma than intact males (hobs).
- The age range for the most common types of skin tumors (tumors of basal cell origin, mast cell tumors, and apocrine gland tumors) is 1 to 12 years.

CONTAGION AND ZOONOSIS

Lymphoma in ferrets has a cutaneous form, which may be associated with a C-type retrovirus.

CLINICAL PRESENTATION

DISEASE FORMS/SUBTYPES

- The most common types of skin tumor in ferrets are tumors of basal cell origin (basal cell tumor, sebaceous adenoma, and sebaceous epithelioma), mast cell tumors, and tumors of apocrine glands.
- Other reported skin tumors of ferrets are squamous cell carcinoma, leiomyosarcoma, lipoma, simple mammary adenoma, anal sac carcinoma, ceruminous gland adenocarcinoma, fibrosarcoma, complex mammary adenoma, fibroma, fibrosarcoma, dermatofibroma, myxosarcoma, histiocytoma, malignant fibrinous histiocytoma, and cutaneous lymphoma.
- Skin tumors represented by one reported case in each of two large surveys are myxoma, leiomyoma, polyp, papilloma, myelosarcoma, sarcoma, and melanoma.

HISTORY, CHIEF COMPLAINT

- Appearance of a mass on the skin or adnexa
- Potential self-trauma or pruritus associated with the mass

PHYSICAL EXAM FINDINGS

- Tumor, solitary or multiple, involving any part of the integument or its adnexa
- Abrasion or ulceration of the mass (more likely if pruritus or self-trauma has occurred)
- Tumors of basal cell origin
  - Basal cell tumors
    - May occur anywhere on the body
    - May be firm, white, pedunculated nodules
    - May present as raised plaques
    - Are sharply demarcated, generally benign
  - Benign sebaceous cell tumors (adenoma, epithelioma, cystadenoma)
    - May occur anywhere on the body
    - Are firm, warty, often multilobular
    - Tan, yellow to brown
    - May be traumatized or ulcerated
  - Sebaceous or squamous adenocarcinomas or carcinomas
    - May be multifocal
    - May be warty or pedunculated
    - May involve the lower jaw or groin among other sites
    - Gray-white to yellow
    - May be ulcerated
- Mast cell tumors
  - May occur anywhere on the body
  - May be multifocal
  - Are firm, flat, well-circumscribed nodules
  - May have a crusty yellow appearance
  - May be ulcerated and denuded of hair
- Apocrine gland tumors
  - Have a predilection for areas of concentration of apocrine glands

(head, neck, prepuce, vulva, perineum)
  - Tumors infiltrate the subcutis.
  - Ulceration may occur.
- Cutaneous (epitheliotropic) lymphoma
  - May occur anywhere on the body (legs and extremities are commonly affected)
  - May wax and wane
  - May be multifocal, spherical, or broad-based
  - Tumors located on the feet may be swollen, hyperemic, and denuded of hair.
  - May ulcerate and crust

ETIOLOGY AND PATHOPHYSIOLOGY

- Tumors of skin and adnexa spontaneously arise; specific genetic, environmental, and infectious influences have not been identified. (Cutaneous lymphomas are of T-cell origin and may be associated with C-type retrovirus.)
- Malignant tumors of apocrine glands may be locally invasive and may metastasize to lymph nodes and viscera.

DIAGNOSIS

DIFFERENTIAL DIAGNOSIS

- Other tumors of skin
- Foreign body reaction/granuloma
- Vaccine reaction
- Furunculosis
- Severe pyoderma/dermatitis
- Cryptococcosis (see Cryptococcosis) affecting the limbs

INITIAL DATABASE

- Complete blood count
- Serum chemistry for older ferrets
- Radiography to determine whether metastasis has occurred

ADVANCED OR CONFIRMATORY TESTING

- Excisional biopsy and histopathologic examination
- Fine-needle aspirates and impression smears may be used in older or debilitated animals, which present as anesthetic risks.

TREATMENT

THERAPEUTIC GOALS

- Removal of tumors
- Preservation of function and adequate defect closure (especially for tumors of the prepuce, vulva, anus, face, or extremities)

ACUTE GENERAL TREATMENT

- Surgical excision is required.
- Wide excision is recommended.
- Submit tumors for histopathologic examination.

POSSIBLE COMPLICATIONS

Resection of apocrine gland tumors of preputial and perineal distribution may result in compromise of the preputial, vaginal, and anal orifices.

RECOMMENDED MONITORING

Ferrets should be evaluated regularly for local occurrence.

PROGNOSIS AND OUTCOME

- Prognosis is good with early resection and wide margins.
- Mast cell tumors, if completely excised, do not recur.
- Resection of cutaneous lymphoma may be associated with prolonged recurrence-free survival.
- Apocrine gland tumors of the preputial gland are commonly malignant. Apocrine gland tumors may be very aggressive.

PEARLS & CONSIDERATIONS

COMMENTS

Topical and systemic chemotherapy in the face of cutaneous lymphoma is generally ineffective.

CLIENT EDUCATION

Clients should be instructed to evaluate excision sites for tumor recurrence.

SUGGESTED READINGS

Antinoff A, et al: Neoplasia. In Quesenberry KE, et al, editors: Ferrets, rabbits, and rodents: clinical medicine and surgery, ed 3, St Louis, MO, 2012, Elsevier, pp 103–121.

Li X, et al: Chapter 18. In Fox JG, editor: Biology and diseases of the ferret, ed 2, Baltimore, 1998, Williams & Wilkins, pp 321–354.

Li X, et al: Neoplastic diseases in ferrets: 574 cases (1968-1997), J Am Vet Med Assoc 212:1402–1406, 1998.

Malik R, et al: Cryptococcosis in ferrets: a diverse spectrum of clinical disease, Aust Vet J 80:749–755, 2002.

CROSS-REFERENCES TO OTHER SECTIONS

Cryptococcosis

AUTHOR: **ROBERT P. MARINI**

EDITORS: **JAMES G. FOX AND ROBERT P. MARINI**

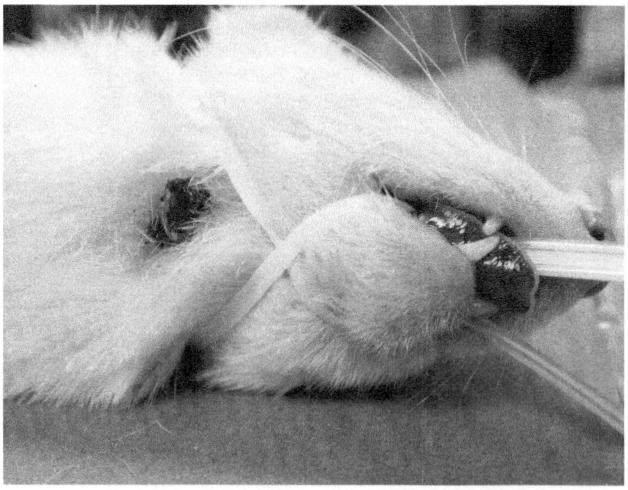

Skin Tumors Mast cell tumor on the neck of a ferret. Note the crusty appearance of the tumor from dried blood. *(Photo courtesy Jörg Mayer, The University of Georgia, Athens.)*

Splenomegaly

BASIC INFORMATION

DEFINITION

Splenomegaly is a nonspecific term that refers to diffuse enlargement of the spleen. The term *splenomegaly* does not imply a particular cause of this enlargement, and as in other species, a range of potential causes should be considered in each case.

SYNONYMS

- Splenic enlargement
- *Hypersplenism* describes splenomegaly together with increased removal of platelets and/or other blood cells by the spleen.

SPECIAL SPECIES CONSIDERATIONS

- The spleen in the ferret is tongue-shaped and follows the visceral surface of the greater curvature of the stomach. In cross-section, it is flat and triangular with a thickness of up to 8 mm at the hilus.
- Normal splenic dimensions in the ferret have been reported as length of 5 to 7 cm and width of approximately 2 cm.
- Splenomegaly is a benign problem in many ferrets.

EPIDEMIOLOGY

SPECIES, AGE, SEX Splenomegaly in the ferret increases in prevalence with age; there is no sex predilection.

ASSOCIATED CONDITIONS AND DISORDERS

- Chronic inflammation, primarily of the gastrointestinal tract, is the most commonly suspected cause.
- Other causes include neoplasms and systemic infections.
- Splenomegaly is a transient result of anesthesia caused by sequestration of blood cells.

CLINICAL PRESENTATION

HISTORY, CHIEF COMPLAINT

- Splenomegaly is most commonly identified as an incidental physical finding at annual or semiannual veterinary visits.
- Severely affected animals may present with clinical signs of lethargy and inappetence.
- Rarely, owners may complain of finding a "lump" or visualizing a dark organ through the abdominal wall.

PHYSICAL EXAM FINDINGS

- Findings are variable owing to the size of the spleen at the time of presentation. Abdominal palpation of the relaxed ferret reveals an oblong firm mass often extending from the left cranial quadrant, along the ventral abdominal wall, to the right caudal quadrant.
- Because of the propensity for capsular rupture, practitioners should always approach palpation of an enlarged spleen with care.

ETIOLOGY AND PATHOPHYSIOLOGY

- A vast majority of cases of splenomegaly may arise as a stereotypical response to chronic inflammation (both clinical and subclinical) in the ferret.
  - Common inflammatory bowel conditions such as proliferative colitis, eosinophilic gastroenteritis, *Campylobacter* spp. infection, or gastric infection with *Helicobacter mustelae* may serve as the inciting factor.
  - Inflammatory mediators result in the marked proliferation of immature red and white blood cells within the splenic red pulp; megakaryocytes are often present.
- Remaining cases of enlarged spleen are due to the presence of a neoplasm:
  - Lymphoma is by far the most common splenic neoplasm in the ferret.
  - Hemangiosarcoma and histiocytic sarcomas are also seen.
- Splenic enlargement is seen in association with hemolytic anemia and is a significant source of red cell removal.
- Congestion due to sequestration of blood during anesthesia will often increase the size of the normal spleen at surgery.
- Splenic infarction may be seen in any case of splenomegaly and can lead to systemic complications and/or rupture.

DIAGNOSIS

DIFFERENTIAL DIAGNOSIS

- Extramedullary hematopoiesis due to chronic systemic inflammatory processes (usually gastrointestinal disease)
- Autoimmune hemolytic anemia
- Splenic lymphoma
- Other splenic neoplasms
- Passive congestion: because no valves are present in the splenic venous system, pressure in the splenic vein reflects the pressure in the portal vein
- Idiopathic hypersplenism

INITIAL DATABASE

- Clinicopathologic changes in splenomegaly are not specific, except for idiopathic hypersplenism, in which a reduction in the number of circulating thrombocytes and occasionally of leukocytes and erythrocytes is seen.
- Persistent lymphocytosis, hypoalbuminemia, and mild elevations in globulins suggest chronic bowel inflammation but are not specific for this condition.
- No significant meaning is attached to an ultrasound finding of splenomegaly. However, if multifocal hypoechoic areas are seen in the parenchyma, the suspicion of lymphosarcoma-associated splenomegaly is justified.

ADVANCED OR CONFIRMATORY TESTING

- Fine-needle aspirate of the spleen may be performed.
  - Several slides should be prepared from each specimen.
  - Cytologic preparations may be stained with Diff-Quik and evaluated in-house; definitive diagnosis should be performed by a pathologist.
  - Benign cases of splenomegaly arising from chronic systemic inflammation are heralded by a bloody aspirate containing peripheral blood elements with large numbers of immature red and white blood cells, and occasional megakaryocytes (located primarily within the feathered edge).
  - Most cases of splenic lymphoma will result in a cellular aspirate with a monomorphic population of lymphocytes.
  - Splenic aspirates from older animals with lymphoma may be falsely negative owing to the mature appearance of the neoplastic lymphocytes.

TREATMENT

THERAPEUTIC GOALS

- The goal of therapy varies according to diagnosis and the predisposing cause of splenomegaly.
  - Splenectomy is performed to extend life expectancy in the case of splenic neoplasms.
  - In cases of extramedullary hematopoiesis due to chronic inflammation, splenectomy is reserved for cases in which marked enlargement predisposes to rupture.

- Splenectomy may be considered early in the progression of hemolytic anemia to extend survival time and the potential for successful treatment of the underlying cause.
- Splenectomy reverses the reduction in the numbers of circulating blood cells (thrombocytes, erythrocytes, leukocytes) seen in idiopathic hypersplenism.

ACUTE GENERAL TREATMENT

- Splenectomy is not considered a difficult procedure in most ferrets.
- Exteriorization of the spleen and ligature of the splenic vessels (performed with care in ferrets with marked abdominal fat) are required.

POSSIBLE COMPLICATIONS

Complications arising from splenectomy have not been reported in ferrets.

RECOMMENDED MONITORING

- If an enlarged spleen is detected during a routine physical examination in a ferret that appears healthy and has no complete blood count or platelet count abnormalities, it should be noted in the record and the ferret monitored by examination once or twice a year with assessment of spleen size.
- If the spleen remains markedly enlarged, repeat the initial database and consider performing a splenic fine-needle aspirate for cytologic evaluation.

PROGNOSIS AND OUTCOME

- The prognosis of splenomegaly is based on the inciting cause.
  - Cases in which histologic or cytologic findings reveal extramedullary hematopoiesis have a good prognosis.
  - The prognosis for nonlymphoid splenic neoplasms is guarded, and for splenic lymphoma, the prognosis is poor.
  - Cases of autoimmune hemolytic anemia warrant a poor long-term prognosis.
  - A 20-month survival time has been reported for cases of idiopathic hypersplenism after splenectomy.

PEARLS & CONSIDERATIONS

COMMENTS

- Splenomegaly is a benign problem in many ferrets.
- In the ferret, it appears that the only significant source of new peripheral blood cells and platelets is the bone marrow, and that proliferating elements in the spleen do not contribute significantly toward ameliorating signs of anemia or myeloid depletion.
- Splenectomy is rarely performed in ferrets with splenomegaly as an incidental finding.
- Splenectomy is commonly performed in animals at risk of splenic rupture, or when the presence of the enlarged spleen results in clinical signs.

SUGGESTED READING

Rakich PM, et al: Cytologic diagnosis of diseases of ferrets, Vet Clin North Am Exot Anim Pract 10:61–78, 2007.

AUTHOR: **BRUCE H. WILLIAMS**

EDITORS: **JAMES G. FOX AND ROBERT P. MARINI**

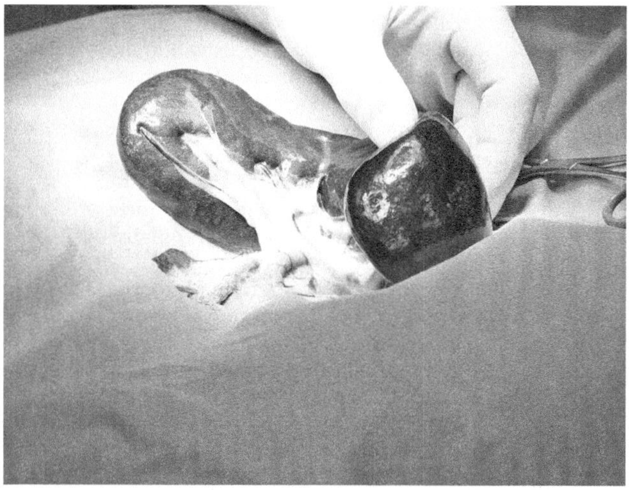

Splenomegaly Exteriorized grossly enlarged spleen of a ferret. A splenectomy usually is not required in the case of splenomegaly. Only in severe cases or with lymphoma or hypersplenism is a splenectomy indicated. *(Photo courtesy Jörg Mayer, The University of Georgia, Athens.)*

FERRETS

Urolithiasis

BASIC INFORMATION

DEFINITION

- Urolithiasis: crystalluria and stone formation that may be associated with lower urinary tract disease and possibly urethral obstruction
- Lower urinary tract infection: bacterial infection and inflammation involving the bladder and the urethra

SYNONYMS

Urinary calculi, cystitis, lower urinary tract infection

SPECIAL SPECIES CONSIDERATIONS

Urolithiasis used to be a common problem in pet ferrets before commercial ferret diets became available.

EPIDEMIOLOGY

SPECIES, AGE, SEX Urinary calculi are most commonly seen in adult males but have also been reported in pregnant females.

GENETICS AND BREED PREDISPOSITION Rare reports have described cystine stones in ferrets (speculated to be caused by a genetic anomaly).

RISK FACTORS Dog food or poor quality (plant protein–based) cat foods promote the development of urolithiasis in ferrets.

CONTAGION AND ZOONOSIS *Staphylococcus aureus, Proteus* spp., and *Escherichia coli* are the most common bacteria associated with cystitis in the ferret.

ASSOCIATED CONDITIONS AND DISORDERS Cystitis

CLINICAL PRESENTATION

DISEASE FORMS/SUBTYPES

- Bacterial cystitis
- Cystitis with crystalluria
- Urinary calculi

HISTORY, CHIEF COMPLAINT Infection initially may be asymptomatic; however, by the time of presentation, most ferrets demonstrate pollakiuria, hematuria, and/or dysuria. Owners may misinterpret the straining observed as "constipation," or tenesmus can lead to diarrhea. Nonspecific signs of illness such as anorexia, lethargy, and depression can be observed in ferrets with urinary calculi and secondary urethral obstruction. Ferrets with urethral obstruction can be observed licking excessively at the preputial region.

PHYSICAL EXAM FINDINGS

- The urinary bladder wall may be palpably thickened, and cystic calculi or sand may be palpable.
- The prepuce may be red from frequent licking.
- The urinary bladder may be distended and painful with urethral obstruction. The overly full bladder may dribble urine, creating a wet, urine-stained ventral abdomen.

ETIOLOGY AND PATHOPHYSIOLOGY

- Magnesium ammonium phosphate (struvite) uroliths are the most common, although other types of stones can be found.
- Dog food or inexpensive, plant protein–based cat foods promote the development of alkaline urine in the ferret.
- Struvite crystals commonly form when urine pH exceeds 6.6.
- Significant crystalluria leads to the development of cystic calculi or to the presence of sandy material in the bladder and the urethra.

DIAGNOSIS

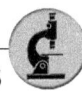

DIFFERENTIAL DIAGNOSIS

- Prostatomegaly or prostatitis associated with adrenocortical disease
- Neoplasia of the urinary tract is rare, but transitional cell carcinoma has been reported and can produce signs similar to chronic cystitis.
- Paraurethral cysts

INITIAL DATABASE

- Urinalysis
  - Obtain a urine sample by cystocentesis using a 23- to 25-gauge needle.
  - Findings consistent with cystitis include hematuria, pyuria, tubular casts, and bacteriuria. Normal ferret urine pH is approximately 6.
- Complete blood count/biochemistry panel results are often unremarkable.
  - An inflammatory leukogram can be seen with an ascending bacterial infection.
  - Urethral obstruction can be associated with azotemia, hyperphosphatemia, metabolic acidosis, and hyperkalemia.
  - Hypoglycemia can be seen with concurrent insulinoma (see Insulinoma).

ADVANCED OR CONFIRMATORY TESTING

- Urine bacterial culture/sensitivity
- Survey radiographs: evaluate the entire length of the urinary tract for radiodense uroliths. Calculi at the os penis can be particularly difficult to detect.
- Abdominal ultrasound: evaluate the urinary tract, prostate, and adrenal glands. Confirm the presence of uroliths or bladder sludge.

TREATMENT

THERAPEUTIC GOALS

- Relieve urethral obstruction.
- Support renal perfusion.
- Manage infection and inflammation.
- Remove urinary calculi, if present.

ACUTE GENERAL TREATMENT

Relieve urethral obstruction

- If the ferret is a good anesthetic risk at the time of presentation, place a urinary catheter under general anesthesia immediately.
  - Provide appropriate analgesia (e.g., buprenorphine 0.01-0.03 mg/kg SC, IM, IV q 8-12 h).
  - Carefully monitor electrocardiogram (ECG) for evidence of hyperkalemia: loss of the P wave, widening of the QRS complex, peaked T waves, and a short QY interval.
  - Relief of obstruction and forced diuresis are usually sufficient in the management of hyperkalemia; however, medical treatment of hyperkalemia is indicated if an arrhythmia is present, in addition to poor perfusion or altered mentation. Give calcium gluconate 50-100 mg/kg slow bolus IV.
  - Use a 24-gauge catheter to identify and dilate the small urethral opening near the tip of the J-shaped os penis.
  - Place a 3 Fr urinary catheter designed for use in ferrets. Alternatively, a 22- to 20-gauge jugular catheter can serve as a makeshift urinary catheter, or a 3.5 Fr red rubber catheter can be placed in a large male.
- If the ferret requires stabilization before anesthetic induction, perform cystocentesis using a 23- to 25-gauge needle to provide temporary relief. Provide fluid therapy and supportive care.
- If a urinary catheter cannot be placed, empty the bladder via cystocentesis and provide supportive care
  - Perform an emergency cystotomy with anterograde flushing of the urethra.
  - Alternatively, tube cystostomy has also been described in the ferret. A 5 or 8 Fr Foley catheter is passed through a ventral paramedian incision and into the bladder lumen, where it is secured with a purse-string suture.
  - In rare instances, an emergency perineal urethrostomy is required.

Support renal perfusion

- Administer fluids first to correct perfusion abnormalities and then rehydrate the patient. Maintenance fluid requirements in ferrets are estimated at 75 mL/kg/d.
- Discontinue any potentially nephrotoxic drugs.

Manage infection and inflammation

- Until culture/sensitivity results are available, use a broad-spectrum antibiotic that reaches high levels in the urinary tract.
- Administer antibiotics for a minimum of 10 to 14 days, continuing treatment several days past resolution of clinical signs.
- Gradually convert the ferret to a high-quality, animal protein–based diet over a period of 1 to 2 weeks.

Remove urinary calculi, if present

- If no urethral obstruction is present, stabilize the patient with fluids, then schedule a cystotomy to remove urinary calculi and flush the bladder.
- Submit calculi for mineral analysis.
- Submit crushed calculi and bladder mucosa for culture and sensitivity.

CHRONIC TREATMENT

- Gradually convert the ferret to a high-quality, animal protein–based diet over a period of 1 to 2 weeks.
- Attempts to feed low-pH cat food (e.g., feline s/d, Hill's Pet Nutrition, Topeka, KS; feline Urinary SO, Royal Canin, St Charles, MO) are generally unsuccessful but have been reported. The protein level of these diets may be inadequate for long-term use in ferrets.
- Because the urine pH of a ferret on a high-quality, meat-based diet is approximately 6.0, urinary acidifiers are usually unnecessary.

POSSIBLE COMPLICATIONS

- Stone formation and subsequent urethral obstruction
- Persistent or recurrent urethral obstruction may require perineal urethrostomy.
- Ascending infection (pyelonephritis) or septicemia is rare but can lead to fever, nonspecific signs of illness (anorexia, depression), and renal failure.

RECOMMENDED MONITORING

- Monitor urine production in catheterized ferrets using a closed line attached to a small (150 to 250 mL) IV bag.
- Monitor patient for signs of cystitis and urethral obstruction.
- Use urinalysis results and urine culture and sensitivity to guide the duration of antibiotic therapy.
- Exacerbation of *Helicobacter mustelae* (see *Helicobacter mustelae*–Associated Gastritis and Ulcers) is not uncommon in ferrets with concurrent illness causing gastritis and possible gastric erosions and ulcers. Monitor ferret for signs of gastrointestinal discomfort such as bruxism (tooth grinding), ptyalism (excessive drooling), pawing at the mouth, anorexia, and diarrhea, including melena.
- Consider prophylactic administration of gastroprotectants in critically ill ferrets (e.g., famotidine 0.5 mg/kg PO, IV, SC q 24 h and/or sucralfate 100 mg/kg PO q 8-12 h).

PROGNOSIS AND OUTCOME

- Good for urethral or bladder calculi if recognized early and managed aggressively
- Recurrence is uncommon after successful treatment and dietary changes.

PEARLS & CONSIDERATIONS

COMMENTS

- Spontaneous urinary tract infections are rare in ferrets. Struvite crystalluria is an important, but much less common, cause of cystitis in the ferret. The most common cause of urinary tract infection in the ferret is underlying adrenocortical disease with associated prostatomegaly.
- Urolithiasis should be the primary differential in ferrets on dog food or an inexpensive, plant protein–based cat food.

PREVENTION

A high-quality, animal protein–based diet will maintain acidic urine and prevent struvite crystal formation.

CLIENT EDUCATION

Educate owners on the importance of feeding a commercial ferret food or a high-quality, animal protein–based cat food.

SUGGESTED READINGS

Fisher PG: Exotic mammal renal disease: diagnosis and treatment, Vet Clin North Am Exot Anim Pract 9:69–96, 2006.

Nolte DM, et al: Temporary tube cystostomy as treatment for urinary obstruction secondary to adrenal disease in four ferrets, J Am Anim Hosp Assoc 38:527–531, 2003.

Pollock CG: Disorders of the urinary and reproductive systems. In Quesenberry KE, et al, editors: Ferrets, rabbits, and rodents: clinical medicine and surgery, St Louis, 2012, Elsevier, pp 44–61.

CROSS-REFERENCES TO OTHER SECTIONS

Adrenal Disease
Helicobacter mustelae–Associated Gastritis and Ulcers
Insulinoma
Prostatic Disease
Renal Disorders

AUTHOR: **CHRISTAL POLLOCK**

EDITORS: **JAMES G. FOX AND ROBERT P. MARINI**

FERRETS

Vaccine Reactions

BASIC INFORMATION

DEFINITION

Vaccination adverse events are usually type I hypersensitivity reactions, or anaphylaxis, in ferrets. Adverse vaccine reactions are most common after distemper vaccination but can occur after rabies vaccination.

SYNONYMS

Type I hypersensitivity reaction, anaphylaxis

SPECIAL SPECIES CONSIDERATION

Canine distemper is the most serious viral infection of ferrets, with mortality rates approaching 100%. Combination canine distemper vaccine and vaccines of ferret cell or low-passage canine cell origin should not be used in ferrets.

EPIDEMIOLOGY

SPECIES, AGE, SEX In one large retrospective study, age, sex, and body weight were not significantly associated with occurrence of adverse vaccine events, but the adverse event incidence rate is increased as the cumulative number of distemper or rabies vaccinations received is increased.

RISK FACTORS Previous exposure (sensitization) increases the chance that the animal may develop a reaction.

CLINICAL PRESENTATION

DISEASE FORMS/SUBTYPES Type I hypersensitivity reaction

HISTORY, CHIEF COMPLAINT Most vaccine reactions occur within 30 minutes of vaccine administration. However, some reactions can be delayed for 24 to 48 hours.

PHYSICAL EXAM FINDINGS Mild vaccine reactions may involve pruritus and skin erythema. More severe vaccine reactions can be associated with hypersalivation, vomiting, diarrhea, piloerection, hyperthermia, cardiovascular collapse, or death.

ETIOLOGY AND PATHOPHYSIOLOGY

- Adverse vaccine reactions are typically type I hypersensitivity reactions.
- Type I hypersensitivity reactions involve lymphoid tissue associated with mucosal surfaces (skin, intestine, lung). Immediate hypersensitivity is mediated by immunoglobulin (Ig) E. The primary cellular component in this hypersensitivity is the mast cell or basophil. The reaction is amplified and/or modified by platelets, neutrophils, and eosinophils.

DIAGNOSIS

DIFFERENTIAL DIAGNOSIS

- Other types of shock
- Trauma

INITIAL DATABASE

Because of the acute nature of the reaction, no tests reliably predict individual susceptibility.

ADVANCED OR CONFIRMATORY TESTING

Lesions vary, depending on severity of reaction.

TREATMENT

THERAPEUTIC GOAL

Provide emergency life support through maintenance of an open airway, prevent circulatory collapse, and reestablish physiologic parameters.

ACUTE GENERAL TREATMENT

- Eliminate inciting antigen if possible (impossible if vaccine was already given).
- Administer an antihistamine (diphenhydramine 0.5-2 mg/kg IV or IM), epinephrine hydrochloride (20 mcg/kg IV, IM, SC, or intratracheally), and/or a short-acting corticosteroid (such as dexamethasone sodium phosphate 1-2 mg/kg IV or IM).
- Administer fluids intravenously at shock dosages to counteract hypotension.
- Administer oxygen or aminophylline (4 mg/kg IM, IV q 12 h) to dyspneic patients.

POSSIBLE COMPLICATIONS

Death in severe reactions

RECOMMENDED MONITORING

Closely monitor hospitalized patient for 24 to 48 hours.

PROGNOSIS AND OUTCOME

If reaction is treated early, prognosis can be good. Death is possible in severe cases.

PEARLS & CONSIDERATIONS

COMMENTS

- Always follow the manufacturer's instructions for vaccine administration.
- Adverse vaccine reactions should be reported to the Center for Biologics, U.S. Department of Agriculture (1-800-752-6255; www.aphis.usda.gov/vs/cvb/adverseeventreport.html).
- Vaccine injection site sarcoma has been described in ferrets.

PREVENTION

Premedication with diphenhydramine 2 mg/kg PO or SC at least 15 minutes before vaccination may help prevent or reduce the severity of the vaccine reaction.

CLIENT EDUCATION

- Before administering the vaccine, inform the owner of the possibility of a vaccine reaction. Have the owner monitor the ferret for adverse reactions in the waiting area for at least 30 minutes after the vaccine is administered.
- Two vaccines are currently approved for canine distemper in ferrets: Fervac-D (United Vaccines, Inc., Madison, WI) and PureVax (Merial, Athens, GA). The incidence of vaccine reaction in ferrets may be less with PureVax compared with other vaccines.
- Rabies vaccines that are available are IMRAB 3 and IMRAB 3 TF (Merial, Athens, GA).

SUGGESTED READINGS

Greenacre CB: Incidence of adverse events in ferrets vaccinated with distemper or rabies vaccine: 143 cases (1995-2001), J Am Vet Med Assoc 223:663–665, 2003.

Moore G, et al: Incidence of and risk factors for adverse events associated with distemper and rabies vaccine administration in ferrets, J Am Vet Med Assoc 226:909–912, 2005.

Munday JS, et al: Histology and immunohistochemistry of seven ferret vaccination-site fibrosarcomas, Vet Pathol 40:288–293, 2003.

CROSS-REFERENCES TO OTHER SECTIONS

Distemper
Rabies (Section VI)

AUTHOR: **JENNIFER GRAHAM**

EDITORS: **JAMES G. FOX AND ROBERT P. MARINI**

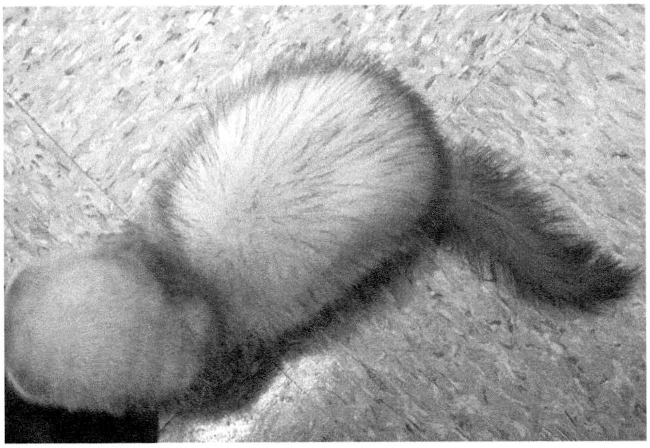

Vaccine Reactions Dorsal aspect of a ferret showed pronounced piloerection. This is an early sign of a vaccine reaction. Piloerection typically occurs 30 to 40 minutes after administration of the vaccine. *(Photo courtesy Jörg Mayer, The University of Georgia, Athens.)*

SECTION II

Procedures and Techniques

EDITOR

Jörg Mayer *DrMedVet, MSc, DABVP (Exotic Companion Mammal), DECZM (Small Mammal)*

INVERTEBRATES

Anesthesia

SYNONYM

Immobilization

OVERVIEW AND GOAL

Gas anesthesia may be the most technically simple and effective method of restraint for terrestrial invertebrates.

INDICATIONS

- Part of the physical exam
- Diagnostic sampling, procedures

EQUIPMENT, ANESTHESIA

- Gloves
- Forceps
- Transparent plastic box (tupperware)
- Anesthesia setup (e.g., isoflurane vaporizer)

ANTICIPATED TIME

10 to 30 minutes depending on the purpose of the procedure

PREPARATION: IMPORTANT CHECKPOINTS

See physical exam procedure for preparation.

PROCEDURE

- Enclose the patient in a gas delivery chamber, and deliver the agent by a direct method or, preferably, with a vaporizer.
- In the tarantula, recommended anesthetic protocols include carbon dioxide at 10% to 20% for 3 to 5 minutes, halothane at 4% for 5 to 10 minutes, methoxyflurane at 4% for 10 to 30 minutes, and isoflurane at 3% to 4% for 10 to 15 minutes.
- For direct delivery, a cotton ball or sponge may be soaked in anesthetic agent and placed in the chamber.
- To ensure that the patient cannot come into contact with the anesthetic agent, a specially built induction chamber is required for the direct method.
- For aquatic species: MS-222 is commonly added to water in a concentration of 100 mg/1 L of water.
  - Buffering MS-222 with the addition of sodium bicarbonate is recommended for use in invertebrates with sensitive skin, such as snails and slugs.
- Benzocaine is probably the best choice of available anesthetics, but it must be made as a stock solution in ethanol and stored away from light.
- Commonly used inhalant anesthetics, such as isoflurane, may be used in aquatic invertebrates by bubbling them through water.
- Immerse the entire patient (or just the foot of gastropods) in the anesthetic solution until it is immobile, then remove it.
- To keep the patient moist and sedate, a misting of anesthetic solution may be applied periodically; by varying this solution's concentration, one can control anesthetic depth.

POST-PROCEDURE

- Determination of depth of anesthesia in invertebrates may be challenging.
- In terrestrial invertebrates, the righting reflex, immobility, and response or lack thereof to gentle prodding or other aversive stimuli are generally used to determine the depth of anesthesia.
- In leeches, attachment to the surface, swimming motion, muscle tone, sucker function, and response to stimulation were assessed for determination of anesthetic depth.
- Reversal of anesthesia in aquatic species is simple and rapid when they are returned to normal water.
- Oxygen supplementation of both terrestrial and aquatic species is recommended for anesthetic recovery or in the event of anesthetic complications.

AUTHOR: **MODIFIED FROM BRAUN ME, HEATLEY JJ, CHITTY J: CLINICAL TECHNIQUES OF INVERTEBRATES, VET CLIN NORTH AM EXOT ANIM PRACT 9:205–221, 2006.**

EDITOR: **JÖRG MAYER**

INVERTEBRATES

Diagnostic Sampling

OVERVIEW AND GOALS

- Proper sampling technique must be observed to obtain diagnostic results.
- Invertebrate patient size demands that sampling be performed with the fewest possible attempts.

INDICATIONS

Quality samples are essential for definitive diagnosis and guidance of treatment.

ANTICIPATED TIME

5 to 10 minutes

PREPARATION: IMPORTANT CHECKPOINTS

- For many procedures, the patient must be anesthetized (see Anesthesia).
- Restraint is sometimes adequate.

PROCEDURE

- Hemolymph collection
  - To assess physiologic parameters, hemolymph samples may be obtained.
  - The small sample amount, not to exceed 10% of patient body weight, can make sampling difficult. In mollusks, hemolymph may be obtained from the heart or the cephalopod sinus by means of a capillary tube or a 25-gauge needle and syringe.
  - To access the heart, a hole may be made in the shell using a dental drill.
  - Alternatively, hemolymph can be sampled from the cephalopedal sinus in anesthetized patients.
  - In bivalve mollusks, once the adductor muscle is transected and the left valve is removed, the heart can be found by its beating.
  - Alternatively, one may file a notch in each valve to create an opening and then insert the needle into the adductor sinus through the adductor muscle.
  - Another method for bleeding snails may be done without shell perforation. Locate the pneumostome (respiratory opening) as a landmark by watching for the appearance of bubbles.
  - In snails weighing less than 50 g, the needle insertion point is approximately 5 mm below the pneumostome, and in snails weighing between 50 g and 200 g, the point is approximately 20 mm below the pneumostome.

- Hemolymph may be aspirated using a 25-gauge needle and syringe.
- Hemolymph can be collected from arthropods by direct withdrawal from the heart, coelom, or legs.
- Methods of hemolymph collection are similar to those described for fluid administration, with aspiration of these sites substituted for injection.
- Integumental diagnostics
  - Integumental lesions may require samples to be taken for isolation of bacterial, fungal, or viral agents.
  - Skin scrapings, swabs, and touch preparations from ulcerated lesions may be used for culture and cytology for diagnosis and identification of bacterial, fungal, and viral infections.
  - Similar diagnostics, along with excision of deeper lesions, may be used for histopathologic examination.
  - Commensal and symbiotic organisms that may live on these animals can make interpretation of results challenging.
  - Culturing techniques need to take into account the ectothermic nature of the host.
  - Standard incubation temperature of 37°C (99°F) may not be optimal for some invertebrate pathogens.
  - After sampling, lesions should be irrigated with saline to minimize dehydration and facilitate healing.
- Fecal examination
  - Fresh samples can simply be collected from the habitat of an individual or taken from a sample of a colony population.
  - Colonies of invertebrates often have to be regarded as a whole organism.
  - In these cases, culling samples of sick and healthy individuals can allow for diagnosis with minimal loss.
  - When the small size of the patient will not allow taking of adequate sample sizes, whole-body extracts may be used diagnostically to determine the causes of dysecdysis and European foulbrood, a disease of honeybees.
  - Samples may be diluted to obtain adequate sample volumes.

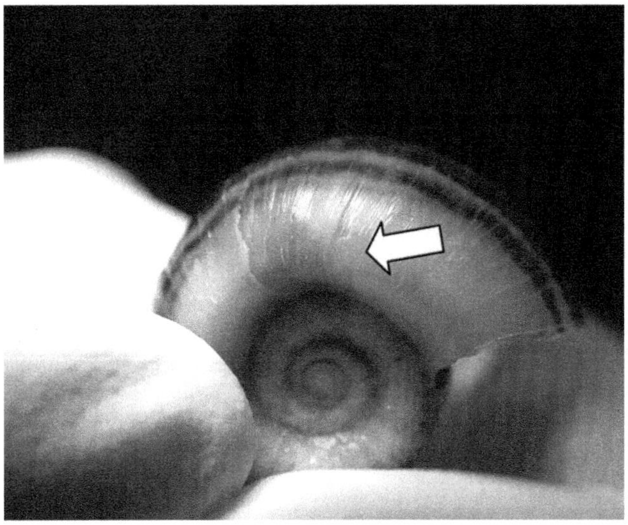

Diagnostic Sampling Pneumostome in the snail may be found by looking for the expulsion of air bubbles. Arrow denotes the light shadow of the air bubbles visualized through the right side of the shell. *(Photo courtesy Braun ME, Heatley JJ, Chitty J: Clinical Techniques of Invertebrates, Vet Clin North Am Exot Anim Pract 9:205–221, 2006.)*

AUTHOR: **MODIFIED FROM BRAUN ME, HEATLEY JJ, CHITTY J: CLINICAL TECHNIQUES OF INVERTEBRATES, VET CLIN NORTH AM EXOT ANIM PRACT 9:205–221, 2006.**

EDITOR: **JÖRG MAYER**

INVERTEBRATES

Dysecdysis/Ectoparasites

SYNONYM

Bad moult

OVERVIEW AND GOALS

- The ability to moult properly is essential for the growth, development, and healing of many species of invertebrates, particularly insects, spiders, centipedes, millipedes, and scorpions.
- Dysecdysis in captive invertebrates occurs in several forms stemming from multiple causes.

INDICATIONS

- The most common causes of dysecdysis are hormonal abnormalities caused by low levels of humidity, overcrowding (i.e., lack of space suitable for moulting), nutritional problems, and infection.
- Dysecdysis can manifest as incomplete or abnormal moulting, inappropriately frequent moulting, or moult arrest.
- For colonial invertebrates with dysecdysis, culling a sample of animals to determine the levels of endogenous ecdysone from total body extracts may be diagnostic.
- Parasitic infestation may cause integumental disorders or dysecdysis.

CONTRAINDICATIONS

- In many species, such as hissing cockroaches and millipedes, the mites and the host form a symbiotic relationship as the mites feed on organic matter gathered in the joints or between the body plates.

- Killing these mites leaves the host vulnerable to bacterial or fungal infection.

EQUIPMENT, ANESTHESIA

- Fine forceps
- Cotton-tipped applicator
- Lubricating gel, oil

ANTICIPATED TIME

5 minutes

PREPARATION: IMPORTANT CHECKPOINTS

Patients often need to be anesthetized for these delicate procedures (e.g., skin or mite removal).

POSSIBLE COMPLICATIONS AND COMMON ERRORS TO BE AVOIDED

- Overzealous traction may damage the underlying exoskeleton.
- Application of a drop of mineral oil onto the spider, to capture the mites as they roam, is not efficacious and may compromise the spider's book lung.
- Bathing a tarantula in a dilute soap solution for mite removal may compromise the book lung.

PROCEDURE

- Apply glycerin to retained epidermis to loosen and remove it by teasing pieces away with forceps or a cotton-tipped applicator.
- Removal is similar to that of the retained spectacle of the snake.
- Treatment of parasitic conditions in arthropods is challenging because of the close taxonomic relationship between the parasite and the host.
- Drugs effective against the mite infestation can also kill the arthropod patient.
- Unlike arthropods, snails with ectoparasite infestation may be safely treated with pyrethroids.
- Manual removal of parasites has the greatest efficacy in arthropods.
- For arthropods such as cockroaches, phasmids, mantids, and scorpions, shaking the arthropod gently in a bag of flour may dislodge the mites.
- Swabbing with a soft paintbrush or cotton ball may dislodge the mites from arthropods.
- Mite removal from spiders may require manual removal with ophthalmic forceps and magnification.
    - A cotton-tipped applicator coated with Vaseline may be used to entrap the mites and lift them from the exoskeleton.
- Anesthesia of the patient may facilitate mite removal by also anesthetizing the mites.
- Flumethrin strips are effective against infestation when placed in the vivarium.

POST-PROCEDURE

- Patients with retained portions of integument that required treatment should undergo review (and correction) of current husbandry practices as necessary.
- Enclosure humidity should be increased to greater than 85% and a thermal gradient should be provided to include the top end of the animal's preferred optimal temperature zone.
- Ectoparasitic mites of spiders and other arthropods are thought to come from food sources such as crickets and mealworms.
- Hence, cleaning debris of past meals from the habitat in a timely manner is recommended.

ALTERNATIVES AND THEIR RELATIVE MERITS

Use of predatory mites, *Hyoaspsis*, can serve as an alternative treatment for mite infestation, but these mites are not universally available owing to certain national environmental policies.

AUTHOR: **MODIFIED FROM BRAUN ME, HEATLEY JJ, CHITTY J: CLINICAL TECHNIQUES OF INVERTEBRATES, VET CLIN NORTH AM EXOT ANIM PRACT 9:205–221, 2006.**

EDITOR: **JÖRG MAYER**

INVERTEBRATES

Euthanasia

SYNONYM

Putting to sleep

OVERVIEW AND GOALS

- Euthanasia is a procedure that must be performed humanely.
- Pain control should be considered when euthanasia of invertebrates is performed.

INDICATIONS

If medical or surgical treatment is unlikely to succeed or is not an option

CONTRAINDICATIONS

Do not freeze the unanesthetized invertebrate patient.

ANTICIPATED TIME

5 to 10 minutes

POSSIBLE COMPLICATIONS AND COMMON ERRORS TO BE AVOIDED

Crushing is an acceptable alternative for euthanasia of snails, but this option does not preserve the carcass for necropsy.

PROCEDURE

- Among accepted options of euthanasia for snails are freezing, immersion in boiling water, and overdosing with the chemical anesthetics outlined (see Handling and Restraint).
- Euthanasia with an anesthetic overdose is the best method for enabling postmortem examination.

ALTERNATIVES AND THEIR RELATIVE MERITS

Further advice is available in the British and Irish Association of Zoo and Aquaria's *Guide to Invertebrate Euthanasia.*

AUTHOR: **MODIFIED FROM BRAUN ME, HEATLEY JJ, CHITTY J: CLINICAL TECHNIQUES OF INVERTEBRATES, VET CLIN NORTH AM EXOT ANIM PRACT 9:205–221, 2006.**

EDITOR: **JÖRG MAYER**

Exoskeleton Repair

SYNONYMS

Exoskeleton or shell trauma

OVERVIEW AND GOALS

- Assessment of an invertebrate integumental injury is important for the patient's appropriate and successful treatment.
- When a traumatic insult occurs to an arthropod's integument from a fall, predation, or surgical intervention, several issues must be addressed to correct the problem.

INDICATIONS

- Prevention of integumental disease relies primarily on the ability of owners to maintain proper environmental conditions for their animals.
- Maintaining both temperature and humidity within optimal limits for a given species may prevent many skin ailments.
- Maintaining appropriate hygiene in the habitat by removing old food, feces, and bedding will reduce the likelihood of parasitic infestation and infectious disease.
- Periodic cleaning of the entire habitat with disinfectants is especially important for the control of myiasis.
- Avoiding overpopulation and providing adequate open space for moulting are essential for maintaining healthy captive invertebrates.
- Treatment of integumental disease can be provided on an emergency basis.
- The break in the protective outer layer may cause hemolymph loss and dehydration and may create an avenue for infection.

CONTRAINDICATIONS

- Soft tissue injury to mollusks can often be fatal because of the large amount of hemolymph that is rapidly lost.
- If immediate treatment is not possible, the patient may be placed in a bowl of normal saline or clean water.
- Any patient exhibiting an exoskeleton or shell injury should be rehydrated and given prophylactic antibiotic therapy.

EQUIPMENT, ANESTHESIA

- Glue
- Wax
- Suture material

ANTICIPATED TIME

5 to 10 minutes

PREPARATION: IMPORTANT CHECKPOINTS

- On injury to the exoskeleton, an increased heart rate increases hemolymph pressure and hence the possibility of hemolymph loss.
- Loss of hemolymph can be immediately fatal, making quick action to repair the defect essential.
- As with other patients, immediate hemolymph stasis may be achieved by direct pressure.
- Other methods used to stop loss of hemolymph include sugar icing, talcum powder, paraffin wax, beeswax, plasticine, and tape to temporarily seal the hole in the exoskeleton.

POSSIBLE COMPLICATIONS AND COMMON ERRORS TO BE AVOIDED

Complete or partial limb loss of an arthropod generally does not require treatment. Although this indicates compromise of the exoskeleton, no great loss of hemolymph generally occurs, and patient survival without ill effects is likely. Many arthropods, especially the young, can regenerate lost limbs as they grow and moult.

PROCEDURE

- The most effective method of exoskeleton repair involves use of a cyanoacrylate adhesive such as tissue adhesive (Vetbond; 3M Animal Care Products, St Paul, MN), Instant Krazy Glue (Elmer's Products, Inc., Columbus, Ohio), or Super Glue (Pacer Technologies, Rancho Cucamonga, CA) to seal wounds or reduce shell fractures.
- Invertebrate patients with exoskeleton repairs should be monitored through the next moult to confirm that dysecdysis has not occurred at the repair site.
- Exoskeleton repair with suture material (Vicryl; Ethicon, Somerville, NJ) has resulted in death of tarantula patients.
    - Suturing may be effective with injury of the prosoma because of the greater tissue density of that body segment; however, dysecdysis may also be likely.
- Risk for hemolymph loss in a mollusk with a damaged shell is dependent on the location of the fracture.
- To repair a compromised shell, reduce fractures and apply an adhesive product, such as cyanoacrylate glue, to maintain the fragments in apposition.
- The shell is then reinforced with scaffolding material that will absorb the adhesive and provide support and stability while the fractures heal.

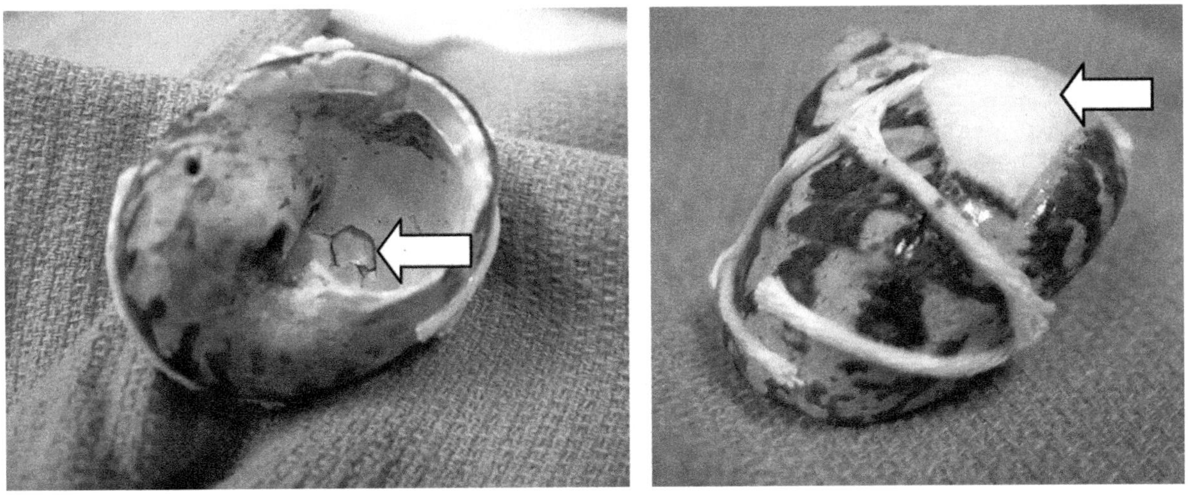

Exoskeleton Repair Should a snail's shell have a defect *(left panel, arrow),* it should be covered as part of the repair *(right panel, arrow).* *(Photo courtesy Braun ME, Heatley JJ, Chitty J: Clinical Techniques of Invertebrates, Vet Clin North Am Exot Anim Pract 9:205–221, 2006.)*

POST-PROCEDURE

- Mollusks with shell injury will benefit from dietary calcium supplementation.
- Persistent shell abnormalities can occur when the mantle of a mollusk is damaged.

AUTHOR: **MODIFIED FROM BRAUN ME, HEATLEY JJ, CHITTY J: CLINICAL TECHNIQUES OF INVERTEBRATES. VET CLIN NORTH AM EXOT ANIM PRACT 9:205–221, 2006.**

EDITOR: **JÖRG MAYER**

INVERTEBRATES

Fluid Administration

OVERVIEW AND GOAL

Hydration status is as important to invertebrate well-being as it is to conventional domestic animals.

INDICATIONS

- Dehydrated arthropods may be sluggish or anorectic or may have a shriveled opisthosoma or abdomen.
- Mollusks will also exhibit sluggishness and anorexia and will have shriveled, desiccated soft tissues.
- Debilitated arthropods can rehydrate themselves but may not be able to obtain water on their own.
- Tarantulas, for instance, are dependent on hemolymph pressure for movement.
- Flexor muscles pulling on the cuticle of the exoskeleton induce flexion of the limbs, but hemolymph pressure is necessary for limb extension.
- Adequate hemolymph pressure in the appendages cannot be achieved when the animal is suffering from volume depletion due to dehydration.

EQUIPMENT, ANESTHESIA

- Water dish
- Syringe
- Cotton ball

ANTICIPATED TIME

5 minutes

PREPARATION: IMPORTANT CHECKPOINTS

A good clinical examination, including a detailed history, is needed to collect evidence of dehydration.

POSSIBLE COMPLICATIONS AND COMMON ERRORS TO BE AVOIDED

- Because of the risk for cardiac laceration with the needle, pericardial or cardiac injection is reserved for immobilized or anesthetized animals.
- All opisthosomal injection sites must be repaired with cyanoacrylate, as described for exoskeleton repair.

PROCEDURE

- The clinician can rehydrate the patient by simply introducing water to its mouthparts.
  - A spoon, a shallow bowl, or a syringe may be used to administer fluids to a tarantula's pharynx. However, care must be taken to not allow the patient, in its compromised state, to become submerged, or it may be unable to remove itself from the water and drown.
  - Mollusks can be rehydrated by submerging the patient in water.
- In severe cases of dehydration, intracoelomic or intracardiac injection may be employed for fluid administration.
- Fluid choices include lactated Ringer's solution, normal saline, and, in the case of tarantulas, spider Ringer's solution consisting of sodium chloride 11.104 g/L, potassium chloride 0.149 g/L, calcium chloride dehydrate 0.588 g/L, magnesium chloride hexahydrate 0.813 g/L, and sodium phosphate heptahydrate 0.268 g/L.
- Fluid is administered through a 27-gauge needle with an insulin syringe.
- The amount administered varies according to the species.
  - In tarantulas, a 10% hydration deficit is approximately 2% to 4% of the spider's body weight.
  - In a 30-g tarantula that is 10% dehydrated, administration of 0.9 mL of fluids is appropriate to replace the deficit.
- The three anatomic options for fluid administration are (1) into the heart, (2) into the coelom of the opisthosoma, and (3) into the ventral joint membranes.
- Pericardial or cardiac injection is accomplished via introduction of the needle on the dorsal midline of the opisthosoma at an angle of 45° to 60° from vertical.
- The intracoelomic injection is administered along the transverse plane in the lateral opisthosoma.
- For injection into the ventral joint membrane of the limbs, the patient need not be anesthetized.
  - Insert a needle shallowly into the ventral joint membrane of any leg. The rate of administration is much slower using this method because of the small space available in the limb.

POST-PROCEDURE

- If damage occurs, the limb may be autotomized and the stump sealed with cyanoacrylate.
- Methods for intracoelomic and ventral joint injection in spiders may be applied to other arthropods.

AUTHOR: **MODIFIED FROM BRAUN ME, HEATLEY JJ, CHITTY J: CLINICAL TECHNIQUES OF INVERTEBRATES, VET CLIN NORTH AM EXOT ANIM PRACT 9:205–221, 2006.**

EDITOR: **JÖRG MAYER**

Handling and Restraint

OVERVIEW AND GOALS

- Techniques for manual restraint must provide safety to the patient and the clinician, as well as adequate patient immobilization.
- Knowledge of defensive or aggressive postures of these species can be helpful to avoid being harmed by these patients.

INDICATIONS

- Part of the physical exam
- Diagnostic sampling

CONTRAINDICATIONS

When handling many invertebrates, one must consider one's safety and the risk for bites and stings.

EQUIPMENT, ANESTHESIA

- Gloves
- Forceps
- Transparent plastic box (tupperware)

ANTICIPATED TIME

5 to 10 minutes depending on the purpose of the procedure

PREPARATION: IMPORTANT CHECKPOINTS

- Urticarial hairs (setae) on tarantulas and some caterpillars may be avoided by wearing latex gloves and eye protection, or by using padded forceps.
- Latex, lightweight leather, or cloth gloves should be worn when handling millipedes, centipedes, and other species that exude noxious, irritant, or venomous secretions.
- Latex gloves used with tarantulas should be rinsed free of powder before handling to protect the spider's book lung, which is a paired organ located in the cranioventral opisthosoma that consists of numerous layers of thin tissue in an air-filled atrium, enabling diffusion of oxygen into the hemolymph.

POSSIBLE COMPLICATIONS AND COMMON ERRORS TO BE AVOIDED

- Direct handling of invertebrates should be done not far above a soft surface.

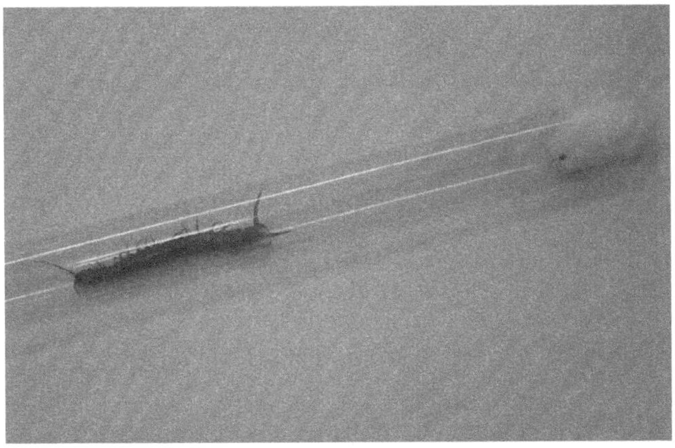

Handling and Restraint Clear plastic tube used to facilitate visual examination of a centipede *Scolopenda* spp. *(Photo courtesy Braun ME, Heatley JJ, Chitty J: Clinical Techniques of Invertebrates, Vet Clin North Am Exot Anim Pract 9:205–221, 2006.)*

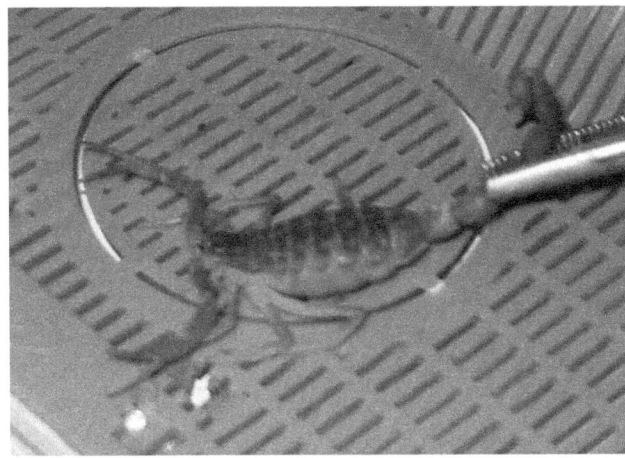

Handling and Restraint Scorpion restraint. The pinchers indicate the hazards of handling this animal. The stinger is gently restrained with forceps, ideally ones that have been padded. *(Photo courtesy Braun ME, Heatley JJ, Chitty J: Clinical Techniques of Invertebrates, Vet Clin North Am Exot Anim Pract 9:205–221, 2006.)*

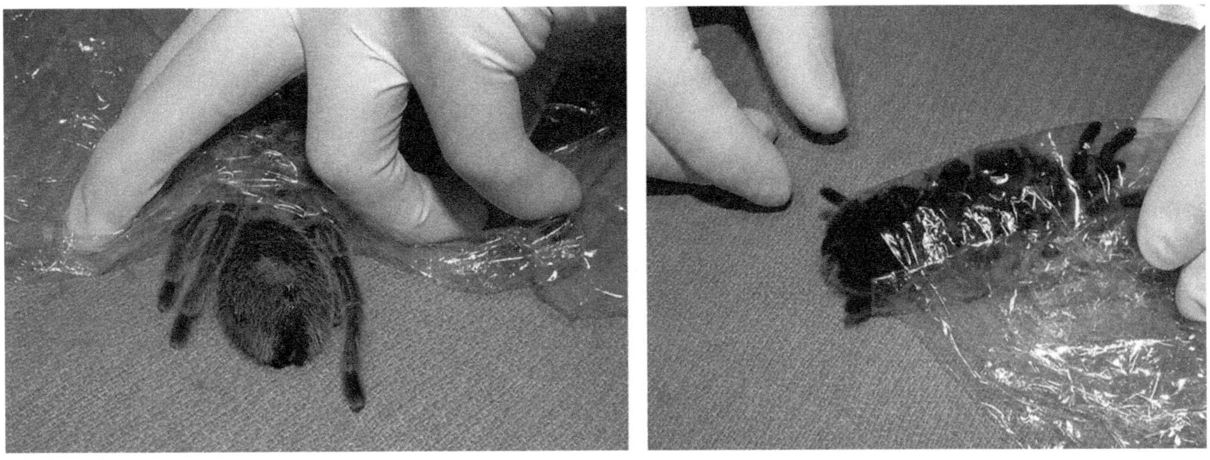

Handling and Restraint Plastic food wrap may be used for restraint of tarantulas. *(Photo courtesy Braun ME, Heatley JJ, Chitty J: Clinical Techniques of Invertebrates, Vet Clin North Am Exot Anim Pract 9:205–221, 2006.)*

- Careless handling resulting in a fall of the patient can damage the invertebrate's exoskeleton, causing loss of hemolymph and even death.

PROCEDURE

- Transparent containers allow close examination with only minor manipulation.
- Clear plastic tubes, such as those used for venomous snakes, and clear plastic boxes are excellent for handling and obtaining external visualization of many species.
- For more invasive restraint, arthropods may be immobilized by using cellophane, transparent plastic, or plexiglass to pin the patient gently in one position.
- Snails, millipedes, and slugs are easily handled by grasping at the midbody or allowing the animal to rest on the gloved hand.
- One should not grasp large spiders but rather should entice them to crawl onto the hand by prodding the abdomen.
- Handling of invertebrates by the extremities is not recommended given the frailty of the limbs, but scorpions may be picked up with padded forceps by the base of the tail.
- Tarantulas will stop moving their legs as they are suspended slightly above the table for this method, which is useful for drawing hemolymph, administering fluid and medications, and examining the ventrum.

ALTERNATIVES AND THEIR RELATIVE MERITS

- Hypothermia is another option for immobilization of terrestrial invertebrates.
- A patient may be placed in a refrigerator for approximately 30 minutes to take advantage of the invertebrate's inability to regulate its body temperature.
  - The patient may then be allowed to warm slowly without ill effects.
  - This method should not be used for surgical procedures or for techniques that cause pain.

AUTHOR: **MODIFIED FROM BRAUN ME, HEATLEY JJ, CHITTY J: CLINICAL TECHNIQUES OF INVERTEBRATES, VET CLIN NORTH AM EXOT ANIM PRACT 9:205–221, 2006.**

EDITOR: **JÖRG MAYER**

FISH

Diagnostic Sampling

SYNONYMS

Wet mount exam, fine-needle aspirate, squash prep, smear, swab, gill snip, skin scrape, fin clip

OVERVIEW AND GOAL

Gain diagnostic information to aid in the management of disease in aquatic animals

INDICATIONS

- Routine part of the minimum database for sick fish (skin scrape, gill snip, fecal wet mount)
- Prepurchase and postpurchase evaluations of new fish
- Annual screening for a fish population

CONTRAINDICATIONS

- Very few contraindications for diagnostic cytologic examination with the following exceptions:
  - Fractious fish that cannot be sedated
  - As in other exotic species, any procedure can be fatal in moribund or debilitated fish patients.
  - Bleeding may hasten death in anemic fish.

EQUIPMENT, ANESTHESIA

Glass slides, glass or plastic cover slips, microscope, small scissors, stains (Gram stain, Diff-Quik, etc.), latex or nonlatex gloves, and water from patient's tank/pond

ANTICIPATED TIME

1 to 5 minutes

PREPARATION: IMPORANT CHECKPOINTS

Prepare sedation container, recovery container, slides with drop of patient's water, cover slips, and gloves (no powder or rinsed).

POSSIBLE COMPLICATIONS AND COMMON ERRORS TO BE AVOIDED

- Skin scrape
  - The possibility of damage to the epithelium exists if excess pressure is used or a large area is scraped, removing the protective mucous coating. Scales may also be lost if excess pressure is used to scrape the body.
  - Samples must be examined promptly on site. Delay in evaluation may result in parasite desiccation or death, rendering identification impossible.
- Fin clip
  - It is important to ask the owner whether the fish is a show fish. Show fish owners will not be happy with a fin defect left by the diagnostic procedure. This is similar to the show dog owner who is very particular about any clipping of the dog's coat.
- Gill snip/scrape
  - Forewarn the owner that there may be some blood secondary to the procedure. The author has seen this event occur most often in gravid female koi.
- Fecal wet mount
  - It is important to use fresh feces. Feces acquired from the bottom of the tank or travel container may be colonized by nonpathogenic organisms.
- Coelomic cavity fluid aspirate
  - It is important the fish be relatively immobile. Sedation may be required. Caution should be taken when attempting to aspirate fluid with very small patients.

PROCEDURE

- Skin scrape
  - A glass or plastic cover slip is scraped at a 45° angle in a cranial-to-caudal direction in small areas of the body.
  - Higher yields of parasites have been reported when areas of low "drag" are scraped, such as immediately distal to the pectoral fins, the "chin," and the caudal peduncle.
  - Place the cover slip with mucus sample on a slide prepared with a drop of the patient's own water.
  - Starting with the lowest power objective, examine under the microscope for parasites, fungal elements, and/or bacteria.
  - Most parasites can be identified by their characteristic movement and size.

- Fin clip
  - Clip a small piece of the end of a fin with small scissors.
  - Place tissue on prepared slide.
  - Examine under microscope for ectoparasites, bacteria, and fungal elements.
- Gill snip
  - The operculum is gently lifted to reveal the gills.
  - With fine scissors such as iris tenotomy or suture removal scissors, snip a tiny section from the end of a few primary lamellae.
  - Place the gill tissue on a slide prepared with a drop of water from the patient's environment.
  - Examine the tissue for various pathogens and secondary lamellar pathology (hyperplasia, hypertrophy, necrosis, lamellar fusion, etc.)
- Fecal wet mount
  - Obtain fresh feces from the patient. Advise owner to place fish in a clean container for travel. Many fish will have defecated en route. With a plastic pipette, the fecal sample can be obtained from the container. Fish may also defecate when sedated. If no fecal material is available, gentle pressure near the vent may yield a sufficient amount for examination.
  - Place on a slide prepared with a drop of water from the patient's tank or pond.
  - Examine for ova or parasites.
- Tissue/Fluid aspirate
  - Similar procedure as with other species for fluid aspirate and tissue aspirate
  - Obtain sample, prepare slide.
  - Stain dried slide with stain of choice, and evaluate.
  - Sample can be used for bacterial, fungal, parasitic, and viral analyses.

POST-PROCEDURE

Monitor fish in recovery container if sedation or anesthesia has been used.

ALTERNATIVES AND THEIR RELATIVE MERITS

Necropsy: More diagnostic information may be obtained when a necropsy is performed and samples are submitted for cytologic and histopathologic examination, but the procedure requires sacrifice of the patient.

AUTHOR: **HELEN E. ROBERTS**

EDITOR: **JÖRG MAYER**

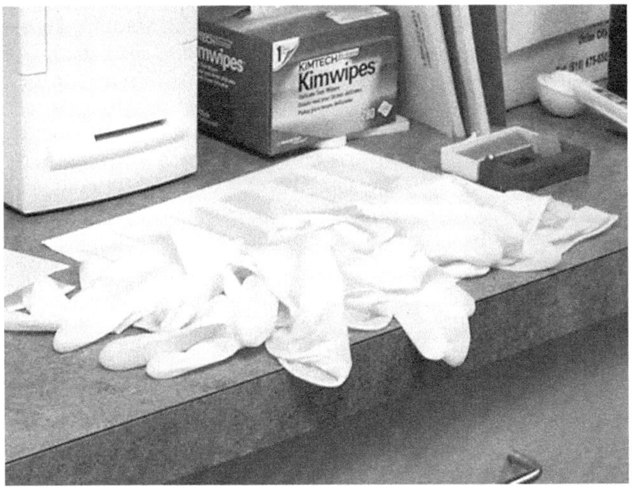

Diagnostic Sampling Materials (slides, cover slips, and gloves) prepared in advance for wet mount cytology on a fish patient. *(Courtesy Helen Roberts.)*

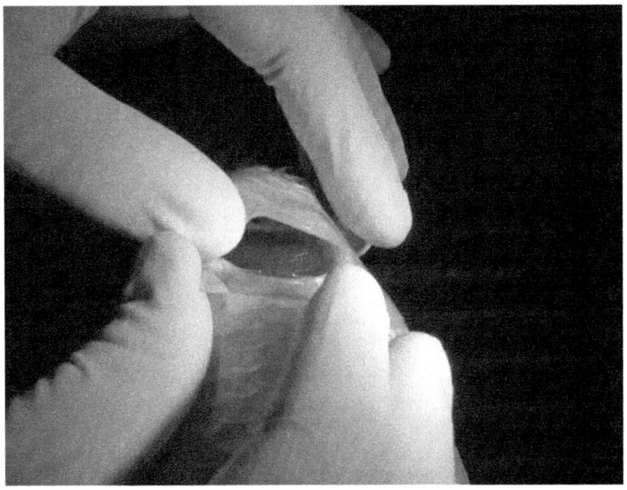

Diagnostic Sampling Use of a cover slip to obtain a gill tissue sample for wet mount cytologic examination. *(Courtesy Helen Roberts.)*

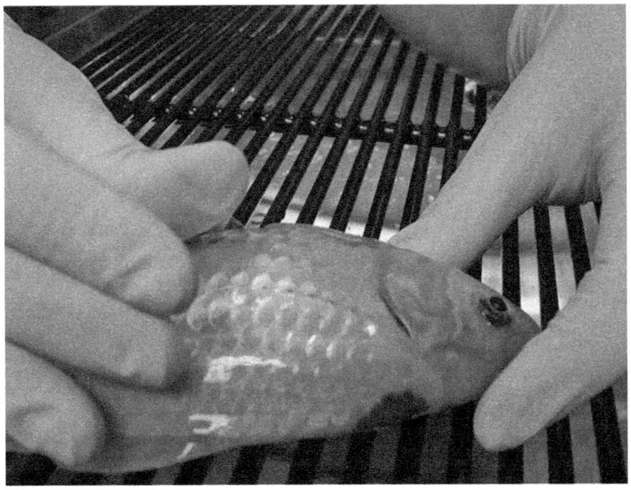

Diagnostic Sampling Use of a cover slip at a 45° angle to obtain a mucus sample from an anesthetized fish for diagnostic wet mount cytology. *(Courtesy Helen Roberts.)*

FISH

Emergency Care

SYNONYM

Resuscitation

OVERVIEW AND GOAL

Many different situations might require the clinician to perform emergency room (ER) treatments on fish.

INDICATIONS

- Trauma
- Cold stunning
- Shock
- Out of pond/tank experience

EQUIPMENT, ANESTHESIA

- Syringe
- Needle
- Table salt or marine salt

ANTICIPATED TIME

30 minutes

PROCEDURE

- Respiration can be assessed as discussed previously, and heart rate can be determined using Doppler or brightness-mode ultrasound and electrocardiography.
- Although the heart may continue to beat after cessation of opercular movement, resuscitation is rarely successful unless the arrest is attributable to an acute stressor or an overdose of anesthetic.
- Airway (A): oxygenated water needs to flow over the gills in a cranial-to-caudal direction to allow respiration (mouth to operculum in teleosts)
  - To clear this pathway, any obstruction in the oral cavity or gill cavity should be removed, including sediment.
- Breathing (B): oxygenation can be improved by promoting water flow over the gills, by forcing water into the oral cavity (by hand, by syringe, or with use of a pump to recirculate the water), or by manually swimming the animal forward through the water column
- Concurrently, oxygen partial pressure in the water should be increased using air stones connected to air pumps or cylinders with compressed room air (1-2 L/h for each liter of water).
- Compressed oxygen can be used, but the increase in partial pressure of oxygen may lead to toxicity, which can present with depressed respiration and neurologic signs. Alternatively, the fish can be placed in a closed container with an oxygen-enriched atmosphere (e.g., bagged with one-third water and two-thirds oxygen).
- Circulation (C): if opercular movement has ceased and the heart is not beating
  - Cardiac compressions are unlikely to be successful because of anatomic features of the area and severe hypoxia.

POST-PROCEDURE

- In freshwater fish, it is often useful to increase salinity to 2 to 3 parts per thousand (ppt; g/L) to decrease osmotic stress.
  - One level tablespoon of sodium chloride per US gallon increases salinity by approximately 3 ppt.
  - Kosher table salt should be used owing to its purity.
  - Some plant and fish species are anecdotally considered sensitive to salinity treatments, but recent evidence suggests that others (e.g., *Corydoras* catfish) may be able to tolerate 0.5 to 2 ppt.
- In marine fish, it is probably most useful to administer fluids to restore volume and acid-base balance.
- Fluids may be given orally into the upper gastrointestinal tract, intracoelomically, or intravenously.
- For oral administration, dechlorinated fresh water can be used. This is the least invasive route and is usually well tolerated in conscious fish; parenteral routes may require chemical restraint.
- For parenteral administration in marine fish, crystalloids such as lactated Ringer's solution (LRS) or 2.5% dextrose and 0.45% saline, potentially together with colloids, can be used.
- For marine elasmobranchs, fluids that more closely match their high plasma osmolality (900 to 1100 mOsm/kg) and high plasma urea, sodium, and chloride are recommended.
  - "Elasmobranch-Ringer's" solution can be made using sodium chloride (10 g/L), $NaHCO_3$ (0.1 g/L), and urea (26 g/L) in LRS to reach an osmolality of 960 mOsm/kg.
  - The solution should be sterilized by passing through a 22-μm filter before intravascular or intracoelomic use.
- In acidotic elasmobranchs, with point-of-care evaluation of acid-base status (e.g., i-STAT chemical analyzers; Abbott Laboratories, East Windsor, NJ) and no improvement after aggressive fluid therapy, sodium bicarbonate or sodium acetate may be used, but these solutions carry a risk of iatrogenic alkalosis.
- Fluid therapy is the recommended treatment for acidosis.
- With acute hemorrhage, blood transfusion from a conspecific may be used.

AUTHOR: **MODIFIED FROM HADFIELD CA, ET AL: EMERGENCY AND CRITICAL CARE OF FISH. VET CLIN NORTH AM EXOT ANIM PRACT 10:647–675, 2007.**

EDITOR: **JÖRG MAYER**

FISH

Injections, Intracoelomic (Ice) and Intramuscular (IM)

Additional Images Available on Website

SYNONYM

Intraperitoneal (IP)

OVERVIEW AND GOAL

Technique for parenteral administration of medications

INDICATIONS

Provide therapy via injections.

CONTRAINDICATIONS

Moribund fish

EQUIPMENT, ANESTHESIA

Injectable drugs, syringes, needles of sufficient size and length

ANTICIPATED TIME

1 to 5 minutes

PREPARATION: IMPORTANT CHECKPOINTS

- Have the drugs drawn and ready for injection.
- Have a separate recovery chamber for fish that may be excessively stressed with capture and therapy.

POSSIBLE COMPLICATIONS AND COMMON ERRORS TO BE AVOIDED

- Overdosing or underdosing due to inadequate estimation of body weight
- Advise the owner that bruising or discoloration may occur at injection sites.
- IP should be restricted to drugs that are nonirritating and capable of crossing endothelial barriers.
- With IM injections, the drug may leak back out the needle track.
- Scale loss

PROCEDURE

- Intraperitoneal injection
  - The technique involves inserting the needle under the scales of the caudal ventral abdomen, then directing it craniodorsally.
  - The bowel will be pushed away from the needle, and the caudal area will prevent penetration of the liver, spleen, and kidney.
- Intramuscular injection
  - Inject into the dorsal muscle mass, halfway between the lateral line and the dorsal fin.
  - Direct the needle cranially under the scales.
  - The volume is 1 to 2 μL/g of body weight (BW).
  - Another IM location might be chosen in show fish owing to possible bruising, such as that affecting the muscles at the base of the pectoral fin.

POST-PROCEDURE

Watch for adverse reactions to the drugs.

ALTERNATIVES AND THEIR RELATIVE MERITS

- It may be possible to use intravenous administration on very large, anesthetized specimens.
- Intracoelomic catheterization has been described for use in koi needing multiple injections over time. (Lewbart GA, Butkus DA, Papich MG, et al: Evaluation of a method of intracoelomic catheterization in koi. J Am Vet Med Assoc 226:784–788, 2005.)

AUTHORS: **DRURY R. REAVILL AND HELEN E. ROBERTS**

EDITOR: **JÖRG MAYER**

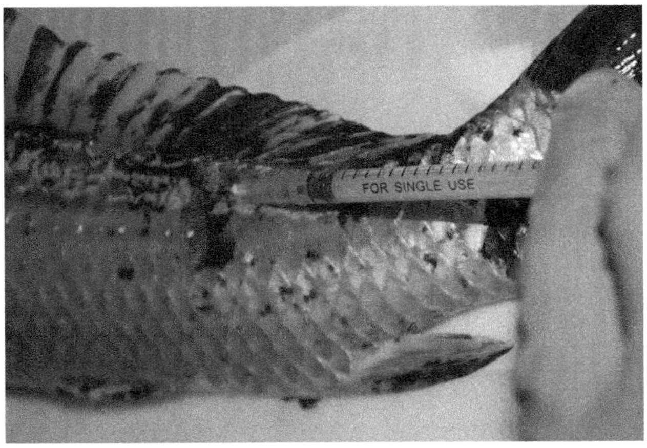

Injections, Intracoelomic (Ice) and Intramuscular (IM) Intramuscular injection in the dorsal epaxial musculature of a koi, *Cyprinus carpio*. *(Courtesy Helen Roberts.)*

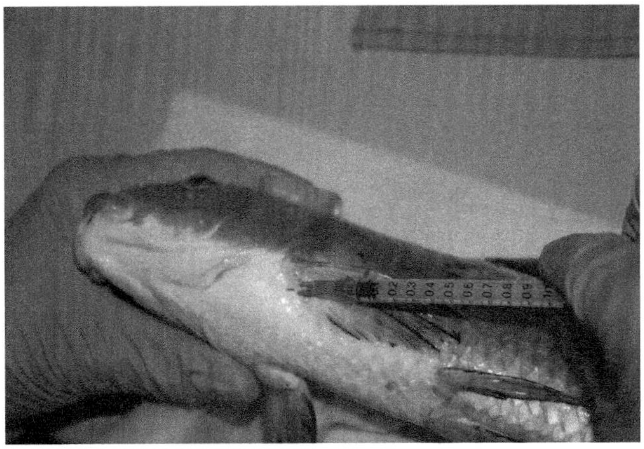

Injections, Intracoelomic (Ice) and Intramuscular (IM) An alternate IM injection site, the muscles at the base of the pectoral fin. *(Courtesy Helen Roberts.)*

FISH

MS 222 Anesthesia

SYNONYMS

- Tricaine methanesulfonate
- TMS
- Finquel (Argent Chemical Laboratories, Redmond, WA)
- Tricaine-S (Western Chemical Inc., Ferndale, WA)

OVERVIEW AND GOALS

- Reduce or eliminate reaction to external stimuli, usually painful stimuli; provide a calmer fish for transport, diagnostic procedures, and physical examination; and reduce clinician injury from aggressive species.
- Sedation of fish for transport reduces oxygen demand, reduces excretion of metabolic wastes, and decreases activity.

INDICATIONS

Physical examination, diagnostic procedures, manual spawning, shipping, minor and major surgical procedures, therapeutic administration (depending on size, temperament of species, and treatment required), and humane euthanasia (with intentional overdose)

CONTRAINDICATIONS

- Moribund fish, species known to be "sensitive" to agent used
- Anesthesia of fish with labyrinth organs (bettas, some gouramis, etc.) should be approached with caution. Owing to the unique anatomy of the labyrinth organ (enables fish to breathe atmospheric oxygen) and the gills of these fish (thick lamellae and decreased lamellar surface area), it is possible to "drown" the fish if an overdose of an anesthetic agent is given.

EQUIPMENT, ANESTHESIA

- Anesthesia/sedation chamber that can hold sufficient volume of water
- Lids/tops for induction and recovery tanks
- Anesthetic powder or stock solution prepared in advance
- Gram scale to weigh anesthetic powder
- Scale to weigh patient
- Fluid volume measuring containers
- Recovery container with fresh water
- Air stone
- Sodium bicarbonate for buffering anesthetic solution

ANTICIPATED TIME

- Time varies with temperature of water, strength of solution, water hardness, salinity, oxygen concentration, and biomass and species of patient.
- Anesthetic effect is slower in very soft water and in colder water temperatures.
- Most species can be safely sedated or anesthetized in 5 to 10 minutes.
- Smaller fish are more sensitive than larger fish within the same species.
- Stress associated with the act of anesthetizing fish can be reduced if the anesthesia takes effect quickly.

PREPARATION: IMPORANT CHECKPOINTS

- Accurate weight (usually in grams) of MS 222 powder (1 part) and sodium bicarbonate (2 parts) for buffering acidic effects in freshwater. Saltwater may not need the addition of sodium bicarbonate because it contains natural buffering agents.
- Use of water from patient's own environment (tank or pond) is strongly recommended.
- Clients should always be advised to bring extra water for sedation/anesthesia and recovery of patient. Plastic gallon jugs are ideal for transport and can be used to provide fresh water for the return trip home.
- With a large group of fish, a small sample can be used as a biotest if the species' reaction is not well known.

POSSIBLE COMPLICATIONS AND COMMON ERRORS TO BE AVOIDED

- Decimal point errors may inadvertently result in iatrogenic overdose.
- Failure to dechlorinate water if treated water (tap, well, etc.) is used
- Failure to monitor fish in the anesthetic solution and during recovery
- The container should be covered to prevent fish jumping out.
- Sick fish tend to be more sensitive to the anesthetic solution. The author starts with a 50% reduction in the recommended concentration of MS 222 and monitors closely for adverse reactions.

PROCEDURE

- Add anesthetic solution to water at desired concentration (see package insert).
- Add fish, cover container.
- Monitor opercular movements and fish behavior until desired plane and stage of anesthesia are reached.
- Most koi are adequately sedated at 50 to 100 ppm (mg/L) in 3 to 5 minutes. Appropriate stage of anesthesia for surgical procedures takes longer.
- Initially, fish may increase opercular movements and become more active.
- This is followed by slower movement of fish, sometimes sinking to the bottom of the container, and loss of equilibrium.
- Some fish do not become laterally recumbent, demonstrating loss of equilibrium, until gently tipped over, so failure to become recumbent is not to be relied on for assessment of depth of anesthesia/sedation.
- For large fish such as sharks, a solution of higher concentration (up to 1 g/L) can be sprayed onto the gills.
- Sterile ophthalmic lubricant should be placed on the eyes, and the eyes should be covered to reduce stimulation.

POST-PROCEDURE

- Place in recovery container with fresh, aerated water.
- Monitor for return to normal (may take up to 30 minutes depending on length of anesthesia/sedation, presence of additional medications, and procedure[s] performed).

ALTERNATIVES AND THEIR RELATIVE MERITS

- Clove oil/eugenol
  - No prescription required; available over the counter at many health food stores and pharmacies
  - Not FDA approved for use in fin fish
  - Slower induction and recovery time than MS 222
  - Concentrations of active ingredients vary in health food store samples.
  - Prohibited for use in food fish
- Aqui-S (isoeugenol)
  - Used in Europe, Australia, and several other countries
  - Not currently approved in United States, but an INAD (investigational new animal drug) has been established for investigational use of isoeugenol as a fish anesthetic
  - A zero day withdrawal in food fish is the main advantage of this drug.
  - Less expensive than tricaine methanesulfonate
- Benzocaine
  - Insoluble in water and must be dissolved in ethanol, methanol, or acetone for use
  - Stock solution can be prepared in advance; store in sealed, dark bottle
  - Not FDA approved for use in fish
  - Long withdrawal time based on high fat solubility and retention in body tissues
  - Less hyperactivity and initial stress than with MS 222
- Metomidate
  - Not FDA approved for use as a fish anesthetic
  - Rapid induction and recovery compared with MS 222, although very long recovery periods have been reported
  - Some color changes (possibly stress induced) have been observed with its use.
  - Varied results with different species; mortalities have been reported in some ornamental species
  - Hyperactivity reported during recovery
  - Anesthetic concentration varies widely with different species.

AUTHOR: **HELEN E. ROBERTS**

EDITOR: **JÖRG MAYER**

FISH

Oral Medication

SYNONYMS

Per os, gastric tubing, medicated food, gavage

OVERVIEW AND GOAL

To administer medications or supportive therapy orally

INDICATIONS

- To provide nutritional and/or fluid support to debilitated fish
- To administer oral medications, utilizing the digestive tract as the portal of entry
- Medicated feed can be used to treat large numbers of fish.

CONTRAINDICATIONS

- Debilitated, frail fish where anesthesia is contraindicated

- Anorectic fish may not eat without being force-fed

EQUIPMENT, ANESTHESIA

- Tube feeding involves a syringe and a metal feeding needle or a soft rubber feeding tube.
- Most fish will require sedation/anesthesia to be tube-fed.

ANTICIPATED TIME

- Days to weeks for forced feedings
- Several minutes per event
- Preparing homemade diet can take up to 1 hour.

PREPARATION: IMPORTANT CHECKPOINTS

- For medications mixed with food items
- Withhold all diets other than the medicated feed.

POSSIBLE COMPLICATIONS AND COMMON ERRORS TO BE AVOIDED

- Medicated foods
  - The fish may refuse to eat the medicated food (unpalatable) or may not eat their entire portion.
  - Not all fish will successfully compete for their portion if this is a multiple-fish treatment.
  - If normal feeding intervals are longer than 24 hours, you may get satiated fish, which will end any effective treatment.
  - Some premedicated feeds may not be stable in water and may disintegrate within a few minutes.
  - One significant problem is that the medication will leach out of the feed material.
- Tube feeding/force feeding
  - Some fish will readily regurgitate gastric contents.
  - The procedure will be stressful for conscious fish; however, sedated fish may regurgitate the material across the gills.
  - Not all fish have a stomach to hold even a small quantity of material, and risk of gastrointestinal tract perforation is present if the tube or needle is placed too vigorously.
  - Fish may have teeth that will complicate passage of the gavage tube.

PROCEDURE

- Medicated foods
  - Commercial medicated diets: products that are commercially prepared with a number of different antimicrobials and are not FDA approved. Aquaflor (Schering-Plough Animal Health Corporation, Summit, NJ), is an FDA-approved aquaculture-medicated feed containing florfenicol and a veterinary feed directive (VFD) drug. Extra-label use in species other than specific approved indications for use in catfish and freshwater-reared salmonids is prohibited.
  - Commercial mixes: a gelatinized diet used to customize drug formulation (e.g., www.mazuri.com, aquatic gel food diet; omnivore, carnivore, and herbivore varieties available). To make the gelatin version, add hot water and let cool. The food can be cut into small pieces and fed. When cool water is used, the mixture will remain a liquid that can be force-fed.
    - Gelatinized diet recipe: a number of recipes have been published:
      - Weigh 35 g of a well-balanced flake food; place in blender.
      - Add 30 g of finely ground vegetables such as fresh or frozen peas.
      - Add 5 mL of food-grade cod liver oil.
      - Add 30 g of cooked oatmeal or wheat germ.
      - Boil water, and then add enough warm water to the above mixture to make slurry.
      - Add vitamin supplements at this time (after cooling because heat will inactivate the vitamins), such as 500 mg of B-complex vitamins or 2-3 g of Brewer's yeast, 250 mg vitamin C, and 50 units of vitamin E; mix well.
      - Add medicants at this time at 0.25% of the mixture; dissolve in warm water before adding to the mixture.
      - Dissolve 5-10 g of powdered unflavored gelatin in approximately 100 mL of boiling water; stir well until the gelatin is dissolved; allow to cool (but not set) for a few minutes, and then add to the mixture.
      - Place mixture in separate bags, and place in the refrigerator. Food should be ready within an hour, or it may be frozen until needed. Food can be broken into bite-size pieces by using a cheese grater or potato peeler. Breaking up the food is important, especially when the food is frozen.
- Tube feeding/force feeding
  - Soak species-appropriate food pellets in warm water; grind live food with water or electrolyte solution; use canned foods such as a/d (Hill's Pet Nutrition Inc., Topeka, KS), Mazuri gel food (PMI Nutrition International LLC, St Louis, MO) mixed with cool water, or Oxbow Critical and Carnivore Care Diets (Oxbow Animal Health, Murdock, NE); or liquefy homemade medicated food. Food must be able to pass through oral syringe or feeding tube.
  - Restrain with sedation (tricaine methanesulfonate) or gentle physical restraint. A wet chamois is helpful to prevent injuries to the skin.
  - Feed approximately 10-30 mL/kg of liquid food.
  - Pass the oral feeding syringe into the upper gastrointestinal tract.
  - Watch for any food particles contaminating/entering the gills.
  - Esophagostomy/gastrostomy tube placement can be used for long-term nutritional support.

POST-PROCEDURE

With medicated diets, watch to see that all food is eaten and all fish requiring treatment had access to the food.

ALTERNATIVES AND THEIR RELATIVE MERITS

- Injectable therapy
  - Stressful for the fish
  - Expensive
  - Involves more handling of the fish
- Tank/pond therapy
  - Inaccurate dosing
  - Not very effective for systemic infection
  - May harm biological filtration
- Top dressing feed
  - Less accurate dosing
  - Can foul the water

AUTHORS: **DRURY R. REAVILL AND HELEN E. ROBERTS**

EDITOR: **JÖRG MAYER**

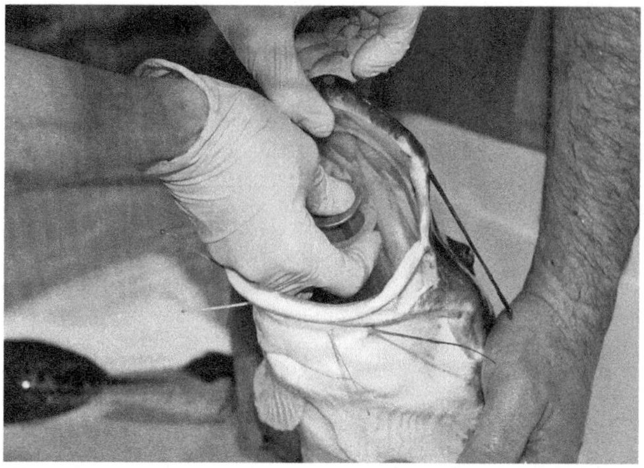

Oral Medication Oral medication administered as a paste via 60 mL oral syringe to a sedated tiger shovelnose catfish, *Pseudoplatystoma fasciatum*. *(Courtesy Helen Roberts.)*

FISH

Surgical Principles

INDICATIONS

Mass removal, exploratory traumatic injury repair, and many other procedures

CONTRAINDICATIONS

Debilitated, anemic, septic, and profoundly lethargic patients are not good surgical candidates.

EQUIPMENT, ANESTHESIA

- Induction container
- Anesthesia delivery system
- Recovery container
- Patient's own water when possible
- Anesthetic (can have stock solution prepared in advance)
- Buffering agent (sodium bicarbonate)
- Gram scale to measure anesthetic
- Surgical instruments appropriate for patient size (ophthalmic instruments may be used on small patients)
- Clear, plastic drape
- Suture material
- Surgical monitoring equipment
- If surgery is to be done pondside or at the client's home, it is best to have lightweight, unbreakable containers such as plastic rather than a glass tank. See Anesthesia for additional details.

ANTICIPATED TIME

Time required varies with procedure.

PREPARATION: IMPORTANT CHECKPOINTS

- Preoperative assessment diagnostics, including blood work, cytologic examination, radiography, and ultrasonographic examinations
- Familiarity with internal anatomy of patient
- Induction chamber containing anesthetic solution (buffered if needed)
- Perioperative surgical container with anesthetic delivery
- Surgical positioning table/shelf (a wedge cut into a piece of 2- to 4-inch upholstery foam works well)
- Instruments, monofilament suture, drape, sterile ophthalmic lubricant
- Preoperative medications if indicated (optional)
  - Analgesics and antiinflammatory agents
    - Rimadyl Injectable (carprofen 50 mg/mL, Pfizer) 2 mg/kg IM
      - Carprofen is not FDA approved for use in fish and should never be used in food fish.
      - Unknown adverse events may occur.
      - The author has used carprofen successfully in a number of species, including koi, goldfish, red-tailed catfish, and orfe.
    - Butorphanol 0.4 mg/kg IM
  - Prophylactic antibiotics
    - Enrofloxacin 10 mg/kg IM
    - Ceftazidime 20 mg/kg IM
- Recovery container with fresh water
- In clinic hospitalization tank if required
- Indoor facility for monitoring recovery if owner has available (winter)

POSSIBLE COMPLICATIONS AND COMMON ERRORS TO BE AVOIDED

- Failure to assess patient risk with anesthesia and surgery
- Failure to have all supplies on hand before administration of patient anesthesia
- Equipment failure
- Use of tissue glue (dermal reactions) for closure
- Failure to monitor patient's anesthetic response during procedure

PROCEDURE

- Wound and ulcer débridement
  - Clean wound gently to remove any necrotic tissue and debris.
  - Irrigate with sterile saline.
  - Apply topical ointment of choice.
  - Can be done pondside or tankside
- Mass removal
  - Dermal masses can extend deep into the muscular layer and may not be amenable to total excision.
  - Surgical wound is left open to heal by second intention because closure is not usually possible.
  - Topical ointment of choice can be applied.
  - May also be done pondside or tankside
- Ophthalmic surgery
  - Enucleation can be used to remove severely traumatized, exophthalmic eyes and neoplasia.
  - The wound is left open to heal by second intention.
  - The excised eye should be submitted for histopathologic examination.
- Exploratory celiotomy
  - Indications: coelomic mass (e.g., gonadal tumor), foreign body obstruction, pneumocystectomy or pneumocystoplasty (partial or complete removal of the swim bladder), etc.
  - Ventral midline is the most common approach with the patient placed in dorsal recumbency. A positioning

device should be used to keep the fish in place.
- To facilitate entry into the coelomic cavity, in large fish, scales along the ventral midline can be gently removed.
- Clean the area gently with sterile saline or dilute povidone-iodine or chlorhexidine. The area should not be scrubbed vigorously because this will damage the epithelium and disrupt the protective mucous layer more than necessary.
- Place sterile, clear plastic drape over the area to be incised. The drape allows the surgeon to monitor the patient and provides some protection against loss of moisture.
- Make the incision, starting caudal to pectoral fins.
- A forceful incision may damage the underlying intestinal tract, so care should be taken to avoid lacerating any organ lying directly beneath the midline.
- The incision can be extended over the pelvic fins, but this requires cutting of the fused pelvic girdle.
- Retractors should be used to increase visibility inside the coelomic cavity.
- Monofilament, absorbable or nonabsorbable suture material such as PDS (Ethicon, Somerville, NJ) and Maxon (Tyco Healthcare, North Haven, CT) and nylon are recommended. Braided suture may provide entry for bacteria. Other sutures may cause excessive reaction in tissues.
- Fish do not readily absorb sutures, so any external sutures need to be removed in 2 to 4 weeks, depending on healing and the presence of secondary infection.
- Closure of the coelomic cavity is generally done with one or two suture layers, depending on the size of the fish.
- Application of a topical ointment is optional.

POST-PROCEDURE

- Patient should be monitored in recovery tank until swimming movements have resumed and fish is ventilating well.
- Addition of salt 1-3 g/L in recovery/hospitalization tank to reduce osmotic stress and as a potential aid in healing surgical incisions
- Antibiotics can be continued postoperatively if indicated.
- Water should be heated to a temperature ideal for wound healing (20°C to 23°C [68°F to 73.4°F]).
- Monitor water quality in hospitalization tank daily.
- Daily water changes may be needed to maintain optimum conditions.
- Tanks should be stripped and disinfected after each use.
- Equipment used should be cleaned, disinfected, and dried after each use.

ALTERNATIVES AND THEIR RELATIVE MERITS

Laparoscopic surgery, currently not widely used (but its use is growing), serves as an alternative to traditional open coelomic surgery. Courses with wet labs and discussion of indications and techniques are available at some veterinary schools.

AUTHOR: **HELEN E. ROBERTS**

EDITOR: **JÖRG MAYER**

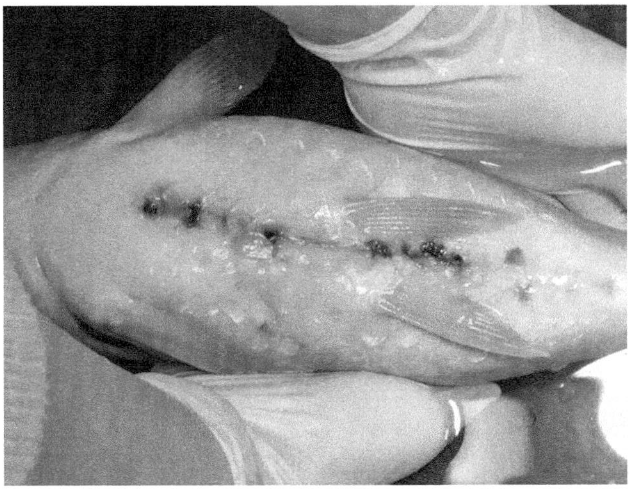

Surgical Principles Exploratory incision on a koi *(Cyprinus carpio)* 4 weeks after surgery. *(Courtesy Helen Roberts.)*

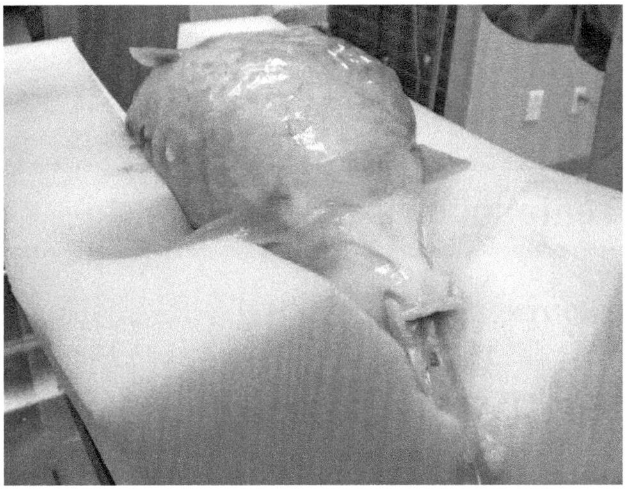

Surgical Principles In preparation for surgery, a koi is held in dorsal recumbency with the use of a piece of upholstery foam. *(Courtesy Helen Roberts.)*

FISH

Tank Pond Therapy

SYNONYMS

Tank treatment, prolonged immersion treatment, dips, baths

OVERVIEW AND GOAL

To administer medications into the water for treatment of various conditions

INDICATIONS

Tank or pond treatment of external parasites or superficial bacteria and/or fungal infections

CONTRAINDICATIONS

- Not for use in conditions requiring systemic therapy

- Cannot be applied if there are sensitive species in the collection that cannot be removed, usually plants or invertebrates
- Systems with low dissolved oxygen or high levels of organic debris

EQUIPMENT, ANESTHESIA

- Calculator
- Measuring devices (dry and liquid volumes)

ANTICIPATED TIME

Days to weeks

PREPARATION: IMPORTANT CHECKPOINTS

- An accurate calculation of the volume of water in the tank or pond in consistent units (metric vs. U.S. Customary System [U.S.C.S.])
- Remember that the "furniture" and the gravel will reduce the water volume.
- Commonly used equations:
  - [Length × Width × Depth (in inches)] ÷ 231 = Gallons water (U.S.C.S.)
  - L × W × D (in cm) ÷ 1000 = Volume in liters for aquaria
  - L × W × Average depth (in feet) × 7.5 = Gallons (U.S.)
  - Average depth (in meters) × W (m) × L (m) × 1000 = Liters

POSSIBLE COMPLICATIONS AND COMMON ERRORS TO BE AVOIDED

- Some drugs will damage the biological filter, resulting in a need to recondition/"restart" the biofilter in the tank/pond and closely monitor water quality.
- Toxic levels of chemical/drugs can be reached in the tank/pond.
- Rapid removal of drug via the filter system or activated charcoal/carbon filter inserts
- Some drugs may bind to the substrates or organic debris and may be rendered inactive.
- Staining of substrate by medications (e.g., Malachite green, methylene blue)
  - Adverse effects on nontarget species, native insects, and amphibians
- Drug having an adverse reaction with the water such as severe pH changes or deoxygenation of the water
- Potential for effluent discharge into native waters from ponds or improper disposal of treated water from aquaria
- Adverse or toxic effects for user or applicator due to improper application

PROCEDURE

- Dips and baths
  - These require immersion of the fish into medicated water for varying lengths of time (dips less than 15 minutes and baths longer than 15 minutes).
  - Watch the fish carefully for signs of distress.
  - After the treatment, place the fish in a clean holding tank for a thorough rinse before replacing in the display tank.
- Indefinite/tank treatment (prolonged immersion)
  - This involves medicating the whole display tank or pond and all inhabitants therein.

POST-PROCEDURE

Watch for adverse reactions to the drugs.

ALTERNATIVES AND THEIR RELATIVE MERITS

- Individual therapy—labor-intensive, more costly
- Involves more handling of the fish

AUTHORS: **DRURY R. REAVILL AND HELEN E. ROBERTS**

EDITOR: **JÖRG MAYER**

FISH

Venipuncture

SYNONYM

Blood collection

OVERVIEW AND GOAL

Acquire a sample of blood that can be used for diagnostic testing

INDICATIONS

Complete blood count, serum chemistry, serologic testing

CONTRAINDICATIONS

Anemia, moribund fish

EQUIPMENT, ANESTHESIA

Syringe 1-3 mL, 22- to 25-gauge needle, ½″ to 1½″ in length

ANTICIPATED TIME

10 seconds

PREPARATION: IMPORTANT CHECKPOINTS

- Patient anesthesia
- Appropriate blood tubes, labeled
- Latex or nonlatex gloves, powder-free
- Syringe can be pretreated with heparin to prevent clotting if serum is not required.

POSSIBLE COMPLICATIONS AND COMMON ERRORS TO BE AVOIDED

- Spinal injury
- Hemolysis of sample if vigorous aspiration is done with syringe
- Bruising at site

PROCEDURE

- Blood samples are best obtained from the caudal vein.
- The technique involves advancing the needle at a cranial-dorsal angle from the ventral surface of the tail, toward the spinal column. The needle is introduced at the ventral midline of the caudal peduncle and caudal to the anal fin. It is possible to collect blood via a lateral approach. The needle is inserted slightly below and perpendicular to the lateral line and cranial to the caudal peduncle. Once the needle tip hits bone, withdraw the needle back slowly with slight pressure on the plunger.
- A 1-mL syringe and a 25-gauge needle can be used on fish as small as 30 g.
- Pretreating the needle with heparin can help prevent coagulation (should not be used in cases where serum is required).
- For larger fish, such as koi, a 3-mL syringe and a 1½″ 22-gauge needle should be used.
- Anesthesia or sedation can facilitate this process.
- Very little information on normal hematology and serum chemistry parameters is available for most pet fish species.
- Example of use: serum can be submitted for KHV serology (antibody test) to confirm previous exposure to cyprinid herpesvirus 3 (CyHV-3)
- Warn owners that a bruise may be evident post venipuncture. The bruise can last several weeks and is more likely to occur on expensive show fish!

POST-PROCEDURE

Place digital pressure on the venipuncture site to minimize bruising.

ALTERNATIVES AND THEIR RELATIVE MERITS

- Cardiocentesis
  - High risk, especially in smaller species, may be impossible.
- Caudal peduncle removal
  - This method is used for fish that have been sacrificed and is seldom, if ever, used in a clinical setting. Blood collected in this fashion most likely would be contaminated with tissue fragments and debris.

AUTHOR: **HELEN E. ROBERTS**

EDITOR: **JÖRG MAYER**

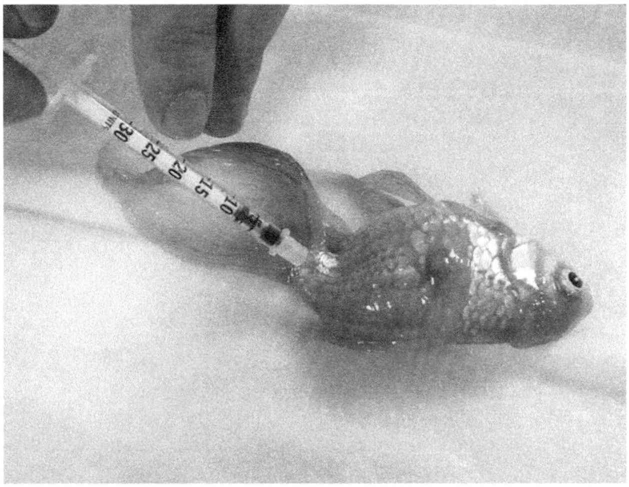

Venipuncture The lateral line in the fish should be used for blood collection; even in this small goldfish, successful collection of blood is possible. *(Photo courtesy Jörg Mayer, The University of Georgia, Athens.)*

AMPHIBIANS

General Emergency Support

Client Education Sheet Available on Website

SYNONYM

Critical care

OVERVIEW AND GOAL

Emergency supportive care as used in mammals can be initiated while a history is being obtained and the prognosis discussed with the owners.

INDICATIONS

Animals often present at the end stage of a chronic disease process, and treatment may not be successful.

CONTRAINDICATIONS

Animals that are obtunded, stuporous, or comatose have a grave prognosis, as do animals in cardiorespiratory arrest.

EQUIPMENT, ANESTHESIA

Basic emergency management of all cases may include appropriate thermal support, fluid support, oxygen administration, and a clean hospital tank.

PROCEDURE

- Antibiotic administration should be started in most cases pending diagnostic results because sepsis is a common finding in ill amphibians.
- Animals that are seizuring (tetany), have muscle fasciculations, or are paretic or paralyzed should be started on calcium administration pending diagnostics because of the prevalence of hypocalcemia resulting from dietary deficiency.
- If toxin exposure is suspected, appropriate antidotes (e.g., atropine for organophosphate toxicity) should be given when possible.
- Amphibians can be easily intubated and ventilation supported with room air or oxygen and an Ambu bag.
- The trachea is very short, and care is needed to maintain the tracheal location and to inflate both lungs.
- Vascular fluid support in anurans can be provided readily with IO fluids.
- In-dwelling IV catheters are difficult to place in most species, but bolus fluids are easily administered into the ventral tail vein of caudatans.
- Although clinicians may apply standard mammalian emergency supportive protocols in amphibian cases, it is important to keep the animal's skin moist at all times and to make sure ambient local temperature around the animal is appropriate.

POST-PROCEDURE

The clinician may have a significant impact on remaining animals in the owner's collection by reviewing husbandry to identify areas for improvement.

AUTHOR: **MODIFIED FROM CLAYTON LA, ET AL: AMPHIBIAN EMERGENCY MEDICINE, VET CLIN NORTH AM EXOT ANIM PRACT 10:587–620, 2007.**

EDITOR: **JÖRG MAYER**

AMPHIBIANS

Handling and Restraint

OVERVIEW AND GOALS

- One should never assume that because someone owns an animal, he or she knows how to handle it properly.
- Therefore, only trained hospital staff should be involved in proper restraint of the animal being examined.
- Experience and preparation facilitate the proper handling of most reptile and amphibian patients.

INDICATIONS

Part of the physical examination

CONTRAINDICATIONS

In severe cases of hyperparathyroidism, handling might cause fracture of bones.

EQUIPMENT, ANESTHESIA

- Gloves
- Water dish (dechlorinated water)
- Fine mesh net
- Magnification device
- Rubber spatula

ANTICIPATED TIME

- With most amphibians, handling should be kept to a minimum to avoid stress to the animal and potential injury.
- 2 to 5 minutes

PREPARATION: IMPORTANT CHECKPOINTS

- Amphibians produce various secretions (e.g., mucus) to protect themselves against opportunistic pathogens.
- Disruption of skin secretions by abrasions caused by mishandling or desiccation of the skin may allow other infectious agents to gain entry.

POSSIBLE COMPLICATIONS AND COMMON ERRORS TO BE AVOIDED

When handling amphibians, one should always use rubber or latex gloves and rinse the gloves to remove the powder or any other coating on the rubber.

PROCEDURE

- First evaluate the animal in the enclosure, noting appearance, position, posture, color or colors, and so forth.
- When this is not possible, the patient may be transferred to a clear plastic container (with or without water, depending on the species).
- Such containers allow for evaluation of many aspects of the animal (primarily external) without actual handling of the patient.
- Always use good lighting and magnifying devices to scan the entire amphibian, including transillumination techniques through the clear plastic.
- When it is difficult to catch the animal, fine mesh nets may be used.
- Large toads, giant salamanders, and hellbenders should have their heads properly yet gently restrained, because they may bite.
- Completely survey the exterior of the animal using magnification and transillumination as needed.
- Palpate the entire animal, assessing all aspects from one end to the other.
- To evaluate the oral cavity, stimulate the animal to open its mouth by gently pressing on the jaws at the soft tissue of the commissure.
  - When this technique is ineffective, a soft, clean rubber spatula may be used gently to open the mouth to examine the oral pharynx and glottis.
- At this point, samples may be collected from the posterior naris and nasal passage.
  - Using a mini-tip, culturette samples for cytologic examination and culture may be collected from the trachea by passing the small swab through the glottis.

POST-PROCEDURE

After the physical examination in the room has been completed, take the animal back to collect the necessary laboratory samples and to measure the body weight and compare it with previously recorded weights.

AUTHOR: **MODIFIED FROM DE LA NAVARRE BJS: COMMON PROCEDURES IN REPTILES AND AMPHIBIANS, VET CLIN NORTH AM EXOT ANIM PRACT 9:237–267, 2006.**

EDITOR: **JÖRG MAYER**

REPTILES

Abscess Removal

OVERVIEW AND GOALS

- Abscessation in reptiles has to be taken seriously because septicemia can occur.
- Look for problems in husbandry because the abscess might be a sign of decreased immune function due to chronic stress.

INDICATIONS

After diagnostic procedure has been performed to diagnose the lesion as an abscess

EQUIPMENT, ANESTHESIA

- Laceration pack
- Depending on lesion, prepare for local or general anesthesia.

ANTICIPATED TIME

5 to 30 minutes

PREPARATION: IMPORTANT CHECKPOINTS

- Most abscesses will not drain owing to the fact that pus is not liquid.
- When possible, surgical removal of the entire abscess in toto is recommended.
  - General or local anesthesia is necessary.
- If the abscess cannot be removed (such as from the mandible), aggressive surgical débridement of the abscess is needed.
  - Marsupializing the abscess wall to the skin will allow important topical/local treatment.

POSSIBLE COMPLICATIONS AND COMMON ERRORS TO BE AVOIDED

- In cases requiring long-term (more than 4 to 6 weeks) systemic antibiotics (such as abscesses with associated osteomyelitis), caution should be used with aminoglycoside antibiotics because of possible nephrotoxicity.
- Recurrence is possible in cases in which the abscess cannot be removed "in toto." Premature closure of the surgical site allows re-formation of the abscess. This is especially true for deeper abscesses or abscesses with concurrent bone involvement, internal abscesses or abscesses involving active glandular tissue such as scent gland

abscesses, and abscesses involving the glands at the commissure of the mouth in chameleons.

PROCEDURE

- Aural abscesses (chelonians)
  - A square or semicircular incision is made (under general or local anesthesia) over the lower half of the tympanum. Remove the skin and part of the tympanum to expose the ear canal to allow removal of caseated material.
  - The large incision will allow continued flushing of the ear canal and second-intention healing after the infection has cleared. The ear canal can be flushed daily with a diluted chlorhexidine solution (as mentioned previously), then packed with 1% silver sulfadiazine cream or Gentocin ophthalmic ointment until all debris is removed and second-intention healing occurs at the incision site.
  - During flushing, the oral cavity may be packed with gauze and /or the head held down to avoid aspiration of the flush material that will empty into the pharyngeal area from the eustachian opening.
  - It is important to evaluate the eustachian opening of both ears while the patient is under anesthesia.
    - If gentle pressure is applied to the normal appearing tympanum, caseated material may be seen from the eustachian opening in the pharyngeal area, indicating the need for bilateral surgery.
- Hemipenal abscesses
  - With the patient under general anesthesia and with use of magnification when possible, abscesses are gently removed or débrided from the hemipenal tissue.
  - Use caution to minimize damage to the vascular supply and architecture of the hemipene. In severe cases, multiple surgeries may be necessary because it may be difficult to safely remove all obvious abscess tissue during the first procedure owing to swelling and inflammation.
  - In severe cases, amputation of the hemipene may be necessary.
- Scent gland abscesses (snakes)
  - With the patient under general anesthesia, scent gland abscesses should be surgically explored.
  - Removal of inspissated material may be possible through a lateral incision over the swollen gland.
  - Open wound or marsupialization of the abscess wall to the skin will allow important topical/local treatment.
  - In severe cases or in recurrent cases, removal of the entire gland may be necessary.
- Subspectacular abscesses
  - With the patient under general anesthesia, a ventral-shaped wedge incision (≈30°) is made in the spectacle (spectaculotomy).
  - Samples for culture and direct mount should be collected immediately. The wedge of spectacle that is removed may be submitted for histopathologic examination.
  - Continued lavage (with saline) and flushing should be performed for several days or weeks (depending on severity).
  - A 24-gauge IV catheter sheath works well to gently flush the subspectacular space.
  - Ensure that the exposed cornea is kept lubricated (2 to 3 times daily) with ophthalmic ointment until the next shed, when the spectacle will be replaced.
  - A broad-spectrum antimicrobial ophthalmic ointment is chosen initially and may be changed on the basis of culture results.
  - Systemic antimicrobials are recommended, especially if the disease is bilateral with high suspicion of general sepsis.
  - Concurrent treatment of infectious stomatitis is necessary in cases in which the subspectacular abscess is the result of an ascending nasolacrimal duct infection. See Stomatitis, Bacterial.

POST-PROCEDURE

- Appropriate initial choices of antibiotics (pending culture and sensitivity results) include amikacin 5 mg/kg IM or SC initial dose, followed by 2.5 mg/kg IM or SC q 72 h; enrofloxacin 5-10 mg/kg IM, SC, or PO q 24-48 h; and ciprofloxacin 11 mg/kg PO q 48-72 h.
- In cases with deep soft tissue, bone involvement, or a poor response to initial therapy, the addition of ceftazidime 20 mg/kg IM or SC q 72 h is recommended to target anaerobic organisms.
- Additionally, in cases in which *Pseudomonas* spp. and other bacteria in the *Pseudomonas* group have been isolated, consider combination therapy such as a quinoline or aminoglycoside and a third- or fourth-generation cephalosporin or penicillin:
  - For example, enrofloxacin 10 mg/kg IM, SC, PO q 24-48 h and ceftazidime 20 mg/kg IM or SC q 72 h; or piperacillin 100-200 mg/kg IM or SC q 24-48 h
  - Or amikacin 5 mg/kg IM or SC initial dose, followed by 2.5 mg/kg IM or SC q 72 h, and ceftazidime 20 mg/kg IM or SC q 72 h; or piperacillin 100-200 mg/kg IM or SC q 24-48 h
- Systemic antimicrobial regimens are continued for a minimum of 4 weeks in mild cases and potentially for 6 to 8 weeks in more severe cases involving bone. The length of treatment will be based on follow-up evaluations, which are critical to ensure progress and complete resolution of lesions.
- Topically, deep abscesses, which may involve bone (e.g., mandibular), can be treated with 1% silver sulfadiazine cream or dimethyl sulfoxide (DMSO)/amikacin solution (8 mL of DMSO is added to 0.25 mL of amikacin 50 mg/mL).
- Depending on culture and sensitivity results, DMSO/enrofloxacin can be used alternatively (add 8 mL of DMSO to 0.5 mL of injectable enrofloxacin 22.7 mg/mL).
  - Depending on severity, a minimum of 21 to 30 days of treatment will be needed.
- In cases of osteomyelitis, patients must be reevaluated frequently for continued curettage and débridement until lesions have resolved.
- Amputation of limbs, digits, or tail may be necessary with severe osteomyelitis (based on radiographs and surgical exploration). Amputation may improve the prognosis for the reptile because it allows more rapid resolution of the infection, reducing the likelihood of hematogenous spread of organisms to other organs in the body.
- In cases of active osteomyelitis in which amputation is not possible or is undesirable, 12 to 16 weeks (or longer) of antibiotic therapy may be necessary. The use of antibiotic-impregnated beads may be useful in these cases, especially in those involving joints and areas for which amputation is not possible.
- In all cases, a follow-up visit is recommended once the systemic course of antimicrobials is near completion to decide whether longer treatment may be necessary.
- Cases with active flushing and second-intention healing should be rechecked before complete closure of the surgery site to ensure that infection has cleared.
- Cases with active osteomyelitis should be rechecked frequently during treatment, with follow-up radiographs used to assess progress with any bone change.

CROSS-REFERENCES TO OTHER SECTIONS

Stomatitis, Bacterial

AUTHOR: **SCOTT J. STAHL**

EDITOR: **JÖRG MAYER**

REPTILES

Assisting Shedding

SYNONYM

Wrongful shed

OVERVIEW AND GOAL

To help the reptile remove old shed skin

INDICATIONS

If animal is not able to remove old shed on its own

CONTRAINDICATIONS

If skin is not ready to shed, shed cycle is not complete.

EQUIPMENT, ANESTHESIA

- Warm water bath
- Towel

ANTICIPATED TIME

30 minutes

POSSIBLE COMPLICATIONS AND COMMON ERRORS TO BE AVOIDED

A dimple or a crease in a spectacle may be present and should not be mistaken for a retained spectacle(s). This crease or dimpling in the single spectacle can be normal for some snakes such as the ball python *(Python regius)*.

PROCEDURE

- Warm water soaks for 15 to 20 minutes (or longer as needed), followed by gentle assisted removal of the skin, may be effective. When assisting with the removal of skin, start cranially and work caudally because this is the normal direction for skin to come off in synchronous shedders such as snakes and geckos.
- Provide warm water soaks at 27°C to 29°C (80°F to 85°F); generally use only water with no additives (antiseptics, soaps, aloe, etc.). Ensure in all, but especially in debilitated, reptile patients to provide shallow baths to prevent drowning.
- Soaking during the veterinary visit followed by gentle removal of retained skin allows the clinician to see whether any associated damage/inflammation may require continued treatment. If all retained shed cannot be removed at this time, the owner can continue to soak daily at home until all skin has come off. Caution owners not to be too aggressive when assisting with skin removal, and inform them that it is best attempted only after/during soaks when the skin is wet.
- Snakes can be placed in pillowcases with warm wet towels to crawl through as a gentle way to assist with retained shed skin.
- Retained spectacles can be gently removed after a warm water soak. A drop of mineral oil or saline solution can be placed over the spectacle. Then, a small, blunt probe can be placed into the periocular space and moved in a circular fashion around the eyes several times. In many cases, this helps loosen or lift the retained spectacle. The probe can then be used to gently tease the retained spectacle from the edge to lift off the underlying spectacle. Caution should be taken to avoid damage to the underlying spectacle. If the spectacle is damaged and the cornea becomes exposed, it must be protected with ophthalmic ointments until the next shed replaces the damaged spectacle. Without aggressive protection, this exposure could lead to irreversible damage to the cornea and loss of the eye.
- Another technique is to place a piece of cellophane tape over the retained spectacle, then attempt to gently lift off the tape. The retained spectacle may be removed with the tape.
- If the spectacle does not come off with any of these techniques, and risk of damage to the current spectacle is a matter of concern, the retained spectacle can be left in place until the next shed cycle. Placement of ophthalmic ointment on the eyes, along with increasing humidity with the next shed cycle, often will result in successful shedding of the retained spectacle.
- Blocked nares from retained skin can be opened gently with a blunt probe. Saline or ophthalmic drops can be placed in the nostrils to loosen the material. The patency of the nares can be checked with the same drops. The same procedure is effective for removal of dried skin around the eyes.

POST-PROCEDURE

- Damaged skin may be protected with 1% silver sulfadiazine cream or hydrogel dressing applied daily until the next shed.
- Severe ulcerated skin lesions may have to be treated initially with topical cleaning/flushing treatments such as dilute chlorhexidine (1 part chlorhexidine to 30 parts saline), followed by topical antimicrobial preparations such as 1% silver sulfadiazine cream. Systemic antimicrobials (based on culture and sensitivity when possible) may be indicated in these cases as well.
- Swollen and/or ulcerated appendages, such as toes and the distal tail, must be treated aggressively to avoid necrosis. Warm water soaks as described earlier can be used to remove dried skin. Topical cleansing followed by application of topical preparations as already described is indicated.
- If osteomyelitis and/or necrosis is present, surgical intervention will be necessary to remove infected bone and necrotic tissue. Radiographs should be used to direct surgery and determine the extent of bone involvement. Amputation of the affected appendage a safe distance above the involved tissue may be necessary. General anesthesia will be necessary for removal of involved bone. Systemic antimicrobials will be necessary in these cases.
- Investigate for problems in husbandry because the problem might be a sign of chronic stress.
- Systemic antibiotic therapy: once the reptile is rehydrated and has an appropriate core body temperature, antibiotic therapy can be initiated. Appropriate initial choices of antibiotics (pending culture and sensitivity results) include amikacin 5 mg/kg IM or SC initial dose, followed by 2.5 mg/kg IM or SC q 72 h; or enrofloxacin 5-10 mg/kg IM, SC, or PO q 24-48 h; or ciprofloxacin 11 mg/kg PO q 48-72 h. In cases with deep soft tissue, bone involvement, or a poor response to initial therapy, the addition of ceftazidime 20-40 mg/kg IM or SC q 72 h is recommended to target anaerobic organisms.

ALTERNATIVES AND THEIR RELATIVE MERITS

- Owners should be encouraged to provide microhabitats for captive reptiles that allow an area of high humidity within their captive environment to prevent shedding issues.
- A humidity box is a good way to provide this microhabitat. A humidity box is a plastic tub or container with a lid that can be removed. The container is filled with an absorbent material that will retain moisture, such as moss, sphagnum, vermiculite, or shredded paper towels. A hole is cut into the container to allow the reptile to go into the box, but the hole is small enough to help retain moisture. Materials in the box are sprayed

routinely with water (and kept clean) to keep the box humid; the reptile can spend time buried in the substrate inside the box, which provides humidity and help with shedding cycles.
- The prognosis is excellent with gentle and appropriate removal of retained skin and protection of damaged skin until healing occurs.
- Cases involving extremities with associated compromise of blood flow and associated osteomyelitis/necrosis have a guarded prognosis. However, with amputation and protection from sepsis with the use of systemic antimicrobials, the prognosis is more favorable.

AUTHOR: **SCOTT J. STAHL**

EDITOR: **JÖRG MAYER**

REPTILES

Blood Pressure

OVERVIEW AND GOAL

Blood pressure can be an aid in monitoring anesthesia and during cardiopulmonary resuscitation (CPR).

INDICATIONS

- Routine surgery
- CPR assessment

EQUIPMENT, ANESTHESIA

- Doppler
- Inflatable cuff
- Invasive monitor
- IV line

ANTICIPATED TIME

5 to 10 minutes

PREPARATION: IMPORTANT CHECKPOINTS

- Blood volume in healthy reptiles varies from 4% to 8%, which is lower than in mammals.
- Osmolarity of reptile plasma is typically lower than that of mammals; consequently, solutions osmotically balanced for mammals (e.g., 0.9% normal saline) are likely to be hypertonic for reptiles and may further deplete the intracellular compartment.

POSSIBLE COMPLICATIONS AND COMMON ERRORS TO BE AVOIDED

Direct pressure monitoring using the carotid and femoral arteries has been shown to be accurate and consistent and to correlate with baroreceptor reflex studies and previously published results, whereas indirect measurements have been highly variable in comparison.

PROCEDURE

- Chelonians tend to have the lowest mean arterial pressure (15 to 40 mm Hg), whereas some lizards (e.g., chameleons) have resting mean arterial pressures similar to those of mammals (60 to 80 mm Hg).
- In the green iguana, the resting systemic arterial pressure is reported to be 40 to 50 mm Hg.
- Snakes have been reported to have an allometric relationship between arterial blood pressure and body mass. As body mass increases, so does blood pressure.
- In chelonians, the cuff is attached at the highest point of the front leg, and the probe detects blood flow on the brachial artery at the palmar aspect of the radius and ulna.
- The cuff is inflated to suprasystolic blood pressure and is slowly released until the first sound is heard.
- The first sound is the measure of indirect systolic blood pressure.
- The caudal artery at the tail can be used in large male chelonians.
- In chameleons, bearded dragons, iguanas, and other lizards, blood pressure can be measured using the front leg as described for chelonians.

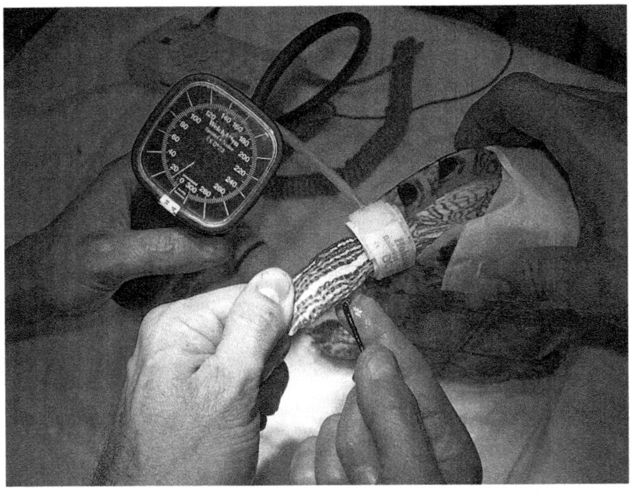

Blood Pressure Indirect blood pressure in a red eared slider. *(From Maria Lichtenberger, Mequon, WI, in Emergency Care of Reptiles, Vet Clin North Am Exot Anim Pract 10:557–585, 2007.)*

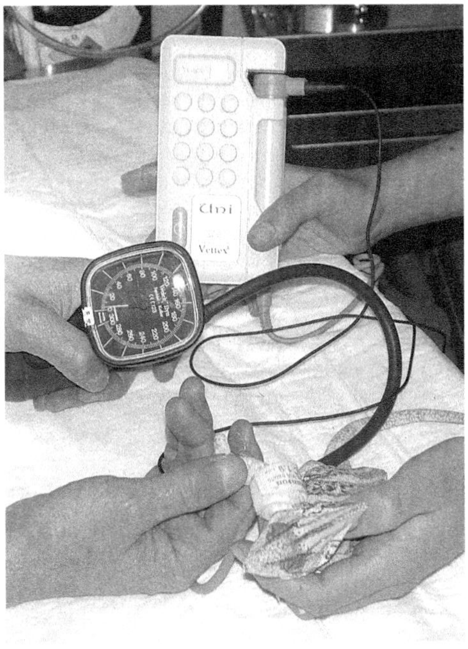

Blood Pressure Indirect blood pressure in a chameleon. *(From Maria Lichtenberger, Mequon, WI, in Emergency Care of Reptiles, Vet Clin North Am Exot Anim Pract 10:557–585, 2007.)*

- In snakes, the cuff is placed just distal to the cloaca, and the probe detects blood flow from the caudal tail artery. Indirect systolic blood pressures between 40 and 90 mm Hg have been reported.
- Direct pressure studies in conscious green iguanas at 28°C (82.4°F), however, have indicated normal resting heart rates of 48 ± 2 bpm and mean arterial blood pressures of 51 ± 2 mm Hg, with a range of 30 to 63 mm Hg.

ALTERNATIVES AND THEIR RELATIVE MERITS

Because direct blood pressure monitoring is likely to be difficult in practice, indirect monitoring using a Doppler monitor (Parks Medical, Aloha, OR) may be the only practical option. Clinicians are advised to be skeptical of the pressure values obtained; as with pulse oximetry, it is probably advisable to pay attention to the trend rather than an individual result.

AUTHOR: **MODIFIED FROM MARTINEZ-JIMENEZ D, ET AL: EMERGENCY CARE OF REPTILES, VET CLIN NORTH AM EXOT ANIM PRACT 10:557–585, 2007.**

EDITOR: **JÖRG MAYER**

REPTILES

Cardiopulmonary-Cerebral Resuscitation

SYNONYM

CPCR

INDICATIONS

Any reptile in crisis, in shock, or considered dead by the owners

CONTRAINDICATIONS

The reptile should be examined for breathing, and when no respiratory excursions are noted, CPCR should be initiated.

EQUIPMENT, ANESTHESIA

Standard cardiopulmonary resuscitation (CPR) equipment

ANTICIPATED TIME

- The clinician should be reminded that reptiles have an ability to convert to anaerobic metabolism; this can result in brain and tissue survival even after many hours of hypoxia.
- Even without a beating heart, the reptile can be warmed and continued on intravenous (IV) or intraosseous (IO) fluids.
- Reports have described reptiles recovering after many hours of arrest with supportive care (i.e., heat, oxygen, and fluids).

PREPARATION: IMPORTANT CHECKPOINTS

Initial assessment should be performed to determine cardiovascular and respiratory stability, mentation, and evidence of trauma or blood loss.

POSSIBLE COMPLICATIONS AND COMMON ERRORS TO BE AVOIDED

- It is common to declare a reptile as dead prematurely.
- Before the official confirmation of death, place the animal in a heated cage and wait for rigor mortis to set in.

PROCEDURE

- The clinician should follow basic life support with the ABC (airway, breathing, circulation) approach of CPCR.
- Secure a patent airway by opening the mouth of the reptile.
- The glottis is located at the base of the tongue in the rostral oral cavity.
- Most reptiles can be easily intubated, and 100% oxygen should be initiated using an Ambu bag (Ridge Medical, Lombard, IL) or ventilator (Small Animal Ventilator, Vetronics, Lafayette, IN) connected to an oxygen outlet or anesthesia machine.
- Positive-pressure ventilation is commenced at a rate of 4 to 6 breaths per minute; peak positive-pressure ventilation should not exceed 8 cm H_2O.
- The heart is not easily auscultated using a standard stethoscope; however, use of electronic stethoscopes and Dopplers is often more rewarding.
- Electrocardiography (ECG) can be used to identify electrical activity and should not be performed in cold reptiles because identification of the boundaries of the waves can be challenging.
- It should be noted that dead reptiles may continue to exhibit cardiac electrical activity for many hours after CNS collapse, whereas mere handling and restraint may induce ECG artifacts.
- Alligator clips from the ECG leads can be attached to hypodermic needles and then placed appropriately through the skin.
- The snake's heart is located in the upper third of the body length, and the leads can be attached cranial and caudal to the heart.

Lead Placement in the Reptilian Patient

Group	Lead Placement	Comment
Ofidia	Self-adhering cutaneous skin electrodes designed for humans are placed approximately two heart-lengths cranial and caudal to the heart.	
Sauria	In lizards with the heart located caudal to pectoral girdle (eg, monitors and tegus), electrodes are placed either in limbs or torso. Lizards with heart located at the level of the pectoral girdle (eg, skinks iguanas, chameleons, and water dragons), electrodes should be placed in the cervical region.	Stainless steel hypodermic needles or loops of stainless steel suture material can be used to attach the alligator clips.
Chelonian	Leads can be placed on limbs; however, placement of the cranial leads on the skin lateral to the neek and medial to the forelimbs is more rewarding. Leads can be attached to dermal bone after drilling holes in the carapace; however, this is a very invasive technique.	Limb lead placement is often adequate but problematic to interpretation because of frequently small surface voltages.
Crocodilian	Use of limb electrodes or torso electrodes is appropriate.	Use same limb lead placement as in lizards.

- In lizards and turtles, the leads can be attached to the front limbs and to the right rear limb, as in dogs and cats.
- The heart is located within the shell of turtles and under the bony sternum in lizards; therefore, heart compressions cannot be performed.
- Except for the crocodile, reptiles lack a functional diaphragm.
- If no heartbeat is detected, epinephrine is administered endotracheally with a catheter inserted down the endotracheal tube if IV or IO access is not possible.
- For endotracheal administration, the dose of emergency drugs should be doubled and diluted with sterile saline to 1 mL/100 g body weight to facilitate delivery of drug to the vascular respiratory tract.
- Doxapram can be administered in cases of severe respiratory depression or arrest; although its effect in reptiles has not been critically assessed, profound and immediate effects have been noted after IV administration.
- Reptiles typically have slow heart rates (30 to 100 bpm); however, in cases of true bradycardia, atropine is likely to be effective.
- If hypovolemia is suspected because of blood loss or severe dehydration, an IV or IO catheter should be placed and fluids administered.
- The effectiveness of resuscitation can be assessed with the use of a Doppler probe placed at the base of the heart or peripherally to detect blood flow.
- The Doppler probe can also be placed over a distal artery to assess pulse quality or to determine systolic blood pressure.

AUTHOR: **MODIFIED FROM MARTINEZ-JIMENEZ D, ET AL: EMERGENCY CARE OF REPTILES, VET CLIN NORTH AM EXOT ANIM PRACT 10:557–585, 2007.**

EDITOR: **JÖRG MAYER**

REPTILES

Collection of Sampling

SYNONYMS

Fecal sample collection, urinalysis, transtracheal sample collection

OVERVIEW AND GOAL

Collecting diagnostic samples is an import part of the physical workup in reptiles.

INDICATIONS

Tests should be routinely run in newly acquired animals and in all sick animals.

EQUIPMENT, ANESTHESIA

- Sterile container
- Catheters
- Gloves
- Culturettes
- Urine test strip

ANTICIPATED TIME

Varies significantly depending on sample from 5 minutes to 30 minutes

PREPARATION: IMPORTANT CHECKPOINTS

- Fecal collection
  - Collecting a fecal sample in a reptile or amphibian can be problematic; most reptiles and amphibians defecate infrequently, especially when they are ill or anorectic.

POSSIBLE COMPLICATIONS AND COMMON ERRORS TO BE AVOIDED

See later.

PROCEDURE

- Fecal collection
  - Evaluation of the feces for protozoal, amoebic, nematode, and other parasites should be considered an essential part of the minimum database.
  - Some species do defecate daily, and a sample may be collected at the next voiding.
  - In some cases, placing the animal in warm water shallow enough for it to keep its head out will stimulate defecation.
  - In sufficiently large patients, a gloved digital cloacal examination is performed.
  - This procedure may stimulate the production of cloacal contents.
  - If no sample can be passively collected, a colonic wash may be performed.
  - The proctodeum, urodeum, and coprodeum are distensible, and the goal is to collect fecal material, so a large-gauge tube is used.
  - The tube is properly lubricated and is inserted into the colon area through the vent.
  - In snakes, care must be taken because the colon is located at the most ventral aspect of the cloaca, and if the tube is directed dorsally, it will enter a blind pocket.
  - Sterile saline at 10 mL/kg is typically injected into the colon; the coelomic cavity is gently massaged before aspiration of the sample.
  - The sample should be evaluated by culture and sensitivity (when indicated), fecal flotation for ova, and a direct wet mount for protozoans.
- Urinalysis
  - Reptilian kidneys lack loops of Henle, so reptiles consistently produce isosthenuric urine with a specific gravity of 1.005 to 1.010, regardless of their hydration status.
  - Urine may be stored in the cloaca or may be refluxed into a bladder; hence microbiological culturing of urine, even by cystocentesis, can lead to erroneous interpretation.
  - The color of reptile urine varies from transparent to brown, depending on the diet and the presence of bile pigments.
  - Glucosuria is abnormal and has been observed in cases of diabetes mellitus.
  - Ketones do not appear in the urine of hyperglycemic, glucosuric chelonians.
  - Although protein may be present in small amounts in the urine of "healthy" domestic mammals, healthy chelonians appear to have only trace amounts of protein in the urine:
    - Contamination with fecal matter, semen, or egg material could introduce proteinaceous materials into the urine, producing a false-positive result.
    - True elevations in urine protein levels may indicate glomerular damage and plasma protein leakage into the urine.
  - Urine pH may be influenced by various factors, including diet, mixture with fecal matter, nutritional status, metabolic or respiratory acidosis, and perhaps urinary tract infection with urease-producing bacteria.
  - Herbivorous reptiles normally produce alkaline urine with a pH of 7 to 8.

- Carnivorous reptiles typically produce urine with a pH of 6 to 7.
- Anorectic tortoises in a state of metabolic acidosis and those emerging from hibernation can produce acidic urine.
- Microscopic analysis is one of the most important aspects of the urinalysis.
- The presence of red and white blood cells is abnormal and may indicate infection of the lower urinary or gastrointestinal tract, or possibly cystic calculi.
- The presence of parasites in the urine indicates the need for treatment using appropriate parasiticides.
- Urate crystals have been reported to take many forms and could be confused with cellular casts.
- However, when a large number of waxy or other cellular casts are found, this is a definite sign that further diagnostic testing is indicated, including plasma biochemical analysis, radiography, and possibly laparoscopy with renal biopsy.

• Transtracheal sample collection
  - Transtracheal collection of material is indicated for optimal evaluation of respiratory disease in reptiles.
  - The sample should be evaluated by aerobic culture and sensitivity testing, direct wet mount, and cytologic examination.
  - Lung worm (order Rhabditida) can be a serious problem in reptiles, and the parasite ova may be observed on a wet mount sample.
  - Sterile saline at 5 to 10 mL/kg is instilled into the trachea/lung after passage of the catheter through the glottis.
    - In chelonians and lizards with unilateral pulmonary lesions, the tip of the catheter must be bent to ensure that the catheter enters the affected lung.
    - Snakes that have one functional lung may have the catheter passed straight down the trachea into the lung.
  - After the sterile saline has been instilled into the lung, the patient is gently rotated to loosen any exudate.
  - Aspiration is then performed, and harvested material is examined using cytologic examination, parasitologic analysis, and bacterial culture and sensitivity.
  - Concerning culture and sensitivity, the best way to ensure a successful culture of pathologic microorganisms is to handle collected specimens properly.

POST-PROCEDURE

- It is important to contact one's laboratory to determine its specific requirements and recommendations for submitting samples.
- Urinalysis
  - Repeated testing is indicated in such cases; consistently high proteinuria, along with other signs of kidney disease, points to the need for further renal evaluation by biochemical testing or biopsy to diagnose the disease process.

AUTHOR: **MODIFIED FROM DE LA NAVARRE BJS: COMMON PROCEDURES IN REPTILES AND AMPHIBIANS, VET CLIN NORTH AM EXOT ANIM PRACT 9:237–267, 2006.**

EDITOR: **JÖRG MAYER**

REPTILES

Dystocia

SYNONYM

Egg binding

OVERVIEW AND GOAL

Surgical removal of follicles or eggs

INDICATIONS

If the normal egg-laying process is interrupted or prolonged

CONTRAINDICATIONS

If animal is severely debilitated

EQUIPMENT, ANESTHESIA

A full surgical procedure should be planned.

ANTICIPATED TIME

1 to 3 hours

PREPARATION: IMPORANT CHECKPOINTS

Surgery can be pursued at any time if the owner prefers to resolve reproductive concerns. Often surgery at this time is a good choice because reptiles are still in good general health, and surgery eliminates the risk of egg yolk coelomitis and the possibility of recurrence of the condition in future seasons.

POSSIBLE COMPLICATIONS AND COMMON ERRORS TO BE AVOIDED

- At surgery, many reptiles may have active egg yolk coelomitis. Removal of any ectopic egg material followed by liberal lavage of the coelom with warm saline is necessary. Patients will require postsurgical broad-spectrum antimicrobials for 3 to 4 weeks.
- In the green iguana, evidence of elevated testosterone values, development of male secondary sexual characteristics, and aggressive behavior have been associated with removal of the ovaries. Owners should be warned of these possible changes.
- For pet reptiles, ovariectomy at an early age is a consideration, to avoid dystocia in mature animals. However, concerns with hormonal changes after ovariectomy, as can be seen with elevations of testosterone in the green iguana, may create new problems.

PROCEDURE

Surgery/manipulation

- Snakes
  - Egg manipulation
    - Use of general anesthesia with propofol (PropoFlo 10 mg/mL) at 5-10 mg/kg IV (tail vein or intracardiac); isoflurane eggs sometimes can be gently manipulated toward the cloaca and removed.
    - Another technique is to gently move the retained egg to the cloaca. The egg then can be visualized through the cloaca and may be aspirated. Often the deflated egg will be easily manipulated out (and the procedure can be repeated for the next egg), or the snake may be allowed to try to pass the deflated egg on its own.
    - Oxytocin can be used to accelerate passing of the deflated egg.

- Cloacoscopy
  - Cloacoscopy can be used in an attempt to manipulate the egg out through the cloaca.
  - The snake is anesthetized as described previously for the egg manipulation technique. A 2.7-mm rigid endoscope with a 5.0-mm Taylor sheath with ports is used to evaluate the cloaca.
  - A continuous warmed saline drip through the port system of the sheath is used to keep the cloaca dilated.
  - The endoscope is gently placed into the cloaca, and the fluid drip is initiated to allow distention of the cloaca.
  - Once the cloaca is dilated, a thorough investigation of the anatomy of the cloaca can be performed.
  - Openings into the oviducts are located dorsally in the urodeum. In some cases, the oviducts may be entered and the ova or retained fetus identified. Gentle manipulation of the ova or fetus with the endoscope or with grasping forceps (along with infusion of warm saline) may allow all or portions of the ova or fetus to be removed.
  - In some cases, entry into the oviduct via the endoscope is not possible because the opening appears to be "sealed closed."
  - Endoscopy when possible allows visualization of the oviduct and the associated obstruction. If severe thickening, hyperemia, obvious infection, or an abnormal ova/fetus is evident, appropriate decisions must be made about next steps.
  - Treatment with antimicrobials and nonsteroidal antiinflammatory drugs such as meloxicam (Metacam) at 0.2-0.3 mg/kg q 24 h can be used to help with active salpingitis.
  - After medical treatment, the endoscopist can repeat the procedure in 10 to 14 days, often with increased success in manipulating the retained ova/fetus.
- Ovocentesis
  - If the egg cannot be manipulated to the cloaca, or if cloacoscopy is unsuccessful or is not available, percutaneous aspiration can be performed.
  - The egg is isolated against the lateral body wall, the area is sterilely prepped, and a 20-gauge needle is inserted between the first and second rows of lateral scales and into the egg.
  - Contents of the egg are aspirated into the syringe using caution to avoid any leakage of egg material into the coelomic cavity.
  - The snake usually will pass the egg within 12 to 24 hours of aspiration.
  - Subsequent eggs behind the first may also have to be aspirated in turn, or they may pass on their own after the first egg has been removed.
  - Eggs that have been retained for longer than a week may not be successfully aspirated because the egg contents may solidify. These eggs will have to be surgically removed.
- Surgery
  - Surgery may be necessary if medical therapy, egg manipulation, and/or ovocentesis has failed.
  - After anesthetizing with propofol and/or isoflurane is done, as described previously, an incision is made between the first and second rows of lateral scales over the retained egg or fetuses.
  - The oviduct is isolated and incised to remove the egg or fetuses.
  - If more than one egg or fetus is present, removal through the same incision may be possible.
  - However, if they are adhered higher up in the oviduct or in the opposite oviduct, multiple incisions may have to be made.
  - The oviduct is closed with a simple continuous pattern using a fine absorbable suture (e.g., 4-0 to 5-0 PDS).
  - The coelom is closed with an absorbable suture, and the skin with a nonabsorbable suture in an everting pattern.

- Lizards
  - Egg manipulation is not a safe or effective option for treating dystocia in lizards.
  - Surgery
    - For preovulatory egg stasis, surgery is often the best option to safely and efficiently solve the problem. Additionally, removal of the ovaries will prevent the problem in the future.
    - In postovulatory cases, if medical management is not indicated or is unsuccessful, or if the lizard is a pet for which reproduction in the future is not desired, surgery is indicated.
    - Anesthesia is initiated with propofol at 10 mg/kg IV into the tail vein; this is followed by intubation and isoflurane.
    - A standard paramedian approach is used by the author to avoid the large ventral midline venous sinus.
    - A large incision is recommended for obtaining good access and visualization of the gonads.
    - The bladder, fat pads, and intestines should be gently retracted out of the way to expose the paired ovaries located dorsally in the mid coelomic cavity.
    - If the lizard is in preovulatory stasis, the large paired ovaries—which resemble a cluster of yellow grapes—will be readily apparent.
    - In preovulatory egg stasis, the surgeon should proceed by removing one of the large ovaries.
    - The left ovary is attached to a branch of the renal vein. The left adrenal gland is located between the left ovary and renal vein.
    - The adrenal gland is pink and elongated and is parallel to the ovary. It is important to not remove or damage this organ while ligating the vessels to the ovary.
    - In preovulatory stasis, the ovary is very large and the vascular supply is easy to expose and ligate.
    - The vessels are double-ligated with suture or vascular clamps.
    - The vessels then are incised between ligatures, laid gently back into the dorsal coelomic cavity, and observed for any hemorrhage.
    - The right ovary is attached directly to the vena cava. The right adrenal gland is located on the opposite side of the vena cava from the right ovary, so it is unlikely to be damaged by ligation of the right ovary.
    - The right and left oviducts should be identified, but it is not necessary to remove them if both right and left ovaries are removed in the preovulatory egg stasis situation.
    - In postovulatory egg stasis, the oviducts are filled with oviductal eggs and will be identified easily upon entry into the abdomen.
    - One oviduct at a time is gently exteriorized from the cranial end (fimbria) to the caudal extent, where the oviduct enters the urodeum.
    - If the lizard is to be maintained for future breeding, a salpingotomy is performed. An incision is made in the oviduct between eggs, and warmed saline is infused into the oviduct to allow the eggs to begin to move freely within the oviduct to increase the number of eggs that can be manipulated through the oviduct incision.
    - Several incisions may be needed in each oviduct for successful

removal of all eggs from the oviducts. Oviduct incisions are closed with a simple continuous pattern using fine absorbable suture (e.g., 4-0 to 5-0 PDS).

- If the lizard is a pet and the owner is not planning to breed the lizard in the future, an ovariosalpingectomy should be performed.
- For an ovariosalpingectomy, the fimbria is ligated with suture or a vascular clamp, and groups of vessels are ligated together by creating windows in the mesosalpinx and ligating them with monofilament absorbable suture or vascular clamps.
- The caudal end of the oviduct is double-ligated with a circumferential and transfixing suture as close as possible to its junction with the urodeum. The procedure is repeated on the opposite oviduct.
- Both oviducts and all eggs are removed.
- This allows access to the small inactive ovaries.
- Caution should be taken when elevating the ovaries because the capsule and vessels may tear and bleed substantially.
- Windows are made in the capsule material between vessels with a pair of blunt-blunt scissors and vascular clips, or suture is used to ligate the vessels.
- It is important to not leave any ovarian tissue attached to the ligated vessels.
- It is necessary to remove both ovaries in postovulatory cases (except if a salpingotomy is performed) because the lizard may ovulate in the future, which could lead to ectopic ova in the coelomic cavity.
- Closure is routinely achieved by gently pulling the musculature of the coelom together with a continuous monofilament absorbable suture.
- The skin (the true holding layer) is closed with an interrupted horizontal mattress suture pattern.
- Nonabsorbable suture (3.0 nylon) or staples can be used to create an everting pattern.

- Chelonians
  - If oxytocin is ineffective, or if eggs are malformed or are too large, surgery may have to be pursued.
  - The plastral approach is invasive, and healing time is extensive. The reader is referred to Hernandez-Divers (2003). Although this procedure may have to be performed in some situations, a much less invasive procedure for egg removal through a prefemoral approach is possible.
  - Prefemoral Coeliotomy
    - The prefemoral surgical approach can be used in chelonians to access the coelomic cavity without invading the plastron. Eggs may have to be aspirated or imploded to allow passage through the prefemoral incision. Additionally, an endoscopically assisted technique has been described that uses the prefemoral site to remove the ovary in preovulatory egg stasis cases (Innis et al., 2007). The prefemoral approach is a less invasive procedure that results in more rapid healing time for the chelonian patient.
    - The chelonian patient is anesthetized (typically with propofol at 10-12 mg/kg IV, followed by intubation and isoflurane) and is placed in dorsal recumbency.
    - The rear limb is pulled back and is secured in place caudally.
    - Surgical retractors or adjustable dental retractors can be used to increase the opening of the prefemoral space.
    - The area is aseptically prepared and draped.
    - An incision is made in the skin midway between the carapace and the plastron in a craniocaudal direction within the fossa.
    - The underlying thin musculature is then bluntly dissected to reveal the coelomic membrane. The membrane is carefully incised, and the coelom is entered. Placing stay sutures in the incision layers can be useful in helping to identify them for proper closure.
    - Once the coelom has been entered, an endoscope can be used to assess the entire coelom.
    - A spay hook works well to retrieve the oviduct (or the ovary in preovulatory cases); it is then gently retracted into the small prefemoral window for inspection.
    - Typically, the oviduct with egg is brought to the incision but cannot pass through. Thus an incision is made in the oviduct, and the egg is aspirated to collapse it, or it is grasped and broken apart.
    - Caution must be used to avoid leakage of egg contents into the coelomic cavity. The oviduct is then closed in one layer with a simple interrupted absorbable suture.
    - The coelom and muscle layers are closed in a simple, interrupted pattern with absorbable suture.
    - The skin is closed with a nonabsorbable suture in an everting pattern such as a horizontal mattress.

POST-PROCEDURE

- Sutures are removed in 6 to 8 weeks.
- Surgery is indicated for resolution of dystocia in many cases.
- Eggs that are removed at surgery and are incubated typically will not successfully hatch.
- It is recommended that reptiles that have had ova/feti removed from the oviduct not be bred the following season but be given a year off to heal.

ALTERNATIVES AND THEIR RELATIVE MERITS

In cases in which dystocia was resolved through medical treatment, the owner must be warned that the reptile patient may present with the same issues in future seasons.

AUTHOR: **SCOTT STAHL**

EDITOR: **JÖRG MAYER**

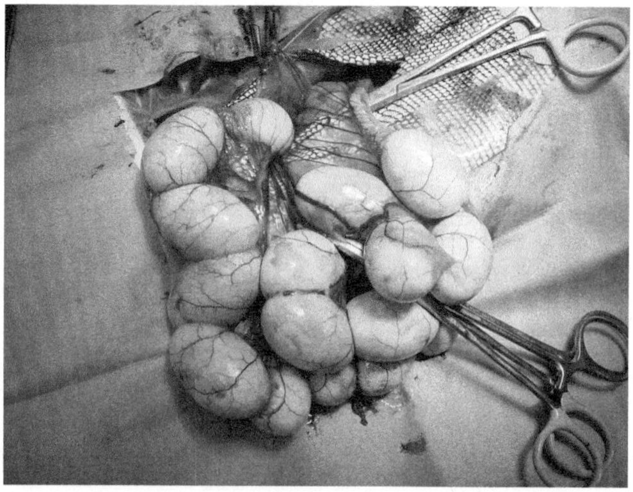

Dystocia Surgical intervention is often needed in cases of egg binding, as with this iguana. *(Photo courtesy Jörg Mayer, The University of Georgia, Athens.)*

REPTILES

Fecal Exam

OVERVIEW AND GOAL

Identification of internal parasites

INDICATIONS

- Diarrhea
- Any signs of GI disease
- Postpurchase wellness exam

EQUIPMENT, ANESTHESIA

Fecal separator, Fecasol fluid, microscope

ANTICIPATED TIME

15 minutes

POSSIBLE COMPLICATIONS AND COMMON ERRORS TO BE AVOIDED

Do not use tap water because this might contain chlorine, which will kill all protozoans immediately.

PROCEDURE

- Gross observation of the stool:
  - Often abnormal in color/appearance (pink, tan, yellow, fluorescent green)
    - Poorly digested prey/food items noted in the stool (bones, skin, etc.)
    - Mucus present or mucoid in appearance
    - Frank blood may be present
    - Fibrinonecrotic tissue evident
  - Malodorous
  - Feces and urine and urates may be bile-stained.
- Direct mounts (fresh mounts)
  - Samples must be collected at the time of the examination; they often will be voided by the patient, or they can be obtained by gently expressing the colon/cloaca or with digital introduction/stimulation of the cloaca.
  - If a fecal sample cannot be gently expressed, a colonic/cloacal wash may be diagnostic.
  - A wash is performed by passing a soft red rubber urinary catheter or metal ball-tipped feeding tube into the cloaca in a caudal-to-cranial fashion.
  - The tube may be lubricated with warm water or, in nonbreeding animals, with a water-soluble lubricant. Attempt to slide the tube into the colon by keeping it along the ventral surface of the cloaca and gently advancing it. If resistance is met, a cloacal wash may be acceptable.
  - Wash a small amount of saline into the cloaca, and gently massage the areas. The fluid then should be aspirated or gently expressed out for examination.
  - After a fecal sample is collected, the feces should be checked immediately for the presence of trophozoites and/or amoebic cysts:
    - Trophozoites of *Entamoeba invadens* are active on fresh mounts with saline and measure approximately 16 to 18 μm.
    - Amoebic cysts are best seen on direct mount or fecal float.
    - Cysts are enhanced by Lugol's iodine stain; they are quadrinucleated and measure approximately 12 to 20 μm.
  - Cloacal or colonic culture (and sensitivity) may be useful to identify opportunistic secondary invaders, such as Gram-negative bacteria, which often colonize the bowel after the amoebae have caused damage.
- Float exam

POST-PROCEDURE

- Monitoring of fecal output macroscopically for improvement (a more normal appearance) and evidence of continued problems (hematochezia, liquid diarrhea, etc.)
- Follow-up fecal evaluations

ALTERNATIVES AND THEIR RELATIVE MERITS

Cloacoscopy can be performed to evaluate the colon, obtain fecal samples, and visualize the response to treatment.

AUTHOR: **SCOTT J. STAHL**

EDITOR: **JÖRG MAYER**

REPTILES

Glomerular Filtration Rate (GFR) Study

OVERVIEW AND GOAL

Iohexol excretion study to determine the glomerular filtration rate (GFR)

INDICATIONS

To rule out kidney disease in reptiles, especially in the green iguana

ANTICIPATED TIME

10 hours

PREPARATION: IMPORANT CHECKPOINTS

- Ensure that the reptile is hydrated and fasted for 24 hours.
- Contact the Diagnostic Center for Population and Animal Health (Michigan State University, East Lansing, MI 48824 USA; telephone: 517-353-1683; http://www.animalhealth.msu.edu/) to check for any changes to the blood collection and submission requirements for iohexol assay and GFR calculation.

POSSIBLE COMPLICATIONS AND COMMON ERRORS TO BE AVOIDED

Intravenous catheterization reduces risks of perivascular injection that would invalidate the results at time 0.

PROCEDURE

- Normal glomerular filtration rates for hydrated iguana are around 15 to 18 mL/kg/h and can be calculated using an iohexol excretion study.
- Weigh the animal accurately, and inject 75 mg/kg iohexol intravenously.

AUTHOR: **STEPHEN J. DIVERS**

EDITOR: **JÖRG MAYER**

REPTILES

Handling and Restraint

Additional Images Available on Website

SYNONYM

Physical exam

OVERVIEW AND GOAL

Appropriate handling and restraint techniques in reptiles are needed because they are part of every physical exam procedure.

CONTRAINDICATIONS

- Dangerous animal
- Do not proceed if you are not familiar with appropriate techniques for safe and easy handling of the animal.
- Do not handle venomous animals without special training or with personnel not trained in handling venomous animals.

EQUIPMENT, ANESTHESIA

Use an appropriately sized towel for each animal.

ANTICIPATED TIME

5 to 10 minutes

PREPARATION: IMPORTANT CHECKPOINTS

Need to know the "weapons" of the animal and special species consideration for evaluating behavior.

POSSIBLE COMPLICATIONS AND COMMON ERRORS TO BE AVOIDED

- Lizards are easily restrained, although one does have to be careful with larger species that pose the potential for injury, as well as with smaller specimens that may escape.
- Tail whipping is common in several lizard species (particularly iguanid species and varanid lizards).
- Biting is another response that may be seen as both a defensive and an aggressive reaction.
  - Never reach over or in front of the mouth of a lizard that is not properly restrained.
- Some snakes (e.g., those that are ill, threatened, or in a preshedding or shedding cycle) may strike out.
- A snake has only one occipital condyle, so dislocation at this joint occurs more easily in snakes than in other species when the head is held too firmly—especially if the snake is fighting to get free.
- Aquatic chelonians may be more likely to bite and scratch, so additional care should be exercised with these animals.

PROCEDURE

- Lizards
  - Always use a towel that is long enough to surround not only the animal's body but also the tail.
    - Unwrap areas for evaluation as needed.
  - Proper control of the head, specifically the mouth, is vital in avoiding possible injury.
    - The head may be controlled by placing a hand or hands behind the mandible and around the neck.
    - The holder must be careful not to damage the large dorsal spines in species in which they are present (e.g., adult male iguanas).
  - To evaluate the oral cavity of lizards, stimulate the animal to open its mouth by gently pressing on the jaws at the soft tissue of the commissure, or by gently pulling down on the tissue below the mandible. (In some species, this is anatomically called the *dewlap*.)
  - Slow, gentle pressure on the dewlap often results in the animal's slowly opening its mouth.
  - In lizards and crocodilians, the vagal-vagal response may be used to help the animal "relax."
  - The vagal-vagal response occurs when pressure, often digital, is applied to both eyes for a period of time as long as a few minutes.
  - When these techniques do not work or do not work completely, a soft, clean rubber spatula may be used to gently open the mouth for examination of the oral pharynx and glottis.
  - When handling Old World chameleons, which typically are most at rest when all four legs and the tail are securely attached to something—preferably a branch—it may be beneficial to incorporate a suitably sized perch to allow the animal to rest during examination.
    - When directly handling these lizards, one should allow them to hold onto the handler's hand with all their feet and the tail; examination and manipulation should proceed one leg at a time while the others remain attached to the handler.
  - In very large lizards that are not cooperating with the physical examination, the best defense is to control head, body, and tail.
    - To control the front feet and arms, hold them gently yet securely against the body of the lizard.
    - To secure the rear legs, if needed, position and grasp them against the tail, just below the pelvis. The tail should be tucked under the arm or between the holder and the table, or it should be wrapped in an appropriately sized towel.
- Snakes
  - Snakes that are not correctly supported or are restrained too tightly will struggle.
  - It is important to locate the head and immobilize it, holding gently but firmly just behind the mandible.
  - To evaluate the oral cavity of snakes, as in lizards, stimulate the animal to open its mouth by gently pressing on the jaws at the soft tissue of the commissure.
  - Gently pulling down on the tissue below the mandible with slight pressure on this skin often results in the animal's slowly opening its mouth.
  - Properly supporting the snake along its entire body may require multiple handlers.

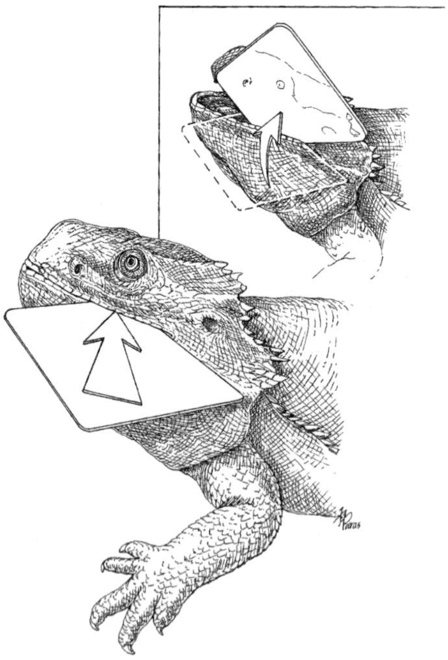

Handling and Restraint To open the mouth, place a plastic credit card or hard rubber spatula at the corner or front of the mouth and use gentle, prolonged pressure combined with a slight wiggling motion. *(From Birchard S, et al: Saunders manual of small animal practice, ed 3, Philadelphia, 2005, Saunders.)*

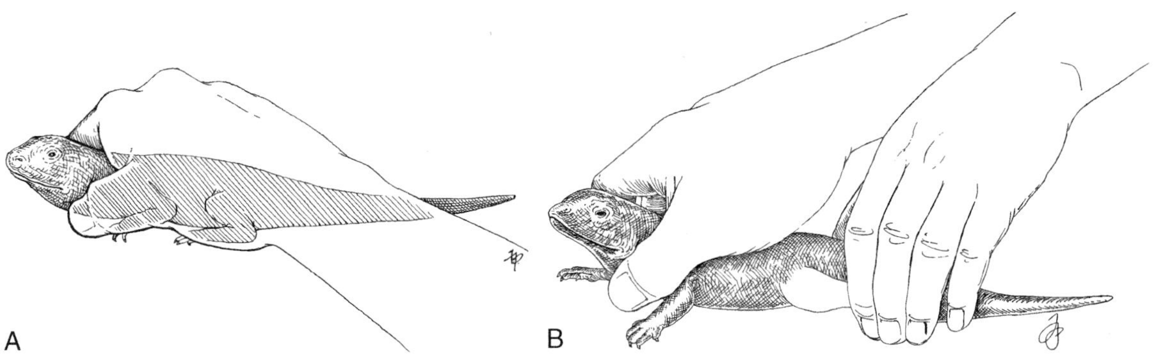

Handling and Restraint A, A one-handed technique for proper restraint of a small lizard. **B,** Proper restraint of a medium lizard. *(From Birchard S, et al: Saunders manual of small animal practice, ed 3, Philadelphia, 2005, Saunders.)*

- Because the vertebrae extend along the entire body, the weight of the hanging snake could dislocate vertebrae or could cause the snake to fight for balance and support.
- Hold the head gently but firmly behind the mandible, and move with the movement of the snake while maintaining control of the head.

- Turtles and tortoises
  - All turtles and tortoises possess strong legs that can be powerful enough to pin or pinch fingers between the shell and the legs.
  - When attempting to evaluate the oral cavity, one first needs to extend and restrain the head.
  - Typically, one person gently immobilizes the exposed and extended forelimbs by holding them directly or pinning them against the shell of the animal.
  - The head then is gently exposed and is held just behind the mandible at about the level of the ears, using the thumb and forefingers.
  - In cases of more resistant turtles, use a pair of closed hemostats placed under the horny upper beak in the area of the premaxilla, and carefully lever the head out into a position from which it may be restrained.
  - One must be gentle when applying pressure on this premaxillary area because the beak can break, especially in unhealthy turtles.
    - Although it most likely will grow back completely, this is a temporary abnormality that may bother the turtle and perhaps may bother the owner even more.
  - In certain turtles, especially larger tortoises, some form of injectable chemical restraint may be required.
    - Trying to mask or box down a turtle to allow performance of a complete physical examination may take hours and typically is not advised.
  - To evaluate the oral cavity of turtles, as in snakes, the animal at times may be stimulated to open its mouth by gentle pressure applied to the jaws at the soft tissue of the commissure.
  - At times, in large enough animals, the tissue below the mandible may be pulled down with gentle pressure; this often results in the animal's slowly opening its mouth.
  - As with lizards, do not reach across or in front of an unrestrained turtle or tortoise. As with all reptiles and amphibians, sedation or anesthesia may be needed, especially in larger, stronger animals.

AUTHOR: **MODIFIED FROM DE LA NAVARRE BJS: COMMON PROCEDURES IN REPTILES AND AMPHIBIANS, VET CLIN NORTH AM EXOT ANIM PRACT 9:237–267, 2006.**

EDITOR: **JÖRG MAYER**

REPTILES

Injections and Medication Administration

Additional Images Available on Website

SYNONYMS

Intravenously, subcutaneously, intramuscularly, intracoelomically, intracardiacally, intraosseously

OVERVIEW AND GOALS

- Administering medications to sick reptiles via different routes
- Routes often vary significantly from those used in treatment routines for other species.

INDICATIONS

For any sick reptilian patient

EQUIPMENT, ANESTHESIA

- Syringe
- Needle
- Catheter
- Spinal needle

ANTICIPATED TIME

5 minutes

PREPARATION: IMPORANT CHECKPOINTS

- Intracardiac injections are generally reserved for situations in which no other vascular access is available.
- Signs of dehydration in reptiles can be similar to those seen in mammals:
  - Loss of skin elasticity and wrinkled appearance progressing to sunken eyes; dry, tacky mucous membranes; and so forth: all must be interpreted with an understanding of normal appearances for that particular species
  - Packed cell volume and total solids can be helpful in evaluating dehydration.

POSSIBLE COMPLICATIONS AND COMMON ERRORS TO BE AVOIDED

- Because of the potential involvement of the renal portal system, some sources recommend that most injections be administered in the cranial half of the body.
- One exception is intracoelomic injections, which typically are given to lizards in the lateral right caudal

quadrant region at a level even with the cranial aspect of the rear leg.

PROCEDURE

- Snakes
  - The jugular veins and the heart are currently the only accepted sites for catheter placement.
  - The right jugular vein is typically larger than the left and thus is the best choice for catheterization.
  - Catheter placement requires that a cut-down incision be made from approximately the fourth to the seventh scute cranial to the heart at the junction of the ventral scutes and the right lateral body scales. The catheter is introduced cranial to caudal.
  - Cardiac catheterization is used in snakes for short-term (as long as 24 hours) or emergency procedures. The technique is the same as that used for cardiocentesis.
  - No accessible intraosseous sites exist in snakes.
- Lizards
  - The cephalic veins are the preferred site for intravenous catheterization.
  - The dorsal (anterior) surface of the antebrachium is prepared for a sterile procedure: cut-down and dissection of the vein is required in most cases.
  - The skin incision should extend from the dorsal proximal limit of the antebrachium medially to allow best visualization of the vein.
  - Intraosseous catheters may be placed in most lizards:
    - The proximal tibia is preferred.
    - Insertion of the catheter into the distal femur has been reported; it is currently recommended that this location be avoided because the stifle joint is invaded and the intercondylar cartilage may be damaged.
  - The proximal tibia is easily accessible; insertion through the craniomedial aspect of the bone avoids invasion of the joint capsule and the articular cartilage.
  - Using a spinal needle (size and length determined by the size of the patient), one drills the needle catheter into the tibia while palpating in the direction of the bone.
  - Placement may be tested by aspirating and obtaining a small flash of blood.
    - If no flashback is observed, a small amount of saline is injected, and the aspiration is attempted again.
    - If the catheter is outside the bone, the muscle will swell with injection of saline.
    - Ultimately, radiographs may be used to confirm the location of catheter placement.
- Chelonians
  - As with venipuncture, the right jugular vein is the preferred site for catheter placement in turtles and tortoises because it is larger than the left in many species.

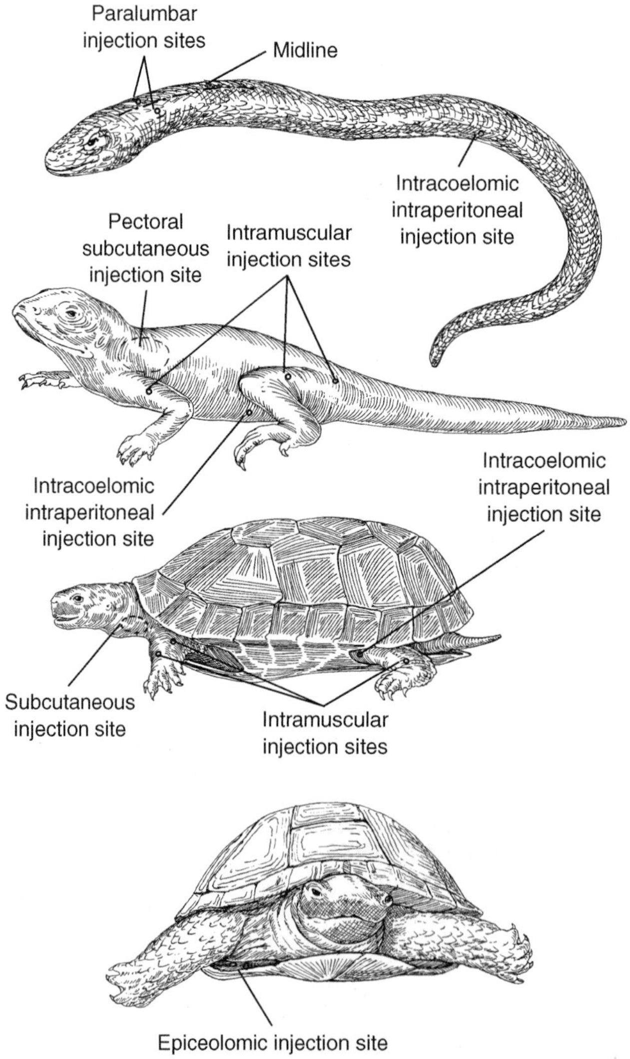

Injections and Medication Administration Common injection sites in a snake *(top)*, lizard *(center)*, and turtle *(bottom)*. *(From Birchard S, et al: Saunders manual of small animal practice, ed 3, Philadelphia, 2005, Saunders.)*

- Animals with thick skin over the jugular vein and those with poor peripheral blood pressure may require cut-down and dissection for identification and catheterization of the vessel.
- An intraosseous catheter can be placed in the cranial or caudal aspect of the bony bridge—the column of bone between the plastron and the carapace.

- Sites and techniques for fluid therapy:
  - Placing the patient in shallow, warm water usually allows some absorption of fluids, moisturizes the skin, and, in some instances, stimulates defecation.
  - Fluid replacement may be done orally in mildly dehydrated, alert patients.
  - Subcutaneous fluids are useful in mildly to moderately dehydrated patients and in patients that will not allow oral access.
  - More rapid routes of fluid delivery for patients with severe dehydration or in shock-type situations are intracoelomic and intravenous ones.
  - With repeated administration of intracoelomic fluids, it is important to aspirate, not only to ensure that the needle is not in a vital organ, but to assess that previously administered fluids have been absorbed.

POST-PROCEDURE

- Reptiles are poikilothermic; therefore, thermal support is vital for optimal maintenance of these patients.
- Properly used radiant heat sources tend to be best at providing a safe temperature gradient. Incubators may be used, but they tend to provide a constant temperature, which generally is adequate only for short-term maintenance.

AUTHOR: **MODIFIED FROM DE LA NAVARRE BJS: COMMON PROCEDURES IN REPTILES AND AMPHIBIANS, VET CLIN NORTH AM EXOT ANIM PRACT 9:237–267, 2006.**

EDITOR: **JÖRG MAYER**

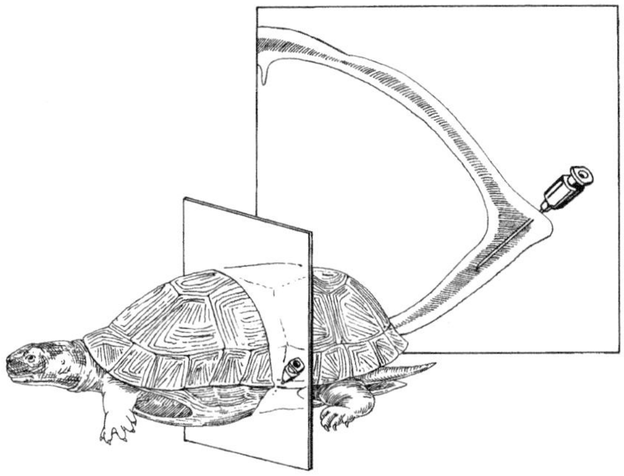

Injections and Medication Administration Intraosseous injection site of the turtle. *(From Birchard S, et al: Saunders manual of small animal practice, ed 3, Philadelphia, 2005, Saunders.)*

REPTILES

Phlebotomy

Additional Images Available on Website

SYNONYMS

Blood collection, venipuncture

INDICATIONS

Part of the physical exam

CONTRAINDICATIONS

Severe anemia

EQUIPMENT, ANESTHESIA

- Syringe and needle
- Vacutainers (heparin lithium, EDTA)

ANTICIPATED TIME

2 minutes

PREPARATION: IMPORTANT CHECKPOINTS

Make sure the animal is warmed to optimal body temperature before phlebotomy.

POSSIBLE COMPLICATIONS AND COMMON ERRORS TO BE AVOIDED

- Access to most venipuncture sites is "blind," and samples may be contaminated with lymph, altering the biochemical parameters.
- When mixed with whole blood, lymph dramatically decreases the white cell count, hematocrit, total solids, and sodium, potassium, and chloride values.

PROCEDURE

- Snakes:
  - Cardiocentesis may be used for blood collection in all snakes.
  - The heart is the first palpable mass, located approximately one-third of the distance from the head, although its location may vary significantly in certain species.
  - Cardiac contractions may be visualized when the snake is placed in dorsal recumbency.
  - After disinfection of the ventral scutes in this area, one slowly inserts into the ventricle a 22- or 25-gauge needle attached to a tuberculin or 3-mL syringe at a 45° angle; with gentle aspiration, blood may be withdrawn.
  - If the aspirant appears transparent, pericardial fluid probably has been collected.
  - The needle should be withdrawn, and another puncture may be performed using a new needle and syringe.

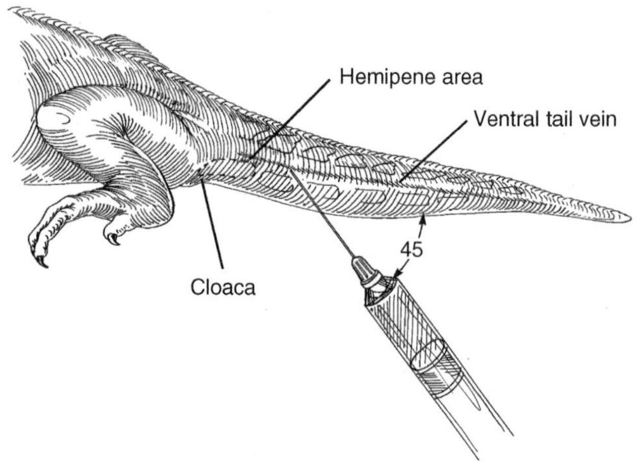

Phlebotomy Venipuncture of ventral tail vein of a lizard. *(From Birchard S, et al: Saunders manual of small animal practice, ed 3, Philadelphia, 2005, Saunders.)*

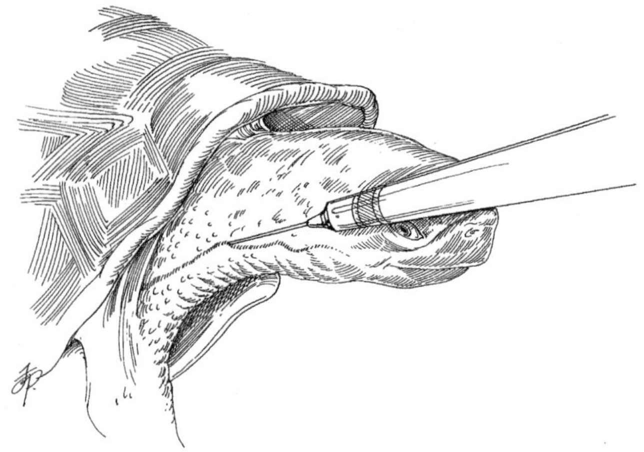

Phlebotomy Jugular venipuncture site in a turtle. *(From Birchard S, et al: Saunders manual of small animal practice, ed 3, Philadelphia, 2005, Saunders.)*

- In larger snakes, an alternative site for blood collection is the ventral coccygeal (tail) vein.
- However, when venipuncture is attempted too close to the vent, one runs the risk of puncturing the hemipenes or the musk glands.

- Lizards:
  - The ventral coccygeal (tail) vein is most commonly used in lizards, although care should be exercised in lizard species that undergo tail autotomy.
  - The venipuncture site is approximately one-fourth the length of the tail caudal to the vent.
    - As in snakes, when venipuncture is attempted too close to the vent, one runs the risk of puncturing the hemipenes or the musk glands.
  - Care must be taken to use a needle long enough to reach the ventral vertebral processes.
  - The needle is inserted between scales at approximately 90° into the midline on the ventral aspect of the tail until it comes in contact with a ventral vertebral process.
  - Gentle aspiration as the needle is advanced often allows one to collect the sample before the needle reaches the vertebral process.
  - If the needle reaches the process, it is slowly withdrawn 1 to 3 mm and is gently aspirated to collect the sample.
  - An alternative approach to the ventral coccygeal vein is a lateral one, in which the needle is inserted from the lateral aspect of the tail between scales and between the two large muscle bodies in the middle of the crease of the tail.
  - When the ventral tail vein is not productive, the ventral abdominal vein may be used.
  - It is suspended in a broad ligament 1 to 2 mm within the coelomic cavity on the ventral midline between the umbilical scar and the pelvic inlet. Again, caution must be exercised because this "blind" venipuncture presents the potential for internal or intracoelomic hemorrhage.
  - Less commonly used is the brachial plexus, which is immediately caudal to the shoulder joint. In diminutive lizards, cardiocentesis with the aid of a Doppler may be required.
- Chelonians
  - The preferred place to collect blood from turtles and tortoises is the jugular veins because these veins have minimal collateral lymphatic vessels.
  - In many specimens, the right vein is larger. Each jugular vein typically runs perpendicular and caudal to the ipsilateral tympanum.
  - Sometimes the jugular veins may be visualized when digital pressure is placed on the thoracic inlet. In some chelonians (e.g., marine turtles), a postoccipital vein or plexus arises from the right jugular vein and is located between the occipital protuberance and the cranial border of the carapace beneath the ligamentum nuchae.
  - The brachial vein or plexus is located behind the elbow joint, under the prominent and palpable tendon of insertion of the biceps brachii.
  - Chelonians have a dorsal midline tail vein that is best approached at the base of the tail. Cardiocentesis may be performed, but a hole must be created in the plastron through which a needle may be introduced.

POST-PROCEDURE

Reptiles sometimes bleed from the phlebotomy site for a prolonged time; make sure bleeding has stopped and the site has been cleaned before returning the pet to the owner.

AUTHOR: **MODIFIED FROM DE LA NAVARRE BJS: COMMON PROCEDURES IN REPTILES AND AMPHIBIANS, VET CLIN NORTH AM EXOT ANIM PRACT 9:237–267, 2006.**

EDITOR: **JÖRG MAYER**

REPTILES

Tracheal or Lung Wash

PROCEDURE

- A sterile red rubber catheter can be passed through the glottis into the trachea and advanced to the lower trachea and /or lungs. Sterile saline (approximately 1% of the reptile's body weight) is then introduced into the respiratory system. It may be helpful to gently roll the patient to increase fluid contact with respiratory surfaces before aspirating the fluid back out for analysis.
- Aerobic and anaerobic culture, cytologic examination, and parasitic examination all can be performed on the fluid recovered. This technique is useful if there has been a poor initial response to therapy or if concurrent parasitic disease is suspected (e.g., wild-caught reptiles).
- In lizards and chelonians, this technique may require sedation.

AUTHOR: **SCOTT J. STAHL**

EDITOR: **JÖRG MAYER**

REPTILES

Wound Care

OVERVIEW AND GOAL

Acute treatment for all traumatic injuries starts with providing supportive care, including warming the patient to the upper limits of its preferred temperatures, assessing hydration status, and initiating fluid therapy if indicated. Once stabilized, broad-spectrum systemic antibiotic therapy may be initiated to protect injured tissues if indicated. This is critical if the injuries involve bite wounds or scratches from cagemates or other animals.

INDICATIONS

Any traumatic open wound

EQUIPMENT, ANESTHESIA

- Bandage material
- Laceration pack (surgical)
- Topical or systemic anesthesia

ANTICIPATED TIME

Depending on wound, 5 to 50 minutes

PREPARATION: IMPORTANT CHECKPOINTS

- Initially stabilize the patient by providing triage and shock therapy:
  - Stop active bleeding.
  - Provide oxygen if necessary.
  - Provide thermal support.
  - Maintain hydration.
- Manage wounds (irrigate, clean, débride, suture, stabilize fractures, bandage).
- Provide antimicrobial coverage as necessary.
- Change husbandry to decrease chance of recurrence.

POSSIBLE COMPLICATIONS AND COMMON ERRORS TO BE AVOIDED

- Bacterial sepsis may occur as the result of severe thermal damage followed by secondary bacterial invasion.
- Deep penetrating puncture wounds (often not obvious at the time of clinical presentation) from bite wounds or scratches from cagemates or other animals may result in bacterial sepsis and death.

PROCEDURE

- Basic wound management
  - Similar to that for higher vertebrates
  - Includes primary closure, second-intention wound healing, and delayed primary healing
  - All wounds initially should be irrigated with copious amounts of warmed physiologic saline. This helps to remove debris and foreign material and helps to demarcate viable from nonviable tissue.
  - After irrigation, débride the wound with sharp dissection of devitalized tissue, and flush again with warm saline. Aggressive débridement will encourage regeneration of the epithelium.
  - At this stage, primary wound closure may be indicated for traumatic wounds that have a known time window of 6 to 12 hours. After irrigation and débridement, wounds may be closed using an everting skin pattern and nonabsorbable suture such as black monofilament nylon or absorbable suture such as polydioxanone. Chromic cat gut should not be used in reptiles because it has been shown to cause an intense inflammatory response.
  - Contaminated or infected wounds are best managed by second-intention healing in reptiles.
  - Daily flushing with warm saline will help to convert a contaminated wound into a healthy granulating wound.
  - After irrigation and débridement of the wound, it should be covered to protect it from desiccation and secondary infection.
  - Contaminated and infected wounds can be managed with wet-to-dry bandages. These are recommended when continued débridement of the wound will be indicated.
  - Gauze may be soaked in chlorhexidine (1 part chlorhexidine:30 parts water) solution or warm saline and placed on the wound. The wet gauze is then covered by dry gauze and is held in place with nonadhesive tape. These wet-to-dry bandages should be changed daily.
  - Wet-to-dry bandages will work to continue débridement of the wound by removal of exudates and any residual foreign material.
  - When changing these bandages, it helps to soak the adhered bandage layer in warm saline before removing it.
  - Wet-to-dry bandages are useful for the first 2 to 5 days, until healthy granulation tissue is present.
  - After this initial period of débridement and treatment, contaminated and infected wounds that will be healing by second intention can be treated with a variety of topical medications to limit or treat infection and to facilitate the healing process.
  - With contaminated or infected thermal wounds, gentle cleansing with dilute chlorhexidine (1 part chlorhexidine:30 parts saline or tap water) may be performed every 1 to 3 days.
  - A thin coating of 1% silver sulfadiazine cream may be applied once daily or every couple of days after gentle cleansing. This antimicrobial

cream is often indicated for topical use on thermal burns and other infected wounds because it has excellent antipseudomonal and antifungal properties.
  - For noninfected and no longer contaminated wounds (healing by second intention), several wound healing products can be used to speed the healing process and to protect these tissues:
    - Hydrogels such as Carravet or Carrasorb (Veterinary Products Laboratories, Phoenix, AZ), which are available in gel, spray, or sponge form. These products encourage healing by containing acemannan (a mannose polymer), which stimulates an increase in cytokine production (from macrophages), resulting in fibroblast and collagen production, angiogenesis, and epidermal growth.
    - Collagen-based products such as Collamand (Veterinary Products Laboratories), which work by providing a template for fibroblast and collagen growth
- Thermal burns
  - Copious warm saline lavage and irrigation is important initially and will help with cleaning the wound and performing the débriding process.
  - Depending on the severity of the burns, damaged skin may need to be gently débrided under anesthesia or sedation.
  - With contaminated or infected thermal wounds, gentle cleansing with dilute chlorhexidine (1 part chlorhexidine:30 parts saline or tap water) may be performed every 1 to 3 days.
  - A thin coating of 1% silver sulfadiazine cream may be applied once daily or every couple of days after gentle cleansing. This antimicrobial cream is often indicated for topical use on thermal burns because it has excellent antipseudomonal and antifungal properties.
- Bite wounds
  - Wounds should be aggressively cleaned with diluted chlorhexidine (1 part chlorhexidine:30 parts saline or tap water).
  - Surgical débridement may be necessary and often requires anesthesia or sedation. If osteomyelitis is evident, based on surgical evaluation or radiographs, surgical removal of involved bone (amputation or curettage) will be necessary.
  - Fresh, noninfected lacerations that can be properly cleaned and irrigated may be sutured using an everting pattern. Leave sutures in place for 6 to 8 weeks; often they will come out by themselves in a subsequent shed.
  - Topical medications such as 1% silver sulfadiazine cream (antibacterial and antifungal) may be applied to wounds that cannot be sutured and that must be left open for second-intention healing. Deep wounds involving bone may benefit from dimethyl sulfoxide (DMSO)/antibiotic preparations such as a DMSO/amikacin solution (8 mL of DMSO is added to 0.25 mL of amikacin 50 mg/mL) given to encourage penetration of local antibiotic deep into the tissues. Depending on culture and sensitivity results, DMSO/enrofloxacin can be used alternatively (add 8 mL of DMSO to 0.5 mL of injectable enrofloxacin 22.7 mg/mL). A minimum of 21 to 30 days of topical treatment may be necessary (in more severe cases, 6 to 8 weeks).
- Rostral abrasions
  - Clean wounds gently with dilute chlorhexidine (1 part chlorhexidine:30 parts saline or tap water), and débride damaged rostral tissue.
  - Remove abscessed material; if osteomyelitis is evident, curettage of affected bone will be necessary. Anesthesia is often required.
  - If nares are blocked, gently attempt to open them with a blunt probe.
  - Apply topical antibiotics such as 1% silver sulfadiazine cream. If deep lesions involving the mandibular and maxillary bones are noted, consider topical treatment with a DMSO/antibiotic solution.

POST-PROCEDURE

- Long-term management of wounds will be necessary because second-intention healing in reptiles is a slow process.
- Systemic antimicrobial regimens may be discontinued after 4 to 6 weeks, but topical wound management may need to continue for months.
- Traumatic injuries including burns or wounds that must heal by second intention require follow-up visits to monitor progress. Reptiles heal slowly compared with other vertebrates, and poor wound management may result in bacterial or fungal invasion and possible sepsis and death.
- Cases that involve damage or loss of bone (including chelonian shells) and osteomyelitis will need follow-up visits that may include radiographs to monitor healing progress.

AUTHOR: **SCOTT J. STAHL**

EDITOR: **JÖRG MAYER**

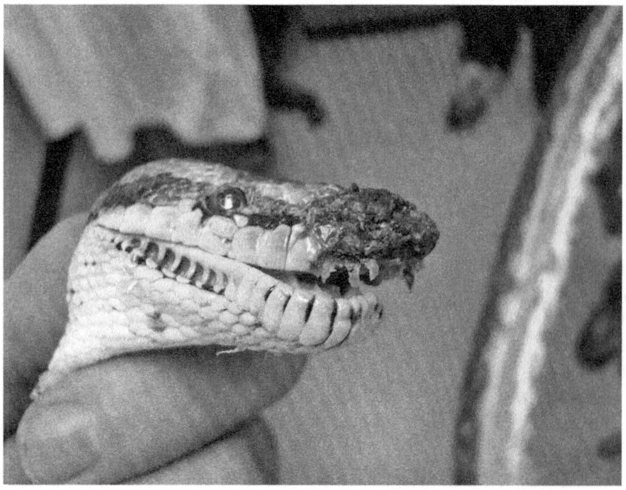

Wound Care A severe case of rostral trauma, which may be due to a prey animal bite. Aggressive débridement is the treatment of choice. *(Photo courtesy Jörg Mayer, The University of Georgia, Athens.)*

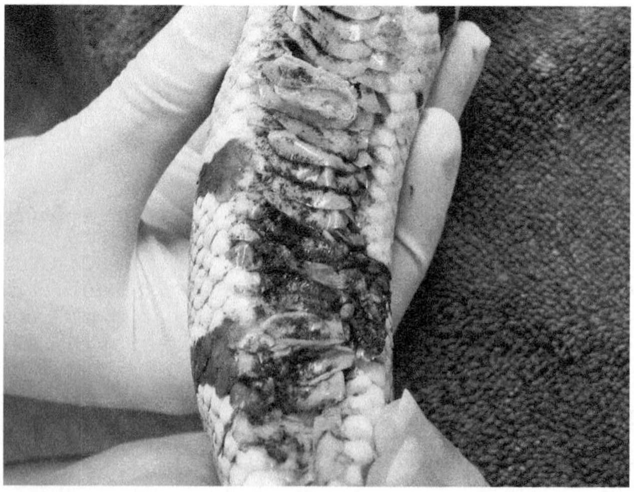

Wound Care Severe ventral burn due to prolonged exposure of the animal to a "hot rock." *(Photo courtesy Jörg Mayer, The University of Georgia, Athens.)*

Air Sac Tube Placement

Additional Images Available on Website

SYNONYM

Abdominal breathing tube

OVERVIEW AND GOAL

In cases of severe upper airway obstruction, such as tracheal aspergillosis or a tracheal foreign body, it becomes necessary to provide an alternate route for ventilation by means of an air sac cannula. Surgical access to the head and neck is easier after placement of an air sac cannula for general anesthesia. Direct application of antimicrobials or nebulization of drugs may be performed through the air sac cannula.

INDICATIONS

- Severe upper airway obstruction
- Surgical access to the head and neck
- Direct instillation of respiratory therapeutics

CONTRAINDICATIONS

Severe pneumonia or severe air sacculitis

EQUIPMENT, ANESTHESIA

The bird should be mask-induced with inhalant anesthesia, although placement may be performed without anesthesia in extreme emergencies.

ANTICIPATED TIME

5 minutes prep time, 1 to 2 minutes for patient prep and air sac cannula placement

PROCEDURE

- More clinicians are comfortable with a left lateral approach because this is the same approach that is used for laparoscopy.
- The upper leg is flexed and abducted to access the space caudal to the last rib or between the last two ribs.
- An incision is made through the skin about one-third of the way down the length of the femur.
- A stab incision is made through the abdominal musculature using sterile mosquito hemostats.
- A red rubber feeding tube or a sterile endotracheal tube of similar diameter to the trachea is guided between the halves of the hemostats into the air sac (which will be the caudal thoracic or abdominal air sac).
- Air flow is checked with a feather or a glass slide held over the opening.
- The tube is butterfly-taped and is sutured to the skin.

POST-PROCEDURE

The tube may be left in place for at least 3 to 5 days. The tip of the cannula can be cultured on removal.

ALTERNATIVES AND THEIR RELATIVE MERITS

The described method also describes the point of entry for coelomic endoscopy.

AUTHOR: **LAUREN V. POWERS**

EDITOR: **JÖRG MAYER**

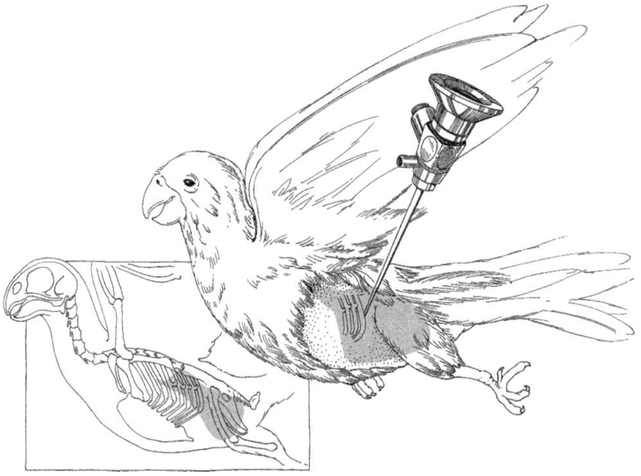

(From Birchard S, et al: Saunders manual of small animal practice, ed 3, Philadelphia, 2005, Saunders.)

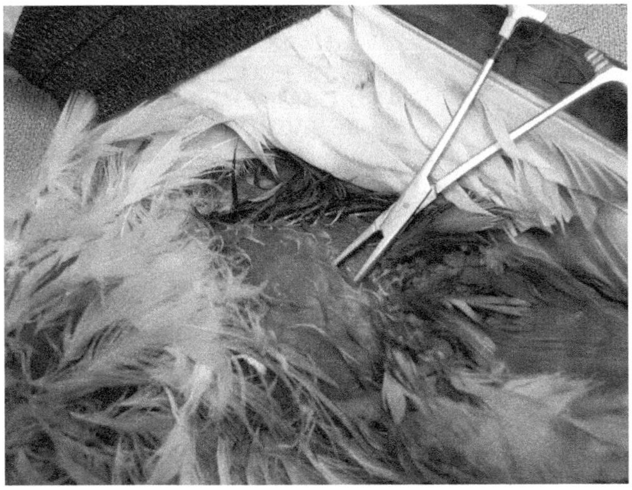

Air Sac Tube Placement Preparation for endoscopy of the abdominal air sac; *inset*, trocar or cannula site.

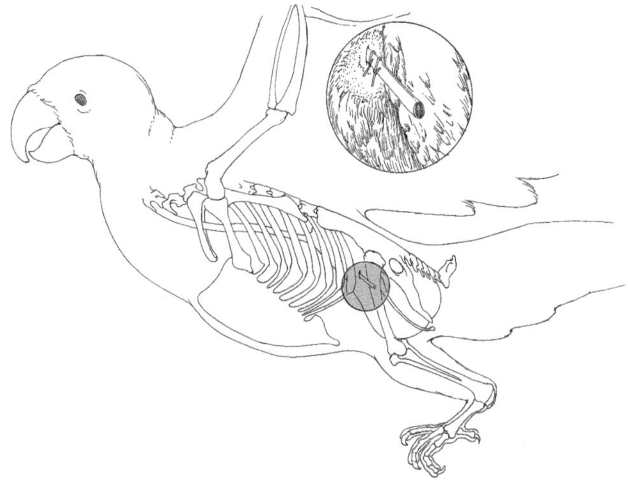

Air Sac Tube Placement Abdominal breathing tube placement; *inset*, enlargement of placement site. *(From Birchard S, et al: Saunders manual of small animal practice, ed 3, Philadelphia, 2005, Saunders.)*

BIRDS

Coelomocentesis

SYNONYM

Abdominocentesis

OVERVIEW AND GOAL

Peritoneal fluid accumulation can occur with certain diseases, such as egg yolk peritonitis and neoplasia. Free peritoneal fluid may be collected for cytologic examination, culture, and biochemical analysis. No single potential coelomic pocket exists in birds. Rather, there are five peritoneal cavities—intestinal, right and left ventral hepatic, and right and left dorsal hepatic. Ascites may accumulate in one or more of these peritoneal spaces. Fluid that accumulates with disease of the female reproductive tract (e.g., egg yolk peritonitis) is generally located in the intestinal peritoneal cavity.

INDICATIONS

- Peritoneal fluid accumulation
    - Egg yolk peritonitis
    - Neoplasia
    - Ascites (e.g., liver failure)

CONTRAINDICATIONS

Critically ill birds may not be stable enough for restraint for sample collection.

EQUIPMENT, ANESTHESIA

- Butterfly or hypodermic needles, 25- to 19-gauge
- 1- to 20-mL syringes

ANTICIPATED TIME

1 to 2 minutes prep time, 1 to 3 minutes for patient preparation and sample collection

PROCEDURE

- For collection, the bird is firmly restrained in an upright and slightly tipped forward position.
- The overlying feathers are plucked, if necessary, and are aseptically prepared with chlorhexidine gluconate or isopropyl alcohol.
- A small-gauge needle (21- to 27-gauge) is inserted through the skin and muscle directly into the pocket of fluid, if it is palpable.
- When an obvious pocket is not palpated, the needle is inserted roughly at the level of the umbilicus to avoid the liver cranially and is directed to the right to avoid the ventriculus on the left.

POST-PROCEDURE

The bird is set down and is monitored closely after sample collection.

AUTHOR: **LAUREN V. POWERS**

EDITOR: **JÖRG MAYER**

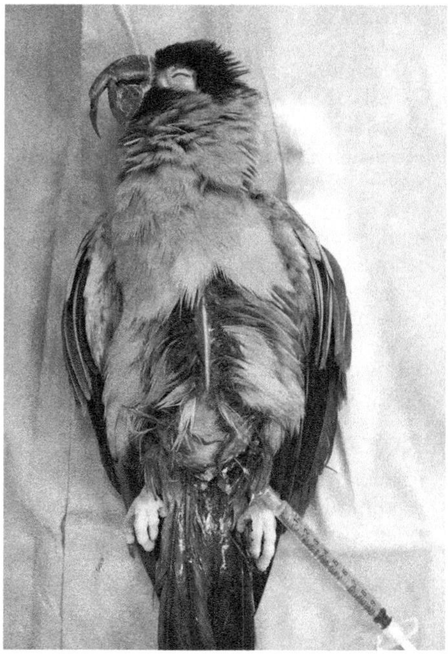

Coelomocentesis Aspiration of free fluid within the intestinal peritoneal cavity of a nanday conure.

BIRDS

Crop Infusion

SYNONYM

Gavage

OVERVIEW AND GOAL

Sick birds are reluctant to eat and usually need nutritional support. If the gastrointestinal tract is functioning well, patients may be force-fed by crop infusion.

INDICATIONS

- Diseases associated with anorexia
- Trauma or deformity of the beak(s) or oral cavity
- Nutritional support or supplementation

CONTRAINDICATIONS

- Gastrointestinal obstruction
- Neurologic or orthopedic impairment that might increase risk of aspiration

EQUIPMENT, ANESTHESIA

- Oral speculum such as nylon dog bone or stainless steel avian oral speculum
- Stainless steel, ball-tipped feeding tube or red rubber feeding tube
- Syringe of suitable size
- Gavage formula

ANTICIPATED TIME

Approximately 5 minutes prep time, and less than 1 minute for crop infusion

POSSIBLE COMPLICATIONS AND COMMON ERRORS TO BE AVOIDED

- The crop should be palpated before infusion, and the residual volume should be considered when infusion volume is determined.
- All other procedures should be completed before tube feeding, in case the bird regurgitates.

PROCEDURE

- A red rubber or stainless steel ball-tipped feeding tube is typically used.

- A safe starting point for fluid volume per feeding has been reported as 30 to 50 mL/kg; however, this author will usually start with 20 to 30 mL/kg and will increase the volume according to what the patient tolerates.
- Enteral nutritional products used include powdered formulas designed for sick birds (e.g., Emeraid Critical Care Diet, Lafeber Co., Cornell, IL) or growing birds (e.g., Exact Hand-Feeding Formula, Kaytee Products, Chilton, WI) and human enteral products.
- Because powdered, rehydrated formulas occasionally clog the feeding tube, use of the largest-diameter feeding tube that is safely feasible is suggested.
- Caloric requirements should be calculated for each bird. The basal metabolic rate (BMR) of the psittacine bird is calculated by the following formula: BMR (kcal) = 78 (body weight [BW]kg$^{0.75}$). The maintenance energy requirement (MER) for adult hospitalized birds is approximately 1.5 times the BMR. Adjustments are made to the MER to accommodate specific illnesses; these have been presented in table form elsewhere.
  - For example, the BMR of a 500-g African gray parrot is about 46 kcal/d. The MER is 1.5 times this figure, or 69 kcal/d. The adjustment factor to use when this bird has mild trauma is 1.0 to 1.2 times the MER, or approximately 76 kcal/d. The caloric concentration of most enteric formulas ranges from 1.5 to 2.0 kcal/mL. If the formula used on this bird is 1.6 kcal/mL, the total volume will be roughly 47 mL/d. Most hospitalized birds are tube-fed 2 to 4 times daily. For our example bird, this amounts to 12 mL every 6 hours, or 16 mL every 8 hours.

POST-PROCEDURE

The patient should be returned to its enclosure as soon as possible after crop infusion.

AUTHOR: **LAUREN V. POWERS**

EDITOR: **JÖRG MAYER**

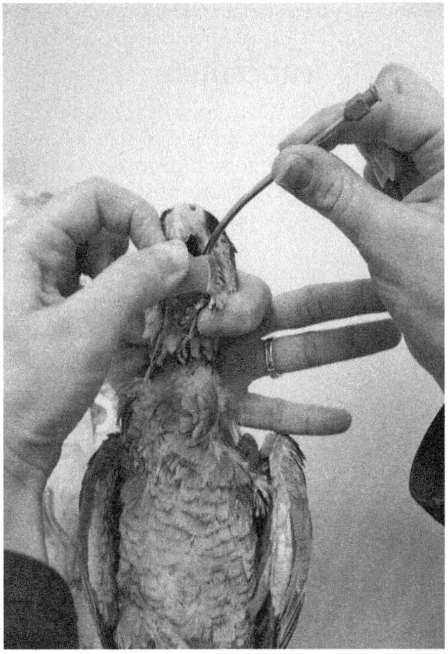

Crop Infusion Placement of ball-tipped stainless steel feeding tube into the crop of a red lored Amazon parrot.

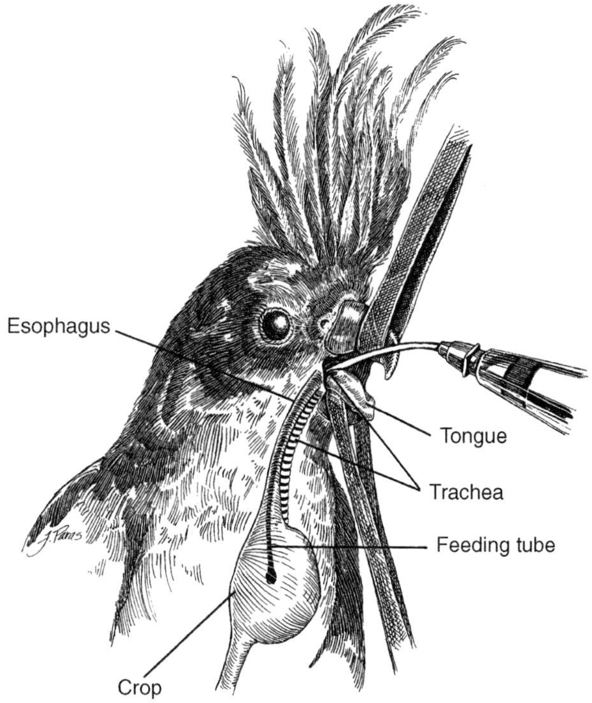

Crop Infusion Forced alimentation. *(From Birchard S, et al: Saunders manual of small animal practice, ed 3, Philadelphia, 2005, Saunders.)*

BIRDS

Duodenostomy

SYNONYM

Intestinal feeding tube placement

OVERVIEW AND GOAL

Nutritional support of the debilitated bird

INDICATIONS

In cases of severe gastric disease, such as proventricular dilatation disease, the stomach can be bypassed by a duodenostomy tube to provide nutritional support.

EQUIPMENT, ANESTHESIA

- Silicone or polyurethane catheter or over-the-needle jugular catheter
- Suture
- Scalpel blade
- Sterile surgical instruments
- General anesthesia is required for tube placement.

ANTICIPATED TIME

10 to 20 minutes prep time, 15 to 30 minutes surgical time

POSSIBLE COMPLICATIONS AND COMMON ERRORS TO BE AVOIDED

Peritonitis

PROCEDURE

- The bird is placed under general anesthesia, and the ventral abdominal area is plucked and aseptically prepared.
- A ventral midline incision is made through skin and the linea.
- A stab incision is made into the ascending limb of the duodenum, and a silicone or polyurethane feeding tube or a 17- to 20-gauge over-the-needle jugular catheter is inserted into the lumen.
- The tube diameter should be no greater than one-third the diameter of the duodenum.
- A second stab incision is made through the body wall, and the tube is fed through this incision and is secured in place with a purse-string or Chinese finger-trap pattern.
- The initial incision is closed routinely.

POST-PROCEDURE

The tube should remain in place for at least 5 days to ensure that a good seal between the intestine and the body wall is formed; this precaution should decrease the chance of peritonitis due to intestinal leakage when the tube is removed.

AUTHOR: **LAUREN V. POWERS**

EDITOR: **JÖRG MAYER**

BIRDS

E-collars

SYNONYM

Elizabethan collar

OVERVIEW AND GOALS

- Prevent birds or mammals from creating further damage by self-mutilation to an existing injury.
- E-collars should be used as the last resort in birds and mammals because the E-collar itself can induce trauma to the patient, and placement can be stressful for the animal.

INDICATIONS

To prevent further injury

CONTRAINDICATIONS

If pet stops eating or drinking, collar may have to be removed.

EQUIPMENT, ANESTHESIA

- Collar fitted for patient
- Foam insulation for waterpipes works well to "stiffen" neck in birds.
- If commercial E-collars are unavailable, one can be made:
  - Radiograph film
    - Cut to size indicated for patient.
    - Add cotton cast padding if needed to soften edges.
  - Soft fabric
    - Depending on location and patient, a t-shirt–like apparatus or a drape (e.g., feather picking) can be prepared.

POSSIBLE COMPLICATIONS AND COMMON ERRORS TO BE AVOIDED

Size patient for correct E-collar to prevent further damage to injury and creation of new injury.

PROCEDURE

- When placing a homemade E-collar around the neck, allow one or two fingerwidths to the neck circumference to ensure proper loose placement.
- Depending on injury and patient:
  - Place E-collar on patient as you would on a dog or a cat.
  - Place E-collar on backward, so the collar bends over the patient's body (to protect thoracic area) and to avoid "blinder" effect.

AUTHOR & EDITOR: **JÖRG MAYER**

BIRDS

Esophagostomy

SYNONYM

Feeding tube placement

OVERVIEW AND GOAL

Nutritional support of the debilitated bird

INDICATIONS

- Esophagostomy tube placement is indicated in cases of severe beak trauma and diseases of the oral cavity or proximal esophagus, such as abscesses and neoplasia.
- Esophagostomy tubes may be directed down the postcrop esophagus, bypassing the crop in cases of severe crop burn.

EQUIPMENT, ANESTHESIA

- Silicone, polyurethane, polyvinylchloride, or red rubber catheter
- Suture or tissue glue
- Scalpel blade
- Sterile hemostats
- Bandage materials
- Sedation is almost always indicated for tube placement.

ANTICIPATED TIME

5 to 10 minutes prep time, 5 to 10 minutes for esophagostomy feeding tube placement

PROCEDURE

- Silicone or polyurethane catheters (e.g., Kendall Argyle Feeding Tube, Kendall Co., Mansfield, MA) are softer

and stiffen less with age than red rubber or polyvinylchloride tubes.
- A stab incision is made through the skin and esophageal wall, directed by a hemostat guided into the precrop esophagus at the cranial to mid portion of the right side of the neck.
- The tube is guided through the crop into the proventriculus and is secured in place with tape butterflied to the catheter and then is secured with acrylic glue or sutures.
- Wrapping of the neck is not always necessary.

POST-PROCEDURE

- The tube should be flushed with water after every feeding and may be left in place for as long as 7 weeks.
- The tube is removed and the opening is allowed to heal by granulation. Surgical closure is not required.

AUTHOR: **LAUREN V. POWERS**

EDITOR: **JÖRG MAYER**

BIRDS

Fluid Therapy

Additional Images Available on Website

OVERVIEW AND GOALS

- Fluid therapy is commonly administered to sick and hospitalized patients.
- Most critically ill birds are presented with moderate to severe (>7%) dehydration, and often in a state of hypovolemic shock.
- Sick birds are reluctant to eat and drink and are at risk for becoming dehydrated.
- The route of delivery is indicated by the severity of dehydration, shock, and anemia.
- Birds that have mild dehydration (<5%) without shock may be hydrated with fluids provided orally or subcutaneously.
- Daily maintenance fluid requirements are estimated at 50 mL/kg/d. Maintenance plus half the fluid deficit is generally administered during the first 12 to 24 hours, with the remainder of the deficit replaced over the following 48 hours.
- Patients with moderate to severe dehydration, hypotension, shock, or severe blood loss or anemia require intravenous (IV) or intraosseous (IO) fluid support.
- Fluid type is selected based on results of biochemical analysis, such as evaluation of electrolytes, glucose, and acid-base status. When these values are not known, a balanced isotonic crystalloid solution, such as lactated Ringer's solution, may be used for rehydration and hemodynamic support.
- For birds with hypotensive shock or hypoproteinemia, a colloidal solution such as hetastarch or Oxyglobin (Biopure, Cambridge, MA) may be used (at 5 to 15 mL/kg) in combination with crystalloids (at 30 to 40 mL/kg) to rapidly restore adequate tissue perfusion.
- In cases of blood loss or severe anemia, whole blood from a suitable donor (ideally one of the same species) may be administered through an IV or IO catheter fitted with a standard small animal blood filter.
- IV and IO catheters may be used to administer dextrose solutions and other components of partial or total parenteral nutrition.

INDICATIONS

- Dehydration, hypovolemia, hypotension, maintenance fluid support, anemia
- Tent eyelid to assess hydration status.

CONTRAINDICATIONS

- Fluids should not be administered or should be used cautiously per os (PO) in birds with regurgitation, gastrointestinal stasis, neurologic diseases, or orthopedic problems of the legs, because of the risk for aspiration.
- Critically ill birds may not tolerate prolonged restraint or sedation for IV or IO catheter placement.

EQUIPMENT, ANESTHESIA

Sedation usually is not required but can be helpful to minimize patient movement during intravenous and intraosseous catheter placement.

ANTICIPATED TIME

Varies depending upon route of administration

PREPARATION: IMPORTANT CHECKPOINTS

Fluids should be warmed before administration; fluids stored at room temperature are 25°C (~75°F).

POSSIBLE COMPLICATIONS AND COMMON ERRORS TO BE AVOIDED

- Fluids administered PO are poorly absorbed in cases of hypovolemic shock as a result of peripheral vasoconstriction.
- Fluids administered subcutaneously, such as PO fluids, are poorly absorbed during hypovolemic shock.

PROCEDURE

- PO fluid administration
- Fluids may be administered PO through a red rubber or stainless steel ball-tipped feeding tube.
  - Using a tube with a diameter greater than that of the trachea reduces the risk of inadvertent tracheal placement.
- The bird is firmly restrained in an upright position with the neck as extended as possible.
- The crop should be palpated before infusion for estimation of fluid volume.
- A speculum, such as a nylon dog bone or a plastic syringe case, should always be used with a red rubber tube to prevent biting and severing of the tube.
- The tube is mildly lubricated, inserted into the left side of the mouth, and guided down the esophagus on the right side of the neck into the crop.
- The neck should be palpated for the presence of both the feeding tube and the trachea, and the oral cavity should be inspected during infusion for the appearance of the fluid.
- Crop capacity may be estimated at roughly 30 to 50 mL/kg, although smaller volumes are often used in sick birds to decrease the risks of regurgitation and aspiration.
- Subcutaneous administration
  - Fluids may be administered subcutaneously in the inguinal, interscapular, or axillary regions.
  - Volumes as great as 20 mL/kg may be administered in one location.
  - The dorsal ventral neck should be avoided owing to the presence of the cervicocephalic air sac.

- Intravenous administration
  - Crystalloid volumes as great as 10 to 15 mL/kg may be safely administered as a single bolus, provided the bird is not critically anemic and repeat administration is not required.
  - When slow or ongoing vascular administration of fluid or medications is required, an IV or IO catheter should be placed.
  - IV catheters are difficult to maintain owing to the thin nature of avian skin.
  - The right jugular and basilic veins are used most frequently, although the medial metatarsal vein may be used in larger birds.
  - A small (24- to 26-gauge) over-the-needle catheter (e.g., 24-gauge, 0.75-inch catheter; Terumo Medical Corporation, Elkton, MD) is guided into the vein, butterflied with tape, and secured to the skin with acrylic glue or sutures.
  - When one is using the basilic vein, the wing is wrapped in a figure-8 bandage.
  - With a jugular catheter, the neck is lightly wrapped in cotton padding and Vetrap (3M, St Paul, MN).
  - A fluid pump that can administer small fluid volumes, such as a syringe pump, should be used. Alternatively, a burette or frequent fluid boluses may be used.
- IO administration
  - Birds are often peripherally vasoconstricted during shock, and vascular access is difficult to impossible. An IO catheter can usually be placed quickly and easily and provides a route for rapid intravascular delivery of fluids and drugs. Sedation reduces the pain of insertion and decreases patient movement but may be risky in critically ill birds.
  - This author has experienced several cases in which a profoundly ill bird died during placement of an IO catheter, perhaps partially because of pain and the resultant sympathetic response. A small volume of 2% lidocaine without epinephrine may be instilled into the skin, subcutaneous tissues, and periosteum before catheter insertion. The author has found that use of lidocaine during IO catheter placement has resulted in a reduced number of deaths in critically ill birds.
  - The distal ulna or the proximal tibia is used most commonly. Potentially pneumatic bones such as the humerus should be avoided.
  - Ideally, a 20- to 25-gauge short spinal needle is used (e.g., 22-gauge, 1.5-inch spinal needle, Sherwood Medical, St Louis, MO). Spinal needles contain a metal stylet that prevents bone coring and needle occlusion.
  - Alternatively, a 22- to 25-gauge hypodermic needle can be used. The lumen may be occluded with sterile surgical wire before insertion. If the lumen remains open during placement and becomes plugged, the needle may be removed and replaced. However, replacement often enlarges the size of the hole and increases leakage around the catheter.
  - Once inserted, the catheter is flushed to check for patency. It is then connected to a preflushed T-port and fluid line and is secured by butterfly taping and acrylic glue or sutures.
  - For the distal ulna, the distal dorsal condyle is palpated and the surrounding site is plucked and aseptically prepared with chlorhexidine gluconate or isopropyl alcohol. The needle is inserted just ventrally to the condyle and is directed proximally toward the elbow along the shaft of the ulna. The catheter is connected to the flushed fluid line and is secured in place; the wing may be wrapped in a figure-8 bandage. Birds occasionally chew at the bandages; covering the catheter and the bandage with flaps of tape or a syringe case can prevent damage to the catheter.
  - For the proximal tibia, the stifle is flexed and the tibial crest is identified. Once the site is plucked and prepared, the needle is advanced through the tibial crest down the shaft of the tibiotarsus toward the hock. The catheter is secured in place and is attached to the flushed fluid line; the leg is lightly padded and bandaged.

POST-PROCEDURE

Radiographic confirmation of intraosseous catheter placement is strongly advised.

AUTHOR: **LAUREN V. POWERS**

EDITOR: **JÖRG MAYER**

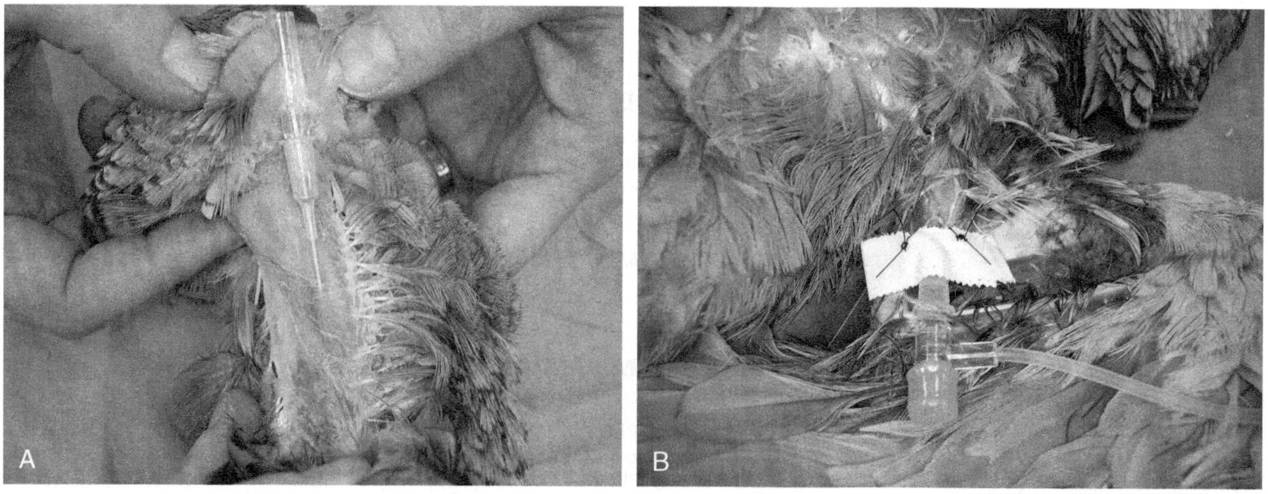

Fluid Therapy A, Placement of an intravenous catheter into the right jugular vein of a red lored Amazon parrot. **B,** Placement of an intravenous catheter into the left ulnar vein of a red lored Amazon parrot.

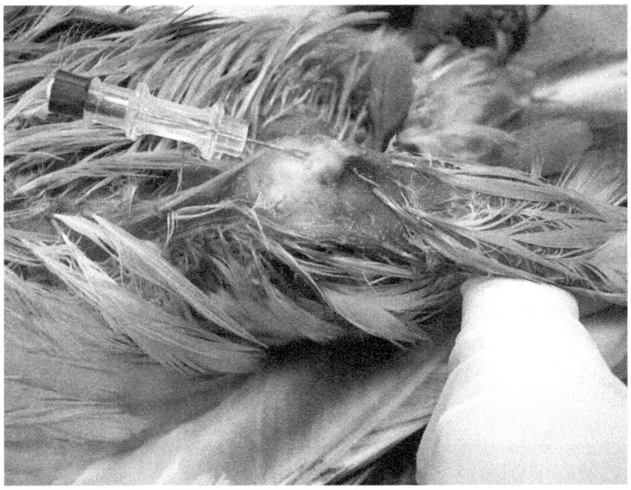

Fluid Therapy Placement of a 22-gauge, 1.5-inch spinal needle intraosseous catheter into the right tibiotarsus of a blue and gold macaw.

BIRDS

Handling and Restraint

OVERVIEW AND GOAL

To safely and quickly secure the avian patient for examination, sample collection, and treatment

INDICATIONS

Examination, sample collection, and patient treatment

CONTRAINDICATIONS

- Before a psittacine is restrained, it should be evaluated within its enclosure.
- Many critically ill birds will panic and may not survive handling.
- If the bird has an increased respiratory rate or effort, or if it appears weak and poorly responsive, it should be placed in a heated (~29.5°C to ~32°C [85°F to 90°F]), oxygenated cage for at least 20 minutes before handling.

EQUIPMENT, ANESTHESIA

- Handcloths are suitable for smaller psittacines, such as budgerigars and cockatiels.
- Thick bath towels are more appropriate for larger birds such as macaws.
- The Avistraint allows the wings to be secured to prevent excessive flapping while allowing access to the rest of the body (see www.avistraint.com).
- Gloves are often used for handling of raptors but are not advised for use with psittacines.
- Sedation may be useful to reduce patient stress and allow a more thorough examination.

ANTICIPATED TIME

As short as possible

PREPARATION: IMPORTANT CHECKPOINTS

- The examination must be brief and limited in critically ill or dyspneic patients. It may be performed in stages, with initial assessment limited to evaluation of the cardiovascular, respiratory, and neurologic systems.
- All equipment needed for examination, sample collection, and treatment should be prepared before restraint of the sick psittacine.

POSSIBLE COMPLICATIONS AND COMMON ERRORS TO BE AVOIDED

- Approaching a bird suddenly from above and behind is generally not advised because the back is a vulnerable location for these prey species.
- Restraint using gloves is not recommended because injury is more likely.
- Birds should not be collected while perched on their owners.
- Capture with bare hands is not recommended because it increases the chance of receiving bites and may lead to a hand phobia in some birds.
- Towel restraint allows better control of the wings but increases the risk for hyperthermia, may restrict motion of the keel and ribs, and prevents complete access for examination.

PROCEDURE

- Untame or panicky birds are best collected from the pet carrier with a towel. The bird may be guided toward an inside wall of the cage and the towel draped around the body.
- Untame breeder birds can be caught from flight cages using a net and can be removed from the cage in a similar fashion.

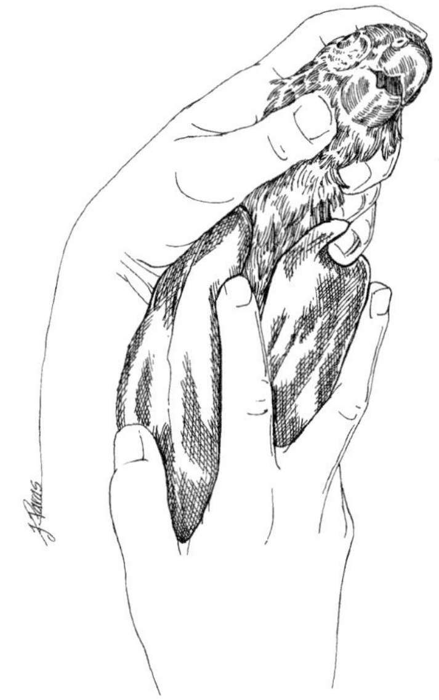

Handling and Restraint Restraint of parrot using a towel. *(From Birchard S, et al: Saunders manual of small animal practice, ed 3, Philadelphia, 2005, Saunders.)*

- Juvenile pet psittacines often allow full examination without restraint.
- Many owners of pet psittacines train their birds to become comfortable with being covered by a towel. These birds may be approached slowly from the front with a towel while they are perched, and the towel may be gently wrapped over and around either side of the body.
- Once secured, the bird's neck is grasped with a free hand, the towel is removed, and the feet (not the feathered legs) are grasped with the other hand. The most important factor in determining whether to use a towel for the avian examination is the individual practitioner's experience and comfort level.

POST-PROCEDURE

Monitoring the bird after the restraining process is important to see how fast the bird recovers from stress. Often chronic underlying respiratory tract problems are masked during routine activity, but a prolonged time of recovery (e.g., tail bobbing for longer than 5 minutes after handling) from the handling might indicate respiratory tract problems.

AUTHOR: **LAUREN V. POWERS**

EDITOR: **JÖRG MAYER**

BIRDS

Nasal Flush

SYNONYM

Nasal irrigation

OVERVIEW AND GOALS

- The nasal flush is a useful tool for collecting samples of material and fluid found between the external nares and the choanal slit—an area that includes the ventral aspect of the middle nasal concha, the suborbital chamber, and occasionally the preorbital diverticulum of the infraorbital sinus.
- Nasal flushing can serve a therapeutic purpose by mechanically flushing out debris from the nasal cavity and can be used to instill therapeutics such as antibiotics.

INDICATIONS

- Clinical signs of upper respiratory disease:
  - Nasal discharge
  - Excessive sneezing
  - Scratching excessively at the nares
  - Excessive head shaking
- Distortion of the nares and/or beak tissue immediately rostral to the nares
- Visible or suspected obstruction of nares and/or nasal cavity
- Nasal foreign bodies, inspissated exudate, debris

CONTRAINDICATIONS

Critically ill birds may not be stable enough for restraint for sample collection.

EQUIPMENT, ANESTHESIA

- Sterile flush solution such as sterile saline or physiologic sterile saline eyewash, preferably warmed
- Suitable size syringe

ANTICIPATED TIME

1 to 2 minutes prep time, less than 1 minute for procedure

PROCEDURE

- The bird is firmly restrained with the head tipped downward to avoid aspiration.
- One to 10 mL of warm sterile saline is infused into each naris and is collected in a sterile container, such as a sterile urine cup, as it exits the oral cavity.

POST-PROCEDURE

The sample may then be submitted for culture, or it may be spun and the sediment examined cytologically.

ALTERNATIVES AND THEIR RELATIVE MERITS

- Choanal swab—indicated with visible lesions of the choana
- Sinus irrigation—indicated for diseases involving the infraorbital sinus; often medication can be used in the flush

AUTHOR: **LAUREN V. POWERS**

EDITOR: **JÖRG MAYER**

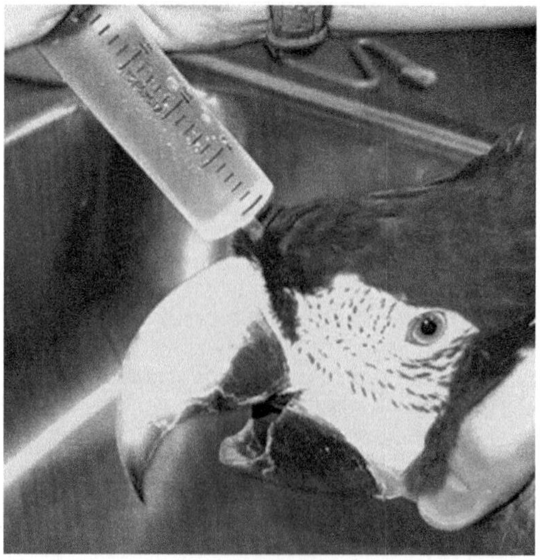

Nasal Flush Instillation of sterile saline into the left nares of a green-winged macaw.

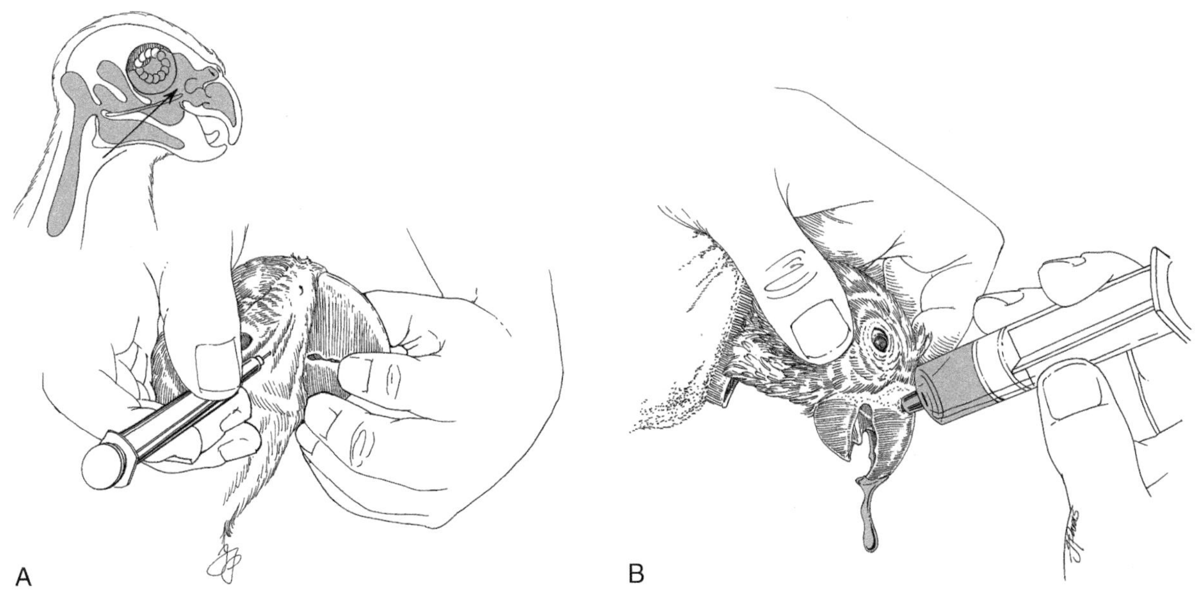

Nasal Flush A, Sinus injection; inset, diagram of sinuses showing injection site (arrow). **B,** Sinus flush.
(From Birchard S, et al: Saunders manual of small animal practice, ed 3, Philadelphia, 2005, Saunders.)

BIRDS

Tracheal or Lung Wash

SYNONYMS

Tracheal irrigation, tracheal aspiration

OVERVIEW AND GOAL

Diagnostic sample collection of lower airway disease

INDICATIONS

- A tracheal wash is indicated in birds with clinical signs or radiographic evidence of lower airway and lung disease:
    - Exercise intolerance
    - Persistent cough
    - Voice change
    - Dyspnea

CONTRAINDICATIONS

Critically ill birds may not be stable enough for restraint for sample collection.

EQUIPMENT, ANESTHESIA

- Oral speculum
- Sterile saline or other isotonic crystalloid solution
- Sterile soft plastic or rubber tube or catheter
- Syringes of suitable sizes

ANTICIPATED TIME

5 minutes prep time, 1 to 2 minutes procedure time or longer, depending upon technique

POSSIBLE COMPLICATIONS AND COMMON ERRORS TO BE AVOIDED

The greatest risk is temporary occlusion of the larger airways with tubing and fluid, which may not be tolerated by birds with severe respiratory compromise without an air sac cannula.

PROCEDURE

- Birds are generally anesthetized with gas anesthesia.
- Ideally, the length of the trachea is measured from survey radiographs.
- A sterile red rubber or other suitable tube is quickly inserted through the glottis or through a sterile endotracheal tube to the tracheal bifurcation at the syrinx.
- Approximately 1 to 2 mL/kg of warm, sterile saline (0.9%) is infused and immediately aspirated.
- The bird may be gently rocked or coupaged to increase sample recovery.
- An endoscope with a port for flushing offers the advantage of visualizing areas of interest before saline infusion.
- An air sac cannula should be placed during endoscope-assisted tracheal washes.

POST-PROCEDURE

The bird should be placed in a heated, oxygenated enclosure and watched closely during recovery.

ALTERNATIVES AND THEIR RELATIVE MERITS

The described method can also be used for tracheal endoscopy.

AUTHOR: **LAUREN V. POWERS**

EDITOR: **JÖRG MAYER**

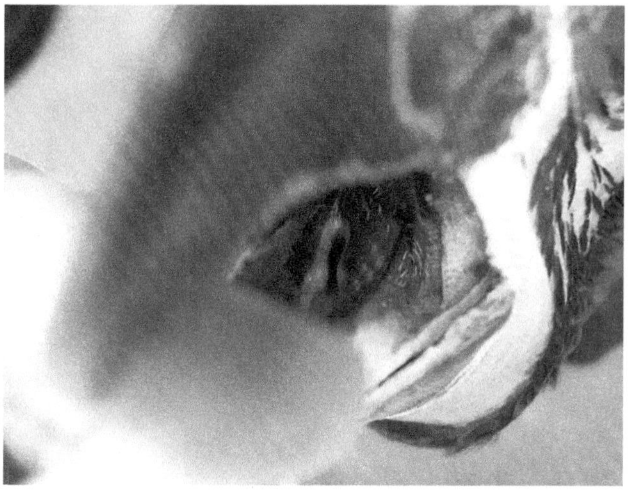

Tracheal or Lung Wash Location of the glottis in a military macaw.

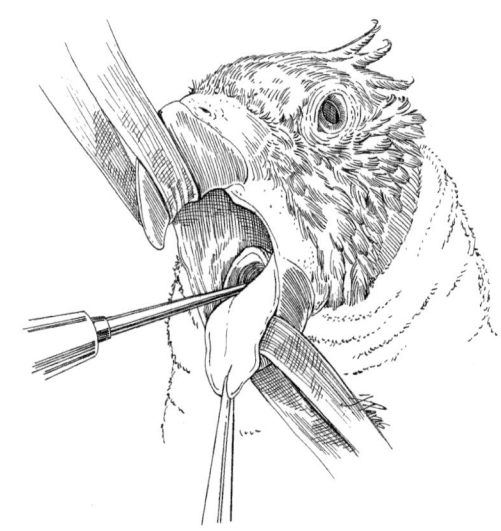

Tracheal or Lung Wash Tracheal injection or wash. *(From Birchard S, et al: Saunders manual of small animal practice, ed 3, Philadelphia, 2005, Saunders.)*

BIRDS

Venipuncture

Additional Images Available on Website

SYNONYMS

Blood collection, phlebotomy

OVERVIEW AND GOAL

To safely and quickly collect a blood sample for diagnostic purposes

INDICATIONS

- Wellness screening
- Evaluation of the sick bird
- Gender identification
- DNA fingerprinting
- Collection of blood for transfusion purposes

CONTRAINDICATIONS

Critically ill birds may not be stable enough for restraint for sample collection.

EQUIPMENT, ANESTHESIA

- The smallest practical needle gauge is advised.
- For birds weighing less than 50 g, this author prefers a 27- or 28-gauge needle (usually that of an insulin syringe).
- For birds between 50 and 100 g, a 26- or 27-gauge needle is used.
- A 22- to 25-gauge needle is used for birds heavier than 100 g.

ANTICIPATED TIME

1 to 2 minutes prep time, less than 1 minute for sample collection (unless larger volumes are collected)

PREPARATION: IMPORTANT CHECKPOINTS

- The diagnostic value of blood collection is limited by the volume that can be collected and the quality of the sample.
- Total blood volume of birds is approximately 60 to 120 mL/kg but is generally estimated at about 10% (100 mL/kg) of body weight.
- As much as 10% of the blood volume (approximately 1% of total body weight) may be safely drawn from healthy-appearing birds for diagnostic testing.
- Smaller samples should be collected in critically ill or anemic birds.

POSSIBLE COMPLICATIONS AND COMMON ERRORS TO BE AVOIDED

- The risks of venipuncture must be weighed against the diagnostic value of the blood sample.
- Coagulopathies may be associated with certain diseases, such as liver failure and aflatoxicosis.

PROCEDURE

- The most common site for blood collection in psittacine birds is the right jugular vein.
  - It is the largest peripheral vein in these birds and is easily accessed in a featherless tract on the right side of the neck.
  - Because no soft tissue covers this vein, the right jugular is prone to hematoma, particularly when the vein is inadvertently lacerated. Serious bleeding can have fatal consequences. The risk for laceration is reduced when the bevel of the needle is facing downward during sample collection.
  - The vein should be punctured directly, rather than approached from the side.
- Blood may be collected from the basilic (wing) vein.
  - Hematoma formation is more common with this vein but is rarely of serious consequence.
- The medial metatarsal vein may also be used.
  - The skin in this location tends to be thicker, and hematoma formation is less likely.
  - This vein is typically smaller than the basilic, which may reduce the sample volume collected.
  - For small sample volumes, a hypodermic needle may be inserted into the vein and blood collected from the needle hub into capillary tubes.
- Although a toenail clip is a quick and easy method of collecting minute blood samples for evaluating hematocrit or blood glucose, it is generally not advised because it may be more painful than venipuncture and often includes tissue artifacts.

POST-PROCEDURE

Pressure is often applied to the venipuncture site for a few seconds to reduce the size or frequency of hematoma formation.

AUTHOR: **LAUREN V. POWERS**

EDITOR: **JÖRG MAYER**

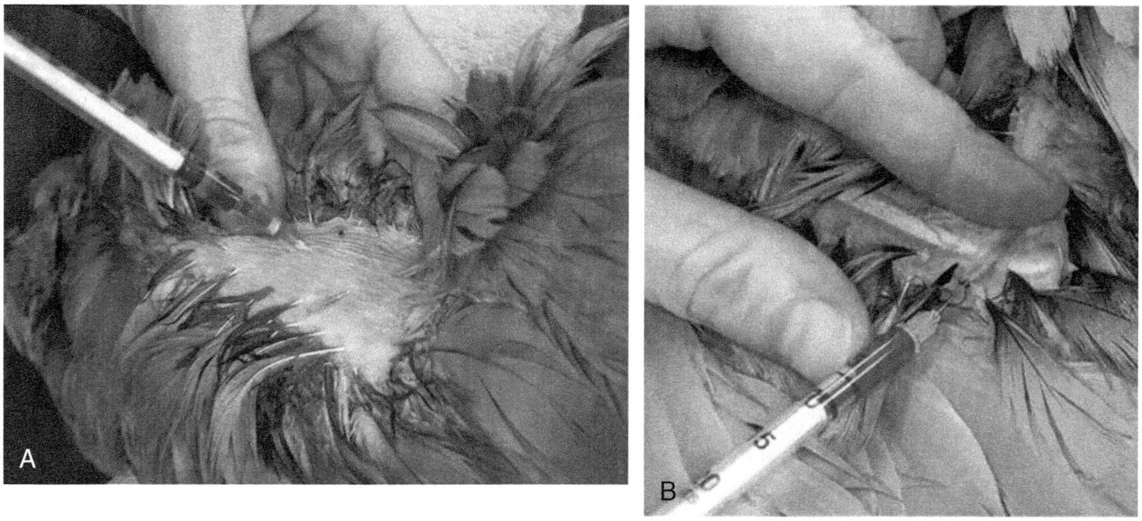

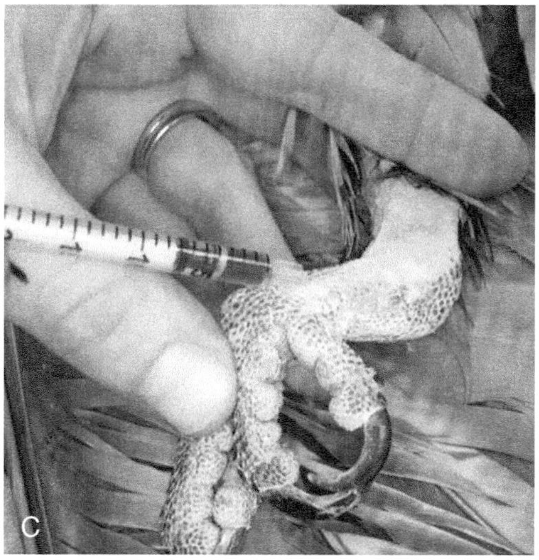

Venipuncture A, Blood collection from the right jugular vein in a military macaw. **B,** Blood collection from the right ulnar vein in a military macaw. **C,** Blood collection from the right medial metatarsal vein in a military macaw.

SMALL MAMMALS

Anesthesia Monitoring in Rabbits and Rodents

OVERVIEW AND GOALS

- The smaller the patient, the less tolerant of hypoxia.
- Small rodents develop irreversible CNS injury within 30 seconds of respiratory arrest.
- Smaller animals have a faster metabolism and often metabolize drugs more quickly. This can explain why the higher dose of drug per kg is required.
- Convective heat loss is rapid; therefore, temperature must be monitored.
- The smaller the patient, the faster the onset of hypothermia if supplemental heat is not provided (see Preventing Hypothermia During Anesthesia).
- Small bodies have a small blood volume. A small amount of blood loss could result in hemorrhagic shock and death.
- Prevent excess and inappropriate restraint in place of adequate tranquilization and anesthesia.

INDICATIONS

- Respiratory depression, hypothermia, airway obstruction, and hypoventilation are common causes of death in rabbits and rodents; therefore, monitoring is essential.
- Anesthetic depth can be monitored by
  - Muscle tone/relaxation
  - Decreased reflex activity

- Absence of limb and body movement
- Jaw tone

CONTRAINDICATIONS

- Anesthesia is rarely contraindicated even in very sick animals. The stress of handling a conscious animal that is sick will often result in death caused by the significant release of catecholamines produced by stress at handling (e.g., conscious radiographs, IV catheter placement).
- Sedation and inhalation anesthesia are mild cardiovascular depressants, and their use is preferred over inducing stress in the sick animal.

EQUIPMENT, ANESTHESIA

- Endotracheal tube
- Non-rebreathing anesthetic system
- Oxygen mask
- Electrocardiography (ECG) monitor
- Esophageal probe with thermometer
- SpO_2, CO_2 monitor
- Pediatric stethoscope
- Circulating hot air blanket or hot water blanket
- Eye lubrication
- Non-rebreathing circuit
- Small balloon

ANTICIPATED TIME

Depends on procedure being performed

PREPARATION: IMPORTANT CHECKPOINTS

- Limit the time under anesthesia by preparing and having all equipment, instruments, and packs and procedures ready before anesthesia is given.
- Have emergency drugs calculated and drawn up before induction of anesthesia.
- Long fasting is not indicated before anesthesia: 1 to 2 hours of fasting is appropriate in attempts to clear the oral cavity of food.
- Remember to remove all paper bedding because the animals often start to chew on it during the fasting time.
- To decrease airway secretions, premedicate with atropine or glycopyrrolate before performing the procedure.
- Evaluate patient carefully before the procedure to make sure that no subclinical problem can complicate the procedure.
  - Full blood work
  - Whole-body radiographs

POSSIBLE COMPLICATIONS AND COMMON ERRORS TO BE AVOIDED

- When an oxygen mask is placed on the head, place the animal's head in extension to facilitate air movement. Assess respiratory rate, pattern, and noise to ensure minimal resistance to breathing. If the pet has problems breathing, move the head to see if the obstruction can be relieved. Use a cotton-tipped applicator to clear the oropharynx and nares, if mucus is plugging the airway.
- Intubate the patient if possible to protect the upper airway and to provide oxygen and anesthesia. Intubation also allows ventilation of the pet, if needed.
- Once intubated, an in-line capnograph is useful in determining correct endotracheal tube placement and as an indirect measurement of $PaCO_2$.
- Use non-rebreathing systems because these systems provide reduced respiratory resistance and mechanical dead space. Use small balloons as breathing bags for extremely small patients to facilitate and monitor air movement.
- Rabbits have a high prevalence of respiratory disease and small chest cavities.
- Rabbits normally develop tachypnea under anesthesia with decreased alveolar ventilation.
- Sudden respiratory and cardiac arrest can occur with hypercapnia and/or hypoxemia.
- Guinea pigs have a small airway and may experience an obstructed airway from regurgitation or profuse salivary secretions.

PROCEDURE

- Endotracheal tube (ET) (see Intubation Technique in Rabbits and Rodents)
  - Several techniques can be used to place an ET. Ensure proper placement by visualizing condensation in the ET (clear ET tubes are recommended) and observing movement in the non-rebreathing bag or with an in-line capnograph.
  - Small-diameter tubes increase the risk of obstruction from saliva and mucus.
- Esophageal probe
  - Use esophageal probes in patients when possible. Esophageal probes that include a thermometer probe are an excellent choice. Esophageal probes are not applicable with rodents and may induce regurgitation in guinea pigs. Therefore, use of a pediatric stethoscope is imperative in these patients.
- ECG
  - Standard lead positions are used; the machine should be able to record at speeds of 100 mm/sec and to amplify signal to at least 1 mV equal to 1 cm.
- Capnography
  - Capnometry is the measurement of CO_2 concentrations in expired gases.
  - Capnography is performed using an in-line analyzer placed between the endotracheal tube and the anesthetic circuit.
  - End-tidal CO_2 ($EtCO_2$) is used to provide a noninvasive estimate of arterial partial pressure of carbon dioxide ($PaCO_2$). $EtCO_2$ usually is less than $PaCO_2$. If the $EtCO_2$ is elevated (above 35 to 45 mm Hg), the patient needs to be ventilated.
- Respiratory rate (RR)
  - An increase in RR may indicate a lighter plane of anesthesia; adjust anesthesia based on time left to complete the procedure.
  - Hypoventilation can be caused accidentally by inadvertent hand placement on the chest, by compression of the respiratory system by the viscera, or by obesity.
  - Watching chest wall for movement can be deceptive in terms of the amount of air movement.
  - Controlled ventilation is advised when the patient is intubated.
  - Mechanical ventilation is ideal, although it is not always practical. If ventilation is possible, 80 breaths per minute is advised, along with a tidal volume of 1.5 mL/100 g of body weight.
  - Use non-rebreathing systems for small animals. Use a small balloon in place of the breathing bag to monitor respirations.
    - Normal HR
      - Rabbits: 180 to 325 bpm
      - Hamsters: 38 to 100 bpm
      - Gerbils: 85 to 160 bpm
      - Mice: 91 to 216 bpm
      - Rats: 71 to 146 bpm
- Temperature
  - Temperature monitoring and regulation are standard of care.
  - Hypothermia is common. Drugs suppress the thermoregulation system, and anesthetic gases are of lower temperature and low humidity.
  - If patient is receiving IV fluids, warm fluids with an IV fluid warmer or place the line in a cup of hot water.
  - To increase temperature, wrap body in towels, circulating water, or air blankets. Do not use heated blankets or hot water bottles next to the skin because they can cause burns. Stockinettes filled with rice and microwaved can serve as a source of heat on the preoperative table, in radiology, or in the cage.
  - Patients should never be left unattended during recovery when wrapped in heating materials:
    - Circulating hot air blankets are a convective heat source.
    - Circulating hot water blankets are a conductive heat source.
    - Heat lamps are a radiant heat source.

- Convective heat sources provide benefit in that they warm the patient rather than preventing loss of heat from the patient (conductive or radiant).
  - Patients can become overheated easily. Monitor temperature constantly.
  - Normal temperature
    - Rabbits: 102.5°F (39.2°C)
    - Guinea pigs: 99°F to 103.1°F (37.2°C)
    - Hamsters: 100°F (37.8°C to 39.5°C)
    - Mice: 99°F (37.2°C)
    - Rats: 100°F (37.8°C)
- Capillary refill time
- Mucous membrane color
- Blood gas
  - Blood gas analysis assesses the patient's oxygenation and acid-base status, as well as adequacy of ventilation. Obtain arterial blood gas from any artery: femoral, metatarsal, or auricular (rabbit). Lidocaine can be infiltrated in the area of the arterial area to prevent reflex vasoconstriction.
- Pulse oximetry
  - Accurate at levels greater than 85% in rabbits and rats
  - Sensors can be placed on the ear, tongue, buccal mucosa, paw, vulva, prepuce, or proximal tail area
  - For rabbits, the base of the tail and the paw are more effective than ears, possibly owing to excessive compression from the sensor clamp.
    - Move the clip frequently owing to compression.
  - Can be inaccurate with decreased blood pressure and vasoconstriction
- Arterial blood pressure (BP)
  - Hypotension can result from poor cardiac output caused by cardiac failure or severe dehydration.
  - Indirect BP can be taken from the legs, forearms, tail, and ears (rabbits).
  - Appropriate cuff size is critical to ensure accurate measurements. The width of the cuff should be 40% of the circumference of the limb. If the cuff is too large, BP reading will be artificially high; if the cuff is too small, BP reading will be artificially low.
  - If a BP monitor is not available and a Doppler is used, clip the hair where the Doppler probe will be placed. Place a small amount of ultrasound gel on the Doppler probe, and apply gently against the artery. Once the flow is detected, increase pressure on the manometer until the flow is no longer heard. Slowly release pressure until the flow is heard again.
  - Decreased volume indicates a decrease in flow or displacement of the probe. Arteries to choose from include the following:
    - Ventral aspect of the tail base
    - Carotid
    - Femoral
    - Auricular arteries
    - Directly over the heart
  - Normal BPs in exotic herbivores do not differ significantly from those of their counterparts in small animal medicine.
  - Normal BP
    - Rabbits: 90 to 120 mm Hg
      - Normal systolic BP in rabbits recorded by telemetry varies between 93 and 99 mm Hg.
      - Normal range of mean arterial pressure in rabbits is 80 to 91 mm Hg; systolic arterial pressure is 92.7 to 135 mm Hg, and diastolic arterial pressure is 64 to 75 mm Hg.
      - However, if the animal is stressed, systolic BP can be as high as 180 mm Hg.
    - Guinea pigs: 80 to 94 mm Hg
    - Hamsters: 150 mm Hg
    - Mice/Rats: 113 to 147 mm Hg
- Fluid therapy
  - Fluid therapy (preoperative and perioperative) is great for patients that may decompensate from blood loss or endotoxemia.
  - Catheters are easier to place preoperatively than perioperatively.
  - Cephalic, saphenous, and auricular (rabbits) veins are easily accessible for intravenous catheters.
  - Intraosseous catheters can be placed in the proximal femur, fibula, or humerus.
  - SC fluids are not adequate to correct deficits or blood loss. Fluid absorption is minimal because tissues are poorly vascularized.
  - Rate of fluid administration depends on hydration status, severity of hemorrhage, type of fluid, and any underlying disease.
  - Standard surgery rate for IV fluids is 10 mL/kg/h.

POST-PROCEDURE

- Pets should be monitored until a full recovery is made. The recovery area should be a warm, quiet environment away from visualization.
- Prolonged recovery can be caused by hypoglycemia, hypothermia, or anesthetic overdose.
- Caution should be used when warming hypothermic patients too fast; warming results in vasodilatation and increased metabolic demand for glucose. This can explain the sudden death that can occur postoperatively.
- Certain types of anesthesia can prolong recovery time.
- Ensure that proper analgesia has been administered, according to the procedure performed.

AUTHOR: **JÖRG MAYER**

EDITOR: **THOMAS M. DONNELLY**

SMALL MAMMALS

Blood Collection, Volume, and Sites

OVERVIEW AND GOALS

- Obtaining samples from mammals is relatively easy and can be done without anesthesia in healthy animals.
- Several sites are easily accessible. The technique and site chosen can depend on the amount of blood needed.
- Anesthesia can be used if assistants are unavailable but may affect hematologic values.
- Ferrets are often distracted by food, but feeding can depend on sample needed.
- Most samples can be run on microtainers, using less than 1.5 mL of blood.
- Collect minimum amount needed for analysis, but you can take 10% (healthy animal) of the blood volume safely (5% of an ill patient):
  - A healthy 750-g ferret generally has 40 mL blood volume.
  - A 1-kg ferret has about 60 mL blood volume.

INDICATIONS

Laboratory analysis for routine health examination or in sick animals

CONTRAINDICATIONS

- Unhealthy animals can be easily stressed; use sedation or anesthesia with caution.
- Stress of blood draw can often be more severe than that seen with sedation or anesthesia.

EQUIPMENT, ANESTHESIA

- Isoflurane/Midazolam
- 22- to 25-gauge needle with a 1-mL or 3-mL syringe
- Microtainers (as indicated by lab)
- Microscope slides
- Alcohol

ANTICIPATED TIME

5 minutes

PREPARATION: IMPORTANT CHECKPOINTS

Before preparing the patient, determine what samples will need to be submitted. Have all required equipment ready before the blood draw.

POSSIBLE COMPLICATIONS AND COMMON ERRORS TO BE AVOIDED

- Complete blood count can be altered starting at induction, with peak alteration 15 minutes after induction.
- In rabbits, the marginal ear vein and the central ear artery are readily accessible. Nothing should be injected into the vessels because thrombosis of the vein can occur, and the area can slough.
  - Bruising and hematomas may occur.

PROCEDURE

- Ferrets
  - Two main techniques: jugular and anterior vena cava
  - Jugular technique: similar to that used in cats
    - Place animal in sternal recumbency, with forelegs extended over table and head extended up.
    - Use a 25-gauge needle with a 1- to 3-mL syringe, or a 22-gauge needle for large males.
    - Shave neck to enhance visibility. The vein is located more laterally than in dogs and cats and can be difficult to visualize in large males.
    - Once the needle is inserted into the vein, blood should flow easily into the syringe. If blood flow is slow, the head may be overextended. Pump the vein by moving the head up and down slowly.
  - Anterior vena cava
    - Restrain ferret on back with forelegs pulled caudally and head and neck extended.
    - Without anesthesia, two assistants will be needed: one to restrain forelegs and head, and the other to restrain rear, cranial to the pelvis.
    - Use a 25-gauge needle with a 3-mL syringe.
    - Insert the needle into the thoracic cavity between the first rib and the manubrium at a 45° angle to the body.
    - Direct the needle to the opposite rear leg or to the most caudal rib, and insert the needle almost to the needle hub. Pull back on the plunger as the needle is slowly withdrawn until blood begins to fill the syringe. If the ferret struggles, withdraw and wait until the ferret is calm to start again.
  - Lateral saphenous and cephalic veins can be used only if a small amount of blood is needed (PCV or GLU).
    - To prevent collapse of the vein, use an insulin syringe or a tuberculin (TB) syringe attached to a 28-gauge needle.
    - The saphenous vein lies just above the hock joint.
    - The cephalic vein lies on the lateral surface of the rear leg.
    - Shave fur for better visualization.
  - Tail vein
    - Rare, but one can use the tail for venipuncture
    - Place ferret in heated environment for several minutes, or use moist heat to promote vasodilatation.
    - Restrain the ferret on the back.
    - Procedure can be painful, so apply topical lidocaine to the area.
    - Insert syringe with a 23- to 25-gauge needle into the groove of the midline, directed toward the body on the ventral side of the tail. The artery is located 2 to 3 mm deep.
    - Once the artery is entered, slowly withdraw the plunger.
    - 3 to 5 mL of blood can be obtained from this site.
    - Apply pressure for 2 to 3 minutes once the needle is removed.
- Rabbits
  - For venipuncture of the ear, pluck the hair and rub the area to dilate the vessel.
    - Clean with warm mild soap or alcohol.
    - Insert a 25- or 27-gauge needle, and allow blood to drip from the hub of the needle into the appropriate tube.
    - Use of a syringe will collapse the vessel.
  - Lateral saphenous
    - Easily accessible: this vein runs medial to lateral, diagonally across the lateral aspect of the tibia
    - Blood can be drawn quickly and easily. Place rabbit in lateral recumbency, and hold off the vein just above the hock joint.
  - Jugular
    - Some sedation may be necessary to reduce stress to the rabbit.
    - Shave and prep the neck midtrachea, cranial to thoracic inlet.
    - Place the rabbit in dorsal recumbency, and have the assistant hold the head over the table with one hand while grasping the body with the other hand.
    - Pull front feet back, toward the rear. Tip the head back to expose the ventral neck region. Jugular should be easily visualized.
    - Without sedation, hold rabbit like a cat, with the front feet over the table, and extend the head up.
    - Pluck or shave hair from the jugular furrow to enhance visualization.
    - Use thumb to hold off vein.
- Once blood is drawn, apply pressure for 2 to 3 minutes.

POST-PROCEDURE

Always apply pressure to the site of venipuncture for several minutes post draw to prevent hematoma formation.

AUTHOR: **JÖRG MAYER**

EDITOR: **THOMAS M. DONNELLY**

SMALL MAMMALS

Blood Transfusion

SYNONYM

Venous transfusion

OVERVIEW AND GOAL

Fresh whole blood is the most commonly used blood product for blood donations because of the limited donor pool and the difficulty associated with storing, making banking difficult. This procedure can be easily successfully completed depending on donor availability, procedure timing, and staff precision. A successful blood transfusion can drastically improve a patient's packed cell volume (PCV) and clotting factors.

INDICATIONS

Blood transfusion in small mammals is generally recommended for acute life-threatening emergencies that result in anemia, such as trauma, internal bleeding (caused by various factors, the most common of which is foreign body ingestion), and/or coagulopathies. It can also be used as postoperative supportive treatment.

CONTRAINDICATIONS

A patient that presents with normal PCV and normal clotting factors should not be receiving blood, and any critically ill patient presented with chronic conditions should be watched closely during the procedure.

EQUIPMENT, ANESTHESIA

In all small mammals, the equipment necessary is very similar, although needle gauge sizes may vary depending on the animal's size and species. Regardless of the species, the entire procedure should be aseptic, and all donors must be sedated or anesthetized.

- For collection:
  - Sterile surgical gloves
  - Butterfly needles
  - Collection syringe with anticoagulant
  - Sedation agents and/or anesthetic agent
- For administration:
  - Intravenous catheter
  - Collection syringe filled with donor's blood mixed with anticoagulant
  - Giving set attached to a filter
  - Syringe driver

ANTICIPATED TIME

- For collection: 20 to 45 minutes
- For administration: maximum of 4 hours (depending on patient's condition)

PREPARATION: IMPORTANT CHECKPOINTS

- The procedure should be aseptic.
- Patient and donor must have their PCV checked before the procedure, and the amount to be transfused should be calculated using the following equation:

$$\text{Anticoagulated blood volume (mL)} = \text{Patient's body weight (BW)} \times 70 \times (\text{PCV desired} - \text{PCV of patient})$$

- Collection syringe should be prepared using the following ratio of anticoagulant agents:
  - 1 mL CPDA-1 (citrate-phosphate-dextrose-adenine) per 7 to 9 mL blood
  - 1 mL CPD (citrate-phosphate-dextrose) or ACD (acid-citrate-dextrose) per 7 mL blood
  - 5 to 10 units heparin per 1 mL blood

ANATOMIC CONSIDERATIONS

Blood should always be collected from the donor using a large vessel. In rabbits, the most common site is the jugular vein, given the amount that a rabbit can donate. In ferrets, the cranial vena cava (CVC) or the jugular vein can be used, and for small rodents, the jugular vein, lateral tail veins, or saphenous vein is used (not recommended is the use of the orbital sinus or submandibular vein because this could compromise the donor's safety and the aseptic technique of the procedure).

POSSIBLE COMPLICATIONS AND COMMON ERRORS TO BE AVOIDED

- Blood groups have not been identified in ferrets or studied in rabbits and rodents. Blood transfusion in these species has been done successfully over the years, and very rarely is a reaction observed. In rabbits, a simple cross-matching test is recommended to identify any incompatibility between donor and patient (to minimize potential complications):
  - Mix 2 drops of plasma from the donor with 1 drop of blood from the patient, and observe for agglutination.
  - Repeat, using 2 drops of plasma from the patient and 1 drop of blood from the donor.
  - If any agglutination is observed, do not transfuse blood from this donor into this patient.

PROCEDURE

- Rabbits
  - For collection:
    - Donor must be sedated (avoid agents that can cause vasoconstriction or hypotension).
    - A healthy rabbit can donate 10 to 20 mL/kg of blood (always provide donor with fluid replacement therapy).
    - Prepare site for collection (jugular vein).
    - Use the butterfly needle with the collection syringe already prepared with anticoagulant agent:
      - 1 mL CPDA-1 (citrate-phosphate-dextrose-adenine) per 7 to 9 mL blood
      - 1 mL CPD (citrate-phosphate-dextrose) or ACD (acid-citrate-dextrose) per 7 mL blood
      - 5 to 10 units heparin per 1 mL blood
- Collection syringe should be vigorously shaken during collection for equal mixture of anticoagulant agent and to avoid coagulation of any blood content.
  - For administration:
    - Venous administration of blood can be provided via jugular, lateral saphenous, marginal ear, or cephalic veins; an intraosseous catheter placed into the femur or tibia can also be used if venous access is limited.
    - Start the infusion at a rate of 1.5 mL/kg/h for the first 20 minutes, then increase to 6 to 12 mL/kg/h if no signs of reaction were observed (total transfusion should not exceed 4 hours).
    - Monitor vital signs of the patient during the procedure.
- Ferrets
  - For collection:
    - Donor must be anesthetized, and blood must be collected immediately after induction (isoflurane anesthesia can decrease many hematology values).
    - A healthy ferret can donate 10% of its body weight of blood (always provide donor with fluid replacement therapy).
    - Prepare site for collection (CVC or jugular vein).
    - Use the butterfly needle with the collection syringe already prepared with anticoagulant agent:
      - 1 mL CPDA-1 (citrate-phosphate-dextrose-adenine) per 7 to 9 mL blood

        - 1 mL CPD (citrate-phosphate-dextrose) or ACD (acid-citrate-dextrose) per 7 mL blood
        - 5 to 10 units heparin per 1 mL blood
    - Collection syringe should be vigorously shaken during collection for equal mixture of anticoagulant agent and to avoid coagulation of any blood content.
  - For administration:
    - Venous administration of blood can be provided via jugular or cephalic veins or by intraosseous placement of a catheter into the femur or tibia.
    - Start the infusion at a rate of 0.5 mL/kg in the first 20 minutes, then increase the rate; transfusion should not exceed 4 hours.
    - Monitor vital signs of the patient during the procedure.
- Rodents
  - For collection:
    - Warming the patient immediately before collection will increase blood flow considerably.
    - Donor must be anesthetized (avoid agents that can cause vasoconstriction or hypotension).
    - A healthy adult rodent can donate 10% of its body weight of blood (always provide donor with fluid replacement therapy).
    - Prepare site (jugular vein, lateral tail veins, or saphenous vein) for collection.
    - Use the butterfly needle with the collection syringe already prepared with anticoagulant agent:
      - 1 mLCPDA-1(citrate-phosphate-dextrose-adenine) per 7 to 9 mL blood
      - 1 mL CPD (citrate-phosphate-dextrose) or ACD (acid-citrate-dextrose) per 7 mL blood
      - 5 to 10 units heparin per 1 mL blood
    - Note that for the smallest patients, an insulin syringe may be ideal for collection and should be prepared in the same way with the anticoagulant agent.
    - The collection syringe should be vigorously shaken during collection for equal mixture of anticoagulant agent and to avoid coagulation of any blood content.
  - For administration:
    - Venous administration of blood can be provided via jugular or cephalic veins or by intraosseous placement of a catheter into the femur or tibia.
    - Start the infusion at a rate of 0.5 mL/kg in the first 20 minutes, then increase the rate; transfusion should not exceed 4 hours.
    - Monitor vital signs of the patient during the procedure.

POST-PROCEDURE

1 to 2 hours after the transfusion, the patient's PCV should be rechecked, together with vital signs. Patient should be monitored and should receive fluid therapy.

ALTERNATIVES AND THEIR RELATIVE MERITS

- Blood is stored using 1 mL CPDA-1 (citrate-phosphate-dextrose-adenine) per 7 to 9 mL blood (it can be stored for 35 days).
- Synthetic colloids can be used when patient is presented with severe anemia or hypovolemia.

REFERENCES

Matos REC, et al: Common procedures in the pet ferret. Vet Clin Exot Anim 9:347–365, 2006.

Siperstein LJ: Ferret hematology and related disorders. Vet Clin Exot Anim 11:535–550, 2008.

AUTHOR: **VIVIANE SILVA RAYMUNDO**

EDITOR: **JÖRG MAYER**

SMALL MAMMALS

Bone Marrow Aspiration and Core Biopsy

OVERVIEW AND GOALS

- A bone marrow sample can help diagnose many diseases, including anemia, thrombocytopenia, pancytopenia, proliferative abnormalities, and suspected hematopoietic malignancy.
- Anesthesia is necessary.
- Samples can be obtained from the proximal femur, iliac crest, and humerus.

INDICATIONS

- Cytopenia
- Unusual blood morphology
- Staging of neoplasia

CONTRAINDICATIONS

- Infection of overlying tissue
- Pet must be stable enough to be anesthetized.

EQUIPMENT, ANESTHESIA

- Anesthesia
- Combinations of agents provide excellent preanesthesia, allowing maintenance with isoflurane or sevoflurane if needed.
- Ferrets
  - PA agents include the following:
    - Midazolam 0.3-1.0 mg/kg IM
    - Ketamine 10-50 mg/kg IM
    - Ketamine/Midazolam 5-10 mg/kg and 0.25-0.5 mg/kg IM
    - Dexmedetomidine 0.02 mg/kg IM
    - Diazepam 1-2 mg/kg IM
    - Diazepam/Ketamine 1-2 mg/kg and 10-20 mg/kg IM
    - Butorphanol 0.05-0.5 mg/kg SC or IM
    - Acepromazine 0.1-0.5 mg/kg SC or IM
- Rabbits
  - PA agents include the following:
    - Ketamine 20-50 mg/kg IM
    - Ketamine/Midazolam 25 mg/kg and 1-2 mg/kg IM
    - Ketamine/Dexmedetomidine 14 mg/kg and 0.07 mg/kg IM
    - Diazepam 1-3 mg/kg IM
    - Diazepam/Ketamine 0.3-0.5 mg/kg and 10-15 mg/kg IM
    - Butorphanol 0.1-1 mg/kg SC or IM
    - Acepromazine 0.5-1 mg/kg SC or IM
- Hair clippers
- Antiseptic scrub
- Surgical blade
- Surgical gloves
- 20-gauge, 1.5-inch spinal catheter
- 6- to 12-mL syringe
- Microscope slides
- Sterile tube with anticoagulant for submission of sample (preferred method depends on lab)
- 10% formalin and container
- Surgical tissue glue

ANTICIPATED TIME

20 minutes

PREPARATION: IMPORTANT CHECKPOINTS

- Consult with lab to ensure that all materials are available and that desired samples can be submitted.
- Have all material ready before anesthesia so patient will be under anesthesia for a minimal amount of time.
- Monitor patient under anesthesia.
- Keep patient warm.
- Provide analgesia before procedure begins.

POSSIBLE COMPLICATIONS AND COMMON ERRORS TO BE AVOIDED

- Clotting of sample
  - Reduce time between collection and smearing of sample.
- Sliding off bone causing soft tissue trauma
  - Use firm but not excessive pressure.

PROCEDURE

- Anesthetize patient.
- Shave and aseptically prep patient in lateral recumbency.
- Proximal femur:
  - Make a small incision through the skin over the greater trochanter with a #15 surgical blade.
  - Hold and stabilize the femur with one hand, while inserting a 20-gauge, 1.5-inch spinal catheter into the bone, medial to the greater trochanter.
  - Use steady pressure and an alternating rotating motion to advance the needle into the marrow cavity.
  - Withdraw the stylet and attach a 6- to 12-mL syringe to the needle.
  - Aspirate the sample into the syringe. As soon as the sample is visible, stop the sucking action to prevent contamination with blood.
  - Once the sample has been collected, close the incision with a small amount of tissue glue.
- Core biopsy:
  - Use the same technique, but use an 18-gauge, 1.5-inch needle in place of the spinal catheter.
  - Collect sample from alternate sides.
  - A white plug of marrow should be obstructing the tip, which can be placed in 10% formalin.

POST-PROCEDURE

- Prepare four to eight slides for cytologic examination. Spray material from syringe onto slide. Place a clean slide on top, allowing the marrow to spread; then slide the slides apart in horizontal fashion.
- Sample also may need to be placed in a purple top lab tube.
- Monitor and recover patient as normal from anesthesia.
- Monitor for pain.
  - Rabbits:
    - Butorphanol 0.1-1.0 mg/kg SC, IM, IV q 4-6 h
    - Buprenorphine 0.01-0.05 mg/kg SC, IM, IV q 6-12 h
    - Morphine 2-5 mg/kg SC, IM q 2-4 h
    - Carprofen 1-2.2 mg/kg PO q 12 h
    - Ibuprofen 2-7.5 mg/kg PO q 12-24 h
    - Meloxicam 0.5 mg/kg SC, PO q 24 h
  - Ferrets:
    - Butorphanol 0.1-0.5 mg/kg SC, IM q 4-6 h
    - Buprenorphine 0.01-0.03 mg/kg SC, IM, IV q 8-12 h
    - Morphine 0.5-5 mg/kg SC, IM q 2-6 h
    - Carprofen 1 mg/kg PO q 12-24 h
    - Ibuprofen 1 mg/kg PO q 12-24 h

AUTHOR: **JÖRG MAYER**

EDITOR: **THOMAS M. DONNELLY**

SMALL MAMMALS

Bronchoscopy

OVERVIEW AND GOAL

To view and assess both the anatomy (mucosal, structural) and the function (dynamic collapse) of the airways from larynx to distal bronchi and to obtain samples from the distal airways for analysis

INDICATIONS

- Diagnostic: evaluation of lower airway and parenchymal disease (culture/cytologic examination, biopsy) and documentation of airway caliber disorders (malacia, collapse, compression, bronchiectasis, bronchial stenosis)
- Therapeutic: foreign body/secretion removal

CONTRAINDICATIONS

- Major: severe hypoxemia, unstable cardiac arrhythmias, heart failure
- Minor: significant resting expiratory effort, bronchomalacia, inexperience

EQUIPMENT, ANESTHESIA

- Equipment
  - Flexible endoscope: 3 to 5 mm in diameter, 55 to 85 cm in length
  - Mouth gag, sterile gauze, suction capabilities
  - Sterile saline
    - Preloaded in three or four 10- to 20-mL syringes for bronchoalveolar lavage (BAL)
    - For rinsing and cleaning
  - Sterile, water-soluble lubricant
  - Forceps: if foreign body removal or mucosal biopsy is required
- Anesthesia
  - Pretreatment with a bronchodilator is recommended, especially in small dogs and all cats; use injectable terbutaline 0.01 mg/kg SC at least 15 minutes before the procedure.
  - IV catheter for administration of a short-acting injectable anesthetic protocol: either atropine 0.02-0.04 mg/kg IM or glycopyrrolate 0.01-0.02 mg/kg IM; in addition, butorphanol 0.05-0.1 mg/kg IM and diazepam 0.1 mg/kg IV, followed by propofol 3-6 mg/kg, slow IV titrated to effect, with repeated miniboluses of propofol (1 mg/kg) as needed over the duration of the procedure to maintain the anesthetized state.
  - Intubation is rarely used for the procedure; an anesthesia T piece is required if the scope will be passed through the tube; jet ventilation can be used if available.
  - Provide oxygen before, during, and after the procedure; insufflate oxygen through the endoscope channel or via a 3 to 8 Fr urinary catheter passed alongside the scope during the procedure; use an endotracheal tube or a face mask for

oxygen administration before and after.
  - Topical 2% lidocaine if needed to decrease pharyngeal/laryngeal sensation, excessive coughing, and movement
  - Doxapram HCl 2.2 mg/kg IV once to assist with the evaluation of intrinsic laryngeal function
  - Electrocardiogram (ECG), oximetry, blood pressure (BP) cuff, and other monitoring equipment

ANTICIPATED TIME

A complete bronchoscopy and bronchoalveolar lavage can be completed within 10 to 20 minutes by an experienced endoscopist; animal recovery time is additional and varies with the type of anesthetic used.

PREPARATION: IMPORTANT CHECKPOINTS

- The bronchoscopist must have a good understanding of normal bronchial mucosa and lung anatomy to diagnose subtle airway abnormalities.
- The bronchoscope should be cleaned and ready for use.
- All supplies and equipment should be available before the procedure is started; anesthetic monitoring and image capture equipment should be turned on and ready to use.
- Antibiotics should be discontinued at least 72 hours before the procedure for accurate culture results.
- Chest radiographs are useful in helping to select specific lung regions for examination and for BAL.

POSSIBLE COMPLICATIONS AND COMMON ERRORS TO AVOID

- Contamination of the BAL sample is possible if care is not taken to avoid touching the upper airways during insertion of the scope. Guarded catheters may be used to decrease the potential for BAL contamination, although catheter cost limits their use.
- Pulmonary barotrauma (tracheobronchial or lung rupture) is possible if the oxygen insufflation rate exceeds the ability of the gas to exit the lungs; this is a matter of concern in smaller animals when the bronchoscope diameter is close to the tracheal size and pressure builds up in the lungs as active insufflation continues.
- Airway collapse during recovery can result in severe hypoxemia; anticipate when active expiratory effort is noted before anesthesia; slow recovery from anesthesia helps minimize this concern.

PROCEDURE

- Sternal recumbency is the recommended position in cats and dogs.
- Topical anesthesia (1% to 2% lidocaine) may be applied to the pharyngeal/laryngeal mucosa to minimize laryngospasm or excessive coughing.
- Provide oxygen as already outlined.
- Evaluate the oropharyngeal/laryngeal region; use IV doxapram HCl (2.2 mg/kg once) to stimulate intrinsic laryngeal motion.
- Insert the bronchoscope into the airways, noting changes in shape (stenosis, stricture), dynamic caliber (malacia, collapse), and mucosa (secretions, erythema, edema, masses).
- In the normal animal, the dorsal tracheal membrane is taut, so there is little if any redundancy (no visible protrusion or collapse into the airway).
- The healthy tracheobronchial mucosa is a smooth, light-pink surface with a rich supply of submucosal capillaries; if these capillaries are not visible, mucosal edema or cellular infiltration is likely present.
- Healthy mucosa has a slightly glistening appearance; mucosal edema is readily apparent because it imparts a gelatinous appearance to the epithelial surface.
- The clinician should examine the carina for abnormalities (widening, compression, mucosal infiltration) before evaluating each lobar and as many segmental and/or subsegmental bronchi as possible (as both the animal and endoscope size will allow).
- Airway bifurcations beyond the carina are referred to simply as *spurs*. Like the carina, these should form a sharp V, but they become widened and appear U shaped with chronic airway inflammation and/or mucosal edema.
- Small polypoid mucosal nodules are commonly encountered in the bronchi of dogs with chronic bronchitis.
- Small amounts of white or slightly opaque mucus may be noted in a healthy animal, but larger accumulations or secretions of unusual color are abnormal.
- The normal monopodial branching system results in gentle, smooth tapering of the airways. Changes may be focal or generalized and include those of shape and size of the airway lumen, such as an intraluminal stricture/tumor, external compression (tumor or lymphadenopathy), bronchiectasis, or dynamic collapse (malacia).
- Whether or not abnormalities are noted, samples should be obtained for culture and cytologic examination. Following the initial airway evaluation, the endoscope is removed from the animal and is cleaned by alternatively suctioning the channel with sterile saline and air immediately before reinsertion.
- The BAL site (lobe and bronchus) is chosen on the basis of radiographic and gross bronchoscopic findings. If no site is clearly abnormal, BALs from both "middle" lung lobes should be collected.
- To perform a BAL, the bronchoscope first is gently wedged into a segmental or smaller bronchus. Aliquots of 10 to 20 mL sterile saline (depending on the size of the animal) are instilled into the airway (via the suction channel or a washing pipette) and then are immediately aspirated using slow, gentle hand suction.
- Ideally, at least two different sites (lung lobes) should be lavaged, with two aliquots per site.
- A 40% to 90% return of the volume instilled is expected. Difficulty in fluid recovery results when a proportionately large endoscope is used (prevents wedging into a small bronchus), and when malacic airways collapse when suction is applied.
- If enough time is available and if anesthetic depth is appropriate, the nasopharynx should also be examined.

POST-PROCEDURE

- Provide supplemental oxygen until fully recovered.
- Crackles are commonly noted on auscultation for a short time following a BAL procedure.
- Process samples immediately.
  - Quantitated aerobic cultures should be made if possible.
  - *Mycoplasma* and anaerobic cultures are processed using Amies transport media, or fluid is submitted in a sterile tube.
  - Cytologic analysis
    - Total white blood cell (WBC) and differential cell counts should be done.
    - The predominant cell in all species should be the alveolar macrophage (70+%), with usually less than 3% to 8% of all other cell types (except the cat, which may have up to 20+% eosinophils and still be normal).
- Handling the scope
  - Immediately rinse/wipe the scope down when finished to prevent secretions from drying.
  - Clean and sterilize the scope as outlined in the manufacturer's manual.
  - Store the scope hanging up (to fully dry it) in a protected space/closet.

ALTERNATIVES AND THEIR RELATIVE MERITS

- Tracheal wash procedures are less expensive and easier to perform,

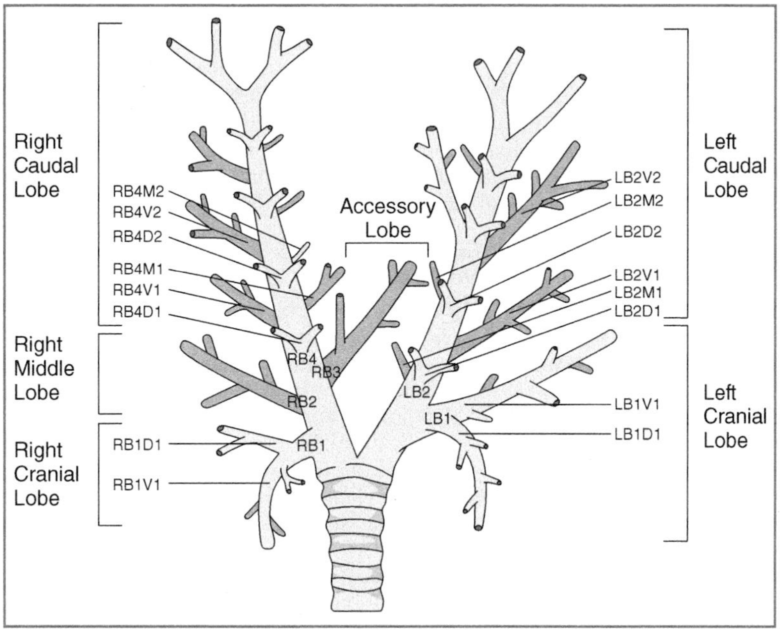

Bronchoscopy Diagrammatic representation of the normal canine tracheobronchial tree. *(Reprinted with permission from Amis T, et al: Systematic identification of endobronchial anatomy during bronchoscopy in the dog, Am J Vet Res 47:2649–2657, 1986. Johnson LR, Drazenovich TL, Hawkins MG: Endoscopic evaluation of bronchial morphology in rabbits, Am J Vet Res Sep;68(9):1022–1027, 2007.)*

but they lack the ability to provide direct sampling into specific sites; also, they provide no information regarding anatomic, structural, or functional airway abnormalities, and they have no therapeutic capability.
- Fine-needle lung aspiration biopsy has been used successfully to sample consolidated lung lobes and larger masses.

AUTHOR: **BRENDAN C. MCKIERNAN**
REPRINTED WITH PERMISSION FROM COTE E: CLINICAL VETERINARY ADVISOR, ED 2, ST. LOUIS, 2011, MOSBY.

AUTHOR & EDITOR: **JÖRG MAYER**

SMALL MAMMALS

Castration

SYNONYM

Orchiectomy (bilateral)

OVERVIEW AND GOAL

Removal of the two testes to sterilize the animal

INDICATIONS

- Control reproduction
- Reduce aggressive and sexual behavior
- Decrease musky odor (ferret)
- Protect against testicular neoplasia

CONTRAINDICATIONS

- When general anesthesia is contraindicated because of severe uncontrolled metabolic disease
- Surgical sterilization in ferrets leads to adrenal disease—consider alternatives (e.g., gonadotropin-releasing hormone [GnRH]-agonist implant such as deslorelin).

EQUIPMENT, ANESTHESIA

- General anesthesia, monitoring, preemptive analgesia, and local anesthesia are used as needed.
- Surgical equipment
  - Surgical drape
  - Scalpel blade (e.g., #11, #15)
  - Artery forceps (e.g., 12.5 cm Halstead Mosquito—straight or curved)
  - Dissecting forceps for intermittent, temporary grasping of soft tissue (e.g., 13 cm Adson, Gillies, or McIndoe plain end; 11.5 cm Continental Standard or Bonney Lane; 15 cm Debakey or Cooley)
  - Scissors (e.g., 14 cm Mayo straight or curved, 14 cm Metzenbaum)
  - Needle holder (e.g., 14 cm Mayo-Hegar)
  - Sutures, absorbable, size (UPS) 3-0 or 4-0 (e.g., Vicryl Rapide [short-term absorption], Vicryl [medium-term absorption], or PDS II [long-term absorption])
  - Tissue adhesive (e.g., Tissue-Glue, Vetbond, Nexabond)

PREPARATION: IMPORTANT CHECKPOINTS

- Perform a full physical examination and hematology/biochemistry analysis (at least urea, PCV, glucose, total protein) to ensure that the patient can undergo general anesthesia.

- The scrotum of rabbits is extremely thin and fragile. Be careful when using clippers to shave scrotal fur that the scrotum is not torn.

ANATOMICAL CONSIDERATIONS

- Ferret
  - The scrotum has two cavities (or sacs), each of which contains a testis and epididymis. Within the scrotal sac on the dorsal aspect of the testis lies the epididymis, which is composed of a mass of convoluted spermatic ducts that are divided into head, body, and tail. The ductus deferens is accompanied by the deferent artery and vein and the main testicular artery and vein, which, with the nerve and lymphatic system vessels, form the spermatic cord.
  - Ferrets are sexually mature between 6 and 9 months and can be castrated at this age.
- Rabbit
  - The inguinal ring is open. The testes descend at 10 weeks, and hairless scrotal sacs can be seen cranial to the penis. The relatively large testes with their large epididymal fat pads can be in an abdominal or scrotal position.
- Rodents
  - In all rodents, the inguinal ring is permanently open, and a functional cremaster muscle allows the testicles to migrate into and out of the abdominal cavity. If the testicles ascend into the abdominal cavity during the procedure, place a little pressure on the abdominal cavity in a cranial-to-caudal direction to make the testicles descend back into a scrotal position.
- Rat
  - In adults, the scrotum is easily visible ventrolateral to the anus. The skin of the scrotum is thin and covered with fine hairs. The testes descend between 30 and 40 days. The testis is oval and measures 20 × 14 mm. The head and tail of the epididymis are often sites of extremely large fat pads.
- Hamster
  - In mature males, a thick fat pad covers the proximal end of the testicle and almost half the epididymis (the dorsomedial side of the testicle). The fat pad gives the hamster a large scrotal silhouette.
- Guinea pig, chinchilla, and degu
  - The scrotum is not well developed, and the testicles are located lateral to the penis in the inguinal region on each side. The scrotum contains the testes, epididymis, and caudal spermatic cord. Caviomorphs have a large epididymal fat pad within the vaginal tunic that helps prevent intestinal hernia. The large seminal vesicles partially occlude the internal inguinal ring, preventing herniation. Most caviomorph rodents have large fat bodies in the abdominal cavity on each side, through which the spermatic cord passes into the inguinal canal.

POSSIBLE COMPLICATIONS AND COMMON ERRORS TO BE AVOIDED

- Hemorrhage if the ligature on the testis pedicle slips. If this occurs, reopen the surgical site to establish where the bleeding is coming from, and replace the ligature.
- Dehiscence of the wound
  - If the wound is clean and is not infected, additional sutures can be placed.
  - If the wound is dirty or infected, it must be cleaned, and secondary intention healing is the preferred method of incisional closure.
- Sutures gnawed or eaten by the patient: this occurs frequently in rats and hamsters
  - If the wound is clean and is not infected, additional sutures and/or tissue adhesive can be used to close the incision. Place an Elizabethan collar on the patient to prevent further chewing of sutures.
  - If the wound is dirty or infected, it must be cleaned and secondary intention healing allowed to occur. Place an Elizabethan collar on the patient to prevent further chewing of sutures.
  - The use of tissue adhesive is recommended in all cases to prevent this situation.
- Inguinal hernia if an open technique is used and the tunica vaginalis is not closed

PROCEDURE

- Open technique
  - With the patient in dorsal recumbency, the fur is clipped around the scrotum, penis, and inner thighs. This area is prepared aseptically.
  - Hold one testis between the thumb and the forefinger.
  - Make a 1.5- to 2-cm-long incision with the blade, through the scrotum parallel to the penis, about in the middle line of the scrotum.
  - Make the same incision on the tunic.
  - Put pressure on the testicle with your thumb and forefinger to exteriorize the testicle, the ductus deferens, their vascular supply, and the epididymal fat pad.
  - The ligament of the tail of the epididymis is broken.
  - A double ligature (4-0 or 3-0 absorbable suture) is placed proximally to the epididymal fat pad.
  - The stump of the fat pad is reentered in the tunic.
  - The tunic is closed with one or two X-shaped sutures using 4-0 or 3-0 absorbable sutures. In ferrets, because the inguinal ring is closed, there is no need to close the tunic.
  - The skin is closed using tissue glue or 4-0 or 3-0 absorbable sutures in a single-interrupted pattern.
- Closed technique
  - The beginning of this technique is the same as the open technique, but the tunica vaginalis is not incised.
  - The tunic is carefully dissected from its attachment to the scrotum.
  - The tunic is exteriorized with the testis and the tail of the epididymis inside.
  - Two ligatures (4-0 or 3-0 absorbable suture) are placed on the cord.
  - The skin is closed using tissue adhesive or 4-0 or 3-0 absorbable sutures in a single-interrupted pattern.
- Abdominal technique
  - In small rodents, some authors describe this technique to prevent the risk of infection because the scrotal incision is close to the anus and the penis and may be contaminated with urine and/or feces. This technique also prevents the risk of hernia through the inguinal ring.
  - Patient in dorsal recumbency: the fur is clipped around the umbilicus. This area is prepared aseptically.
  - An abdominal incision of 1 cm is made medially, 1 cm caudal to the umbilicus.
  - The testicle is gently pushed cranially by applying pressure on the scrotum.
  - The testicle is exteriorized by grasping the fat pad or the epididymis with nontraumatic dissecting forceps.
  - The ligament of the tail of the epididymis is broken.
  - Two ligatures (4-0 or 3-0 absorbable suture) are placed proximally to the epididymal fat pad.
  - The same technique is used with the second testicle.
  - The abdominal wall is closed with a continuous pattern using 3-0 or 4-0 absorbable sutures.
  - The skin is closed with an intradermal continuous pattern using 4-0 absorbable sutures and tissue adhesive, or with 4-0 or 3-0 absorbable cutaneous sutures in a single-interrupted pattern.

POST-PROCEDURE

- Analgesia for 3 to 5 days

- Remove cage bedding, litter, and substrate for 1 week; place paper towels on the bottom of the cage instead.
- Recheck the surgical wound 10 days after surgery.

ALTERNATIVES AND THEIR RELATIVE MERITS

- Deslorelin implants (GnRH agonist) can be used in ferrets to achieve chemical castration and reduce the musky odor.
- The implant is active for 2 to 2.5 years and is placed subcutaneously.
- Data on other exotic mammal species are not available.

REFERENCES

Jenkins JR: Surgical sterilization in small mammals, spay and castration. Vet Clin North Am Exot Anim Pract 3:617–627, 2000.
Ludwig L, et al: Soft tissue surgery. In Quesenberry KE, et al, editors: Ferrets, rabbits, and rodents: clinical medicine and surgery, ed 2, New York, 2004, Elsevier, pp 132–133.
O'Malley B: Section 4, Small mammals. In O'Malley B, editor: Clinical anatomy and physiology of exotic species: structure and function of mammals, birds, reptiles, and amphibians, St Louis, 2005, Saunders Elsevier, pp 163–261.
Pignon C, et al: Stérilisation de convenance des petits mammifères. In Bulliot C, editor: Chirurgie des tissus mous et dentisterie des petits mammifères de compagnie, Le Point Vétérinaire, 2009, Numéro spécial, pp 35–41.
Redrobe S: Soft tissue surgery of rabbits and rodents. Semin Avian Exot Pet Med 11:231–245, 2002.

AUTHOR: **CHARLY PIGNON**

EDITOR: **JÖRG MAYER**

SMALL MAMMALS

Echocardiography

SYNONYM

Cardiac ultrasound

OVERVIEW AND GOALS

- Echocardiography gives valuable information about cardiac anatomy and function, the presence of abnormal communications between cardiac chambers or vessels, and cardiac blood flow.
- Diagnostic choice for diagnosing structural and functional cardiac abnormalities
- Can detect mediastinal masses and can help detect heartworm disease
- Used in conjunction with good quality radiographs to identify severity of cardiac disease and presence of congestive heart failure (CHF)
- A complete echocardiograph can reveal congenital or acquired cardiac lesions.
- Evaluate valvular function
- Quantify systolic and diastolic functions
- Estimate chamber size

INDICATIONS

- Congenital or acquired cardiac disease
- Radiographs in combination with an echocardiogram should be performed to evaluate cardiac size if concern exists.

CONTRAINDICATIONS

- Should be stable enough to handle manual restraint
- Heavy sedation (e.g., midazolam) is suggested if animal is stressed or diseased.

EQUIPMENT, ANESTHESIA

- Ultrasound machine
- Ultrasound gel
- Isopropyl alcohol
- Hair clippers

ANTICIPATED TIME

5 to 10 minutes

PREPARATION: IMPORTANT CHECKPOINTS

- Fasting is not needed.
- Clip hair where ultrasound probe will be used.

POSSIBLE COMPLICATIONS AND COMMON ERRORS TO BE AVOIDED

Use high-frequency transducers to obtain quality images.

PROCEDURE

- Obtain with or without sedation (sedation may affect values).
- Place patient in right and left lateral recumbency.
- Place electrocardiograph (ECG) clips on patient, as recommended by the manufacturer.
- Two-dimensional ECG provides assessment of cardiac size and function.
- Standard M-mode measurements are obtained, including chamber dimensions, wall thickness, and indices of systolic function.
- Spectral Doppler imaging is used to quantify the velocity of normal and abnormal blood flow.
- Color flow Doppler echocardiography allows visual inspection of blood flow direction and detection of turbulent flow, including valvular regurgitation.
- As in most mammals, the left atrial diameter is 1.0 to 1.5 times the diameter of the aorta, left and right atria are comparable in size, the aorta and the main pulmonary artery have the same diameter, and the left ventricular free wall thickness is similar to the interventricular septum thickness in healthy exotic herbivores.
- The thickness of the right ventricular free wall and the diameter of the right ventricular chamber are one-third to one-half of their counterpart in the left ventricle.

POST-PROCEDURE

- Remove ECG clips.
- Remove remaining ultrasound gel from animal.

AUTHOR: **JÖRG MAYER**

EDITOR: **THOMAS M. DONNELLY**

Table Reference Echocardiographic Measures of Small Exotic Herbivores

Parameter, mm	Rabbit	Guinea Pig	Chinchilla
LVIDd	12.88-15.86	6.49-7.21	5.1-6.9
LVIDs	8.83-11.27	4.18-4.52	2.3-4.3
LVPWd	1.91-2.41	1.44-2.06	2.0-2.8
LVPWs	2.93-4.03	1.91-2.61	—
IVSd	1.66-2.40	1.88-2.68	1.5-2.3
IVSs	2.60-3.5	2.22-3.38	—
LA	8.52-10.80	4.61-5.29	4.3-5.9
AO	7.50-9.02	4.40-4.90	3.7-6.0

Range derived from mean ± 1 SD; animals anesthetized in most instances.
Abbreviations: *AO,* Aorta; *d,* diastolic; *IVS,* internal ventricular septum; *LA,* left atrium; *LVID,* left ventricular internal diameter; *LVPW,* left ventricular posterior wall; *s,* systolic.

SMALL MAMMALS

E-Collars

SYNONYM

Elizabethan collar

OVERVIEW AND GOALS

- Prevent birds or mammals from creating further damage by self-mutilation to an existing injury
- E-collars should be used as the last resort in birds and mammals because the E-collar itself can induce trauma to the patient, and placement can be stressful for the animal.

INDICATIONS

To prevent further injury

CONTRAINDICATIONS

If pet stops eating or drinking, collar may have to be removed.

EQUIPMENT, ANESTHESIA

- Collar fitted for patient
- Foam insulation for waterpipes works well to "stiffen" neck in birds.
- If commercial E-collars are unavailable, one can be made:
  - Radiograph film
    - Cut to size indicated for patient
    - Add cotton cast padding if needed to soften edges.
  - Soft fabric
    - Depending on location and patient, a t-shirt–like apparatus or a drape can be prepared (e.g., feather picking).

POSSIBLE COMPLICATIONS AND COMMON ERRORS TO BE AVOIDED

Size patient for correct E-collar to prevent further damage to injury or creation of new injury.

PROCEDURE

- When placing a homemade E-collar around the neck, allow one or two fingerwidths to the neck circumference to ensure proper loose placement.
- Depending on injury and patient:
  - Place E-collar on patient as you would on a dog or cat
  - Place E-collar on backward, so the collar bends over the patient's body (to protect thoracic area) and to avoid "blinder" effect

AUTHOR: **JÖRG MAYER**

EDITOR: **THOMAS M. DONNELLY**

SMALL MAMMALS

Electrocardiography

SYNONYMS

ECG, EKG

OVERVIEW AND GOALS

- Electrocardiogram (ECG) should be used most often for the diagnosis of arrhythmias when an irregular rhythm is detected on auscultation.
- To obtain tracings of heart rhythm
- To identify abnormal rhythm and conduction disturbances
- Optimal choice for evaluating cardiac arrhythmias

INDICATIONS

- To confirm cardiac disease
- Part of general monitoring during anesthesia
- Monitoring of cardiac arrhythmias
- Little is known about the electrocardiographic changes associated with cardiac disease in exotic herbivores; therefore, the use of P wave and QRS complex morphology changes to assess cardiac chamber dilatation or hypertrophy is not recommended.
- The ECG is usually recorded with the patient gently restrained in sternal recumbency using alligator clips.

CONTRAINDICATIONS

- Should be stable enough to handle manual restraint

- Heavy sedation (e.g., midazolam) is suggested if animal is stressed or diseased.

EQUIPMENT, ANESTHESIA

- Standard ECG machine
- Alcohol or ultrasound gel

ANTICIPATED TIME

5 minutes

PREPARATION: IMPORTANT CHECKPOINTS

- Because ferrets and rabbits object to alcohol on their skin, ultrasound gel can be used.
- Clips can pinch the skin, so ECG clips can be flattened to reduce discomfort.
- Distract ferrets with Nutrical.

POSSIBLE COMPLICATIONS AND COMMON ERRORS TO BE AVOIDED

- Minimize artifact by:
  - Using enough gel for conduction between skin and clips
  - Preventing patient/metal contact
  - Choosing a quiet, comfortable environment
  - Minimizing movement that can mimic abnormal events
- Second-degree atrioventricular (AV) block can be seen in normal healthy ferrets.

PROCEDURE

- Lay patient in lateral recumbency.
- Offer ferrets food as a distraction.
- Place alcohol or gel on the patient at the site of the ECG clips.
- Apply clips as indicated by the manufacturer.
- Monitor ECG for 4 minutes.
- Remove clips and gel from the animal.
- Normal cardiac activity of exotic herbivores results in a positive P wave followed by a primarily upright QRS complex in lead II.
- The T wave is usually positive, which reflects ventricular repolarization.
- The ECG of normal rabbits includes a pointed P wave in some breeds, peaked T waves, and a relatively long ST segment.
- The guinea pig ECG tracing more closely mimics that of humans when compared with other exotic herbivores because of the similarity of ion channels.

POST-PROCEDURE

Incorporate data from examination and radiographic findings with ECG measurements.

AUTHOR: **JÖRG MAYER**

EDITOR: **THOMAS M. DONNELLY**

Table **Reference Electrocardiographic Measurements of Small Exotic Herbivores**

Parameter, units	Guinea Pig	Rabbit
P wave duration, sec	0.015-0.035	0.01-0.05
P wave amplitude, mV	0.01	0.04-0.12
P-R interval, sec	0.048-0.060	0.04-0.08
QRS duration, sec	0.008-0.046	0.02-0.06
R wave amplitude, mV	1.1-1.9	0.03-0.39
QT interval, sec	0.106-0.144	0.08-0.16
T wave amplitude, mV	0.062	0.05-0.17
Mean electrical axis, degrees	120 to 180	−43 to +80

SMALL MAMMALS

Feeding Tube Placement in Rabbits and Rodents

OVERVIEW AND GOALS

- Feeding critically ill patients that cannot eat or refuse to eat is essential to the recovery of the pet.
- Enteral nutrition facilitates administration of the correct nutrition and medication needed to meet requirements.
- Nasogastric tubes seem to be tolerated better by patients than orogastric tubes; however, the smaller tube size limits the products that can be fed to the patient.
- Liquid diets must be prepared that are high calorie, to help overcome the nutritional deficit that the patient will experience.
- Pharyngostomy tubes can be surgically placed, allowing commercially prepared diets to be delivered.

INDICATIONS

Anorectic rabbits and rodents

CONTRAINDICATIONS

- This procedure may require some sedation in smaller patients.
- Animals with recurrent vomiting or regurgitation
- Semiconsciousness or unconsciousness
- Severe coagulopathies
- If GI stasis already caused stomach bloat
- Stomach outflow obstruction

EQUIPMENT, ANESTHESIA

- Nasogastric
  - Proparacaine
  - Flexible infant nasogastric tube
  - Marker to mark length of tube required
  - Lubricating jelly
  - Butterfly tape
  - Suture material
  - E-collar
  - Radiograph machine
  - High-calorie liquid nutrition
    - Critical HN (Mead Johnson Nutritionals, Evansville, IN)
    - Canned pumpkin to add fiber

ANTICIPATED TIME

5 minutes

PREPARATION: IMPORTANT CHECKPOINTS

- Select the largest tube that will fit through the nares.

- Premeasure feeding tube by placing against the animal and determining the length from the nasal opening to the stomach; mark the tube.

POSSIBLE COMPLICATIONS AND COMMON ERRORS TO BE AVOIDED

- Excessive use of proparacaine
- Tube obstruction with food particles
- Rhinitis
- Esophageal reflux
- Vomiting or regurgitation
- Aspiration of vomit or regurgitated material
- Aspiration pneumonia

PROCEDURE

- Nasogastric tube
  - Place several drops of proparacaine ophthalmic anesthetic onto nasal membrane.
  - Lubricate the tube with jelly.
  - After 3 minutes, introduce the nasogastric tube into the nasal meatus, directing it caudally and ventrally. If patient objects, withdraw and apply more proparacaine.
  - After passing the tube, secure the tube by placing butterfly tape and suturing it to the top of the patient's head, between the ears.
    - It can also be recommended to preplace these sutures so that the animal does not dislodge the tube when trying to suture in place.
  - Check for correct placement with
    - A lateral radiograph
    - Injection of air into the tube and auscultation of the stomach for gurgling sounds
    - DO NOT INJECT WATER in case of incorrect tube placement.
  - Place E-collar to prevent patient from pulling out the tube.
  - Feed patient a liquid diet designed for rabbits or rodents.
- Pharyngostomy
  - Procedure is exactly the same as for dogs and cats.

POST-PROCEDURE

- The maximum tolerable amount of food should be 5 to 6 mL/ 100 g body weight per meal. Split the daily diet amount into two meals (at noontime and in the evening) because this can help prevent reflux.
- Ensure that the tube does not migrate out.
- Flush the tube with water (greater than the volume of the tube itself) before and after feeding to prevent obstruction.
- Food should be administered slowly to prevent distention in the stomach.

AUTHOR: **JÖRG MAYER**

EDITOR: **THOMAS M. DONNELLY**

SMALL MAMMALS

Fluid Therapy in Rabbits and Rodents

OVERVIEW AND GOALS

- Perfusion deficits are corrected based on
  - Capillary refill time (CRT)
    - Decreased refill time
  - Mucous membranes
    - Mucus membranes become tacky and pale.
  - Blood pressure
    - Decreased blood pressure
  - Dehydration
    - Decreased skin turgor
- Any deficit greater than 12% can cause perfusion abnormalities:
  - Cold extremities
  - Decreased urine output
  - Tachycardia
  - Bradycardia
  - Weak pulses
- The goal should be to give the least amount of fluid to reach desired goals (and prevent fluid overload).

INDICATIONS

- Dehydration
- Surgery
- Trauma/injury

EQUIPMENT, ANESTHESIA

- Fluid of choice
- Administration set
- IV fluid pump

POSSIBLE COMPLICATIONS AND COMMON ERRORS TO BE AVOIDED

- With any fluid administration, observe for signs of overhydration.
  - Serous nasal discharge
  - Chemosis
  - Tachycardia
  - Cough
  - Pulmonary crackles and edema
  - Dyspnea
- Remove catheter after 72 hours.
- Complications associated with long-term catheter placement:
  - Bacterial endocarditis
  - Thrombophlebitis
  - Thromboembolism

PROCEDURE

Fluid choice

- Crystalloids
  - Can be chosen based on clinical findings
  - Primarily water with sodium and glucose base, with some additional electrolytes
  - Crystalloids distribute to all body compartments.
  - Replace interstitial and intravascular fluid losses
  - Rehydrate over 12 to 24 hours
  - Surgery rate: 10 mL/kg/h
  - Maintenance rate is 80-120 mL/kg/d.
    - 0.9% NaCl
      - Treat for:
        - Hyperkalemia
        - Hypercalcemia
        - Hypochloremic metabolic alkalosis
    - Contents of normal saline
      - Na = 154 mEq/L
      - Cl = 154 mEq/L
      - pH = 5.4
    - Lactated Ringer's solution (LRS)
      - Used to correct acidosis
      - Do not use the same line to administer blood products.
      - Contents of LRS:
        - Na = 130 mEq/L but total cations of 137 mEq/L (still is isotonic)
        - Cl = 109 mEq/L
        - Lactate = 28 mEq/L
        - K = 4 mEq/L
        - CA = 3 mEq/L
    - Normosol (is NOT just normal saline)
      - Normosol contains added K and Mg, which may be unsuitable for some patients such as patients with renal failure.
      - Contents of Normosol:
        - Na = 140 mEq/L

- Cl = 98 mEq/L
- K = 4 mEq/L
- Mg = 3 mEq/L
- Acetate = 27 mEq/L
- Gluconate = 23 mEq/L
- pH = 6.6
- 5% dextrose
  - Rarely indicated
  - Once dextrose is metabolized, only water remains.
- Plasmalyte
  - Contents of Plasmalyte A
    - Na = 140 mEq/L
    - Cl = 98 mEq/L
    - K = 5 mEq/L
    - Mg = 3 mEq/L
    - Acetate = 27 mEq/L
    - Gluconate = 23 mEq/L
    - pH = 7.4 (Plasmalyte 148: pH = 5.5)
- Hypertonic saline
  - A hyperosmolar crystalloid used to treat hypovolemia
  - Leads to rapid intravascular volume expansion
    - 5 mL/kg over 5 to 10 minutes
  - Expansion is transient, and additional colloids must be added.
  - Observe for the following:
    - Hypernatremia
    - Hyperchloremia
    - Hypokalemia
    - Dehydration
    - Avoid using in dehydrated patients.
- Perioperative
  - 5% to 10% blood loss: crystalloid
  - Administer at 3 times the volume of estimated blood loss.

- Colloids
  - Can be chosen for critical and hypotensive cases
  - Contain large molecules that do not pass through the capillary membranes
  - Aid in the expansion of intravascular fluid volume and oncotic pressure
    - Whole blood
      - 5-10 mL/kg/h
    - Plasma
      - Observe for potential reactions.
        - Swollen head and limbs
    - Hetastarch
      - 10-20 mL/kg/d
      - Hetastarch with crystalloids: reduces the need for crystalloids 33% to 50%
      - In shock, administer a Hetastarch bolus 5 mL/kg over 15 minutes.
      - Can be repeated; dose cannot exceed 20 mL/kg/d
      - Increases activated clotting time
    - Dextran 70
      - May prolong bleeding times
    - Albumin
      - Observe for potential reactions:
        - Swollen head and limbs
  - Can use in conjunction with crystalloid therapy, reducing by 40% to 60% the volume needed
  - Perioperative
    - 10% to 20% loss: choose hetastarch or plasma
    - 20% to 30% whole blood
- Subcutaneous fluid administration
  - Not ideal in critically ill patients, but may be the only way to administer fluids
    - Adult rabbits: 100-150 mL/kg/24 h
    - Guinea pig and chinchilla: 100 mL/kg/24 h
    - Rodents: 10 mL/kg
  - Divide total daily dose into three administrations given q 8 h.
  - Administer fluids under the loose skin, over the shoulders and back.

AUTHOR: **JÖRG MAYER**

EDITOR: **THOMAS M. DONNELLY**

SMALL MAMMALS

Intraosseous Catheters

OVERVIEW AND GOAL

It may be difficult to place an IV catheter in patients in critical condition with low blood pressure. Fluids and some medications may be given intraosseously until an intravenous catheter can be established.

INDICATIONS

Critically ill patients

CONTRAINDICATIONS

This is a very painful procedure; therefore, appropriate analgesia has to be used.

EQUIPMENT, ANESTHESIA

- Anesthesia (if needed; many critically ill patients will not need sedation)
  - Use isoflurane only.
- Spinal needle
  - Ideal to prevent bone plugs
- Teflon catheter, 18 to 23 gauge, 1 to 1.5 inches in length
  - If spinal needle is not available
- Saline
- Lidocaine for topical analgesia
- Surgical blade
- Betadine and alcohol to prepare area aseptically
- Male adapter
- Tape to secure catheter.
- Antimicrobial ointment
- Fluids
- E-collar

ANTICIPATED TIME

10 minutes

PREPARATION: IMPORTANT CHECKPOINTS

Best location is in the greater trochanter of the femur or tibial crest.

PROCEDURE

- Sedate or anesthetize.
- Clip hair over selected site and prepare aseptically.
- If indicated, inject lidocaine as a local anesthetic.
- Glove.
- Palpate top of the greater trochanter or the tibial crest with your finger.
- Create a stab incision with a surgical blade.
- Pass the needle (size is patient dependent: 18 to 23 gauge and 1 to 1.5 inches in length).
- Insert needle anterograde, parallel to the long axis of the femur and into the medullary cavity.
  - Once the needle is in the marrow cavity, no resistance should be noted. If you meet resistance, you are hitting the cortical bone. Withdraw the needle and redirect it.
- Flush needle gently with saline and attach a male adapter.
- Apply antimicrobial ointment to the insertion site, and place dressing over the entire unit.
- Replacement fluids can be administered by slow drip. When the patient is rehydrated, replace with IV catheter and remove IO catheter.
- Place an E-collar on the patient to prevent IO removal.

POST-PROCEDURE

- Fluid requirements: 20-25 mL/d plus deficit correction
- Shock: 25-40 mL/kg/24 h
- Pain medication

- Rabbits
  - Butorphanol 0.1-1.0 mg/kg SC, IM, IV q 4-6 h
  - Buprenorphine 0.01-0.05 mg/kg SC, IM, IV q 6-12 h
  - Morphine 2-5 mg/kg SC, IM q 2-4 h
  - Carprofen 1-2.2 mg/kg PO q 12 h
  - Ibuprofen 2-7.5 mg/kg PO q 12-24 h
  - Meloxicam 0.5 mg/kg SC, PO q 24 h
- Ferrets
  - Butorphanol: 0.05-0.5 mg/kg SC, IM, IV q 8-12 h
  - Buprenorphine 0.01-0.03 mg/kg SC, IM, IV q 8-12 h
  - Morphine: 0.5-5 mg/kg SC, IM q 2-6 h
  - Carprofen: 1.0 mg/kg PO q 12-24 h
  - Ibuprofen: 1 mg/kg PO q 12-24 h

- Remove catheter within 72 hours.

AUTHOR: **JÖRG MAYER**

EDITOR: **THOMAS M. DONNELLY**

SMALL MAMMALS

Intubation Technique in Rabbits and Rodents

OVERVIEW AND GOALS

- Respiratory depression, obstruction, and hypoventilation are common causes of death in rabbits and rodents. Intubation allows ventilation and prevents aspiration of vomit.
- Patients must be adequately sedated before intubation, decreasing the risk of injury from the technique.

INDICATIONS

Endotracheal intubation is indicated for upper airway protection, administration of oxygen and inhalant anesthesia, and assisted ventilation when needed.

CONTRAINDICATIONS

- Smaller endotracheal tubes (ETs) increase the risk of obstruction from mucus or saliva secretions.
- Can create trauma to larynx
- Analyze risk versus benefit with length of procedure, ensuring that ET intubation is indicated.

EQUIPMENT, ANESTHESIA

- Clear ETs are recommended, allowing visualization of obstructions or mucous plugs in the tubes.
- Endotracheal tubes
  - Rabbits 2 to 3 mm
  - Rats, guinea pigs: 14 to 16 gauge, over-the-needle catheter
- Pediatric laryngoscope
- Polyurethane catheters (to use as a guide)
- Topical anesthesia
  - Lidocaine

ANTICIPATED TIME

Less than 5 minutes

PREPARATION: IMPORTANT CHECKPOINTS

- Premeasure endotracheal tube or over-the-needle catheter to see how far the device should be inserted.
- Rabbits and rodents should not be fasted before anesthesia because high metabolism and small glycogen reserves predispose patients to hypoglycemia.

POSSIBLE COMPLICATIONS AND COMMON ERRORS TO BE AVOIDED

- Check the patient's oral cavity (especially guinea pigs) before intubation because food is often left in the mouth.
- Intubation is difficult in these species and in some cases may be unachievable.
- Patient should be adequately sedated before intubation is attempted, to prevent damage from the procedure.
- Stop attempts to intubate after 1 minute, or if trauma occurs to the site.

PROCEDURE

- Rabbits
  - Head and neck should be extended to align the pharynx and trachea with the oropharynx. Be careful to not hyperextend because this can cause spinal injury.
  - Because rabbits are nasal breathers, you must displace the epiglottis ventral to the soft palate to visualize the glottis.
  - Rabbits must be adequately relaxed before intubation. This is indicated by the absence of response to a toe or ear pinch.
  - Polyurethane catheters can be used as a guide for ET.
  - Dilute lidocaine and apply to glottis.
  - Two techniques are used to intubate rabbits: blind and direct visualization
    - Blind visualization: requires spontaneous respiration for accurate endotracheal placement and relies on respiratory noise. Place rabbit in sternal recumbency and have assistant grasp head from above and behind with the fingers under the lower jaw. Insert ET tube into the space between the incisors and the first premolar, and pass caudally over the tongue. Slightly hyperextend the head and pass the tube into the glottis, listening for respiratory sounds. Gurgling indicates that the tube is in the esophagus. Withdraw the ET until respiratory noise is heard again, and advance into the trachea. It may help to rotate the tube 180°. The rabbit may cough out the tube; therefore, be sure to secure it immediately. Do not continue for longer than 1 minute, and stop if hemorrhage or laryngeal edema occurs. Secure the tube with tie gauze, behind the ears. Verify tube placement with lung sounds; ensure that the ET is not in a single bronchus.
    - Direct: have assistant open the jaw with gauze around upper and lower incisors. Grasp tongue with gauze and pull aside. Insert laryngoscope with pediatric tip into oropharynx. Hyperextend the head and displace the glottis. Insert tube into trachea. You may need to use a small-diameter catheter as a guide, passing the ET over top. You can also place the rabbit in dorsal recumbency to facilitate visualization of the glottis. Do not continue for longer than 1 minute, and stop if hemorrhage or laryngeal edema occurs. Secure the tube with tie gauze, behind the ears. Verify tube placement with lung sounds; ensure that the ET is not in a single bronchus.
- Guinea pigs
  - Use blind technique as already described. Place rodent in lateral recumbency with head and neck moderately extended
  - Guinea pigs can be difficult and will regurgitate if the oropharynx is stimulated. The cheeks of guinea pigs

generally contain food, and they produce salivary secretions profusely. Secretions can be controlled with glycopyrrolate.
   - The soft palate of guinea pigs is fused to the base of the tongue, and entry to the glottis is made through a small opening called the *palatal ostium.* This is easily traumatized, which can result in profuse bleeding. Therefore, guinea pigs can be difficult to intubate; however, it can be accomplished by placing the patient in a dorsally recumbent position and using a 14-gauge over-the-needle catheter. Verify tube placement with lung sounds; ensure that the ET is not in a single bronchus.
- Rats
   - Direct visualization of the glottis requires magnification and a direct light source.
   - Use an ear speculum that has the distal two-thirds removed along the right side.
   - Place the rat in dorsal recumbency, and use a 14-gauge or 16-gauge over-the-needle catheter.
   - The assistant can use gauze to open the upper and lower jaw. Use a cotton-tipped applicator to clear secretions and grasp the tongue. Apply topical anesthetic to the glottis to reduce laryngospasm.
   - Insert catheter into trachea and secure a surgical suture to the catheter. Secure suture to prevent excess insertion of catheter into trachea. Mucous obstruction does occur, so you may need to change catheter frequently.
   - Verify tube placement with lung sounds; ensure that the ET is not in a single bronchus, skin, over the shoulders, and back.

POST-PROCEDURE

- Monitor postoperatively for heart rate, respiratory rate, and temperature.
- Ensure that pain medication is administered, if indicated.

AUTHOR: **JÖRG MAYER**

EDITOR: **THOMAS M. DONNELLY**

SMALL MAMMALS

Nasolacrimal Cannulation of Rabbits

OVERVIEW AND GOALS

- The nasolacrimal drainage system is a means of transport for tears from the lacrimal lake to the nasal cavity.
- The rabbit eye has a single punctum, located midway between the margin of the lower palpebrum and the nictitans near the medial canthus. The opening measures 2 to 4 mm and, depending on the size of the patient, may be pigmented.
- Dacrocystitis and nasal duct obstruction can cause epiphora, which is one of the most common ocular problems for rabbits.
- Common pathogens associated with obstructed lacrimal ducts include *Pasteurella, Bacillus subtilis, Staphylococcus aureus, Bordetella, Pseudomonas, Haemophilus, Treponema paraluiscuniculi, Mycoplasma,* chlamydiae, and myxoma virus.

INDICATIONS

- Chronic conjunctivitis is common; flushing is required to clear the infection.
- Dental disease and sinusitis can cause an obstruction in the nasolacrimal duct.

CONTRAINDICATIONS

- Rabbits have powerful hind legs and kick violently. Without proper restraint, rabbits can fracture their vertebrae.
- Never pick rabbits up by their ears.
- Avoid repeated or forceful flushing because iatrogenic trauma can worsen the situation.

EQUIPMENT, ANESTHESIA

- Examination gloves
- Proparacaine
- Standard lacrimal cannula or a 24-gauge Teflon catheter without the stylet
- Tranquilization can be used; assess the temperament of the rabbit because many will allow the procedure to be completed without sedation.
- Chemical restraint may be used when rabbits become stressed and fractious:
   - Midazolam 1 mg/kg IM can be used as a preanesthetic.
   - Ketamine 5-15 mg/kg IM can be used as a preanesthetic.
   - Ketamine/Midazolam 25 mg/kg and 1 mg/kg IM produces excellent relaxation.
- Isoflurane and sevoflurane are easy to administer, and pets recover well.
- Warmed sterile saline
- Sterile syringe if culture is indicated
- Sterile red top tube to collect sample
- Medication to flush duct, if indicated

ANTICIPATED TIME

5 minutes, depending on severity of obstruction

PREPARATION: IMPORTANT CHECKPOINTS

Wear gloves to prevent contamination and spread of potential pathogens

POSSIBLE COMPLICATIONS AND COMMON ERRORS TO BE AVOIDED

Metal cannulas are available but must be sterilized between patients and can cause iatrogenic trauma.

PROCEDURE

- Apply proparacaine to the eye, and allow to sit for 3 minutes.
- Restrain the patient:
   - Scruff the patient with one hand and support the hind quarters with the other. Do not allow rabbits to kick because they can fracture their vertebrae.
   - If needed, wrap a towel around the rabbit (like a burrito) to aid in restraint.
- To assess patency of the duct, fluorescein dye can be placed into the eye and the rabbit can be observed for the presence of dye at the nasal aperture of the duct.
- A standard lacrimal cannula or a Teflon intravenous catheter without the stylet can be used to enter the punctum to flush the duct with a saline solution or medication of choice.
- Saline can be warmed to decrease discomfort.
- If a culture is required, flush sterile saline into the catheter with a sterile syringe. Place a collection cup beneath the rabbit's nose, and lavage.

POST-PROCEDURE

- Recurrence is common; flushing may have to be performed every 2 or 3 days or weekly until consecutive clear flushings occur.
- In chronic and severe infections, ophthalmic and oral antibiotics may be flushed into the duct.

AUTHOR: **JÖRG MAYER**

EDITOR: **THOMAS M. DONNELLY**

SMALL MAMMALS

Ovariohysterectomy

SYNONYMS

- Spay
- Ovariectomy—removal of the ovary: not done
- Ovariohysterectomy—removal of ovaries and uterus: typical
- Ovariohysterovaginectomy—when neutering a female rabbit, the surgical procedure consists of an incision made through the vagina distal to the vaginal fornix.

OVERVIEW AND GOAL

Removal of the female gonads and part of the genital tract to sterilize the animal

INDICATIONS

- Control reproduction
- Dystocia
- Infection of the genital tract
- Uterine prolapse (chinchilla)
- Decrease the musky odor in ferrets
- Prevent life-threatening bone marrow suppression caused by chronically high estrogen levels in ferrets
- Prevent neoplasia of the genital tract, the mammary gland (rats), and the pituitary gland (rats)

CONTRAINDICATIONS

- When general anesthesia is contraindicated because of severe uncontrolled metabolic disease
- Ferrets in estrus with a low packed cell volume (PCV) (<20%)
- Surgical sterilization in ferrets leads to adrenal disease.

EQUIPMENT, ANESTHESIA

- General anesthesia, monitoring, preemptive pain control, and local anesthesia are used as needed.
- Surgical equipment:
    - Surgical drape
    - A #11 or #15 scalpel blade
    - Mosquito forceps, nontraumatic forceps, needle holder, scissors, grooved directors, lone star retractor
    - Gauzes
    - 3-0 or 4-0 absorbable sutures (PDS, Vicryl)
    - Tissue glue

ANTICIPATED TIME

About 10 minutes of preparation and 20 minutes of surgery

PREPARATION: IMPORTANT CHECKPOINTS

- Perform a full physical examination and blood work (at least urea, PCV, blood glucose, total protein) to make sure that the patient can undergo general anesthesia.
- If, during the physical examination, abdominal palpation of the uterus reveals an abnormal shape, or if any vulvar discharges are noted, perform an abdominal ultrasound to control the uterus.
- The bladder needs to be emptied manually before surgery is begun.

ANATOMIC CONSIDERATIONS

- Ferret: average size of the ovary is 0.45 cm long by 0.55 cm wide and 0.21 cm thick. When mature, the left ovary lies caudal to the middle of the 14th rib and caudal to the left kidney. The right ovary is caudal to the middle of the last rib (15th) and caudal to the right kidney. The ovaries are suspended by ligaments from the abdominal wall and are surrounded by some fat tissue. The ferret uterus is bicornuate, comprising two long, tapering uterine horns that combine immediately in front of the cervix to form a short uterine body. Mature uterine horns are about 4.3 cm long and 0.22 cm wide, and the body is 1.7 cm long and 0.25 cm wide. Blood supply is provided by the companion ovarian and uterine arteries and veins; sympathetic innervation comes from the aortic and renal plexuses.
- Rabbit: ovaries are elongated and are located more caudally than in cats and dogs. The oviducts are very long and coiled. The uterus is duplex, being separate along its length, and forms two cervices, uniting only to form a long vagina. It is bright pink and lies dorsal to the urinary bladder. The mesometrium is a site of fat storage and, even in young does, builds up fat tissue rapidly. The suspensory ligaments are long, making exteriorization of the uterus easy. The urethra enters the vagina via the vestibule.
- Rodents
    - Rats: right ovary is located at the level of L4-5 just caudal to the right kidney. The left ovary lies at L5-6 caudal to the left kidney. The left ovary is nearer the midline than the right. Both are embedded in fat. The oviduct is convoluted and winds around the ovary in 10 to 12 garland-like loops. The uterus is duplex. An anastomosis between the ovarian artery (a branch of the aorta) and the uterine artery (a branch of the internal iliac) occurs in the uterine mesentery. The mesovarium and the mesometrium contain voluminous amounts of fat. In the female rat, the urethra and the vaginal orifice are completely separate.
    - Hamster: ovaries are oval, situated dorsolateral to the kidneys, and are completely enclosed in a fat-filled ovarian bursa. The oviduct is long and tightly coiled. The uterine artery in the hamster provides a major portion of the blood supply to the ovary. In some hamsters, coils of the ovarian and uterine arteries anastomose close to the ovary. The uterus is duplex and leads into two cervices, with the undivided part being 7 to 8 mm long.
    - Guinea pig, chinchilla, degus: ovaries are located caudolateral to the kidneys and are supported by a short mesovarium. The oviduct lies in close contact within the ovarian bursa. A pink bicornuate uterus is noted with a short uterine body and a single cervix opening into the

vagina. The broad ligament (mesovarium, mesosalpinx, and mesometrium) contains a lot of fat, which makes identification of the ovarian pedicle difficult during ovariohysterectomy. As in most mammals, an anastomosis between the ovarian artery (a branch of the aorta) and the uterine artery (a branch of the internal iliac) occurs in the uterine mesentery. The uterine artery provides the main blood supply to the ovary.

POSSIBLE COMPLICATIONS AND COMMON ERRORS TO BE AVOIDED

- Hemorrhage if ligatures on the ovarian pedicle or on the uterus slip. If this occurs, reopen the surgical site to identify where the bleeding is coming from, and replace the ligatures.
- Dehiscence of the wound: if the wound is clean and not infected, some other sutures can be placed; placement of an Elizabethan collar on the patient can be attempted. If the wound is dirty or infected, it must be cleaned, and second intention healing is preferred.
- Sutures eaten by the patient: This can occur frequently in rats and hamster. If the wound is clean and is not infected, some other sutures can be placed; placement of an Elizabethan collar on the patient can be attempted. If the wound is dirty or infected, it must be cleaned, and second intention healing is preferred. Use of tissue glue is recommended in all cases to prevent this situation.

PROCEDURE

Ferrets

- The patient is placed in dorsal recumbency, and the fur is clipped from the xiphoid process to the pubis. This area is prepared aseptically. It is not recommended to use alcohol, to minimize evaporative cooling.
- A skin incision of 4 to 5 cm is made with the blade, beginning cranially 1 cm under the umbilicus.
- The subcutaneous tissue is dissected with Metzenbaum scissors until the linea alba is visualized.
- The linea alba is grasped with a nontraumatic forceps and is punctured. The grooved director is inserted by the puncture site and is used to perform a 4- to 5-cm incision of the linea alba.
- Most of the time, the uterus can be visualized just after opening of the abdominal cavity. If this is not the case, it is searched dorsally to the bladder.
- The ovarian pedicle is relatively loose, so exteriorization of the ovaries is not difficult. The ovary is manipulated with a nontraumatic forceps; when all anatomic structures are identified, a mosquito is placed on the ovarian pedicle.
- The ovaries need to be perfectly visualized before the mosquito is placed. In older ferrets, the fat tissue surrounding the ovary has to be dissected to prevent any ovarian remnant.
- Two ligatures with a PDS 3-0 or with two hemostatic clips are placed on the ovarian pedicle. The pedicle is then sectioned caudally to the ligature, and hemostasis is checked before the ovarian pedicle is released by opening the mosquito.
- The same procedure is performed for the other ovary.
- When the two ovaries are removed, the large ligament is dissected to exteriorize the uterus.
- The cervix is identified by taxis. A mosquito is placed cranially to the cervix.
- A transfixating ligature and a classic ligature (PDS 3-0) are placed between the cervix and the mosquito.
- The uterus is sectioned and hemostasis is checked before the mosquito is removed.
- The muscular layer is closed by a continuous pattern with monofilament resorbable sutures (PDS 3-0). Suturing is started on the caudal area to visualize the bladder without puncturing it.
- A subcutaneous continuous pattern is performed with resorbable sutures (the author's best choice is Vicryl Rapide 4-0, which is soft, causes very little irritation, and is well tolerated).
- Then a continuous intradermic pattern can be performed with the use of tissue or tissue glue. If tissue glue is not available, one can close the skin using an interrupted pattern. Most of the time, skin sutures are well tolerated and a bandage is not useful.

Rabbits

- A 3- to 4-cm incision is made centered midway between the umbilicus and the pubis.
- The narrow linea alba needs to be lifted from the abdominal contents as a stab incision is made into the abdomen; be very careful when entering the abdominal wall because the thin-walled cecum and the bladder are often pressed firmly against the ventral abdomen.
- The uterus typically can be seen because it lies cranial and dorsal to the cranial pole of the bladder and may be lifted through the incision with forceps.
- The oviduct is coiled in a large loop that is several times longer than that of a dog or cat; when sutures are placed around the ovarian pedicle, attention should be focused on not leaving any portion of it.
- The mesovarium could be full of fat tissue in mature does. This fat tissue is fragile and is irrigated by multiple vessels. Dissection of the mesovarium needs to be performed carefully. To perform this dissection without major bleeding, a bipolar forceps could be useful.
- The uterus is ligated just caudal to the cervices, and the vagina is closed using a second ligature.
- Closure of the abdomen is routine.

Rats

- A 2-cm ventral midline incision is made between the umbilicus and the pubis. Gerbils of both sexes have a sebaceous gland located midventrally on the abdomen near the umbilicus. The incision need to be diverted to one side and the skin undermined to expose the linea alba.
- The uterine horns are identified dorsal to the apex of the bladder.
- The ovaries are removed as described previously.
- It has been recommended that the uterus be ligated cranial to the cervix to prevent urine from spilling into the abdomen when the uterus is transected.
- Care must be taken to avoid damaging the urinary bladder, which lies immediately dorsal to the uterus. Gentle tissue handling and avoidance of manipulation of the gastrointestinal tract are important because rodents, especially hamsters, are likely to develop adhesions.
- It is recommended that after the abdominal wall is closed, an intradermic continuous pattern should be performed and the skin closed with tissue glue. Hamsters and rats are used to remove skin sutures.

Guinea Pig, Chinchilla, and Degu

- A 4- to 5-cm incision is made centered midway between the umbilicus and the pubis. Usually little subcutaneous tissue is present and the linea alba is broad, making it easy to identify. Immediately dorsal (deep) to the body wall is the thin-walled cecum, and the bladder (also thin-walled) is just caudal to the cecum. It is vital to avoid iatrogenic injury to these structures, especially the cecum.
- A blunt instrument or a finger could be used to move the cecum and the bladder to the side on which the surgeon is standing, allowing visualization of the uterine horn on the opposite side.
- The ovaries are supported by a short mesovarium, and they are difficult to exteriorize. It may be necessary to extend the incision cranially to avoid accidental tearing of the friable,

fat-filled ovarian ligament. The broad ligaments also contain a large amount of fat, which can make identification of ovarian vessels difficult.
- A single artery and vein run medial to each ovary and the uterine horn. Most of the time, gentle blunt dissection is needed to create an opening in the mesovarium to allow placement of two hemostatic clips or two ligatures of an absorbable suture.
- The end of the technique is similar to the one described in ferrets.

POST-PROCEDURE

- Pain medication for 5 days
- Remove the litter and the substrate for 1 week, and place paper towels or newspaper instead.
- Recheck the surgical wound 10 days after surgery is performed.

ALTERNATIVES AND THEIR RELATIVE MERITS

- A deslorelin implant can be used in the ferret to achieve a chemical spay, which decreases the musky odor.
- The implant is working for 2 to 2.5 years and prevents adrenal disease.
- No data on other exotic mammal species are available.

REFERENCES

Jenkins JR: Surgical sterilization in small mammals, spay and castration, Vet Clin North Am Exot Anim Pract 3:617–627, 2003.

O'Malley B: Section 4, Small mammals. In O'Malley B, editor: Clinical anatomy and physiology of exotic species: structure and function of mammals, birds, reptiles, and amphibians, St Louis, 2005, Saunders Elsevier, pp 163–261.

Pignon C, et al: Stérilisation de convenance des petits mammifères. In Bulliot C, editor: Chirurgie des tissus mous et dentisterie des petits mammifères de compagnie, Le Point Vétérinaire, Numéro spécial 35–41, 2009.

Redrobe S: Soft tissue surgery of rabbits and rodents, Semin Avian Exot Pet Med 11:231–245, 2002.

AUTHOR: **CHARLY PIGNON**

EDITOR: **JÖRG MAYER**

SMALL MAMMALS

Preventing Hypothermia During Anesthesia

OVERVIEW AND GOALS

- Temperature regulation is the standard of care and must be monitored. Hypothermia is common because drugs suppress the thermoregulation system.
- Anesthetic gas is of a lower temperature and has less humidity than the body.
- Convective heat loss is rapid; therefore, temperature must be monitored.
- It is ideal to use a thermometer probe attached to an esophageal probe. To increase temperature, wrap the body in towels, circulating water, or air blankets. Do not use heated blankets or hot water bottles because they can cause burns.

INDICATIONS

Any animal undergoing anesthesia

EQUIPMENT, ANESTHESIA

- Thermometer
- Circulating water blanket
- Circulating warm air blanket
- Stockinette filled with rice
- Towels and blankets

ANTICIPATED TIME

Determined by the length of the procedure and postoperative recovery

PREPARATION: IMPORTANT CHECKPOINTS

Be prepared to monitor temperature preoperatively, perioperatively, and postoperatively.

POSSIBLE COMPLICATIONS AND COMMON ERRORS TO BE AVOIDED

- It is easier to maintain temperature than to increase the temperature of a patient under anesthesia.
- Placing animals directly on a heat source such as a heating pad can cause significant burns to the patient. Always place a towel between hot water bottles or heating pads and the patient.
- A patient's core body temperature can continue to drop for a time after the onset of rewarming. This condition, referred to as the "afterdrop," is caused by the return of cold peripheral blood to the body core and movement of blood from the warmer core to the periphery. A second important complication to anticipate is the development of rewarming shock. Rapid rewarming will cause a great metabolic burden on patients and significant vasodilatation, which can overwhelm an already compromised circulatory system.
- Circulating hot air blankets are a convective heat source.
- Circulating hot water blankets are a conductive heat source.
- Heat lamps are a radiant heat source.
- Convective heat sources provide benefit as they warm the patient, rather than preventing loss of heat (conductive or radiant) from the patient.
- Primary and secondary types of hypothermia commonly occur during surgery or general anesthesia. Intubation prevents nasal warming of inspired air, and cold, dry air is delivered directly to the lungs. Application of antiseptic agents will increase heat loss because they evaporate, and cold table surfaces and open body cavities will cause further heat loss via conduction and radiation.
- Anesthetic agents widen the thermoregulatory threshold; therefore, thermogenic responses are not initiated until low temperatures are reached. Anesthetic agents inhibit centrally mediated thermoregulatory vasoconstriction, resulting in peripheral vasodilatation and redistribution of core heat to the cooler periphery.
- Anesthesia decreases the basal metabolic rate by 15% to 40% and inhibits muscular activity, leading to decreased heat production. Hypothermia delays anesthetic and surgical complications such as arrhythmias, hypotension, respiratory depression, bradycardia, coagulopathy, blood sludging, and anesthetic drug overdose. The duration of surgery and of anesthetic procedures should be minimized to prevent secondary hypothermia.

PROCEDURE

- Use circulating hot air blankets.
- Use a circulating hot water blanket under the patient for surgery and recovery (with a towel in between patient and table).
- Place hot water bottles or examination gloves filled with hot water around the patient (with a towel in between).

- Use hot towels pulled directly from the dryer.
- Draping the patient as soon as possible in surgery decreases heat loss.
- If the patient is on IV fluids, warm fluids to body temperature with an IV fluid warmer or a hot cup of water.
- Make "rice bags": fill a stockinette with rice and place in microwave. Place next to the patient.
- Patients can become overheated easily. Monitor temperature constantly.
    - Normal temperature
        - Rabbits: 102.5°F (39.2°C)
        - Guinea pigs: 99°F to 103.1°F (37.2°C to 39.5°C)
        - Hamsters: 100°F (37.8°C)
        - Mice: 99°F (37.2°C)
        - Rats: 100°F (37.8°C)

POST-PROCEDURE

- Continue monitoring until patient has made a full recovery.
- Place patients in a warm, well-oxygenated, quiet environment, away from stimulation.

AUTHOR: **JÖRG MAYER**

EDITOR: **THOMAS M. DONNELLY**

SMALL MAMMALS

Recognition of Pain in Rabbits and Rodents

OVERVIEW AND GOALS

- Pain should be assumed based on evaluation of stress, injury, or surgery that the animal has experienced.
- Rabbits and rodents are generally underdosed with pain medication.
- Rabbits appear to be more sensitive to visceral than to orthopedic pain.

INDICATIONS

- Rabbits
    - Inactive
    - Anorectic
    - Poor response
    - Grinding of the teeth
    - Change in posture and/or gait (especially hunched position and reluctance to move)
- Rodents
    - Increased heart rate and respiratory rate
    - Anorectic
    - Trembling
    - Grinding of the teeth
    - Change in posture and/or gait (especially hunched position and reluctance to move)

EQUIPMENT, ANESTHESIA

Sedation with benzodiazepines (e.g., midazolam 0.5-2 mg/kg IM) is often indicated when rabbits are presented in stressed or poor condition. If rabbits experience situational stress at the veterinarian's clinic, in addition to underlying disease problems, release of catecholamines due to stress of the physical examination or procedure (e.g., IV catheter placement, radiographs) can often be fatal.

PREPARATION: IMPORTANT CHECKPOINTS

- Multimodal analgesia targets different pathways and may be of benefit to the patient.
- Preemptive analgesia should be implemented when possible—prevent the pain before performing the procedure.

POSSIBLE COMPLICATIONS AND COMMON ERRORS TO BE AVOIDED

- Untreated pain leads to:
    - Tachycardia
    - Arrhythmias
    - Vasoconstriction
    - Increased myocardial demand
    - Delayed wound healing
    - Death

PROCEDURE

- Rabbits
    - Butorphanol 0.1-1.0 mg/kg SC, IM, IV q 4-6 h
    - Buprenorphine 0.01-0.05 mg/kg SC, IM, IV q 6-12 h
    - Morphine 2-5 mg/kg SC, IM q 2-4 h
    - Carprofen 1-2.2 mg/kg PO q 12 h
    - Ibuprofen 2-7.5 mg/kg PO q 12-24 h
    - Meloxicam 0.5 mg/kg SC, PO q 24 h
    - Oxymorphone 0.2 mg/kg SC, IM q 4 h
- Rats
    - Butorphanol 2 mg/kg SC q 4-6 h
    - Buprenorphine 0.01-0.05 mg/kg SC q 8-12 h
    - Morphine 2-5 mg/kg SC, IM q 2-4 h
    - Carprofen 4 mg/kg PO q 12 h
    - Ibuprofen 10-30 mg/kg PO q 4 h
    - Meloxicam 1 mg/kg SC, PO q 24 h
- Mice
    - Butorphanol 0.1-0.5 mg/kg IM, SC q 4-6 h
    - Buprenorphine 0.05 mg/kg SC q 8-12 h
    - Morphine 2-5 mg/kg SC q 2-4 h (not suitable for hamsters)
    - Meloxicam 1 mg/kg PO q 12 h
    - Ibuprofen 7-15 mg/kg PO q 4 h

POST-PROCEDURE

Observe for vomiting, diarrhea, anorexia due to medications.

AUTHOR: **JÖRG MAYER**

EDITOR: **THOMAS M. DONNELLY**

SMALL MAMMALS

Rectal Prolapse and Intussusception Treatment in Hamsters, Mice, and Guinea Pigs

OVERVIEW AND GOALS

- Rectal prolapse can occur in rodents owing to constipation or diarrhea. If diagnosed and treated quickly, the prolapse can be retained by a purse-string suture.
- Inflammation or edema of the tissue may worsen the prolapse.
- Prolapsed tissue can become traumatized, resulting in necrosis of the tissue.
- Intussusception can occur with chronic cases of constipation or gastroenteritis.
- Prolapsed intussusception generally requires a laparotomy, whereas rectal prolapse does not.
- Intussusception produces partial or complete intestinal obstruction.
- Necrosis of the bowel wall can be the result of an intussusception, increasing the risk for peritonitis to develop.

INDICATIONS

- Rectum is protruding.
- Animal is hunched up and stretches out or rolls in an attempt to decrease pain.

CONTRAINDICATIONS

Animal is unstable for anesthesia.

EQUIPMENT, ANESTHESIA

- Anesthesia
- Saline
- Dextrose
- Empty syringe casing
- Suture material

ANTICIPATED TIME

20 minutes

PREPARATION: IMPORTANT CHECKPOINTS

- Try to manually reduce if possible.
- Treat underlying cause to prevent recurrence.
- Provide pain medication before manipulation.

POSSIBLE COMPLICATIONS AND COMMON ERRORS TO BE AVOIDED

- Recurrent prolapse
- Hematochezia
- Dehiscence and stricture of resection
- If an anastomosis is performed, peritonitis

PROCEDURE

- Rectal prolapse
  - Anesthetize patient to prevent tenesmus during reduction.
    - Guinea pigs: dexmedetomidine/ketamine 0.025 mg/kg and 5 mg/kg IM
    - Hamsters: isoflurane
    - Mice: isoflurane
  - Lavage prolapsed tissue with saline, and inspect viability.
  - If tissue is edematous, soak it in a dextrose solution to reduce swelling.
  - Insert a syringe casing (size of casing depends on size of patient) into the rectum to prevent overtightening of purse-string
  - Place purse-string suture around rectum at the mucocutaneous junction.
  - Resect necrotic tissue if needed.
- Intussusception
  - Try to reduce if possible. If bowel damage is present, anastomosis is indicated.
  - Perioperative antibiotics, if indicated

POST-PROCEDURE

- Prolapse
  - Provide postoperative analgesia
    - Guinea pigs:
      - Buprenorphine 0.05 mg/kg SC q 8-12 h
      - Butorphanol 0.2-4 mg/kg SC q 4 h
      - Carprofen 1-2 mg/kg PO q 12-24 h
      - Ibuprofen 10 mg/kg PO q 4 h
      - Ketoprofen 1 mg/kg SC q 12-24 h
    - Hamsters
      - Buprenorphine 0.1-0.5 mg/kg SC q 8-12 h
      - Butorphanol 1-5 mg/kg SC q 4 h
    - Mice
      - Buprenorphine 0.02-0.5 mg/kg SC q 8-12 h
      - Butorphanol 1-2 mg/kg SC q 4 h
      - Carprofen 5-10 mg/kg PO q 12-24 h
  - Clean area after each defecation.
  - Observe for straining.
  - Hot pack the area to decrease swelling.
  - Use a warm washcloth or gauze compress for 5 minutes.
  - Offer patient a bland, soft diet of baby food and cereals (except rice cereal) for 10 days.
  - Stool softeners may be indicated.
  - Slowly introduce normal diet after sutures are removed (3 to 5 days).
- Intussusception
  - Observe for clinical signs to recur.

AUTHOR: **THOMAS M. DONNELLY**

EDITOR: **JÖRG MAYER**

SMALL MAMMALS

Restraint and Carrying, How to Pick up Rabbits and Rodents

OVERVIEW AND GOALS

- To facilitate minor, minimally painful procedures
  - Initial exam, blood draw, skin scrape, etc.
- Minimize stress and injury to the animal while preventing the veterinary technician and the veterinarian from being bitten
  - Hold patient steady, don't squeeze.
- When restraining rabbits and rodents, it is important to be gentle, yet firm, with restraint.
- Rabbits have massive strength in their hind legs; therefore, the hind

quarters must be supported, preventing injury.
- Consider tranquilization to prevent excessive restraint.

INDICATIONS

- Physical examination
- Diagnosis and treatment of appropriate diseases

CONTRAINDICATIONS

- Use caution in stressed or debilitated animals.
- Warn owners of critically ill patients and consider supportive care before examination or diagnostics.

EQUIPMENT, ANESTHESIA

- Towel
- Cat bag
- Chemical restraint may be used when rabbits become stressed and fractious, or when diagnostics, physical exams, or treatments may induce pain or discomfort.
  - Midazolam 0.5-2 mg/kg IM can be used as a preanesthetic when used alone.
  - Midazolam 0.25-0.5 mg/kg IM when used with an opioid
  - Ketamine 1 mg/kg IM can be used as a preanesthetic.
  - Ketamine/Midazolam 1 mg/kg and 0.25-0.5 mg/kg IM produces excellent relaxation.
  - Dexmedetomidine 0.1-0.2 mg/kg IM or IV: can be used in conjunction with ketamine and reversed with atipamezole
- Isoflurane and sevoflurane are easy to administer, and pets recover well.

ANTICIPATED TIME

Depends on procedure

POSSIBLE COMPLICATIONS AND COMMON ERRORS TO BE AVOIDED

- Rabbits have powerful hind legs and kick violently. Without proper restraint, rabbits can fracture their vertebrae.
- Never pick up rabbits by the ears.
- Gerbils can slough their tails when grasped incorrectly. This is common in young animals, or when injuries occur to the distal end of the tail.
- Hamsters may jump from hands or tables without warning. Prepare for the pet to jump.
- Hamsters are known to bite. Scoop them up in the palm of the hand to prevent startling. When hamsters are touched suddenly on the back, this may induce a threatening behavior.
  - When hamsters roll on their back, they are showing signs of defensive behavior and may become fear aggressive.
- Mice often jump from the restrainer, and they do bite. Be prepared to prevent injury.
- If any rabbit or rodent becomes stressed, take a short break.
- Over-restraint can cause respiratory distress or injury. Gloves can prevent the restrainer from knowing how much force is being used. It is advised not to use gloves, but rather to use a correct restraint method.

PROCEDURE

- Rabbits
  - Grasp the scruff with one hand and use the other hand to support the hind quarters.
  - Tuck the head under your arms as if carrying a football. Rabbits will relax when the head and eyes are covered.
  - For physical exams, cover the table with a towel to prevent the rabbit from slipping.
  - The rabbit may be placed in a cat bag to aid in restraint for drawing blood or for injections or medication administration
  - To examine the abdomen, roll the rabbit onto the rump, and then roll onto the back, as if cradling a baby. This also aids in taking the temperature.
  - When returning the rabbit to the cage, place the caudal end in the cage first. This can decrease the chance that the rabbit will kick when released.
- Gerbils
  - Scruff technique: using the thumb and the forefinger, scruff the excess skin at the shoulder blades. Cradle the gerbil in the palm, and use the pinkie of the same hand to stabilize the tail; this provides additional support.
  - Over-the-back technique: approach the animal from behind, and place the forefinger and index finger on either side of the mandible to immobilize the head. Hold the remaining body with the palm of the hand.
  - A small, light towel can be placed over/around the gerbil. This allows the patient to have something to chew on and protects the handler's fingers.
- Hamsters
  - Hamsters have an abundance of loose skin over the shoulders. Grasp the skin with all four fingers and the thumb. Stabilize the hamster in the palm of the hand.
  - Use a light towel, as described previously.
- Mice
  - Initially grab the mouse by the tail; then use the scruff technique as previously described.
  - Use a small light towel, as described earlier.
- Rats
  - Scruff the rat with the thumb and forefingers over the shoulders and neck. Use the palm of your hand to support the body.
- Guinea pigs
  - Guinea pigs enjoy being picked up and cupped in the hand. They require minimal restraint; place one hand on the rump to prevent the animal from backing away.
- Chinchillas
  - Most chinchillas are easy to hold and do not bite. Scoop the pet up from the bottom of the cage. Use one hand to support the abdomen and the other to support the hind quarters.
- Team members can use a variety of homemade devices to help with restraint or treatment of rodents.
- Place the rodent in a stockinette. This allows the pet to breathe while confined. A hole can be cut in the stockinette if blood needs to be drawn, etc.
- The rodent can be placed in a syringe casing. Cut a small hole in the opposite end to allow air into the casing.
- The rodent can be fit into a clear plastic bag. Cut a hole in the corner, allowing air to enter the sack, and remove remaining space around the rodent. This is a great tool for administering injections.

POST-PROCEDURE

Observe patient for respiratory rate, heart rate, and stress. If needed, place patient in an oxygen cage until patient has calmed down.

AUTHOR: **JÖRG MAYER**

EDITOR: **THOMAS M. DONNELLY**

SMALL MAMMALS

Urethral Catheterization of Ferrets

OVERVIEW AND GOALS

- Urethral catheterization is common in male ferrets.
- Urethral blockage is a common sequela of adrenal disease in male ferrets. Hormonal influence causes the prostate gland to enlarge, which constricts the urethra.
- Catheterization in female ferrets is rare and can be difficult.

INDICATIONS

To allow the passage of urine

CONTRAINDICATIONS

Urethral obstruction can be life threatening, and the risk of recurrence depends on the cause of the obstruction. Owners must be given the long-term prognosis.

EQUIPMENT, ANESTHESIA

- Combinations of agents provide excellent preanesthesia, allowing maintenance with isoflurane or sevoflurane if needed.
  - PA agents include the following:
    - Midazolam 0.3-1.0 mg/kg IM
    - Ketamine 10-50 mg/kg IM
    - Ketamine/Midazolam 5-10 mg/kg and 0.25-0.5 mg/kg IM
    - Diazepam 1-2 mg/kg IM
    - Diazepam/Ketamine 1-2 mg/kg and 10-20 mg/kg IM
    - Butorphanol 0.05-0.5 mg/kg SC or IM
    - Acepromazine 0.1-0.5 mg/kg SC or IM
- Sterile gloves
- Vaginal speculum (females)
- 3.5 Fr red rubber urethral catheter or 3.0 Fr ferret urinary catheter
- Sterile lubrication
- 24-Gauge catheter
- Saline
- Suture
- Tape
- Sterile empty IV bag with administration set, to use as a closed urinary system
- E-collar

ANTICIPATED TIME

Varies, depending on severity of obstruction

PREPARATION: IMPORTANT CHECKPOINTS

- Freezing catheters before insertion can increase stiffness and aid in insertion.
- Use of a stylet or a sterile metal guitar string can stiffen the catheter, aiding in insertion.
- Monitor ferrets under anesthesia. Maintain body temperature; monitor heart and respiratory rates.

POSSIBLE COMPLICATIONS AND COMMON ERRORS TO BE AVOIDED

- Urethral tear/laceration
- Urinary bladder rupture
- Lactic urinary tract infection
- Urethral stricture

PROCEDURE

- Female
  - Tranquilize or place the ferret under anesthesia.
  - Measure the desired length of catheter needed to reach the bladder.
  - Place the ferret in ventral recumbency and elevate rear quarters with a towel.
  - Prep area aseptically and use sterile gloves.
  - A vaginal speculum may be used to locate the urethral opening in the floor of the urethral vestibule, which is approximately 1 cm cranial to the clitoral fossa.
  - Introduce a 3.5 Fr red rubber urethral catheter fitted with a wire stylet into the urethral orifice.
  - Advance to the bladder and secure with butterfly tape strips around the catheter just where it enters the vulva, and at another point 3 to 5 cm distal (on the tail), and suture to the skin.
  - Tape the catheter to the tail to assist with support and comfort.
  - Attach a urine collection device (such as a sterile, empty IV fluid bag, attached to an administration set).
  - Place an E-collar on the ferret to prevent removal of the catheter.
- Male
  - Tranquilize or place the ferret under anesthesia.
  - Measure the desired length of the catheter needed to reach the bladder.
  - Place the ferret in ventral recumbency, and elevate rear quarters with a towel.
  - Prep area aseptically using sterile gloves.
  - Dilate the urethral opening by passing a 24-gauge IV catheter just inside the tip of the urethra, and flush with saline.
  - Slip the tip of the lubricated urinary catheter into the dilated opening alongside the IV catheter, and while gently flushing with saline, pass the catheter into the bladder.
  - Resistance can occur at the pelvic flexure; therefore, try repeated flushings and re-lubricate the catheter as needed until it passes.
  - Once in place, secure the catheter with butterfly tape strips around the catheter just where it enters the penis, and at another point 3 to 5 cm distal, and suture to the skin.
  - Tape the catheter to the tail to assist with support and comfort.
  - Attach a urine collection device (such as a sterile, empty IV fluid bag, attached to an administration set).
  - Place an E-collar on the ferret to prevent removal of the catheter.

POST-PROCEDURE

- Monitor patients recovering from anesthesia. Hypothermia and hypoglycemia can occur, causing postprocedural death.
- Monitor bladder size frequently.
- Repeat urinalysis and culture 1 week after the catheter is removed.

ALTERNATIVES AND THEIR RELATIVE MERITS

A cystocentesis may be performed in an emergency when a catheter cannot be placed. Patient may then be transferred to a referral hospital.

AUTHOR: **JÖRG MAYER**

EDITOR: **THOMAS M. DONNELLY**

SECTION III

Differential Diagnosis

EDITOR

Jörg Mayer *DrMedVet, MSc, DABVP (Exotic Companion Mammal), DECZM (Small Mammal)*

Acute Respiratory Distress Syndrome

- Check immediately for mechanical obstruction; take radiographs if possible.
- Take good history to exclude exposure to inhalation toxin or recent trauma.

<table>
<tr><th>Reptile</th><th>Bird</th><th>Mammal</th></tr>
<tr><td></td><td colspan="2">Noxious gas inhalation</td></tr>
<tr><td></td><td colspan="2">Smoke inhalation</td></tr>
<tr><td colspan="3">Trauma</td></tr>
<tr><td colspan="3">Pneumonia, infectious or aspiration</td></tr>
<tr><td colspan="3">Parasites (e.g., pentastomes)</td></tr>
<tr><td colspan="3">Neoplasms (e.g., chondroma in trachea)</td></tr>
<tr><td colspan="3">Congestive heart failure</td></tr>
<tr><td></td><td>Sarcocystosis</td><td></td></tr>
<tr><td colspan="3">Coagulopathy (rare)</td></tr>
<tr><td colspan="3">Atherosclerosis (ruptured pulmonary blood vessels)</td></tr>
<tr><td colspan="3">Excess environmental heat</td></tr>
<tr><td colspan="3">Sepsis</td></tr>
<tr><td colspan="3">Pain</td></tr>
<tr><td colspan="3">Upper airway obstruction (e.g., fungal granuloma, tracheal or bronchial foreign body)</td></tr>
<tr><td colspan="3">Electrocution</td></tr>
<tr><td colspan="3">Neurologic insult</td></tr>
<tr><td colspan="3">Strangulation</td></tr>
</table>

Alopecia

Alopecia	Mammal
Ectoparasites	Lice, mites, fleas, leading to severe pruritus
Hormonal imbalances	Hyperestrogenism with retained ovary or adrenal disease
Self-mutilation	In stressful situations, fur is often short or is licked off.
Aggression from superior animal	Barbering by superior animal often starts with "loss" of whiskers.
Nutrient deficiency	Zinc, vitamin A deficiency can cause hair loss.
Irritant or contact dermatitis	Allergic dermatitis
Infectious agents (pyoderma)	Dermatitis due to a variety of bacteria
Chemotherapy	Rarely observed (whiskers are first to fall out)
Cushing's disease	Common in the hamster
Fungal infection	*Trichophyton* and *Microsporum* are common.
Sebaceous adenitis	Described in rabbits
Burn	Especially after surgical procedure, burn by heat element
Sebaceous gland hyperplasia	Gland can get impacted or, in cases of hyperactivity, can irritate surrounding areas.
Pregnancy	Physiologic response to high estrogen levels (often bilateral flank alopecia)
Age-related alopecia	Very old animals can become bald or get a thin hair coat.
Hypothyroidism	Especially in the guinea pig
Post-clipping alopecia	Will not regrow after shaving
Drug-induced	Prolonged steroid therapy

Anemia

- Perform a full complete blood count to rule out systemic infection and to characterize the nature of the anemia. Look for evidence of regenerative or nonregenerative anemia.
- Care needs to be taken when blood is collected from small patients to avoid artificially causing anemia in a sick patient.
- Severe anemia is considered if packed cell volume is less than 20%.
- Consider bone marrow collection in cases of severe, nonregenerative anemia.

<table>
<tr><th>Reptile</th><th>Bird</th><th>Mammal</th></tr>
<tr><td colspan="3">Chronic disease</td></tr>
<tr><td colspan="3">Trauma (hemorrhage)</td></tr>
<tr><td colspan="3">Internal bleeding</td></tr>
<tr><td colspan="3">Chronic renal failure</td></tr>
<tr><td colspan="3">Chronic malnutrition (protein deficiency)</td></tr>
<tr><td colspan="3">Iatrogenic (phlebotomy)</td></tr>
<tr><td colspan="3">Zinc toxicosis</td></tr>
<tr><td colspan="3">Hemolysis</td></tr>
<tr><td colspan="3">Hemoparasites (e.g., Plasmodium, Leucocytozoon)</td></tr>
<tr><td colspan="3">Iron/Vitamin B deficiency</td></tr>
<tr><td colspan="3">Bone marrow suppression (e.g., lymphoma, iatrogenic [e.g., fenbendazole, chemotherapeutics])</td></tr>
<tr><td colspan="3">Ectoparasites</td></tr>
<tr><td colspan="3">Endoparasites</td></tr>
<tr><td colspan="3">Neoplasia (hemangiosarcoma)</td></tr>
<tr><td colspan="3">Drug induced</td></tr>
<tr><td colspan="3">Irradiation</td></tr>
<tr><td colspan="3">Hemolytic anemia</td></tr>
<tr><td colspan="3">Hyperestrogenism</td></tr>
<tr><td colspan="3">Hypothyroidism</td></tr>
</table>

Anorexia

- Anorexia is a nonspecific clinical sign that is often noted with various disease processes.
- Anorexia can be due to pathologic causes but also may be due to physiologic events. One has to make sure to be able to differentiate between the two so as not to administer treatment when not needed and not to delay treatment when needed.
- Always perform a complete physical examination when evaluating the patient.

<table>
<tr><th></th><th>Reptile</th><th>Bird</th><th>Mammal</th></tr>
<tr><td>Pathologic</td><td colspan="3">Acute disease</td></tr>
<tr><td></td><td colspan="3">Chronic disease</td></tr>
<tr><td></td><td colspan="3">Toxicity (environmental or iatrogenic)</td></tr>
<tr><td></td><td colspan="3">Sepsis</td></tr>
<tr><td></td><td colspan="3">Mass occupying problem (e.g., egg binding, tumor in abdomen/coelom)</td></tr>
<tr><td></td><td colspan="3">Trauma</td></tr>
<tr><td></td><td colspan="3">Parasitism</td></tr>
<tr><td>Functional</td><td colspan="3">Central Nervous System problem</td></tr>
<tr><td></td><td colspan="3">Pain</td></tr>
<tr><td></td><td colspan="3">Gastrointestinal (GI) obstruction</td></tr>
<tr><td></td><td colspan="3">GI inflammatory disease</td></tr>
<tr><td></td><td colspan="2">Severely overgrown beak (turtles and tortoises)</td><td></td></tr>
<tr><td></td><td colspan="3">Respiratory distress</td></tr>
<tr><td></td><td colspan="2">Preparing for breeding/egg laying</td><td></td></tr>
<tr><td></td><td colspan="2">Resorption of ovarian follicles</td><td></td></tr>
<tr><td></td><td>Preparation for hibernation/brumation</td><td></td><td></td></tr>
<tr><td></td><td colspan="2"></td><td></td></tr>
<tr><td>Environmental</td><td>Husbandry-related problem</td><td></td><td></td></tr>
<tr><td></td><td colspan="3">Stress (cagemate aggression, competition)</td></tr>
<tr><td></td><td colspan="3">Introduction of new foods</td></tr>
</table>

Ascites

- Called *dropsy* in animals without diaphragm
- Care needs to be taken when fluid is collected in avian patients to avoid artificially causing a connection to the lungs and drowning the bird.
- Renal failure is common in freshwater fish.

Fish/Amphibian	Reptile	Bird	Mammal
Renal failure (osmotic pressure draws water into animal)			
Egg binding			
Idiopathic edema in amphibians	Egg yolk peritonitis		
Liver cirrhosis/malfunction			
		Hemochromatosis	Lymphatic accumulation
Coelomitis/peritonitis			
Abdominal/Coelomic neoplasia or masses			
Hypoproteinemia			
Organomegaly			
Cardiovascular insufficiency			
Viral infection			
Amyloidosis			
Trauma (hemoperitoneum)			
Parasitic infestation			
Ovarian cysts			

Azotemia

- Blood urea nitrogen (BUN) usually is not of diagnostic value in avians and reptilians.
- Azotemia in mammals might be considered as gout in birds and reptiles.
- Monitor for increase in uric acid in avians and reptilians.

	Reptile/Amphibian	Bird	Mammal
Prerenal causes	Postprandial		
	High-protein diet		
	Hypovolemia		
	Heart failure		
	Dehydration		
	Stomach ulcers		
	Poor nutrition (vitamin A deficiency)		
	Inactivity		
	Decreased blood circulation		
Postrenal causes			Urolith
			Prostatitis
			Cystitis
Renal	Toxins (hypervitaminosis D_3)		
	Infectious disease		
	Glomerulonephritis		
	Renal failure		

Clinical Parameter	Prerenal	Primary Renal	Postrenal
Creatinine	Increased	Increased	Increased
BUN	Increased	Increased	Increased
Urine specific gravity	Increased	Decreased	Increased
Urine sediment	Normal	Abnormal	Abnormal
Urine production	Decreased	Variable	Decreased
Hematocrit	Increased	Variable	Increased
Potassium	Normal or low	Variable	Increased
Phosphorus	Normal	Variable	Increased
Metabolic acidosis	Mild	Mild to severe	Mild to severe

Bleeding Disorder

<table>
<tr><th>Reptile</th><th>Bird</th><th>Mammal</th></tr>
<tr><td></td><td>“Conure bleeding syndrome”</td><td></td></tr>
<tr><td colspan="3">Toxicity</td></tr>
<tr><td></td><td>Heavy metal toxicosis (bloody urates in Amazon species)</td><td></td></tr>
<tr><td colspan="3">Excessive supplementation with vitamin E (e.g., fish-eating birds)</td></tr>
<tr><td colspan="3">Rodenticide toxicosis (e.g., snakes, owls, ferrets)</td></tr>
<tr><td colspan="3">Aflatoxicosis, mycotoxicosis</td></tr>
<tr><td colspan="3">Severe hypocalcemia</td></tr>
<tr><td colspan="3">Severe liver failure</td></tr>
<tr><td colspan="3">Sepsis</td></tr>
<tr><td colspan="3">Disseminated intravascular coagulation</td></tr>
<tr><td colspan="3">Drug-induced (NSAIDs, chemotherapy)</td></tr>
<tr><td colspan="3">Chronic malnutrition</td></tr>
<tr><td colspan="3">Coagulation disorder</td></tr>
<tr><td colspan="3">Rodenticide toxicosis</td></tr>
<tr><td colspan="3">Metabolic disorder (liver failure)</td></tr>
<tr><td colspan="3">Neoplasm (Hemangiosarcoma)</td></tr>
<tr><td colspan="3">Clotting disorder</td></tr>
<tr><td colspan="3">Vitamin K deficiency</td></tr>
</table>

NSAIDs, Nonsteroidal antiinflammatory drugs.

Bronchial Disease

<table>
<tr><th>Reptile/Amphibian</th><th>Bird</th><th>Mammal</th></tr>
<tr><td></td><td></td><td>Allergic reaction</td></tr>
<tr><td>Hypervitaminosis D_3 plus hypercalcemia</td><td></td><td>Heartworm disease</td></tr>
<tr><td colspan="3">Cardiac disease</td></tr>
<tr><td colspan="3">Fungal disease (aspergillosis)</td></tr>
<tr><td colspan="3">Primary airway infection (Bordetella, Pasteurella, Mycoplasma, Chlamydia)</td></tr>
<tr><td colspan="3">Inhalation of toxic substances (fumes)</td></tr>
<tr><td colspan="3">Parasitic disease (pentastomes, crenosoma, capillaria, filaroides, etc.)</td></tr>
<tr><td colspan="3">Viral disease (herpes, influenza)</td></tr>
<tr><td colspan="3">Aspiration of food or foreign material</td></tr>
<tr><td colspan="3">Inflammatory disease</td></tr>
</table>

Central Nervous System (CNS) Disorders, Multifocal/Diffuse

DISEASES THAT TYPICALLY RESULT IN MULTIFOCAL OR DIFFUSE CNS SIGNS

DEGENERATIVE

- Storage disease
- Multineuronal degeneration

ANOMALOUS

- Hydrocephalus/syringomyelia/hydromyelia complex

METABOLIC

- Hepatic
- Renal
- Hypoglycemia
- Hyperthyroidism
- Hypothyroidism
- Hyperadrenocorticism
- Hyperosmolar syndromes
  - Adipsia

NEOPLASTIC

- Lymphoma
- Leukemias
- Metastatic tumors

NUTRITIONAL

Thiamine

INFLAMMATORY DISEASES

INFECTIOUS

- Viral
  - Distemper
  - Herpes
  - Parvovirus
  - Parainfluenza

- Feline infectious peritonitis (FIP)
- Feline immunodeficiency virus (FIV)
- Bacterial
  - Bacterial encephalitis
  - Tetanus
- Fungal
  - Cryptococcosis
  - Blastomycosis
  - Coccidioidomycosis
  - Candidiasis
  - Aspergillosis
- Protozoal
  - Toxoplasmosis
  - Neosporosis
- Parasitic
  - *Toxocara*
  - *Cuterebra*
- Rickettsial
  - Rocky Mountain spotted fever
  - *Ehrlichia*
- Unclassified
  - Protothecosis

NONINFECTIOUS

- Granulomatous meningoencephalomyelitis (GME)
- Breed-associated CNS inflammation (necrotizing encephalitis): Pug, Maltese, Yorkshire terrier
- Spinal cord vasculitis
- Nonclassified
  - Steroid-responsive meningoencephalitis

IDIOPATHIC

- Dysautonomia

VASCULAR DISEASE

- Intracranial hemorrhage
- Thromboembolism
- Hypertension
- Spinal hemorrhage

Modified from Ettinger S, Feldman E: Textbook of veterinary internal medicine, ed 6, St Louis, 2005, Saunders.

Central Nervous System (CNS) Signs

- Seizures are very common in the avian patient.
- Treat seizure immediately before working on the differential diagnosis.

	Reptile	Bird	Mammal
Physical	Trauma		
	Heatstroke		
	Vascular (e.g., atherosclerosis)		
	Emboli (parasite, yolk)		
	Freeze damage during hibernation		
Infectious	Sepsis		
		Proventricular dilatation disease	*Encephalitozoon cuniculi* infestation
	Viral encephalitis (herpes)		
	Visceral larval migrans (e.g., *Balisascaris*)		
			Ectoparasites in guinea pigs
	Fungal abscess		
	Cryptococcus		
Metabolic	Hypernatremia ("salt poisoning," severe water deprivation)		
	Nutritional causes and deficiencies		
	Metabolic problems (e.g., hypocalcemia, hypoglycemia)		
	Cholesterol deposits		
Iatrogenic	Ivermectin, amphotericin B, dimetronidazole, insulin		
Toxicity	Heavy metal, mycotoxins, toxic plant ingestion		
		Teflon toxicity	
Other	Idiopathic		
	Degenerative		
	Idiopathic epilepsy		
	Vestibular disease		
	Behavioral abnormality		
		Neoplasia	

Conjunctivitis

<table>
<tr><th>Reptile</th><th>Bird</th><th>Mammal</th></tr>
<tr><td colspan="3">Bacterial infection (Chlamydia, Mycoplasma, mycobacteriosis, etc.)</td></tr>
<tr><td colspan="3">Fungal infections (Candida)</td></tr>
<tr><td colspan="3">Trauma</td></tr>
<tr><td colspan="3">Exposure to high doses of ultraviolet light</td></tr>
<tr><td colspan="3">Vitamin A deficiency</td></tr>
<tr><td colspan="3">Sinusitis</td></tr>
<tr><td colspan="3">Viral infection (pox, herpes, distemper)</td></tr>
<tr><td></td><td colspan="2">Allergic reaction</td></tr>
<tr><td colspan="3">Foreign body</td></tr>
<tr><td colspan="3">Irritant/Toxin</td></tr>
<tr><td colspan="3">Congenital (e.g., microophthalmia of cockatiels)</td></tr>
<tr><td></td><td>Lovebird eye disease</td><td></td></tr>
</table>

Constipation

- Never try to massage the content out of the coelomic cavity.
  - Iatrogenic trauma is a very common sequel.
- See Constipation algorithm, Sec. V.

<table>
<tr><th>Reptile</th><th>Bird</th><th>Mammal</th></tr>
<tr><td colspan="2">Egg binding</td><td>Anal or rectal inflammation</td></tr>
<tr><td colspan="3">Impaction (substrate ingestion)</td></tr>
<tr><td>Cold stunning</td><td></td><td></td></tr>
<tr><td colspan="3">Gastrointestinal (GI) parasites</td></tr>
<tr><td></td><td colspan="2">Abdominal hernia</td></tr>
<tr><td colspan="3">GI mycobacteriosis</td></tr>
<tr><td colspan="3">Dehydration</td></tr>
<tr><td colspan="2">Cloacolith</td><td>Prostate problems: hyperplasia, neoplasm, abscess</td></tr>
<tr><td colspan="3">Foreign body ingestion</td></tr>
<tr><td colspan="3">Renal failure</td></tr>
<tr><td colspan="3">Neoplasia (abdominal mass)</td></tr>
<tr><td colspan="3">Obesity</td></tr>
<tr><td colspan="3">Spinal disorder</td></tr>
<tr><td></td><td colspan="2">Anxiety disorder</td></tr>
<tr><td></td><td></td><td>Hypothyroidism</td></tr>
<tr><td></td><td></td><td>Cecal impaction</td></tr>
<tr><td></td><td></td><td>Megacolon</td></tr>
<tr><td></td><td></td><td>Stress</td></tr>
<tr><td></td><td></td><td>Ileus</td></tr>
<tr><td colspan="3">Postsurgical</td></tr>
<tr><td colspan="3">Intraabdominal sepsis</td></tr>
<tr><td colspan="3">Diet: dry, less fiber</td></tr>
<tr><td colspan="3">Hypocalcemia</td></tr>
<tr><td colspan="3">Intestinal strictures</td></tr>
<tr><td colspan="3">Lumbosacral disease, spinal cord injury</td></tr>
<tr><td colspan="3">Pain</td></tr>
<tr><td colspan="3">Hospitalization</td></tr>
</table>

Conversion Factors

Component	Conventional Unit	Conversion Factor	SI Unit
Alanine aminotransferase (ALT)	units/L	1	U/L
Albumin	g/dL	10	g/L
Alkaline phosphatase	units/L	1	U/L
Ammonia (as NH_3)	µg/dL	0.587	µmol/L
Amylase	units/L	1	U/L
Androstenedione	ng/dL	0.0349	nmol/L
Anion gap	mEq/L	1	mmol/L
Antidiuretic hormone	pg/mL	0.923	pmol/L
Aspartate aminotransferase (AST)	units/L	1	U/L
Bicarbonate	mEq/L	1	mmol/L
Bilirubin	mg/dL	17.1	µmol/L
Blood gases (arterial)			
$Paco_2$	mm Hg	1	mm Hg
pH	pH units	1	pH units
Pao_2	mm Hg	1	mm Hg
Calcitonin	pg/mL	1	ng/L
Calcium	mg/dL	0.25	mmol/L
	mEq/L	0.5	mmol/L
Carbon dioxide	mEq/L	1	mmol/L
Chloride	mEq/L	1	mmol/L
Cholesterol	mg/dL	0.0259	mmol/L
Copper	µg/dL	0.157	µmol/L
Corticotropin (ACTH)	pg/mL	0.22	pmol/L
Cortisol	µg/dL	27.59	nmol/L
Creatine	mg/dL	76.26	µmol/L
Creatine kinase (CK)	units/L	1	U/L
Creatinine	mg/dL	88.4	µmol/L
Creatinine clearance	mL/min	0.0167	mL/sec
Dehydroepiandrosterone (DHEA)	ng/mL	3.47	nmol/L
Diazepam	µg/mL	3.512	µmol/L
Digoxin	ng/mL	1.281	nmol/L
Estradiol	pg/mL	3.671	pmol/L
Estriol	ng/mL	3.467	nmol/L
Ethanol (ethyl alcohol)	mg/dL	0.217	mmol/L
Ethylene glycol	mg/L	16.11	µmol/L
Ferritin	ng/mL	2.247	pmol/L
Fibrinogen	mg/dL	0.0294	µmol/L
Fluoride	µg/mL	52.6	µmol/L
Follicle-stimulating hormone	mIU/mL	1	IU/L
Fructose	mg/dL	55.5	µmol/L
Galactose	mg/dL	55.506	µmol/L
Glucagon	pg/mL	1	ng/L
Glucose	mg/dL	0.0555	mmol/L
Glutamine	mg/dL	68.42	µmol/L
Gamma glutamyl transferase (GGT)	units/L	1	U/L
Hematocrit	%	0.01	Proportion of 1.0
Hemoglobin (whole blood)	g/dL	10	g/L
• Mass concentration		0.6206	mmol/L
High-density lipoprotein cholesterol (HDL-C)	mg/dL	0.0259	mmol/L
Histidine	mg/dL	64.45	µmol/L
Homocysteine (total)	mg/L	7.397	µmol/L
Human chorionic gonadotropin (hCG)	mIU/mL	1	IU/L
Hydroxyproline	mg/dL	76.3	µmol/L
Immunoglobulin A (IgA)	mg/dL	0.01	g/L
Immunoglobulin D (IgD)	mg/dL	10	mg/L
Immunoglobulin E (IgE)	mg/dL	10	mg/L

Component	Conventional Unit	Conversion Factor	SI Unit
Immunoglobulin G (IgG)	mg/dL	0.01	g/L
Immunoglobulin M (IgM)	mg/dL	0.01	g/L
Insulin	μIU/mL	6.945	pmol/L
Iron, total	μg/dL	0.179	μmol/L
Iron binding capacity, total	μg/dL	0.179	μmol/L
Isopropanol	mg/L	0.0166	mmol/L
Lactate (lactic acid)	mg/dL	0.111	mmol/L
Lactate dehydrogenase	units/L	1	U/L
Lactate dehydrogenase	%	0.01	Proportion of 1.0
Lead	μg/dL	0.0483	μmol/L
Leucine	mg/dL	76.237	μmol/L
Lipase	units/L	1	U/L
Lipids (total)	mg/dL	0.01	g/L
Lipoprotein (a)	mg/dL	0.0357	μmol/L
Lithium	mEq/L	1	mmol/L
Low-density lipoprotein cholesterol (LDL-C)	mg/dL	0.0259	mmol/L
Luteinizing hormone (LH, leutropin)	IU/L	1	IU/L
Magnesium	mg/dL	0.411	mmol/L
Manganese	ng/mL	18.2	nmol/L
Methemoglobin	% of total hemoglobin	0.01	Proportion of total hemoglobin
Methionine	mg/dL	67.02	μmol/L
Nicotine	mg/L	6.164	μmol/L
Nitrogen, nonprotein	mg/dL	0.714	mmol/L
Norepinephrine	pg/mL	0.00591	nmol/L
Osmolality	mOsm/kg	1	mmol/kg
Oxalate	mg/L	11.1	μmol/L
Parathyroid hormone	pg/mL	1	ng/L
Phenobarbital	mg/L	4.31	μmol/L
Phosphorus	mg/dL	0.323	mmol/L
Plasminogen	mg/dL	0.113	μmol/L
	%	0.01	Proportion of 1.0
Plasminogen activator inhibitor	mIU/mL	1	IU/L
Platelets (thrombocytes)	$\times 10^3/\mu L$	1	$\times 10^9/L$
Potassium	mEq/L	1	mmol/L
Progesterone	ng/mL	3.18	nmol/L
Prolactin	μg/L	43.478	pmol
Proline	mg/dL	86.86	μmol/L
Protein, total	g/dL	10	g/L
Prothrombin	g/L	13.889	μmol/L
Prothrombin time (protime, PT)	Sec	1	Sec
Pyruvate	mg/dL	113.6	μmol/L
Quinidine	μg/mL	3.08	μmol/L
Red blood cell count	$\times 10^6/\mu L$	1	$\times 10^{12}/L$
Renin	pg/mL	0.0237	pmol/L
Reticulocyte count	% of RBCs	0.01	Proportion of 1.0
Serotonin (5-hydroxytryptamine)	ng/mL	0.00568	μmol/L
Sodium	mEq/L	1	mmol/L
Somatostatin	pg/mL	0.611	pmol/L
Taurine	mg/dL	79.91	μmol/L
Testosterone	ng/dL	0.0347	nmol/L
Theophylline	μg/mL	5.55	μmol/L
Thyroglobulin	ng/mL	1	μg/L
Thyrotropin (thyroid-stimulating hormone, TSH)	mIU/L	1	mIU/L
Thyroxine, free (T_4)	ng/dL	12.87	pmol/L
Thyroxine, total (T_4)	μg/dL	12.87	nmol/L
Transferrin	mg/dL	0.01	g/L
Triglycerides	mg/dL	0.0113	mmol/L

Continued

Component	Conventional Unit	Conversion Factor	SI Unit
Triiodothyronine			
Free (T_3)	pg/dL	0.0154	pmol/L
Total (T_3)	ng/dL	0.0154	nmol/L
Tryptophan	mg/dL	48.97	μmol/L
Tyrosine	mg/dL	55.19	μmol/L
Urea nitrogen	mg/dL	0.357	mmol/L
Uric acid	mg/dL	59.48	μmol/L
Valine	mg/dL	85.5	μmol/L
Vitamin A (retinol)	μg/dL	0.0349	μmol/L
Vitamin B_6 (pyridoxine)	ng/mL	4.046	nmol/L
Vitamin B_{12} (cyanocobalamin)	pg/mL	0.738	pmol/L
Vitamin C (ascorbic acid)	mg/dL	56.78	μmol/L
Vitamin D			
1,25-Dihydroxyvitamin D	pg/mL	2.6	pmol/L
25-Hydroxyvitamin D	ng/mL	2.496	nmol/L
Vitamin E	mg/dL	23.22	μmol/L
Vitamin K	ng/mL	2.22	nmol/L
Warfarin	μg/mL	3.247	μmol/L
White blood cell count	$\times 10^3/\mu L$	1	$\times 10^9/L$
White blood cell differential count (number fraction)	%	0.01	Proportion of 1.0
Zinc	μg/dL	0.153	μmol/L

Corneal Ulcer

- Ulcers should be classified by depth (superficial, deep stromal, descemetocele) and by cause.
- The ulcers can also be classified as nonhealing, sterile, infected, or rapidly progressive.

<table>
<tr><th>Reptile/Amphibian</th><th>Bird</th><th>Mammal</th></tr>
<tr><td>Post hibernation</td><td></td><td></td></tr>
<tr><td>Corneal lipidosis</td><td>“Mynah bird keratitis”</td><td>Entropion</td></tr>
<tr><td colspan="2">Following transport</td><td>Lid defects</td></tr>
<tr><td colspan="3">Trauma/Scratch</td></tr>
<tr><td colspan="3">Cranial nerve defects (CN V, VII)</td></tr>
<tr><td colspan="3">Foreign body</td></tr>
<tr><td colspan="3">Herpesvirus</td></tr>
<tr><td></td><td></td><td>Chinchilla: prolonged exposure to dustbath</td></tr>
<tr><td></td><td></td><td>Ferrets: exposure keratitis secondary to exophthalmos</td></tr>
<tr><td></td><td></td><td>Young kangaroos: dehydration</td></tr>
<tr><td></td><td></td><td>Keratoconjunctivitis sicca</td></tr>
<tr><td colspan="3">Glaucoma with progressive buphthalmos</td></tr>
<tr><td colspan="3">Uveitis</td></tr>
<tr><td colspan="3">Exophthalmos from orbital abscess</td></tr>
<tr><td colspan="3">Severe debilitation</td></tr>
</table>

Cranial Nerve Deficits

Nerve	Clinical Signs	Clinical Tests	Normal Response	Abnormal Response
I. Olfactory	Hyposmia or anosmia	Smell of food or nonirritating, volatile substance	Interest in food; sniff, recoil, or nose lick with volatile substance	No response
II. Optic	Visual impairment and hesitancy in moving	1. Obstacle test 2. Visual placing reaction 3. Menace reaction 4. Following movement test	1. Avoidance of obstacle 2. Visual placement of limbs 3. Eye blink 4. Eyes following objects	1. Bumping objects 2-4. No response
III. Oculomotor	1. Ventrolateral strabismus 2. Paralysis of upper eyelid (ptosis), mydriasis	1. Ocular movement in horizontal and vertical planes 2. Point source of light in each eye	1. Normal ocular excursion 2. Direct and consensual pupillary light reflexes	1. Impaired movements of affected eye 2. On affected side, direct pupillary reflex absent, consensual reflex present; on normal side, direct pupillary reflex present, consensual reflex absent
Sympathetic control of pupillary function	Constricted pupil (miosis), enophthalmos, prolapse of third eyelid, ptosis of upper lid			
IV. Trochlear	Usually not noted			
V. Trigeminal (motor and sensory)	1. Atrophy of masticatory muscles 2. Inability to close mouth	1. Jaw tone 2. Palpate and observe masticatory muscles 3. Palpebral reflex 4. Corneal reflex 5. Probe nasal mucosa 6. Touch face	1. Resistance to opening jaws 2. Normal muscle contour and resilience 3. Eye blink 4. Eye blink and globe retraction 5. Recoil 6. No reaction	1. Lack of resistance 2. Atrophy, hypotonia 3-5. No response 6. Intense discomfort
VI. Abducent	Medial strabismus	Ocular movements in horizontal plane	Normal ocular excursion	Impaired lateral movement of affected eye
VII. Facial	1. Asymmetry of facial expression 2. Inability to close eyelids 3. Lip commissure paralysis 4. Ear paralysis	1. Palpebral reflex 2. Corneal reflex 3. Menace reaction 4. Tickle ear	1-3. Eye blink 4. Ear flick	1-4. No response
VIII. Vestibulocochlear vestibular	Nystagmus, head tilt, circling Falling and rolling	1. Ocular movements in horizontal and vertical planes 2. Caloric and rotatory test 3. Righting reactions	1-2. Normal physiologic nystagmus 3. Normal righting	1-3. No response, ventrolateral strabismus on dorsal extension of head
Cochlear	Deafness	Hand clap	Startle reaction, blink ear contraction	No response
IX. Glossopharyngeal	Dysphagia	Gag reflex	Swallowing response	No response
X. Vagus	1. Dysphagia 2. Abnormal vocalizing 3. Inspiratory dyspnea 4. Megaesophagus	1. Gag reflex 2. Laryngeal reflex 3. Oculocardiac reflex	1. Swallow 2. Cough 3. Bradycardia	1-3. No response
XI. Spinal accessory	Usually not noted			
XII. Hypoglossal	Deviation of tongue	1. Tongue stretch 2. Nose rub	1. Retraction 2. Lick response	1-2. No response

With permission from Braund KG: Clinical syndromes in veterinary neurology, St Louis, 1994, Mosby.

Dangerous Antibiotics

Reptile/ Amphibian	Bird	Mammal	Reptile/ Amphibian	Bird	Mammal
	Carnidazole	**Guinea Pig**			Tylosin
	Cephaloridine	Amoxicillin			Vancomycin
Chloramphenicol		Ampicillin			
	Dimetridazole	Aureomycin			**Hamster**
	Ivermectin	Bacitracin			Ampicillin
	Levamisole	Cefadroxil			Carbenicillin
	Lincomycin	Cephalexin/Cefadroxil			Cephalosporins
Metronidazole		Cephalosporins			Chloramphenicol
	Polymyxin B	Cephazolin			Clindamycin
	Praziquantel	Chlortetracycline			Erythromycin
	Procaine penicillin	Clindamycin			Gentamicin
	Quinacrine HCl	Dihydrostreptomycin			Lincomycin
	Selenium sulfide	Erythromycin			Neomycin
	Sulfachlorpyridazine	Lincomycin			Penicillin
	Ticarcillin	Oxytetracycline			Streptomycin
		Penicillin			Tetracycline
		Procaine			Ticarcillin
		Streptomycin	Chlorhexidine (ingestion during soaking)		Trimethoprim-sulfamethoxazole
		Tetracycline			
			Ivermectin in tortoises		Vancomycin
		Rabbit			
		Erythromycin	Use with extreme caution:		
		Spiramycin			
		Ampicillin	Amikacin, gentamicin		
		Cephalexin	Fenbendazole		
		Clindamycin	Amphotericin B		
		Lincomycin	Griseofulvin		
		Minocycline	Vitamins A, D, E		
		Penicillin (PO)	Pyrethrins and pyrethroids		
		Spectinomycin	Organophosphates and carbamates		

Dermatosis

- A detailed history is extremely important to exclude husbandry/management-related causes of the dermatoses. In the avian patient, rule out systemic disease before addressing behavioral aspects of self-mutilation.
- Often a biopsy is needed as part of the diagnostic process.

	Reptile	Bird	Mammal
Parasitic	Ectoparasites (mites, fleas, lice)		
		Giardia in cockatiels	
Fungal	Dermatophytosis, yeasts		
Bacterial/Viral	Sepsis (blister disease in snakes)	Circovirus in lovebirds	Staphylococcal
		PBFD	
Behavioral	Cagemate aggression		
		Self-mutilation	
	Normal behavior (e.g., male bites female during courtship)		
Neoplasia	Cutaneous lymphoma, lipoma, papilloma		
		Xanthoma	
		Endoparasites	

	Reptile	Bird	Mammal
Systemic disease		Allergy	
	Metabolic disease		
	Liver disease		
	Regional neurologic disease		
	Pain		
	Diabetes mellitus		
		Food allergies	
		Hypothyroid	
Husbandry-related	High or low humidity, wrong substrate, small enclosure, burn wound, frost bite		
	Topical irritant (cleaning solution/chemical irritation)		
	Trauma		
	Predation from prey animal		
Nutritional deficiencies	General malnutrition		
	Vitamin A/B/E, Se, zinc deficiency		
Other		Feather cyst	

PBFD, Psittacine beak and feather disease.

Diabetes Mellitus

Reptile/Amphibian	Bird	Mammal
Iatrogenic hypoglycemia		
Pancreatitis		
Hepatic lipidosis		
Hypoinsulinemia		
		Ferret: sequel after insulinoma surgery
Water dragon appears predisposed	Toco toucans, budgerigars, and cockatiels frequently develop it	Many lab animals (e.g., degus, chinchilla, mice, rats) are prone to it
Egg-related peritonitis		
Islet cell carcinomas		
Pituitary adenoma		
Renal carcinomas		
Stress		

Diarrhea

- Diarrhea is an excess amount of water in the feces. Often the patient is dehydrated. Check cloacal area for staining, which often indicates a chronic problem.
- Examine appearance and odor of feces because this might indicate nature of problem (anaerobic bacteria, blood).
- Perform occult blood test on fecal material.
- Make sure that presentation is not polyuria mixed with normal fecal deposit.
- See Diarrhea algorithm, Sec. V.

<table>
<tr><th>Reptile</th><th>Bird</th><th>Mammal</th></tr>
<tr><td colspan="3">Bacterial/Viral enteritis (Gram-negative, Salmonella, Chlamydophila, Clostridium)
Mycobacteriosis (gastrointestinal [GI])</td></tr>
<tr><td colspan="3">Malnutrition or sudden food change</td></tr>
<tr><td colspan="3">Toxicoses (heavy metal, mycotoxin)</td></tr>
<tr><td colspan="3">Systemic disease (hepatic, renal, pancreatic)</td></tr>
<tr><td colspan="3">Poor-quality food (low-fiber, high-fat foods)</td></tr>
<tr><td colspan="3">Fungal (Candida)</td></tr>
<tr><td colspan="3">Parasitic (coccidia, tapeworm, protozoa)</td></tr>
<tr><td colspan="3">Stress</td></tr>
<tr><td></td><td>Viral disease (herpes, polyoma, proventricular dilatation disease)</td><td>Inflammatory bowel disease</td></tr>
<tr><td colspan="3">Intussusception</td></tr>
<tr><td colspan="3">Antibiotic-induced</td></tr>
<tr><td></td><td>Impending egg laying</td><td></td></tr>
<tr><td colspan="2">Egg binding/Coelomitis</td><td></td></tr>
<tr><td colspan="3">GI lymphoma</td></tr>
<tr><td></td><td>Cloacal papilloma</td><td></td></tr>
</table>

Distended Coelom

- Radiographs are often unrewarding in diagnosing the origin or nature of the distention; coelomic ultrasound exams often can shed light on the nature of the distention.
- An ultrasound-guided fine-needle aspiration can also aid in the diagnostic process and carries less risk of iatrogenic trauma than a blind stick.

<table>
<tr><th>Reptile</th><th>Bird</th><th>Mammal</th></tr>
<tr><td colspan="2">Egg binding</td><td></td></tr>
<tr><td colspan="3">Ascites (hepatic failure, cardiac failure, hypoproteinemia)</td></tr>
<tr><td colspan="3">Ovarian cysts, retained follicles</td></tr>
<tr><td colspan="3">Organomegaly</td></tr>
<tr><td colspan="3">Trauma (hemoperitoneum)</td></tr>
<tr><td colspan="3">Neoplasia</td></tr>
<tr><td colspan="2">Peritonitis (e.g., egg yolk)</td><td></td></tr>
<tr><td colspan="3">Obesity</td></tr>
<tr><td colspan="3">Parasitic infestation (extraluminal)</td></tr>
<tr><td colspan="3">Amyloidosis</td></tr>
<tr><td colspan="3">Hypoproteinemia</td></tr>
<tr><td colspan="3">Uroliths or fecoliths</td></tr>
<tr><td colspan="3">Normal egg laying or gestation</td></tr>
<tr><td colspan="3">Rupture of abscess</td></tr>
<tr><td colspan="3">Gastrointestinal perforation</td></tr>
<tr><td></td><td></td><td>GDV (guinea pigs)</td></tr>
<tr><td></td><td></td><td>Cushing's disease (hamster)</td></tr>
<tr><td></td><td></td><td>Heartworm</td></tr>
<tr><td></td><td></td><td>Hypothyroidism</td></tr>
<tr><td></td><td></td><td>Myopathy: abdominal muscle weakness</td></tr>
<tr><td colspan="3">Pneumoperitoneum/coelom</td></tr>
<tr><td></td><td></td><td>Pyometra</td></tr>
</table>

GDV, Gastric dilatation and volvulus.

Dyspnea

<table>
<tr><th>Infectious Causes</th><th>Reptile/Amphibian</th><th>Bird</th><th>Mammal</th></tr>
<tr><td>Bacterial</td><td colspan="3">Gram-negative and Gram-positive agents</td></tr>
<tr><td></td><td colspan="2">Chlamydial</td><td>Mycoplasma</td></tr>
<tr><td>Fungal agents</td><td></td><td>Aspergillosis</td><td></td></tr>
<tr><td></td><td></td><td colspan="2">Cryptococcus</td></tr>
<tr><td>Viral agents</td><td>Herpes</td><td></td><td></td></tr>
<tr><td></td><td></td><td colspan="2">Influenza</td></tr>
<tr><td></td><td></td><td>Infectious laryngotracheitis</td><td></td></tr>
<tr><td>Parasitic</td><td></td><td>Capillaria (gape worm)</td><td></td></tr>
<tr><td></td><td colspan="2">Mites</td><td></td></tr>
<tr><td></td><td>Pentastomites</td><td></td><td></td></tr>
<tr><td>Metabolic</td><td colspan="3">Organ failure</td></tr>
<tr><td></td><td></td><td>Hemochromatosis</td><td></td></tr>
<tr><td></td><td colspan="3">Anemia</td></tr>
<tr><td></td><td colspan="2">Gout</td><td></td></tr>
<tr><td></td><td colspan="3">Acidemia</td></tr>
<tr><td></td><td colspan="3">Pain</td></tr>
<tr><td>Toxins</td><td></td><td>Teflon</td><td></td></tr>
<tr><td></td><td></td><td colspan="2">Smoke</td></tr>
<tr><td>Physical</td><td colspan="3">Aspiration pneumonia</td></tr>
<tr><td></td><td colspan="3">Foreign body inhalation</td></tr>
<tr><td></td><td colspan="3">Mass occupying abdomen</td></tr>
<tr><td></td><td colspan="3">Ascites</td></tr>
<tr><td></td><td colspan="3">Trauma</td></tr>
<tr><td></td><td colspan="2">Coelomitis</td><td>Peritonitis</td></tr>
<tr><td></td><td colspan="2">Egg binding</td><td>Gravid</td></tr>
<tr><td></td><td>Constrictive cartilage growth</td><td></td><td></td></tr>
<tr><td></td><td colspan="3">Nasal obstruction</td></tr>
<tr><td></td><td></td><td></td><td>Diaphragmatic hernia</td></tr>
<tr><td></td><td colspan="3">Obesity</td></tr>
<tr><td>Other</td><td colspan="3">Bronchial disease</td></tr>
<tr><td></td><td colspan="3">Pulmonary edema</td></tr>
</table>

Dystocia

Under no circumstances should the egg or the fetus manipulated to be expelled. Trauma to the reproductive tract is a common sequel to manipulation and can often lead to fatal consequences.

<table>
<tr><th></th><th>Reptile/Amphibian</th><th>Bird</th><th>Mammal</th></tr>
<tr><td>Husbandry-related</td><td colspan="3">Malnutrition (Ca, vitamin A or E def)</td></tr>
<tr><td></td><td colspan="3">Lack of exercise</td></tr>
<tr><td></td><td colspan="3">Lack of suitable substrate</td></tr>
<tr><td></td><td colspan="3">Old age</td></tr>
<tr><td></td><td colspan="3">Stress</td></tr>
<tr><td></td><td colspan="3">Poor physical condition</td></tr>
<tr><td></td><td>Low temperature</td><td></td><td></td></tr>
</table>

Continued

	Reptile/Amphibian	Bird	Mammal
Anatomic	Oviduct/uterine infection		
	Oviduct/uterine rupture or other pathology		
	Egg is located in bladder (common after oxytocin injections)		Abnormalities of the fetus
			Guinea pig: bred too late, after pelvis fused
	Concurrent disease		
	Oversized fetus/egg		
	Inadequate muscular contractions		
	Obstruction of the birth canal		

Emaciation

See Weight Loss algorithms, Sec. V.

Reptile/Amphibian	Bird	Mammal
Parasitic infestation		
Cagemate aggression		
Nutrient absorption problem		
Organ failure		
Nutrient deficiency/underfeeding		
Stress		
Poor husbandry (cool temperature)	Proventricular dilatation disease	Inflammatory bowel disease
Cancer (gastrointestinal lymphoma)		
	Avian gastric yeast	
Oral/dental disease		
Nephropathy		
Gastroenteropathy		
Cardiac disease		
		Hyperthyroidism
		Chronic fever
End-stage renal failure		
Neoplasia		
Chronic infection/inflammation		
Anemia		
Chronic diarrhea		

Gastric Stasis

Reptile/Amphibian	Bird	Mammal
Cold temperature		Hairball
Stress		
Foreign body ingestion		
Bloat		
Constipation		
Gastrointestinal torsion		
Abdominal pain		
Oral problems	Beak problems	Dental problems
Poor husbandry		
Preparation for hibernation	Atypical proventricular dilatation disease	Hypertrophic pylorus
Dehydration		
Intraabdominal abscess		

Hematuria

Care has to be taken to correctly diagnose hematuria because urine or urates often can be colored reddish owing to other causes.

Reptile/Amphibian	Bird	Mammal
	Renal pathology	
	Blunt trauma	
	Neoplasia of urinary tract or reproductive tract	
	Post renal biopsy	
	Inflammatory disease	
	Bleeding disorder	
		Estrus
		Uroliths
	Amazons: lead toxicity	Parasites (bladder worms)
		Pseudohematuria: porphyrins
		Cystitis
	Warfarin toxicity	
	DIC	
	Food coloring	

DIC, Disseminated intravascular coagulation.

Hepatic Failure

Reptile/Amphibian	Bird	Mammal
	Trauma	
	Toxins/Mycotoxins	
	Drug-induced	
	Infectious agents (ascending bowel infection)	
	Peritonitis/Coelomitis	
	Pancreatitis	
	Hepatic lipidosis	
	Chronic congestive heart failure	
	Hemochromatosis	Biliary obstruction
	Hepatic fibrosis	
	Hepatic cirrhosis	
	Hepatic neoplasia	
	Viral hepatitis (adeno-, herpes, polyoma-, paramyxo-)	
	Parasitic hepatitis (coccidiosis, *Toxoplasma,* Microsporidium, trematodes, etc.)	
		Heatstroke

Hypercalcemia

- Significant elevation can be seen in females during folliculogenesis and during egg laying.
- Rabbits usually have higher calcium levels than other mammals.

Reptile	Bird	Mammal
Vitamin A or D toxicosis		
Normal ovulation		
Dehydration/Hemoconcentration		
Toxicosis (drugs, plant, rodenticide)		
Hyperparathyroidism		
Neoplasia (paraneoplastic syndrome, e.g., lymphoma)		
	Cystic ovarian disease	
Normal ovulation		Growing animals
Hyperproteinemia, lipemia		
Environmental hypothermia		
Laboratory error/Detergent contamination of sample		
		Chronic kidney disease
	Osteomyelitis	
Hypertrophic osteodystrophy		
Excessive Ca supplementation		
Granulomatous disease		

Hyperkalemia

- Use green top tube (heparinized) to collect blood to avoid lysis of blood cells.
- If very small needles (25 gauge, 27 gauge) are used for blood collection, lysis of blood cells is common, causing elevation in Ka.

Reptile	Bird	Mammal
Severe tissue damage		
Renal failure (decreased excretion)		
Adrenal disease		
Dehydration		
Hemolytic anemia		
Phlebotomy (lysis of red blood cells)		
Iatrogenic (excess Ka in fluids, nonspecific β-blockers, spironolactone, enalapril)		
Ruptured urinary bladder		Ruptured urinary bladder
	Thrombocytosis	
	Insulin deficiency	
	Acute tumor lysis syndrome	
Drug-induced (spironolactone, amiloride, prostaglandin inhibitor, heparin)		

Hyperlipidemia

- Nutritional causes appear to account for the vast majority of hyperlipidemia cases.
- Hospitalize patient for a few days before repeat blood check to rule out husbandry-related causes of hyperlipidemia.

Reptile	Bird	Mammal
Nutritional (excess fat in diet)		
Starvation		
Post hibernation		
Liver disease		
Bile duct obstruction		
Hypothyroidism (see References)		
	Atherosclerosis	
Normal reproductive activity in the female		
Lipid metabolism disorder		
Pancreatic disease		
Egg yolk coelomitis		
Postprandial blood sample		

REFERENCES

Carter JK, et al: Rapid induction of hypothyroidism by an avian leukosis virus, Infect Immun 40:795–805, 1983.
Frye FL, et al: Hypothyroidism in turtles and tortoises, Vet Med Small Anim Clin 69:990–993, 1974.
Ramachandran AV, et al: Local and systemic alterations in cyclic 3′,5′ AMP phosphodiesterase activity in relation to tail regeneration under hypothyroidism and T4 replacement in the lizard, *Mabuya carinata*, Mol Reprod Dev 45:48–51, 1996.

Incontinence, Urinary

Reptile/Amphibian	Bird	Mammal
		Renal calculi
		Spinal cord compression
		Spinal cord trauma
		Pyelonephritis
		Spinal epidural abscess
Neoplasms, brain		
		Urinary obstruction
Neoplasms, spinal cord		
		Urinary tract infection
		Prostatitis/Vaginitis
Loss of cloacal sphincter tone		Loss of urethral sphincter tone
	PU/PD stress	
Hyperhydration		

PD, Polydipsia; *PU*, polyuria.

Inflammatory Bowel Disease

Reptile/Amphibian	Bird	Mammal
		Antibiotic-associated colitis
		Colon cancer
		Fever of unknown origin
		Intestinal lymphoma
		Ischemic colitis
		Pseudomembranous colitis
		Radiation-induced colitis
		Food allergies
Parasitic infestation (e.g., *Giardia, Coccidia, Toxoplasma,* etc.)		
Chronic bacterial infection		
Ascending infection from cloaca		Eosinophilic syndrome

Lameness

- Always observe for movements of legs and pain sensation, swelling, or skin lesions, etc.
- Lack of movement or response to pain indicates a neurologic problem.

Reptile	Bird	Mammal
Trauma		
Neoplasia (e.g., osteosarcoma)		
Severe constipation (especially Chelonians)	Renal tumors (impingement on the ischiatic nerve)	
Toxicoses		
Gout		
Neurologic problems (e.g., peripheral neuropathy from proventricular dilatation disease, lead toxicosis, egg binding)		
Nutritional/Husbandry mistakes		
Congenital/developmental defects		
Chronic disease		
Pain (e.g., osteoarthritis)		
Metabolic (e.g., hypocalcemia)		
Infectious (e.g., arthritis due to *Mycoplasma* or *Salmonella*)		

Liver Failure

- Liver biopsy is the most accurate way to diagnose and characterize the nature of liver failure.
- Bile acids appear fairly sensitive and specific in the avian patient to diagnose liver failure.

Reptile	Bird	Mammal
Nutritional (hepatic lipidosis)		
Infectious (bacterial, viral, fungal) local or general mycobacteriosis, chlamydophilosis Herpesvirus, polyomavirus, adenovirus, etc.		
Chronic disease (e.g., fibrosis, cirrhosis)		
Neoplasia (e.g., lymphoma, metastatic disease, primary liver tumors)		
Amyloidosis		
Parasitic (coccidian, *Toxoplasma,* trematodes, *Plasmodium, Histomonas,* etc.)		
Post hibernation	Hemochromatosis	
Toxicosis (e.g., mycotoxicosis)		
Trauma		

Nasal Discharge

Reptile/Amphibian	Bird	Mammal
Rhinitis		
Bacterial infections		
Neoplasia		
Viral infections		
Fungal infections		
Parasitic infestations		
Food aspiration		
	Sinusitis	
	Inhalation of toxins/irritants	
Vitamin A deficiency		
Iatrogenic: prolonged antibiotic therapy		
Lower respiratory tract pathology		
		Nasal polyps
		Megaesophagus
		Oronasal fistula
Foreign body inhalation		
Trauma		

Neurologic Signs

RELATIONSHIP OF CLINICAL SIGNS TO ANATOMIC SITE OF LESION

Clinical Signs	Functional System	Anatomic Location
Inability to prehend	Masticatory and tongue muscles	CN V, XII, pons-medulla
Dysphagia	Tongue; palatal, pharyngeal, and esophageal muscles	CN IX, X, XI, XII, medulla
Drooling	Facial paralysis, dysphagia	CN VII, middle ear, medulla
		CN IX, X, medulla
Head tilt, nystagmus, loss of balance, rolling	Vestibular system	CN VIII: inner ear, medulla, cerebellum
Strabismus	CN to extraocular muscles, vestibular system	CN III, IV, VI, midbrain-medulla
		Inner ear-medulla-cerebellum
Circling		
With loss of balance	Vestibular system	Inner ear, medulla, cerebellum
Without loss of balance	Limbic system (?)	Frontal lobe, rostral thalamus
Head and eye deviation—turning to one side	Limbic system (?)	Frontal lobe, rostral thalamus
Pacing, head pressing	Limbic system	Frontal lobe, rostral thalamus
Opisthotonos	Upper motor neuron	Rostral cerebellum, midbrain
Blindness	Visual system	
	Dilated unresponsive pupils	Eyeball, optic nerves
	Normal pupils	Visual cortex-cerebrum, (midbrain)
Depression, semicoma, coma	Ascending reticular activating system	Pons to thalamus-cerebral cortex
Seizures	Cerebrum, thalamus-hypothalamus	
Hyperesthesia, hyperactivity to external stimuli	Ascending reticular activating system	Thalamus, cerebrum
Aggressive behavior, mania-hysteria, odontoprisis	Limbic system	Thalamus, cerebrum
Tremor		
Associated with movements, head, and neck	Cerebellar system	Cerebellum
Associated with movements, head, trunk, limbs	Multiple systems	Diffuse CNS
Episodic, not associated with movements, head, trunk, limbs		Thalamus, cerebrum
Bradycardia, hypothermia, hyperthermia	UMN for general visceral efferent system	Hypothalamus
Irregular-ataxic respirations	UMN for respiratory muscle LMN	Pons-medulla

From de Lahunta A: Veterinary neuroanatomy and clinical neurology, St Louis, 1983, Saunders.

CN, Cranial nerve; *CNS,* central nervous system; *LMN,* lower motor neuron; *UMN,* upper motor neuron; ?, may occur with lesion in this location.

Polyphagia

	Reptile/ Amphibian	Bird	Mammal
Neoplastic disorders			Insulinoma/Islet cell tumor
	Cancer		
Infectious disorders	Parasitic infestation		
Metabolic, storage disorders	Hypoglycemia		
	Diabetes mellitus, poorly controlled		
	Diabetic ketoacidosis/coma		
	Gouty attack		
	Increased exercise		
	Poor-quality food		
	Obesity		
	Hypothalamic lesion, hypothalamic dysfunction		
			Pregnancy
			Lactation
			Cold environment
	Malabsorption syndrome		
Psychological disorders	Stress		
	Competition		
	Highly palatable food		
	Boredom		
Endocrine disorders			Hyperthyroidism
Iatrogenic	Thyroid administration/Toxicity		
	Hypoglycemia, diabetic/treatment		
	Insulin (Humulin/Novulin) administration/Toxicity		
			Phenobarbitone
			Benzodiazepines

Polyuria/Polydipsia

Although polyuria is relatively common in the avian patient, it is uncommon in the reptilian patient.

PHYSIOLOGIC

Reptile	Bird	Mammal
Stress		
	Egg laying	
	Feeding chicks	
Hot and dry environments		Cold environments
	Hand-fed chicks	
Diet with high water content		

PATHOLOGIC

<table>
<tr><th>Reptile</th><th>Bird</th><th>Mammal</th></tr>
<tr><td colspan="3">Diabetes mellitus</td></tr>
<tr><td></td><td colspan="2">Diabetes insipidus</td></tr>
<tr><td colspan="3">Renal disease, gout</td></tr>
<tr><td colspan="3">Liver disease</td></tr>
<tr><td colspan="3">Peritonitis</td></tr>
<tr><td colspan="3">Nutritional (excess protein, vitamin A def, hypervitamin D_3, excess salt)</td></tr>
<tr><td colspan="3">Toxins (heavy metal, salt, mycotoxin, ethylene glycol, etc.)</td></tr>
<tr><td colspan="3">Neoplasia</td></tr>
<tr><td></td><td colspan="2">Behavioral (fear, psychogenic)</td></tr>
<tr><td colspan="3">Iatrogenic (aminoglycosides, steroids, progesterone, etc.)</td></tr>
<tr><td colspan="3">Hypothalamic thirst center defect</td></tr>
<tr><td></td><td></td><td>Hyperthyroidism</td></tr>
<tr><td colspan="3">Hyperglycemia</td></tr>
<tr><td colspan="3">Nephropathy, hypokalemic</td></tr>
<tr><td colspan="3">Glucosuria</td></tr>
<tr><td colspan="3">Hypercalciuria</td></tr>
<tr><td></td><td></td><td>Pheochromocytoma</td></tr>
<tr><td colspan="3">Primary polydipsia</td></tr>
<tr><td></td><td></td><td>Leptospirosis</td></tr>
<tr><td></td><td></td><td>Diabetes insipidus</td></tr>
<tr><td></td><td></td><td>Postobstructive diuresis</td></tr>
<tr><td></td><td></td><td>Hyperadrenocorticism</td></tr>
<tr><td></td><td></td><td>Antidiuretic hormone resistance (nephrogenic diabetes insipidus)</td></tr>
<tr><td></td><td></td><td>Antidiuretic hormone deficiency (central diabetes insipidus)</td></tr>
<tr><td></td><td></td><td>Pyelonephritis</td></tr>
<tr><td></td><td></td><td>Pyometra</td></tr>
</table>

Regurgitation/Vomiting

- Although regurgitation in snakes is fairly common and does not have to be related to systemic disease, in lizards and turtles, it is highly pathologic, and often the prognosis is poor to grave.
- In the avian patient, always do a thorough behavioral analysis to rule out behavioral regurgitation versus pathologic causes.

<table>
<tr><th>Reptile</th><th>Bird</th><th>Mammal</th></tr>
<tr><td colspan="3">Systemic infection (especially Gram-negative)</td></tr>
<tr><td colspan="3">Liver disease (lipidosis, hepatitis)</td></tr>
<tr><td></td><td colspan="2">Toxicosis (heavy metal, mycotoxins, etc.)</td></tr>
<tr><td></td><td>Iatrogenic (doxycycline, etc.)</td><td></td></tr>
<tr><td>Stress (snakes being handled after eating)</td><td>Behavioral (courtship, breeding)</td><td>Megaesophagus</td></tr>
<tr><td colspan="3">Systemic fungal infections</td></tr>
<tr><td colspan="3">Gastrointestinal obstruction (volvulus, intussusception, stricture, etc.)</td></tr>
<tr><td colspan="3">Gastrointestinal neoplasia</td></tr>
<tr><td>Low environmental temperatures</td><td>Husbandry mistakes</td><td>Hypothyroidism</td></tr>
<tr><td></td><td>Parasitic infection</td><td></td></tr>
<tr><td></td><td>Fungal (e.g., Macrorhabdus ornithogaster, proventricular zygomycosis)</td><td></td></tr>
<tr><td></td><td>Proventricular dilatation disease</td><td></td></tr>
<tr><td colspan="3">Viral infection</td></tr>
<tr><td colspan="3">CNS disease</td></tr>
<tr><td colspan="3">Pancreatitis</td></tr>
<tr><td colspan="3">Overfeeding</td></tr>
<tr><td colspan="3">Motion sickness</td></tr>
<tr><td colspan="3">Peritonitis/coelomitis</td></tr>
</table>

Renal Failure

Permanent uric acid elevations are commonly seen once 70% to 80% of the glomerular filtration rate is decreased.

Reptile	Bird	Mammal
Infectious (bacterial, fungal, viral)		
Metabolic (gout, amyloidosis, hemochromatosis)		
Toxic (hypercalcemia, vitamin D, hemoglobin, drugs, etc.)		
Environmental mistakes (low humidity, etc.)	Neoplasia	
Chronic disease (immune complexes)		
Fibrosis		
Urolith obstruction		
Neoplasia (e.g., renal lymphoma)		
Nutritional (e.g., excessive dietary protein, inadequate vitamin A)		
Parasitic (*Isospora, Microsporidium,* coccidia, etc.)		
Hypertension		
Pancreatitis		
Iatrogenic (drug-induced)		
		Leptospirosis
		Pyelonephritis
Decreased cardiac output		
Hypovolemia		

Seizures

CAUSES

EXTRACRANIAL

Hypoglycemia
- Glycogen storage diseases
- Beta-cell neoplasm of pancreas/insulinoma
- Youth and malnutrition (especially small or toy breeds)
- Youth and GI disease (especially small or toy breeds)
- Insulin excess during treatment for diabetes mellitus
- Intestinal leiomyosarcoma

Hypoxemia
- Cardiorespiratory disease (e.g., severe bradycardia or severe tachycardia, disorders producing polycythemia)

Hepatoencephalopathy

Renal disease, especially nephrotic syndrome (embolism)

Hypocalcemia

Hyperkalemia

Hyperlipoproteinemia

GI disease
- Parasitism
- "Garbage intoxication"

Polycythemia
- Right-to-left shunt (e.g., reversed patent ductus arteriosus, tetralogy of Fallot, atrial or ventricular septal defect with concurrent pulmonic stenosis or pulmonary hypertension)
- Renal neoplasm (erythropoietin-producing)
- Chronic lung disease
- Polycythemia vera

INTRACRANIAL

Inflammation
- Canine distemper encephalitis, toxoplasmosis, cryptococcosis, neosporosis
- Other viral encephalitides: rabies
- Feline infectious peritonitis (FIP) meningoencephalitis in cats

Neoplasia
- Primary or metastatic

Malformation
- Hydrocephalus, lissencephaly-pachygyria

Injury

Degeneration
- Thiamine deficiency in cats
- Cerebral infarction in cats
- Intoxications: lead, mercury, arsenic, chlorinated hydrocarbons, organophosphates, hexachlorophene, ethylene glycol, radiopaque media for myelography, metaldehyde, tremorgenic mycotoxins (penitrem A, roquefortine), blue-green algae, chocolate, marijuana, ethanol/methanol/fermented materials (e.g., bread dough), prescription human medications

IDIOPATHIC EPILEPSY

Modified from de Lahunta A: Veterinary neuroanatomy and clinical neurology, St Louis, 1983, Saunders.

SEIZURES: CAUSES GROUPED ACCORDING TO AGE

PREVALENCE OF COMMON SEIZURE DISORDERS IN RELATION TO PATIENT'S AGE AT TIME OF ONSET OF FIRST SEIZURE

Age at onset: before 8 months

Rare: idiopathic epilepsy

Mainly
- Developmental disorders (e.g., malformations, hydrocephalus)
- Encephalitis or meningitis
- Trauma
- Extracranial causes
  - Hepatic encephalopathy (e.g., portacaval shunt)
  - Hypoglycemia
  - Intoxications
  - Intestinal parasitism

Age at onset: 8 months to 4 years
Mainly: idiopathic epilepsy
Seldom
- Developmental disorders (e.g., malformations, hydrocephalus)
- Trauma
- Encephalitis or meningitis
- Acquired hydrocephalus
- Neoplasia
- Extracranial causes
  - Hepatic encephalopathy (e.g., portacaval shunt, liver disease)
  - Hypocalcemia
  - Electrolyte disturbances
  - Hypothyroidism
  - Intoxications

Age at onset: after 4 years
Seldom
- Idiopathic epilepsy
- Trauma
- Encephalitis or meningitis
- Acquired hydrocephalus
- Extracranial causes
  - Hepatic encephalopathy (e.g., serious liver disease)
  - Hypocalcemia
  - Electrolyte disturbances
  - Hypothyroidism

Increasing
- Neoplasia
- Degenerative disorders
- Vascular disorders
- Extracranial causes
  - Hypoxia
  - Hypoglycemia

Modified with permission from Braund KB: Clinical syndromes in veterinary neurology, St Louis, 1994, Mosby, p 242.

SEIZURES: CHARACTERISTICS AND DIFFERENTIATION

Seizures, Differentiation from Other Events

	Seizure (Grand Mal)	Seizure (Partial)	Syncope	Episodic Weakness	Narcolepsy/ Cataplexy
Precipitating event	Usually none	Usually none	Exertion, pain, micturition, defecation, cough, stressful event	Exertion or none	Excitement, feeding
Prodrome	Minutes to days; atypical behavior (e.g., anxious, more withdrawn, attention-seeking) ± vomiting		Seconds; acute weakness, staggering, vocalization, autonomic stimulation	None (disorder is neuromuscular)	None
Aura	None	Marks onset of partial seizure	None	None	None
Event features	Chomping, hypersalivation, tonic-clonic limb motion; duration often 1-2 minutes; duration >5 minutes is consistent with seizure and highly inconsistent with syncope	Localized signs	Motionlessness; flaccid or rigid extension of limbs; opisthotonos possible; no tonic-clonic activity; duration generally transient (<1 minute)	Gradual or sudden loss of muscle tone, causing recumbency; mentation and consciousness remain normal; no tonic-clonic activity	Instantaneous loss of muscle tone; animal is immobile (sleeping) but appears to be aware of its surroundings
Recovery	Slowness returning to consciousness; disorientation (commonly 10 minutes or longer); blindness, circling, and other signs of central nervous system dysfunction common	Varies	Rapid recovery of normal mentation; often able to walk (and considered back to normal by owner) within minutes	Highly variable; generally reflective of course of onset (gradual onset associated with slow recovery); in some cases, rapid-onset disorders may have a protracted course	Fairly rapid (several seconds to 1 minute), with appearance of waking from sleep

Modified from Ettinger SJ, Feldman EC: Textbook of veterinary internal medicine, ed 6, St Louis, 2005, Saunders, p 27.
Convulsive syncope (anoxic) and anoxic-epileptic seizures are syncopal events generally caused by cardiac arrhythmias that produce profound syncope, temporary cerebral hypoxia, and seizures. Therefore, clarification of the type of event observed by the owner (syncope vs. seizure) may be difficult and generally rests on the observation of an episode, the presence of heart disease, and the documentation of a severe bradycardia or tachycardia during the event. Videotaping of an episode by the owner and cardiac event monitoring (pager-size portable electrocardiographic [ECG] unit that is triggered by the owner when an event occurs) can be invaluable in clarifying whether an animal is experiencing seizures versus syncope.

SEIZURES, REFRACTORY OR POORLY CONTROLLED

FACTORS RESPONSIBLE FOR INADEQUATE CONTROL OF SEIZURES

Medication and dosage
- Improper choice of drug
- Insufficient drug dosage
- Delayed increase in dosage
- Inadequate increase in dosage
- Too rapid change of medication
- Too rapid reduction of dosage
- Excessive fluctuations in serum concentrations
- Inappropriately combined drugs
- Failure to monitor serum levels
- Noncompliance
- Drug-drug interactions

Other precipitating factors
- Additional medications
- Additional diseases
- Physical or psychological stress

Diagnostic failures
- Extracerebral causes of seizures
- Progressive brain lesions
- Misidentification of episodes
- Syncope
- Myasthenia gravis
- Narcolepsy/cataplexy

Modified with permission from Kirk RW, Bonagura JD, editors: Kirk's current veterinary therapy XI: small animal practice, St Louis, 1993, Saunders, p 986.

Undigested Food in Droppings

Reptile	Bird	Mammal
Stress (frequent handling, etc.)	Proventricular dilatation disease	
	Dehydration	
Low environmental temperature	Ventricular koilin disorder	
Other husbandry-related problems (e.g., inappropriate food)	Fungal infections (*Candida*, zygomycosis, *Macrorhabdus ornithogaster*)	
	Recently weaned	
	Lack of grit	
	Neoplasia (e.g., proventricular or ventricular adenocarcinoma)	
Toxin (e.g., heavy metal)		
Gastrointestinal (GI) foreign body		
Enteritis		
GI lymphoma		
Parasitic disease		
Systemic disease (liver disease)		

Urate Coloration

For reptiles and birds:

- Normal color of urates is white to light beige.
- Abnormal is red, yellow, brown, and green.

For rabbits:

- Reddish discoloration of urine is very common.

	Reptile	Bird	Mammal
Infectious	Bacterial infection		
		Chlamydial (green)	
Viral		Acute PBFD	
		Herpesvirus	
Metabolic	Liver disease (yellow to green)		Porphyrins
		Hemochromatosis	Crystalluria
	Hemolysis		
			Myoglobinuria
Nutritional	Hypervitaminosis B		
	From food coloring (natural or artificial)		
	Berries, beets		
Toxic		Lead toxicity (hematuria in amazons)	
Physical		Cloacal papilloma	
	Bleeding from reproductive or urinary tract		
Iatrogenic			Azo dyes
	Drug-induced		
Other		Conure bleeding syndrome	

PBFD, Psittacine beak and feather disease.

Uric Acid Elevation

Permanent uric acid elevations are commonly seen once 70% to 80 % of the glomerular filtration rate is decreased.

Reptile	Bird
Renal disease	
Excess protein in diet	
Tissue necrosis	
Starvation	
Severe dehydration	
Toxicoses (e.g., heavy metal)	
Infections (e.g., polyomavirus, ascending or hematogenous bacterial infection)	
	Contamination during collection (toenail clip)
Postprandial (e.g., hawks, penguins)	

Weakness/Ataxia

Reptile	Bird	Mammal
Husbandry-related (low temperature, etc.)	Proventricular dilatation disease	Fever
	Atherosclerosis	
	Psychological disorders	
Abdominal/coelomic effusion		
Anemia		
Cardiovascular disease/low output		
Chronic overactivity		
Chronic systemic disease		
Chronic wasting diseases (e.g., mycobacteriosis)		
Drug-related		
Electrolyte disorder		
Encephalitis (bacterial, viral, fungal)		
Endocrine disorder (addisonian)		
Head or spinal trauma		
Liver disease (lipidosis, hepatitis)		
Metabolic disease (e.g., hypoglycemia, hypocalcemia)		
Neoplasia (e.g., brain or spinal tumor)		
Nutritional deficiency (poor-quality food)		
Skeletal disease		
Toxins (e.g., heavy metal toxicosis, salt, insecticide, Teflon)		
Vestibular disease (e.g., otitis media/interna)		
Viral disease		

Weight Loss

- Weight loss greater than 10% of body weight should be considered abnormal, and a careful investigation into the case should be initiated.
- It is good custom to recommend to pet owners that pets should be weighed on a regular basis because weight loss is often an early warning sign in cases of systemic disease.

<table>
<tr><th>Reptile</th><th>Bird</th><th>Mammal</th></tr>
<tr><td colspan="3">Infections (Gram-negative bacterial, viral, fungal)</td></tr>
<tr><td colspan="3">Parasites (endo- and ecto-)</td></tr>
<tr><td colspan="3">Metabolic problems (maldigestion/malabsorption)</td></tr>
<tr><td colspan="3">Nutritional problems (inadequate diet/amount/poor diet)</td></tr>
<tr><td colspan="3">Toxins</td></tr>
<tr><td colspan="3">Neoplasia</td></tr>
<tr><td colspan="3">Functional abnormalities (oral/dental disease, protein-losing disease)</td></tr>
<tr><td colspan="3">Stress, pain, competition</td></tr>
<tr><td colspan="3">Geriatric cachexia</td></tr>
<tr><td>Post hibernation</td><td colspan="2">During weaning (normal)</td></tr>
<tr><td colspan="3">Cardiac disease</td></tr>
<tr><td></td><td></td><td>Hyperthyroidism</td></tr>
<tr><td></td><td></td><td>Chronic fever</td></tr>
<tr><td colspan="3">End-stage renal disease</td></tr>
<tr><td colspan="3">Chronic inflammation of any cause</td></tr>
</table>

Laboratory Tests

EDITOR

Jörg Mayer *DrMedVet, MSc, DABVP (Exotic Companion Mammal), DECZM (Small Mammal)*

Adrenal Panel, Ferret

DEFINITION

- The ferret adrenal panel is a test used in the diagnosis of adrenal disease in the ferret. This condition is a primary disease of the cortex of the adrenal gland, and the panel tests levels of steroid hormones produced by the stratum reticularis of the adrenal cortex. Hormones measured in the panel include 17-OH progesterone, estradiol, and androstenedione.
- This test measures blood baseline levels and suggests that significant elevation in the concentrations of one or all hormones is suggestive of adrenal gland pathology.

SYNONYMS

- 17-OH progesterone (17-hydroxyprogesterone; progesterone-17-OH)
- Estradiol (estrogen)
- Androstenedione (4-androstenedione)

PHYSIOLOGY

- The pathophysiology of ferret adrenal-associated endocrinopathy shows hyperplasia of the adrenal cortex zona reticularis layer, which produces these sex hormones. Increased levels of circulating estrogens can cause bone marrow suppression, which can result in a normocytic normochromic anemia, leukopenia, and/or thrombocytopenia. Chronic high estrogen levels (i.e., estrogen toxicity) suppress the anagen phase of the growing hair, resulting in telogenic hair follicles and alopecia and pruritus. Spayed female ferrets may exhibit estrus-like symptoms of vulvar enlargement, clear mucoid vulvular discharge, and male attraction behavior. Male ferrets (intact and neutered) can develop a cystic prostate enlargement with urethral compression and may develop a sexual behavior with marked aggression. Some studies suggest that a genetic background or early neutering/spay is a contributing factor for having adrenal cortical disease (ACD).
- This adrenalocrinopathy is unlike Cushing's syndrome seen in dogs and cats, which occurs in the zona fasciculata, where excess cortisol is produced. This major difference in the pathophysiology of adrenal disease has implications for both diagnosis and treatment.
- Many causes have been suggested for the disease, from early age neutering to extended photoperiods to genetics to food sources and husbandry.
- Ferret adrenal disease is a primary pathology of the adrenal gland, and the histopathology of the disease can be divided into three categories: adrenal hyperplasia, adenoma, and adenocarcinoma.
- At this point in time, surgical removal of an affected adrenal gland is the only curative treatment for ferrets with adrenal gland disease. Removal of one gland does not result in atrophy of the remaining and so also differs from what is seen in dogs and cats.
- Bilateral removal of the adrenal glands is indicated only when both adrenals are shown to be pathologic; with sufficient ectopic adrenal tissue, no hypoadrenocorticism phase (i.e., addisonian crisis) is reported postoperatively.

TYPICAL NORMAL RANGE

Ferret Adrenal Panel Values

Steroid	SI Units	Mean ± SD	Upper Normal Cutoff Value
Cortisol	nmol/L	53 ± 42	140
17 OH progesterone	nmol/L	0.2 ± 0.3	0.8
Estradiol	pmol/L	107 ± 38	180
Androstenedione	nmol/L	6.6 ± 4.1	15
DHEAS	nmol/L	10 ± 9	28

Source: Rosenthal KL, Peterson ME: *J Am Vet Med Assoc* 209:1097–1102, 1996.
DHEAS, Dehydroepiandrosterone.

CLINICAL APPLICATIONS

CAUSES OF ABNORMALLY HIGH LEVELS

- Pathologic
  - Adrenal disease (adrenal hyperplasia, adenoma, adenocarcinoma)
- Physiologic
  - 17-OH progesterone increases in the third trimester of pregnancy, primarily owing to fetal adrenal production, and drops abruptly before delivery; low values must be interpreted in light of breeding dates.
  - Changes in estradiol levels in serum may occur with skin disease and neoplasia and can indicate the presence or absence of a functional ovarian tissue.
  - This test is sensitive to circadian rhythms (the natural highs and lows that the body experiences during a day).
  - Some seasonal changes can be seen initially with an increase in androgen levels in the spring, but with time, levels are steadily high year-round.

NEXT DIAGNOSTIC STEPS TO CONSIDER IF LEVELS ARE HIGH

- Abdominal ultrasound exam performed to measure the size of the adrenal glands and to check for ovarian remnants or the uterine stump
- Exploratory surgery
- Urine cortisol:creatinine ratio (UCCR)
  - Reference range for the UCCR: $>1.6 \times 10^{-6}$ (1); 2.1×10^{-6} (2)

CAUSES OF ABNORMALLY LOW LEVELS

- Hypoadrenocorticism (Addison's disease)
- Insufficiency

NEXT DIAGNOSTIC STEPS TO CONSIDER IF LEVELS ARE LOW If clinical signs of ACD are present but with no supportive diagnostic test results, consideration should be given to performing an abdominal ultrasound and repeating the adrenal panel in 3 months if clinical signs persist.

SPECIMEN AND PROCESSING CONSIDERATIONS

DRUG EFFECTS ON LEVELS Ketoconazole: inhibits cholesterol metabolism

SAMPLE FOR COLLECTION AND ANY SPECIAL SPECIMEN HANDLING NOTES

- Proper sample collection and handling are essential for accurate test results:
  - Do not send whole blood.
  - Do not send samples in serum-separator tubes (polymer gel tubes). This causes hemolysis of samples, and the gel is known to precipitate drugs.
  - Please label sample containers adequately.
    - Owner's name
    - Animal's name
    - Test desired
    - Time of collection
  - Collect baseline serum sample (0.5 mL).
    - Clot at room temperature, centrifuge within 1 hour, separate serum, and freeze.
    - Alternatively, store blood samples in the refrigerator for 2 to 4 hours to clot, centrifuge, remove serum, and freeze.
    - Do not send immediately before a holiday!
    - Be sure to include a brief history of the case, especially the sex status and age of the animal.
    - Ship frozen samples, preferably in a styrofoam container, for next day delivery, along with one or two cool packs (add insulating materials [peanuts, paper], and seal styrofoam seams with tape).
- The following hormones will be assayed: estradiol, androstenedione, and 17- hydroxyprogesterone. (Dehydroepiandrosterone [DHEAS] is no longer available.)

PEARLS

Remember that the size of the adrenal gland and hormone production do not have to be correlated. It is possible to get significantly elevated hormone levels without a significant increase in size of the gland, making exact identification of the diseased gland problematic during surgery. Medical treatment might be indicated in these cases, with an abdominal ultrasound performed 3 month later to document the change in size of the adrenal gland before surgery is performed.

REFERENCES

Gould WJ, et al: Evaluation of urinary cortisol:creatinine ratios for the diagnosis of hyperadrenocorticism associated with adrenal gland tumors in ferrets. J Am Vet Med Assoc 206:42–46, 1995.

Schoemaker NJ, et al: Urinary glucocorticoid excretion in the diagnosis of hyperadrenocorticism in ferrets. Domestic Anim Endocrinol 27:13–24, 2004.

AUTHOR: **DAVID ESHAR**

EDITOR: **JÖRG MAYER**

Alanine Aminotransferase

DEFINITION

Alanine aminotransferase (ALT) is an enzyme primarily located in hepatocyte cytoplasm.

SYNONYM

Serum glutamic-pyruvic transaminase (SGPT)

PHYSIOLOGY

- ALT, like other aminotransferase enzymes, catalyzes the interconversion of amino acids by transferring amino groups.
- In most species, ALT is found primarily in hepatocyte cytoplasm and leaks into the blood when hepatocyte cell membrane injury occurs.
- Low concentrations of ALT in erythrocytes and skeletal muscle may cause minor ALT increases in hemolytic diseases, muscle wasting, or muscle injury.

TYPICAL NORMAL RANGE

The typical normal range for this laboratory test varies greatly among species. The reader is referred to the following Elsevier publications for additional information:

Carpenter J: Exotic animal formulary, ed 4, St Louis, 2013, Saunders.

Mader D: Reptile medicine and surgery, ed 2, St Louis, 2006, Saunders.

CLINICAL APPLICATIONS

CAUSES OF ABNORMALLY HIGH LEVELS

- Active hepatocellular damage causes an increase in ALT in some species.
  - End-stage liver disease does not typically cause an increase in ALT because liver cells are not actively being destroyed.
- ALT increases slightly in gastrointestinal disease with associated mild liver inflammation or bacterial infection.
- Fever causes a slight increase in ALT.
- Drug induction of cytochrome P450 system
- Myocarditis
- Rats on a high-protein diet have shown a significant increase in this enzyme.

NEXT DIAGNOSTIC STEPS TO CONSIDER IF LEVELS ARE HIGH

- In species in which ALT is specific for liver damage, if elevations greater than 2 times the upper limit of the reference range persist, assess history for exposure to hepatotoxins, including medications. If none, begin to assess hepatic structure (e.g., abdominal radiographs, ultrasound) and function (e.g., serum bile acids, alkaline phosphatase).
- Consider liver biopsy if values remain elevated or are increased.
- In rats, evaluate diet for high protein content.

IMPORTANT INTERSPECIES DIFFERENCES

- In the ferret, ALT is highly liver specific, and the activity of ALT in hepatocytes is 3 to 10 times higher than in other tissues.
- In the rabbit, ALT is not specific for liver damage.
- In birds, ALT is not specific for liver damage and is not useful when the avian chemistry profile is evaluated.
- In reptiles, ALT has little tissue specificity.

SPECIMEN AND PROCESSING CONSIDERATIONS

DRUG EFFECTS ON LEVELS Anticonvulsants (primidone and phenytoin), glucocorticoids, mebendazole, and thiacetarsamide can lead to increased ALT levels by induction of the cytochrome P450 enzyme system, not necessarily by toxicity.

LAB ARTIFACTS THAT MAY INTERFERE WITH READINGS OF LEVELS OF THIS SUBSTANCE

- Lipemia will artificially increase ALT.
- Hemolysis will cause a false increase in ALT.

SAMPLE FOR COLLECTION AND ANY SPECIAL SPECIMEN HANDLING NOTES

- Serum (red top tube): allow to clot, centrifuge, and separate serum from clot.

- For small animals and/or small blood samples (<200 μL), use heparinized plasma (green top tube) for biochemistry and hematology.

PEARLS

Distinguishing between physiologic drug-induced cytochrome P450 elevations of ALT and pathologic hepatocyte damage elevations of ALT can be challenging because enzyme induction displays marked individual-to-individual variability. Correlate the finding with other clinical pathology abnormalities, and inquire about drug administration history.

AUTHOR: **CARRIE A. PHELPS**

EDITOR: **JÖRG MAYER**

Albumin

DEFINITION

Water-soluble proteins found in egg whites, blood, lymph, and other tissues and fluids. Serum albumin is the most abundant protein in the blood and is measured.

PHYSIOLOGY

- Albumin is produced in the liver.
- It is important in maintaining colloidal osmotic pressure and transporting large organic molecules.
- The most accurate measurement is performed using a spectrophotometer.

TYPICAL NORMAL RANGE

The typical normal range for this laboratory test varies greatly among species. The reader is referred to the following Elsevier publications for additional information:

Carpenter J: Exotic animal formulary, ed 4, St Louis, 2012, Saunders.

Mader D: Reptile medicine and surgery, ed 2, St Louis, 2006, Saunders.

CLINICAL APPLICATIONS

CAUSES OF ABNORMALLY HIGH LEVELS

- A true increase in albumin is pathognomonic for dehydration.
  - An associated increase in globulin and total protein also occurs with dehydration.
- In egg-laying species (birds, reptiles, monotremes), albumin increases during egg formation as the egg yolk is floating in albumin.
- Consider laboratory error, especially in rabbits, when the bromcresol green method is used to determine serum albumin levels.

NEXT DIAGNOSTIC STEPS TO CONSIDER IF LEVELS ARE HIGH

- Rule out dehydration; if normal hydration, recheck albumin level.
- Evaluate reproductive status of female egg-laying animals.

CAUSES OF ABNORMALLY LOW LEVELS

- Decreased production
  - Liver disease (cirrhosis/fibrosis, neoplasia, portosystemic shunt, amyloidosis)
- Increased loss
  - Intestinal loss (malabsorption, maldigestion, mycobacterial disease, endoparasites)
  - Renal loss (glomerulonephritis and glomerulosclerosis)
  - Severe malnutrition (common in rabbits)
  - Exudative skin diseases (burns, large wounds, vasculitis, frostbite)
  - Blood loss (chronic)
  - Inflammatory disease (septicemia or viremia): increase in globulins is also seen
  - Polyuria and polydipsia

NEXT DIAGNOSTIC STEPS TO CONSIDER IF LEVELS ARE LOW

- Review history with special attention to intestinal, renal, and hepatic disease.
- Assess in conjunction with hematocrit, total protein, serum globulin, liver enzymes, and renal function.
- If a cause is not determined, additional testing to be considered includes bile acids, fecal flotation, and fecal occult blood.
- Additional tests (radiographs, ultrasound, biopsy) should be dictated by history, physical examination, and previous test results.

IMPORTANT INTERSPECIES DIFFERENCES

- A mild increase in serum albumin occurs in birds during egg laying.
- Chicks have lower albumin levels than adult birds

SPECIMEN AND PROCESSING CONSIDERATIONS

DRUG EFFECTS ON LEVELS Long-term treatment with hepatotoxic drugs (e.g., phenobarbital) or renal toxic drugs (e.g., amikacin) might cause levels to decrease.

LAB ARTIFACTS THAT MAY INTERFERE WITH READINGS OF LEVELS OF THIS SUBSTANCE

- Lipemia can cause an artificially low albumin.
- Hemolysis will lead to a falsely elevated albumin.
- In rabbits, the albumin value is often erroneous when the bromcresol green method is used to determine serum albumin levels. Determine the method of analysis when the albumin value is higher than the total protein value.

SAMPLE FOR COLLECTION AND ANY SPECIAL SPECIMEN HANDLING NOTES

- Serum (red top tube): allow to clot, centrifuge, and separate serum from clot.
- For small animals and/or small blood samples (<200 μL), use heparinized plasma (green top tube) for biochemistry and hematology.

PEARLS

In birds, normal levels of albumin can be low.

AUTHOR: **CARRIE A. PHELPS**

EDITOR: **JÖRG MAYER**

Alkaline Phosphatase

DEFINITION

Alkaline phosphatases (ALPs) are membrane-associated enzymes found in most tissues of the body that hydrolyze monophosphates at an alkaline pH.

SYNONYMS

Alk phos, AP, SAP

PHYSIOLOGY

Numerous isoenzymes of ALP are found in the blood. Recognition of the occurrence of these isoenzymes is critical for interpreting ALP measurements in disease diagnosis. In most mammalian species, two genes encode for ALP: one for intestinal ALP and the other for hepatic, renal, osseous, and other tissue ALPs. Isoenzymes of ALP identified from different tissues, which are the result of the same gene expression, arise from organ-specific posttranslational modification. In exotic pets, hepatic, bone, intestinal, and placental ALP isoenzymes are diagnostically important. Most routine assays measure total serum ALP; electrophoresis, sensitivity to heat, and reactivity with antiserum are required to identify the various isoenzymes. ALP is useful primarily in diagnosing hepatobiliary disease. However, because serum ALP also arises from nonhepatic tissues in most species and is sensitive to drug induction, it has limited specificity for hepatobiliary disease in most animals. Increases in serum ALP derived from bone are generally associated with osteogenesis in young, growing animals.

TYPICAL NORMAL RANGE

The typical normal range for this laboratory test varies greatly among species. The reader is referred to the following Elsevier publications for additional information:

Carpenter J: Exotic animal formulary, ed 4, St Louis, 2013, Saunders.
Mader D: Reptile medicine and surgery, ed 2, St Louis, 2006, Saunders.

CLINICAL APPLICATIONS

CAUSES OF ABNORMALLY HIGH LEVELS

- Hepatic necrosis or hepatocyte swelling may lead to impaired bile flow, resulting in biliary stasis.
- Growing animals or animals with bone disease: in birds, increases in ALP are associated mainly with increased osteoblastic activity.

NEXT DIAGNOSTIC STEPS TO CONSIDER IF LEVELS ARE HIGH

- Disregard in young animals if no other abnormalities are found.
- Evaluate hepatobiliary structure and function.
- Ultrasound and biopsy of the liver are necessary to determine the exact nature of hepatic disease.
- Evaluate bone in radiographs of birds for potential osteoblast/osteoclast activity.

CAUSES OF ABNORMALLY LOW LEVELS No significant causes of decreased ALP are known. However, low levels can be seen with diarrhea and in pregnancy.

IMPORTANT INTERSPECIES DIFFERENCES

- Birds and reptiles
  - In birds, elevations of ALP are commonly associated with osteoblastic/osteoclastic activity seen in bone growth and repair, osteomyelitis, nutritional secondary hyperparathyroidism, and ovulatory activity.
  - In reptiles, elevations of ALP do not occur with renal disease because ALP is excreted by damaged renal cells and does not enter the plasma.
- Small mammals
  - In rats, ALP increases rapidly after a meal and thus cannot be reliably employed to detect cholestasis. On a per gram basis, intestinal mucosa in the rat has higher ALP activity than mucosa in the liver.
  - Rabbits are unique in having two hepatic isoenzymes separable by diethylaminoethyl (DEAE-)cellulose chromatography.
  - The corticosteroid-induced isoenzyme of ALP due to endogenous stress, adrenal hyperplasia, hyperadrenocorticism, and corticosteroid administration is unique to the dog and has not been reported in other species.

SPECIMEN AND PROCESSING CONSIDERATIONS

DRUG EFFECTS ON LEVELS Elevated levels of ALP can result from cytochrome P450 induction associated with administration of phenobarbital, phenytoin, theophylline, thyroxine, and primidone.

LAB ARTIFACTS THAT MAY INTERFERE WITH READINGS OF LEVELS OF THIS SUBSTANCE Increased ALP is associated with marked hemolysis.

SAMPLE FOR COLLECTION AND ANY SPECIAL SPECIMEN HANDLING NOTES

- Serum (red top tube): allow to clot, centrifuge, and separate serum from clot
- For small animals and/or small blood samples (<200 μL), use heparinized plasma (green top tube) for biochemistry.

AUTHOR: **CANDACE HERSEY-BENNER**

EDITOR: **JÖRG MAYER**

Ammonia

DEFINITION

Ammonia is formed in the body during decomposition of nitrogen-containing organic materials in a large number of metabolically important reactions. It is generated primarily in the gastrointestinal tract by bacterial degradation of amines, amino acids, and purines, by the action of bacterial ureases on urea, and by catabolism of glutamine in the intestines.

SYNONYMS

- Ammonium: NH^{4+}
- Ammonia: NH_3
- Total ammonia nitrogen (TAN)

PHYSIOLOGY

- Ammonia is produced in the gastrointestinal tract, diffuses through the intestinal mucosa, and is carried by the

portal circulation to the liver. Detoxification by hepatocytes occurs through enzymatic conversion of ammonia to urea or uric acid by mitochondria or through consumption of ammonia in the production of glutamine. Any ammonia that escapes hepatic metabolism enters the systemic circulation, where skeletal muscle and other tissues detoxify ammonia by forming glutamine. Ammonia is highly neurotoxic, causing neurotransmitter abnormalities and inducing injury to astrocytes.
- High circulating ammonium concentrations have been considered as a marker of hepatic dysfunction.
- Many aquatic species will excrete ammonia as their main nitrogenous waste. Excretion occurs not only by the kidneys but also by the gills and the skin.

TYPICAL NORMAL RANGE

Normal ammonia levels are not reported for exotic species.

CLINICAL APPLICATIONS

CAUSES OF ABNORMALLY HIGH LEVELS

- Blood
  - Hepatic disease: failure of the liver to detoxify ammonia (cirrhosis, neoplasia, polyomavirus in birds) or shunting of portal blood away from the liver
  - Artifactual: hemolysis due to improper sample handling; use of ammonium heparin as anticoagulant; deterioration of blood sample before analysis or centrifugation
- Water
  - Check water quality in aquatic species.
  - Improper husbandry is often the cause of ammonia accumulation (overfeeding, infrequent cleaning, overstocking).

NEXT DIAGNOSTIC STEPS TO CONSIDER IF LEVELS ARE HIGH

- Blood
  - Rule out sample error. Review history, examination, complete blood count, serum chemistry panel, and abdominal imaging results to assess for signs of hepatobiliary disease and portal circulation abnormalities.
- Water
  - In aquatic systems, change water and check water filtration system. Investigate sources of ammonia buildup.

IMPORTANT INTERSPECIES DIFFERENCES Ammonia is produced by aquatic species and is a significant toxin. Always measure ammonia levels when analyzing water quality.

SPECIMEN AND PROCESSING CONSIDERATIONS

LAB ARTIFACTS THAT MAY INTERFERE WITH READINGS OF LEVELS OF THIS SUBSTANCE Red blood cells contain 2 to 3 times the amount of ammonia found in plasma. Delayed harvesting of plasma, specimen processing, and the presence of hemolysis will result in increased ammonia levels.

SAMPLE FOR COLLECTION AND ANY SPECIAL SPECIMEN HANDLING NOTES Cleanly draw blood into a cold, ammonia-free heparin (green) tube; separate plasma from cells immediately using temperature-controlled (refrigerated) centrifuge; store on ice and test within 1 hour, or freeze (–20°C [–4°F]) and test within 49 hours.

PEARLS

- Because of difficulties in proper specimen handling, measurement of serum bile acids and urine bile acid-to-creatinine ratio has replaced ammonium measurement.
- Aquatic systems should be free of ammonia. The toxicity of ammonia in water intensifies with increasing pH and water temperature.

AUTHOR: **CARRIE A. PHELPS**

EDITOR: **JÖRG MAYER**

Amylase

DEFINITION

Amylase is an enzyme that catalyzes the hydrolysis of complex carbohydrates in the gastrointestinal tract.

SYNONYMS

Alpha-amylase, Amy, AM, AMS

PHYSIOLOGY

- Amylase is found in high concentration in the pancreas of virtually all animals. However, it is also found in the liver, salivary glands, and small intestinal mucosa of many species; the quantity of amylase in these organs varies considerably with different species. Removal of amylase from blood in all species is relatively rapid, but the mechanism of clearance is species-specific. In many animals, amylase is excreted by the kidney; the liver appears to be involved in other animals. Amylase produced by the pancreas enters the small intestine to assist in digestion by hydrolyzing complex carbohydrates; ionized calcium is required for this process.
- Serum amylase levels increase substantially during acute bouts of pancreatitis, but because of its lack of organ specificity in exotic species, the diagnostic value of amylase levels is minimal.

TYPICAL NORMAL RANGE

To convert from U.S. units (units/L) to S.I. units (U/L), multiply by 1.

	Units/L
Birds	
Psittacines	
African grey	210-530
Amazon parrot	205-510
Budgerigar	200-500
Cockatiel	205-490
Cockatoo	200-510
Conure	100-450
Eclectus parrot	200-645
Lovebird	90-400
Macaw	150-550
Quaker parrot	100-400
Senegal parrot	190-550
Passeriformes	
Canary	190-485
Mammals	
Hedgehogs	510 ± 170 (244-858)
Rabbit	200-500

CLINICAL APPLICATIONS

CAUSES OF ABNORMALLY HIGH LEVELS Pancreatic duct obstruction, pancreatic disease/neoplasia/necrosis, renal insufficiency (decreased glomerular filtration), intestinal obstruction, enteritis, zinc toxicity, hepatic disease, or diabetic ketoacidosis.

NEXT DIAGNOSTIC STEPS TO CONSIDER IF LEVELS ARE HIGH

- Correlate with history, examination findings, complete blood count and remainder of serum chemistry panel.
- If consistent with pancreatitis, consider abdominal ultrasonography to assess further (serum lipase elevation is not specific for pancreatitis, and pancreatic lipase immunoreactivity is not developed for exotic species).
- If renal disease is present owing to reduced glomerular filtration, creatinine and blood urea nitrogen will be elevated.
- In birds, measure blood zinc levels for toxicity.

CAUSES OF ABNORMALLY LOW LEVELS

- Exocrine pancreatic insufficiency
- Hepatotoxicity in some rodents

NEXT DIAGNOSTIC STEPS TO CONSIDER IF LEVELS ARE LOW

- Assess for pancreatic insufficiency (serum trypsin–like immunoreactivity is not developed for exotic species).
- Fecal protease test will also have low enzymatic activity.
- Assess for hepatotoxicity in rodents.

IMPORTANT INTERSPECIES DIFFERENCES

- Birds and reptiles
  - Circulating serum levels of amylase have not been validated in reptiles.
  - The salivary glands of some birds produce amylase to aid in the digestion of carbohydrates. Whether salivary isoamylase contributes significantly to serum levels is unknown.
- Small mammals
  - In rabbits, serum amylase levels are lower than in other mammalian species because the liver produces little or no amylase, and cecal microorganisms contribute to amylase production.
  - The salivary glands of rats and mice have amylase activity nearly as high as that seen in the pancreas. Whether salivary isoamylase contributes significantly to serum levels is unknown.

SPECIMEN AND PROCESSING CONSIDERATIONS

SAMPLE FOR COLLECTION AND ANY SPECIAL SPECIMEN HANDLING NOTES

- Serum (red top tube): allow to clot, centrifuge, and separate serum from clot
- For small animals and/or small blood samples (<200 μL), use heparinized plasma (green top tube) for biochemistry and hematology.
- Amylase is fairly stable compared with other analytes measured in routine chemistry panels.
- U.S. units (units/L) and S.I. units (U/L) are the same.

AUTHOR: **CANDACE HERSEY-BENNER**

EDITOR: **JÖRG MAYER**

Aspartate Aminotransferase

DEFINITION

Aspartate aminotransferase (AST) is found in a wide variety of tissues but has high concentrations in skeletal muscle, cardiac muscle, and red blood cells, and in the liver. An increase in AST alone is not suggestive of damage to any particular organ or tissue.

SYNONYM

AST

PHYSIOLOGY

AST, like other aminotransferase enzymes, catalyzes the interconversion of amino acids by transferring amino groups.

TYPICAL NORMAL RANGE

The typical normal range for this laboratory test varies greatly among species. The reader is referred to the following Elsevier publications for additional information:

Carpenter J: Exotic animal formulary, ed 4, St Louis, 2013, Saunders.

Mader D: Reptile medicine and surgery, ed 2, St Louis, 2006, Saunders.

CLINICAL APPLICATIONS

CAUSES OF ABNORMALLY HIGH LEVELS

- Hemolyzed samples can cause elevated AST owing to the presence of the enzyme in red blood cells.
- High levels of AST are suggestive of damage to the liver or skeletal muscle and can be suggestive of cardiac muscle disorders or hemolysis.
- Severe exertion can also increase AST levels.
- Muscle damage
  - Seizures
  - Trauma
  - Capture myopathy (exertional rhabdomyolysis)
  - Intramuscular injection
- Hepatic damage
  - Drugs
  - Hemochromatosis (iron storage disease) in birds
  - Endocrine disease (diabetes mellitus, hyperthyroidism)
  - Hypoxia (cardiopulmonary origin)
  - Lipidosis (severe)
  - Inflammation/infection
  - Toxic
  - Neoplasia

NEXT DIAGNOSTIC STEPS TO CONSIDER IF LEVELS ARE HIGH

- Complete blood count, chemistry panel, bile acids, radiographs, abdominal ultrasound ± liver biopsy.
- Ruling out traumatic muscular injury is important, and creatine kinase (CK) levels can help to assess muscle damage.

IMPORTANT INTERSPECIES DIFFERENCES In pigeons, AST is highly sensitive in detecting hepatocellular damage caused by ethylene glycol ingestion.

SPECIMEN AND PROCESSING CONSIDERATIONS

DRUG EFFECTS ON LEVELS

- Some drugs such as anticonvulsants and estrogens have been shown to increase AST activity in small animals.
- Metronidazole toxicity in reptiles can lead to a significant increase in AST in the face of a mild increase in CK.
- In birds, cephalosporins, metronidazole, trimethoprim-sulfa, and

dexamethasone can cause an increase in AST.

LAB ARTIFACTS THAT MAY INTERFERE WITH READINGS OF LEVELS OF THIS SUBSTANCE

- Hemolyzed samples can lead to erroneously elevated levels of AST owing to release of AST from the red cells.
- Lipemia will artifactually increase AST.

SPECIMEN Serum

REFERENCES

Bush BM: Interpretation of laboratory results for small animal clinicians, Ames, IA, 1992, Blackwell.

Carpenter JW: Exotic animal formulary, ed 3, St Louis, 2004, Elsevier.

Harrison GJ, et al: Clinical avian medicine, vol II, South Palm Beach, FL, 2006, Spix Publishing, pp 443, 616, 619.

Mader DR: Reptile medicine and surgery, ed 2, St Louis, 2006, Elsevier, pp 464, 651.

Yin SA: The small animal veterinary nerdbook, ed 2, Davis, CA, 1988, CattleDog Publishing, pp 4.4, 4.7.

AUTHOR: **CARRIE A. PHELPS**

EDITOR: **JÖRG MAYER**

Azurophil Count

DEFINITION

A mononuclear, phagocytic leukocyte that resembles a monocyte but has fine eosinophilic cytoplasmic granules, which give the overall cytoplasm a red or purple color.

SYNONYM

Azurophilic monocyte

PHYSIOLOGY

Little is known about azurophils. They seem to occur most commonly in iguanas and in many species of snakes. They resemble monocytes, and it is assumed that they have a similar origin and play a similar role in immune function.

CLINICAL APPLICATIONS

CAUSES OF ABNORMALLY HIGH LEVELS *Reptiles:* Azurophilia occurs secondarily to antigenic stimulation, especially as the result of viral or bacterial infection. In boas and pythons, an inclusion body will commonly cause an azurophilia. Hepatazoon infections have also been shown to cause an increase in azurophils. In reptiles as well, chronic granulomatous conditions will produce azurophilia.

NEXT DIAGNOSTIC STEPS TO CONSIDER IF LEVELS ARE HIGH

- Reptiles
  - After an azurophilia is detected, a hunt for the source of infection should be conducted. This can include serum antibody titers or PCR testing based on clinical findings. Hepatazoon should be detected with a manual differential count.
  - Radiographs should be performed to look for granulomas. A laparoscopic exam of the coelomic cavity can be done to look for smaller granulomas.

CAUSES OF ABNORMALLY LOW LEVELS In most reptiles, the lower limit of the reference range for azurophils is zero; therefore, azuropenia has little to no diagnostic significance.

SPECIMEN AND PROCESSING CONSIDERATIONS

SAMPLE FOR COLLECTION AND ANY SPECIAL SPECIMEN HANDLING NOTES

- Reptiles
  - Use heparinized (green top) tubes when collecting complete blood count (CBC) samples.
- Amphibians
  - Use heparinized (green top) tubes when collecting CBC samples. Owing to the small volumes often collected, use a heparinized syringe to collect the sample, and make slides immediately after collection whenever possible.
- Fish
  - Samples for differential cell counts should be prepared immediately after collection. It is important to rapidly dry slides because slow drying may alter morphology. Diff-Quik stain can be used, but it is not optimal for differential counts. If necessary to collect samples in tubes, use heparinized tubes. ETDA causes hemolysis in fish anesthetized with tricaine.

REFERENCES

Fudge AM: Laboratory medicine: avian and exotic pets, ed 1, Philadelphia, 2000, WB Saunders, pp 9–27, 193–204.

Salakij C, et al: Hematology, morphology, cytochemical staining, and ultrastructural characteristics of blood cells in king cobras *(Ophiophagus hannah)*, Vet Clin Pathol 31:116–126, 2002.

AUTHOR: **JONATHAN W. BALL**

EDITOR: **JÖRG MAYER**

Basophil Count

DEFINITION

- A granular leukocyte with a pale-staining nucleus and a cytoplasm containing coarse bluish-black granules. Basophils of mammals usually have a lobed nucleus. In lower vertebrates, the nucleus is often nonlobed.
- In reptiles, basophils are described as small, variably sized cells with numerous dark metachromatic-staining round granules, which often make it difficult to visualize the nucleus. Turtles and crocodiles have larger basophils (8 to 15 μm) compared with lizards (95 to 10 μm).

PHYSIOLOGY

- Basophils are granulocytes; they develop in the bone marrow through a process similar to that seen with neutrophils and eosinophils. Basophils develop from myeloid stem cells under the influence of a variety of cytokines, most notably interleukin (IL)-3, but also IL-5 and granulocyte-monocyte colony-stimulating factor (GM-CSF). They then progress through several stages of development over the course of approximately 2 to 3 days in the marrow before they are released into the bloodstream. The basophils then travel in the bloodstream for an average of 6 hours before entering the tissues. Migration into the tissues is promoted by IL-1, tumor necrosis factor (TNF)-α, and endotoxin. Basophils can remain in the tissues for up to 2 weeks unless until they are activated or they degenerate.
- Basophils are activated by IL-3 or immunoglobulin (Ig)E binding to receptors on the cell membrane. This causes cells to release the content of their granules as a mixture of vasoactive chemicals, including histamine. The granules also contain chemotactic factors, which stimulate the migration of eosinophils to the tissues. Therefore, it is thought that basophils take part in the early immune response.

TYPICAL NORMAL RANGE

The typical normal range for this laboratory test varies greatly among species. The reader is referred to the following Elsevier publications for additional information:

Carpenter J: Exotic animal formulary, ed 4, St Louis, 2013, Saunders.

Mader D: Reptile medicine and surgery, ed 2, St Louis, 2006, Saunders.

CLINICAL APPLICATIONS

CAUSES OF ABNORMALLY HIGH LEVELS

- Mammals
  - A common cause of basophilia in mammals is an allergic reaction—immediate or delayed. The source of the allergic reaction can be any common allergen, including drugs, foods, inhalants, and insect stings/bites. Parasites are another common cause of basophilia. Parasites that have been associated with a basophilia include fleas, GI parasites, and vascular parasites.
  - Neoplasia can lead to increased basophil counts. Mast cell tumors lead to a basophilia because of the chemotactic factors released when mast cells degranulate. Basophil leukemia leads to a basophilia, often with an increase in the number of morphologically abnormal cells. Other, less common neoplastic conditions, including lymphomatoid granulomatosis, essential thrombocythemia, and polycythemia vera, may lead to basophilia.
  - Basophilia up to 30% has been observed in the clinically normal rabbit.
- Birds
  - Early inflammatory responses associated with histamine release will cause a basophilia because histamine attracts basophils. A common infectious cause of basophilia associated with inflammation is the presence of *Escherichia coli* endotoxin. Noninfectious agents, including turpentine, trypan blue, bovine serum albumin, saline, and *Staphylococcus aureus*, have also been shown to cause a basophilia.
  - Stress, especially from starvation, heat, or induced moulting, has been associated with basophilia. Tissue damage will cause a transient increase in basophils.
  - Respiratory disease can lead to increased basophil levels as well, although this finding has been inconsistent. The presence of air sac mites has been inconsistently associated with basophilia.
  - In some species of birds, especially Budgerigars and Amazon parrots, active chlamydial infection will cause a basophilia.
  - Basophilia has also been associated with cutaneous basophile hypersensitivity in birds sensitized to phytohemagglutinin.
  - Unlike the case in mammals, basophilia in birds has no association with internal or external parasites, other than possibly air sac mites.
- Reptiles
  - In reptiles, the basophilia is often associated with chronic illness or intestinal parasitism. It can occur in the presence of blood parasites (e.g., hemogregarines).
  - Pirhemocyton virus infections have also been shown to cause basophilia.

NEXT DIAGNOSTIC STEPS TO CONSIDER IF LEVELS ARE HIGH

- Basophils make up such a small population of the white blood cells (WBC) that caution must be taken not to overinterpret a basophilia. A marked increase or a persistent mild increase in the basophil count should be noted before extensive diagnostics are pursued.
- Mammals
  - To work up a basophilia, a thorough search for parasites should be conducted. This should include a direct fecal smear and a fecal float. A smear of whole blood should be done to demonstrate red blood cell (RBC) or WBC parasites. A smear of the buffy coat can be done for a better chance of seeing WBC parasites. Serum antibody titers or PCR tests can also be done if clinical signs warrant. The skin and the hair coat should be examined for signs of fleas.
  - Any cutaneous or subcutaneous masses found during the physical exam should be aspirated and submitted for cytologic examination.
  - A careful examination of the environment should be performed for possible allergens. In small mammals, the bedding is often a cause of allergies, possibly because of the type of bedding, or because the bedding is changed too infrequently. If no parasitic or allergic cause of basophilia can be found, a bone marrow aspirate can be done.
- Birds
  - After basophilia is detected in a bird, a thorough examination should be done to look for signs of inflammation or infection.
  - Serum antibody titers or PCR tests for chlamydia should be done, especially in Budgerigars and Amazon parrots.
  - A careful examination should be done to detect any signs of respiratory disease, including air sac mites. This can include radiographs, tracheal transillumination to look for mites, a tracheal wash, or possibly laparoscopic examination of the lungs and air sacs.
  - Examine the environment for possible allergens, causes of stress, or sources of toxin exposure.
  - If no parasitic or allergic cause of basophilia can be found, a bone marrow aspirate can be done.
- Reptiles
  - After basophilia is detected in a reptile, a blood smear should be done to look for the presence of blood parasites or pirhemocyton viral inclusions in erythrocytes.
  - A buffy coat smear can also be done to increase the chances of finding WBC parasites. Serum antibody titers or PCR tests can be done if clinical signs warrant.
  - In some turtle species (especially aquatic turtles), a high basophil count might be a normal finding.

CAUSES OF ABNORMALLY LOW LEVELS

- In most animals, the lower limit of the reference range for basophils is zero; therefore, basopenia has no diagnostic significance.
- Birds: evidence suggests that as birds age, the number of circulating

basophils decreases; juveniles generally have a much greater circulating basophil population.

SPECIMEN AND PROCESSING CONSIDERATIONS

SAMPLE FOR COLLECTION AND ANY SPECIAL SPECIMEN HANDLING NOTES

- Mammals
  - Use EDTA (purple top) tubes to collect for complete blood count (CBC).
- Birds and reptiles
  - For differential counts, it is best if slides can be made from fresh whole blood.
  - Use heparinized tubes to collect for CBC in most species. ETDA may cause RBC hemolysis in some species. If the volume of collected blood is large enough, submit one sample of each, and let the clinical pathologist decide which one is better suited.
- Amphibians
  - Use heparinized tubes for collecting CBC samples. Because of the small volumes often collected, use a heparinized syringe to collect the sample, and make slides immediately after collection whenever possible.
- Fish
  - Samples for differential cell counts should be prepared immediately after collection. It is also important to rapidly dry slides because slow drying may alter the morphology. Slides can be stained with LG or WLG stain. Diff-Quik stain can be used, but it is not optimal for differential counts. If it is necessary to collect samples in tubes, use heparinized tubes. ETDA causes hemolysis in fish anesthetized with tricaine.

PEARLS

- Birds
  - Monocytosis and basophilia are often the only hematologic abnormalities seen in Budgerigars with a chlamydial infection.
  - In Amazon parrots, especially Mexican red-headed parrots *(Amazonia viridigonalis)*, the granules of basophils appear to be larger and more prominent than in other psittacines.
- Reptiles
  - A large degree of normal variability in basophil populations is seen between reptile species. Normal values can range from 0 to 40% of the total WBC count.
  - Some species of turtles, especially snapping turtles and Reeve's turtles, generally have higher concentrations of basophils.

REFERENCES

Carpenter JW, et al: Exotic animal formulary, ed 2, Philadelphia, 2001, WB Saunders, pp 36, 80–86, 195–208, 213, 256, 268, 292, 320, 344, 363, 386–387.

Fudge AM: Laboratory medicine: avian and exotic pets, ed 1, Philadelphia, 2000, WB Saunders, pp 9–27, 193–204.

Groff JM, et al: Hematology and clinical chemistry of cyprinid fish, Vet Clin North Am 2:741–776, 1999.

Hoegeman S: Diagnostic sampling of amphibians, Vet Clin North Am 2:731–740, 1999.

Jones MP: Avian clinical pathology, Vet Clin North Am 2:663–688, 1999.

Redrobe S, et al: Sample collection and clinical pathology of reptiles, Vet Clin North Am 2:709–730, 1999.

Stockham SL, et al: Fundamentals of veterinary clinical pathology, ed 1, Ames, IA, 2002, Iowa State Press, pp 50–83.

AUTHOR: **JONATHAN W. BALL**

EDITOR: **JÖRG MAYER**

Bile Acids

DEFINITION

The bile acids are a collection of detergent-like compounds (predominantly cholic acid and chenodeoxycholic acid in mammals). The primary bile acids are synthesized from cholesterol in the liver and are secreted in bile to aid in digestion and absorption of fat and fat-soluble vitamins.

PHYSIOLOGY

- Bile acid synthesis in mammals and birds occurs in the liver and is the primary pathway in the metabolism of cholesterol, which is the precursor molecule for bile acid synthesis.
- Bile acids are conjugated in the liver, to glycine or taurine, to inhibit intestinal bile acid resorption and promote lipid metabolism. Bacteria in the intestine further modify bile acids.
- Bile acids are secreted via the bile duct into the small intestine and emulsify ingested fats to be solubilized for digestion and absorption.
- In birds (with or without a gallbladder), secretion of bile acids is continuous.

TYPICAL NORMAL RANGE

- Reptiles
  - <60 μmol/L—great interspecies variation
- Birds
  - Although reference ranges for bile acid concentrations have not been established for all avian species, bile acid concentrations are considered to be elevated in pigeons and psittacine species if they are greater than 70 mmol/L in fasted (12-hour) samples. Postprandial bile acid concentrations vary between bird species and are challenging to interpret.
- As an indicator of the severity of a liver disease, avian values for enzymatic (spectrophotometer) methods are as follows (radioimmunoassay shows lower values):

Liver Disease Severity	Bile Acid Values, μm/l
Minimal	50-150 μM/L
Mild	150-250 μM/L
Moderate	250-500 μM/L
Severe	500-700 μM/L

CLINICAL APPLICATIONS

CAUSES OF ABNORMALLY HIGH LEVELS

- Increased bile acid values can be observed with portosystemic shunts, liver failure (especially in chronic or vascular disease), and cholestasis.
- In birds, elevated values are seen postprandially and in liver disease such as fibrosis, lipidosis, hepatic vacuolation, cholangitis, bile duct proliferation, steroid hepatopathy, chlamydial infection, and mycobacteriosis. Iron storage disease and neoplasia of the liver have inconsistent effects on bile acid values.

Bile Acid Values of Selected Avian Species as Measured by Radioimmunoassay (RIA) and the Enzymatic Method (Spectrophotometer) in μMol/L

	RIA	Colorimetric
Birds		
Psittacines		
African grey parrot	18-71	12-96
Amazon parrots	19-144	33-154
Budgerigar parakeet	20-65	32-117
Caique	12-112	
Cockatiel	25-85	15-139
Cockatoos	34-112	8-11
Conure	32-105	8-15
Eclectus parrot	30-110	8.8-9.8
Grey-cheek parakeet	15-96	
Lory	20-97	
Lovebird	25-95	12-90
Macaw	7-100	
Pionus parrot	15-92	
Quaker parrot	21-90	
Senegal parrot	0-85	20-94
Passeriformes and Columbiformes		
Canary	23-90	
Pigeon	22-60	
Piciformes		
Toucan	20-40	
Emu	6-45	
Ostrich	4-40	
Raptors		
Peregrine falcon	20-118	
Mammals		
Guinea pig	57 μg/mL	
Rat	56.0 ± 6.6 μmol/L (male) 27.7-41.1 μmol/L (female)	
Ferret	0.0-8.0 μmol/L 1-28 μmol/L (mean, 9.1 μmol/L) for males 2-14 μmol/L (mean, 4.4 μmol/L) for females	

NEXT DIAGNOSTIC STEPS TO CONSIDER IF LEVELS ARE HIGH Assess for liver disease (serum chemistry profile, imaging, liver biopsy).

CAUSES OF ABNORMALLY LOW LEVELS Decreased bile acids usually are attributable to delayed gastric emptying or an ileal abnormality, acute/early liver disease, liver cirrhosis, microhepatica, and fasting.

IMPORTANT INTERSPECIES DIFFERENCES In birds, bile acids are considered sensitive and specific for liver disease. However, a great interspecies difference has been noted between preprandial and postprandial values.

SPECIMEN AND PROCESSING CONSIDERATIONS

LAB ARTIFACTS THAT MAY INTERFERE WITH READINGS OF LEVELS OF THIS SUBSTANCE

- Decrease: lipemia, hemolysis, and icterus give decreased bile acid values when the enzymatic method is used (spectrophotometer). Radioimmunoassays (RIAs) are not affected.
- Increase: hypertriglyceridemia gives increased bile acid values when the enzymatic method is used (spectrophotometer). RIAs are not affected.

SAMPLE FOR COLLECTION AND ANY SPECIAL SPECIMEN HANDLING NOTES

- Blood
  - Serum (red top tube): allow to clot, centrifuge, and separate serum from clot
  - For small animals and/or small blood samples (<200 μL), use heparinized plasma (green top tube) for biochemistry and hematology.
  - Store at 2°C to 8°C (35.6°F to 46.4°F) (refrigeration).
- Urine
  - Obtain fresh urine. Avoid blood contamination.

PEARLS

A single preprandial value exceeding normal limits can be due to spontaneous gallbladder contraction.

AUTHOR: **DAVID ESHAR**

EDITOR: **JÖRG MAYER**

Bilirubin

DEFINITION

Bilirubin is a breakdown product of heme, derived primarily from senescent erythrocytes. It is carried by albumin to the liver, where it is detoxified by the glucuronic acid pathway, conjugated, and excreted into the bile. Biliverdin produced in reptiles and birds also undergoes this detoxification in the liver and is excreted into the bile.

SYNONYM

Bili

PHYSIOLOGY

Three forms of bilirubin have been identified: conjugated, unconjugated, and a fraction that is irreversibly bound to protein. Unconjugated bilirubin is the most clinically significant fraction because it is the form that is most likely to cause tissue damage.

TYPICAL NORMAL RANGE

The typical normal range for this laboratory test varies greatly among species. The reader is referred to the following Elsevier publications for additional information:

Carpenter J: Exotic animal formulary, ed 4, St Louis, 2013, Saunders.

Mader D: Reptile medicine and surgery, ed 2, St Louis, 2006, Saunders.

CLINICAL APPLICATIONS

CAUSES OF ABNORMALLY HIGH LEVELS

- Prehepatic
  - Hemolytic crisis
- Hepatic
  - Hepatic disease (decreased ability to conjugate and excrete bilirubin)
  - Intrahepatic cholestatic disease
- Post-hepatic
  - Bile duct obstruction results in an accumulation of conjugated bilirubin.

NEXT DIAGNOSTIC STEPS TO CONSIDER IF LEVELS ARE HIGH Complete blood count, chemistry panel, urinalysis, bile acids, radiographs ± abdominal ultrasound

IMPORTANT INTERSPECIES DIFFERENCES

- Birds have an enzyme called *heme oxygenase*, which converts the protoporphyrin in heme to biliverdin. Both birds and reptiles have decreased hepatic production of biliverdin reductase, which converts biliverdin to bilirubin. Although decreased, biliverdin reductase is still present in some birds. Bacteria in the intestine may produce biliverdin reductase as well, and bilirubin can be absorbed from the gastrointestinal tract.
- Bilirubin is found only in small quantities in the avian and reptilian plasma, making it a relatively useless clinical parameter in these species.
- Rabbits also produce biliverdin as the primary heme metabolite, but in contrast to birds and reptiles, bilirubin is present in the blood of rabbits at measurable levels.
- Although the rabbit produces significantly more bile than a dog of equal size, rabbits have low activity of biliverdin reductase, and only about 30% is converted.

SPECIMEN AND PROCESSING CONSIDERATIONS

LAB ARTIFACTS THAT MAY INTERFERE WITH READINGS OF LEVELS OF THIS SUBSTANCE

- Hemolysis interferes with measurement. The value can be increased or decreased, depending on the method of analysis.
- Lipemia will artifactually increase bilirubin levels.
- Light will degrade bilirubin (up to 50% in 1 hour under fluorescent light).

SAMPLE FOR COLLECTION AND ANY SPECIAL SPECIMEN HANDLING NOTES

- Serum separator tube
- Protection from light
- Storage of sample in fridge

PEARLS

- Yellow discolored urates in birds have been linked to excessive bilirubin due to a potential hepatopathy.
- In most cases where avian plasma is yellow, this is not due to an increased bilirubin level but rather to carotenoids in food.

REFERENCES

Carpenter JW: Exotic animal formulary, ed 3, St Louis, 2004, Elsevier.

Harrison GJ, et al: Clinical avian medicine, vol 2, South Palm Beach, FL, 2006, Spix Publishing, pp 620–621.

Yin SA: The small animal veterinary nerdbook, ed 2, Davis, CA, 1988, CattleDog Publishing, pp 4.4–4.7.

AUTHOR: **CARRIE A. PHELPS**

EDITOR: **JÖRG MAYER**

Blood Urea Nitrogen (BUN)

DEFINITION

Blood urea nitrogen (BUN) measures the amount of urea nitrogen, a waste product of protein metabolism, in the blood.

SYNONYMS

Urea nitrogen, BUN

PHYSIOLOGY

- Urea is formed in the liver as a derivative of protein catabolism; urea then is released into the circulation, where it is excreted by the kidney. Excretion is a passive process that does not require energy, and urea is freely filtered through the glomerular basement membrane of the kidney. The BUN concentration is inversely proportional to the glomerular filtration rate. Tubular reabsorption can occur and is directly related to urine flow. With a high urine flow, reabsorption is minimal; however, if urine outflow is decreased, tubular reabsorption of urea can be significantly increased. Other routes of excretion include saliva, the gastrointestinal (GI) tract, and sweat.

- BUN serum levels are influenced by protein levels in the diet, liver function, intestinal bleeding and subsequent nitrogen absorption, and the state of hydration. Creatinine generally serves as a better indicator of renal function because BUN can be influenced by many nonrenal factors. It is important to remember that increases in serum concentrations of both substances do not occur until an estimated 75% of renal function has been lost, making early diagnosis of many renal diseases difficult.

TYPICAL NORMAL RANGE

BUN*

Species	mg/dL	mmol/L
Fish		
Carp	1.9-3.6	0.7-1.3
Reptiles		
Boa constrictor	<1-10	0.4-3.6
Ball python	0-3	0-1
Gopher snake	2 (1-5)	0.7 (0.4-1.8)
Yellow rat snake	4 (0-20)	1.4 (0-7.1)
Bearded dragon	3 (3-4)	1 (1-1.4)
Iguanid lizard	2 (1-5)	0.7 (0.4-1.8)
Green iguana	2 (0-11)	0.7 (0-3.9)
Common box turtle	49 (20-102)	17.5 (7.1-36.4)
Red-eared slider	23 (4-54)	8.2 (1.4-19.3)
Desert tortoise	46 (30-62)	16.4 (10.7-22.1)
Gopher tortoise	30 (1-130)	10.7 (0.4-46.4)
Radiated tortoise	16 (2-90)	5.7 (0.7-32.1)
Aldabra tortoise	33 (21-57)	11.8 (7.5-20.3)
Alligator	2 (0-13)	0.7 (0-4.6)
Mammals		
Sugar gliders	17 ± 7	6.1 ± 2.5
Hedgehogs	27 ± 9 (13-54)	9.6 ± 3.2 (4.6-19.3)
Mouse	17-28	6.1-10
Rat	15-21	5.4-7.5
Gerbil	17-27	6.1-9.6
Hamster	12-26	4.3-9.3
Guinea pig	9-32	3.2-11.4
Chinchilla	17-45	6.1-16.1
Prairie dog	21-44	7.5-15.7
Rabbit	15-30	5.4-10.7
Ferret	22 (10-45)	7.8 (3.6-16.1)

*To convert from U.S. units (mg/dL) to S.I. units (mmol/L), multiply by 0.357.

CLINICAL APPLICATIONS

CAUSES OF ABNORMALLY HIGH LEVELS An increase can be due to prerenal, renal, or postrenal problems. Elevated protein catabolism can result from GI bleeding, starvation, extreme exercise, infection, fever, and steroid use. Additional increases can occur with decreased renal perfusion due to dehydration, cardiac disease, and loss of renal mass.

NEXT DIAGNOSTIC STEPS TO CONSIDER IF LEVELS ARE HIGH Creatinine will be low to normal in nonrenal disease and high in renal and postrenal disease. Serum phosphorus will be high in renal disease. Albumin will be low with glomerulopathy. Urine examination (dipstick, specific gravity, production) is indicated in cases with high BUN.

CAUSES OF ABNORMALLY LOW LEVELS Decreased values may be seen with hepatic insufficiency/disease, a low-protein diet, and anabolic steroid use. Young animals might have a low BUN owing to high anabolic metabolism. Diuretics can also decrease BUN. Certain drugs such as aminoglycosides, amphotericin B, and chloramphenicol can also decrease blood levels of BUN. In cases of polyuria/polydipsia (PU/PD), urinary excretion of urea is increased. Urine examination (dipstick, specific gravity, production) and measurement of water intake are indicated in cases of low BUN; in addition, serum electrolytes and calcium need to be checked.

NEXT DIAGNOSTIC STEPS TO CONSIDER IF LEVELS ARE LOW Serum bile acids will be high with hepatic disease.

IMPORTANT INTERSPECIES DIFFERENCES

- Birds and reptiles: BUN has relatively little diagnostic value because urea is present only in small amounts in avian and reptile serum. An increase in BUN level might reflect a stage of dehydration. This has been suggested to be a useful parameter for assessment of hydration in tortoises and pigeons deprived of water.
- Small mammals: In general, rodents concentrate urine very well. BUN therefore is a reliable indicator of severe renal compromise. In rats, an age-dependent decrease in the BUN value has been reported. Different mouse strains can show different normal levels. In the hamster, the female appears to have higher values than the male. The guinea pig appears to have higher levels than other rodents. The ferret commonly presents with increased levels of BUN caused by prerenal or postrenal events. Common prerenal causes of elevation include a high-protein diet and GI hemorrhage due to ulcers or foreign bodies; postrenal factors include decreased excretion due to prostatitis and cystitis due to adrenal disease.
- Rabbits have a limited capacity to concentrate urea in the face of dehydration; this results in elevated values of BUN and creatinine and may be associated with renal disease in other species.
- Fish: The primary end-product of protein metabolism in fish in ammonia (NH_3), which is excreted mainly via the gills. Urea makes up only about 10% of the nitrogenous waste in fish. The level of BUN in fish does not appear to have significant diagnostic value. Increased values have been reported with infectious disease processes, along with increased environmental concentrations of ammonia.

SPECIMEN AND PROCESSING CONSIDERATIONS

DRUG EFFECTS ON LEVELS

- Increased levels: drugs such as steroids or nonsteroidal antiinflammatory drugs (NSAIDs) may cause GI ulcers, thereby increasing the BUN value
- Decreased levels: levels have been shown to decrease with administration of diuretics, aminoglycosides, amphotericin B, and chloramphenicol

SAMPLE FOR COLLECTION AND ANY SPECIAL SPECIMEN HANDLING NOTES Heparinized plasma or serum: collect in a green top tube for reptiles and avian species, and in a red top tube for mammal species

PEARLS

High BUN levels should always be interpreted along with a combination of other factors before a diagnosis of prerenal or postrenal disease is made. Bacteria in the gut may produce urea, which can be absorbed from the GI tract.

AUTHOR: **CANDACE HERSEY-BENNER**

EDITOR: **JÖRG MAYER**

Body Surface Area Conversions Using the Meeh Coefficients

DEFINITION

Many drugs used in chemotherapy are given as mg/M^2 (mg per body surface area) instead of as mg/kg. Debate continues as to whether this is a more adequate and accurate way to dose drugs; however, we would like to provide the reader with the basic concepts and a formula that can be used to calculate body weight into surface area for different species.

TYPICAL NORMAL RANGE

The basic formula is as follows:

$$M^2 = \text{Body weight (g)}^{2/3} \times K \times 10^{-4}$$

where $\mathbf{M^2}$ equals the body surface area, and **K** is the Meeh coefficient for the targeted species. Remember that because of various body shapes and forms, the coefficients vary slightly between certain species. We list here a few species for which this Meeh coefficient has been established:

- Hedgehog = 7.5
- Mouse, guinea pig, swine = 9.0
- Rat = 9.1
- Marmot = 9.3
- Rabbit = 9.75
- Bird, fish, turtle = 10.0
- Sloth = 10.4
- Frog = 10.6
- Porcupine = 10.8
- Monkey = 11.8
- Snake = 12.5
- Bat = 57.5

REFERENCE

Schmidt-Nielsen K: Scaling, why is animal size so important? New York, 1984, Cambridge University Press.

AUTHOR & EDITOR: **JÖRG MAYER**

Calcium

DEFINITION

Calcium (Ca) is the most abundant chemical (mineral) element in the animal body; it is an essential constituent of the skeleton and of teeth. In addition, Ca is a cation in intracellular and extracellular fluid, making it an integral component of living cells and tissue fluids.

SYNONYMS

Ca, Ca^{2+}

PHYSIOLOGY

- Within body fluids, Ca is present in three forms:
  - Complexed Ca (≈6%): associated with phosphate, citrate, and other anions
  - Protein-bound Ca (≈47%): most bound to albumin within the plasma
  - Ionized Ca (≈47%)
- The protein-bound Ca within plasma is involved in coagulation of blood. The plasma of mammals usually contains 80 to 120 mg Ca/L (30 mmol/L), but that of laying hens contains more than that (between 300 and 400 mg/L) (75 to 100 mmol/L).
- Ionized Ca is physiologically active; one of its most important physiologic functions is control of the permeability of cell membranes.
- Parathyroid hormone, which causes transfer of exchangeable Ca from bone into the bloodstream, and calcitriol maintain Ca homeostasis by preventing Ca deficit or excess.

TYPICAL NORMAL RANGE

The typical normal range for this laboratory test varies greatly among species. The reader is referred to the following Elsevier publications for additional information:

Carpenter J: Exotic animal formulary, ed 4, St Louis, 2013, Saunders.

Mader D: Reptile medicine and surgery, ed 2, St Louis, 2006, Saunders.

CLINICAL APPLICATIONS

CAUSES OF ABNORMALLY HIGH LEVELS

- Reptiles
  - Typically iatrogenic owing to oversupplementation of Ca and vitamin D_3
  - Osteolytic bone disease (rare)
  - Primary hyperparathyroidism (rare)
  - Pseudohyperparathyroidism (rare)
  - Female reptiles exhibit features of Ca metabolism similar to those of birds during egg production.
    - During egg development, female reptiles have hypercalcemia in response to estrogen and reproductive activity.
- Birds
  - Reproductive physiologic and/or pathologic increase in females
  - Hypervitaminosis D
  - Primary hyperparathyroidism
  - Renal secondary hyperparathyroidism
  - Nutritional secondary hyperparathyroidism
  - Neoplasia
    - Lymphoma, osteosarcoma
  - Osteomyelitis
  - Granulomatous disease
- Mammals
  - Neoplastic: carcinoma, pseudohyperparathyroidism
  - Rabbits with chronic renal failure and impaired Ca excretion
  - Hypercalcemia in rabbits is often falsely diagnosed because of high total serum calcium levels in comparison with other animals:
    - Affected by age and reproductive status
    - Increased calcium intake resulted in higher total plasma Ca concentrations only in adult rabbits, not in young ones (5 to 19 weeks of age).

NEXT DIAGNOSTIC STEPS TO CONSIDER IF LEVELS ARE HIGH

- Obtain a thorough dietary and supplementation history.
- Determine sex and reproductive status.
- Determine Ca, ionized calcium (iCa), and phosphorus (P) levels.
- Correct Ca concentration if albumin is low (iCa unaffected).
- Determine Ca-to-P ratio and product (suspected renal disease).

- Measure vitamin D metabolites (excess).
- Evaluate urine specific gravity and azotemia to assess for renal impairment.
- Perform a serum parathyroid hormone (PTH) assay.
- Primary hyperparathyroidism, pseudohyperparathyroidism = High Ca (high iCa), low P.
- Secondary renal hyperparathyroidism = High Ca (low iCa), high P, high BUN.
- Vitamin D toxicity = High Ca, high P, normal BUN.
- Assess for neoplasia with complete blood count, abdominal and skeletal radiographs, or ultrasound.
- Assess bone mineral density on radiographs (hyperparathyroidism).
- Repeat sample to rule out hemolysis or another artifact.

CAUSES OF ABNORMALLY LOW LEVELS

- Reptiles
  - Dietary Ca and vitamin D_3 deficiencies, excessive dietary phosphorus
  - Alkalosis, hypoalbuminemia, or hypoparathyroidism
  - Secondary nutritional hyperparathyroidism is a common disorder of herbivorous reptiles.
  - Lack of proper exposure to ultraviolet light predisposes reptiles to hypocalcemia.
- Birds
  - Nutritional
    - Excess dietary phosphorus (seed)
    - Hypovitaminosis D
    - Dietary deficiency (severe)
  - Chronic egg laying—egg-bound hen
  - Hypomagnesemia
  - Hypoparathyroidism
  - Pancreatitis
  - Malabsorption
  - Alkalosis
- Mammals
  - Demand for Ca during late pregnancy (hypocalcemic tetany)
  - Protein-binding properties of Ca, albumin levels can affect total Ca concentrations.

NEXT DIAGNOSTIC STEPS TO CONSIDER IF LEVELS ARE LOW

- Obtain thorough dietary and supplementation history.
- Determine sex and reproductive status.
- Determine Ca, iCa, and P levels.
- Correct Ca concentration if albumin is low (ionized Ca unaffected).
- Measure vitamin D metabolites (deficiency).
- Measure serum alkaline phosphatase (elevated in nutritional secondary hyperparathyroidism [NSHP]).
- Determine serum magnesium.
- Perform serum PTH assay.
- Assess bone mineral density on radiographs.
- Assess for osteoblastic tumor with skeletal radiographs.
- Repeat sample to rule out artifact.

IMPORTANT INTERSPECIES DIFFERENCES

- Fish
  - Water is a readily available source of Ca, and the plasma Ca concentration of fish is influenced by the environmental Ca concentration. Because fish have access to a continuous supply of Ca, they must limit their calcium intake, unless environmental Ca levels are low.
- Reptiles
  - The Ca-to-P ratio is extremely important in determining renal disease and/or chronic malnutrition in reptilian species.
- Small mammals
  - The plasma Ca concentration of rabbits is closely proportional and varies with levels of dietary Ca.

SPECIMEN AND PROCESSING CONSIDERATIONS

DRUG EFFECTS ON LEVEL

- Birds
  - Vitamin D–type rodenticide: reported to lead to high plasma Ca.
  - Sample collected immediately after parenteral Ca therapy leads to high plasma Ca.
  - Calcitonin therapy reported to lead to low plasma Ca.

LAB ARTIFACTS THAT MAY INTERFERE WITH READINGS OF LEVELS OF THIS SUBSTANCE

- In general,
  - Hemolysis can result in falsely increased or decreased amounts of Ca owing to increasing amounts released from erythrocytes or through dilution.
  - Lipemia causes visible clouding of serum. This can lead to dilution of normal substances in the aqueous component of serum, resulting in falsely decreased concentrations.
- Reptiles
  - When quantifying Ca, the laboratory measures only the protein-bound Ca.
- Birds
  - Ca assays are sensitive to artifacts and dilution and may be falsely low:
    - Controversy continues regarding adjustment of plasma Ca (as is done in small animal clinical pathology) made for low albumin because Ca is largely protein bound.
    - High Ca levels are common in reproductively active females, in which plasma Ca values can be as high as 25 mg/dL (3.1 mmol/L).

SAMPLE FOR COLLECTION AND ANY SPECIAL SPECIMEN HANDLING NOTES

- Reptiles
  - Plasma is preferred over serum for chemistries because clot formation may be prolonged in reptiles and may change serum electrolyte and glucose values.
- Birds
  - Lithium heparin is the anticoagulant of choice for most avian blood samples, and biochemistries that are evaluated are most commonly obtained from plasma.
- Small mammals
  - Small blood samples (<2 mL) should be placed in microtainers. Heparin microtainers are preferred because more plasma can be obtained from small samples.
    - All samples should be centrifuged and plasma/serum separated from cells as soon as possible; tests should be run immediately or the specimens transported frozen.

PEARLS

- Fish
  - In freshwater teleosts, Ca ions enter cells through passive diffusion along an electrochemical gradient via Ca channels when transported to the blood by chloride cells in the gills. Stanniocalcin is a hormone that is unique to certain fish (e.g., teleosts); it acts as a Ca channel blocker to prevent the development of hypercalcemia.
  - Fish do not possess parathyroid glands or a PTH-like hormone. It is not yet known how fish that do not produce stanniocalcin regulate their blood Ca concentration.
- Reptiles
  - Ca:P is often the first biochemical indicator of renal disease. Animals commonly present with weakness, anorexia, and lethargy, and may exhibit muscle tremors or fasciculations.
  - In the healthy reptile, Ca:P is typically greater than 1. In cases of renal disease, it often falls to less than 1.
  - The solubility index is a useful calculation that enables the clinician to make therapeutic decisions concerning the need for calcium therapy, vitamin D_3, phosphorus restriction or binders, and diuresis.
    - This index is calculated as Ca × PO_4 (in mmol/L or mg/dL) and normally is less than 55 mg/dL (<9 mmol/L). If the solubility index increases to between 55 and 70 mg/dL (9 and 12 mmol/L), mineralization of diseased tissue, including kidneys, may occur. If the solubility index increases to

above 70 mg/dL (>12 mmol/L), mineralization of healthy tissue occurs.
- Small mammals
  - Ca metabolism in the rabbit is slightly different from that in other domestic species. Dietary Ca is readily absorbed from the intestine, and total plasma values reflect dietary intake. Therefore, total blood Ca levels are higher and can vary over a wider range than in other species.

AUTHOR: **CARRIE A. PHELPS**

EDITOR: **JÖRG MAYER**

Chloride

DEFINITION

Major extracellular anion that helps regulate acid-base and fluid balance

PHYSIOLOGY

Chloride (Cl) is a major extracellular anion. It is the biggest component of gastric juices. Changes in Cl independent of sodium usually occur with changes in acid-base status. Cl is considered an acid, meaning that an increase equals acidosis and a decrease is consistent with alkalosis. The concentration of Cl usually parallels that of sodium and is related to bicarbonate. Cl levels can be corrected for changes in serum sodium to determine whether or not the change is independent of sodium. If the change in Cl is parallel to a change in sodium, the Cl will correct. If the change is independent, the corrected value will remain decreased or elevated. A common cause of independent Cl change is gastrointestinal disease. Cl is regulated by the kidneys; it is filtered out by the glomeruli and is reabsorbed in the tubules, where it follows water and sodium.

TYPICAL NORMAL RANGE

The typical normal range for this laboratory test varies greatly among species. The reader is referred to the following Elsevier publications for additional information:

Carpenter J: Exotic animal formulary, ed 4, St Louis, 2013, Saunders.

Mader D: Reptile medicine and surgery, ed 2, St Louis, 2006, Saunders.

CLINICAL APPLICATIONS

CAUSES OF ABNORMALLY HIGH LEVELS

- Metabolic acidosis caused by diarrhea, shock, renal failure, ketoacidotic diabetes mellitus, severe muscular exertion, excessive use of carbonic anhydrase inhibitors, or poisoning with ethylene glycol or metaldehyde can cause hyperchloremia.
- Increases can also be due to increased sodium levels from increased sodium intake (diet, IV fluids), excessive water loss, and reduced intake of water (water deprivation, inability to drink).
- Other causes include ammonium Cl therapy (urinary acidifier) and renal disease.
- Hyperchloremia is rarely found in avian species.

NEXT DIAGNOSTIC STEPS TO CONSIDER IF LEVELS ARE HIGH

- Urine specific gravity: evaluate the relationship to sodium to help rule out differential diagnosis
- Corrected Cl to determine whether relationship to sodium is changed: Cl (corrected) = Cl (measured) × (Na [normal]/Na [measured])

CAUSES OF ABNORMALLY LOW LEVELS

- Hypochloremia can be caused by metabolic alkalosis (vomiting or regurgitation), decreased sodium levels (absolute or relative overhydration), Cl-losing diuretics (chlorothiazide, furosemide, and ethacrynic acid), renal disease, and congestive heart failure (due to water retention).
- Iatrogenic overhydration with IV fluids that are low in sodium

NEXT DIAGNOSTIC STEPS TO CONSIDER IF LEVELS ARE LOW

- Evaluate the relationship to sodium to help to rule out differential diagnosis. Corrected Cl to determine whether relationship to sodium is changed: Cl (corrected) = Cl (measured) × (Na [normal] /Na [measured])
- Urine fractional excretion of Cl
- Blood gas (metabolic alkalosis)

SPECIMEN AND PROCESSING CONSIDERATIONS

DRUG EFFECTS ON LEVELS

- Amphotericin, lithium, acetazolamide, ammonium chloride, and androgens can elevate Cl levels.
- Falsely elevated levels can be caused by iodide or bromide.
- Depressed levels can be caused by furosemide, thiazides, bicarbonate, and laxatives.

LAB ARTIFACTS THAT MAY INTERFERE WITH READINGS OF LEVELS OF THIS SUBSTANCE

- Ion-specific electrodes will measure and report other halides as Cl, causing artificial elevation.
- Hemoglobin and bilirubin can falsely elevate levels if a colorimetric test is used.
- Lipemia and hyperproteinemia can falsely lower Cl serum levels if ion-specific electrodes are not used.

SAMPLE FOR COLLECTION AND ANY SPECIAL SPECIMEN HANDLING NOTES

- Reptiles: plasma is preferred over serum for chemistries because clot formation may be prolonged in reptiles and may change serum electrolyte and glucose values. Also, a greater volume per unit of blood can be obtained.
- Birds: lithium heparin is the anticoagulant of choice for most avian samples if used for both hematology and chemistry
- Small mammals: small blood samples (<2 mL) should be placed in microtainers. Heparin microtainers are preferred because more plasma can be obtained from small samples.
- All samples should be centrifuged and plasma/serum separated from cells as soon as possible; tests should be run immediately or the specimen transported frozen.

PEARLS

- Some reptiles have nasal salt glands to eliminate salt from their system. In rare cases of disorders of the salt gland, the electrolyte balance might be affected.
- Cl is considered to be of low diagnostic value in reptiles.

REFERENCES

Campbell TW: Clinical pathology. In Mader DR, editor: Reptile medicine and surgery, Philadelphia, 1996, WB Saunders.

Carpenter JW: Exotic animal formulary, ed 3, Philadelphia, 2004, WB Saunders.

Fudge AM, editor: Laboratory medicine: avian and exotic pets, Philadelphia, 2000, WB Saunders.
Jones MP: Avian clinical pathology, Vet Clin North Am Exot Anim Pract 2:663–687, 1999.
Stoskopf MK, editor: Fish medicine, Philadelphia, 1993, WB Saunders.

AUTHOR: **CARALEE MANLEY**

EDITOR: **JÖRG MAYER**

Cholesterol

DEFINITION

Major lipid found only in the body and important precursor of steroids, bile acids, and cholesterol esters

PHYSIOLOGY

Cholesterol is the precursor of all steroid hormones, cholesterol esters, and bile acids, and is a component of the plasma membrane of cells. Total cholesterol consists of free cholesterol and cholesterol esters. Serum cholesterol is derived from the diet and is synthesized in the liver. Low-density lipoproteins (LDLs) consist mostly of protein, are rich in cholesterol, and are derived from the breakdown of very low-density lipoproteins (VLDLs). High-density lipoproteins (HDLs), the smallest particles, consist mostly of cholesterol, protein, and phospholipids, with only a small quantity of triglycerides. LDLs are a source of cholesterol for peripheral cells, such as the adrenal gland; HDLs transport cholesterol from peripheral cells back to the liver. LDLs and HDLs do no contribute to visible lipemia. Excess cholesterol is excreted via the bile, where it is esterified. Cholesterol measurements can provide supportive evidence in some diseases.

TYPICAL NORMAL RANGE

The typical normal range for this laboratory test varies greatly among species. The reader is referred to the following Elsevier publications for additional information:

Carpenter J: Exotic animal formulary, ed 4, St Louis, 2013, Saunders.
Mader D: Reptile medicine and surgery, ed 2, St Louis, 2006, Saunders.

CLINICAL APPLICATIONS

CAUSES OF ABNORMALLY HIGH LEVELS

- Hypercholesterolemia results from increased levels of cholesterol-rich lipoproteins (LDLs and HDLs). Postprandial hyperlipidemia (very common) may occur after a fatty meal, but values should return to normal within 12 hours; increased levels can occur even if the animal is fasted.
- Endocrine disorders such as hypothyroidism and diabetes mellitus can cause hypercholesterolemia. Thyroid hormones stimulate cholesterol synthesis and degradation to bile acids. Diabetes mellitus causes an increase in triglycerides (VLDLs), which degrade to LDLs, both of which are rich in cholesterol. Hepatic breakdown of cholesterol is decreased.
- Acute pancreatitis causes elevations resulting from increases in both LDLs and HDLs.
- Severe trauma causes an increase in catecholamines and increased lipolysis. Insulin secretion is suppressed, causing elevated cholesterol levels (within 48 hours).
- Starvation can cause fat mobilization and degradation in obese animals along with hypercholesterolemia.
- Primary liver damage (hepatic lipidosis) and bile duct obstruction can cause increased levels because cholesterol is excreted in the bile and can accumulate owing to cholestasis; mild increases can be caused by acute hepatitis.
- Renal loss of protein through primary glomerular diseases (glomerulonephritis and renal amyloidosis) and subsequent nephrotic syndrome cause a compensatory response of increased serum cholesterol levels (increased VLDLs) in an attempt to maintain plasma oncotic pressure in the face of hypoalbuminemia.
- Atherosclerosis can cause hypercholesterolemia in birds.
- During the active phase of reproduction (folliculogenesis), high values can be observed in reptiles and birds. It is important to avoid interpreting these values as a pathologic process.

NEXT DIAGNOSTIC STEPS TO CONSIDER IF LEVELS ARE HIGH

- If possible, obtain fasting levels to avoid postprandial hyperlipidemia.
- Abdominal ultrasound can be used to evaluate the reproductive status of the animal.
- In female birds, consider taking a radiograph; check for physiologic hyperostosis, which occurs in the reproductive phase.
- Evaluate diet and try to reduce cholesterol intake.

CAUSES OF ABNORMALLY LOW LEVELS

- Hepatic insufficiency—acquired (cirrhosis) or congenital (portosystemic shunts)—would result in decreased cholesterol synthesis (as well as hypoalbuminemia and usually decreased blood urea nitrogen [BUN]).
- Hypocholesterolemia can also result from a low-fat diet or malnutrition.
- Hyperthyroidism affects the clearance of cholesterol and triglycerides and may result in mild decreases.
- Protein-losing enteropathy and possible fat malabsorption/digestion may cause decreased cholesterol levels.
- Aflatoxicosis, *Escherichia coli*, endotoxemia, and spirochetosis can cause depressed levels in avian species.

NEXT DIAGNOSTIC STEPS TO CONSIDER IF LEVELS ARE LOW

- Evaluate albumin and BUN for evidence of hepatic insufficiency.
- Request bacterial culture.
- Rule out starvation.

IMPORTANT INTERSPECIES DIFFERENCES

- Amphibians: high cholesterol findings have been associated with lipid keratopathy—a common disease in captive amphibians that is thought to be linked to a high-fat diet
- In fatty liver disease, elevations of cholesterol can be associated with lipemia.
- Rabbits: male rabbits appear to have lower levels than females. In addition, a diurnal variation has been observed, with higher levels in the late afternoon.

SPECIMEN AND PROCESSING CONSIDERATIONS

DRUG EFFECTS ON LEVELS

- Corticosteroids can cause fat mobilization and increased levels.
- Other drugs that may alter results include phenytoin, prochlorperazine, thiazides, and phenothiazines.

LAB ARTIFACTS THAT MAY INTERFERE WITH READINGS OF LEVELS OF THIS SUBSTANCE

- Falsely elevated values can be caused by hemolysis or phenytoin.
- Falsely depressed values can be caused by high levels of vitamin C that interfere with cholesterol estimation.

SAMPLE FOR COLLECTION AND ANY SPECIAL SPECIMEN HANDLING NOTES

- Reptiles: plasma is preferred over serum for chemistries because clot formation may be prolonged in reptiles and may change serum electrolyte and glucose values. Also, a greater volume per unit of blood can be attained.
- Birds: lithium heparin is the anticoagulant of choice for most avian blood samples; evaluation of biochemistries is most commonly performed on plasma.
- Small mammals: small blood samples (<2 mL) should be placed in microtainers. Heparin microtainers are preferred because more plasma can be obtained from small samples.
- All samples should be centrifuged and plasma/serum separated from cells as soon as possible. Tests should be run immediately or the specimen transported frozen.

PEARLS

A high-cholesterol diet for birds might induce renal failure, in addition to other health problems.

REFERENCES

Campbell TW: Clinical pathology. In Mader DR, editor: Reptile medicine and surgery, Philadelphia, 1996, WB Saunders.

Carpenter JW: Exotic animal formulary, ed 3, Philadelphia, 2004, WB Saunders.

Fudge AM, editor: Laboratory medicine: avian and exotic pets, Philadelphia, 2000, WB Saunders.

Jones MP: Avian clinical pathology, Vet Clin North Am Exot Anim Pract 2:663–687, 1999.

AUTHOR: **CARALEE MANLEY**

EDITOR: **JÖRG MAYER**

Creatine Kinase

DEFINITION

Creatine kinase (CK) exists as three isozymes in skeletal muscle, in cardiac muscle, and in the brain. CK is considered to be specific for muscle cell damage and is used primarily for the diagnosis of skeletal muscle injury. CK has a relatively short half-life (<72 hours).

SYNONYMS

CK, creatine phosphokinase, CPK

PHYSIOLOGY

CK is a magnesium-dependent dimeric enzyme that is responsible for catalyzing the reaction that converts adenosine diphosphate (ADP) and creatine phosphate to adenosine triphosphate (ATP) and creatinine in skeletal, cardiac, and smooth muscle, as well as in the brain. CK is present in the cytosol and mitochondria of myocytes. Therefore, CK is critical for energy production in muscle tissue for contraction. Serum CK activity is primarily of muscle origin. In many species, it is considered a sensitive indicator of skeletal or cardiac muscle damage.

TYPICAL NORMAL RANGE

The typical normal range for this laboratory test varies greatly among species. The reader is referred to the following Elsevier publications for additional information:

Carpenter J: Exotic animal formulary, ed 4, St Louis, 2013, Saunders.

Mader D: Reptile medicine and surgery, ed 2, St Louis, 2006, Saunders.

CLINICAL APPLICATIONS

CAUSES OF ABNORMALLY HIGH LEVELS

- Skeletal muscle damage, severe exertion, capture myopathy (exertional rhabdomyolysis), hypothyroidism (mammals), and CNS disorders (e.g., seizure activity)
- Myositis, hyperthermia, hypothermia, vitamin E/selenium deficiency, trauma/surgical, ischemia

NEXT DIAGNOSTIC STEPS TO CONSIDER IF LEVELS ARE HIGH Evaluate for muscle disease or injury or muscle catabolism.

SPECIMEN AND PROCESSING CONSIDERATIONS

LAB ARTIFACTS THAT MAY INTERFERE WITH READINGS OF LEVELS OF THIS SUBSTANCE

- Hemolysis and hyperbilirubinemia will artificially increase CK levels. Release of CK after intramuscular injection and traumatic venipuncture can also increase CK levels. False increases in CK generally are 2 to 3 times the upper normal limit.
- Dilution of the serum or plasma sample during the assay reduces the concentrations of natural inhibitors and can result in greatly increased CK activity.

PEARLS

Elevations in plasma CK can often be seen in reptiles or birds that have struggled to resist restraint during blood collection.

REFERENCES

Bush BM: Interpretation of laboratory results for small animal clinicians, Ames, IA, 1991, Blackwell.

Carpenter JW: Exotic animal formulary, ed 3, St Louis, 2004, Elsevier.

Harrison GJ, et al: Clinical avian medicine, vol 2, South Palm Beach, FL, 2006, Spix Publishing, pp 617, 622–623.

Mader DR: Reptile medicine and surgery, ed 2, St Louis, 2006, Elsevier, p 652.

AUTHOR: **CARRIE A. PHELPS**

EDITOR: **JÖRG MAYER**

Creatinine

DEFINITION

Creatinine is a nitrogenous waste product produced by the breakdown of creatine, which is an important part of muscle. A serum creatinine test measures the amount of creatinine in the blood; it is an indirect indicator of renal glomerular filtration rate and can estimate renal function.

SYNONYM

Creat

PHYSIOLOGY

Creatinine, the waste product produced via the catabolism of phosphocreatine, is filtered mainly by the kidney, although a small amount is actively secreted. Some tubular reabsorption of creatinine occurs, but this is compensated by a roughly equivalent degree of tubular secretion. Any changes in levels of creatinine in the blood are related to excretion and therefore reflect kidney function. However, in cases of severe renal dysfunction, creatinine clearance will be overestimated owing to active secretion of creatinine, which accounts for a larger fraction of the total creatinine cleared. Higher than normal creatinine and blood urea nitrogen (BUN) can be indicative of dehydration.

TYPICAL NORMAL RANGE

The typical normal range for this laboratory test varies greatly among species. The reader is referred to the following Elsevier publications for additional information:

Carpenter J: Exotic animal formulary, ed 4, St Louis, 2013, Saunders.

Mader D: Reptile medicine and surgery, ed 2, St Louis, 2006, Saunders.

CLINICAL APPLICATIONS

CAUSES OF ABNORMALLY HIGH LEVELS Severe dehydration, egg yolk peritonitis, septicemia, renal disease/trauma, prolonged exercise, and nephrotoxic drugs can cause elevated levels of creatinine. Any prerenal, renal, or postrenal processes that cause a decrease in glomerular filtration rate (GFR) can result in abnormally high levels. Other conditions include pyometra, gastric dilatation/torsion, diabetes mellitus, hypercalcemia of malignancy, and a high-protein diet, which may result in elevated levels.

NEXT DIAGNOSTIC STEPS TO CONSIDER IF LEVELS ARE HIGH BUN should be checked for elevation when creatinine levels are elevated. Urine creatinine-to-serum creatinine and urine specific gravity are useful in the differentiation of prerenal from renal azotemia. In chronic renal disease, hyperphosphatemia and hypocalcemia or hypercalcemia can be seen. Urine analysis (dipstick and specific gravity) should be performed. To differentiate prerenal from postrenal azotemia in birds, the urea-to-creatinine ratio (Urea [mmol/L] × 1000/Creatinine [μmol/L]) and the urea-to-uric acid ratio (Urea [mmol/L] × 1000/Uric acid [μmol/L]) can be calculated. These ratios will be high during dehydration or ureteral obstruction because reabsorption of urea is disproportionately higher than that of both creatinine and uric acid.

CAUSES OF ABNORMALLY LOW LEVELS Muscle disease or wasting decreases the amount of phosphocreatine available for conversion, thereby decreasing the serum creatinine concentration. A decreased serum creatinine value is not recognized as clinically significant, but low levels can be seen when renal blood flow is decreased and in cases with body condition loss.

NEXT DIAGNOSTIC STEPS TO CONSIDER IF LEVELS ARE LOW

- A decreased serum creatinine value is not recognized as clinically significant.
- Check for chronic weight loss.

IMPORTANT INTERSPECIES DIFFERENCES

- Birds and reptiles: creatinine is a poor indicator of renal function in avian species because birds reportedly excrete creatine before it is converted to creatinine. In reptiles, creatinine production is variable and virtually nonexistent, and measurement is unreliable. However, blood levels may be diagnostic for renal disease in some reptile species.
- Small mammals: It has been demonstrated that creatinine is an insensitive indicator of renal failure in ferrets, perhaps in part because of their capacity for extrarenal elimination of creatinine. Ferrets have a considerably lower and narrower range of creatinine in the blood compared with other mammals.

SPECIMEN AND PROCESSING CONSIDERATIONS

DRUG EFFECTS ON LEVELS Elevated levels: cephalosporins, gentamicin, oxytetracycline, amphotericin B, trimethoprim-sulfadiazine, and furosemide

LAB ARTIFACTS THAT MAY INTERFERE WITH READINGS OF LEVELS OF THIS SUBSTANCE

- Elevated levels: false-high serum test values can result when Jaffe's reaction is used; a chromagen color reaction is seen when the sample contains noncreatinine chromagens, such as ketones, glucose, fructose, ascorbic acid, protein, urea, and ascorbic acid.
- Decreased levels: creatinine deteriorates in plasma samples older than 24 hours, leading to unreliable results. Bilirubin can cause sampling errors.

SAMPLE FOR COLLECTION AND ANY SPECIAL SPECIMEN HANDLING NOTES Heparinized plasma or serum: collect in a green top for reptiles and avian species, and in a red top for mammal species

PEARLS

Three-fourths of renal function must be lost before abnormalities in creatinine concentration are seen. Creatinine is not influenced by diet or GI ulcers.

AUTHOR: **CANDACE HERSEY-BENNER**

EDITOR: **JÖRG MAYER**

Eosinophil Count

DEFINITION

- Mammals
  - A granular leukocyte with a cytoplasm containing coarse, round, or rod-shaped orange/red (eosinophilic) granules of uniform size
- Birds
  - A granular leukocyte with a bluish cytoplasm containing round orange/red (eosinophilic) granules. A large degree of variation of size, shape, and color has been noted among species. Some birds may have granules, which stain bluish.
- Reptiles
  - A granular leukocyte with a cytoplasm containing a variable number of round orange/red (eosinophilic) granules. In some species, the granules may stain blue-green.
- Cyprinid fish
  - A granular leukocyte with a pale blue-to-pink cytoplasm and round-to-oval bright red–staining granules. They also have a small eccentric, condensed nucleus that may vary in shape.

SYNONYM

Eos

PHYSIOLOGY

- Eosinophils are granulocytes; they develop in a similar pattern to neutrophils and basophils. Eosinophil differentiation from myeloid stem cells is promoted by interleukin (IL)-5 and granulocyte-monocyte colony-stimulating factor (GM-CSF) (released by mast cells, macrophages, and lymphocytes). Eosinophils then progress through various stages of maturity within the bone marrow and are released into the bloodstream. Similar to neutrophils, eosinophils have a circulating and marginated pool. Eosinophils spend only a short time in the bloodstream passing through circulating and marginated pools before they enter the tissues. At any given time, most eosinophils are found in the tissues rather than in the bloodstream. Migration of eosinophils into the tissues and to sites of infection is promoted by various chemotactic agents, especially histamine and eotaxin. Eosinophils can survive in the tissues for an undetermined length of time—possibly for weeks.
- Eosinophils have limited phagocytic abilities; most of their antibacterial and antiparasitic effects are mediated by the contents of their granules. Degranulation releases a variety of cytotoxic proteins, including major basic protein and proinflammatory cytokines and peroxidase. In addition to the presence of bacteria or parasites, eosinophil degranulation can be promoted through binding of immunoglobulin (Ig)E antibodies to the cell membrane. This is part of the inflammatory mechanism associated with allergic disease. Eosinophils can reduce hypersensitivity reactions by inhibiting chemical mediators released by mast cells.

TYPICAL NORMAL RANGE

The typical normal range for this laboratory test varies greatly among species. The reader is referred to the following Elsevier publications for additional information:

Carpenter J: Exotic animal formulary, ed 4, St Louis, 2013, Saunders.

Mader D: Reptile medicine and surgery, ed 2, St Louis, 2006, Saunders.

CLINICAL APPLICATIONS

CAUSES OF ABNORMALLY HIGH LEVELS

- Mammals
  - In mammals, one of the most common causes of eosinophilia is parasitism—internal or external. Intracellular blood parasites do not cause an eosinophilic response. Allergic reactions, such as fleabite dermatitis, asthma, hypersensitivity to staphylococcal or streptococcal infection, and milk allergy in ruminants, are common causes of eosinophilia.
  - Neoplasia can cause eosinophilia as a primary or a secondary response. Mast cell tumors lead to eosinophilia owing to the chemotactic agents released by degranulating mast cells. Eosinophilia can also occur as a paraneoplastic condition. Eosinophilic leukemia will lead to elevated eosinophil counts, often with an increase in the number of cells with abnormal morphology.
  - Tissue damage can cause an eosinophilia. Several idiopathic causes of eosinophilia, including eosinophilic gastroenteritis, are known.
  - Hypoadrenocorticism will cause abnormally high levels of eosinophils. Eosinophilia alone should not be considered a sign of hypoadrenocorticism; rather, it is part of a constellation of hematologic changes that occur along with a decrease in glucocorticoid production.
- Birds
  - In birds, it is not established if eosinophilia is related to parasitism—internal or external. Intracellular blood parasites do not cause an eosinophilic response. Hypersensitivity reactions, specifically, delayed type IV reactions, can cause eosinophilia. Similar to the case in mammals, tissue damage can result in eosinophilia.
- Reptiles
  - In reptiles, a potential cause of eosinophilia is parasitism—internal or external. Intracellular blood parasites do not cause an eosinophilic response. Allergic reactions and other hypersensitivity reactions can cause eosinophilia. Tissue damage causes an eosinophilia as well.
  - Variations in eosinophil numbers have been associated with activity level. With low activity, especially hibernation, they are associated with eosinophilia.

NEXT DIAGNOSTIC STEPS TO CONSIDER IF LEVELS ARE HIGH

- Mammals
  - After an eosinophilia is detected, a thorough search for parasite infection should be conducted. This should include a direct fecal smear, as well as a fecal float. The skin and hair coat should be examined for external parasites, and a skin scraping performed as needed. Both superficial and deep skin scrapings may have to be performed.
  - If any cutaneous or subcutaneous masses are detected during the physical examination, they should be aspirated and the samples submitted for cytologic examination.
  - With persistent eosinophilia, a complete examination of the animal's environment—directly or via questioning of the owner—should be done to look for possible causes of allergic hypersensitivity. With small animals, the bedding is often a source of inhalant allergies owing to the type of bedding or the buildup of waste products from infrequent changes. If inhalant allergies or asthma is suspected, thoracic radiographs should be taken. An interstitial-to-bronchiolar radiographic pattern is a common finding with chronic asthma or allergic hypersensitivity.
  - If no other obvious causes of eosinophilia are noted, a bone marrow biopsy should be conducted.

- Birds and reptiles
  - After an eosinophilia is detected, a thorough search for parasitic infection should be conducted as the role of parasites in eosinophilia is not 100% clear to this date. This should include a direct fecal smear, as well as a fecal float. Skin/feathers or scales should be examined for external parasites.
  - With persistent eosinophilia, a complete examination of the animal's environment—directly or via questioning of the owner—should be performed to look for possible causes of trauma, stress, or allergic hypersensitivity.

CAUSES OF ABNORMALLY LOW LEVELS

- In most animals, the lower limit of the reference range for eosinophils is zero; therefore, eosinopenia has little to no diagnostic significance.
- An eosinopenia with elevated glucocorticoid levels (exogenous or endogenous) may be noted, but a neutrophilia combined with a lymphopenia is a much stronger diagnostic sign.
- Reptiles
  - Activity levels and season can affect eosinophil counts. High activity levels and the summer months have been associated with a decrease in eosinophil levels.

SPECIMEN AND PROCESSING CONSIDERATIONS

DRUG EFFECTS ON LEVEL Glucocorticiods can cause abnormally low levels.

SAMPLE FOR COLLECTION AND ANY SPECIAL SPECIMEN HANDLING NOTES

- Mammals
  - Use EDTA (purple top) tubes to collect for complete blood count (CBC).
- Birds
  - For differential counts, it is best if slides can be made from fresh whole blood.
  - Use EDTA (purple top) tubes to collect for CBC in most species. ETDA may cause red blood cell (RBC) hemolysis, especially in Brush turkeys, Corvidaie, Crowned cranes, Currasows, and Hornbills.
- Reptiles
  - Use heparinized (green top) tubes when collecting CBC samples.
- Amphibians
  - Use heparinized (green top) tubes when collecting CBC samples. Because of the small volumes often collected, use a heparinized syringe to collect the sample, and make slides immediately after collection whenever possible.
- Fish
  - Samples for differential cell counts should be prepared immediately after collection. It is important to rapidly dry the slides because slow drying may alter the morphology. Slides can be stained with LG or WLG stain. Diff-Quik stain can be used, but it is not optimal for differential counts. If it is necessary to collect samples in tubes, use heparinized tubes. ETDA causes hemolysis in fish anesthetized with tricaine.

PEARLS

- Reptiles
  - Most snakes, including Yellow rat snakes and Ball pythons, have no eosinophils. Species that have eosinophils are generally larger than other reptiles.
  - Turtles generally have larger eosinophil populations compared with other reptiles.
  - Lizard species generally have smaller eosinophil populations compared with other reptiles.

REFERENCES

Carpenter JW, et al: Exotic animal formulary, ed 2, Philadelphia, 2001, WB Saunders, pp 36, 80–86, 195–208, 213, 256, 268, 292, 320, 344, 363, 386–387.

Fudge AM: Laboratory medicine: avian and exotic pets, ed 1, Philadelphia, 2000, WB Saunders, pp 9–27, 193–204, 269–274.

Groff JM, et al: Hematology and clinical chemistry of cyprinid fish, Vet Clin North Am 2:741–776, 1999.

Hoegeman S: Diagnostic sampling of amphibians, Vet Clin North Am 2:731–740, 1999.

Jones MP: Avian clinical pathology, Vet Clin North Am 2:663–688, 1999.

Redrobe S, et al: Sample collection and clinical pathology of reptiles, Vet Clin North Am 2:709–730, 1999.

Stockham SL, et al: Fundamentals of veterinary clinical pathology, ed 1, Ames, IA, 2002, Iowa State Press, pp 50–83.

AUTHOR: **JONATHAN W. BALL**

EDITOR: **JÖRG MAYER**

Gammaglutamyl Transferase (GGT)

DEFINITION

Gammaglutamyl transferase (GGT) catalyzes the transfer of the gammaglutamyl group from a donor peptide to an acceptor compound. The biliary system is the primary source of plasma GGT.

SYNONYM

α-Glutaryltransferase

PHYSIOLOGY

GGT is present in serum and in low levels in the cell membranes of all cells, except muscle in mammals. GGT may be involved in the metabolism and detoxification of glutathione. In addition to biliary GGT, which is the main source of GGT, significant levels of renal epithelial GGT can be found in the urine.

TYPICAL NORMAL RANGE

The typical normal range for this laboratory test varies greatly among species. The reader is referred to the following Elsevier publications for additional information:

Carpenter J: Exotic animal formulary, ed 4, St Louis, 2013, Saunders.

Mader D: Reptile medicine and surgery, ed 2, St Louis, 2006, Saunders.

CLINICAL APPLICATIONS

CAUSES OF ABNORMALLY HIGH LEVELS

- Increased serum GGT levels are most commonly associated with cholestatic disorders, as well as with increased de novo synthesis and membrane elution.
- Biliary (obstruction/damage)
  - Neoplasia (biliary carcinoma)
  - Inflammation
  - Cholelithiasis
  - Cholestasis (intrahepatic or extrahepatic)
  - Other biliary compromise

NEXT DIAGNOSTIC STEPS TO CONSIDER IF LEVELS ARE HIGH Complete blood count, chemistry panel, abdominal radiographs, abdominal ultrasound, ± liver biopsy

CAUSES OF ABNORMALLY LOW LEVELS Artifactual owing to hemolysis

IMPORTANT INTERSPECIES DIFFERENCES

- GGT in the rabbit is found primarily in the bile duct of the epithelium and therefore is more diagnostic for hepatobiliary disease than for hepatocellular damage.
- Increased GGT was found in most pigeons with experimentally induced liver disease. However, GGT activity in the avian liver is reported as very low, making it a parameter with low sensitivity but high specificity for liver disease.
- Increases in GGT activity have been noted in birds with bile duct carcinoma, sometimes in association with papilloma or herpesvirus infection.
- Tissue values of GGT may be very low in reptiles but are still considered liver specific.

SPECIMEN AND PROCESSING CONSIDERATIONS

DRUG EFFECTS ON LEVEL Increases have been seen with long-term anticonvulsant and corticosteroid therapies.

LAB ARTIFACTS THAT MAY INTERFERE WITH READINGS OF LEVELS OF THIS SUBSTANCE

- Lipemia may erroneously increase or decrease the GGT.
- Heparin (used as treatment or as anticoagulant) can artificially increase the value.

REFERENCES

Bush BM: Interpretation of laboratory results for small animal clinicians, Ames, IA, 1992, Blackwell.

Carpenter JW: Exotic animal formulary, ed 3, St Louis, 2004, Elsevier.

Ettinger SF, et al: Textbook of veterinary internal medicine, ed 6, vol 2, St Louis, 2005, Elsevier, pp 1425.

Harrison GJ, et al: Clinical avian medicine, vol II, South Palm Beach, FL, 2006, Spix Publishing, pp 624.

Mader DR: Reptile medicine and surgery, ed 2, St Louis, 2006, Elsevier, pp 807.

AUTHOR: **CARRIE A. PHELPS**

EDITOR: **JÖRG MAYER**

Globulins

DEFINITION

Globulins are proteins that are mostly involved in the immune defense system. Any protein that is not albumin is classified as a globulin. In birds, globulins are regarded as anything that is not transthyretin (prealbumin).

SYNONYM

Glob

PHYSIOLOGY

- Acute phase proteins are produced in the liver in response to inflammatory cytokines. These proteins, such as α_2-macroglobulin and immunoglobulins, increase in inflammatory states, but albumin will decrease because albumin is a negative acute phase protein. This will result in a decreased albumin-to-globulin ratio.
- Globulins usually are separated into five fractions by electrophoresis.
- In birds, plasma globulins that have been identified are α_1-antitrypsin (α_1-globulin fraction) and α_2-macroglobulin (α_2-globulin fraction). Fibrinogen, β-lipoprotein, transferrin, complement, and vitellogenin make up the β-globulin fraction; immunoglobulins and complement degradation products constitute the gamma (γ)-globulin fraction. Most of the immunoglobulins are synthesized in the lymphoid tissue.
- Examining banding patterns by plasma gel electrophoresis can help the practitioner determine whether a decreased albumin-to-globulin ratio is due to inflammation or to egg formation in birds.

TYPICAL NORMAL RANGE

The typical normal range for this laboratory test varies greatly among species. The reader is referred to the following Elsevier publications for additional information:

Carpenter J: Exotic animal formulary, ed 4, St Louis, 2013, Saunders.

Mader D: Reptile medicine and surgery, ed 2, St Louis, 2006, Saunders.

CLINICAL APPLICATIONS

CAUSES OF ABNORMALLY HIGH LEVELS

- Chronic immune stimulation/inflammation (e.g., inflammatory bowel disease [IBD], Aleutian disease)
- Dehydration (albumin will increase as well)
- Lymphoma or multiple myeloma
- Egg formation

NEXT DIAGNOSTIC STEPS TO CONSIDER IF LEVELS ARE HIGH

- Complete blood count (CBC), chemistry panel, urinalysis
- Check for increased albumin to rule out dehydration.

CAUSES OF ABNORMALLY LOW LEVELS

- Decreased globulins are generally the result of decreased production (e.g., liver failure), decreased uptake/transfer (in neonates), or increased loss.
- Causes include the following:
  - Liver failure
  - Neonatal
  - Protein-losing enteropathy
  - Blood loss (subacute to chronic)
  - Immunodeficiency

NEXT DIAGNOSTIC STEPS TO CONSIDER IF LEVELS ARE LOW CBC, chemistry panel, urinalysis, radiographs, abdominal ultrasound ± liver biopsy, endoscopy ± intestinal biopsy, bile acids

IMPORTANT INTERSPECIES DIFFERENCES

- In birds, oviparous females may have a decreased albumin-to-globulin ratio owing to an increase in the globulin fraction during the reproductive period. This increase is due to production of vitellogenin and other proteins used in egg formation.
- In ferrets, the globulin value is often encountered as high in chronic subclinical forms of inflammatory diseases such as IBD. In cases of Aleutian disease, values are often greater than 6 g/dL. To differentiate enteral forms of inflammation and other chronic inflammatory disease processes, a lipase level is useful because the GI tract in the ferret appears to produce more lipase than is produced by the pancreas.

SPECIMEN AND PROCESSING CONSIDERATIONS

LAB ARTIFACTS THAT MAY INTERFERE WITH READINGS OF LEVELS OF THIS SUBSTANCE Globulin levels are calculated by subtracting albumin from total protein. Any error in measurements of albumin or total protein will yield erroneous globulin levels.

REFERENCES

Carpenter JW: Exotic animal formulary, ed 3, St Louis, 2004, Elsevier.

Harrison GJ, et al: Clinical avian medicine, vol II, South Palm Beach, FL, 2006, Spix Publishing, pp 625.

Yin SA: The small animal veterinary nerdbook, ed 2, Davis, CA, 1988, CattleDog Publishing, pp 4.5.

AUTHOR: **CARRIE A. PHELPS**

EDITOR: **JÖRG MAYER**

Glucose

DEFINITION

- A simple sugar, C6H12O6, found in most foodstuffs
- It is the only monosaccharide present in significant amounts in blood and body fluids.
- Glucose is the major source of energy through the process of oxidative metabolism.

SYNONYMS

D-Glucose, $C_6H_{12}O_6$, glycogen (storage form)

PHYSIOLOGY

- Glucose in the blood is derived from three main sources:
  - Intestinal absorption
    - Glucose is the end-product of carbohydrate digestion, absorbed by enterocytes.
    - Increased blood glucose concentrations occur 2 to 4 hours after a meal in simple-stomached animals.
  - Hepatic production
    - Gluconeogenesis and glycogenolysis within hepatic cells produce glucose when metabolically necessary.
      - Gluconeogenesis converts noncarbohydrate sources, primarily amino acids (from protein) and glycerol (from fat), in simple-stomached animals.
      - Glycogenolysis converts glycogen (poly-glucose) stored in hepatocytes to glucose through hydrolysis.
  - Kidney production
    - Gluconeogenesis and glycogenolysis within renal epithelial cells can result in the formation of glucose when metabolically necessary.
- The plasma concentration of glucose is controlled by a number of hormones, in particular, insulin and glucagon. The physiology of glucose homeostasis is controlled primarily by insulin release in response to elevated glucose levels (postprandial), although in birds, glucagon appears to serve as the primary regulator. Significant species variations in glucose levels have been noted. In general, levels are lowest in reptiles (60 to 100 mg/dL) and highest in birds (200 to 500 mg/dL), with mammals in between (100 to 200 mg/dL).

  Glucose that is not needed for energy is stored in the form of glycogen as a source of potential energy, readily available when needed. Most glycogen is stored in the liver and in muscle cells. When these and other body cells are saturated with glycogen, excess glucose is converted to fat and is stored as adipose tissue.

TYPICAL NORMAL RANGE

The typical normal range for this laboratory test varies greatly among species. The reader is referred to the following Elsevier publications for additional information:

Carpenter J: Exotic animal formulary, ed 4, St Louis, 2013, Saunders.

Mader D: Reptile medicine and surgery, ed 2, St Louis, 2006, Saunders.

CLINICAL APPLICATIONS

CAUSES OF ABNORMALLY HIGH LEVELS

- Hyperglycemia
  - Postprandial hyperglycemia
  - Diabetes mellitus
  - Increased glucocorticoid concentrations
    - Hyperadrenocorticism
    - Stress
    - Therapeutic corticosteroids
- Catecholamine release
  - Exertion
  - Pain
  - Excitement
  - Pheochromocytoma
- Increased growth hormone (growth hormone–producing tumor)
- Increased glucagon (glucagon-producing tumor)
- Increased progesterone production (diestrus in female)
- Pancreatitis
- Drugs (see later)
- Hyperthyroidism
- Moribund animals
- Birds
  - Hyperglycemia is generally defined by blood glucose concentrations exceeding 500 mg/dL.
  - Hyperglycemia most often results from catecholamine release from stress, glucocorticosteroid excess from administration of corticosteroids, and diabetes mellitus.
  - Exertion, excitement, and extreme temperatures stimulate the release of catecholamines, resulting in a mild to moderate increase in the blood glucose concentration. Stress hyperglycemia can occasionally produce a strong positive on urine glucose dipstick, similar to diabetes mellitus.
  - Excess glucocorticosteroids normally cause a mild to moderate increase in the blood glucose concentration (≤600 mg/dL) in birds.
  - Concentrations greater than 700 mg/dL are suggestive of diabetes mellitus in birds.
  - The pathophysiology of diabetes mellitus in birds is variable, however, and appears to be associated with excess glucagon in the presence of hyperglycemia. In psittacine birds, pancreatitis and pancreatic islet cell tumors are known causes. In some species (e.g., tucans [*Ramphastidae*]), diabetes occurs commonly and may be related to diets rich in fruits. Budgerigars and cockatiels are predisposed to diabetes associated with hepatic lipidosis. Birds suffering from diabetes mellitus demonstrate polyuria and urinary glucose concentrations exceeding 1 mg/dL.
  - Reproductively active cockatiel hens can present with "pseudodiabetes."

Plasma glucose levels are elevated but remain under 1000 mg/dL. The cause appears to be reduced pancreatic function from inflammation associated with yolk peritonitis.

- Reptiles
  - The normal blood glucose concentration of most reptiles ranges between 60 and 100 mg/dL, but this is subject to marked physiologic variation.
  - The most common cause of hyperglycemia is iatrogenic delivery of excessive glucose.
  - Although a persistent, marked hyperglycemia and glucosuria are suggestive of diabetes mellitus, the disorder is rarely observed in reptiles.
  - Hyperglycemia also occurs with glucocorticosteroid excess.
- Ferrets
  - Hyperglycemia most often is transient and due to postprandial increases.
  - Glucocorticoid excess (e.g., chronic stress, exogenous corticoids, hyperadrenocorticism) produces mild elevations in glucose concentration (150 to 200 mg/dL).
  - Stress-induced catecholamine release can result in higher elevations of glucose (200 to 300 mg/dL) and simulates diabetes mellitus.
  - Diabetes mellitus is relatively rare in ferrets and most often is iatrogenic and associated with surgical removal of pancreatic insulin-secreting neoplasms, or may be associated with use of drugs such as megestrol acetate. Glucose concentrations are greater than 400 mg/dL and frequently are greater than 1000 mg/dL.
- Rabbits
  - Hyperglycemia is a relatively common finding in rabbits and can be accompanied by glycosuria.
  - Stress-induced catecholamine release is believed to be the most common cause. Handling pet rabbits or warm temperatures result in increased blood glucose.
  - Glucocorticoid excess (e.g., stress induced, exogenous corticoids, hyperadrenocorticism) is also possible.
  - Hyperglycemia is associated with severe gastrointestinal distress ranging from acute obstruction to chronic stasis.
  - Diabetes mellitus is rarely a cause of hyperglycemia in rabbits and is rarely diagnosed in pet rabbits. Rare hereditary diabetes occurs in some populations. Herbivorous animals withstand the absence of insulin more readily than carnivorous ones. Management of hyperglycemia in herbivorous animals is done via diet modification.

NEXT DIAGNOSTIC STEPS TO CONSIDER IF LEVELS ARE HIGH

- Obtain a thorough evaluation of the patient, including dietary and supplementation history.
- Determine sex and reproductive status.
- Focus on laboratory evaluation of pancreatic function and glucose metabolism:
  - Blood glucose analysis
  - Urine glucose analysis
  - Oral vs. intravenous glucose tolerance test
  - Pancreatic enzyme serum levels
  - Serum insulin assay
  - Serum or plasma fructosamine concentration

CAUSES OF ABNORMALLY LOW LEVELS

- Hypoglycemia
  - Artifact/laboratory error
  - Decreased glucose absorption (starvation or malabsorption)
  - Increased insulin production (beta-cell tumors)
  - Therapeutic insulin overdose
  - Hypoadrenocorticism
  - Hypothyroidism
  - Growth hormone deficiency
  - Hepatic failure
  - Portosystemic shunt
  - Extreme exertion
  - Sepsis
  - Glycogen storage diseases
  - Neonatal hypoglycemia
  - Neoplasia (paraneoplastic insulin production from non–beta-cell tumors)
- Birds
  - Hypoglycemia is associated with starvation and malnutrition and, less likely, with sepsis and multiorgan failure.
  - In pet birds, starvation hypoglycemia can be observed in 1 to 3 days—earlier for birds with poor health or nutritional status. Carnivorous birds are able to maintain glucose homeostasis longer owing to larger glycogen stores and greater capacity for hepatic gluconeogenesis.
- Reptiles
  - Hypoglycemia most often results from starvation and malnutrition.
  - Severe hepatobiliary disease and septicemia are additional causes.
- Ferrets
  - Insulin-secreting pancreatic neoplasms (i.e., insulinomas) are common in ferrets.
  - Starvation/malnutrition and chronic hepatic disease are also causes of hypoglycemia.
  - Septicemia should also be considered.
- Rabbits
  - Hypoglycemia is more significant than hyperglycemia in rabbits and most often is associated with starvation and malnutrition.
  - Hepatic dysfunction and disturbances in digestion and absorption of carbohydrates are also observed.
  - Insulin-secreting pancreatic neoplasms or Addison's disease has not been reported in pet rabbits, although such conditions could potentially occur.

NEXT DIAGNOSTIC STEPS TO CONSIDER IF LEVELS ARE LOW

- Consider artifactual hypoglycemia (see later).
- Obtain a thorough physical examination for evidence of malnutrition or chronic disease.
- Obtain a thorough dietary and supplementation history.
- Assess for potential environmental stressors (noise/lighting, temperature, other pets).
- Determine sex and reproductive status.
- Laboratory evaluation of pancreatic function and glucose metabolism:
  - Blood and urine glucose analysis
  - Serum insulin and glucagon assays
  - Glucose tolerance testing
  - Pancreatic and liver enzyme analysis
- Laboratory assessment of nutritional status (electrolytes, albumin/protein, red blood cells [RBCs])
- Laboratory assessment of chronic disease (leukogram)

IMPORTANT INTERSPECIES DIFFERENCES

- Birds
  - The blood glucose concentration in normal birds ranges from 200 to 500 mg/dL. The plasma glucose concentration varies according to a circadian rhythm; however, this variation is clinically insignificant in healthy birds.
  - Unlike in mammals, glucagon is the primary regulator of blood glucose levels in birds. This is especially true for granivorous birds, which have an abundance of pancreatic alpha cells and normally lower insulin-to-glucagon ratios. Normal avian plasma glucagon concentrations are 1 to 4 ng/mL—10- to 50-fold greater than normal mammalian concentrations. Diabetes mellitus in pet birds most often is a result of excess glucagon rather than insufficient insulin action.
  - Short-term fasting in birds does not decrease glucose utilization per unit body weight as it does in fasted mammals owing to extensive hepatic glycogenolysis. Avian glucagon concentrations normally increase by 200% to 400% during a short-term fast. During fasting, the

greatest energy loss is associated with fat depletion and protein mobilization, thereby resulting in loss of body weight in birds, best observed as a reduction in the pectoral muscle mass. Glucose concentrations are more stable in fasting carnivorous birds owing to increased glycogen stores. Hypoglycemia can be observed in granivorous birds after several days of fasting.

- Reptiles
  - The normal blood glucose concentration of most reptiles ranges between 60 and 100 mg/dL; however, marked physiologic variation in levels is seen, as well as differences due to nutritional status, environmental conditions (temperature), and species.
  - Species differences can represent fundamental differences in physiology. For example, an increase in temperature produces hypoglycemia in turtles and hyperglycemia in alligators. In aquatic reptiles, hypoxia associated with diving produces a physiologic hyperglycemia because of anaerobic glycolysis.
  - Laboratory results and tolerance curves must be interpreted with regard to species, nutritional status, and environmental conditions.
  - Clinical signs associated with hypoglycemia in reptiles include tremors, loss of righting reflex, torpor, and dilated, nonresponsive pupils.
- Ferrets
  - The normal plasma glucose concentration of ferrets varies with the genetic type, with most between 90 and 150 mg/dL. Normal serum reference ranges for serum immunoreactive insulin and the insulin-to-glucose ratio have been reported as 4.6 to 43.3 IU/mL (S.I. units, 33 to 311 pmol/L) and 3.6 to 34.1 IUmg (S.I. units, 4.6 to 44.2 pmol/mmol), respectively.
  - Hypoglycemia is commonly the result of an insulin-producing pancreatic endocrine tumor. A 4- to 5-hour fasting plasma glucose level often is used to screen ferrets for insulinomas. Fasting plasma glucose concentrations less than 60 mg/dL are supportive of a presumptive diagnosis of insulinoma, whereas concentrations between 60 and 90 mg/dL are suggestive of an insulinoma, and those greater than 90 mg/dL are considered to be normal.
- Rabbits
  - The normal plasma glucose concentration of rabbits (75 to 100 mg/dL) is influenced by genetics, age, and diet.
  - Hyperglycemia most often is due to a significant stress response with catecholamine release. Diabetes is rare in rabbits and is almost never observed in pet rabbits. As a result, a diagnosis of diabetes mellitus cannot be made on a single blood sample and requires serial blood and urine sampling (time of day, phase of digestion, anesthesia, and influence of handling can all affect glucose levels). Mild glycosuria is common in rabbits and is not a significant finding.
  - As herbivores, rabbits graze for long periods of the day and are continually absorbing nutrients from the digestive tract. Volatile fatty acids produced through bacterial fermentation in the cecum serve as a continual energy source and allow maintenance of plasma glucose concentrations during short-term (<16 hours) fasting.
  - Mucoid enteropathy, a common digestive disorder in rabbits, is associated with hyperglycemia early owing to stress-induced glycogenolysis, followed by hypoglycemia late secondary to anorexia.
- Rodents
  - The plasma glucose concentration in rats and mice decreases with age, with an average decrease of 2 mg/dL per month in mice.
  - Many strains of mice as well as the Chinese hamster and the Wistar BB rat are used as animal models for diabetes mellitus; therefore, glucose tolerance tests have been developed for mice. Certain strains of rodents, such as ob/ob obese mice, the Zucker fatty rat (falfa), and the LA/N corpulent rat, are used as animal models for non–insulin-dependent diabetes mellitus.
  - In guinea pigs, insulin-dependent diabetes is believed to result from an infectious agent that causes fatty degeneration of the pancreas, affecting both exocrine and endocrine pancreatic functions. Affected guinea pigs have hyperglycemia, glucosuria, ketonuria, and beta-cell hypoplasia.
  - Immunoassays for determination of insulin and glucagon in rats can be calibrated to measure plasma levels in mice, but guinea pig insulin and glucagon are immunologically distinct and cannot be determined by using rat antibodies.
- Nonhuman primates
  - A fasting plasma glucose concentration greater than 115 mg/dL is suggestive of impaired glucose metabolism; concentrations greater than 140 mg/dL are suggestive of diabetes mellitus. The intravenous glucose tolerance test (IVGTT) is used more frequently than the oral glucose tolerance test, and it is indicated for use in primates that are mildly hyperglycemic. Prediabetic primates have prolonged hyperglycemia after administration of glucose.
  - Decreased insulin response and glucose intolerance can occur with hemorrhage, stress, pregnancy, and use of certain pharmacologic agents, such as atropine and barbiturates.
  - Hypoglycemia in nonhuman primates is indicated by serum glucose concentrations less than 50 mg/dL.

SPECIMEN AND PROCESSING CONSIDERATIONS

DRUG EFFECTS ON LEVELS

- Hypoglycemia may be caused by insulin, antihistamines, beta-blockers (e.g., propranolol), sulfonylureas (e.g., chlorpropamide), ethanol, salicylates, and anabolic steroids.
- Hyperglycemia can result from administration of glucocorticoids/corticosteroids, adrenocorticotropic hormone, ketamine, morphine, L-asparaginase, beta-adrenergic drugs, diazoxide, furosemide, acetazolamide, thiazides, salicylates, phenothiazines, nitrofurantoin, heparin, glucagon, thyroxine, progestins, medroxyprogesterone (Depo-Provera), and estrogens. Fluids that contain high glucose concentrations can also produce hyperglycemia.

LAB ARTIFACTS THAT MAY INTERFERE WITH READINGS OF LEVELS OF THIS SUBSTANCE

- Collection
  - Serum or plasma should be separated from whole blood within 30 minutes of collection to minimize consumption of glucose by cellular components. Glucose shows a decrease of approximately 10% every 30 to 60 minutes in whole blood in a room temperature specimen with normal cell counts. Loss is accelerated by increased temperatures and excessive cellularity (leukemia, bacteremia).
- Reagent strip methods
  - With reagent strips, extremely increased or decreased packed cell volumes (PCVs) may alter the measured value. The reagent pad must be fully covered with blood to avoid false low values. Reagent strips are less accurate at high glucose concentrations (i.e., >300 mg/dL). Proper calibration of handheld instruments is essential, especially for low and high values.

SAMPLE FOR COLLECTION AND ANY SPECIAL SPECIMEN HANDLING NOTES

- Glucose is measured in whole blood, serum, or plasma.

- Portable glucose monitors use small amounts (3 to 5 microliters) of whole blood.
- Chemistry analyzers require separation of whole blood to remove cellular components. Separation must be performed as soon as possible while excessive temperatures are avoided to prevent consumption of glucose by red and white blood cells and bacteria.

PEARLS

- Birds
  - Stress hyperglycemia is common; although glucose levels tend to be lower than those in patients with diabetes, stress hyperglycemia is often associated with a positive urine dipstick, indistinguishable from diabetes mellitus.
  - Starvation/malnutrition is a common cause of hypoglycemia in pet birds. Hypoglycemia can be seen in 1 to 3 days in granivorous birds versus much longer in carnivorous birds owing to lower glycogen stores.
- Reptiles
  - Most alterations in glucose concentrations are iatrogenic. Reptile glucose concentrations exhibit wide physiologic variation. Diabetes mellitus is rare in reptiles.
- Ferrets
  - Diabetes mellitus is rarely seen. Prolonged hypoglycemia should prompt investigation for a possible insulin-producing pancreatic endocrine tumor.
- Rabbits
  - Hyperglycemia with glucosuria is common in rabbits, most often caused by stress-induced catecholamine release. Diabetes mellitus is not commonly seen in pet rabbits. Hypoglycemia is more serious and frequently is due to malnutrition or starvation.

REFERENCES

Blood DC, et al: Saunders comprehensive veterinary dictionary, ed 2, New York, 1999, WB Saunders.

Campbell TW: Clinical pathology. In Mader DR, editor: Reptile medicine and surgery, ed 2, Philadelphia, 1996, WB Saunders.

Carpenter JW: Exotic animal formulary, ed 3, Philadelphia, 2004, WB Saunders.

Fudge AM: Laboratory medicine: avian and exotic pets, Philadelphia, 2000, WB Saunders.

Harcourt-Brown F: Textbook of rabbit medicine, Boston, 2002, Butterworth-Heinemann.

Harrison GJ, et al: Clinical avian medicine, South Palm Beach, FL, 2006, Spix Publishing.

Quesenberry KE, et al: Ferrets, rabbits, and rodents: clinical medicine and surgery, ed 2, St Louis, 2004, Elsevier.

Thrall MA, et al: Veterinary hematology and clinical chemistry, Philadelphia, 2004, Lippincott Williams & Wilkins.

Willard MD, et al: Small animal clinical diagnosis by laboratory methods, St Louis, 2004, WB Saunders.

AUTHOR: **JULIE DECUBELLIS**

EDITOR: **JÖRG MAYER**

Hematocrit

DEFINITION

- The fraction of whole blood that is composed of red blood cells (RBCs). Hematocrit (HCT) does NOT include white blood cells (WBCs) or platelets. Electronic analyzers use the following formula to calculate HCT: HCT = (Mean corpuscular volume [MCV] × RBC)/10.
- Automated analyzers cannot be used for species with nucleated red blood cells.

SYNONYMS

Packed red cells, packed cell volume (PCV), HCT

PHYSIOLOGY

- HCT values are slightly less than PCV because there is no trapped plasma in an automated hematocrit calculation, as can occur with spun, packed cell values.
- Sources of variation
  - Owing to variable MCV in different species, values for HCT may be erroneous if the instrument is not calibrated for specific species. A manual determination (centrifugation) is suggested in most cases.
  - Abnormal plasma osmolality and electrolyte balance may result in a difference between HCT and PCV.
- Although PCV measures change in red cell volume as they occur in vivo, dilution of red cells with normal saline and standing in hematology instruments may cause red cells to return to their normal volume.

TYPICAL NORMAL RANGE

The typical normal range for this laboratory test varies greatly among species. The reader is referred to the following Elsevier publications for additional information:

Carpenter J: Exotic animal formulary, ed 4, St Louis, 2013, Saunders.

Mader D: Reptile medicine and surgery, ed 2, St Louis, 2006, Saunders.

CLINICAL APPLICATIONS

CAUSES OF ABNORMALLY HIGH LEVELS

- Polycythemia (an increase in PCV) can be relative or absolute and can be caused by a variety of processes.
- Relative polycythemia is the result of a change in the proportion of circulating RBCs to blood plasma without any change in the size of the red cell itself.
- Splenic contraction
- Dehydration
- High PCV is usually relative and is often the result of dehydration. This represents an increased proportion of RBCs caused by decreased fluid volume in the vascular space. With dehydration, you will often see an associated increase in total protein levels as well.
- Absolute polycythemia is an actual increase in the size of the red cell; it can be primary (polycythemia vera or erythropoietin-producing tumors) or secondary (resulting from disease in another organ system). Absolute polycythemia generally is associated with a very high PCV.
- Increased oxygen demand
- Chronic obstructive pulmonary disease
- Obstructive airway disease
- Chronic respiratory disease

NEXT DIAGNOSTIC STEPS TO CONSIDER IF LEVELS ARE HIGH

- Old samples can cause RBCs to swell, leading to a false increase in PCV.

- A total protein level from a chemistry panel or a total protein obtained from a serum sample using a refractometer is useful in evaluating hydration status.
- A pulse oximeter can be used to evaluate blood oxygen saturation.

CAUSES OF ABNORMALLY LOW LEVELS

- Abnormally low PCV in the absence of lab error indicates anemia and can be the result of a variety of events:
    - Hemorrhage
    - Hemolysis
    - Lack of production
    - Parasitism
    - Coagulopathies
    - Gastrointestinal bleeding
    - Destruction of red blood cells
    - Bacterial septicemia
    - Aflatoxicosis
    - Chronic inflammatory disease
    - Mycobacteriosis, chlamydiosis, aspergillosis, chronic hepatitis
    - Neoplasia
    - Lymphoid leukemia
    - Overhydration

NEXT DIAGNOSTIC STEPS TO CONSIDER IF LEVELS ARE LOW If sample error is ruled out, a blood smear can be prepared and scanned for evidence of polychromasia or reticulocyte count; it can be prepared for bone marrow biopsy (regenerative/nonregenerative), fecal examination (direct/float), endoscopy or fecal occult blood testing to rule out gastrointestinal bleeding, and ultrasound examination for neoplasia, radiographs, blood chemistry panel, and complete blood count to rule out other causes of anemia.

IMPORTANT INTERSPECIES DIFFERENCES

- Ferrets can have a higher HCT than most other mammals (sometimes up to 60% is normal).
- It has been suggested that HCT is one of the best diagnostic parameters in avian and rabbit medicine.
- RBCs are nucleated in birds and reptiles.
- PCV in reptiles is often lower than in mammals (≈20% to 30%).

SPECIMEN AND PROCESSING CONSIDERATIONS

DRUG EFFECTS ON LEVELS

- Long-term use of metronidazole in reptiles (>6 doses) has been shown to lower PCV.
- Use of inhalation anesthesia (isoflurane) in ferrets has been shown to decrease HCT significantly but temporarily owing to splenic pooling.

LAB ARTIFACTS THAT MAY INTERFERE WITH READINGS OF LEVELS OF THIS SUBSTANCE

- Nucleated RBCs as found in birds and reptiles may not be counted accurately by automated cell counters. This may lead to a falsely decreased automated RBC count.
- Hemolysis from traumatic venipuncture can lead to a falsely decreased PCV, especially when small needles are used (smaller than 25 gauge).
- Underfilling of blood tubes can cause RBCs to shrink and can lead to a falsely decreased PCV.
- Autoagglutination causes a falsely low PCV.
- Lymphatic contamination, especially in reptiles, can artificially lower PCV.
- Old samples can cause RBCs to swell, leading to a false increase in PCV.

SAMPLE FOR COLLECTION AND ANY SPECIAL SPECIMEN HANDLING NOTES

- In some avian and reptile species, RBCs lyse in EDTA. When in doubt, collect the sample in heparin, or submit samples in both anticoagulants.
- A PCV percentage can be obtained by spinning down a sample of whole blood in a microcapillary tube. The cell column can then be measured and PCV evaluated. PCV can also be obtained on automated machines, often with heparinized blood, although these counts may sometimes be inaccurate.
- Follow directions with respect to the amount needed when filling the vacutainer to avoid artificial dilution with liquid anticoagulant followed by lowering of HCT.

PEARLS

If the animal has received oxyglobin, determination of HCT can be difficult owing to coloration of the serum.

REFERENCES

Bush BM: Interpretation of laboratory results for small animal clinicians, Ames, IA, 1991, Blackwell.

Carpenter JW: Exotic animal formulary, ed 3, St Louis, 2004, Elsevier.

Harrison GJ, et al: Clinical avian medicine, vol 2, South Palm Beach, FL, 2006, Spix Publishing, p 606.

AUTHOR: **CARRIE A. PHELPS**

EDITOR: **JÖRG MAYER**

Lead

DEFINITION

Lead is a nonessential element that is absorbed from the environment, usually by ingestion, into the blood system, affecting a variety of body systems. The lead test measures amounts of the heavy metal lead in peripheral blood (Pb).

SYNONYMS

Pb, plumbism (lead toxicity)

PHYSIOLOGY

- Lead can be found in numerous sources in the environment as metallic salts or organoleads. Sources of lead include paints, metallic objects (e.g., wires, sinkers, weights, gun pellets), toys, contaminated pastures, and urban gas emissions.
- Lead toxicokinetics depends on the lead compound and the exposure route. Lead absorption usually requires ionization; for this reason, gun pellets, embedded deep in muscle tissue, are poorly absorbed. About 90% of the lead absorbed will be bound to red blood cells, which use it as a vehicle for multiorgan distribution, with the bone as a major reservoir. Blood levels may be elevated for 1 to 2 months after a single exposure.
- Lead affects the normal body chemistry by competing with some enzymatic groups (mainly sulfhydryl) and cations, inhibiting membranous enzymes and disrupting vitamin D metabolism.
- Lead interferes with hemoglobin synthesis and suppresses bone marrow and red blood cell formation in all species. In mammals, it commonly causes basophilic stippling and ballooning of erythrocytes, which can

result in intravascular hemolysis and macrocytic hypochromic anemia.
- Lead toxicity is commonly associated with the central nervous system (CNS) and causes brain edema and demyelination of nerves, encephalopathy, and peripheral neuropathy with clinical presentation of excitation and intermittent depression. Lead toxicity can also cause hepatocellular necrosis, myocardial degeneration, arterioles, fibrinoid necrosis, gizzard myonecrosis, renal tubular cell necrosis, and gastrointestinal (GI) stasis.
- Subclinical and chronic levels can be detected, but clinical signs are usually present when measured levels are above threshold values. Intoxications are relatively common in birds and can also be observed in mammals and reptiles.

TYPICAL NORMAL RANGE

- Most species
  - Blood levels >0.3 to 0.35 ppm (30 to 35 µg/dL) highly suggestive
  - Blood levels >0.6 ppm (60 µg/dL) definitive
- Avian
  - Blood levels >0.2 ppm (20 µg/dL) suggestive
  - Blood levels >0.5 ppm (50 µg/dL) definitive
- Rabbits
  - Blood levels >0.1 ppm (10 µg/dL) with clinical signs
- Chinchilla
  - Blood level >0.25 ppm (25 µg/dL) definitive, levels >0.15 ppm (15 µg/dL) are suspicious

CLINICAL APPLICATIONS

CAUSES OF ABNORMALLY HIGH LEVELS Absorption (usually ingestion) of a lead-containing foreign body or chronic accumulation from water/food sources

NEXT DIAGNOSTIC STEPS TO CONSIDER IF LEVELS ARE HIGH
- Whole-body radiographs to rule out foreign body ingestion/chronic toxicity or, in very rare cases, lead outside the GI tract
- Blood lead test

CAUSES OF ABNORMALLY LOW LEVELS Lead is a nonessential element; low levels should be a normal finding.

NEXT DIAGNOSTIC STEPS TO CONSIDER IF LEVELS ARE LOW
- Check for other heavy metals such as zinc.
- Ca-EDTA urinary postchelation test

IMPORTANT INTERSPECIES DIFFERENCES
- Birds are highly sensitive to lead toxicity; lead toxicity should be considered with every bird showing CNS signs.
- Rabbits presented for GI stasis and depression that are allowed to free-roam the house should be lead-tested if supportive treatment does not show an expected result.

SPECIMEN AND PROCESSING CONSIDERATIONS

LAB ARTIFACTS THAT MAY INTERFERE WITH READINGS OF LEVELS OF THIS SUBSTANCE Do not use tubes containing interfering substances that are often present in some glass tubes (such as the SST tube with silica clot activator, polymer gel, and silicone-coated interior).

SAMPLE FOR COLLECTION AND ANY SPECIAL SPECIMEN HANDLING NOTES
- Heparinized whole blood is preferred; testing can be done on EDTA in whole blood. A minimum of 250 µL is required. Do not spin this blood. For birds, it is possible to use 100 µL; do not send in capillary tubes; do use heparin tubes (green top).
- Lead levels can be determined from tissue samples (kidney, liver, bone, hair, etc.).

PEARLS

- A quick in-house blood lead test is available on the market; it requires only 50 µL of whole blood and delivers results in 3 minutes (see http://www.esainc.com).
- Quick lead-check strips to check material for lead content are available in most hardware stores.

REFERENCES

Plumlee KH: Clinical veterinary toxicology, St Louis, 2004, Mosby, p 208.

Quesenberry KE, et al: Ferrets, rabbits and rodents: clinical medicine and surgery, ed 2, St Louis, 2004, WB Saunders.

AUTHOR: **DAVID ESHAR**

EDITOR: **JÖRG MAYER**

Lipase

DEFINITION

Enzyme that breaks down triglycerides into monoglycerides and free fatty acids by hydrolyzing them

PHYSIOLOGY

Lipase is produced primarily in the pancreas, with a small amount produced by the gastric mucosa. It is a cytosolic enzyme that breaks down triglycerides into monoglycerides and free fatty acids. It is inactivated and excreted by the kidney. Lipase is considered a more sensitive indicator of pancreatic necrosis than amylase (fewer false negatives) but can be normal with pancreatitis.

TYPICAL NORMAL RANGE

- To convert U/dL to IU/L, multiply by 280.
- Ferret
  - 0 to 200 U/L
- Bird
  - For reference values of selected species, see chart below.
- Reptile
  - *Testudo hermanni*, 15 to 99 IU/L

SPECIES	VALUE, U/L
African grey	35-350
Amazon	35-225
Budgerigar	30-300
Canary	29-255
Cockatiel	30-280
Cockatoo	25-275
Conure	30-290
Eclectus	35-275
Lovebird	30-320
Macaw	30-250
Parakeet	30-220
Pionus	30-250
Quaker	25-225
Senegal	35-250

CLINICAL APPLICATIONS

CAUSES OF ABNORMALLY HIGH LEVELS
- Acute pancreatitis, pancreatic neoplasia, pancreatic abscesses, and pancreatic duct obstruction can result in high levels of lipase and usually are 2 to 3 times the upper limit of normal.
- Rarely, renal insufficiency can cause a mild increase in lipase associated with decreased renal clearance. Mild

increases have also been reported with liver disease.
- Lipase can be elevated by peritonitis, gastritis, and intestinal manipulation: ferrets with inflammatory bowel disease (IBD) or enteric glia cells (EGC) and other generalized gastrointestinal (GI) pathologies
- Diets rich in fats can increase lipase.

NEXT DIAGNOSTIC STEPS TO CONSIDER IF LEVELS ARE HIGH
- Rule out pancreatitis and renal disease (decreased elimination).
- Perform an abdominal ultrasound and scan for other signs of GI problems (e.g., large mesenteric lymph nodes).
- Consider biopsy of the pancreas for histopathologic assessment.
- In ferrets, consider biopsy of the GI tract at multiple locations (stomach and small intestines).
- Run zinc levels in birds.

CAUSES OF ABNORMALLY LOW LEVELS Exocrine pancreatic insufficiency

NEXT DIAGNOSTIC STEPS TO CONSIDER IF LEVELS ARE LOW Rule out pancreatic insufficiency.

IMPORTANT INTERSPECIES DIFFERENCES
- Very little information is available on avian species and correlation with pancreatic disease.
- It appears that the ferret produces more lipase in the stomach than is produced by other species. Therefore, elevated lipase levels might be more diagnostic for pathologies of the GI tract than for those of the pancreas.

SPECIMEN AND PROCESSING CONSIDERATIONS

DRUG EFFECTS ON LEVELS Glucocorticoid administration can elevate levels due to lipemia.

LAB ARTIFACTS THAT MAY INTERFERE WITH READINGS OF LEVELS OF THIS SUBSTANCE Lipemia, hemolysis, and icterus can artificially decrease lipase levels.

SAMPLE FOR COLLECTION AND ANY SPECIAL SPECIMEN HANDLING NOTES
- Reptiles: plasma is preferred over serum for chemistries because clot formation may be prolonged in reptiles and may change serum electrolyte and glucose values. Also, a greater volume per unit blood can be obtained.
- Birds: lithium heparin is the anticoagulant of choice for most avian blood samples; evaluation of biochemistries is most commonly performed on plasma.
- Small mammals: small blood samples (<2 mL) should be placed in microtainers. Heparin microtainers are preferred because more plasma can be obtained from small samples.
- All samples should be centrifuged and plasma/serum separated from cells as soon as possible; tests should be run immediately or the specimen transported frozen.

PEARLS

- Increased lipase and globulin levels in ferrets might be suggestive of a chronic GI problem such as IBD or EGC. Offer GI biopsies to diagnose these often subclinical problems. Consider harvesting GI biopsies every time you perform abdominal surgery in a ferret.
- Azathioprine has been used for medical management in confirmed or suspected cases.

REFERENCES

Campbell TW: Clinical pathology. In Mader DR, editor: Reptile medicine and surgery, Philadelphia, 1996, WB Saunders.

Carpenter JW: Exotic animal formulary, ed 3, Philadelphia, 2004, WB Saunders.

Fudge AM, editor: Laboratory medicine: avian and exotic pets, Philadelphia, 2000, WB Saunders.

Jones MP: Avian clinical pathology, Vet Clin North Am Exot Anim Pract 2:663–687, 1999.

AUTHOR: **CARALEE MANLEY**

EDITOR: **JÖRG MAYER**

Lymphocyte Count

DEFINITION

A mononuclear, nongranular leukocyte having a deeply staining nucleus with dense chromatin and sparse, pale-staining cytoplasm

SYNONYMS

Lymphs, B cells, T cells

PHYSIOLOGY

- Lymphocytes are mononuclear cells that may develop in peripheral lymph tissue, such as lymph nodes (mammals), thymus (mammals, birds, reptiles, amphibians), spleen (mammals, birds, reptiles, amphibians), gut-associated lymph tissues (mammals, birds, reptiles, amphibians) and bursa of Fabricius (birds), or in bone marrow (mammals, birds, reptiles, amphibians). Two major types of lymphocytes have been identified: B cells, which provide the humoral immune response, and T cells, which provide the cell-based immune response. T and B cells develop from a common stem cell, which is distinct from cell lines that produce granulocytes. Differentiation into B or T cells is influenced by various cell mediators.
- After development in bone marrow or lymph tissue, lymphocytes can enter the peripheral circulation. Similar to neutrophils, they are divided into circulating and marginated pools. The presence of these two pools serves as the basis for a phenomenon known as a "physiologic shift"—lymphocytosis due to a shift of lymphocytes from the marginated pool into the circulating pool in response to endogenous release of epinephrine caused by extreme excitement. This increases the lymphocyte count because only cells in the circulating pool are collected for a differential count. Unlike neutrophils, they can travel freely—not just between peripheral pools but also between blood and tissues. Migration into tissues occurs in response to various chemotactic agents. Lymphocytes have a lifespan that ranges from hours to years.
- The development of lymphocytes in fish has not been completely worked out. They may originate in the thymus and finish their development in the kidneys and the spleen.
- Two important morphologic variations in lymphocytes are of clinical relevance: reactive lymphocytes and lymphoblasts. Reactive lymphocytes have a dark blue–staining cytoplasm, often with small, clear perinuclear areas known as *Golgi zones.* They occur as a result of antigenic stimulation. Lymphoblasts usually are larger than normal lymphocytes, and their nuclei have nucleoli and pale-staining

chromatin. The finding of lymphoblasts in the peripheral circulation is often a sign of lymphoid neoplasia.

TYPICAL NORMAL RANGE

The typical normal range for this laboratory test varies greatly among species. The reader is referred to the following Elsevier publications for additional information:

Carpenter J: Exotic animal formulary, ed 4, St Louis, 2013, Saunders.

Mader D: Reptile medicine and surgery, ed 2, St Louis, 2006, Saunders.

CLINICAL APPLICATIONS

CAUSES OF ABNORMALLY HIGH LEVELS

- Lymphocytosis is most commonly caused by chronic antigenic stimulation. This can occur as the result of bacterial, viral, fungal (usually systemic), or protozoal infection. Neoplasia, especially lymphocytic leukemia or lymphoma, can also lead to lymphocytosis. In this condition, it is often possible to find lymphoblasts in circulation or soft tissue masses.
- Mammals
  - Epinephrine, whether endogenous as part of the fight-or-flight reaction, or exogenous, will cause a physiologic shift of lymphocytes from the marginated pool into the circulating pool, resulting in lymphocytosis.
  - Hypoadrenocorticism can lead to lymphocytosis, possibly caused by a decrease in glucocorticoid hormones. Glucocorticoids normally suppress lymphocyte production or lead to lymphocyte redistribution, as in the lymphopenia found with a stress leukogram.
  - Lymphoma or lymphocytic leukemia should be considered with persistently high counts or extremely high values.
  - Lymphocyte numbers can vary in certain species based on the season.
- Birds
  - Lymphocytosis is not commonly found in birds. It does occur in response to chronic antigenic stimulation but most often is due to viral causes. Other causes include lymphocytic leukemia and blood parasites.
- Reptiles
  - In reptiles, lymphocytosis is most commonly caused by chronic antigenic stimulation or inflammation. This can be due to bacterial, viral, fungal (usually systemic), parasitic, or protozoal infection. Wound healing can also cause a lymphocytosis.
  - Some seasonal variation in the lymphocyte population has been noted, including an increase in the summer months.
- Fish
  - In fish, increased temperature to a maximum of 25°C (77°F) can lead to lymphocytosis.

NEXT DIAGNOSTIC STEPS TO CONSIDER IF LEVELS ARE HIGH

- Mammals
  - After the presence of lymphocytosis is detected, a thorough search for the source of antigenic stimulation should be conducted. This should include appropriate bacterial and fungal cultures based on clinical findings. Serum antibody titers or PCR tests can be done if clinical signs warrant.
  - If any masses or enlarged lymph nodes are present concurrently with a lymphocytosis, they should be aspirated and submitted for cytologic examination. With lymph nodes, this is important, to distinguish between antigenic stimulation and neoplasia. If no obvious infections or palpable masses are identified, an ultrasound of the abdomen or abdominal radiographs should be performed to look for enlarged abdominal lymph nodes, abdominal masses, or changes to the gastrointestinal (GI) tract. Any masses, enlarged lymph nodes, or abnormal GI tissue found should be aspirated if possible. If not, surgical exploration with mass removal or biopsy should be considered.
  - The bone marrow should also be biopsied, especially if neoplasia is suspected.
- Birds and reptiles
  - After the presence of lymphocytosis is detected, a thorough search for the source of antigenic stimulation should be conducted, especially with the presence of reactive lymphocytes. This should include appropriate bacterial and fungal cultures based on clinical findings. Serum antibody titers or PCR tests can also be done if clinical signs warrant. Survey coelomic radiographs should be performed to look for masses. Laparoscopic examination of the coelomic cavity to look for fungal infiltrates or other masses should also be considered. Any masses found should be biopsied.
  - The bone marrow should also be biopsied, especially if neoplasia is suspected.
- Fish
  - Lymphocytosis in fish, as with many other hematologic abnormalities, should be followed by a comprehensive analysis of their environment, especially water temperature. It may also by helpful to aspirate the spleen or the kidneys.

CAUSES OF ABNORMALLY LOW LEVELS

- Lymphopenia can be caused by excessive production of corticosteroids. Corticosteroids cause lymphopenia via two mechanisms: in the short term, they shift lymphocytes out of the circulating pool; over the long term, they decrease lymphopoiesis. The source of the excess could be physiologic such as secondary to stress, or it may be due to hyperadrenocorticism. Exogenous corticosteroids can cause lymphopenia through a similar mechanism as endogenous corticosteroids.
- Severe infection (bacterial or viral) can cause lymphopenia because lymphocytes move from the circulating pool into the tissues. Endotoxemia and septicemia can lead to lymphopenia, mostly as a result of the increase in corticosteroids that occurs in response to inflammation.
- Decreased production of lymphocytes can also lead to lymphopenia. This can occur secondarily to immune suppressive drug administration or to neoplasia affecting lymphopoietic tissue, including the bone marrow or the bursa of Fabricius in birds. If the animal is young, congenital hypoplasia of lymphatic tissue should also be considered.
- Mammals
  - Loss of lymphatic fluid can lead to a lymphopenia. This can be seen with chylothorax that is idiopathic or secondary to trauma. It is also noted with lymphatic loss into the GI tract, or as the result of GI lymphoma, other GI neoplasia, enteritis (granulomatous or ulcerative), paratuberculosis, protein-losing enteropathy, or lymphangiectasia.
- Birds
  - Lymphopenia in birds may be secondary to infection but is usually of viral origin.
- Reptiles
  - Severe acute viral infection can cause lymphopenia in reptiles because lymphocytes move from the circulating pool into the tissues.
  - Several noninfectious causes of lymphopenia in reptiles are known. During winter hibernation, reptiles often experience a decrease in circulating lymphocytes. Even reptiles that do not hibernate show a decrease in lymphocytes in the winter. Malnutrition can also lead to a lymphopenia.
- Fish
  - Lymphopenia in fish can be caused by increased water temperatures (>25°C [>77°F]). Stress can also cause lymphopenia in fish, probably

through a mechanism similar to that seen in other animals.
  - Certain infectious diseases have been shown to cause lymphopenia in some species of fish. They include *Ichthyophthirius multifiliis* (mirror carp), *Aeromonas hydrophila* (common carp, goldfish), and *Pseudomonas fluorescens* (common carp goldfish).

NEXT DIAGNOSTIC STEPS TO CONSIDER IF LEVELS ARE LOW

- The first step when detecting lymphopenia is to rule out a physiologic stress response. If the collection was very stressful and only a mild lymphopenia was noted, a stress response should be considered and the sample redrawn after the animal calms down. The presence of exogenous drugs that may be causing the lymphopenia should be ruled out.
- Once artifact is eliminated as a cause of lymphopenia, infection should be considered, and appropriate cultures, including blood cultures, should be done based on other clinical findings. Serum antibody titers or PCR tests can also be done if clinical signs warrant.
- Mammals
  - If no obvious infections are noted, an abdominal ultrasound should be performed to examine the adrenal glands. It may be helpful to perform lymph node or bone marrow biopsies to look for lymphopoietic hypoplasia or evidence of neoplasia.
- Birds
  - It may also be helpful to perform a biopsy of the bursa of Fabricius to look for lymphopoietic hypoplasia or other evidence of tissue damage.
- Reptiles
  - Lymphopenia in reptiles should prompt a comprehensive examination of signs of viral infection. A bone marrow biopsy may also be warranted if no obvious signs of infection are noted. Serum antibody titers or PCR tests can be done if clinical signs warrant.
- Fish
  - Lymphopenia in fish, as with many other hematologic abnormalities, should be followed by a comprehensive analysis of their environment, especially water temperature. Culture for *Ichthyophthirius multifiliis, Aeromonas hydrophila*, or *Pseudomonas fluorescens* should be performed.

SPECIMEN AND PROCESSING CONSIDERATIONS

DRUG EFFECTS ON LEVELS

- Epinephrine or norepinephrine can cause lymphocytosis.
- Immune suppressive drugs may cause lymphopenia.
- Glucocorticoids also may cause lymphopenia.

LAB ARTIFACTS THAT MAY INTERFERE WITH READINGS OF LEVELS OF THIS SUBSTANCE *Avian:* Variability in size and staining characteristics of avian lymphocytes can make them difficult to distinguish from monocytes, so inexperienced laboratories can falsely report populations of either cell line. Because monocytes generally are much rarer than lymphocytes, a false monocytosis may be reported.

SAMPLE FOR COLLECTION AND ANY SPECIAL SPECIMEN HANDLING NOTES

- Mammals
  - Use EDTA (purple top) tubes to collect for complete blood count (CBC).
- Birds
  - For differential counts, it is best if slides can be made from fresh whole blood. Use EDTA (purple top) tubes to collect for CBC in most species. ETDA may cause red blood cell (RBC) hemolysis, especially in Brush turkeys, Corvidae, Crowned cranes, Currasows, and Hornbills.
- Reptiles
  - ETDA may cause RBC hemolysis in some species. Use heparinized (green top) tubes when collecting CBC samples. If plenty of blood is available, submit a paired sample (one EDTA and one heparin) and let the clinical pathologist decide which sample is appropriate.
- Amphibians
  - Use heparinized (green top) tubes when collecting CBC samples. Because of the small volumes often collected, use a heparinized syringe to collect the sample, and make slides immediately after collection whenever possible.
- Fish
  - Samples for differential cell counts should be prepared immediately after collection. It is important to rapidly dry the slides because slow drying may alter the morphology. Diff-Quik stain can be used, but it is not optimal for differential counts. If it is necessary to collect samples in tubes, use heparinized tubes. ETDA causes hemolysis in fish anesthetized with tricaine.

PEARLS

- Mammals
  - The Kurloff cell is a unique cell found only in guinea pigs that resembles a lymphocyte, except that it contains round or oval inclusions. Little is currently known about the origin or function of this cell. Some researchers believe that it may be a type of T lymphocyte that possibly originates from the thymus or the spleen.
  - Kurloff cells are found in low numbers in young male guinea pigs. They can be found in greater numbers in females. They seem to respond to estrogen stimulation; thus the number of cells varies with the estrous cycle. Their highest concentration occurs during pregnancy. This led some researchers to hypothesize that they play a role in the physiologic barrier between mother and fetus.
  - Chinchillas show a decrease in lymphocytes in the summer months and an increase in lymphocytes in the fall and spring.
  - Lead toxicity can cause a lymphocytosis in rabbits.
- Birds
  - Reactive lymphocytes most often are associated with severe viral infection, chlamydial infection, *Aspergillus* infection, *Salmonella* infection, or tuberculosis infection.
- Reptiles
  - Female reptiles of some species have greater circulating lymphocyte counts than males.

REFERENCES

Carpenter JW, et al: Exotic animal formulary, ed 2, Philadelphia, 2001, WB Saunders, pp 36, 80–86, 195–208, 213, 256, 268, 292, 320, 344, 363, 386–387.

Fudge AM: Laboratory medicine: avian and exotic pets, ed 1, Philadelphia, 2000, WB Saunders, pp 9–27, 193–204, 269–274.

Groff JM, et al: Hematology and clinical chemistry of cyprinid fish, Vet Clin North Am 2:741–776, 1999.

Hoegeman S: Diagnostic sampling of amphibians, Vet Clin North Am 2:731–740, 1999.

Jones MP: Avian clinical pathology, Vet Clin North Am 2:663–688, 1999.

Redrobe S, MacDonald J: Sample collection and clinical pathology of reptiles, Vet Clin North Am 2:709–730, 1999.

Stockham SL, et al: Fundamentals of veterinary clinical pathology, ed 1, Ames, IA, 2002, Iowa State Press, pp 50–83.

AUTHOR: **JONATHAN W. BALL**

EDITOR: **JÖRG MAYER**

Monocyte Count

DEFINITION

A mononuclear, phagocytic leukocyte, with an oval or kidney-shaped nucleus and blue cytoplasmic granules

PHYSIOLOGY

- Monocytes develop from common precursor cells with neutrophils (colony-forming unit granulocyte-monophage [CFU-GM]). Cytokines act on these precursor cells to shunt develop down the neutrophil or monocyte pathway. Monocytes pass through several developmental stages in the bone marrow, and once mature, they enter the bloodstream. Unlike in neutrophils, there is no bone marrow storage pool for monocytes. In the bloodstream, they enter the circulating or the marginated pool. After approximately 1 day in circulation, monocytes leave the bloodstream and enter the tissues. In the tissues, monocytes become macrophages.
- In the tissues, the main role of monocytes, or macrophages, is the phagocytosis of bacteria, debris, degenerate cells, infected cells, and neoplastic cells. They also process antigens and present them to T lymphocytes, thus stimulating cellular immunity. Macrophages promote immune function through release of a variety of chemotactic agents. Macrophages are not as good at destroying ingested bacteria; thus some organisms, most notably *Mycobacterium* spp., can replicate inside the cell.
- A subtype of macrophage is the multinucleated giant cell. This cell is of diagnostic significance because it forms in response to an antigen that is too large for phagocytosis by a single cell. Most often, it is a foreign body, a large parasite, or a fungus.

TYPICAL NORMAL RANGE

The typical normal range for this laboratory test varies greatly among species. The reader is referred to the following Elsevier publications for additional information:

Carpenter J: Exotic animal formulary, ed 4, St Louis, 2013, Saunders.

Mader D: Reptile medicine and surgery, ed 2, St Louis, 2006, Saunders.

CLINICAL APPLICATIONS

CAUSES OF ABNORMALLY HIGH LEVELS

- Mammals
  - In mammals, one of the most common causes of monocytosis is inflammation, which can be due to infection (bacterial, fungal, protozoal), neoplasia, or tissue damage (necrosis, hemorrhage, hemolysis, infarction, trauma).
  - Excessive corticosteroids, whether from endogenous or exogenous sources, can also cause a monocytosis. This is likely similar to the neutrophil stress response, in which cells shift from the marginated pool into the circulating pool. Stress can cause a monocytosis via an increase in corticosteroids. Hyperadrenocorticism should be considered as a cause of monocytosis, especially with a concurrent neutrophilia.
  - Monocytic leukemia can directly cause a monocytosis. In this condition, the number of morphologically abnormal monocytes should be increased.
  - Monocytosis can develop secondary to immune neutropenia. Because monocytes and neutrophils share a common stem cell, ineffective neutrophil production may lead to an increase in monocyte production.
- Birds
  - In birds, chronic infection is the most common cause of monocytosis. Bacterial infections, including *Mycobacterium*, *Chlamydia* (active or chronic), and *Salmonella*, are common causes of monocytosis. Fungal infection, especially aspergillosis and parasitism, is also associated with monocytosis. Chronic bacterial dermatitis can also cause monocytosis.
  - Monocytosis is associated with the formation of individual granulomas or granulomatosis. This can result from bacterial or fungal causes.
  - As in mammals, tissue damage, especially necrosis, can lead to an increase in monocytes.
- Reptiles
  - In reptiles, chronic infection of bacterial, fungal or viral origin is the most common cause of monocytosis. Granuloma formation secondary to a bacterial (especially mycobacterial) or parasitic infection also results in a monocytosis.
- Fish
  - In cyprinid fish, the most common cause of monocytosis is stress or infectious disease.

NEXT DIAGNOSTIC STEPS TO CONSIDER IF LEVELS ARE HIGH

- Mammals
  - The first step after monocytosis is detected is to determine whether it is an artifact. If the increase is mild, consider retesting after the animal has calmed down, especially with a concurrent mild neutrophilia. Also rule out exogenous sources of corticosteroids.
  - Next, examine the animal carefully for signs of infection, and do appropriate bacterial or fungal cultures. Serum antibody titers or PCR tests can be done if clinical signs warrant. Thoracic and abdominal radiographs should be performed to look for the presence of granulomas.
  - Any enlarged lymph nodes should be aspirated and submitted for cytologic examination.
  - If possible, blood cortisol levels should be measured to test for hyperadrenocorticism. In ferrets, it is possible to do an ACTH stimulation test. An abdominal ultrasound can also be performed to examine the adrenal glands and look for granulomas.
  - If there are no obvious signs of infection, a bone marrow biopsy should be considered.
- Birds and reptiles
  - Because infection is the most common cause of monocytosis in birds, a comprehensive search for the source of infection should be performed. Appropriate cultures should be performed based on clinical findings, including serum antibody titers or a PCR test for *Chlamydia* (avian) or other diseases based on clinical signs. A fecal float should be performed to check for parasites.
  - Radiographs should be performed to look for granulomas. Laparoscopic examination of the coelomic cavity and air sacs can also be done to look for smaller granulomas.
- Fish
  - In fish with monocytosis, a comprehensive search for the source of infection should be performed. Appropriate bacterial testing should be performed based on clinical findings.

CAUSES OF ABNORMALLY LOW LEVELS

- In most animals, the lower limit of the reference range for monocytes is zero; therefore, monocytopenia has little to no diagnostic significance.
- *Birds:* Some authors feel that in birds, monocytopenia can be due to acute

infection or inflammation. But again, for most avian species, zero is the lower limit of the reference range; therefore, caution should be used in placing too much emphasis on a finding of monocytopenia.

SPECIMEN AND PROCESSING CONSIDERATIONS

DRUG EFFECTS ON LEVELS Corticosteroids can cause abnormally high levels.

LAB ARTIFACTS THAT MAY INTERFERE WITH READINGS OF LEVELS OF THIS SUBSTANCE Variability in the size and staining characteristics of avian lymphocytes can make them difficult to distinguish from monocytes, so inexperienced laboratories can falsely report populations of either cell line. Because monocytes generally are much rarer than lymphocytes, this can lead to a false monocytosis.

SAMPLE FOR COLLECTION AND ANY SPECIAL SPECIMEN HANDLING NOTES

- Mammals
  - Use EDTA (purple top) tubes to collect for complete blood count (CBC).
- Birds
  - For differential counts, it is best if slides can be made from fresh whole blood.
  - Use EDTA (purple top) tubes to collect for CBC in most species. ETDA may cause RBC hemolysis, especially in Brush turkeys, Corvidae, Crowned cranes, Currasows, and Hornbills.
- Reptiles
  - Use heparinized (green top) tubes when collecting CBC samples.
- Amphibians
  - Use heparinized (green top) tubes when collecting CBC samples. Because of the small volumes often collected, use a heparinized syringe to collect the sample, and make slides immediately after collection whenever possible.
- Fish
  - Samples for differential cell counts should be prepared immediately after collection. It is important to rapidly dry slides because slow drying may alter the morphology. Diff-Quik stain can be used, but it is not optimal for differential counts. If it is necessary to collect samples in tubes, use heparinized tubes. ETDA causes hemolysis in fish anesthetized with tricaine.

PEARLS

- Mammals
  - Monocytosis rarely occurs in sick ferrets.
- Birds
  - Monocytosis and basophilia are often the only hematologic abnormalities seen in Budgerigars with chlamydial infection.
- Reptiles
  - Monocytes have been reported to be absent in healthy rat snakes but to occur in sick snakes.

REFERENCES

Carpenter JW, et al: Exotic animal formulary, ed 2, Philadelphia, 2001, WB Saunders, pp 36, 80–86, 195–208, 213, 256, 268, 292, 320, 344, 363, 386–387.

Groff JM, et al: Hematology and clinical chemistry of cyprinid fish, Vet Clin North Am 2:741–776, 1999.

Hoegeman S: Diagnostic sampling of amphibians, Vet Clin North Am 2:731–740, 1999.

Jones MP: Avian clinical pathology, Vet Clin North Am 2:663–688, 1999.

Redrobe S, et al: Sample collection and clinical pathology of reptiles, Vet Clin North Am 2:709–730, 1999.

Stockham SL, et al: Fundamentals of veterinary clinical pathology, ed 1, Ames, IA, 2002, Iowa State Press, pp 50–83.

AUTHOR: **JONATHAN W. BALL**

EDITOR: **JÖRG MAYER**

Neutrophil-Heterophil Count

DEFINITION

- Neutrophil: a granular leukocyte with a multilobed nucleus connected by threads of chromatin and cytoplasm, which contains pale-staining granules
- Heterophil: a granular leukocyte with multilobed nucleus and similar physiologic activities as neutrophils, but with granules that vary in size and stain characteristics. Found in fish, amphibians, reptiles, birds, and some mammals.

SYNONYMS

- Neutrophil-polymorphonuclear cells (PMNs), segs
- Heterophil

PHYSIOLOGY

- Neutrophils and heterophils are distinguished on the basis of their different morphologic and staining characteristics, but they serve similar functions—killing of bacteria through opsonization, ingestion, and lysis. The granules that are responsible for the unique staining pattern of neutrophils-heterophils contain a variety of proteins and enzymes, which facilitate the destruction of bacteria and can damage host tissue.
- Neutrophils develop in the bone marrow from myeloid stem cells. Cytokines such as interleukin (IL)-1, IL-3, IL-6, and granulocyte-macrophage colony-stimulating factor (GM-CSF) stimulate the granulocyte colony-forming cell to develop into the neutrophil precursor cell. The population continues to progress through several stages in the bone marrow and is known as the *proliferating pool.* Neutrophil populations are controlled at this stage by programmed cell death, which is decreased in response to chemotactic signals for neutrophil production. Generally, cells are in this stage for approximately 3 days, and then they enter maturation, or the postmitotic pool. In the postmitotic pool, neutrophils develop into bands and then into mature segmented neutrophils, which are stored in the sinusoids of the bone marrow. From here, neutrophils are released into the bloodstream. Release of neutrophils is increased by a variety of cytokines (IL-1, IL-6, tumor necrosis factor [TNF]-α, TNF-β, granulocyte colony-stimulating factor [G-CSF], GM-CSF) and chemotactic agents.
- Neutrophils in the blood are divided into two pools: the circulating pool and the marginated pool. The marginated pool consists of neutrophils temporarily adhered to or rolling along the endothelium. The ratio between the two pools is approximately 1:1 in many mammals. The presence of two blood pools of neutrophils is clinically

significant because the marginated pool can enter the circulating pool in response to stimuli, most notably exogenous or endogenous corticosteroids. This is the physiologic basis of the neutrophilia found in response to stress, because only the cells in the circulating pool are collected for a differential count. Neutrophils usually circulate in the blood for about 10 hours.

- Eventually, neutrophils pass through both blood pools and enter the tissues. Inflammatory cytokines stimulate alterations in endothelial cell production; this encourages adhesion and extravasation of neutrophils.
- In mammals, neutrophils survive for a few days in healthy tissue before they degenerate and are phagocytized by macrophages.
- In fish, neutrophils are produced in the kidney and in the spleen. The maturation process includes progranulocytes and proneutrophils. The size, shape, and stain characteristics of the granules vary among species of fish.
- Several morphologic and developmental changes in neutrophils, when present, provide clues regarding the nature of the current pathology. When there is a great demand in the body for neutrophils, most often in acute severe inflammation, a condition known as a *left shift* may occur. In a left shift, premature neutrophils from the developing population, usually bands but occasionally even more immature cells if the demand is great, are released into the bloodstream. Band cells have granule staining patterns similar to those of mature neutrophils, but the nucleus is unsegmented and generally is kidney- to horseshoe-shaped.
- Toxic changes can also be detected in neutrophils. These changes reflect damage to the neutrophil during maturation in the bone marrow. The source of the damage most often is endotoxemia, but other toxins or infections that affect the marrow can create toxic neutrophils. Toxic neutrophils generally have increased basophilic staining cytoplasm, vacuoles, Döhle bodies (irregularly shaped blue cytoplasmic inclusions), nuclear swelling, and occasionally toxic granules.
- Degenerate neutrophils have swollen, pale-staining nuclei. They represent cells that have been damaged by bacteria or by the cytotoxic substance released by other neutrophils. They are most commonly found in tissues at the site of an infection.
- It is important to distinguish degenerate neutrophils from senile neutrophils, which also can be present in tissues. Neutrophils that age normally in tissues have hypersegmented nuclei—generally five or more segments. If these hypersegmented neutrophils are seen in the blood, this can be a sign of increased endogenous or exogenous corticosteroids or myelodysplasia, or it can be an artifact of prolonged storage of samples.

TYPICAL NORMAL RANGE

The typical normal range for this laboratory test varies greatly among species. The reader is referred to the following Elsevier publications for additional information:

Carpenter J: Exotic animal formulary, ed 4, St Louis, 2013, Saunders.

Mader D: Reptile medicine and surgery, ed 2, 2006, St Louis, Saunders.

CLINICAL APPLICATIONS

CAUSES OF ABNORMALLY HIGH LEVELS

- Mammals
  - A major rule-out for neutrophilia in mammals is acute or chronic inflammation. Infections of bacterial, viral, fungal, or protozoal origin should be considered a major rule-out for neutrophilia. Other noninfectious sources of inflammation can also lead to increased neutrophil counts. These include tissue damage, as seen in infarcts or necrosis. Hemolysis, whether a primary immune-mediated condition or a secondary response, can also cause neutrophilia. Foreign bodies will produce inflammation, which can lead to neutrophilia.
  - Another common cause of neutrophilia in mammals is excessive glucocorticoid levels resulting from endogenous or exogenous sources. Glucocorticoids cause an increase in neutrophils through two mechanisms: (1) they shift cells from the marginated pool to the circulating pool, and (2) they promote the release of neutrophils from the bone marrow. Stress causes an increase in glucocorticoid release, which leads to mild to moderate neutrophilia with no left shift. This is often known as a *physiologic stress response.* Hyperadrenocorticism is another source of elevated glucocorticoids that will lead to a neutrophilia, which often is more pronounced than a stress response. Of course, administration of steroid-containing medications can lead to a neutrophilia through the same mechanism as endogenous glucocorticoids.
  - Neoplasia is another important rule-out for neutrophilia. Neutrophilia can develop in response to inflammation caused by neoplasia or as a paraneoplastic condition. It can also be a direct result of neoplasia, as in myelogenous leukemia, which usually is characterized by an increase in the numbers of morphologically abnormal cells, such as band cells and other promyelocytes.
- Birds
  - A major cause of heterophilia in birds is acute or chronic inflammation. Infections of bacterial (including chlamydial), fungal, or parasitic origin should be considered a major rule-out for heterophilia. Other noninfectious sources of inflammation can also lead to increased heterophil counts. These include tissue damage, as seen in trauma, hemorrhage, infarcts, or necrosis. Hemolysis can also cause heterophilia. Foreign bodies will produce inflammation, which can lead to heterophilia.
  - Another important cause of heterophilia in birds is excessive glucocorticoids from endogenous or exogenous sources. Glucocorticoids cause an increase in heterophils through two mechanisms: (1) they shift cells from the marginated pool to the circulating pool, and (2) they promote the release of heterophils from the bone marrow. Stress causes an increase in glucocorticoid release, which leads to mild to moderate heterophilia with no left shift. This is often known as a *physiologic stress response.* Hyperadrenocorticism is another source of elevated glucocorticoids that will lead to a heterophilia, which often is more pronounced than a stress response. Of course, administration of steroid-containing medications can lead to a heterophilia through the same mechanism as endogenous glucocorticoids.
  - Neoplasia is another important rule-out for heterophilia. Heterophilia can develop in response to inflammation caused by neoplasia or as a paraneoplastic condition. It can also be a direct result of neoplasia, as in myelogenous leukemia, which usually is characterized by an increase in the numbers of morphologically abnormal cells.
- Reptiles
  - A major cause of heterophilia in reptiles is acute or chronic inflammation. Infections of bacterial, viral or fungal origin should be considered a major rule-out for heterophilia. Other noninfectious sources of inflammation can also lead to increased heterophil counts. These include tissue damage, as seen in

trauma, hemorrhage, infarcts, or necrosis. Foreign bodies will produce inflammation, which can lead to neutrophilia.

- Stress can lead to neutrophilia through an increase in glucocorticoid release, which in turn causes a shift of neutrophils from the marginated pool into the circulating pools. Metabolic disease can lead to a neutrophilia, likely through increases in glucocorticoid release.
- Neoplasia is another important rule-out for heterophilia. Heterophilia can develop in response to inflammation caused by neoplasia or as a paraneoplastic condition. It can also be a direct result of neoplasia, as in myelogenous leukemia, which usually is characterized by an increase in the numbers of morphologically abnormal cells.

- Amphibians
  - A major cause of heterophilia in amphibians is acute or chronic inflammation. Infections of bacterial, viral, or fungal origin should be considered a major rule-out for heterophilia. Other noninfectious sources of inflammation can also lead to increased heterophil counts. These include tissue damage, as seen in trauma, hemorrhage, infarcts, or necrosis. Foreign bodies will produce inflammation, which can lead to neutrophilia.
- Fish
  - The most common causes of neutrophilia in fish are stress, increased temperature (up to 25°C [77°F]), and infectious diseases.

NEXT DIAGNOSTIC STEPS TO CONSIDER IF LEVELS ARE HIGH

- Mammals
  - After a neutrophilia is recognized, the first step is to determine whether it is due to the stress of collecting the sample. If the animal was obviously stressed, or if the complete blood count (CBC) shows a mild neutrophilia without a left shift and a lymphopenia, consider retesting after the animal calms down. Any exposure to steroids should be ruled out.
  - Once you have determined that neutrophilia is not due to stress, a thorough examination should be done for infection. This should include a direct fecal smear and a fecal float to check for the presence of protozoa or their eggs. Appropriate bacterial and fungal cultures should be performed on the basis of clinical findings. Serum antibody titers or PCR tests can be done if clinical signs warrant. Thoracic and abdominal radiographs can be done to look for the presence of neoplasia or granulomas that may be contributing to the neutrophilia.
  - If no obvious signs of infection are noted, the functional adrenal glands should be examined for the presence of hyperadrenocorticism. If possible, blood cortisol levels should be measured. In ferrets, it is possible to do an ACTH stimulation test. An abdominal ultrasound can be performed to examine the adrenal glands. This is also helpful in the search for enlarged lymph nodes or intraabdominal masses, which could be responsible for the neutrophilia.
  - A bone marrow biopsy can be performed to look for signs of damage to the bone marrow or neoplasia.
- Birds
  - After a heterophilia is recognized, the first step is to determine whether it is due to the stress of collecting the sample. If the animal was obviously stressed, or if the CBC shows a mild heterophilia without a left shift and a lymphopenia, consider retesting after the animal calms down. Any exposure to steroids should be ruled out.
  - Once you have determined that heterophilia is not due to stress, a thorough examination should be done for infection. This should include a direct fecal smear and float to check for signs of parasitism. Appropriate bacterial and fungal cultures should be performed on the basis of clinical findings. Serum chlamydial titers or chlamydial PCR tests can also be done if clinical signs warrant, especially in the presence of a degenerative left shift. Other serum antibody titers or PCR tests can be done as appropriate. Coelomic radiographs can be taken to look for the presence of neoplasia or granulomas that may be contributing to the heterophilia.
  - Because increased levels of glucocorticoids can lead to heterophilia, laparoscopic examination of adrenal glands can be performed to look for any neoplastic changes.
  - A bone marrow biopsy can be performed to look for signs of myelogenous leukemia.
- Reptiles
  - After a heterophilia is recognized, the first step is to determine whether it is due to the stress of collecting the sample. If the animal was obviously stressed, or if the CBC shows a mild heterophilia without a left shift and a lymphopenia, consider retesting after the animal calms down. Any exposure to steroids should be ruled out.
  - Once you have determined that heterophilia is not due to stress, a thorough examination should be done for infection. This should include a direct fecal smear and float to check for signs of parasitism. Appropriate bacterial and fungal cultures should be performed on the basis of clinical findings. Serum antibody titers or PCR tests can be done if clinical signs warrant. Coelomic radiographs can be taken to look for the presence of neoplasia or granulomas that may be contributing to the heterophilia.
  - Because increased levels of glucocorticoids can lead to heterophilia, laparoscopic examination of adrenal glands can be performed to look for any neoplastic changes.
  - A bone marrow biopsy can be done to look for signs of myelogenous leukemia.
- Amphibians
  - After a heterophilia is identified in an amphibian, a thorough examination should be done for infection. This should include a direct fecal smear and float to look for signs of parasitism. Appropriate bacterial and fungal cultures should be performed based on clinical findings. Serum antibody titers or PCR tests can be done if clinical signs warrant. Coelomic radiographs can be taken to look for the presence of neoplasia or granulomas that may be contributing to the heterophilia.
- Fish
  - Heterophilia in fish, similar to many other hematologic abnormalities, should be followed by a comprehensive analysis of their environment, especially water quality, temperature, and oxygen levels.

CAUSES OF ABNORMALLY LOW LEVELS

- Mammals
  - A common cause of neutropenia in mammals is severe infection, most often of bacterial or viral origin. The presence of severe infection creates an increased demand for neutrophils in the tissue, which causes migration of neutrophils out of the circulating and marginated pools, resulting in a neutropenia on CBC.
  - Anything that decreases the production of neutrophils can lead to neutropenia. Injury to the bone marrow of infectious (bacterial, viral, fungal), neoplastic, or toxic causes can lead to neutropenia as a result of direct damage to neutrophil precursors. Certain drugs can lead to neutropenia via damage to the bone marrow in dose-dependent toxicity or as an idiosyncratic reaction. Some of the more common

myelosuppressive drugs include estrogen, chloramphenicol, griseofulvin (idiosyncratic), phenylbutazone (idiosyncratic), and many of the chemotherapy drugs. The toxic effects of estrogen on bone marrow are a major concern in unspayed ferrets, which will continually secrete high levels of estrogen if they fail to conceive during their heat cycle. Myelofibrosis can also cause neutropenia through loss of neutrophil precursor cells. Certain immune-mediated conditions will destroy bone marrow in general or neutrophil cell lines specifically and can also result in neutropenia.

- Birds
  - A common cause of heteropenia in birds is severe infection, most often of bacterial or viral origin. This includes bacterial septicemia or endotoxemia. The presence of severe infection creates an increased demand for heterophils in the tissue, which causes migration of neutrophils out of the circulating and marginated pools, resulting in a neutropenia on CBC. If a degenerative left shift is noted, chlamydiosis should be suspected.
  - Anything that decreases the production of heterophils can lead to heteropenia. Injury to the bone marrow of infectious (bacterial, viral, fungal, protozoal), neoplastic, or toxic causes can lead to heteropenia as a result of direct damage to heterophil precursors. Certain drugs can lead to heteropenia via damage to the bone marrow in dose-dependent toxicity or as an idiosyncratic reaction. Some of the more common myelosuppressive drugs include estrogen, chloramphenicol, griseofulvin (idiosyncratic), phenylbutazone (idiosyncratic), and many of the chemotherapy drugs. Myelofibrosis can cause heteropenia through loss of heterophil precursor cells.
- Reptiles
  - A common cause of heteropenia in reptiles is severe infection, most often of bacterial or viral origin. The presence of severe infection creates an increased demand for heterophils in the tissue, which causes migration of neutrophils out of the circulating and marginated pools, resulting in a neutropenia on CBC.
  - Anything that decreases the production of heterophils can lead to heteropenia. Injury to the bone marrow of infectious (bacterial, viral, fungal, protozoal), neoplastic, or toxic causes can lead to heteropenia as a result of direct damage to heterophil precursors. Certain drugs can lead to heteropenia via damage to the bone marrow in dose dependent toxicity or as an idiosyncratic reaction. Some of the more common myelosuppressive drugs include estrogen, chloramphenicol, griseofulvin (idiosyncratic), phenylbutazone (idiosyncratic), and many of the chemotherapy drugs. Myelofibrosis can cause heteropenia through loss of heterophil precursor cells.
- Amphibians
  - A common cause of heteropenia in amphibians is severe infection, most often of bacterial or viral origin. The presence of severe infection creates an increased demand for heterophils in the tissue, which causes migration of the neutrophils out of the circulating and marginated pools, resulting in a neutropenia on CBC.
  - Anything that decreases the production of heterophils can lead to heteropenia. Injury to the bone marrow of infectious (bacterial, viral, fungal, protozoal), neoplastic, or toxic causes can lead to heteropenia as a result of direct damage to heterophil precursors. Certain drugs can lead to heteropenia via damage to the bone marrow in dose-dependent toxicity or as an idiosyncratic reaction. Some of the more common myelosuppressive drugs include estrogen, chloramphenicol, griseofulvin (idiosyncratic), phenylbutazone (idiosyncratic), and many of the chemotherapy drugs. Myelofibrosis can cause heteropenia through loss of heterophil precursor cells.
- Fish
  - In fish, *Aeromonas salmonicida* infection has been shown to reduce granulocyte numbers.

NEXT DIAGNOSTIC STEPS TO CONSIDER IF LEVELS ARE LOW

- Mammals
  - After a neutropenia is detected, the first step is to begin a thorough search for infection or inflammation. This should include appropriate bacterial cultures, including blood cultures, serum antibody titers, or PCR tests based on clinical findings.
  - A bone marrow biopsy should also be considered. This is especially relevant if toxic neutrophils or other morphologically abnormal neutrophils are present in the circulation.
- Birds
  - After a heteropenia is detected, the first step is to begin a thorough search for infection or inflammation. This should include appropriate bacterial cultures, including blood cultures, serum antibody titers, or PCR tests based on clinical findings. If a degenerative left shift is noted, serum chlamydial titers or chlamydial PCR tests should be done.
  - A bone marrow biopsy should be considered. This is especially relevant if toxic heterophils or other morphologically abnormal heterophils are present in the circulation.
- Reptiles
  - After a heteropenia is detected, the first step is to begin a thorough search for infection or inflammation. This should include appropriate bacterial cultures, including blood cultures, serum antibody titers, or PCR tests based on clinical findings.
  - A bone marrow biopsy should be considered. This is especially relevant if toxic heterophils or other morphologically abnormal heterophils are present in the circulation.
- Amphibians
  - After a heteropenia is detected, the first step is to begin a thorough search for infection or inflammation. This should include appropriate bacterial cultures, including blood cultures, serum antibody titers, or PCR tests based on clinical findings.
  - A bone marrow biopsy should be considered. This is especially relevant if toxic heterophils or other morphologically abnormal heterophils are present in the circulation.
- Fish
  - After a heteropenia or a granulocytopenia is detected in fish, *Aeromonas salmonicida* cultures should be included in the general workup.

SPECIMEN AND PROCESSING CONSIDERATIONS

DRUG EFFECTS ON LEVELS

- Glucocorticoids cause an increase in neutrophils/heterophils in mammals and birds.
- Estrogen, chloramphenicol, griseofulvin (idiosyncratic), phenylbutazone (idiosyncratic), and many of the chemotherapy drugs can cause neutropenia/heteropenia via damage to the bone marrow.

LAB ARTIFACTS THAT MAY INTERFERE WITH READINGS OF LEVELS OF THIS SUBSTANCE *Mammals:* Prolonged time before examination can lead to falsely elevated numbers of aged neutrophils.

SAMPLE FOR COLLECTION AND ANY SPECIAL SPECIMEN HANDLING NOTES

- Mammals
  - Use EDTA (purple top) tubes to collect for CBC.

- Birds
  - For differential counts, it is best if slides can be made from fresh whole blood.
  - Use EDTA (purple top) tubes to collect for CBC in most species. ETDA may cause RBC hemolysis, especially in Brush turkeys, Corvidae, Crowned cranes, Currasows, and Hornbills.
- Reptiles
  - Use heparinized (green top) tubes when collecting CBC samples.
- Amphibians
  - Use heparinized (green top) tubes when collecting CBC samples. Because of the small volumes often collected, use a heparinized syringe to collect the sample, and make slides immediately after collection whenever possible.
- Fish
  - Samples for differential cell counts should be prepared immediately after collection. It is important to rapidly dry slides because slow drying may alter the morphology. Diff-Quik stain can be used, but it is not optimal for differential counts. If it is necessary to collect samples in tubes, use heparinized tubes. ETDA causes hemolysis in fish anesthetized with tricaine.

PEARLS

- Mammals
  - Two morphologic subtypes of neutrophils indicate a severe infection. They can occur with a neutrophilia or a neutropenia. The first subtype consists of toxic neutrophils, whose presence is commonly associated with endotoxemia; however, other toxins or infections that affect the marrow can create toxic neutrophils. The second subtype is band cells, which are immature neutrophils. When they are released into the circulation in higher numbers than normal, this is a condition known as *a left shift*. It often indicates a severe inflammatory response with a high demand for neutrophils. In a degenerative left shift, band cells or other immature neutrophils are present in greater quantities than mature neutrophils. This is a sign of severe acute inflammation or infection. Degenerative left shift is a sign of acute chlamydial infection or overwhelming disease.
- Birds
  - Two morphologic subtypes of heterophils indicate a severe infection. They can occur with a heterophilia or a heteropenia. The first subtype consists of toxic heterophils, whose presence is commonly associated with endotoxemia; however, other toxins or infections that affect the marrow can create toxic heterophils. The second subtype is band cells, which are immature neutrophils. When they are released into the circulation in higher numbers than normal, this is a condition known as *a left shift*. It often indicates a severe inflammatory response with a high demand for heterophils. In a degenerative left shift, band cells or other immature heterophils are present in greater quantities than mature heterophils. This is a sign of severe acute inflammation or infection. Degenerative left shift is a sign of acute chlamydial infection or overwhelming disease.
- Reptiles
  - Two morphologic subtypes of heterophils indicate a severe infection. They can occur with a heterophilia or a heteropenia. The first subtype consists of toxic heterophils, whose presence is commonly associated with endotoxemia; however, other toxins or infections that affect the marrow can create toxic heterophils. The second subtype is band cells, which are immature neutrophils. When they are released into the circulation in higher numbers than normal, this is a condition known as *a left shift*. It often indicates a severe inflammatory response with a high demand for heterophils. In a degenerative left shift, band cells or other immature heterophils are present in greater quantities than mature heterophils. This is a sign of severe acute inflammation or infection.
- Amphibians
  - Differential blood counts should be stained with Natt-Herrick solution.

REFERENCES

Carpenter JW, et al: Exotic animal formulary, ed 2, Philadelphia, 2001, WB Saunders, pp 36, 80–86, 195–208, 213, 256, 268, 292, 320, 344, 363, 386–387.

Groff JM, et al: Hematology and clinical chemistry of cyprinid fish, Vet Clin North Am 2:741–776, 1999.

Hoegeman S: Diagnostic sampling of amphibians, Vet Clin North Am 2:731–740, 1999.

Jones MP: Avian clinical pathology, Vet Clin North Am 2:663–688, 1999.

Redrobe S, et al: Sample collection and clinical pathology of reptiles, Vet Clin North Am 2:709–730, 1999.

Stockham SL, et al: Fundamentals of veterinary clinical pathology, ed 1, Ames, IA, 2002, Iowa State Press, pp 50–83.

AUTHOR: **JONATHAN W. BALL**

EDITOR: **JÖRG MAYER**

pH

DEFINITION

pH is a measure of the degree to which a solution is acidic or alkaline. pH is measured by the activity of H^+ ions and is commonly represented as $-\log_{10}[H^+]$. An acid is a substance that can give up a hydrogen ion (H^+). A solution with a pH less than 7.0 (water, neutrality) is considered acidic. A base is a substance that can accept a hydrogen ion. A solution with a pH greater than 7.0 is considered basic/alkaline.

SYNONYM

Blood gas analysis is the method used to determine blood pH.

PHYSIOLOGY

- Maintaining pH within a narrow range is vital to any living organism, so that chemical reactions may proceed at physiologic rates and electrolyte concentration gradients can be maintained. The goal of the body's buffer systems is to "neutralize" excess acid or base until those excess ions can be eliminated by the renal (urine) or the respiratory (gas) system. Primary buffers are bicarbonate (HCO_3^-) and carbon dioxide (CO_2). They are interrelated in the blood via the generation of carbonic acid, according to the following equation:

$$CO_2 + H_2O \rightleftharpoons H_2CO_3 \rightleftharpoons HCO_3^- + H^+$$

- Bicarbonate concentration is regulated primarily by renal elimination, and carbon dioxide concentration by respiratory elimination. Increased HCO_3^- (metabolic alkalosis) or decreased CO_2 (respiratory alkalosis) will drive the equation to the left, buffering more H^+ and raising the pH. Decreased HCO_3^- (metabolic acidosis) or increased CO_2 (respiratory acidosis) will drive the equation to the right, liberating more H^+ and lowering the pH. The formal relationship between the two buffers is represented in the modified Henderson-Hasselbalch equation:

$$pH = pKa + \log\frac{[HCO_3^-]}{0.03\ P_{CO_2}}$$

- Often the body will attempt to compensate for a metabolic or respiratory derangement by altering the nonaffected system. For example, a primary metabolic acidosis is compensated by increased ventilation to reduce P_{CO_2} to counter the decreased HCO_3^-. Likewise, a metabolic alkalosis would be compensated by decreased ventilation. A primary respiratory acidosis would be compensated by decreased renal elimination of HCO_3^-, and a respiratory alkalosis by increased renal elimination.

TYPICAL NORMAL RANGE

The typical normal range for this laboratory test varies greatly among species. The reader is referred to the following Elsevier publications for additional information:

Carpenter J: Exotic animal formulary, ed 4, St Louis, 2013, Saunders.

Mader D: Reptile medicine and surgery, ed 2, St Louis, 2006, Saunders.

CLINICAL APPLICATIONS

CAUSES OF ABNORMALLY HIGH LEVELS

- Metabolic alkalosis
  - Increased pH and HCO_3^-
  - Often accompanied by a compensatory increase in P_{CO_2}
  - Chloride responsive (low urine chloride)
    - Vomiting of gastric contents or aggressive nasogastric tube (NGT) suctioning
    - Diuretic therapy (e.g., loop diuretics, thiazides)
    - Contraction alkalosis
    - Oral administration of sodium bicarbonate or other organic anions (e.g., lactate, citrate, gluconate, acetate)
    - Post hypercapnia
  - Chloride resistant
    - Hyperadrenocorticism
    - Primary hyperaldosteronism
    - Exogenous steroids
    - Licorice toxicity (glycyrrhizic acid)
- Respiratory alkalosis
  - Increased pH, decreased P_{CO_2}
  - Often accompanied by a compensatory decrease in HCO_3^-
  - Result of tachypnea ("primary hypocapnia")
  - Hypoxia from chronic pulmonary disease, pulmonary thromboembolism, congestive heart failure, severe anemia
  - Direct stimulation of the medullary respiratory center from neurologic or liver disease, fever/sepsis, heatstroke, or drugs (salicylate and xanthine toxicity)
  - Excessive mechanical ventilation

NEXT DIAGNOSTIC STEPS TO CONSIDER IF LEVELS ARE HIGH

- Perform a detailed physical examination and history, including diet and medications.
- Inquire and assess for potential drug/toxin exposure.
- Examine the blood gas components to evaluate the primary disorder and the degree of compensation. Confirm the source of the gas (arterial or venous). The primary disturbance in metabolic alkalosis is an elevation of HCO_3^-. Adequate respiratory hypoventilation should result in a 0.7-mm Hg increase in P_{CO_2} for each 1-mEq/L increase in HCO_3^-. The primary disturbance in respiratory alkalosis is a decrease in P_{CO_2}. Adequate metabolic compensation should result in a 2.5-mEq/L decrease in HCO_3^- (acute respiratory conditions) or a 5.5-mEq/L decrease in HCO_3^- (chronic respiratory conditions) for each 10-mm Hg decrease in P_{CO_2}. Inadequate compensation should prompt consideration of a complex disorder or underlying renal or respiratory disease.
- Evaluate respiratory rate for elevation (primary respiratory) or depression (compensation of metabolic alkalosis).
- Perform clinical and laboratory assessment of fluid status (dehydration with metabolic alkalosis) and electrolytes (dehydration concentration, reduced chloride with vomiting). Use electrolyte as a quality control to assess for potential errors with the blood gas.
- Assess for fever and evidence of sepsis. Obtain blood cultures.

CAUSES OF ABNORMALLY LOW LEVELS

- Metabolic acidosis
  - Decreased pH and HCO_3^-
  - Usually accompanied by a compensatory decrease in P_{CO_2}
  - Caused by addition of acid, failure to excrete acid, loss of HCO_3^-, or a combination thereof
  - Normochloremic (increased anion gap)
    - Ethylene glycol intoxication
    - Diabetic ketoacidosis
    - Uremic acidosis
    - Lactic acidosis
    - Salicylate intoxication
    - Methanol ingestion
  - Hyperchloremic (normal anion gap)
    - Hypoadrenocorticism
    - Diarrhea
    - Carbonic anhydrase inhibitory (e.g., acetazolamide)
    - Dilutional acidosis
    - Ammonium chloride
    - Cationic amino acids (lysine, arginine, histidine)
    - Renal tubular acidosis
    - Posthypocapnic metabolic acidosis
- Respiratory acidosis
  - Decreased pH, increased P_{CO_2}
  - Usually associated with a compensatory increase in HCO_3^-
  - Primarily due to hypoventilation ("primary hypercapnia")
  - Airway obstruction
    - Aspiration
  - Respiratory center depression
    - Neurologic disease (e.g., brainstem, high cervical spinal cord lesion)
    - Drugs (e.g., narcotics, sedatives, barbiturates, inhalation anesthetics)
    - Toxemia
  - Cardiopulmonary arrest
  - Neuromuscular defects
    - Tetanus, botulism, polyradiculoneuritis, polymyositis, tick paralysis
    - Drug induced (succinylcholine, pancuronium, aminoglycosides with anesthetics, organophosphates)
  - Restrictive diseases
    - Diaphragmatic hernia, pulmonary fibrosis, pleural effusion, hemothorax, pyothorax
    - Chest wall trauma, pneumothorax
  - Pulmonary disease
    - Respiratory distress syndrome, pneumonia, severe pulmonary edema, diffuse metastatic disease, smoke inhalation, pulmonary thromboembolism, chronic obstructive pulmonary disease, pulmonary mechanical ventilation
  - Inadequate ventilation

NEXT DIAGNOSTIC STEPS TO CONSIDER IF LEVELS ARE LOW

- Perform a detailed physical examination and history, including diet and medications.
- Inquire and assess for potential drug/toxin exposure.
- Evaluate respiratory rate for elevation depression in primary respiratory acidosis or elevation in compensation of a metabolic acidosis.
- Examine the blood gas components to evaluate the primary disorder and the degree of compensation. Confirm the

source of the gas (arterial or venous). The primary disturbance in metabolic acidosis is a decrease in HCO_3^-. Adequate respiratory hyperventilation should result in a 0.7-mm Hg decrease in P_{CO_2} for each 1-mEq/L decrease in HCO_3^-. The primary disturbance in respiratory acidosis is an increase in P_{CO_2}. Adequate metabolic compensation should result in a 1.5-mEq/L increase in HCO_3^- (acute respiratory conditions) or a 3.5-mEq/L increase in HCO_3^- (chronic respiratory conditions) for each 10-mm Hg increase in P_{CO_2}. Inadequate compensation should prompt consideration of a complex disorder or underlying renal or respiratory disease.

- For respiratory acidosis, assess for underlying pulmonary or cardiac disease with radiographs. Evaluate for potential airway obstruction. Perform a detailed neurologic examination to look for underlying CNS or neuromuscular disease. Consider drugs and toxins.
- For metabolic acidosis, assess electrolytes (chloride), glucose (ketoacidosis), and renal function (renal tubular acidosis). Calculate the anion gap ($[Na^+] - ([Cl^-] + [HCO_3^-])$). Remember that a falsely low anion gap can be caused by hypoalbuminemia, hypermagnesemia, hypercalcemia, and hypophosphatemia. With a normal anion gap, first consider renal disease, dilutional, and assess for signs of hypoadrenocorticism. With an elevated anion gap, check blood and urine glucose and ketones for evidence of diabetic ketoacidosis (DKA), urine for crystals (ethylene glycol), and blood urea nitrogen (BUN) and lactate for common sources of acidosis.

IMPORTANT INTERSPECIES DIFFERENCES

- Fish
  - Acid-base regulation in fish is more challenging compared with that in terrestrial animals because the composition of water varies to a greater degree than that of air. Large and rapid changes in oxygen and carbon dioxide (CO_2) levels, electrolyte concentrations, and temperature are significant challenges to acid-base regulation. The branchial epithelium is the site of gas exchange and principal ion regulation in fish; ions readily transfer across the gill surface. Changes in water ionic composition affect the ionic transfer process across the branchial epithelium, which in turn affects osmotic and acid-base regulation.
  - Fish have a low blood CO_2 concentration compared with that of terrestrial animals.
  - This results from the high rate of gill ventilation and the much larger capacity of water for carbon monoxide (CO) dissolution. The small environmental and arterial CO_2 gradient and gill system limit the ability of fish to compensate for changes in arterial CO_2 by hyperventilation or hypoventilation. As a result, changes in CO_2 are too small to contribute significantly to the acid-base balance in fish.
  - Fish have more significant metabolic regulation and a larger epithelial ionic transfer capacity than air-breathing mammals, in addition to a capacity for gain of bicarbonate from the environment to facilitate normalization of acid-base status. Epithelial ionic transfer is a function of the chloride cells located in juxtaposition to the secondary circulatory system of the central venous gill sinus.
- Reptiles
  - The normal blood pH of turtles and most other reptiles ranges between 7.5 and 7.7 at 23°C to 25°C (73.5°F to 77°F). The normal blood pH of some snakes and lizards may fall below 7.4. The blood pH of reptiles is labile and fluctuates with temperature and physiologic state. An increase in temperature or excitement may cause the blood pH to decrease. The blood pH often increases with anesthesia, from a normal value of 7.5 to 7.6 to a new value of 7.7 to 7.8. The buffering systems that regulate blood pH in mammals most likely are the same in reptiles, with the bicarbonate/carbonic acid buffer system being the most important because of the rapid rate of CO_2 elimination via the lungs after conversion from H_2CO_3. Total plasma CO_2 or bicarbonate concentrations are reported rarely in reptiles; however, normal total CO_2 values for most reptiles are expected to range between 20 and 30 mmol/L.
  - Therefore, a postprandial metabolic alkalosis accompanied by a decrease in chloride and an increase in bicarbonate is observed in alligators as the result of extensive gastric hydrochloric acid secretion.
- Birds
  - The normal avian anion gap is 15 mEq/L for most species. Respiratory acidosis is a common complication of anesthesia in birds, but it is rarely assessed.

SPECIMEN AND PROCESSING CONSIDERATIONS

DRUG EFFECTS ON LEVELS

- Acetazolamide, NH_4Cl, and $CaCl_2$ have the potential to cause acidosis.
- Antacids, sodium bicarbonate, potassium citrate or gluconate, and loop diuretics have the potential to cause alkalosis.
- Salicylates (aspirin, component of Pepto-Bismol) may cause metabolic acidosis, respiratory alkalosis, or both.

LAB ARTIFACTS THAT MAY INTERFERE WITH READINGS OF LEVELS OF THIS SUBSTANCE

- Blood gas assessment is extremely dependent on technique. A small syringe is required to eliminate the possibility of air contamination. If the blood sample is exposed to air (including bubbles in the sample), P_{CO_2} decreases and P_{O_2} increases, artificially increasing the pH.
- If analysis is delayed and the tube sits at room temperature, P_{CO_2} will increase and P_{O_2} will decrease from aerobic metabolism by white blood cells (WBCs), resulting in an artificially decreased pH. This artifact is minimized by keeping the sample on ice. Prolonged venous stasis during venipuncture increases P_{CO_2} and decreases pH. Preservative can also affect results. Citrate, oxalate, or EDTA can decrease pH. Excessive heparin (>10% of the sample volume) may decrease the pH, P_{CO_2}, and HCO_3^-.

SAMPLE FOR COLLECTION AND ANY SPECIAL SPECIMEN HANDLING NOTES

- Arterial blood is required to evaluate P_{O_2} for pulmonary function, but free-flowing jugular blood is acceptable for acid-base analysis. Pulmonary artery, jugular vein, and cephalic vein samples usually have similar values, whereas arterial blood has a slightly lower HCO_3^- and a significantly lower P_{CO_2}. For routine blood gas analysis, a 3-mL syringe with a 25-gauge needle is used to collect 0.5 to 1.5 mL of blood. The interior of the syringe is filled with heparin (1000 U/mL), and the contents are expelled to coat the tube with heparin and eliminate air contents. After blood collection, the needle is stopped, and any air bubbles must be expelled to prevent gas exchange. The sample is rolled in the palms for mixing and is placed on ice.
- Prevent exposure to room air (insert needle into a rubber stopper). Analysis should occur within 15 to 30 minutes of collection, or within 2 hours of immersion of the sample in an ice water bath.
- Handheld devices have been developed for cage-side measurement and provide rapid blood gas with accurate results.

PEARLS

- Fish

 - Acid-base regulation in fish is more challenging. The composition of water varies to a greater degree than that of air, so large and rapid changes in oxygen and carbon dioxide (CO_2) levels, electrolyte concentrations, and temperature are significant challenges to acid-base regulation. Carbon dioxide uploading is so efficient in the gills that respiratory effects are minimal. Fish have more significant metabolic regulation via epithelial ionic transfer capacity, as well as the ability to take up bicarbonate from the aqueous environment.
- Reptiles
  - The blood pH of reptiles is labile and fluctuates with temperature and physiologic state. An increase in temperature or excitement may cause the blood pH to decrease. The blood pH frequently increases with anesthesia.

REFERENCES

Blood DC, et al: Saunders comprehensive veterinary dictionary, ed 2, Philadelphia, 1999, WB Saunders.

Campbell TW: Clinical pathology. In Mader DR, editor: Reptile medicine and surgery, ed 2, Philadelphia, 1996, WB Saunders.

Carpenter JW: Exotic animal formulary, ed 3, Philadelphia, 2004, WB Saunders.

Fudge AM: Laboratory medicine: avian and exotic pets, Philadelphia, 2000, WB Saunders

Harcourt-Brown F: Textbook of rabbit medicine, Boston, 2002, Butterworth-Heinemann.

Harrison GJ, et al: Clinical avian medicine, South Palm Beach, FL, 2006, Spix Publishing.

Quesenberry KE, et al: Ferrets, rabbits, and rodents: clinical medicine and surgery, ed 2, St Louis, 2004, Saunders.

Thrall MA, et al: Veterinary hematology and clinical chemistry, Philadelphia, 2004, Lippincott Williams & Wilkins.

Willard MD, et al: Small animal: clinical diagnosis by laboratory methods, St Louis, 2004, Saunders.

AUTHOR: **JULIE DECUBELLIS**

EDITOR: **JÖRG MAYER**

Phosphorus

DEFINITION

Phosphorus is a major intracellular anion, and most intracellular phosphorus is organic. Most inorganic phosphate is located extracellularly.

SYNONYM

Phosphate

PHYSIOLOGY

- Phosphorus is derived mainly from the diet, especially from meat and dairy products. Phosphorus is an important constituent of bone and teeth and plays an important role in storage, release, and transfer of energy and acid-base metabolism. Phosphorus is regulated largely by parathyroid hormone (PTH), which promotes phosphate release from bone and excretion by the kidney by decreasing renal tubular reabsorption. PTH is not very responsive to phosphorus levels and acts secondarily on these levels. Calcitonin decreases renal tubular reabsorption of phosphorus to promote phosphaturia. Vitamin D is stimulated by hypophosphatemia and must be hydroxylated in the liver, then in the kidney, to produce the active form. Vitamin D acts to increase intestinal resorption of phosphorus and calcium. Serum levels are determined by a balance between intake and loss but do not necessarily reflect total body stores. Calcium is commonly assessed concurrently because of their physiologic relationship. Assays measure total inorganic phosphate concentrations in serum or plasma. Abnormalities in phosphorus levels are often complex problems and are interdependent with other parameters.
- A change in phosphorus is not always consistent with disease, so its diagnostic value can be considered poor.

TYPICAL NORMAL RANGE

The typical normal range for this laboratory test varies greatly among species. The reader is referred to the following Elsevier publications for additional information:

Carpenter J: Exotic animal formulary, ed 4, St Louis, 2013, Saunders.

Mader D: Reptile medicine and surgery, ed 2, St Louis, 2006, Saunders.

CLINICAL APPLICATIONS

CAUSES OF ABNORMALLY HIGH LEVELS

- Young, growing animals can have increased phosphorus levels.
- High-phosphate diets can lead to nutritional secondary hyperparathyroidism. However, phosphate values can be within normal range because of increased amounts of parathyroid hormone and adjustment to the phosphate level.
- Renal failure results in a reduced ability to excrete phosphate and in phosphate accumulation within the plasma. There tends to be a reciprocal fall in plasma calcium concentrations, stimulating parathyroid hormone and demineralization of bone (renal secondary hyperparathyroidism). This releases more calcium and more phosphate into the plasma. Decreased renal glomerular filtration rate and decreased filtration of phosphorus also result in hyperphosphatemia and can be associated with prerenal, renal, or postrenal causes of azotemia.
- Bladder rupture results in retention of urine in the peritoneal cavity and equilibrium with phosphorus in the circulation. Phosphorus-rich urine moves down its concentration gradient into the circulation. Failure to excrete phosphate ions causes elevated plasma phosphorus levels.
- Hypervitaminosis D caused by excessive dietary supplementation, calciferol poisoning, or plant toxicity elevates phosphorus and calcium levels.
- Hypoparathyroidism caused by deficient hormone production results in increased tubular reabsorption of phosphate and high plasma levels, but low serum calcium.
- Neoplastic bone tumors stimulating osteoclast activity and osteolysis cause release of phosphorus.
- Trauma or muscle necrosis can cause release of phosphate from muscle.
- Postprandial testing can demonstrate transient elevations.
- Leakage from devitalized intestinal mucosa can also elevate levels.
- In egg-laying species, an increase in phosphorus can be seen in females during egg production.

NEXT DIAGNOSTIC STEPS TO CONSIDER IF LEVELS ARE HIGH

- Evaluate urine specific gravity and azotemia to determine degree of renal impairment.
- Serum PTH
- Determine ionized calcium

- Compare with calcium level. Use calcium-to-phosphorus ratio and product.
- Abdominal radiographs and/or ultrasound
- Radiography of long bones for evidence of neoplasia and to document skeletal status
- Renal biopsy
- Repeat sample to rule out artifact.
- Determine sex and reproductive status.

CAUSES OF ABNORMALLY LOW LEVELS

- Malabsorption/digestion of phosphate is usually due to use of oral phosphate-binding agents (e.g., aluminum hydroxide), low-phosphate diets, anorexia, starvation, or nutritional imbalance.
- Hypovitaminosis D or low dietary calcium levels can depress phosphorus levels.
- Primary hyperparathyroidism and pseudohyperparathyroidism lead to increased production of parathyroid hormone. This results in lower plasma phosphorus levels because of its increased excretion. Parathyroid hormone inhibits tubular phosphate reabsorption.
- Diuresis causes increased excretion of water and lower phosphate values.
- Depressed levels can be caused by renal disease with impaired renal tubular phosphorus reabsorption, intracellular shift of phosphate into cells from alkalosis (especially respiratory), metabolic acidosis, insulin administration, or hyperglycemia.

NEXT DIAGNOSTIC STEPS TO CONSIDER IF LEVELS ARE LOW

- PTH assay
- Measurement of vitamin D metabolites (vitamin D deficiency)
- Radiology (poor bone quality, pathologic fractures)

IMPORTANT INTERSPECIES DIFFERENCES

- *Reptiles:* calcium-to-phosphorus ratio (Ca:P) less than 2:1 is suggestive of renal disease or chronic malnutrition.
- Calcium phosphorus product: if Ca × P ≤ 50, no renal problem is suspected; if Ca × P ≥ 70, suspect renal disease (Be careful with interpretation of these values because during active reproduction, Ca value can go above 20 mg/dL.)

SPECIMEN AND PROCESSING CONSIDERATIONS

DRUG EFFECTS ON LEVELS

- Oral phosphate-binding agents may depress phosphate levels.
- Aluminum (antacids), diuretics (furosemide, thiazides, and acetazolamide), bicarbonate, insulin, and anticonvulsant drugs can cause hypophosphatemia.
- Glucocorticoids stimulate urinary excretion of phosphate and hypophosphatemia.
- Anabolic steroids, furosemide, IV supplementation, vitamin D supplementation, tetracyclines, and phosphate-containing enemas can cause hyperphosphatemia.

LAB ARTIFACTS THAT MAY INTERFERE WITH READINGS OF LEVELS OF THIS SUBSTANCE

- Hemolysis and lipemia will falsely elevate phosphate values.
- EDTA can falsely decrease phosphorus levels in birds.
- Mannitol can falsely depress serum phosphorus levels.
- Oxalate or citrate may interfere with phosphorus assay.

SAMPLE FOR COLLECTION AND ANY SPECIAL SPECIMEN HANDLING NOTES

- *Reptiles:* plasma is preferred over serum for chemistries because clot formation may be prolonged in reptiles and may change serum electrolyte and glucose values. Also, a greater volume per unit blood can be obtained.
- *Birds:* lithium heparin is the anticoagulant of choice for most avian blood samples; evaluation of biochemistries is most commonly obtained from plasma.
- *Small mammals:* small blood samples (<2 mL) should be placed in microtainers. Heparin microtainers are preferred because more plasma can be obtained from small samples.
- All samples should be centrifuged and plasma/serum separated from cells as soon as possible; tests should be run immediately or the specimen transported frozen.

PEARLS

- See Calcium, Sec. IV on using phosphorus to evaluate renal status in reptiles.
- A seed-based diet for birds can be significantly low in phosphorus.

REFERENCES

Campbell TW: Clinical pathology. In Mader DR, editor: Reptile medicine and surgery, Philadelphia, 1996, WB Saunders.

Carpenter JW: Exotic animal formulary, ed 3, Philadelphia, 2004, WB Saunders.

Fudge AM, editor: Laboratory medicine: avian and exotic pets, Philadelphia, 2000, WB Saunders.

Jones MP: Avian clinical pathology, Vet Clin North Am Exot Anim Pract 2:663–687, 1999.

Stoskopf MK, editor: Fish medicine, Philadelphia, 1993, WB Saunders.

AUTHOR: **CARALEE MANLEY**

EDITOR: **JÖRG MAYER**

Platelet Count

DEFINITION

Platelets (thrombocytes) are the smallest of all the formed elements in the blood. Counting may be performed directly (in a hemocytometer chamber) or indirectly (estimating from the stained blood smear by number per field or in comparison with the number of white blood cells), or by a quantitative buffy coat (QBC) method, expressed as the number of cells per liter of blood. Automated methods generally are not accurate in exotic species, especially for avian and reptile thrombocytes. The Natt-Herrick method is most common for manual counting. Blood is diluted 1:200 and is applied to a charged Neubauer-ruled hemocytometer. The number of platelets/thrombocytes is counted in the large central grid on both sides, and this value is multiplied by 1000 to obtain the number per µL of blood.

SYNONYM

Thrombocyte count (birds, reptiles)

PHYSIOLOGY

Platelets are cytoplasmic fragments formed from megakaryocytes in the bone marrow. They are the smallest of the cellular components of the blood in mammals and contain numerous cytosolic organelles and granules, including lysosomes, alpha granules (thromboglobulin, von Willebrand factor, fibrinogen), and dense bodies (adenine, serotonin, calcium). Avian and reptile patients lack platelets but contain thrombocytes—small nucleated cells believed to be derived from the monocyte lineage. The main function of both platelets and thrombocytes involves primary hemostasis. This process is best understood in platelets, whereby vascular damage exposes subendothelial basement membrane collagen, creating a surface for platelet adhesion via surface receptors (glycoprotein 1b) in association with von Willebrand factor. Binding causes activation of platelets with release of cytoplasmic granules and conformational changes to allow additional platelet-platelet bridges to form via fibrinogen and additional surface receptors (glycoprotein IIb/IIIa). This primary hemostatic plug is then stabilized from activation of coagulation with the ultimate formation of cross-linked fibrin. Thrombocytes are believed to function in a similar manner and are also capable of phagocytosis. Because platelets are consumed during the clotting process, conditions accompanied by excessive clotting (sepsis with disseminated intravascular coagulation) are associated with acute reductions in platelet numbers (thrombocytopenia). Platelets and thrombocytes can be destroyed by immune-mediated mechanisms that target their surface receptors. Absolute increases in platelet numbers (thrombocytosis) normally reflect excessive production through nonspecific bone marrow stimulation, sometimes resulting from malignancy.

TYPICAL NORMAL RANGE

The typical normal range for this laboratory test varies greatly among species. The reader is referred to the following Elsevier publications for additional information:

Carpenter J: Exotic animal formulary, ed 4, St Louis, 2013, Saunders.

Mader D: Reptile medicine and surgery, ed 2, St Louis, 2006, Saunders.

CLINICAL APPLICATIONS

CAUSES OF ABNORMALLY HIGH LEVELS

- Thrombocytosis results from excessive platelet production. It can occur with malignancies such as myeloproliferative disorders and leukemias, anemias, infectious or inflammatory diseases, or endocrinopathies (diabetes mellitus, hyperadrenocorticism). The mechanism is believed to be due to nonspecific bone marrow stimulation, with cross-stimulation of platelet production from elevation of cytokines, including interleukin (IL)-3, IL-6, granulocyte-monocyte colony-stimulating factor (GM-CSF), and erythropoietin.
- Thrombocytosis is also seen with splenic contracture or splenectomy.
- Immune suppressive therapy results in increased platelet counts.
- Essential thrombocythemia (platelet leukemia) is not well documented in exotic animals.

NEXT DIAGNOSTIC STEPS TO CONSIDER IF LEVELS ARE HIGH

- Perform a detailed history and physical examination, including medication history, possible toxic exposures, and recent/current illness.
- Perform a manual count and examination of the peripheral smear.
- Examine the leukocyte count, differential, and peripheral smear morphology for evidence of leukocyte abnormalities (left shift with infection, excess leukocytes or blasts with malignancy) or anemia.
- If current or recent infection is evident, reassess count after resolution of illness.
- Consider evaluation for endocrinopathy.
- If thrombocytosis persists, or if the cause is unclear, perform a bone marrow examination.

CAUSES OF ABNORMALLY LOW LEVELS Decreased platelet/thrombocyte numbers (thrombocytopenia) result from impaired production or increased rate of destruction. Isolated defects in platelet production are rare and usually are drug induced (alcohols, carbamazepine). More commonly, platelet production is reduced as part of trilineage marrow suppression. This can result from aplastic anemia, myelodysplasias or hematopoietic malignancies, granulomatous diseases, or marrow suppression from chemotherapy or radiation. Accelerated loss is commonly due to consumption from disseminated intravascular coagulation (DIC) or severe blood loss/anemia, but it is also seen with immune-mediated destruction (autoimmune [ITP], alloimmune, drug-induced) or microangiopathic destruction (thrombotic thrombocytopenic purpura [TTP]).

NEXT DIAGNOSTIC STEPS TO CONSIDER IF LEVELS ARE LOW

- Perform a detailed history and physical examination, including medication history, possible toxic exposures (alcohol), and recent/current illness. If the animal is septic/toxic appearing, assess for DIC by obtaining fibrin degradation product levels (D-dimer).
- Perform a manual count and examination of the peripheral smear.
- Assess for possible aggregation causing pseudothrombocytopenia.
- Estimate platelet size and morphology.
- Larger, immature platelets or reactive thrombocytes with nuclear pleomorphism are associated with increased production due to rapid peripheral destruction. Assess for DIC, acute hemorrhage, or coagulopathy due to liver disease, vitamin K deficiency, or toxic exposure (warfarin). If the animal is stable, consider drug-induced or other immune-mediated destruction. Perform coagulation assays (prothrombin time [PT], partial thromboplastin time [PTT]).
- Small, rare platelets prompt consideration of decreased production. Examine the leukocyte count, differential, and peripheral smear morphology for evidence of myelodysplasia or leukemia.
- Consider bone marrow examination if thrombocytopenia does not appear because of sepsis/DIC, to help differentiate between production and destruction origins.

IMPORTANT INTERSPECIES DIFFERENCES

- Birds
    - The avian clotting cell is the thrombocyte, a nucleated cell likely derived from a monocyte precursor. The cell is small and oval with a dense, basophilic nucleus and pale cytoplasm containing a few red granules and possibly phagocytic vacuoles. On activation, the cytoplasm becomes intensely eosinophilic with irregular margins.
    - Avian thrombocytes normally are present at a concentration of 20,000 to 30,000/µL. Automated thrombocyte counts normally are not performed because the cells are nucleated and resemble lymphocytes in size. The thrombocytes tend to clump, also hindering accurate counts. A crude estimate can be performed by counting the number in 5 oil immersion fields, dividing by 1000 (corrected to number of erythrocytes), and multiplying by 3,500,000 (average number of erythrocytes per microliter of blood) for birds with normal hematocrits.

- As occurs with mammalian platelets, activated thrombocytes aggregate and form a primary plug of hemostasis. Low or deficient thrombocytes are associated with reduced formation of primary vascular plugs and are clinically observed as mucosal and superficial ecchymotic and petechial bleeding. Psittacines frequently display periorbital edema and petechial hemorrhages. Bleeding into body cavities and potential spaces is more common with a coagulopathy due to disorders of the coagulation cascade, including vitamin K deficiency and warfarin.
- Thrombocytopenia in birds (<20,000/μL) is rare and is most often due to peripheral consumption, usually severe septicemia. This has been well documented with *Salmonella* and *Escherichia coli* infections in chickens. Viral infections, such as circovirus in African grey parrots and reovirus and polyomavirus in psittacines, are also a cause of abrupt thrombocytopenia. Thrombocytopenia with infection is believed to be due to DIC, although laboratory documentation in birds is rare. Chronic infection can lead to marrow suppression and decreased platelet production.

- Ferrets
  - The mammalian platelet is derived from megakaryocytes in the bone marrow and is anuclear. The cytoplasm contains numerous granules, including alpha and dense granules, both necessary for platelet function. Ferret platelets average 8.7 ± 0.8 μm^3 in size. The platelets aggregate in response to adenosine diphosphate (ADP) and collagen as in humans, but not with ristocetin. Platelet counts are approximately 100×10^3/μL higher in females. Thrombocytopenia is most commonly seen in hyperestrogenism, where counts can be below 20×10^3/μL. Lymphoma is a less common cause of thrombocytopenia.
- Rabbits
  - Compared with humans, rabbits have higher platelet counts and a more active intrinsic coagulation system. Rabbit platelets have an unusually high serotonin content—20 to 25 times that of human platelets. They clot in response to ADP, collagen, and serotonin, but not with epinephrine. The rabbit platelet is approximately 6.1 ± 1.1 μm^3 in size. Counts do not demonstrate a sex difference, as in ferrets. Thrombocytopenia in rabbits is most often due to septicemia. Rabbits are 10 times more sensitive to endotoxin than humans and respond with a brisk DIC.
- Reptiles
  - The reptile thrombocyte is an elliptical nucleated cell measuring 8 to 16 μm in length by 5 to 9 μm in width. It has pale cytoplasm with occasional azurophilic granules and vacuoles and abundant microtubules on ultrastructural analysis. The nucleus is dense and round with extensive lobulations on ultrastructural analysis. Thrombocytopenia is most often associated with septicemia *(Salmonella)* and DIC. Reactive thrombocytes with polymorphic nuclei are frequently observed in these conditions.

SPECIMEN AND PROCESSING CONSIDERATIONS

DRUG EFFECTS ON LEVELS

- Elevated platelet counts are caused by immune suppressive agents such as prednisolone and vincristine.
- Decreased platelet counts are caused by ethanol, carbamazepine, and many chemotherapeutic agents.
- Other drugs, including aspirin, ibuprofen, and indomethicin, do not affect platelet numbers but interfere with platelet function.

LAB ARTIFACTS THAT MAY INTERFERE WITH READINGS OF LEVELS OF THIS SUBSTANCE

- Both platelets and thrombocytes tend to aggregate, which can result in decreased automated and manual counts. Manual analysis should include examination for large platelet clumps on peripheral smears, especially if the count is reduced.
- Thrombocytes are nucleated and have a size and nuclear-to-cytoplasmic ratio similar to lymphocytes. As a result, automated counters tend to group them with these leukocytes, resulting in an artificially depressed count.

SAMPLE FOR COLLECTION AND ANY SPECIAL SPECIMEN HANDLING NOTES Blood should be collected into a tube with anticoagulant (EDTA, heparin, citrate) to prevent platelet aggregation. Thrombocytes tend to aggregate with heparin.

PEARLS

- Birds
  - Thrombocytes are nucleated and are best assessed manually. Thrombocytopenia should prompt investigation for a bacterial or viral infection.
- Ferrets
  - Platelet counts are higher in females. Thrombocytopenia is commonly seen with hyperestrogenism in unspayed females.
- Rabbits
  - Thrombocytopenia should raise concern for septicemia/DIC.
- Reptiles
  - Thrombocytopenia is most commonly due to sepsis *(Salmonella)* and is associated with reactive, pleomorphic thrombocytes.

REFERENCES

Blood DC, et al: Saunders comprehensive veterinary dictionary, ed 2, Philadelphia, 1999, WB Saunders.

Campbell TW: Clinical pathology. In Mader DR, editor: Reptile medicine and surgery, ed 2, Philadelphia, 1996, WB Saunders.

Carpenter JW: Exotic animal formulary, ed 3, Philadelphia, 2004, WB Saunders.

Fudge AM: Laboratory medicine: avian and exotic pets, Philadelphia, 2000, WB Saunders.

Harcourt-Brown F: Textbook of rabbit medicine, Boston, 2002, Butterworth-Heinemann.

Harrison GJ, et al: Clinical avian medicine, South Palm Beach, FL, 2006, Spix Publishing.

Quesenberry KE, et al: Ferrets, rabbits, and rodents: clinical medicine and surgery, ed 2, St Louis, 2004, Saunders.

Thrall MA, et al: Veterinary hematology and clinical chemistry, Philadelphia, 2004, Lippincott Williams & Wilkins.

Willard MD, et al: Small animal clinical diagnosis by laboratory methods, St Louis, 2004, Saunders.

AUTHOR: **JULIE DECUBELLIS**

EDITOR: **JÖRG MAYER**

Potassium

DEFINITION

A predominantly extracellular mineral necessary for proper function of all cells, especially muscle and nerve cells

SYNONYM

K^+

PHYSIOLOGY

- Potassium is largely—approximately 98%—found extracellularly. The proper concentration is maintained at the cellular level by the Na^+/K^+-ATPase (sodium/potassium–adenosine triphosphatase) pump, located on cell membranes, which removes 3 Na^+ ions from the cell in exchange for 2 K^+ ions. This is especially vital in nerve cells for maintaining the proper electrochemical membrane potential.
- The potassium concentration can be affected at the cellular level by a number of factors. The pH of the extracellular environment is one of the major influences on potassium serum concentration. Acidotic conditions promote cellular uptake of H^+ to maintain homeostasis. For each H^+ taken up by the cells, a K^+ is moved extracellularly to preserve electroneutrality. Alkalosis has the opposite effect, promoting cellular uptake of K^+ in exchange for H^+, although this effect is not as strong as the response to acidosis. Increases in sodium bicarbonate cause a decrease in potassium, both directly and by creating an alkalotic environment. Insulin causes cells to take up K^+. Insulin increases the activity of the membrane-bound Na^+/H^+ exchanger, causing an increase in intracellular Na, which increases the activity of the Na^+/K^+-ATPase pump, leading to a decrease in extracellular K^+. Catecholamines decrease K^+ concentrations by B_2 activation of adenylate cyclase, which stimulates the action of the Na^+/K^+-ATPase pump. Elevations in thyroid hormones can decrease potassium by upregulating the Na^+/K^+-ATPase pump.
- The body maintains potassium concentration primarily through the action of the kidneys. Potassium is freely filtered by the glomerulus. It is actively reabsorbed in the proximal tubules, but regulation occurs mostly at the collecting ducts. Both aldosterone and antidiuretic hormone (ADH) increase potassium loss into the urine. Alkalotic urine also promotes potassium loss due to decreased resorption. Increased dietary intake of potassium leads to increased urinary loss.

TYPICAL NORMAL RANGE

The typical normal range for this laboratory test varies greatly among species. The reader is referred to the following Elsevier publications for additional information:

Carpenter J: Exotic animal formulary, ed 4, St Louis, 2013, Saunders.

Mader D: Reptile medicine and surgery, ed 2, St Louis, 2006, Saunders.

CLINICAL APPLICATIONS

CAUSES OF ABNORMALLY HIGH LEVELS

- One of the most common causes of hyperkalemia is acidosis, whether it results from metabolic or respiratory causes. To maintain pH in the face of acidosis, cells take up H^+ in exchange for K^+, to maintain electrical neutrality within the cell. This exchange results in hyperkalemia. Because all cells contain potassium, cellular damage, especially hemolysis or muscle damage, can be a source of hyperkalemia.
- Mammals
  - The kidney is the major organ involved in potassium homeostasis, so anything that affects its function can cause hyperkalemia. Acute renal failure can be an important cause in mammals. Dehydration, and thus a decrease in glomerular filtration rate (GFR), can contribute to elevated potassium. Urinary tract obstruction, which causes a decrease in GFR, will have a similar effect. Hypoadrenocorticism can lead to increased potassium, primarily by decreasing aldosterone release. Aldosterone promotes potassium loss into the kidneys; therefore, primary hypoaldosteronism can lead to hyperkalemia.
  - Urine contains a high concentration of potassium relative to blood. Therefore, rupture anywhere along the urinary tract (ureter, bladder, urethra) can cause hyperkalemia as potassium enters the bloodstream from the peritoneal cavity along its concentration gradient.
  - Several miscellaneous processes can cause hyperkalemia via undetermined mechanisms. These include peritoneal effusion and repeated drainage of chylous thoracic effusion.
  - Administration of fluids with a high concentration of potassium can cause hyperkalemia.
- Birds
  - As with mammals, the kidneys are the major organs involved in potassium homeostasis. Anything that affects renal function, whether disease or dehydration, can cause hyperkalemia, although not as consistently as in mammals.
  - Dietary supplementation of potassium can lead to hyperkalemia.
- Reptiles
  - Hyperkalemia is associated with acute renal disease in reptiles.
- Consider oversupplementation with a vitamin/mineral supplement.
- Fish
  - In fish, several causes of hyperkalemia are known. They include hemolysis, hypoxia, strenuous activity, stress, and nitrate toxicity.

NEXT DIAGNOSTIC STEPS TO CONSIDER IF LEVELS ARE HIGH

- In mammals, the first diagnostic step is to rule out hemolysis or other disease processes with a complete blood count (CBC). It may be helpful to run a blood lactate level and a blood gas analysis to look for metabolic or respiratory acidosis. Urinalysis should be done to assess kidney and urinary tract function. If abnormalities are found in the blood work, the abdomen should be examined next via ultrasound. Ultrasound can be used to examine the bladder, ureters, and urethra for patency to rule out an obstruction or rupture. It can also be used to examine the health of the kidneys (signs of renal failure) or adrenal glands. If any abnormalities or masses are found, ultrasound can be used to guide biopsies (especially of the kidneys). Because hypoadrenocorticism can cause hyperkalemia, it may be beneficial to measure ACTH levels, although normal values are known for very few species. In ferrets, it is possible to do an ACTH stimulation test.
- Birds and reptiles
  - The next diagnostic step should consist of complementary blood work, including CBC, lactate, uric acid levels to check for kidney function, and possibly blood gas analysis to check for respiratory or metabolic acidosis. Additionally, the kidneys and adrenal glands can be examined using coelomic radiographs or, if possible, laparoscopic

techniques. If warranted by visual inspection, a renal biopsy can be performed with a laparoscope.

- Fish
  - The metabolic function of a fish is much more dependent on environmental factors compared with the species previously discussed; therefore, the environment should be the first area of focus in attempts to ascertain the cause of any metabolic disorder. Water quality, including pH, oxygen content, and the presence of nitrates or other pollutants, should be carefully assessed. A CBC can be done to look for hemolysis and signs of concurrent disease.

CAUSES OF ABNORMALLY LOW LEVELS

- Hypokalemia can occur as the result of alkalosis of metabolic or respiratory origin. In alkalosis, cells release H^+ to maintain pH, and K^+ ions are taken up to maintain electrical neutrality. Insulin also causes cells to take up potassium. Therefore, increased insulin, whether from exogenous (e.g., overdosing of insulin) or endogenous (e.g., an insulinoma) sources, can cause hypokalemia.
- A major iatrogenic cause of hypokalemia is excessive diuretic therapy, especially with loop and thiazide diuretics. Dietary deficiency or overhydration can also be a cause of hypokalemia.
- Another major cause of hypokalemia is increased loss via the GI tract. This most commonly occurs through vomiting or diarrhea. Loss of potassium through the kidneys may also be increased.
- Mammals
  - See General Comments.
- Birds
  - Any metabolic disease that affects homeostasis, including diseases of the adrenal glands, can lead to hypokalemia.
  - Alterations in serum chemistry values such as hypoproteinemia or hyperlipemia can also lead to reduced potassium levels.
- Reptiles
  - Hypokalemia in reptiles is associated with similar conditions as in other animals, although metabolic diseases seem to be less important.
- Fish
  - Major causes of hypokalemia in fish include environmental acidity and the presence of infectious disease. In common carp, Gram-negative bacterial infection and some viral infections have been shown to cause hypokalemia.

NEXT DIAGNOSTIC STEPS TO CONSIDER IF LEVELS ARE LOW

- Mammals
  - The first step after diagnosis of hypokalemia is to obtain further blood work, including blood glucose. Sustained hypoglycemia is suspicious for elevated insulin levels, which could be causing the hypokalemia. If hypoglycemia is sustained, this may be beneficial for measurement of blood insulin levels. A blood gas can be done to look for signs of metabolic and respiratory alkalosis. If possible, it may be helpful to measure blood cortisol levels or the sodium-to-potassium ratio to check for hypoadrenocorticism. With hypoadrenocorticism, the cortisol level should be low, and hypernatremia and hypokalemia should be noted.
  - A urinalysis can be performed for examination of kidney function.
  - An abdominal ultrasound can be done to examine the adrenal glands for signs of hypoplasia and the pancreas for signs of an insulinoma. The kidneys should also be examined for signs of renal disease or failure.
- Birds and reptiles
  - After hypokalemia has been diagnosed in a bird, further blood work should be done to assess metabolic status. This should include a blood gas to check for metabolic or respiratory alkalosis, uric acid levels to examine renal function, and albumin and glucose levels.
  - Endoscopic examination of the adrenal gland and the kidneys can be performed to look for signs of renal disease; biopsy specimens can be taken from these organs at the same time.
- Fish
  - The metabolic function of a fish is much more dependent on environmental factors compared with the species previously discussed; therefore, the environment should be the first area of focus in attempts to ascertain the cause of any metabolic disorder. Water quality, including pH, oxygen content, and the presence of nitrates or other pollutants, should be carefully assessed. Cultures for Gram-negative infection should be considered, especially in carp.

SPECIMEN AND PROCESSING CONSIDERATIONS

DRUG EFFECTS ON LEVELS

- Angiotensin-converting enzyme (ACE) inhibitors can cause hyperkalemia, especially in patients with compromised renal function.
- Trimethoprim can cause hyperkalemia by decreasing renal potassium excretion.
- Insulin causes a decrease in serum potassium levels.
- Loop and thiazide diuretics can cause hypokalemia.

LAB ARTIFACTS THAT MAY INTERFERE WITH READINGS OF LEVELS OF THIS SUBSTANCE

- Birds
  - Hemolysis increases potassium levels.
  - ETDA may cause red blood cell (RBC) hemolysis, especially in Brush turkeys, Corvidae, Crowned cranes, Currasows, and Hornbills; this may lead to hyperkalemia.
  - Intracellular shift caused by samples allowed to sit at room temperature may cause hypokalemia.
  - Serum potassium concentration is higher than plasma concentration because of release from thrombocytes during coagulation.
  - In pigeons, plasma potassium is decreased by approximately 60% within 2 hours of the sample being drawn.
  - In chickens, plasma potassium is decreased by approximately 30% within 2 hours of the sample being drawn.
  - In macaws, plasma potassium concentrations are increased approximately 30% within 4 hours.
- Reptiles
  - EDTA can cause RBC lysis, which leads to hyperkalemia.
  - Lymphodepletion from sampling a site other than the jugular can result in decreased potassium.
- Fish
  - Improper or prolonged storage of whole blood can increase potassium levels.
  - Refrigeration of samples for 1 to 3 hours elevates potassium.
  - Major changes in plasma electrolyte concentrations occur when whole blood is stored at room temperature for longer than an hour.

SAMPLE FOR COLLECTION AND ANY SPECIAL SPECIMEN HANDLING NOTES

- *Birds:* biochemistries should be collected in lithium heparinized tubes and then centrifuged to separate serum
- *Reptiles:* use heparinized tubes for chemistry analysis
- *Amphibians:* use heparinized tubes for chemistry analysis
- *Fish:* lithium heparin tubes are preferred for plasma electrolyte analysis

PEARLS

- In case of a urinary blockage, the potassium level should be checked before anesthesia if the animal is scheduled for emergency surgery. It is important to lower the potassium

before anesthesia to avoid cardiac arrest.
- *Fish:* ETDA causes hemolysis in fish anesthetized with tricaine.

REFERENCES

Carpenter JW, et al: Exotic animal formulary, ed 2, Philadelphia, 2001, WB Saunders, pp 36, 80–86, 195–208, 213, 256, 268, 292, 320, 344, 363, 386–387.

Fudge AM: Laboratory medicine: avian and exotic pets, ed 1, Philadelphia, 2000, WB Saunders, pp 63, 218, 317–318.

Groff JM, et al: Hematology and clinical chemistry of cyprinid fish, Vet Clin North Am 2:741–776, 1999.

Hoegeman S: Diagnostic sampling of amphibians, Vet Clin North Am 2:731–740, 1999.

Jones MP: Avian clinical pathology, Vet Clin North Am 2:663–688, 1999.

Redrobe S, et al: Sample collection and clinical pathology of reptiles, Vet Clin North Am 2:709–730, 1999.

Stockham SL, et al: Fundamentals of veterinary clinical pathology, ed 1, Ames, IA, 2002, Iowa State Press, pp 350–357.

AUTHOR: **JONATHAN W. BALL**

EDITOR: **JÖRG MAYER**

Protein, Total

DEFINITION

- Total serum protein levels measure the total amount of protein in serum (serum is the fluid portion of blood, without fibrinogen). Total plasma protein levels measure the protein in plasma (fluid portion of blood with fibrinogen).
- Proteins in the serum are composed of albumin, antibodies, complement, different enzymes, coagulation factors, and transport proteins, with albumin and globulins making up the vast majority.

SYNONYMS

TPP, TP, serum protein, total solids

PHYSIOLOGY

Serum or plasma proteins are primarily synthesized in the liver; a smaller percentage due to immunoglobulins is produced by lymphocytes and plasma cells. Total protein consists of albumin, globulins, and fibrinogen (in plasma only). Proteins function to control oncotic pressure, transport substances (hemoglobin, lipids, calcium), and promote inflammation and the complement cascade. Changes in total protein levels are due mostly to changes in albumin concentration. More information concerning protein can be found in Albumin, Sec. IV. Electrophoresis is a common diagnostic tool used to track and identify abnormalities in different blood proteins.

TYPICAL NORMAL RANGE

The typical normal range for this laboratory test varies greatly among species. The reader is referred to the following Elsevier publications for additional information:

Carpenter J: Exotic animal formulary, ed 4, St Louis, 2013, Saunders.

Mader D: Reptile medicine and surgery, ed 2, St Louis, 2006, Saunders.

CLINICAL APPLICATIONS

CAUSES OF ABNORMALLY HIGH LEVELS
- Values can vary by breed and by age, but increased levels are consistent with dehydration, hypovolemia (albumin), chronic disease, neoplasia (lymphosarcoma and hepatic carcinoma) (globulin), acute inflammation (globulin), infection, prolonged hyperthermia, and anabolic steroids.
- In female birds, a higher level of total protein can be observed during egg laying.

NEXT DIAGNOSTIC STEPS TO CONSIDER IF LEVELS ARE HIGH Rule out dehydration by checking packed cell volume (PCV) or hematocrit. A concurrent elevation in PCV and TPP suggests dehydration. Rule out parasitism with a direct fecal smear and float and a CBC to determine whether an underlying infectious process is occurring. Perform an electrophoresis to determine which protein fraction is causing the elevation.

CAUSES OF ABNORMALLY LOW LEVELS Panhypoproteinemia can be seen with renal (glomerular) or hepatic disease in which increased loss and decreased production are occurring respectively. Lower levels can be a consequence of overhydration/hemodilution, hemorrhage, intestinal parasitism, young animals (<6 months old), and starvation/malnutrition. Specific causes of hypoalbuminemia include decreased protein intake, decreased absorption/pancreatic dysfunction, gastrointestinal loss, renal disease, hepatic disease, septicemia, dermatopathies (burns—excessive serum exudates), and congestive heart failure.

NEXT DIAGNOSTIC STEPS TO CONSIDER IF LEVELS ARE LOW An equally low PCV is suggestive of overhydration. An elevated bile acid level and reduced urea are consistent with hepatic disease. Check for proteinuria if renal involvement is suspected. Effects of hemorrhage will be apparent 2 to 3 hours post blood loss and will be accompanied by a low PCV. Perform an electrophoresis.

IMPORTANT INTERSPECIES DIFFERENCES
- *Birds and reptiles:* avian total protein is about half the value of mammalian species. Lymphoid hypoplasia, aplasia, and psittacine circovirus infections (psittacine beak and feather disease [PBFD]) can contribute to decreased protein levels. Elevated levels can be seen with lymphoproliferative conditions such as *Chlamydophila* infection, egg yolk peritonitis, and tuberculosis. *Raptor* species typically have higher total protein, and the value tends to increase with the overall size of the raptor. Egg-laying females have been shown to have an increase in total protein.
- *Fish:* changes in TPP can occur with stress, seasonal effects on temperature and metabolic activity, size, sex, nutritional status, and composition of feed. Low protein levels have been associated with starvation, chronic stress, hepatic disease, and infectious disease. Bacterial skin disease can result in passive loss of protein and influx of water, leading to hemodilution, which can lower total plasma protein.

SPECIMEN AND PROCESSING CONSIDERATIONS

DRUG EFFECTS ON LEVELS None specifically known in exotic pets. In dogs and cats, an increase is reported with testosterone, estrogens, and growth hormone, and a decrease has been associated with thyroxine and cortisol.

LAB ARTIFACTS THAT MAY INTERFERE WITH READINGS OF LEVELS OF THIS SUBSTANCE Chromagens (hemolysis), lipids, and glucose can artificially increase values when measured with a refractometer or by chemical measurement. High levels of solutes such as urea, glucose, cholesterol, sodium, or dextran can artificially increase TPP. Total plasma protein levels are more accurate than total serum protein levels taken with a refractometer. Protein electrophoresis is a reliable method for determining protein levels.

SAMPLE FOR COLLECTION AND ANY SPECIAL SPECIMEN HANDLING NOTES Heparinized plasma or serum: collect in a green top for reptiles and avian species, in a red top for mammal species.

AUTHOR: **CANDACE HERSEY-BENNER**

EDITOR: **JÖRG MAYER**

Red Blood Cell (RBC) Count

DEFINITION

- The number of blood cells in a given sample of blood; usually expressed as the number of cells per liter of blood (RBCs [red blood cells] × 10^{12}/L, vs. WBCs and platelets × 10^9/L).
- Measurement is often performed with a differential white cell count to determine the numbers of various types of leukocytes in the sample. Cell counts are useful in the diagnosis of various blood dyscrasias, anemias, infections, and other abnormal conditions of the body. This is one of the tests most commonly done on blood.
- Packed cell volume (PCV) or hematocrit (HCT) is an indirect measure of RBC numbers, expressed as a percentage of the total volume of blood. PCV, by common usage, has become synonymous with HCT. Traditionally, PCV is obtained by centrifuging an anticoagulated blood sample; with automated counters, this value is calculated from measurements of mean cell volume (MCV) and RBC count. As a result, automated laboratory values may differ slightly from in-clinic manual values.

SYNONYMS

- Blood count
- Packed cell volume (PCV) and hematocrit (HCT) are used to represent the RBC count, but they reflect both cell count and volume (MCV).

PHYSIOLOGY

- RBCs derive from erythroblasts in the bone marrow. Clones of dividing blasts and maturing erythroid precursors occupy discrete erythroid islands in the marrow, interspersed between more diffuse myeloid elements. Precursor red cells engage in continual production of hemoglobin from heme and globin. Iron is an integral component of each heme molecule, and the process is dependent on the production of erythropoietin in the kidney. In mammals, the red cell nucleus undergoes degeneration and is extruded before the reticulocyte and mature cell stages. In these species, nucleated red cells should not be observed in the peripheral blood. In avians, amphibians, fish, and reptiles, the nucleus is retained in the mature red cell. Red cells are normally circulated at the mature or reticulocyte stage. This represents a cell that has not yet lost cytoplasmic ribosomes and thus is still engaging in protein synthesis for several days in the periphery. Ribosomes and RNA impart a basophilic staining to the erythrocyte cytoplasm and sometimes can be observed on hematoxylin and eosin (H&E) as polychromatic cells. More specific dyes are used for reticulocyte counting. Mature red cells vary in size according to species. In birds, red cell size is proportional to species size. Reptiles have very large erythrocytes. Lifespan varies. It is shortest in avians (28 days in chickens) and longest in reptiles (up to 800 days).
- Red cell numbers are regulated by hemoglobin mass and oxygenation. The percentage of blood volume containing red cells—the PCV or hematocrit—is fairly stable between species, such that smaller red cells are normally associated with higher concentrations. Counts vary normally with life stage and environmental conditions (altitude, hibernation), as well as pathologically from primary or secondary phenomena. An abnormal increase in red cell numbers is called *polycythemia.* It can be primary from excessive production or, more commonly, secondary from impaired oxygenation or drug effects. A reduction in red cell numbers is called *anemia.* Anemia can be due to failure in red cell or hemoglobin production from nutritional disorders, chronic diseases and infections, and malignancy. Anemia can also result from premature destruction of cells by hemolysis of infected or self-targeted cells, or by blood loss from trauma or internal (gastrointestinal) losses. Depending on the nutritional and physical condition of the host, a response to anemia can be seen with increased immature reticulocytes in the periphery.

TYPICAL NORMAL RANGE

The typical normal range for this laboratory test varies greatly among species. The reader is referred to the following Elsevier publications for additional information:

Carpenter J: Exotic animal formulary, ed 4, St Louis, 2013, Saunders.

Mader D: Reptile medicine and surgery, ed 2, St Louis, 2006, Saunders.

CLINICAL APPLICATIONS

CAUSES OF ABNORMALLY HIGH LEVELS

- Increased concentration of RBCs or PCV with normal plasma protein suggests primary or secondary polycythemia. Primary polycythemia results from increased bone marrow production of RBCs. Secondary polycythemia is a compensatory, erythropoietin-dependent increase in RBC mass due to decreased oxygen levels, most commonly resulting from lung disease. Secondary polycythemia can also result from drugs that elevate erythropoietin, including androgens, corticosteroids, and prostaglandins. Paraneoplastic production of erythropoietin from renal cell carcinomas and lymphosarcomas has been reported in mammals.
- Increased concentration of RBCs or PCV accompanied by an increase in plasma protein suggests dehydration, hemoconcentration, or hypovolemia (relative polycythemia).
- Splenic contracture from a significant stress response can cause elevations in RBCs in mammals, but this is rare in birds.

NEXT DIAGNOSTIC STEPS TO CONSIDER IF LEVELS ARE HIGH

- Perform a careful physical examination and history, including medications. Assess for potential causes of the stress response.
- Clinically assess patient for evidence of dehydration (mucous membranes, skin turgor). Examine the electrolytes for evidence of hemoconcentration (prerenal azotemia, uremia, hypercalcemia, and hyperglycemia with elevated total plasma protein). Repeat studies after replacement of the fluid deficit.
- Examine red cell morphology (schistocytes, target cells) and indices (microcytosis) to rule out compensatory erythrocytosis resulting from impaired hemoglobin production.
- If levels remain elevated, assess for secondary polycythemia from impaired oxygenation (pneumonia, pulmonary hypersensitivity) marked by hypoxia, tachypnea, dyspnea, and x-ray abnormalities. Check for potential drug causes or renal tumors.
- If these findings are negative, consider bone marrow biopsy to assess for increased production from malignancy (primary polycythemia).

CAUSES OF ABNORMALLY LOW LEVELS

- Anemia occurs when the red cell mass falls below the reference range for the age, sex, and breed of the species concerned. Laboratory assessment reveals low values for PCV, hemoglobin, and RBC count. Mean corpuscular volume (MCV), mean corpuscular hemoglobin concentration (MCHC), and red cell distribution width percentage (RDW) vary according to the underlying cause.
- Anemias are most often classified using red cell indices rather than by specific cause.
- Hypochromic microcytic anemias
  - Indices
    - Decreased MCV
    - Decreased MCHC
    - Increased polychromasia
    - Normal to increased RDW
  - Causes
    - Nutritional deficiencies (iron)
    - Chronic, indolent hemorrhage
    - Parasites (blood-sucking ectoparasites)
- Hypochromic macrocytic anemias
  - Indices
    - Increased MCV
    - Decreased MCHC
    - Increased polychromasia
    - Normal to increased RDW
  - Causes
    - Acute blood loss with marrow response
    - Chronic gastrointestinal bleeding with response
    - Hemolytic anemias with marrow response
    - Early response to lead toxicity
    - Nutritional deficiencies in mammals (folate, B_{12})
    - Toxins (rapeseed in birds)
- Normochromic normocytic anemias
  - Indices
    - Normal MCV
    - Normal MCHC
    - Slight or no polychromasia
    - Normal or slightly increased RDW
  - Causes
    - Anemia of chronic disease and neoplasms
    - Bacterial infections (tuberculosis, chlamydiosis)
    - Systemic fungal infections (aspergillosis)
    - Viral illnesses
    - Hyperestrogenism from prolonged estrus
    - Starvation/malnutrition
- Anemias are also classified by response (nonregenerative or regenerative).
- Nonregenerative anemias lack reticulocytosis to replace red cell losses. During the first 2 to 3 days after hemorrhage or hemolysis, anemia may be nonregenerative. When no response is seen for several days, this suggests a primary or secondary bone marrow disorder. Nonregenerative anemias are characterized by decreased RDW and polychromasia, indicating lack of larger, more basophilic reticulocytes.
- Regenerative (responsive) anemias occur when the bone marrow is actively responding to losses or destruction by increasing production of RBCs. Findings that indicate regenerative anemia include polychromasia, reticulocytosis, and hypercellular bone marrow with a low myeloid-to-erythroid ratio. Regenerative anemias require sufficient time for regeneration to occur (2 to 3 days), adequate blood-forming elements (iron, appropriate vitamins, protein), sufficient erythrocytic colonies in the bone marrow, and adequate kidney function to form erythropoietin.

NEXT DIAGNOSTIC STEPS TO CONSIDER IF LEVELS ARE LOW

- Perform a careful physical examination and history, including diet and medications. Assess for potential chronic/underlying disease causes of anemia.
- Assess for clinical signs of anemia (pale mucous membranes, etc.).
- Laboratory assessment of RBC count, PCV, hemoglobin, MCV, RDW, MCHC, and reticulocyte count. Obtain electrolytes to examine for dehydration/dilution effects and a leukogram to rule out diminished red cell production from bone marrow replacement by leukemia.
- Perform a manual analysis of the blood smear to assess RBC size, shape (spherical, targetoid, schistocytes), nucleation, and staining characteristics (polychromasia suggestive of reticulocytosis, stippling suggestive of metal toxicity). Assess for parasites in the red and white cells. Examine platelets and white cells for additional abnormalities.
- Perform a urinalysis for possible hematuria/hemoglobinuria.
- Perform a fecal examination for occult gastrointestinal blood loss.

IMPORTANT INTERSPECIES DIFFERENCES

- Birds
  - Mature avian erythrocytes generally are larger than mammalian erythrocytes but smaller than reptilian erythrocytes. RBC size varies from 135 femtoliters (fL) in the cockatiel to 165 fL in the macaw to 220 fL in the ostrich. RBC counts show a broader range of normal values among different birds. A general rule of thumb is that PCV is similar between species, so smaller avian species will have smaller erythrocytes and higher total RBC counts. The avian erythrocyte half-life is much shorter than in mammals (chickens, 28 days). Mature avian erythrocytes are elliptical and have an elliptical, centrally positioned nucleus. The nuclear chromatin is uniformly clumped and becomes increasingly condensed with age. A slight degree of anisocytosis is considered to be normal for birds.
  - Macaws of the *Ara* genus, particularly blue and gold macaws (*Ara arauna*), are susceptible to respiratory hypersensitivity marked by interstitial pneumonitis with fibrosis. Secondary polycythemia commonly develops, and PCV often exceeds 60%. Primary polycythemia is very rare in pet birds.
  - In addition to the causes of anemia already listed, specific entities are found in some birds. Conures (*Aratinga* spp.) can have spontaneous bleeding associated with coagulopathy of unknown origin. Acute somnolence, hemoptysis, and possible internal bleeding are accompanied by a regenerative anemia. Yolk peritonitis is associated with a normochromic, normocytic anemia of chronic disease.
- Amphibians
  - Erythrocytes of amphibians are nucleated, elliptical discs with homogeneous cytoplasm and a distinct nuclear bulge and irregular nuclear margins. The mean size of a variety of frog and toad erythrocytes is 22 × 14 μm. Salamanders

and newts complete their erythrocyte maturation in the peripheral circulation. As a result, the cytoplasm is heterogeneous and on ultrastructural examination contains clusters of granular and vacuolar bodies. Some amphibians, such as the slender salamander *(Batrachoceps attenuatus)*, lack nuclei in most of their erythrocytes.

- Reptiles
  - Mature erythrocytes in reptiles generally are larger than those in birds and mammals and have extremely long lifespans of up to 600 to 800 days. RBC counts are highest just before hibernation and lowest immediately after hibernation. Males generally have higher counts than females. Reptilian erythrocytes are ellipsoidal cells with centrally positioned, oval to round nuclei, dense purple chromatin, and often irregular margins. Slight to moderate anisocytosis is common, and immature red cells and mitotic red cells are frequently observed in the periphery, especially during shedding and post hibernation. Anemias are usually accompanied by minimal response owing to the long life span of red cells. Reptilian reticulocytes, similar to avian reticulocytes, have a distinct ring of aggregated reticulum that encircles the red cell nucleus. Hemoparasites are common in reptiles and can result in hemolytic anemias. Common organisms include trypanosomes, *Hemogregarina* spp., *Hepatozoan* spp., *Karyolysis* spp., *Plasmodium* spp., *Hemoproteus* spp., *Schellackia* spp., *Babesia* spp., *Aegyptianella* spp., *Sauroplasma* spp., *Serpentoplasma* spp., and *Leishmania* spp. Certain viruses are associated with inclusions and hemolysis (iridovirus). Neoplasms are rare causes of anemia in reptiles.
- Rabbits
  - Rabbit erythrocytes are anucleate biconcave discs with an average volume of 65 fL and a half-life of 57 to 67 days. Regenerative anemias most often are the result of lead toxicity because gastrointestinal ulcers and bleeding are infrequent in rabbits. A hypochromic macrocytic anemia with basophilic stippling is observed. Sources of lead in the home (paint) and the cage should be sought. Nonregenerative anemias are seen with infection (*Pasteurella*, chronic otitis, abscesses, cellulitis, pneumonia, pyometra, mastitis), renal disease, or neoplasms (uterine adenocarcinoma, lymphosarcoma). High-dose ivermectin therapy is associated with a microcytic nonregenerative anemia.
- Ferrets
  - Ferret RBCs are anucleate biconcave discs with an average volume of 50 fL. The half-life is believed similar to cats. Anemia is common and in unspayed females results from hyperestrogenism from prolonged estrus. Gastrointestinal losses are most common overall and result from gastric and duodenal ulcers, foreign bodies, and colitis. Flea infestations are also associated with blood loss and anemia. Hemolytic anemia can result from Aleutian disease virus infection. Lead and zinc toxicosis are seen and result in hypochromic regenerative anemias. Nonregenerative anemias are seen most frequently with chronic renal disease and less often with hemolytic anemias and lymphoma.

SPECIMEN AND PROCESSING CONSIDERATIONS

DRUG EFFECTS ON LEVELS

- Drugs that decrease RBCs
  - Corticosteroids, cyclophosphamide, high-dose ivermection (bone marrow suppression)
  - Phenylhydrazine (hemolytic anemia)
- Lead toxicity (macrocytic hypochromic anemia)
- Anesthetic agents such as isoflurane, enflurane, and halothane can result in significant (up to 33%) and rapid decreases in RBC count, hematocrit, and hemoglobin concentration (ferrets).
- Drugs that increase RBCs
  - Erythropoietin, androgens, corticosteroids, epinephrine, and prostaglandins

LAB ARTIFACTS THAT MAY INTERFERE WITH READINGS OF LEVELS OF THIS SUBSTANCE

- Erythrocyte clumping or agglutination (observed in autoimmune disease, malignancies) can cause falsely depressed red cell counts.
- Hemolysis can occur during traumatic venipuncture or post collection with prolonged intervals before analysis, resulting in low counts.
- Whole blood collected in additive-free tubes (red top) without anticoagulant or in slow collections is prone to clot and can result in low counts.
- Excessive hemoconcentration from fluid loss can produce artificially elevated red cell counts.
- Atypical erythrocytes occasionally are present in the peripheral blood of normal birds; such erythrocytes may represent artifacts associated with preparation.

SAMPLE FOR COLLECTION AND ANY SPECIAL SPECIMEN HANDLING NOTES

- Birds
  - Laboratory evaluation of avian erythrocytes involves the same routine procedures as those used in mammalian hematology, but with a few modifications. The standard manual technique for using microhematocrit capillary tubes and centrifugation (12,000*g* for 5 minutes) can be used to obtain a PCV, but this is not optimal because of microclots and sludging. Hemoglobin concentration is determined by the cyanmethemoglobin method; however, free nuclei from lysed erythrocytes must be removed by centrifugation of the cyanmethemoglobin reagent–blood mixture before the optical density value is obtained, to avoid overestimation of the hemoglobin concentration. The total erythrocyte concentration in birds can be determined using the same automated or manual methods as are used for determining total erythrocyte counts in mammalian blood. Two manual methods for obtaining total red blood cell count in birds are the erythrocyte unopette (Becton-Dickinson, Franklin Lakes, NJ) method used in mammalian hematology and the Natt-Herrick method, which involves preparation of Natt-Herrick solution to be used as stain and diluent.
- Ferrets
  - Ferrets are commonly anesthetized for blood collection. Anesthetics such as isoflurane, enflurane, and halothane can produce significant (up to 33%) and rapid decreases in red blood cell count, hematocrit, and hemoglobin concentration, especially with prolonged use.
- Amphibians
  - The microhematocrit method is used for obtaining a PCV; this is the method used most commonly for evaluating the red cell mass of amphibians. The cyanmethemoglobin method is used commonly to determine hemoglobin concentration in amphibian blood. As with hemoglobin determinations in birds, reptiles, and fish, the procedure requires centrifugation of the blood-cyanmethemoglobin mixture to remove free erythrocyte nuclei before optical density is measured. Total erythrocyte count in amphibians can be determined by manual counting with a hemocytometer or with use of an electronic cell counter.

PEARLS

- Birds
  - Because PCV is generally preserved across species, the smaller the avian species, the smaller the erythrocytes (MCV) and the higher the total RBC count. Avian erythrocytes are nucleated.
  - Anemia is a common clinical finding in pet birds because of the short half-life of the avian erythrocyte.
- Amphibians
  - Salamanders and newts complete their erythrocyte maturation in the peripheral circulation; some lack nuclei in most circulating red cells.
- Reptiles
  - Reptilians have large red cells with long lifespans. Anemias are commonly associated with parasitic infection and often have a blunted, prolonged marrow response.
- Rabbits
  - Regenerative anemias can be associated with environmental lead toxicity. Nonregenerative anemias are commonly due to chronic infection or to high-dose ivermectin therapy.
- Ferrets
  - Gastrointestinal blood losses are the most common causes of anemia. Prolonged estrus in females also is commonly observed. Use caution with inhaled anesthetics because they are associated with rapid decreases in RBC count, hematocrit, and hemoglobin concentration, especially with prolonged use.

REFERENCES

Blood DC, et al: Saunders comprehensive veterinary dictionary, ed 2, Philadelphia, 1999, WB Saunders.

Campbell TW: Clinical pathology. In Mader DR, editor: Reptile medicine and surgery, ed 2, Philadelphia, 1996, WB Saunders.

Carpenter JW: Exotic animal formulary, ed 3, Philadelphia, 2004, WB Saunders.

Fudge AM: Laboratory medicine: avian and exotic pets, Philadelphia, 2000, WB Saunders.

Harcourt-Brown F: Textbook of rabbit medicine, Boston, 2002, Butterworth-Heinemann.

Harrison GJ, et al: Clinical avian medicine, South Palm Beach, FL, 2006, Spix Publishing.

Quesenberry KE, et al: Ferrets, rabbits, and rodents: clinical medicine and surgery, ed 2, St Louis, 2004, Saunders.

Thrall MA, et al: Veterinary hematology and clinical chemistry, Philadelphia, 2004, Lippincott Williams & Wilkins.

Willard MD, et al: Small animal clinical diagnosis by laboratory methods, St Louis, 2004, Saunders.

AUTHOR: **JULIE DECUBELLIS**

EDITOR: **JÖRG MAYER**

Reticulocyte Count

DEFINITION

Reticulocytes are precursors to erythrocytes that have expelled the nucleus. They are larger in volume but have less hemoglobin than mature erythrocytes.

SYNONYM

Polychromatophilic erythrocyte

PHYSIOLOGY

- A regenerative response by the bone marrow is best indicated by increased numbers of immature erythrocytes, better known as *reticulocytes.*
- These are cells that have recently entered the peripheral circulation; increases are seen along with polychromasia.
- A reticulocyte has decreased hemoglobin content in relation to increased volume as compared with a mature red blood cell (RBC).
- Reticulocytes are larger and contain ribosomes, which disappear when the RBC is fully mature.
- In species with a nucleated RBC, immature erythrocytes are seen as rounder cells with a bluer cytoplasm, and the nuclear chromatin appears as more dense and scattered.
- In some species, small quantities of reticulocytes are a normal finding. A regenerative response to anemia should result in a greater number of reticulocytes than are seen during health.
- It typically takes 3 to 5 days before you can see a response to anemia, with a peak response noted after 7 to 10 days. Reticulocyte counts are expressed as a percentage of red cells, thus they can be falsely elevated by decreased numbers of red blood cells. Reticulocytosis can be indicative of hemolysis or hemorrhage. Reticulocytosis can be present with or without the presence of anemia.

TYPICAL NORMAL RANGE

- Birds
  - Most birds: 2% to 8%
- Small mammals
  - Majority of small mammals: 1% to 2%
  - Rabbits: 2% to 4%
  - Hedgehogs: 8% to 14%
  - Albino male ferrets: 1% to 20% (mean, 4.0%)

CLINICAL APPLICATIONS

CAUSES OF ABNORMALLY HIGH LEVELS

- Hemorrhagic: blood loss due to trauma, gastrointestinal parasitism, coagulation disorders, ulceration, and some viral diseases
- Hemolytic anemia: parasites (*Plasmodium* spp. in birds), bacterial septicemia, acute toxicosis (oil ingestion, lead), burns, and immune-mediated conditions

NEXT DIAGNOSTIC STEPS TO CONSIDER IF LEVELS ARE HIGH

- Evaluate RBC morphology.
- Reevaluate in 3 to 5 days to allow bone marrow to mount a sufficient regenerative response.
- Perform bone marrow aspirate/biopsy.
- Determine and correct the cause of regenerative anemia.

CAUSES OF ABNORMALLY LOW LEVELS

- Nonregenerative anemia by a primary marrow disorder or by a systemic disease resulting in suppression of erythropoiesis
- Decreased levels of erythropoietin
- Iron deficiency

NEXT DIAGNOSTIC STEPS TO CONSIDER IF LEVELS ARE LOW

- Perform bone marrow aspirate or biopsy.
- Determine cause of nonregenerative anemia.

IMPORTANT INTERSPECIES DIFFERENCES Reptilian reticulocytes usually are smaller and rounder than mature erythrocytes.

SPECIMEN AND PROCESSING CONSIDERATIONS

SAMPLE FOR COLLECTION AND ANY SPECIAL SPECIMEN HANDLING NOTES

- Small mammals

- Small blood samples (<2 mL) should be placed in microtainers. Heparin microtainers are preferred because more plasma can be obtained from small samples.
- New methylene blue stain is incubated 15 minutes with whole blood before preparation for a reticulocyte count.

- Birds
  - For differential counts, it is best if slides can be made from fresh whole blood.
  - Use EDTA (purple top) tubes to collect for complete blood count (CBC) in most species.
  - ETDA may cause RBC hemolysis, especially in Brush turkeys, Corvidae, Crowned cranes, Currasows, and Hornbills.
- Reptiles
  - ETDA may cause RBC hemolysis in some species.
  - Use heparinized (green top) tubes when collecting CBC samples.
  - Heparin may create a blue tinge to blood smears and clumping of thrombocytes and leukocytes.
  - If plenty of blood is available, submit paired sample (one EDTA and one heparin), and let the clinical pathologist decide which sample is of superior quality.
  - Blood smears for staining may best be made from blood containing no anticoagulant.

PEARLS

- Age, sex, nutritional status, season, and environmental conditions may affect the results of biochemical assays in reptiles.
- Best seen with new methylene blue stain, which stains the characteristic clumps of residual cytoplasmic RNA
- The reticulocyte count is considered the gold standard in determining whether an anemia is considered regenerative or nonregenerative.
- The reticulocyte count usually is not included in a normal CBC and must be ordered separately.
- Note that the healthy ferret can have a relatively high reticulocyte count in comparison with other species.

AUTHOR: **CARALEE MANLEY**

EDITOR: **JÖRG MAYER**

Sodium

DEFINITION

Sodium is the primary cation (positive ion) in extracellular fluids in animals.

SYNONYMS

Na, Na^+

PHYSIOLOGY

Sodium, which is present mainly in the extracellular fluid (ECF), aids in determining the volume of the ECF and its osmotic pressure. Changes in serum sodium concentration always reflect changes in water balance. Serum sodium concentration indicates the amount of sodium relative to the amount of water in the extracellular fluid and provides no direct information about the total body sodium content. Increased serum sodium concentration indicates hyperosmolality and develops when water intake has been inadequate, when fluid lost is hypotonic to ECF, or when an excessive amount of sodium has been ingested or administered. Cell membranes are relatively impermeable, and a "sodium pump" is needed to return sodium that does enter the ECF. The amount of sodium is regulated primarily by the kidney. Decreased serum sodium occurs when hypo-osmolality is developing, when an animal is unable to excrete ingested water, or when urinary and insensible losses have combined osmolality greater than that of ingested or parenterally administered fluids. Water and sodium are controlled by atrial natriuretic peptide (ANP) (causes natriuresis by increasing glomerular filtration rate [GFR], inhibiting tubular sodium reabsorption, and decreasing the production of renin). The renin-angiotensin-aldosterone system (RAAS) is stimulated by decreased renal perfusion pressure in the afferent arteriole and ultimately produces angiotensin II, which leads to increased tubular sodium reabsorption. Antidiuretic hormone (ADH) is synthesized in the hypothalamus and is stimulated by the hypertonicity of the plasma, which is sensed by osmoreceptors in the hypothalamus. A change in serum sodium concentration as small as 1% to 2% can cause release of ADH. Hypernatremia always reflects a free water deficit.

TYPICAL NORMAL RANGE

The typical normal range for this laboratory test varies greatly among species. The reader is referred to the following Elsevier publications for additional information:

Carpenter J: Exotic animal formulary, ed 4, St Louis, 2013, Saunders.

Mader D: Reptile medicine and surgery, ed 2, St Louis, 2006, Saunders.

CLINICAL APPLICATIONS

CAUSES OF ABNORMALLY HIGH LEVELS

- Hypernatremia can be caused by increased sodium intake from a highly salty diet or seawater, or from salt poisoning.
- Administration of sodium-containing IV fluids (e.g., isotonic saline solution) and primary hypoaldosteronism can elevate levels.
- Dehydration from vomiting or regurgitation, diarrhea, increased water deprivation from panting due to heatstroke, fever, or hyperventilation may cause hypernatremia.
- High-protein diets cause a marked urea-induced diuresis and resultant hypernatremia.
- Decreased water intake may result from water not being provided or from insufficient intake of water; this also may be caused by an inability to drink (CNS damage, brain tumor, senility, pharyngeal problems), by being comatose or debilitated, or as the result of prolonged postop anesthesia.
- Hypoadrenocorticism might possibly cause hypernatremia.

NEXT DIAGNOSTIC STEPS TO CONSIDER IF LEVELS ARE HIGH

- Evaluate packed cell volume (PCV) and total protein for status of hydration.
- Determine urine specific gravity.
- Check for diseases already listed.

CAUSES OF ABNORMALLY LOW LEVELS

- GI losses from severe diarrhea or vomiting may cause hyponatremia. Initially, sodium concentration is maintained in the ECF by allowing a corresponding water loss to occur. Eventually, the fall in ECF, cardiac output, and blood pressure triggers increased ADH secretion, and water is replaced and conserved, resulting in

further sodium loss (increased PCV and total plasma protein are noted).
- End-stage chronic renal failure causes sodium excretion to remain high (look for increased urea, creatinine, and phosphate levels).
- Diuretic therapy: "loop" diuretics (furosemide) inhibit active reabsorption of sodium in the ascending limb of the loop of Henle. Benzothiadiazines act in the convoluted part of the distal tubule to block sodium reabsorption. An aldosterone antagonist (e.g., spironolactone) limits sodium in the distal tubule by competing with aldosterone for receptor sites. Use of hypertonic dextrose and mannitol induces an osmotic diuresis.
- Overhydration from excessive water intake (psychogenic polydipsia; look for low urinary specific gravity), acute renal failure (polyuric phase), and administration of sodium-free or low-sodium solutions (0.45% saline or isotonic 5% dextrose solution). The response stimulates ADH secretion, thirst, and subsequent water retention.
- Reduced renal perfusion from edema, ascites, and hydrothorax and resultant increased blood pressure (e.g., congestive heart failure) may cause hyponatremia.
- Third space loss from pleural effusion, abdominal effusion, or obstructive bowel disease may cause hyponatremia.
- Patients with a ruptured bladder with subsequent uroabdomen have a low sodium concentration in their abdomen. Because of the small size of the sodium ion, it rapidly diffuses across the peritoneal lining, down its concentration gradient from the plasma, and into the abdominal fluid. This also occurs with ascites from liver failure.
- Depressed sodium levels can result from congestive heart failure, which causes inappropriate water retention in excess of sodium, extensive dermatitis or burns, milk (mastitis), salivary losses, sweating, end-stage liver disease, and hypoadrenocorticism.
- Juvenile levels are low in avian species.

NEXT DIAGNOSTIC STEPS TO CONSIDER IF LEVELS ARE LOW
- Evaluate PCV and total protein for evidence of dehydration.
- Evaluate urea, creatinine, and phosphate levels for evidence of renal failure.
- Evaluate specific gravity for evidence of overhydration or renal failure.
- Calculate plasma osmolality; if normal or high, can rule out renal failure or pseudohyponatremia (e.g., hyperlipidemia, hyperproteinemia, mannitol)
- Urine osmolality
- Urine sodium concentration

IMPORTANT INTERSPECIES DIFFERENCES Some marine avian species have nasal salt or supraorbital glands that enable them to secrete large amounts of sodium in response to osmotic changes.

SPECIMEN AND PROCESSING CONSIDERATIONS

DRUG EFFECTS ON LEVELS
- Elevated serum levels can be caused by lithium, demeclocycline, and amphotericin.
- Mannitol can falsely depress sodium levels.

LAB ARTIFACTS THAT MAY INTERFERE WITH READINGS OF LEVELS OF THIS SUBSTANCE
- Hyperlipidemia and hyperproteinemia will result in falsely depressed levels of sodium. This occurs when the plasma has a high proportion of lipids or proteins, which dilute the sodium.
- Mishandling (dehydration) of the blood sample can artifactually increase levels.

SAMPLE FOR COLLECTION AND ANY SPECIAL SPECIMEN HANDLING NOTES
- *Reptiles:* plasma is preferred over serum for chemistries because clot formation may be prolonged in reptiles and may change serum electrolyte and glucose values. Also, a greater volume per unit of blood can be obtained.
- *Birds:* lithium heparin is the anticoagulant of choice for most avian blood samples; evaluation of biochemistries is most commonly obtained from plasma.
- *Small mammals:* small blood samples (<2 mL) should be placed in microtainers. Heparin microtainers are preferred because more plasma can be obtained from small samples.
- All samples should be centrifuged and plasma/serum separated from cells as soon as possible; tests should be run immediately or the specimen should be transported frozen.

REFERENCES

Campbell TW: Clinical pathology. In Mader DR, editor: Reptile medicine and surgery, Philadelphia, 1996, WB Saunders.

Carpenter JW: Exotic animal formulary, ed 3, Philadelphia, 2004, WB Saunders.

Fudge AM, editor: Laboratory medicine: avian and exotic pets, Philadelphia, 2000, WB Saunders.

Jones MP: Avian clinical pathology, Vet Clin North Am Exot Anim Pract 2:663–687, 1999.

Stoskopf MK, editor: Fish medicine, Philadelphia, 1993, WB Saunders.

AUTHOR: **CARALEE MANLEY**

EDITOR: **JÖRG MAYER**

Thyroid Hormones

DEFINITION
- Thyroxine (T_4) is the major storage form of iodine-containing thyroid hormone.
- Free T_4 (fT_4) is the biologically available, non–protein-bound form of the hormone able to enter cells.
- T_3 is the active form of the thyroid hormone.
- Chief function is to increase rate of cell metabolism.

SYNONYMS
T_4, T_3

PHYSIOLOGY
- Up to 99.9% of T_4 is protein bound in the circulation and therefore is not biologically active.
- Thyroxine is deiodinated to the active form of the hormone (T_3) in cells. It binds to receptor proteins in cells, inducing DNA translation and production of proteins associated with cell growth, oxidative phosphorylation, and membrane transport of electrolytes, resulting in an increase in metabolic rate and growth stimulation.

TYPICAL NORMAL RANGE

Chemistry	U.S. Units	→	S.I. Units
Thyroxine (T_4)	1 μg/dL	Converts to	13.00 nmol/L
Chemistry	**S.I. Units**	**→**	**U.S. Units**
Thyroxine (T_4)	1 nmol/L	Converts to	0.07 μg/dL

1 nmol/L of Total (T3) Triiodothyronine converts to 64.94 ng/dL. 1 ng/dL of Total (T3) Triiodothyronine converts to 0.02 nmol/L.

Mammals		
Rat	T_4: 3-7 μg/dL	T_3: 25-100 ng/dL
Mouse	T_4: 4-7 μg/dL	T_3: 65-140 ng/dL
Hamster	T_4: 3-7 μg/dL	T_3: 30-80 ng/dL
Guinea pig	T_4: male, 2.9 ± 0.6 μg/dL	T_3: male, 39 ± 17 ng/dL
	T_4: female, 3.2 ± 0.7 μg/dL	T_3: female, 44 ± 10 ng/dL
	Free T_4: male, 1.26 ± 0.41 ng/dL	Free T_3: female, 260 ± 59 pg/dL
Ferret	T_4: male, 3.24 ± 1.65 μg/dL	T_4: female, 1.87 ± 0.79 μg/dL
	T_3: male, 58 ± 9 ng/dL	T_3: female, 53 ± 13 ng/dL
Chicken	T_4: 9.43 ± 73.2 ng/mL	T_3: 1.5 ± 0.58 ng/mL

CLINICAL APPLICATIONS

CAUSES OF ABNORMALLY HIGH LEVELS

- Hyperthyroidism
- Exogenous T_4, thyroid-stimulating hormone (TSH), or thyrotropin-releasing hormone (TRH)
- Administration of iodine (or compounds containing iodine)

NEXT DIAGNOSTIC STEPS TO CONSIDER IF LEVELS ARE HIGH

- If hyperthyroidism is suspected: other thyroid tests (fT_4, TSH)
- Evaluate diet, supplements for iodine content.
- Imaging (ultrasound, scintigraphy)

CAUSES OF ABNORMALLY LOW LEVELS

- Hypothyroidism
- Euthyroid sick syndrome

NEXT DIAGNOSTIC STEPS TO CONSIDER IF LEVELS ARE LOW TSH: evaluate for nonthyroidal disease

IMPORTANT INTERSPECIES DIFFERENCES

- Birds have very low levels of thyroid hormones.
- A thyroid stimulation test must be performed to evaluate the function of the thyroid.

SPECIMEN AND PROCESSING CONSIDERATIONS

DRUG EFFECTS ON LEVEL Glucocorticoids, sulfonamides, phenobarbital, nonsteroidal and antiinflammatory drugs may decrease concentrations.

LAB ARTIFACTS THAT MAY INTERFERE WITH READINGS OF LEVELS OF THIS SUBSTANCE

- Moderate to marked hemolysis decreases T_3.
- Artifactual increase in free T_4 if sample is not kept cold
- Artifactual increase in free and total T_4 if stored in glass tubes at 37°C (98.6°F)

SAMPLE FOR COLLECTION AND ANY SPECIAL SPECIMEN HANDLING NOTES

- Serum (red top tube) or EDTA acid plasma (purple top tube)
- Separate serum or plasma from red blood cells as soon as possible.
- Store in refrigerator at 2°C to 8°C (35.6°F to 46.4°F).

PEARLS

- Total T_4 is a good screening test because of its sensitivity to disease, but it is a poor confirmatory test because of its low specificity.
- Free T_4 is not as likely to be affected by nonthyroidal illness or drugs.
- Free T_4 is also measured by radioimmunoassay, which is cheaper but of no apparent benefit over total T_4 and is less accurate than free T_4 by equilibrium dialysis.
- In domestic species, the T_3 test is of little diagnostic value.

AUTHOR & EDITOR: **JÖRG MAYER**

LABORATORY TESTS

Uric Acid

DEFINITION

Uric acid is the major breakdown product of protein in birds and reptiles in which plasma levels can be measured.

SYNONYM

UA

PHYSIOLOGY

In birds and reptiles, uric acid is the major end-product of protein metabolism. It is produced by the liver and excreted by kidney tubules; impaired elimination is an indication of renal disease. However, normal levels can be seen in early disease states. Approximately 90% of uric acid is secreted by the proximal tubules in avian species. Excreted UA passes through the cloaca and is retropulsed back into the rectum and cecum, where is it broken down by bacteria and is reabsorbed. At least 60%

of renal function must be lost for an elevation in uric acid to be seen; therefore, it is not a sensitive indicator of renal disease. The definition of *hyperuricemia* is as follows: "plasma uric acid concentration higher than the calculated limit of solubility of sodium urate in plasma." For most birds and reptiles, this theoretical limit of solubility usually is estimated to be about 10.8 mg/dL (600 μmol/L).

TYPICAL NORMAL RANGE

The typical normal range for this laboratory test varies greatly among species. The reader is referred to the following Elsevier publications for additional information:

Carpenter J: Exotic animal formulary, ed 4, St Louis, 2013, Saunders.

Mader D: Reptile medicine and surgery, ed 2, St Louis, 2006, Saunders.

CLINICAL APPLICATIONS

CAUSES OF ABNORMALLY HIGH LEVELS Dehydration, gout, severe tissue damage/renal disease, nephrocalcinosis, septicemia, bacteremia, starvation, shock, and hypovitaminosis A–induced damage to renal tubular epithelium, as shown in the macaw, can cause elevated levels of uric acid in plasma. Significant dehydration that affects glomerular filtration rate (GFR) and results in lack of movement of uric acid through the tubules will contribute to elevated levels. Herbivorous reptiles fed high-protein diets can also cause hyperuricemia.

NEXT DIAGNOSTIC STEPS TO CONSIDER IF LEVELS ARE HIGH A 24-hour fasting sample should be taken if postprandial elevations are suspected in *Raptor* species. Consider having a kidney biopsy performed along with histopathologic examination to document the health of the kidneys.

CAUSES OF ABNORMALLY LOW LEVELS Lower uric acid levels can occur with younger birds; however, hypouricemia is infrequently seen and if seen may indicate severe hepatic disease or starvation.

IMPORTANT INTERSPECIES DIFFERENCES

- *Birds and reptiles:* carnivorous birds and reptiles have a higher normal level of circulating uric acid. Postprandial elevations have been seen in raptors and reptiles. 24-Hour fasting samples can be taken to rule out postprandial elevations. Terrestrial reptiles tend to excrete as much as 90% of their nitrogenous waste as uric acid, whereas aquatic species excrete as little as 10% as urea and ammonia. Amphibians secrete urea, not uric acid.
- *Small mammals:* uric acid is not significantly produced in most mammalian species
- *Fish:* increased values of urea and uric acid can be seen with infectious disease processes

SPECIMEN AND PROCESSING CONSIDERATIONS

DRUG EFFECTS ON LEVEL Colchicine, allopurinol, furosemide, and other diuretics are commonly used to lower high uric acid levels.

SAMPLE FOR COLLECTION AND ANY SPECIAL SPECIMEN HANDLING NOTES Heparinized plasma or serum: collect in a green top for reptiles and avian species, in a red top for mammal species.

AUTHOR: **CANDACE HERSEY-BENNER**

EDITOR: **JÖRG MAYER**

Zinc

DEFINITION

- Zinc is an essential trace mineral that serves as a cofactor for enzymes in many tissues. It is involved in regulation of the immune response and is involved in cell replication and in the development of cartilage and bone, as well as modulation of keratogenesis, wound healing, maintenance of normal reproductive function, and acuity of taste and smell, among other physiologic functions.
- The zinc test measures the level of the essential heavy metal zinc in the peripheral blood using a flame atomic absorption assay.
- Elevated blood zinc levels may indicate recent exposure or chronic intake.

SYNONYMS

Zn, galvanize, blue powder, asarco L15, merrillite, jasad

PHYSIOLOGY

- Zinc is an essential element for both mammals and birds and has a major role in growth, skeleton development, collagen formation, skin (hair and feathers), wound healing, and reproduction.
- Zinc can be found mainly in alloys and galvanized objects but also in some medications and rubber products. American pennies minted after 1983 contain about 99% zinc. Animals absorb zinc mainly by ingesting zinc-containing objects and high-content food pellets. Absorption takes place mainly at the small intestines; zinc is taken by plasma albumin and β_2-macroglobulin, metabolized in the liver, and exported to peripheral tissues, where it is deposited in various body organs.
- The exact mechanism of zinc toxicity is still unclear and is attributed to its divalent character and competition with similar elements in the body (e.g., copper, iron).
- Clinical presentation is mainly of lethargy, diarrhea, and anemia. In birds, it seems that zinc toxicity mainly affects the pancreas (necrosis). Common clinical signs of zinc intoxication in birds include anorexia, acute gastroenteritis, yellow feces, vomiting, extreme loss of plumage, and hepatomegaly; these are similar to the clinical signs of lead toxicity.
- The key clinical sign of a zinc deficiency is usually dermatosis. In birds, signs of zinc deficiency include relatively nonspecific clinical presentations such as a reduction in the immune response, early embryonic death, fetal abnormalities, weak chicks at hatching, retarded growth, alopecia, dermatitis, delayed sexual development, and abnormal skeletal formation.

TYPICAL NORMAL RANGE

- Whole blood levels greater than >2 ppm are usually considered diagnostic for zinc toxicosis when accompanied by appropriate clinical signs.
- Normal Eclectus parrots can have higher physiologic Zn concentrations

of up to 2.5 ppm. In cockatoos, Zn concentrations of up to 3.0 ppm may be normal.

	SERUM/PLASMA, MEAN ± SD, ppm*	
Genus	Normal	Toxic
Macaw	1.23 ± 0.55	8.22 ± 5.74
Cockatoo	2.01 ± 0.78	4.58 ± 3.10
Cockatiel	1.58 ± 0.48	7.86 ± 6.89
Conure	1.25 ± 0.59	9.43 ± 4.82
Amazon	1.48 ± 0.40	2.82 ± 0.64
Lories/lorikeet	1.71, 2.62	—
Lovebird	2.33	—
Poicephalus	1.43 ± 0.52	—
Eclectus parrot	1.60 ± 0.90	2.92 ± 0.20
African grey	1.34 ± 0.48	3.14 ± 0.77

From Puschner B, et al: Normal and toxic zinc concentrations in serum/plasma and liver of psittacines with respect to genus differences, J Vet Diagn Invest 11:522–527, 1999.

*Normal and toxic zinc concentrations in serum/plasma and liver of psittacines with respect to genus differences.

CLINICAL APPLICATIONS

CAUSES OF ABNORMALLY HIGH LEVELS Ingestion of high zinc content food pellets, pennies (minted after 1983), and galvanized objects

NEXT DIAGNOSTIC STEPS TO CONSIDER IF LEVELS ARE HIGH

- Test for blood and urine zinc levels.
- Obtain whole-body radiographs.
- Test (biopsy or necropsy) zinc levels from liver, kidney, and pancreas.

CAUSES OF ABNORMALLY LOW LEVELS Malnutrition, malabsorption, animals on total parenteral nutrition. Although this does not appear to be a problem in exotic pets, zinc deficiency can happen in species used for commercial production (e.g., poultry) or that graze on pastures with zinc-deficient soil.

NEXT DIAGNOSTIC STEPS TO CONSIDER IF LEVELS ARE LOW Perform a skin biopsy because a zinc-deficient dermatosis (hyperkeratosis) is a common clinical sign in animals with a zinc deficiency.

IMPORTANT INTERSPECIES DIFFERENCES Birds tend to show great diurnal variations in zinc blood levels: early morning samples might show toxic levels that drop to normal at around noon and remain so throughout the evening.

SPECIMEN AND PROCESSING CONSIDERATIONS

LAB ARTIFACTS THAT MAY INTERFERE WITH READINGS OF LEVELS OF THIS SUBSTANCE Some rubber stoppers on blood collection tubes and syringes may contain zinc, which may affect the sample. Plastic stoppers are preferred in these samples. The serum should be separated from the blood clot.

SAMPLE FOR COLLECTION AND ANY SPECIAL SPECIMEN HANDLING NOTES Trace element–free tubes and syringes made of glass or all-plastic syringes should be used for sampling. Use only royal blue top tubes with plastic stopper.

PEARLS

Caution: phosphine gas (faint garlic or rotten fish odor; gas is liberated in the breath of animals with zinc phosphide intoxication, as during gastric lavage) is a public health hazard and may cause severe/permanent respiratory injury to veterinary personnel or to bystanders. If a psittacine patient died with clinical signs suggestive of Zn toxicosis, determination of the Zn levels in the liver and histopathologic examination of pancreas are necessary in order to establish an accurate diagnosis.

REFERENCES

Puschner B, et al: Normal and toxic zinc concentrations in serum/plasma and liver of psittacines with respect to genus differences, J Vet Diagn Invest 11:522–527, 1999.

AUTHOR: **DAVID ESHAR**

EDITOR: **JÖRG MAYER**

SECTION V

Clinical Algorithms

EDITOR

Jörg Mayer *DrMedVet, MSc, DABVP (Exotic Companion Mammal), DECZM (Small Mammal)*

AMPHIBIANS

Sudden Death

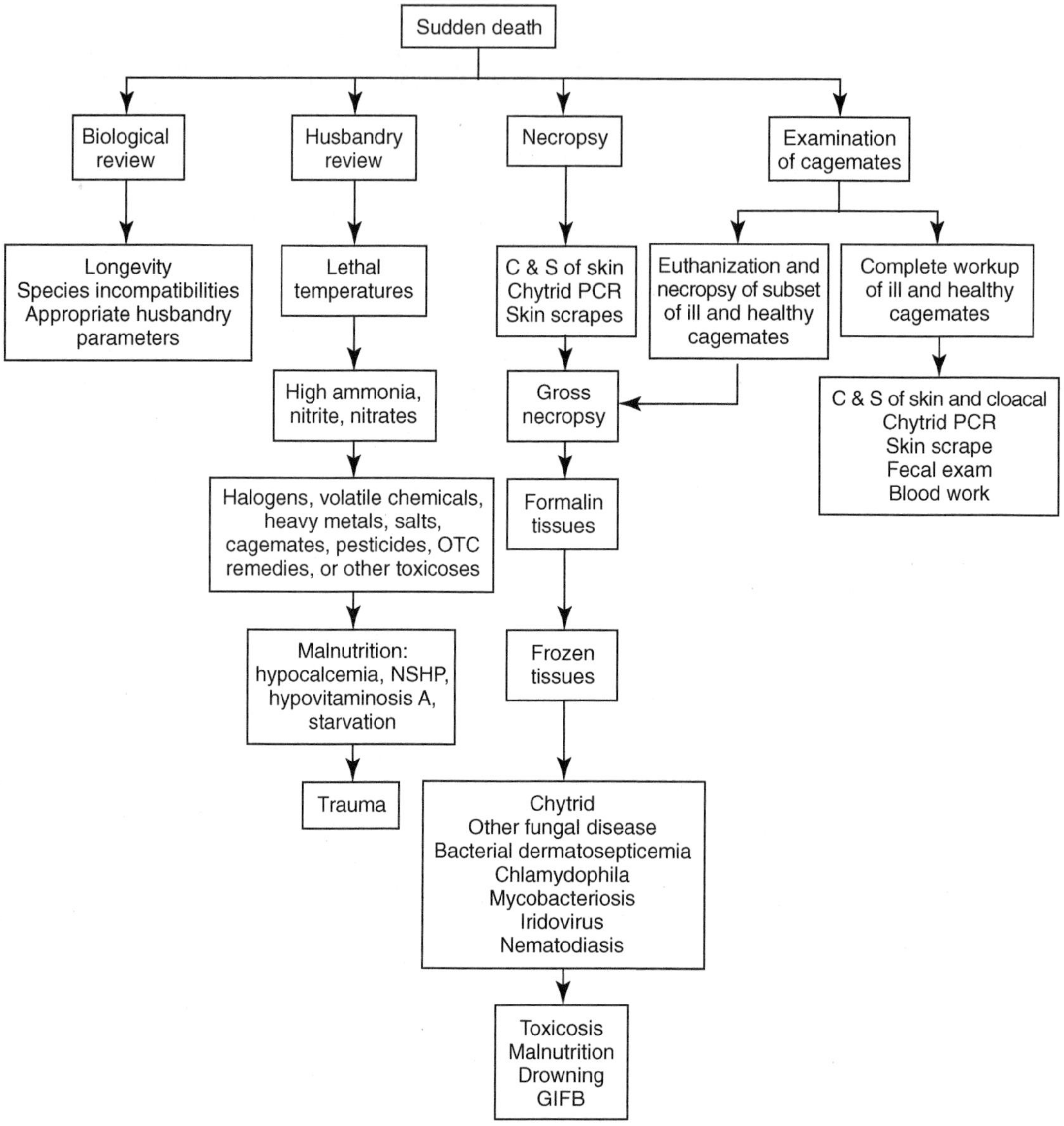

AUTHOR: **KEVIN M. WRIGHT**

AMPHIBIANS

Weight Loss

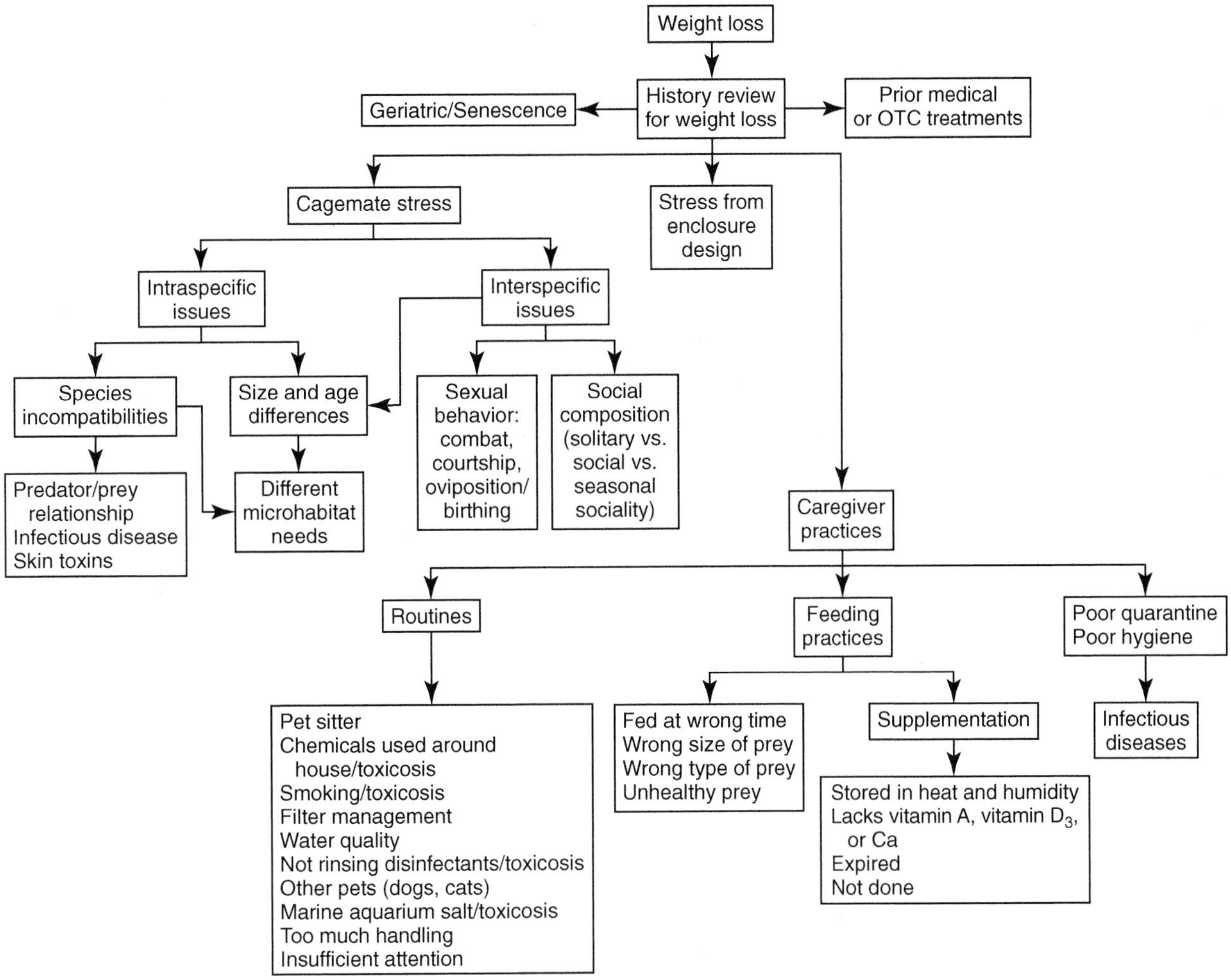

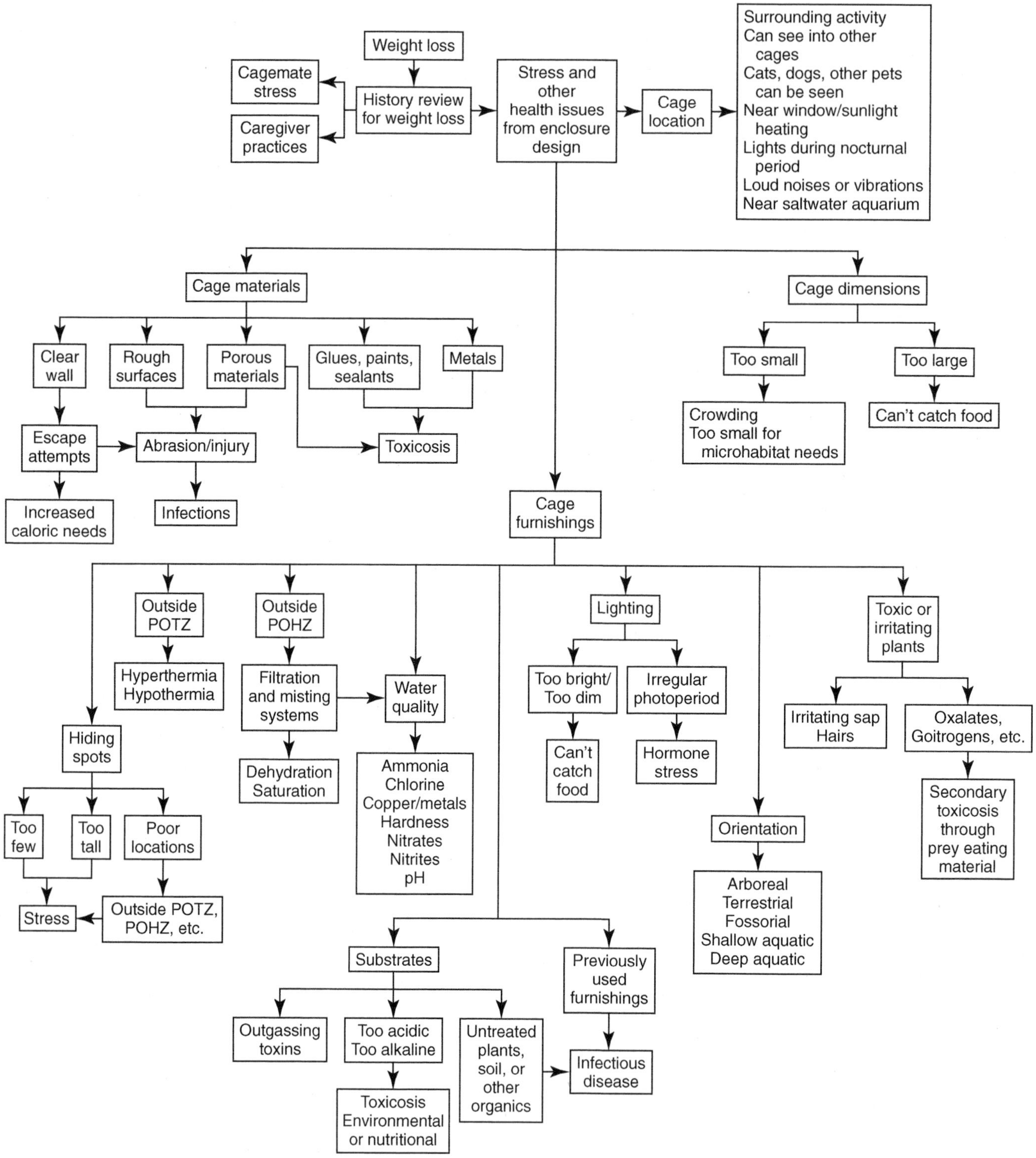
Weight loss
History review for weight loss
Cagemate stress
Caregiver practices
Stress and other health issues from enclosure design
Cage location
Surrounding activity
Can see into other cages
Cats, dogs, other pets can be seen
Near window/sunlight heating
Lights during nocturnal period
Loud noises or vibrations
Near saltwater aquarium
Cage materials
Clear wall
Rough surfaces
Porous materials
Glues, paints, sealants
Metals
Escape attempts
Abrasion/injury
Toxicosis
Increased caloric needs
Infections
Cage dimensions
Too small
Too large
Crowding
Too small for microhabitat needs
Can't catch food
Cage furnishings
Outside POTZ
Outside POHZ
Hyperthermia
Hypothermia
Filtration and misting systems
Water quality
Dehydration
Saturation
Ammonia
Chlorine
Copper/metals
Hardness
Nitrates
Nitrites
pH
Hiding spots
Too few
Too tall
Poor locations
Stress
Outside POTZ, POHZ, etc.
Lighting
Too bright/ Too dim
Irregular photoperiod
Can't catch food
Hormone stress
Toxic or irritating plants
Irritating sap
Hairs
Oxalates, Goitrogens, etc.
Secondary toxicosis through prey eating material
Orientation
Arboreal
Terrestrial
Fossorial
Shallow aquatic
Deep aquatic
Substrates
Outgassing toxins
Too acidic
Too alkaline
Untreated plants, soil, or other organics
Toxicosis
Environmental or nutritional
Previously used furnishings
Infectious disease

REPTILES

CNS Chelonia

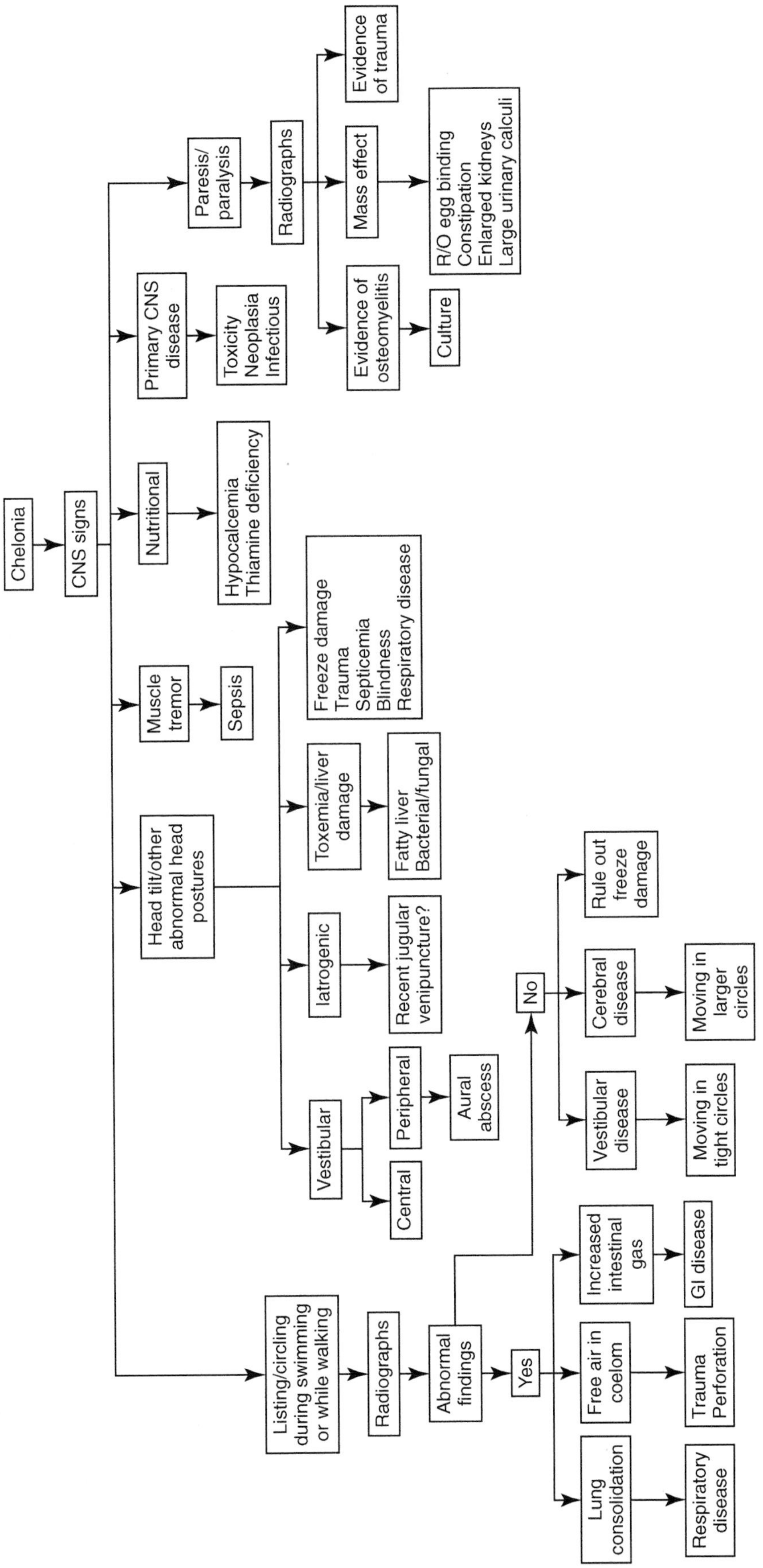

REPTILES

CNS Lizard

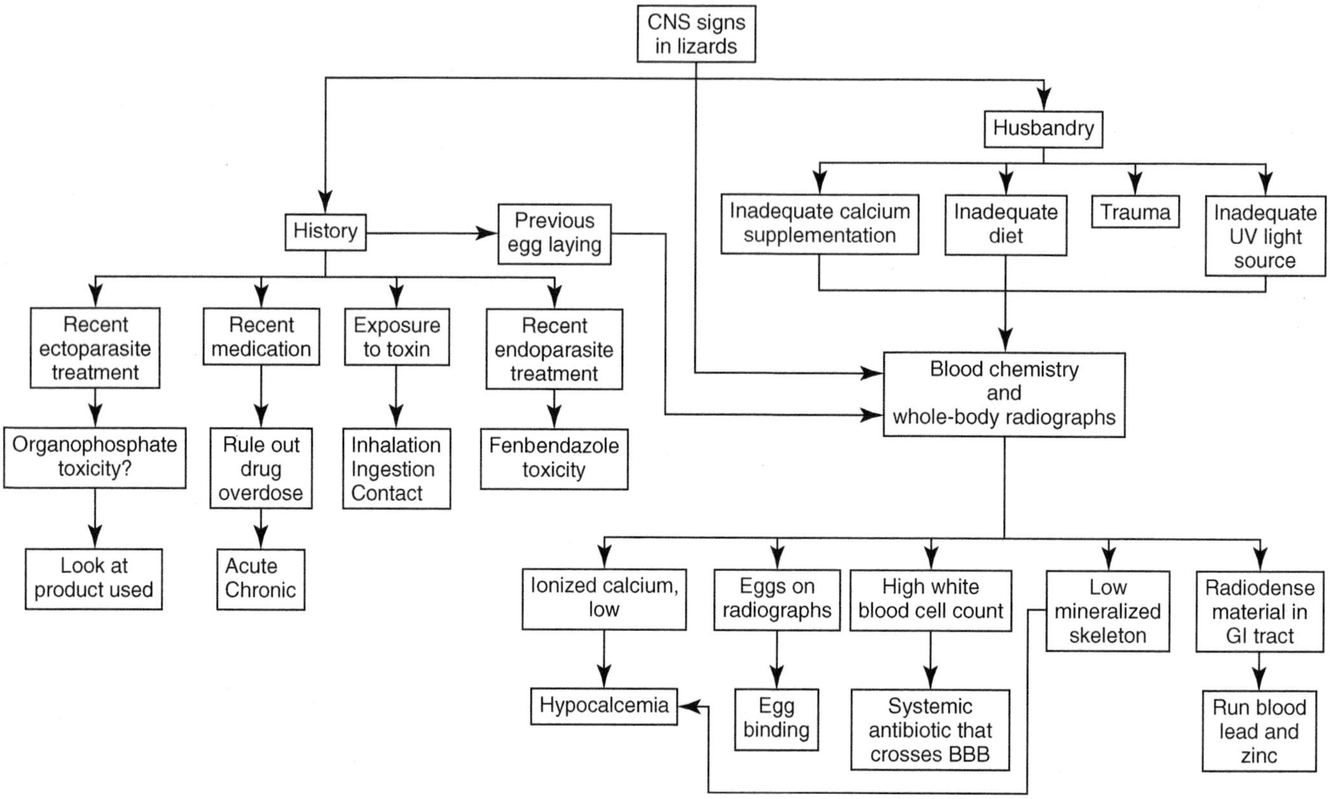

REPTILES

CNS Snakes

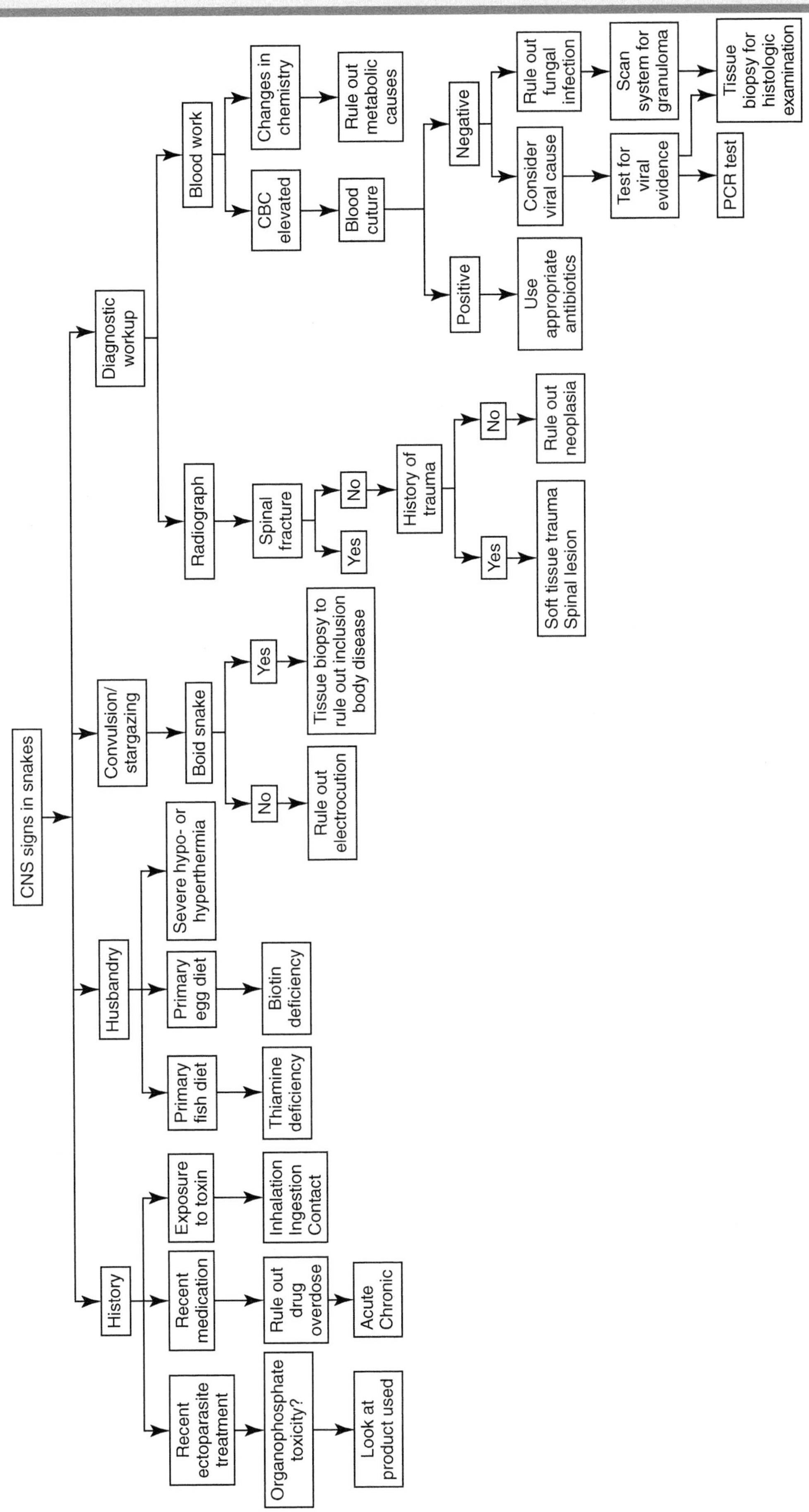

CLINICAL ALGORITHMS
REPTILES

Constipation

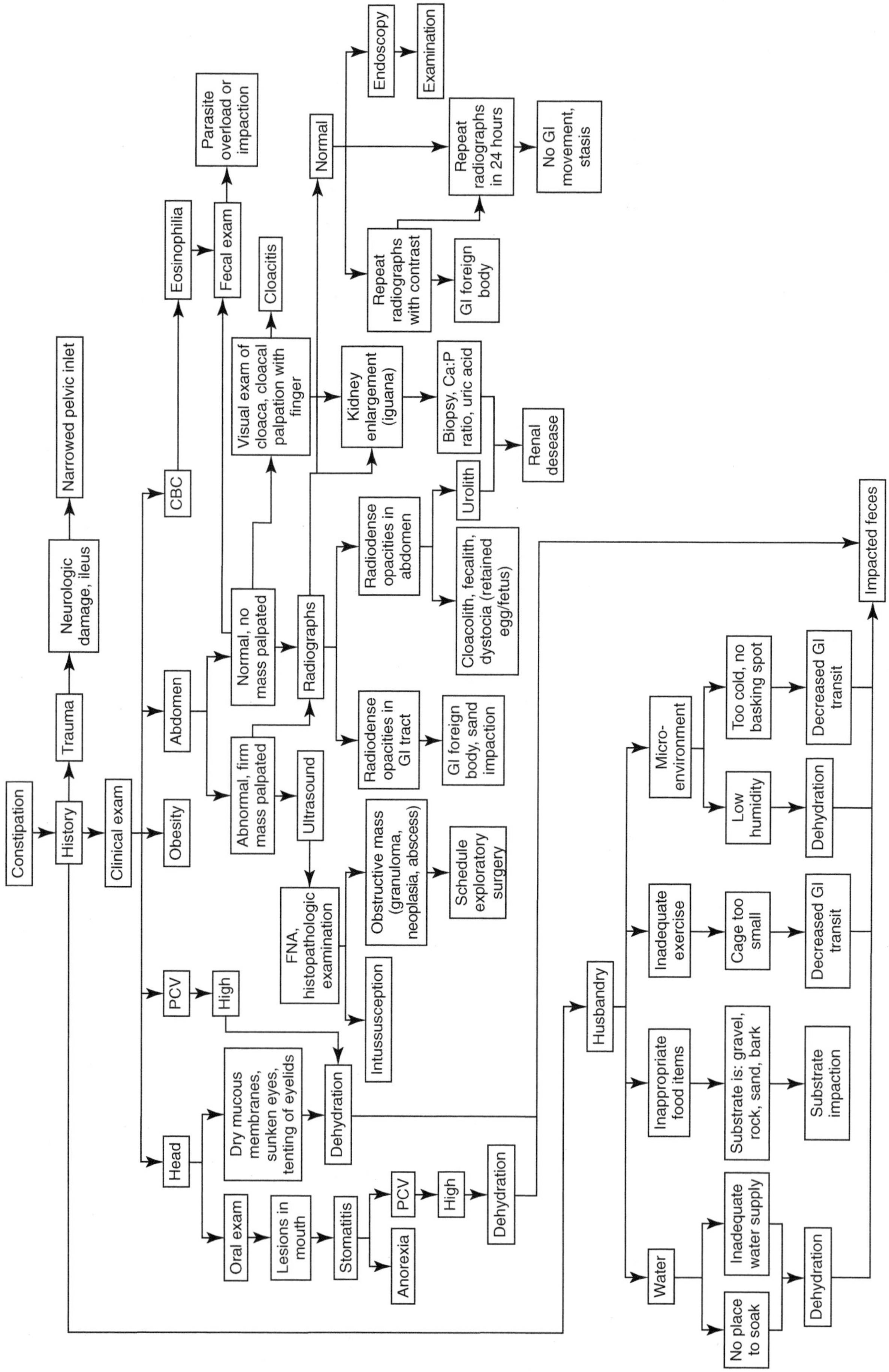

REPTILES

Diarrhea

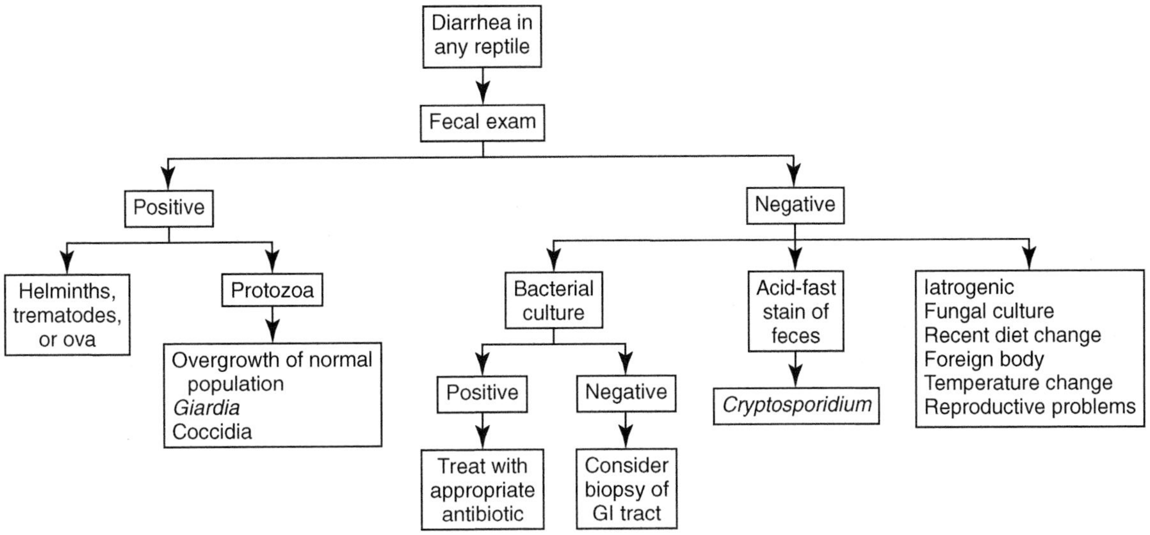

REPTILES

Parasites

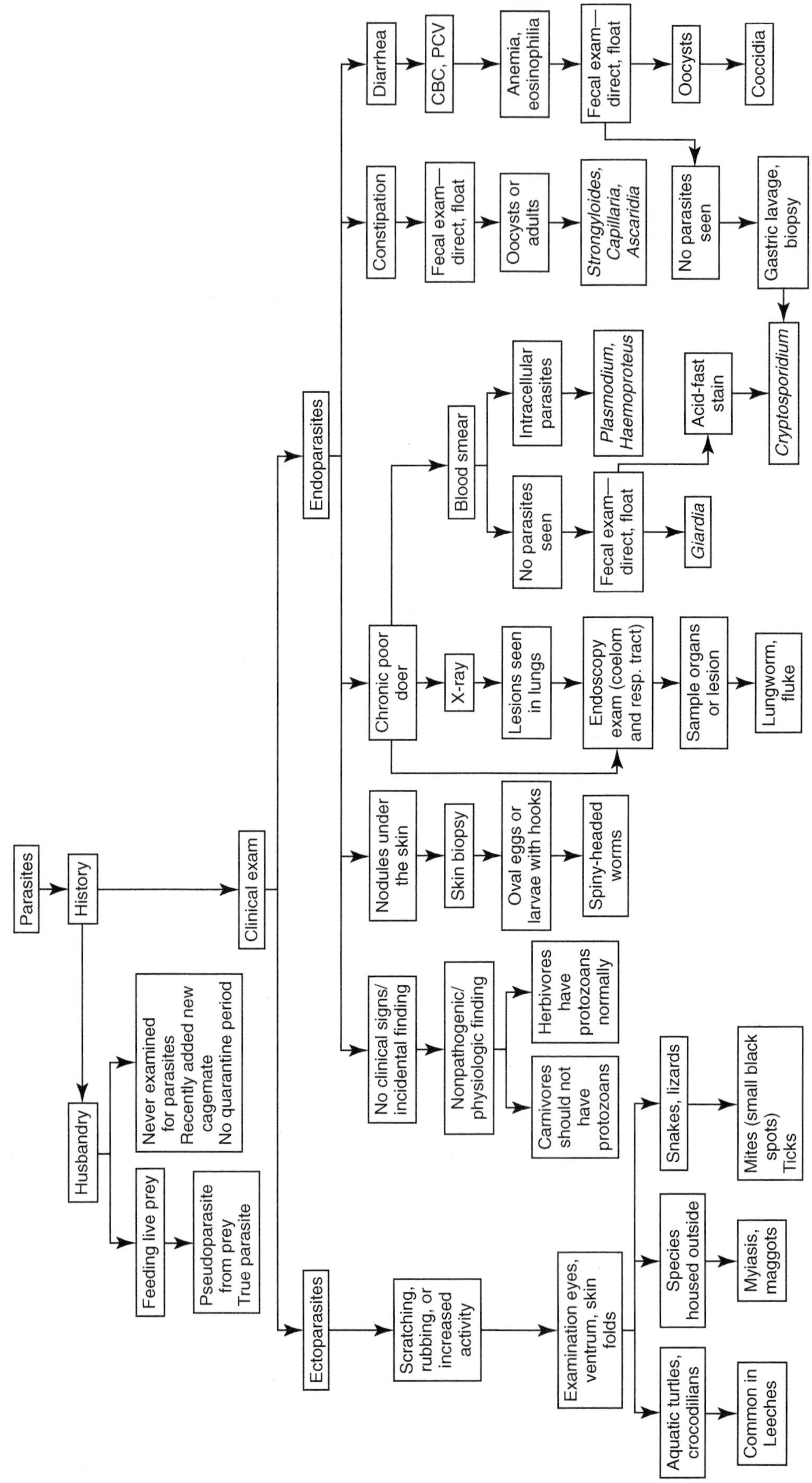

REPTILES

Prolapse

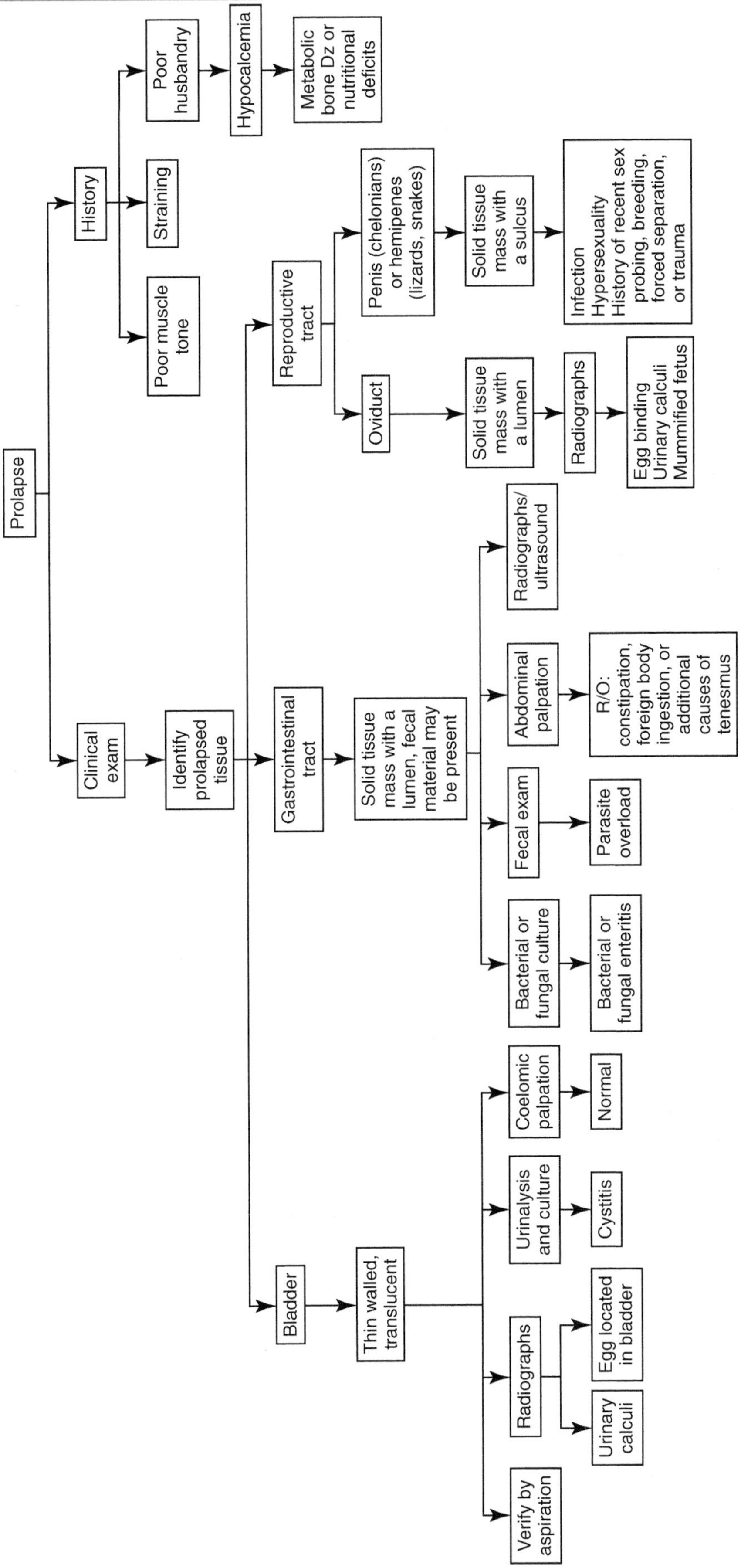

REPTILES

Regurgitation

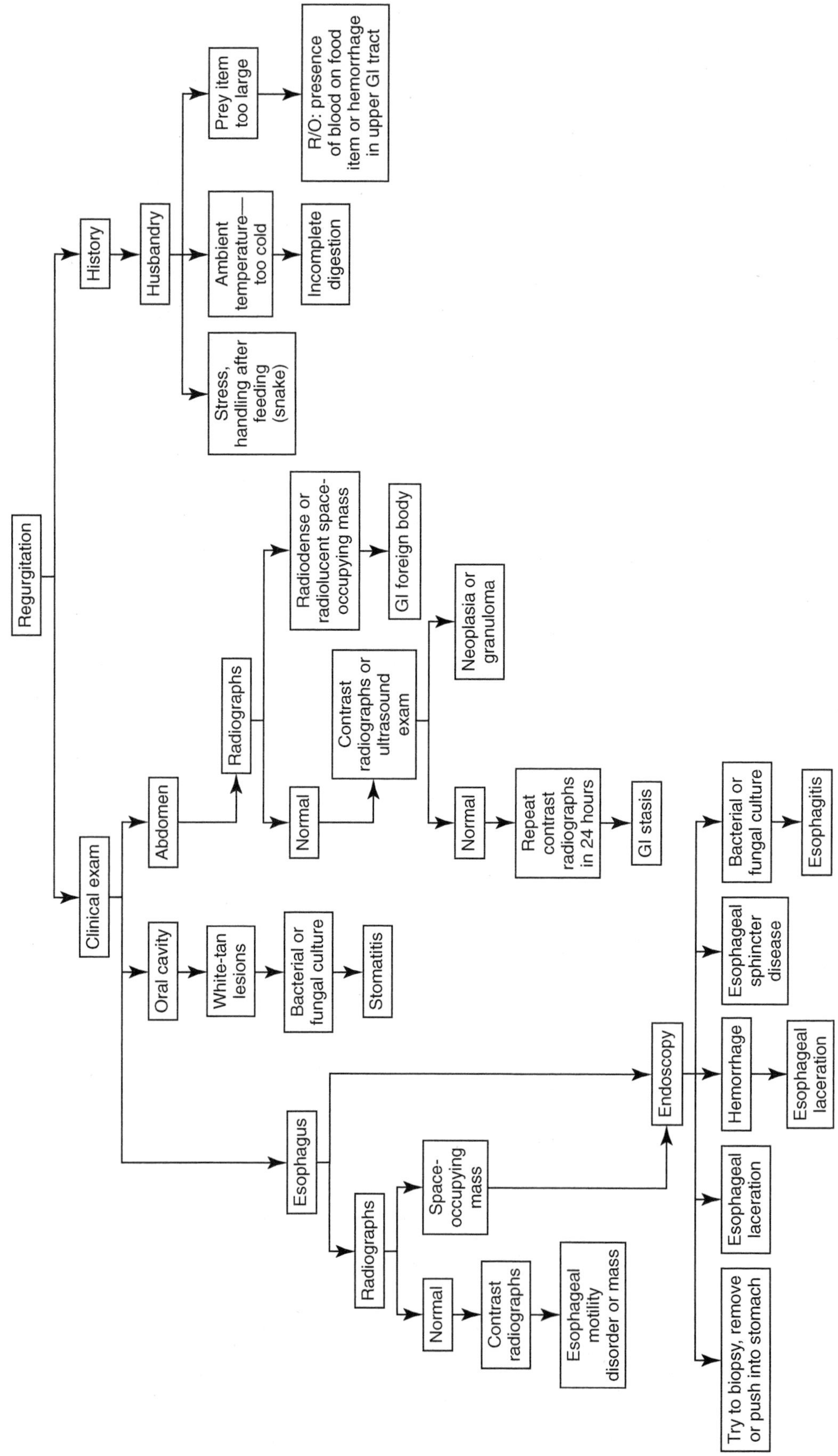

Swellings

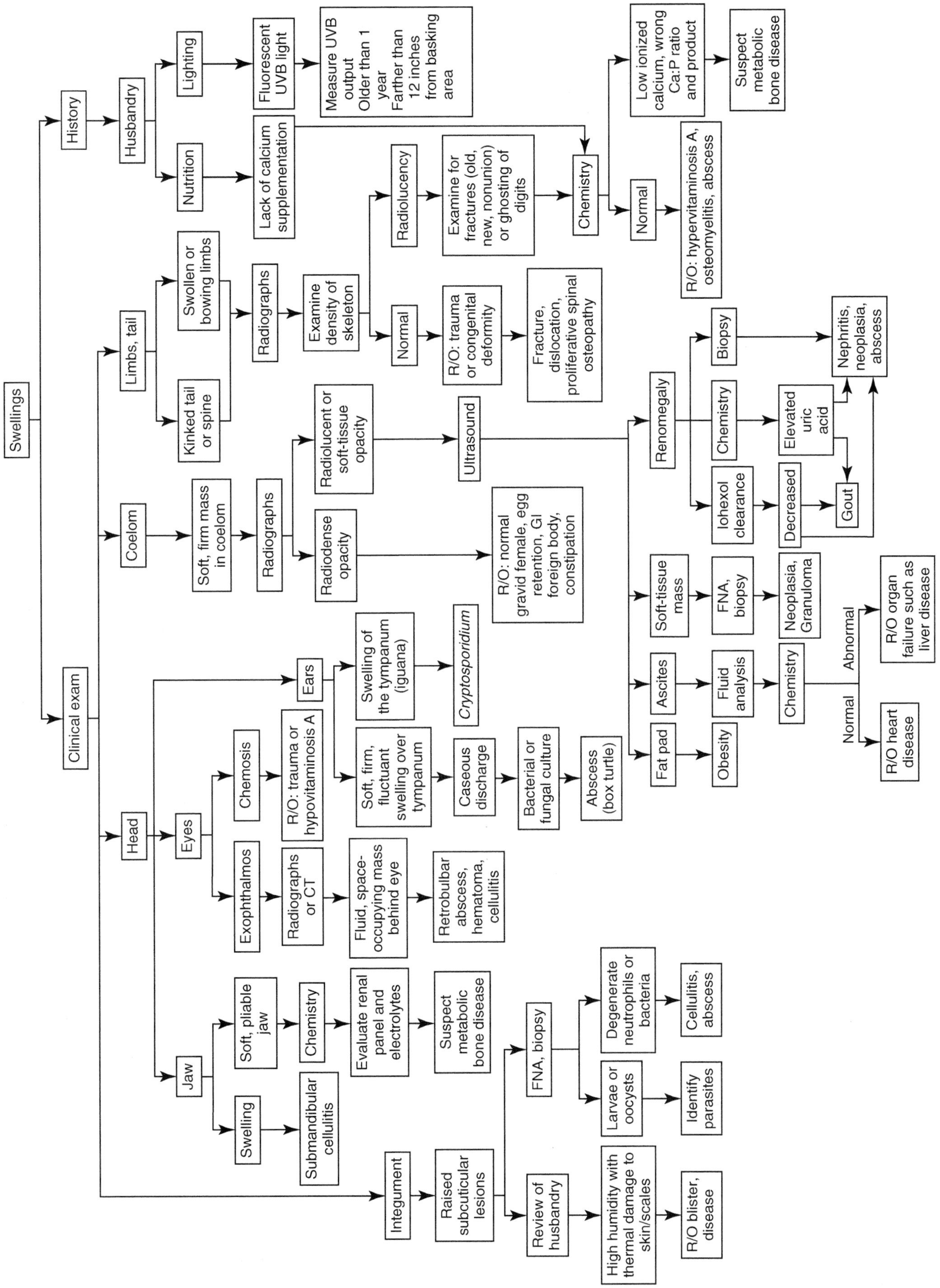

Swellings
History
Husbandry
Lighting
Fluorescent UVB light
Measure UVB output
Older than 1 year
Farther than 12 inches from basking area
Nutrition
Lack of calcium supplementation
Chemistry
Low ionized calcium, wrong Ca:P ratio and product
Suspect metabolic bone disease
Normal
R/O: hypervitaminosis A, osteomyelitis, abscess
Clinical exam
Limbs, tail
Swollen or bowing limbs
Kinked tail or spine
Radiographs
Examine density of skeleton
Radiolucency
Examine for fractures (old, new, nonunion) or ghosting of digits
Normal
R/O: trauma or congenital deformity
Fracture, dislocation, proliferative spinal osteopathy
Coelom
Soft, firm mass in coelom
Radiographs
Radiolucent or soft-tissue opacity
Ultrasound
Radiodense opacity
R/O: normal gravid female, egg retention, GI foreign body, constipation
Renomegaly
Biopsy
Chemistry
Elevated uric acid
Iohexol clearance
Decreased
Gout
Nephritis, neoplasia, abscess
Soft-tissue mass
FNA, biopsy
Neoplasia, Granuloma
Ascites
Fluid analysis
Chemistry
Abnormal
R/O organ failure such as liver disease
Normal
R/O heart disease
Fat pad
Obesity
Head
Ears
Swelling of the tympanum (iguana)
Cryptosporidium
Soft, firm, fluctuant swelling over tympanum
Caseous discharge
Bacterial or fungal culture
Abscess (box turtle)
Eyes
Chemosis
R/O: trauma or hypovitaminosis A
Exophthalmos
Radiographs or CT
Fluid, space-occupying mass behind eye
Retrobulbar abscess, hematoma, cellulitis
Jaw
Soft, pliable jaw
Chemistry
Evaluate renal panel and electrolytes
Suspect metabolic bone disease
Swelling
Submandibular cellulitis
Integument
Raised subcuticular lesions
FNA, biopsy
Degenerate neutrophils or bacteria
Cellulitis, abscess
Larvae or oocysts
Identify parasites
Review of husbandry
High humidity with thermal damage to skin/scales
R/O blister, disease

Unspecific Problem/Not Doing Well

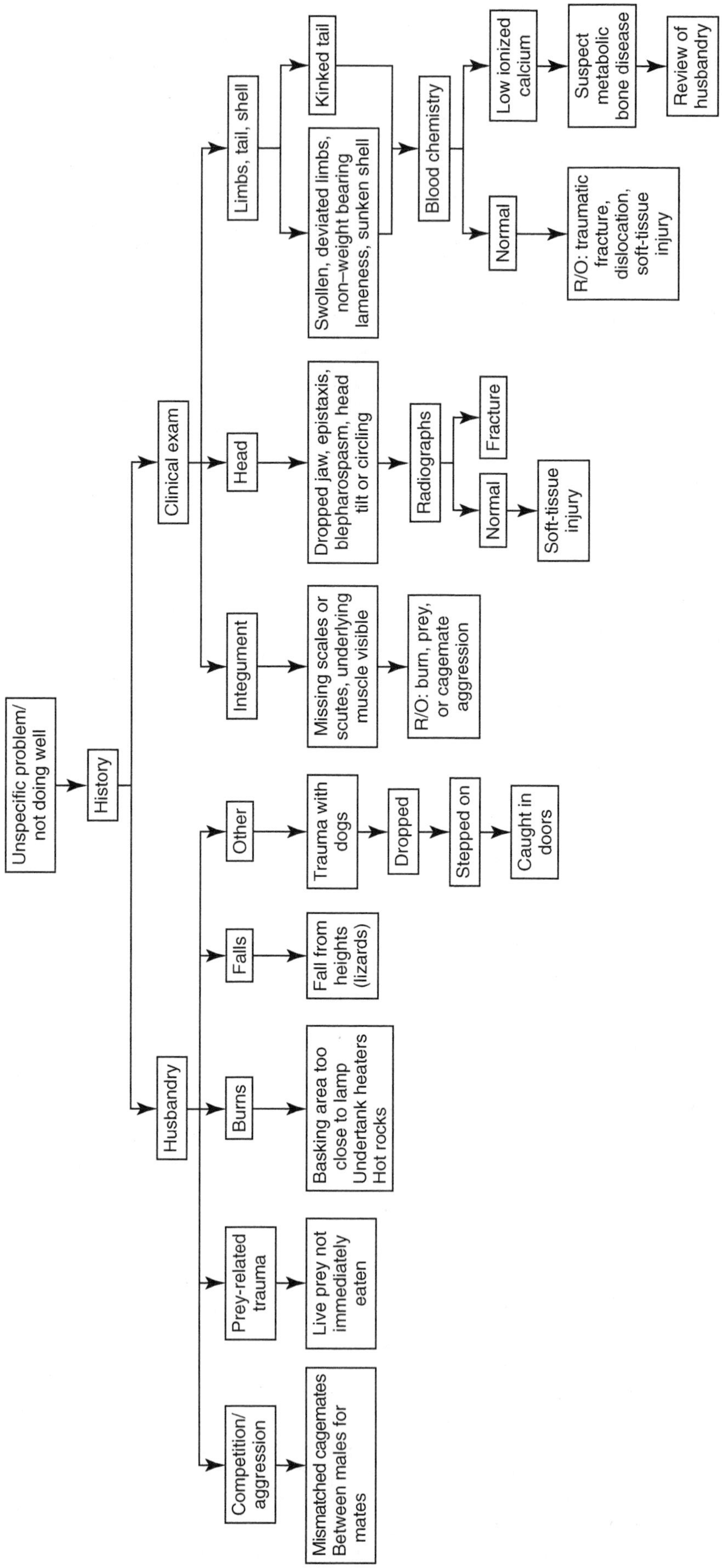

REPTILES

Vomiting

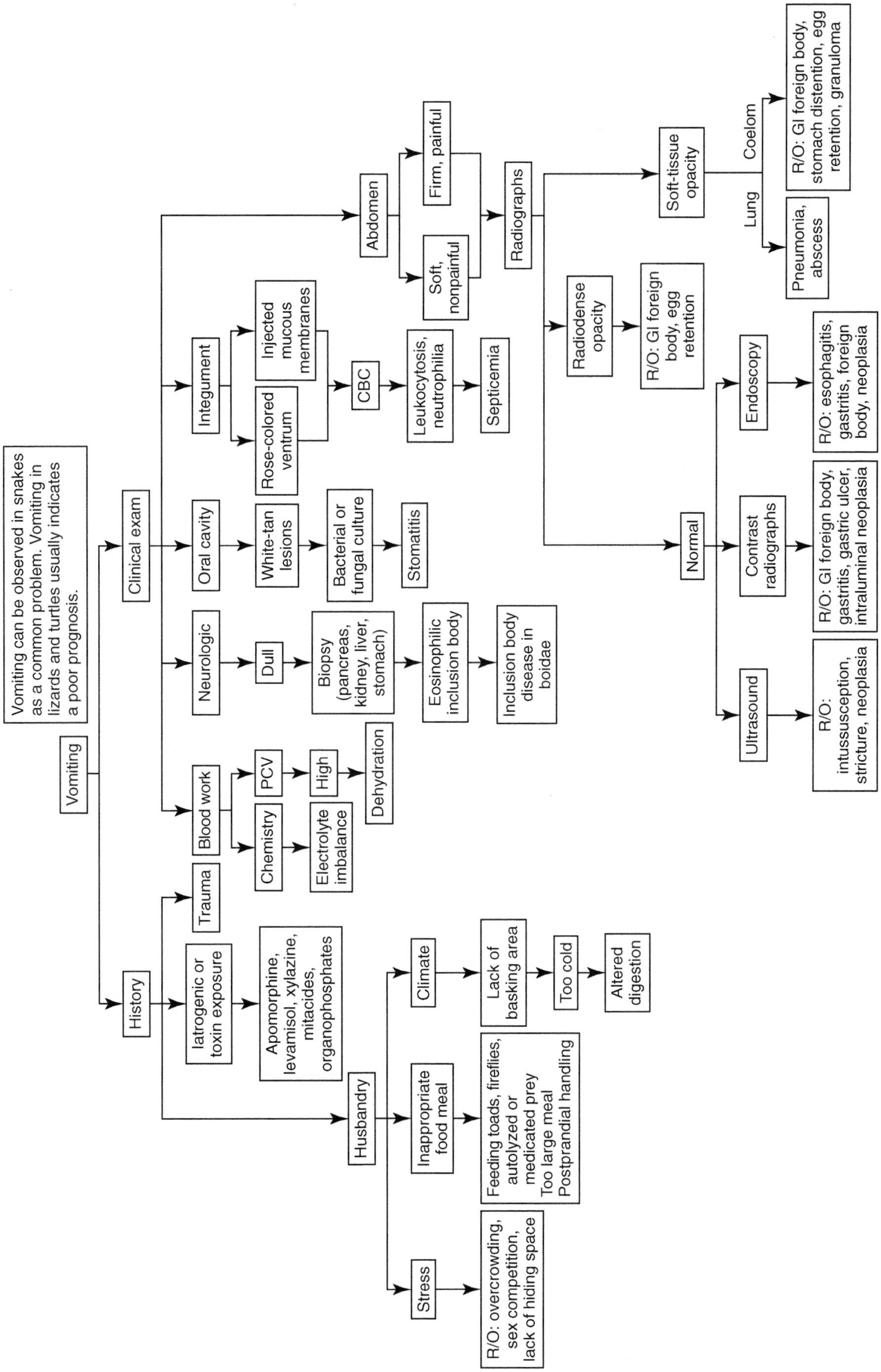

Weight Loss

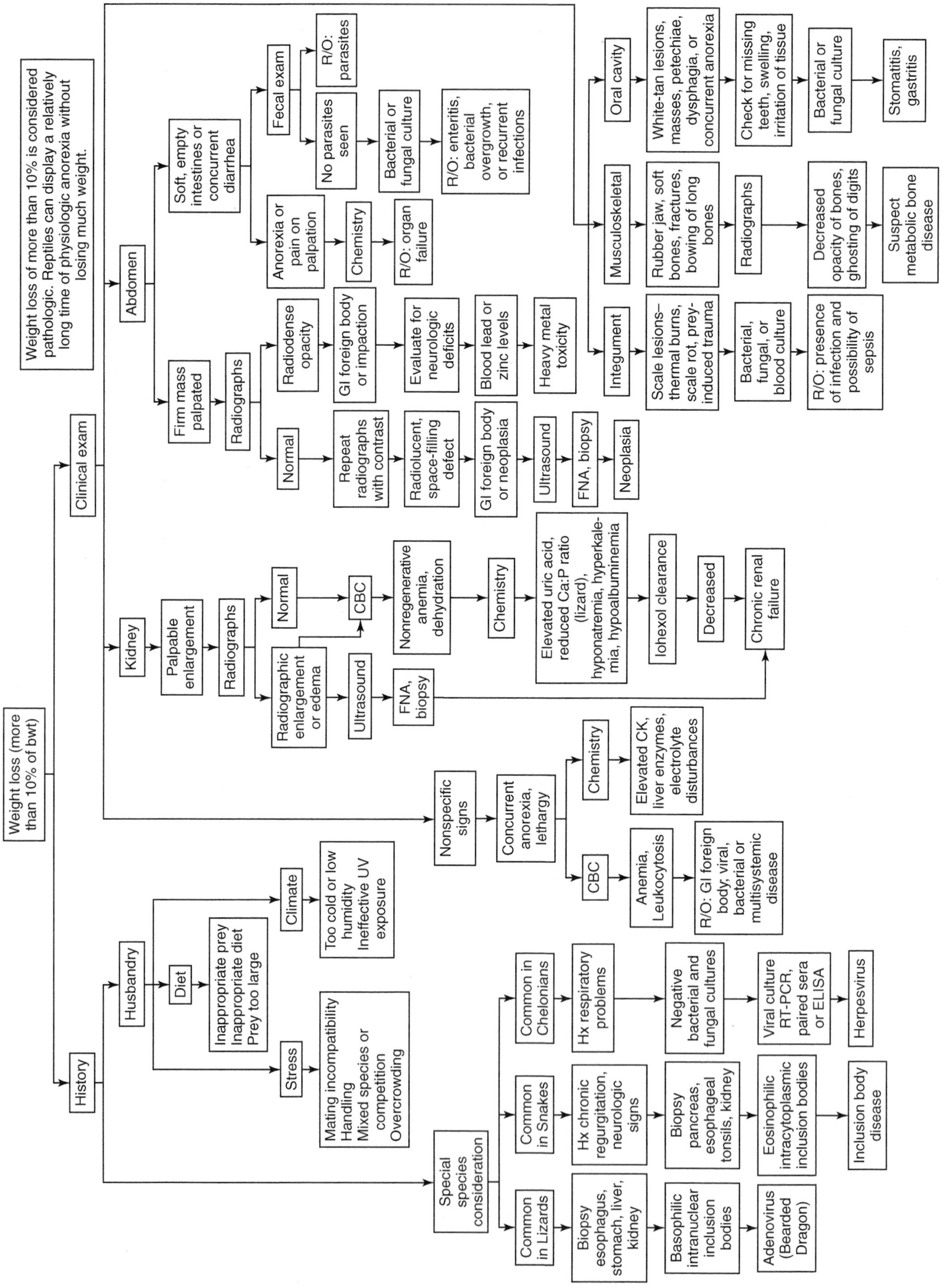
Weight loss of more than 10% is considered pathologic. Reptiles can display a relatively long time of physiologic anorexia without losing much weight.
Weight loss (more than 10% of bwt)
History
Clinical exam
Husbandry
Diet
Inappropriate prey
Inappropriate diet
Prey too large
Climate
Too cold or low humidity
Ineffective UV exposure
Stress
Mating incompatibility
Handling
Mixed species or competition
Overcrowding
Special species consideration
Common in Lizards
Biopsy esophagus, stomach, liver, kidney
Basophilic intranuclear inclusion bodies
Adenovirus (Bearded Dragon)
Common in Snakes
Hx chronic regurgitation, neurologic signs
Biopsy pancreas, esophageal tonsils, kidney
Eosinophilic intracytoplasmic inclusion bodies
Inclusion body disease
Common in Chelonians
Hx respiratory problems
Negative bacterial and fungal cultures
Viral culture RT-PCR, paired sera or ELISA
Herpesvirus
Nonspecific signs
Concurrent anorexia, lethargy
CBC
Anemia, Leukocytosis
R/O: GI foreign body; viral, bacterial or multisystemic disease
Chemistry
Elevated CK, liver enzymes, electrolyte disturbances
Kidney
Palpable enlargement
Radiographs
Radiographic enlargement or edema
Ultrasound
FNA, biopsy
Normal
CBC
Nonregenerative anemia, dehydration
Chemistry
Elevated uric acid, reduced Ca:P ratio (lizard), hyponatremia, hyperkalemia, hypoalbuminemia
Iohexol clearance
Decreased
Chronic renal failure
Abdomen
Firm mass palpated
Radiographs
Normal
Repeat radiographs with contrast
Radiolucent, space-filling defect
GI foreign body or neoplasia
Ultrasound
FNA, biopsy
Neoplasia
Radiodense opacity
GI foreign body or impaction
Evaluate for neurologic deficits
Blood lead or zinc levels
Heavy metal toxicity
Soft, empty intestines or concurrent diarrhea
Anorexia or pain on palpation
Chemistry
R/O: organ failure
Fecal exam
No parasites seen
Bacterial or fungal culture
R/O: enteritis, bacterial overgrowth, or recurrent infections
R/O: parasites
Integument
Scale lesions–thermal burns, scale rot, prey-induced trauma
Bacterial, fungal, or blood culture
R/O: presence of infection and possibility of sepsis
Musculoskeletal
Rubber jaw, soft bones, fractures, bowing of long bones
Radiographs
Decreased opacity of bones, ghosting of digits
Suspect metabolic bone disease
Oral cavity
White-tan lesions, masses, petechiae, dysphagia, or concurrent anorexia
Check for missing teeth, swelling, irritation of tissue
Bacterial or fungal culture
Stomatitis, gastritis

SMALL MAMMALS

Alopecia

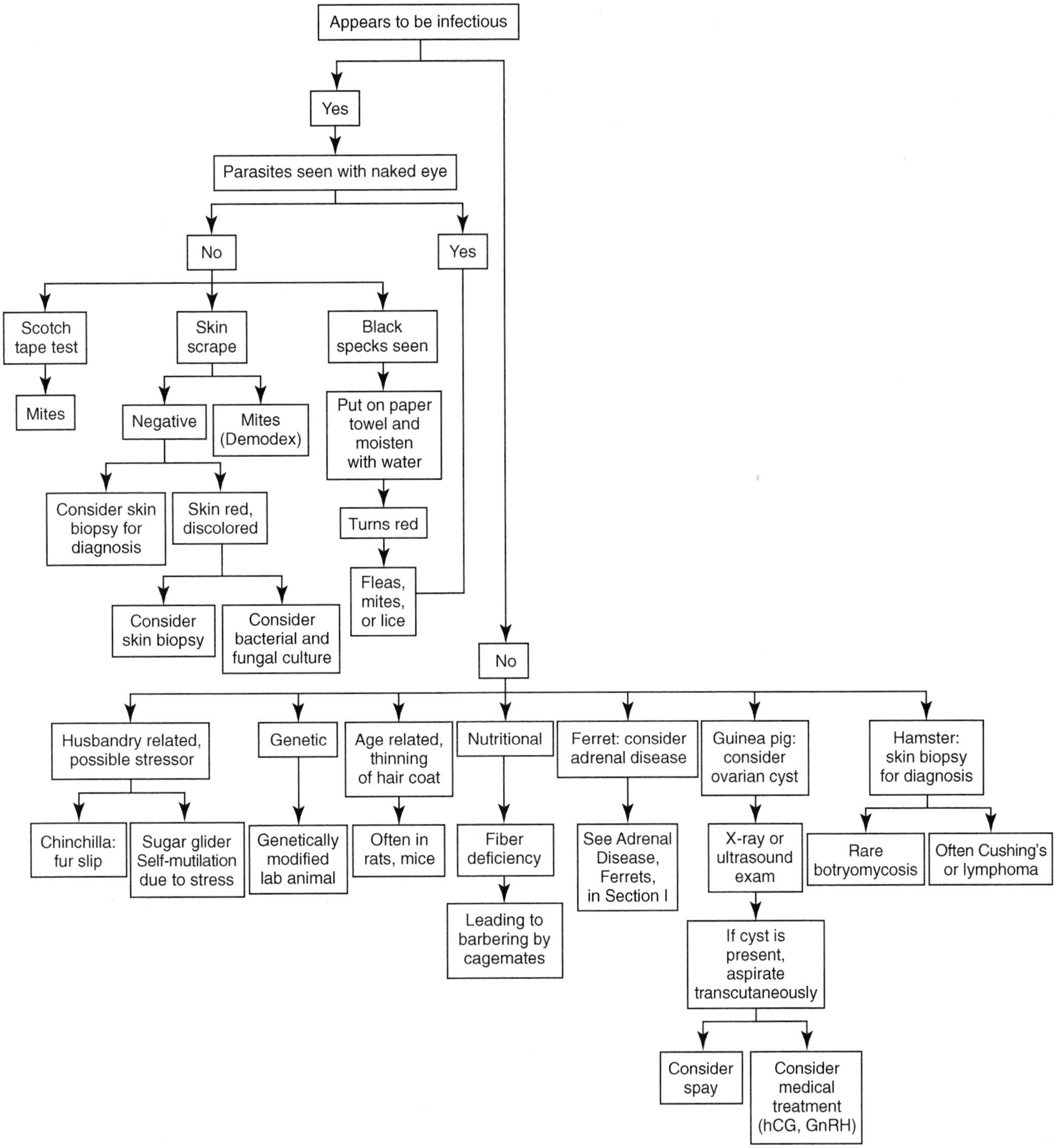

SMALL MAMMALS

Anorexia

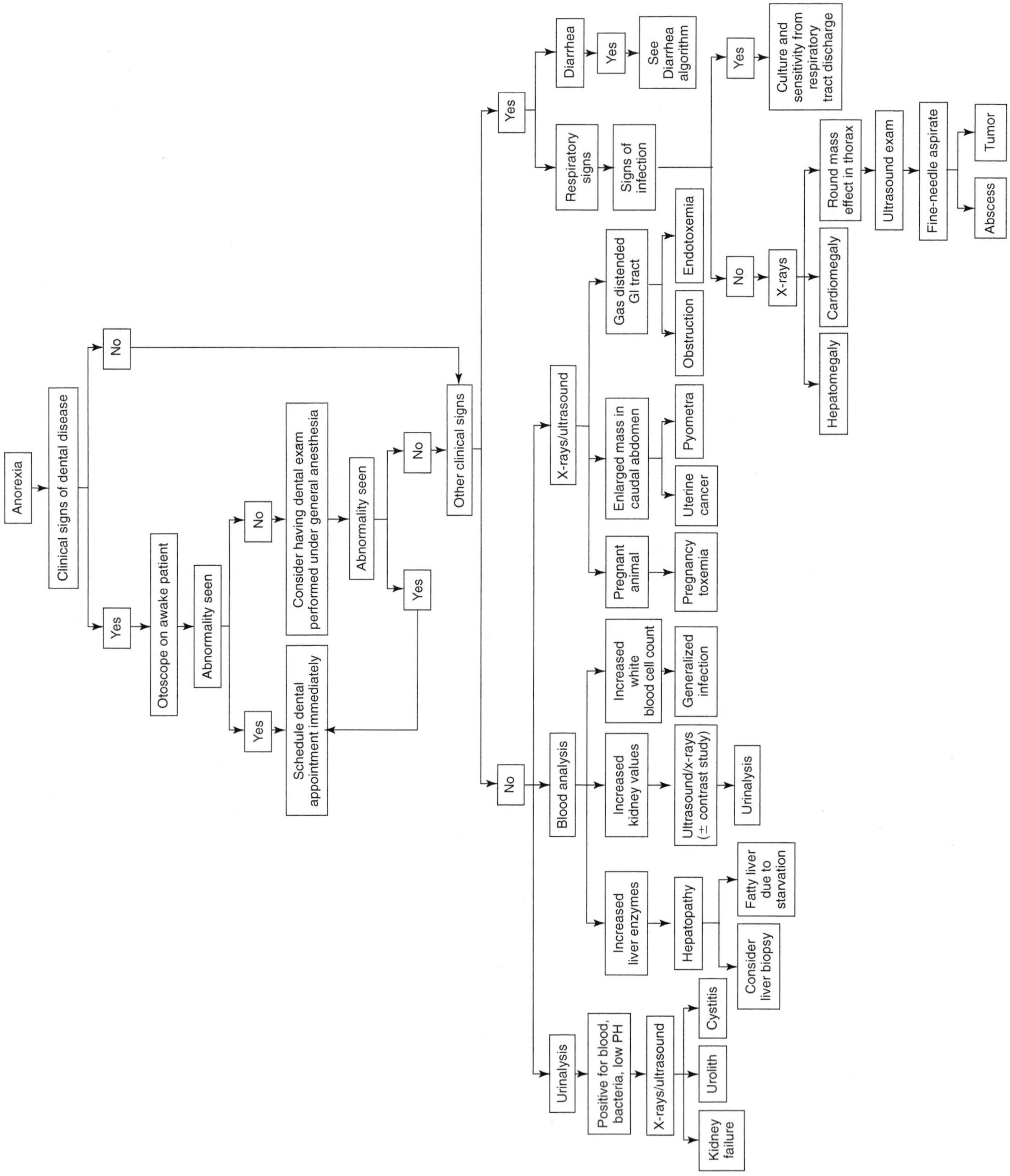

CNS Signs

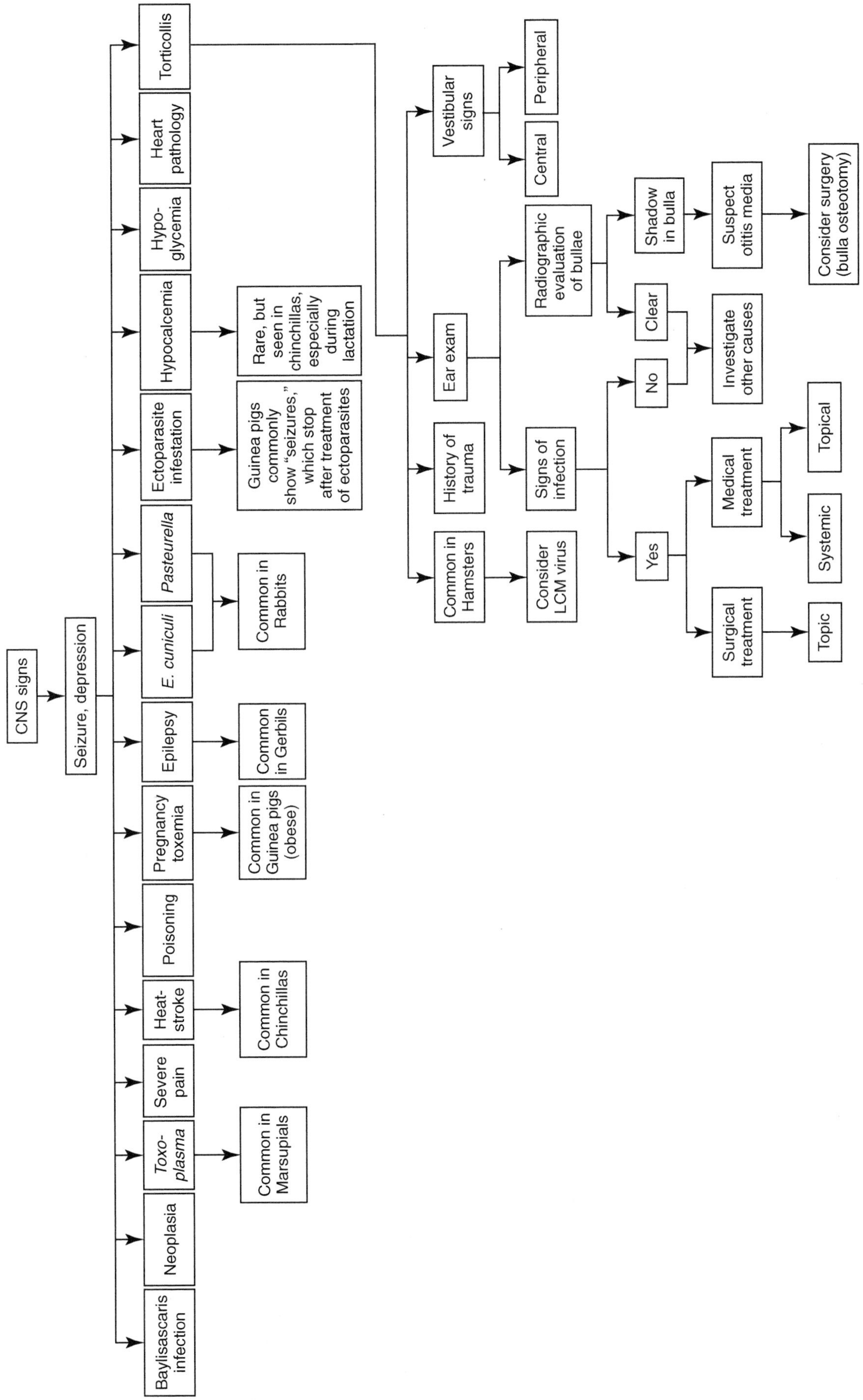
CNS signs
Seizure, depression
Baylisascaris infection
Neoplasia
Toxoplasma
Common in Marsupials
Severe pain
Heat-stroke
Common in Chinchillas
Poisoning
Pregnancy toxemia
Common in Guinea pigs (obese)
Epilepsy
Common in Gerbils
E. cuniculi
Pasteurella
Common in Rabbits
Ectoparasite infestation
Guinea pigs commonly show "seizures," which stop after treatment of ectoparasites
Hypocalcemia
Rare, but seen in chinchillas, especially during lactation
Hypo-glycemia
Heart pathology
Torticollis
Common in Hamsters
Consider LCM virus
History of trauma
Ear exam
Vestibular signs
Central
Peripheral
Signs of infection
Yes
No
Surgical treatment
Topic
Medical treatment
Systemic
Topical
Radiographic evaluation of bullae
Clear
Shadow in bulla
Investigate other causes
Suspect otitis media
Consider surgery (bulla osteotomy)

SMALL MAMMALS

Diarrhea

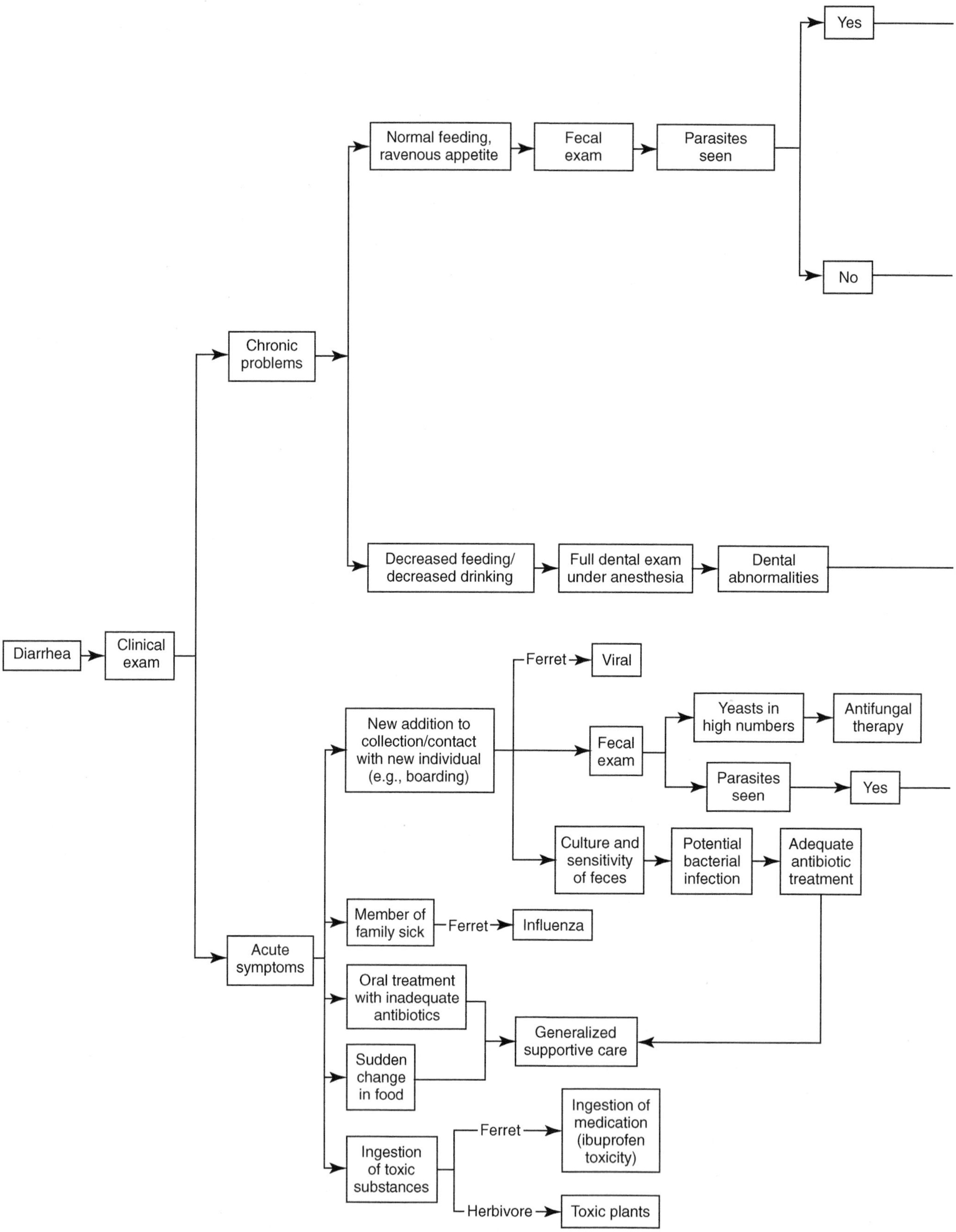

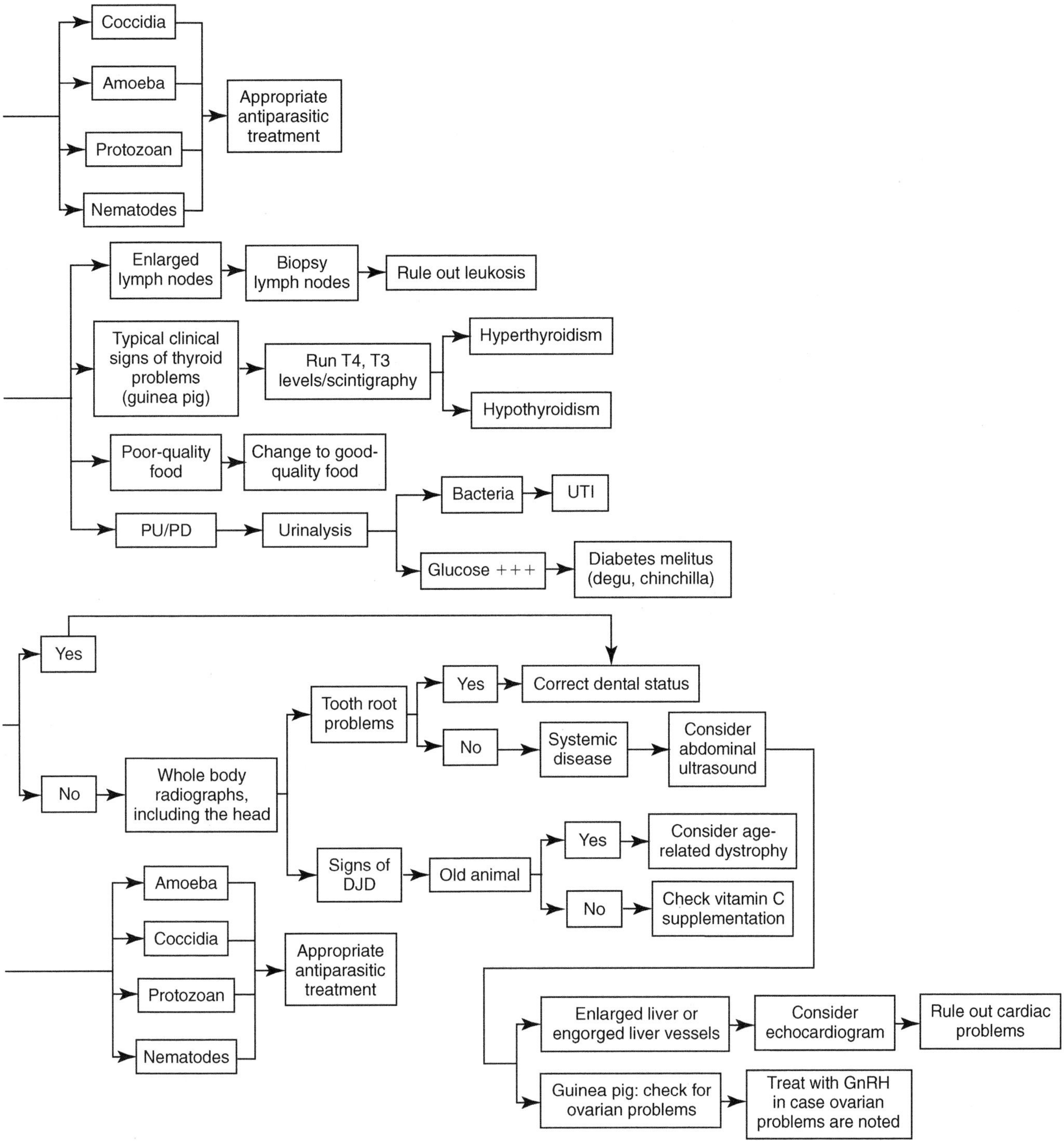
Coccidia
Amoeba
Protozoan
Nematodes
Appropriate antiparasitic treatment
Enlarged lymph nodes
Biopsy lymph nodes
Rule out leukosis
Typical clinical signs of thyroid problems (guinea pig)
Run T4, T3 levels/scintigraphy
Hyperthyroidism
Hypothyroidism
Poor-quality food
Change to good-quality food
PU/PD
Urinalysis
Bacteria
UTI
Glucose +++
Diabetes melitus (degu, chinchilla)
Yes
No
Whole body radiographs, including the head
Tooth root problems
Yes
Correct dental status
No
Systemic disease
Consider abdominal ultrasound
Signs of DJD
Old animal
Yes
Consider age-related dystrophy
No
Check vitamin C supplementation
Amoeba
Coccidia
Protozoan
Nematodes
Appropriate antiparasitic treatment
Enlarged liver or engorged liver vessels
Consider echocardiogram
Rule out cardiac problems
Guinea pig: check for ovarian problems
Treat with GnRH in case ovarian problems are noted

SMALL MAMMALS

Dyspnea

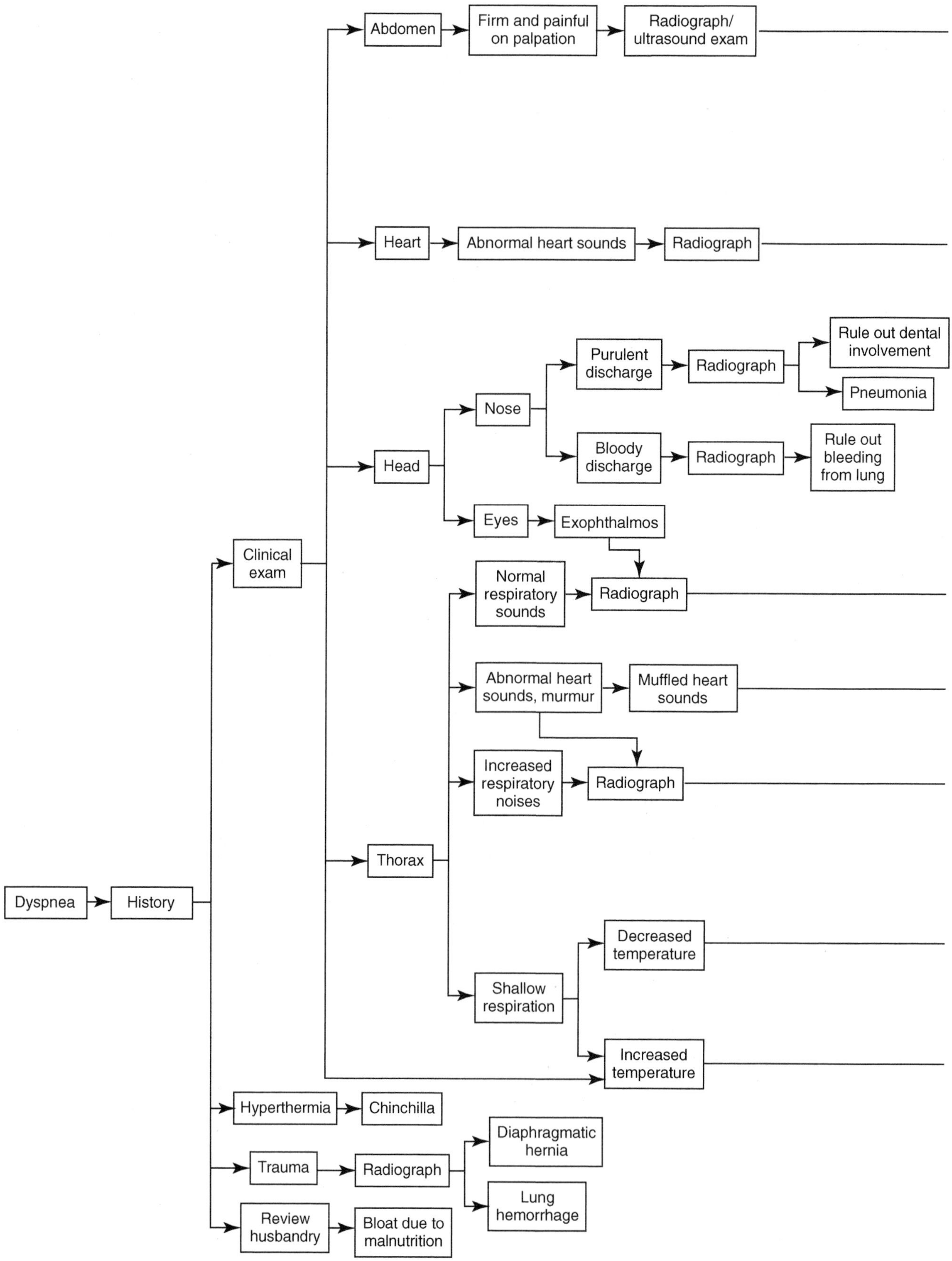

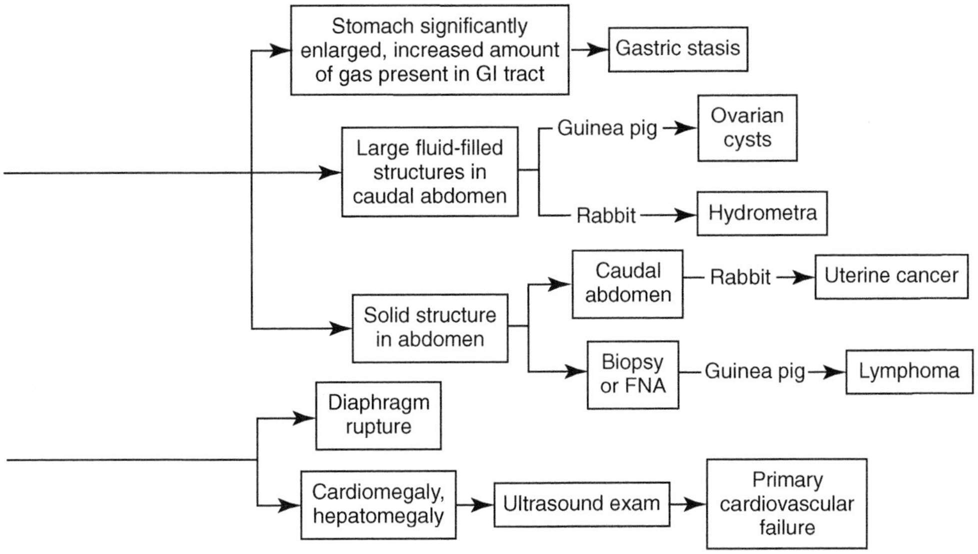
Stomach significantly enlarged, increased amount of gas present in GI tract
Gastric stasis
Large fluid-filled structures in caudal abdomen
Guinea pig
Ovarian cysts
Rabbit
Hydrometra
Solid structure in abdomen
Caudal abdomen
Rabbit
Uterine cancer
Biopsy or FNA
Guinea pig
Lymphoma
Diaphragm rupture
Cardiomegaly, hepatomegaly
Ultrasound exam
Primary cardiovascular failure

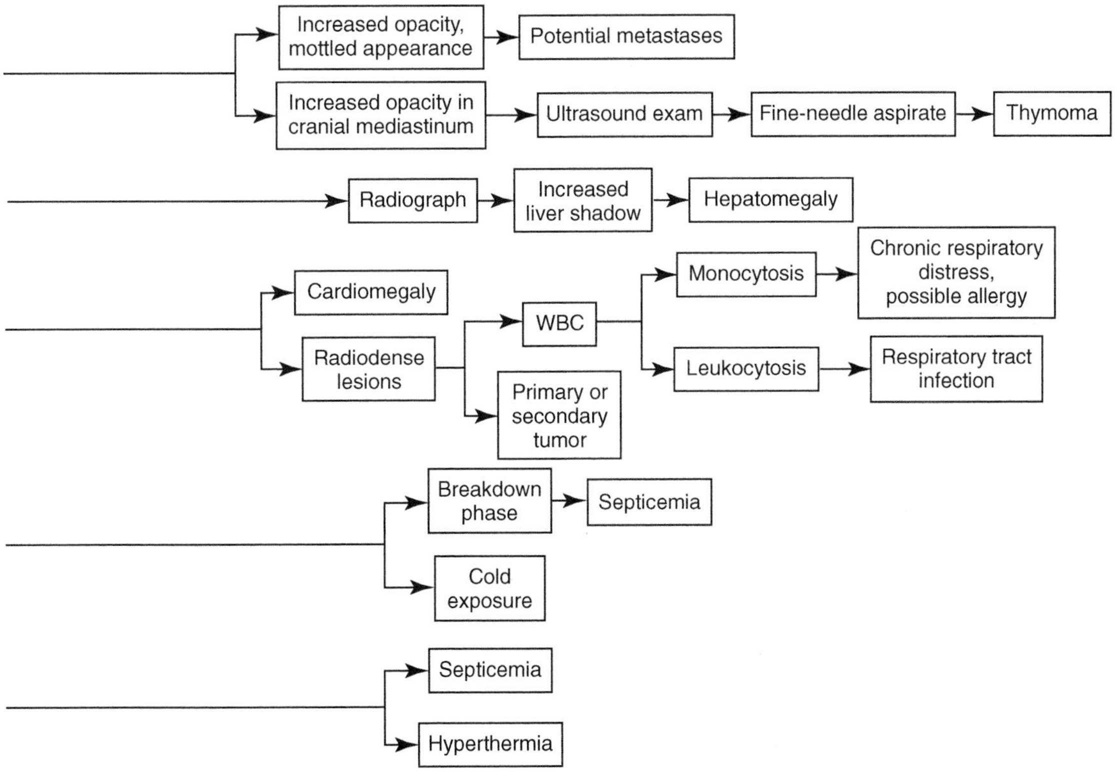
Increased opacity, mottled appearance
Potential metastases
Increased opacity in cranial mediastinum
Ultrasound exam
Fine-needle aspirate
Thymoma
Radiograph
Increased liver shadow
Hepatomegaly
Cardiomegaly
Radiodense lesions
WBC
Monocytosis
Chronic respiratory distress, possible allergy
Leukocytosis
Respiratory tract infection
Primary or secondary tumor
Breakdown phase
Septicemia
Cold exposure
Septicemia
Hyperthermia

SMALL MAMMALS

Lameness

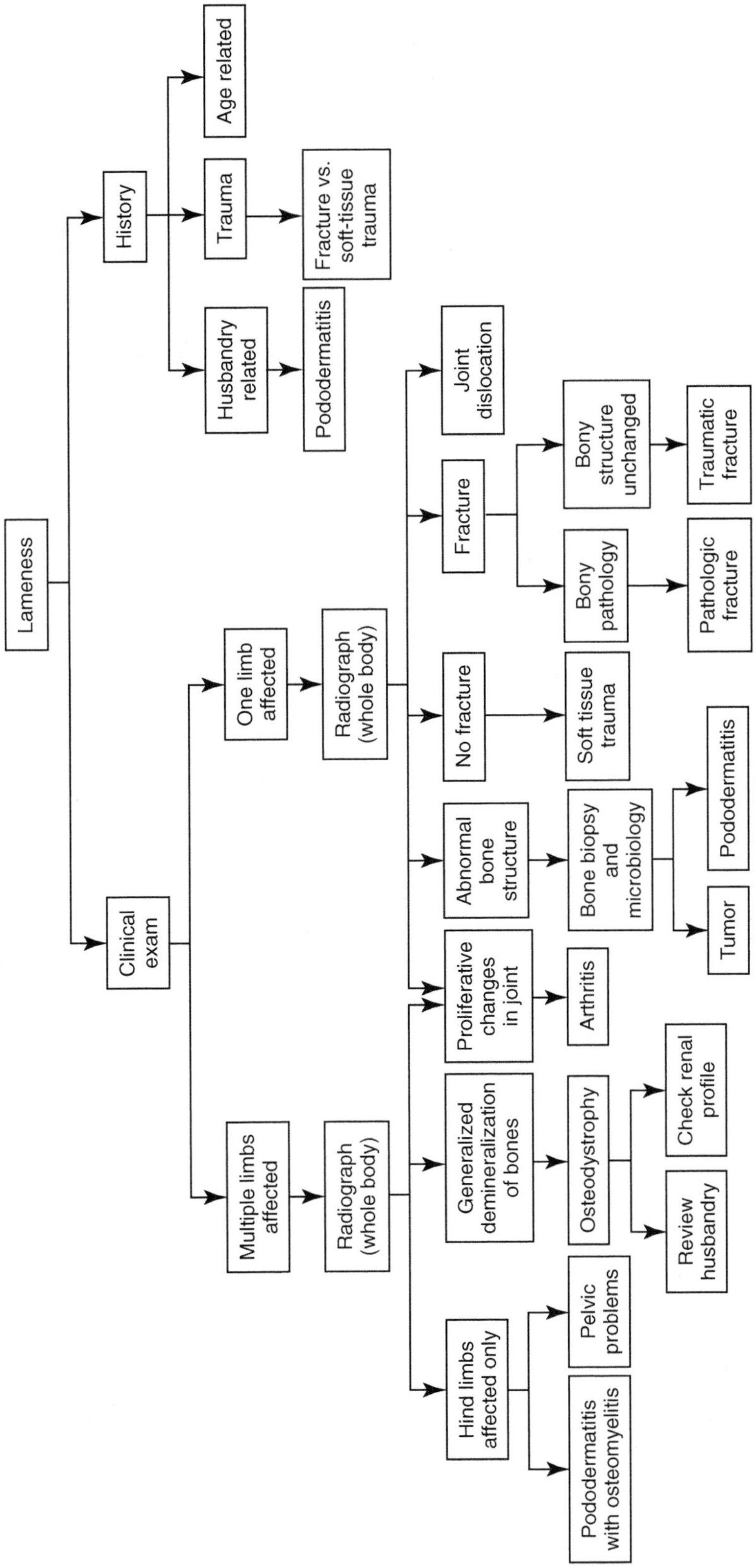

Lumps and Bumps

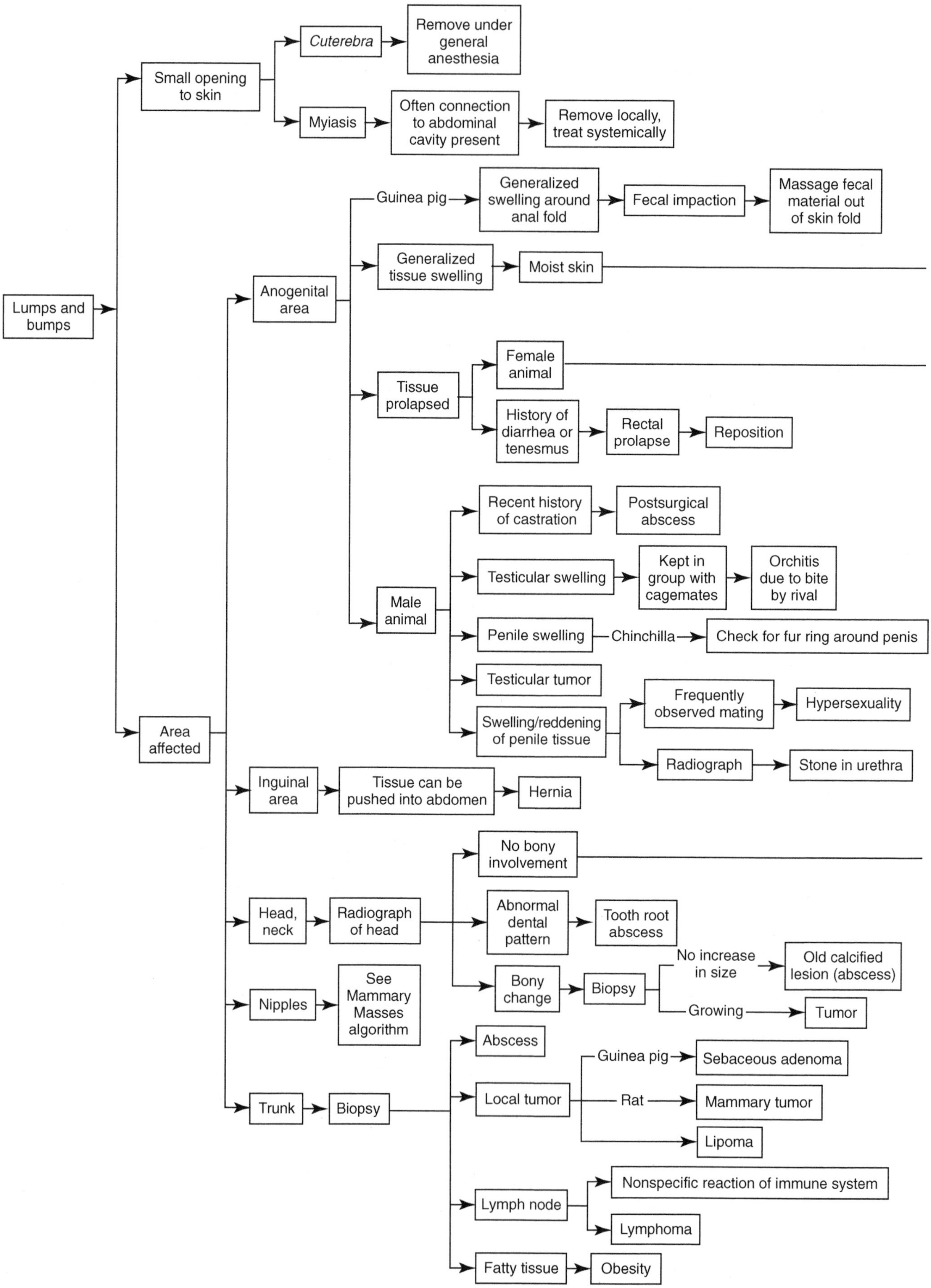

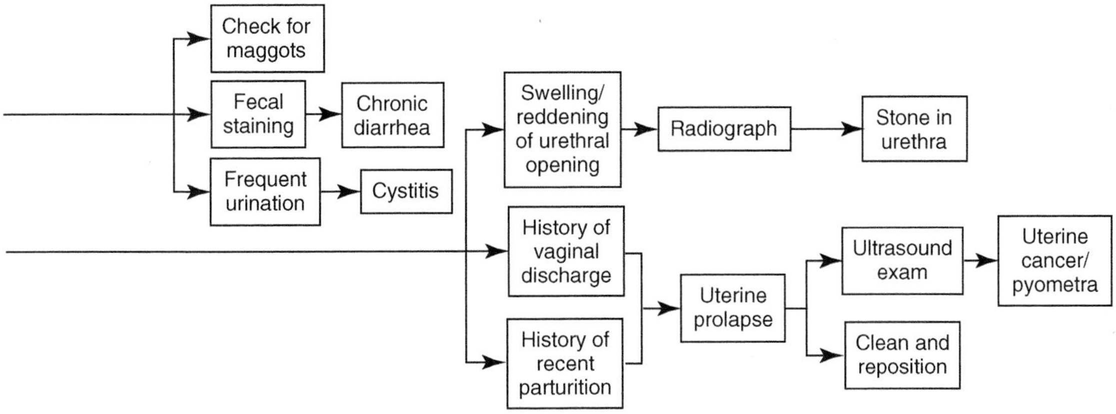

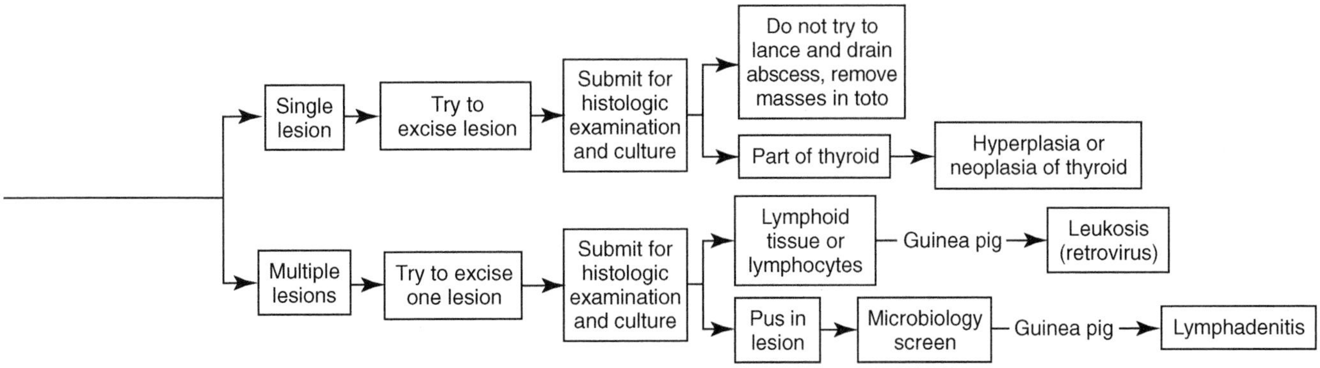

CLINICAL ALGORITHMS

SMALL MAMMALS

SMALL MAMMALS

Mammary Mass

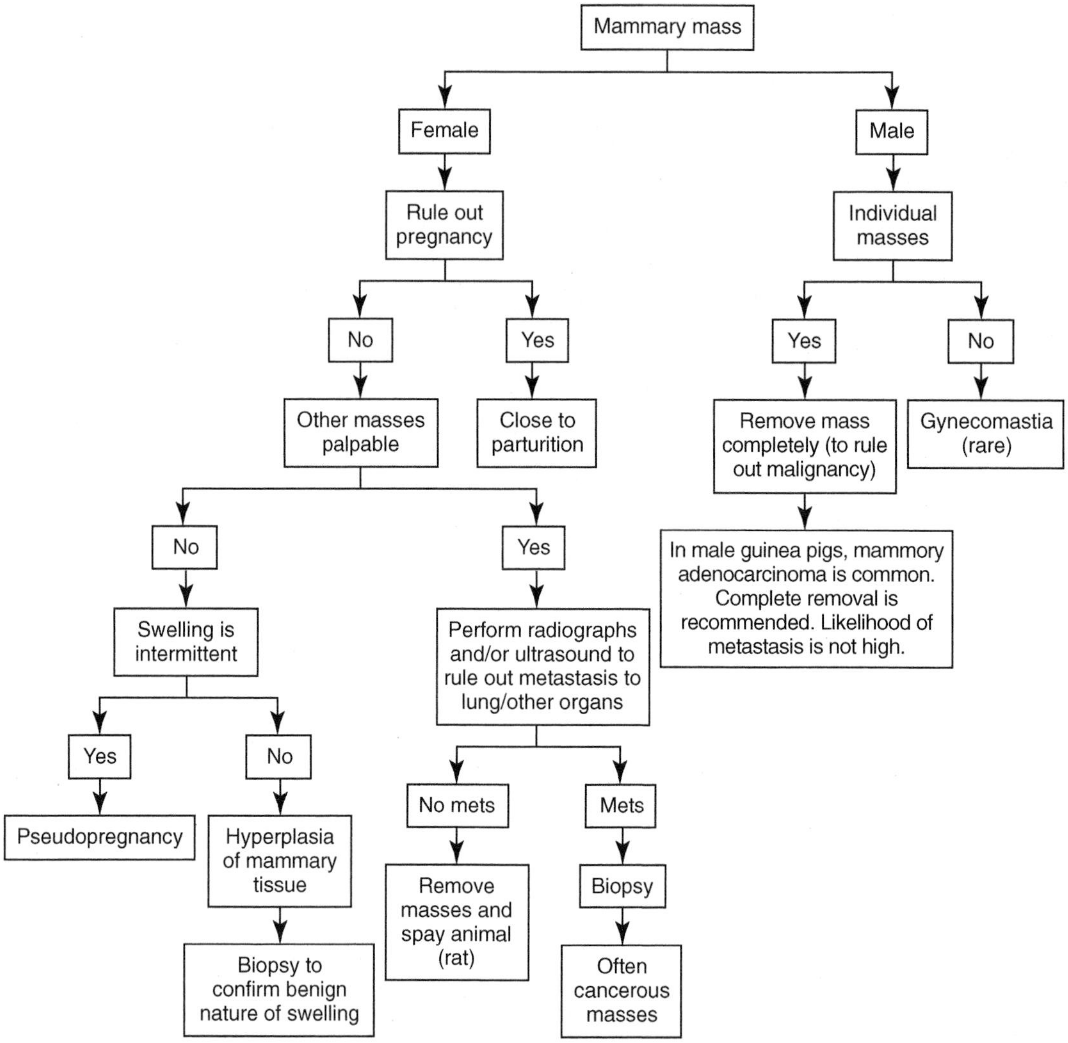

Ocular Changes

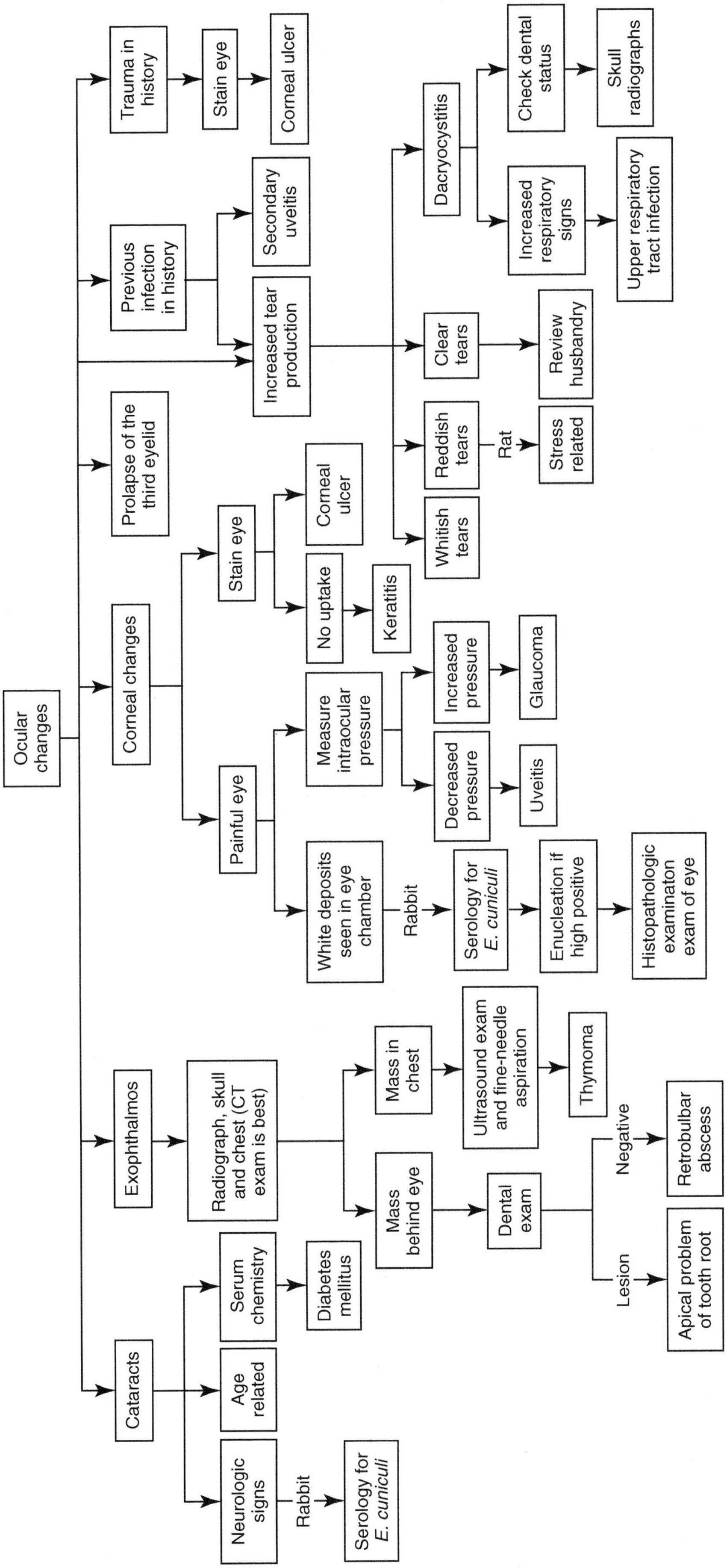

SMALL MAMMALS

Painful Abdomen

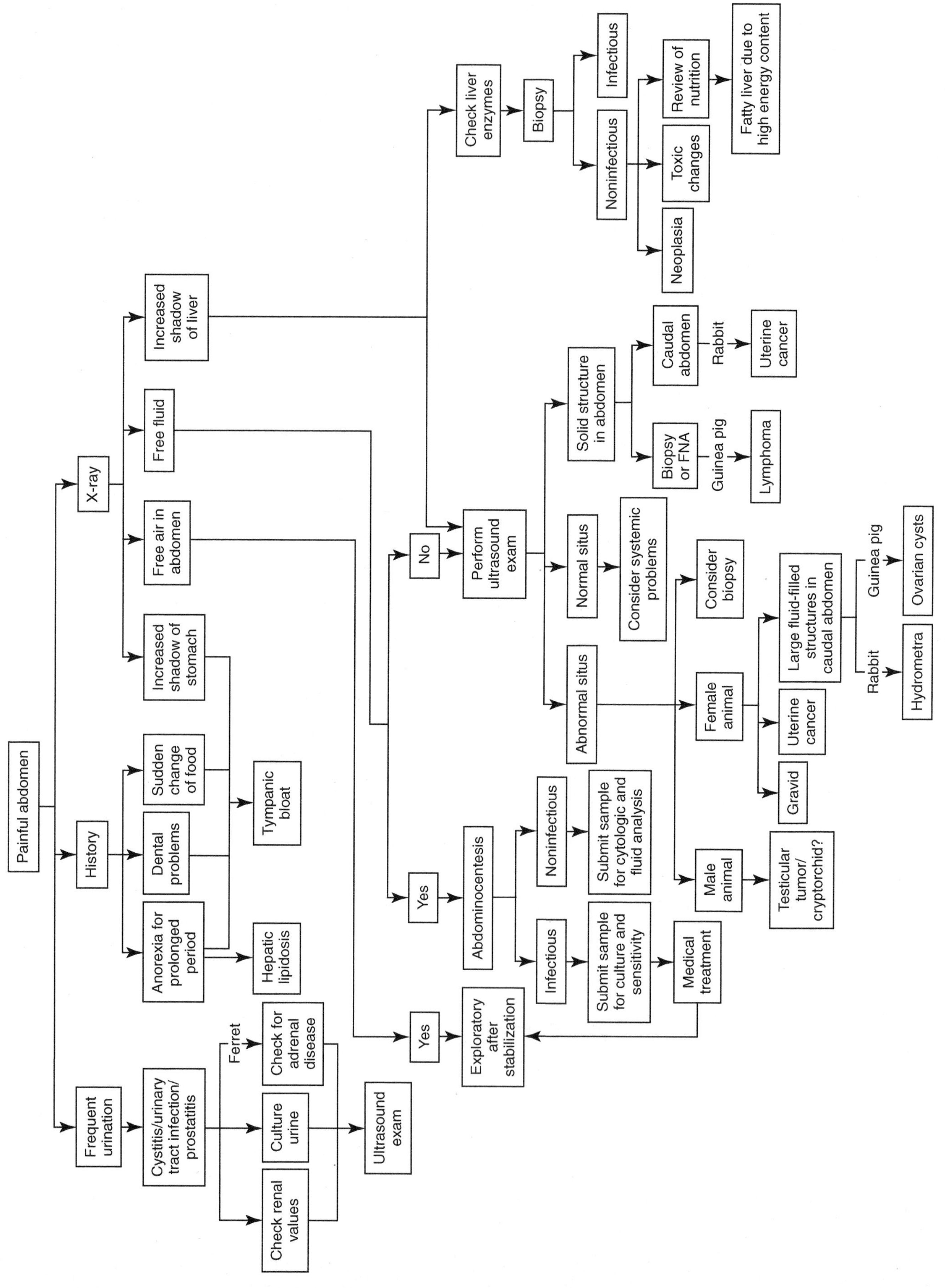

Paresis

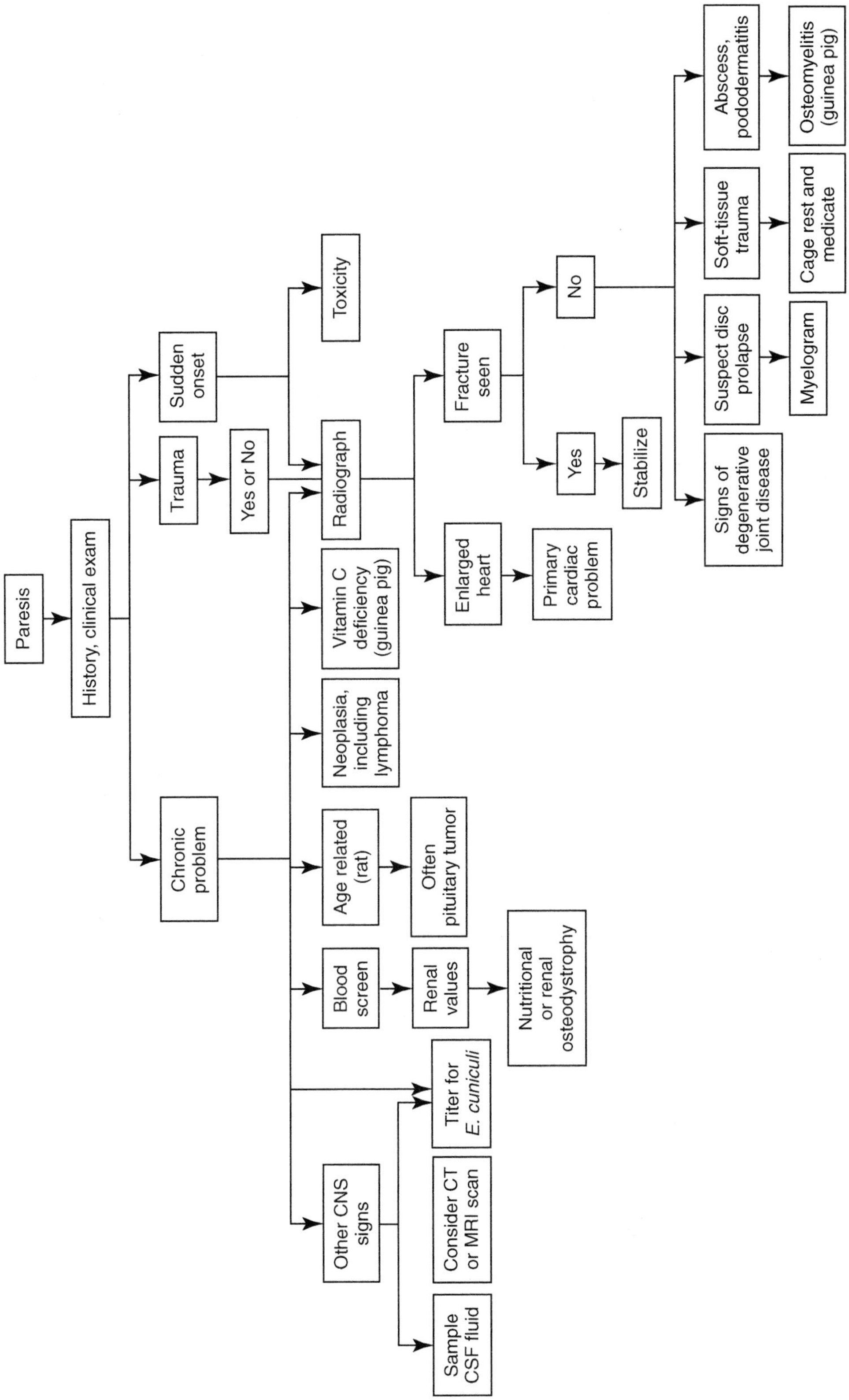
Paresis
History, clinical exam
Sudden onset
Trauma
Chronic problem
Yes or No
Toxicity
Radiograph
Vitamin C deficiency (guinea pig)
Neoplasia, including lymphoma
Age related (rat)
Often pituitary tumor
Blood screen
Renal values
Nutritional or renal osteodystrophy
Titer for E. cuniculi
Other CNS signs
Consider CT or MRI scan
Sample CSF fluid
Fracture seen
Enlarged heart
Primary cardiac problem
Yes
Stabilize
No
Signs of degenerative joint disease
Suspect disc prolapse
Myelogram
Soft-tissue trauma
Cage rest and medicate
Abscess, pododermatitis
Osteomyelitis (guinea pig)

SMALL MAMMALS

Skin/Fur Changes

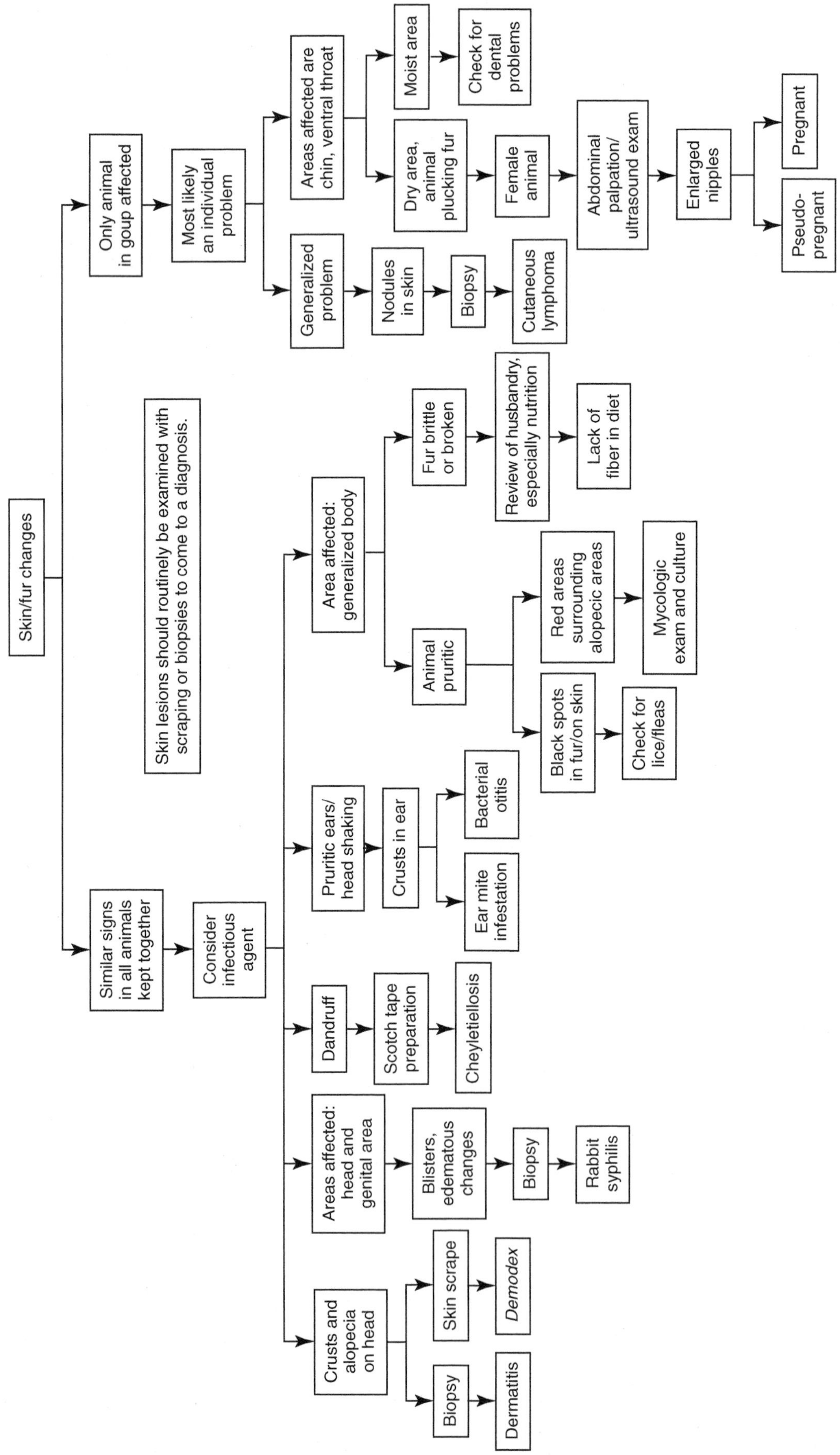

Vaginal Discharge

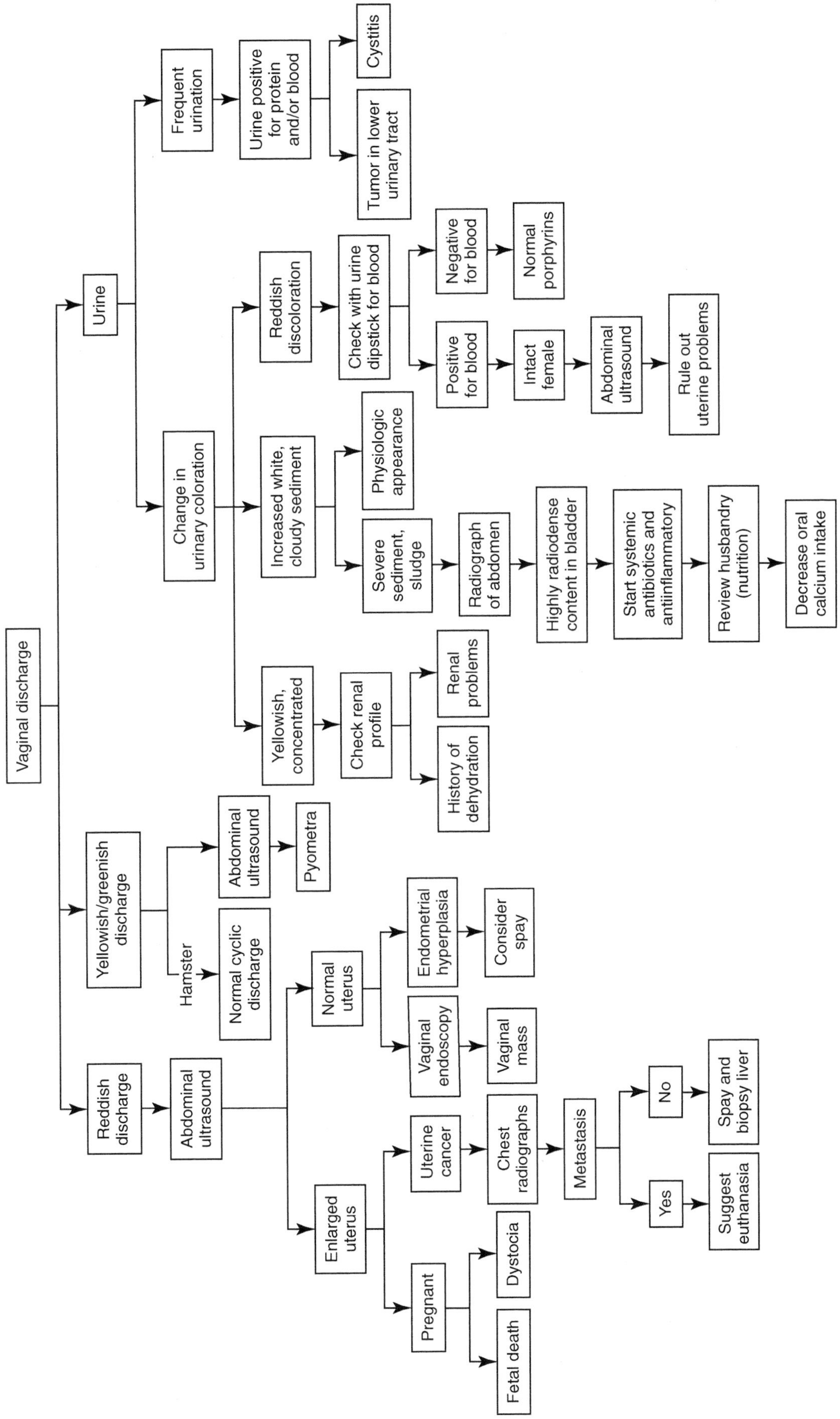

SMALL MAMMALS

Weight Loss, Chronic

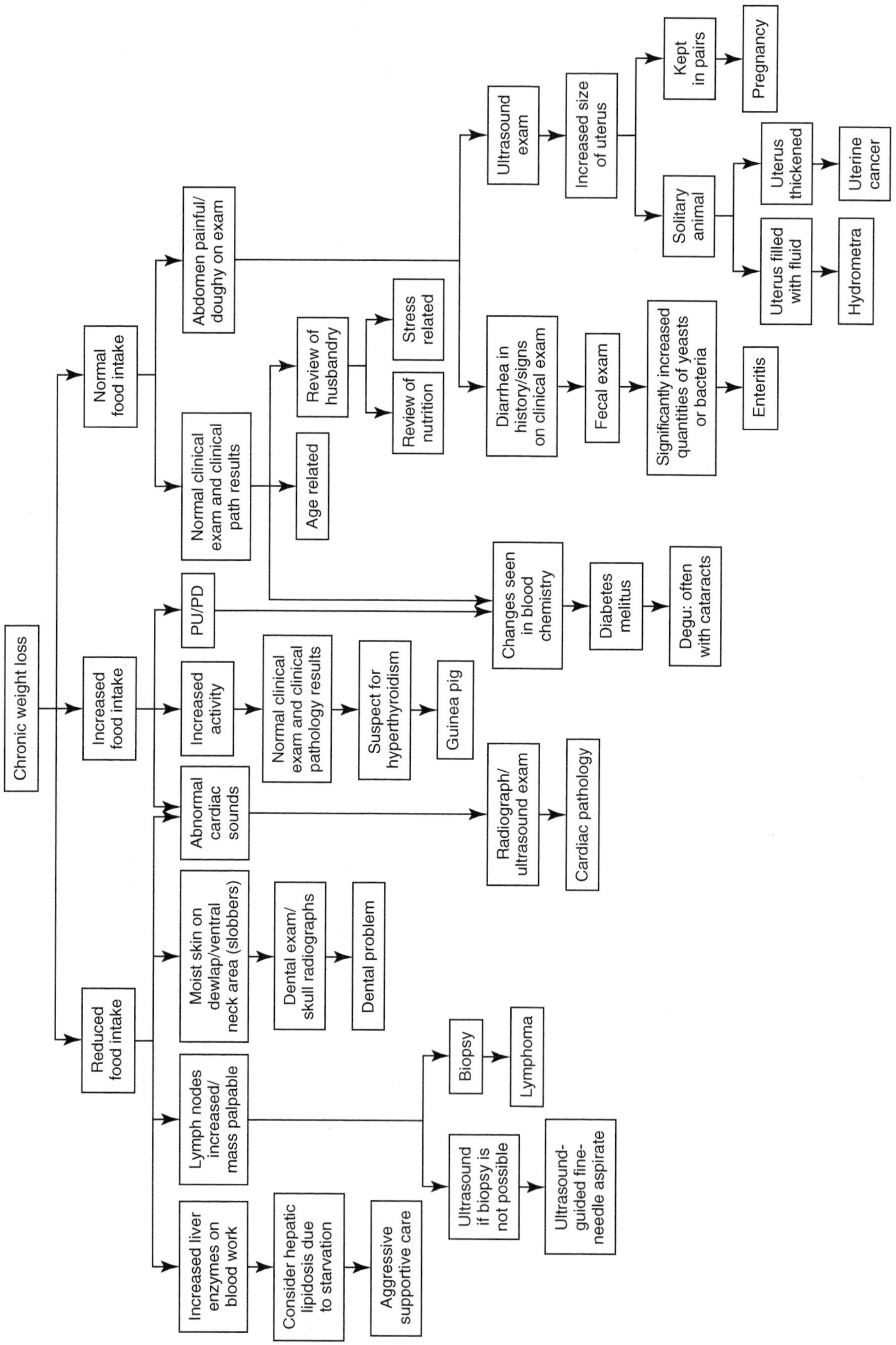

RABBITS

Urinary Changes

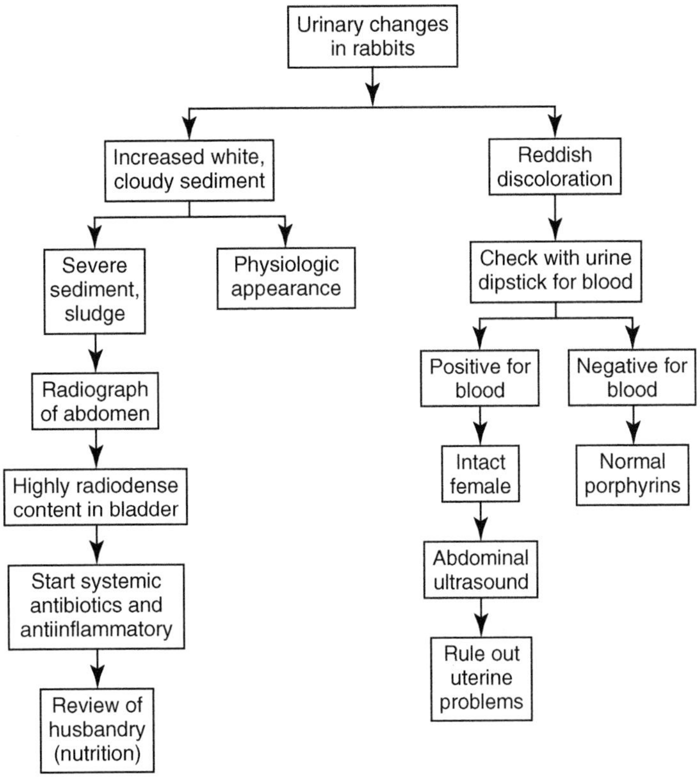

Zoonoses

EDITORS

Thomas M. Donnelly, BVSc, DipVetPath, DACLAM

Simon R. Starkey, BVSc, PhD, DABVP

Acariasis

BASIC INFORMATION

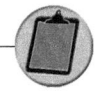

DEFINITION AND INFECTIOUS AGENT

- Mites of the order Acari are arachnids, which are responsible for acariasis in both humans and animals. Three clinically significant suborders of mites are seen in animals, each containing several different families.
- Most acariases are highly contagious in susceptible species, but they usually are highly species specific and are not capable of reproducing on aberrant hosts.
- Despite the vast number of different mite species, only a few can be successfully transmitted to humans, and zoonotic infections are predominantly self-limiting.
- *Cheyletiella* spp. (family Cheyletiellidae) are members of the suborder Prostigmata. They are highly contagious parasites of some mammal species.
- *Dermanyssus* spp. (family Dermanyssidae) are members of the suborder Mesostigmata that primarily parasitize birds, but are also seen in mammals. These mites normally reside in the environment (nests and roosts) during the day, but feed on sleeping birds during the night. Another member of the family Dermanyssidae is *Liponyssoides sanguineus*, which is a parasite of rodents.
- *Ornithonyssus* spp. (family Macronyssidae) are also parasites of the suborder Mesostigmata. They look similar to dermanyssid mites and have also been found on birds and rodents. These parasites differ from dermanyssids in that they spend most of their time on their hosts. Other similar genera include *Ophionyssus* and *Chiroptonyssus*.
- Mites of the family Sarcoptidae (within the suborder Astigmata) are a significant problem in a wide range of host species, but their degree of species specificity makes them less of a zoonotic concern. Genera included in this family are *Sarcoptes*, *Notoedres*, and *Trixacarus*. These mites have been known to parasitize many domestic and exotic animal species, and some may be passed transiently to humans. However, the variant of *Sarcoptes scabiei* that is found primarily in humans (*S. scabei* var. *hominis*) is not a zoonotic disease in that humans are the primary host.
- Members of the family Trombiculidae are parasitic in their larval stage (chiggers). They also belong to the suborder Prostigmata. These mites have been detected in a variety of wild and domestic animals and birds.

SYNONYMS

Disease

- In humans
  - *Dermanyssus* and *Ornithonyssus* infestations are also known as gamasoidosis, avian mite dermatitis, and bird mite rash.
  - Zoonotic infestation with members of the family Sarcoptidae is usually called *pseudoscabies* but has also been named "cavalryman's itch" and "pig-handler's itch."
- In animals
  - *Cutaneous acariasis* and *mange* are general terms for mite infestation.
  - Cheyletiellosis is widely known as "walking dandruff" because of its appearance.
  - Infestation of animals with Sarcoptidae is commonly called *sarcoptic mange* or *scabies*.

Organism

- *Cheyletiella* spp. are also known as "walking dandruff mites" or "fur mites."
- *Dermanyssus gallinae* is also known as the "red poultry mite," "chicken mite," or "pigeon mite." The common name of *Dermanyssus americanus* is the "American bird mite." *Liponyssoides sanguineus* is known commonly as the "house mouse mite."
- *Ornithonyssus bacoti* is also known as the "tropical rat mite." *Ornithonyssus bursa* and *O. sylviarum* are commonly called the "tropical fowl mite" and the "northern fowl mite," respectively. Other mites of this family are the snake mite *(Ophionyssus natricis)* and the free-tailed bat mite *(Chiroptonyssus robustipes)*.
- *Sarcoptes*, *Trixacarus*, and *Notoedres* spp. are known as "mange mites" or "scabietic mites."
- The common name of Trombiculidae larvae is *chiggers*. They are also known as "harvest mites," "mower's mites," and "red bugs."

EPIDEMIOLOGY

ANIMAL SPECIES—HOSTS AND/OR CARRIERS

Mammals

- *Cheyletiella parasitivorax* (rabbit), *Cheyletiella yasguri* (dog), and *Cheyletiella blackei* (cat) are fairly host specialized.
- *Dermanyssus* spp. may infest small rodents such as mice and gerbils.
- *Liponyssoides sanguineus* is most often associated with the house mouse, but has also been seen in gerbils.
- *Ornithonyssus* spp. affect bats, rats, and other rodents. Reports have described cases of *O. bacoti* in hamsters and gerbils leading to potential zoonoses.
- *Sarcoptes scabiei* variants are specialized to many wild and domestic species. In the wild, sarcoptic mange has been associated with foxes. Exotic mammals that have been shown to carry *S. scabiei* include ferrets and rarely young hedgehogs. *Trixacarus caviae* is the most common mite of the guinea pig. *Notoedres* spp. are usually parasites of cats and rodents. *Notoedres muris* is the "mange ear mite of rats." Sarcoptid mites may also affect rabbits but are seen less frequently than *Cheyletiella* spp., and their zoonotic potential remains questionable.
- Chiggers may infest small mammals, dogs, cats, and ungulates.

Birds

- *Dermanyssus gallinae* has been found in pet birds, poultry, and wild birds. It is the most common mite of pigeons.
- *Ornithonyssus sylviarum* and *Ornithonyssus bursa* affect a variety of wild and domestic birds, including ducks, finches, pigeons, starlings, psittacines, and canaries.
- Chiggers can be found on the wings and vents of affected birds.

Reptiles

- *Ophionyssus natricis* is a Macronyssid mite that has rarely been reported in snakes.
- Chiggers may also be seen rarely in reptiles.

MODES OF TRANSMISSION

- Transmission of mites occurs by physical contact with infested individuals or by contact with mites in the environment.
- *Cheyletiella* spp. most often are transmitted by direct contact, but they can also be picked up from the environment, especially in sleeping areas. These mites can survive off the host for longer than other mites (females up to 10 days, maybe longer), making it possible to come into contact with

them for some time after the host has left.

- *Ornithonyssus* and *Dermanyssus* spp. are transmitted by contact with affected animals, as well as by infested bedding material and bird roosts. These mites have the ability to survive for months in the environment after birds have been removed.
- *Trixacarus*, *Sarcoptes*, and *Notoedres* spp. are spread largely by direct skin-to-skin contact with infested individuals. Humans may be exposed by holding, petting, and grooming animals. Indirect transmission via fomites is rare, but when the disease is in a crusted, hyperkeratotic form, mites may persist in sloughed epidermis for days. Survival rate is decreased by higher ambient temperature and humidity.
- Chiggers, because of their life cycle, are not directly transmitted from animals to humans, but the presence of animals does pose an indirect risk to humans. These mites lay eggs on leaves and grass blades, which hatch in 1 to 2 weeks. Larvae cling onto animals that brush against them and begin to feed.
- In all zoonotic acariases, a common characteristic is self-limiting infestation of humans. Because these mites are incapable of reproducing on unusual hosts, they cannot complete their life cycle on or be transmitted by humans.

CLINICAL PRESENTATION OF ANIMALS

Rabbits

- *Cheyletiella parasitivorax* may present as mild alopecia, heavy (walking) dandruff, loose body fur, thick red-brown crusts on the ears, or scaly, red, oily patches on the dorsum and head. Additionally, infection is often asymptomatic, reports have described large percentages of rabbits in commercial colonies as carriers.

Ferrets

- *Sarcoptes scabiei* usually presents as intense pruritus and generalized alopecia, often localized to the toes and feet. It is most prominent on sparsely haired skin and eventually may lead to lichenification, exudation, and crusting. Toenails may become deformed and may slough.

Guinea pigs

- *Trixacarus caviae* is also intensely pruritic, to the point that it has been associated with self-trauma, seizures, and abortions. Lesions appear on the shoulders, dorsum, and flank. Alopecia may progress to lichenification, hyperpigmentation, crusting, and scaling as the infestation becomes more chronic. Secondary bacterial infection is also common. A subclinical carrier state can exist in guinea pigs for some time until a period of immune compromise.

Small rodents

- *Ornithonyssus* and *Dermanyssus* spp. may manifest as papules, but some species can cause anemia, debility, weakness, pruritus, and death in small rodents. Subclinical carriers may also exist. *O. bacoti* is a vector of the rodent filarial nematode *Litomosoides carinii*.
- *Notoedres muris* in rats affects the pinnae, nose tail, and sometimes external genitalia and paws, causing a pruritic and papular, crusting dermatitis. Typical pinna lesions are papillomas such as horny excrescences with thick yellow crusts. Those on the nose are wartlike and horny, but tail and dermal lesions are erythematous and vesicular and are often associated with alopecia. Rarely, hamsters are infested with *N. muris*. Infestation is similar to rats. *N. muris* is not known to infest humans.

Birds

- *Ornithonyssus* infestation most commonly causes blackened feathers, cracks and scabs around the cloaca, and decreased productivity in birds.
- *Dermanyssus* spp. cause anemia and decreased production in poultry. In pet birds, signs include restlessness, excessive preening, pruritus, anemia, and death.
- Large burdens of chiggers can lead to anorexia, lethargy, and death.

RISK FACTORS

Rabbits

- *Cheyletiella* spp. are highly contagious. Risk factors include exposure to infested animals and infestation of the environment.

Ferrets

- Risk of infestation by *Sarcoptes scabiei* is directly related to the amount of contact with infested animals. Young or immune compromised ferrets may be at greater risk.

Guinea pigs

- Guinea pigs are most likely to become carriers of *Trixacarus caviae* when kept in close contact with severely affected cagemates. Risk factors for the development of clinical disease in carriers include stressors such as old age and concurrent disease (e.g., hypovitaminosis C).

Small rodents

- Risk of *Ornithonyssus* spp. and *Dermanyssus* spp. infection is directly related to environmental exposure to the mites.
- *Notoedres* spp. risk, similar to the risk of any sarcoptid mites, is related to the amount of physical contact with infested individuals.

Birds

- Risk of *Ornithonyssus* spp. and *Dermanyssus* spp. exposure in pet birds is related to the degree of environmental exposure, as well as to proximity to wild birds (such as pigeons) and recently abandoned or fledgling nests. Nestlings may be predisposed because of their stationary lifestyle.
- The risk of picking up chiggers is related to the environmental burden. Birds that are kept outside may be at greater risk.

GEOGRAPHY AND SEASONALITY

- Most zoonotic mites are found worldwide.
- *Ornithonyssus* spp. are present worldwide, with some predominating in tropical areas (*O. bursa*), and others in Australia, New Zealand, and the temperate Northern Hemisphere (*O. sylviarum*). *Dermanyssus* spp. are found worldwide.
  - Most cases involving these mites take place in late spring or early summer, when fledglings are leaving the nest and the mites are searching for another food source.
- Chiggers are found worldwide and are more prevalent in late summer and early autumn. Large numbers are present in some parts of Asia.

PATHOBIOLOGY

- *Cheyletiella* spp. are hair-clasping, nonburrowing mites that live on the keratin layer of the epidermis, feeding on debris, tissues, and body fluids. They usually stay on one host for life but often will move transiently to other hosts to feed.
- *Ornithonyssus* spp. and *Dermanyssus* spp. are nonburrowing, blood-sucking mites. In animals, pathogenesis is often linked to blood loss, in addition to dermatologic effects. Additionally, *Ornithonyssus bursa* can carry Western equine encephalitis, and *Ornithonyssus bacoti* is a potential vector of several pathogens (i.e., murine typhus [*Rickettsia typhi*], rickettsialpox [*R. akari*], Q fever [*Coxiella burnetii*], Lyme disease [*Borrelia burgdorferi*], hantavirus [hemorrhagic fever with renal syndrome], and plague [*Yersinia pestis*]). *Liponyssoides sanguineus* can be a vector of rickettsialpox in humans.
- *Trixacarus*, *Sarcoptes*, and *Notoedres* spp. live in tunnels in the skin, starting at hairless patches. A hyperkeratosis often results from their presence. These mites leave the skin susceptible to secondary bacterial infection, often with *Streptococcus pyogenes* or *Staphylococcus aureus*.
- Chiggers form a stylostome (feeding tube) through the epidermis, which is

lined by necrotic cells. The mouth parts of these mites may remain in the skin after the mites are scratched off, leaving the host highly pruritic for days after removal. In Asia, chiggers are also vectors of the rickettsial bacterium *Orientia tsutsugamushi*, the cause of scrub typhus, a disease characterized by fever, papular rash, various signs of malaise, and lymphadenopathy in humans. They are also suspected to be vectors for various other arthropod-borne diseases.

CLINICAL PRESENTATION OF HUMANS

INCIDENCE IN HUMANS

- *Cheyletiella* spp. are the most common zoonotic mites of exotic pets, although owners are more likely to be infected by dogs and cats. *Cheyletiella* spp. are highly contagious, and having infested pets poses a high risk to humans. Up to 20% of pet owners with infested animals will become infected.
- *Ornithonyssus* spp. and *Dermanyssus* spp. pose the greatest risk to people with occupational exposure to birds or a history of contact with wild birds, pigeons, poultry, or nest material. Handling of wild or pet rodents (especially those with dermatologic problems) may be a source of exposure. Especially after fledglings have left a nest or after rodent extermination, these mites may be seeking a new host. Reports have described *Dermanyssus* spp. and *Ornithonyssus* spp. biting people exposed to caged birds and pet gerbils. *Liponyssoides sanguineus* is unlikely to seek a human host, but this may occur in urban areas where the mouse population has been eradicated.
- Infrequent reports have documented transmission of *Trixacarus*, *Sarcoptes*, and *Notoedres* spp. from exotic pets to humans. The human variant or scabies (*Sarcoptes scabiei* var. *hominis*) is a much more significant public health concern because it can be transmitted between humans. Farmers, veterinarians, wildlife rehabilitators, and pet owners may be at risk of infestation with *Trixacarus*, *Sarcoptes*, and *Notoedres* species. Zoonotic transmission of these mites is seen mostly from dogs, cats, and livestock, but reports have discussed transmission from a variety of infested small mammals. According to some reports, reverse zoonotic transmission (from humans to animals) may also be possible.
- Chiggers are not directly zoonotic in that they are transmitted only from animals to humans via the environment. These mites pose a threat to people who spend more time in outdoor areas where wild or free-ranging animals are present, and can be a significant problem in infested areas. The risk of obtaining chiggers is increased by living near an area that has a high parasite burden.
- Humans might be particularly susceptible to acariases of any kind if they are in a state of immune compromise (e.g., post transplantation surgery, HIV infection, frail and elderly persons).
- People living in crowded, unsanitary conditions in close proximity to host species have a greater chance of contracting these zoonoses.
- Poor sensory perception (e.g., neurologic disease, leprosy) may predispose people to acariasis.

DISEASE FORMS/SUBTYPES

Dermatologic acariasis

- Acariasis normally manifests as a dermatologic condition.

Systemic reactions

- Systemic reactions to mites are rare and often involve a component of allergic response.
  - One case of systemic response to *Cheyletiella* infection has been reported and involved peripheral eosinophilia and circulating immune complexes.
- Chiggers have been reported to cause hypersensitivity reactions.

Vector-borne diseases

- Some zoonotic mite species transmit bacterial or viral pathogens.

HISTORY, CHIEF COMPLAINT

History

- The history of affected individuals usually involves close contact with the animal host species or presence within an environment known to have a heavy mite burden. However, reports have described zoonotic mite infestation with no known exposure to affected animals.

Chief complaint

- The predominant chief complaint of humans with zoonotic acariases is of pruritus and nonspecific idiopathic dermatitis.

PHYSICAL FINDINGS IN INFECTED HUMANS

- *Cheyletiella* infestation in humans usually will cause a mildly pruritic dermatitis on the abdomen, chest, arms, legs, and buttocks. Small urticarial papules and vesicles may develop into an erythematous rash or into yellow crusted lesions that can be intensely pruritic. An area of central necrosis is often noted. Rare bullous eruptions and systemic reactions have been reported, especially in people with concurrent autoimmune disease.
- *Ornithonyssus* and *Dermanyssus* infestations often present as painful, localized nonspecific dermatitis. They usually manifest as an erythematous papular rash that often excoriates because of intense pruritus. Occasionally, vesicles, urticarial plaques, diffuse erythema, or hemorrhage is seen. Affected areas of the skin are those usually covered by clothing (such as arms and trunk); the face and webs of fingers are usually spared. *Liponyssoides sanguineus* usually causes a small, painless eschar or dark crust resolving in 2 to 3 weeks, but mites of this species may carry rickettsialpox *(R. akari)*, which causes fever, and a self-limiting maculopapular rash that scabs over within a few days.
- *Trixacarus*, *Sarcoptes*, and *Notoedres* spp. cause pruritus and a papular rash over the shoulders, axillae, abdomen, and legs and in the spaces between fingers. As with most zoonotic acariases, infestation is self-limiting, lasting 1 to 3 weeks. Burrowing may be absent in zoonotic scabies.
- Chiggers can cause a dermatitis characterized by small red papules with intense pruritus or wheals that may bleed and progress to pustules. Affected sites may remain painful for weeks and most often are located on feet, ankles, and borders of constricting clothing. Allergic reactions and concurrent scrub typhus in endemic areas can add to the clinical picture.

INCUBATION PERIOD The incubation period varies depending on the mite species, but it is usually fairly short. The life cycle of *Cheyletiella* spp. takes approximately 35 days, but these mites normally infest humans only transiently, quickly biting without burrowing and then returning to the animal host. Dermanyssid and Macronyssid mites may also bite humans while they are transiently present. For sarcoptid mites, the incubation period can be 2 to 6 weeks, but mites may begin to bite humans within hours of contact. Signs of chiggers may appear within 3 to 4 days of infestation.

DIAGNOSIS

DIFFERENTIAL DIAGNOSIS

HUMANS

- Human scabies
- Bedbug bites
- Psoriasis
- Lice
- Insect bites
- Chicken pox
- Contact dermatitis
- Folliculitis
- Bacterial cellulitis
- Atopic dermatitis

ANIMALS

- Other arthropod infestation
- Ringworm
- Yeast infection
- Bacterial dermatitis

- Endocrine disease
- Nutritional deficiency
- Barbering
- Allergic reaction

INITIAL DATABASE

- Obtaining a thorough history is often the most important step in diagnosing acariasis in both humans and animals. Information about interaction with host species and the degree of pruritus may be highly suggestive of specific diseases.
- A basic physical examination is also very important. The distribution and appearance of the dermatitis may provide valuable information.
- Blood work may help to identify an inflammatory response, but it is unlikely to be diagnostic.

ADVANCED OR CONFIRMATORY TESTING

- Skin scraping, the most common means of diagnosis, can be used to detect mites, eggs, or scybala (brown-gold–colored feces). A scalpel blade, possibly coated with mineral or immersion oil, is held at a right angle to the skin surface and is used to remove debris, along with the stratum corneum. The skin is scraped until pink but not hemorrhaging, and material is placed onto a microscope slide with additional oil as needed. The sample is normally examined as a wet mount under low power.
- Unfortunately, skin scrapings are often negative, leading to diagnosis by exclusion of other diseases that takes into consideration history, clinical presentation, and distribution pattern.
- Other techniques include epidermal biopsy and the burrow ink test, in which blue or black ink is applied to the skin and is pulled into burrows by capillary action; when excess ink is removed by alcohol, ink-colored burrows are revealed.
- An adhesive tape test can be used for superficial mites such as *Cheyletiella* spp. Tape is pressed onto areas of dermatitis to collect mites and eggs. These mites may also be obtained by using a fine-toothed comb or toothbrush after applying a rapid-acting insecticidal spray. If crusts are placed in alcohol, mites may be detected floating to the top.
- Sarcoptid mites are 0.3 to 0.5 mm and circular, with four pairs of legs. *Cheyletiella* spp. measure approximately 0.6 × 0.3 mm and are easily identified by their large palpal claws.
- Ornithonyssid mites may be detected more easily in the environment than on the animal. These gray mites turn red after feeding on blood.
- Chiggers may be found only in the environment. They are free-living in nymphal and adult stages, and larvae are most easily recognized by their bright red/orange color and scutum pattern.
- Diagnosis of most zoonotic acariases in humans is made difficult by the fact that most mites will only transiently remain on the human host, unable to persist to life cycle completion. Additionally, human and animal variants of *Sarcoptes scabiei* are physically indistinguishable, making this species difficult to assess.

TREATMENT

HUMANS

- Because human infestations are normally self-limiting, the most important step is to remove the source of zoonotic infection. This is best accomplished by treating or avoiding contact with the host animal and disinfecting the environment.
- *Cheyletiella* spp. zoonoses should resolve within 3 weeks of treatment of the infested pet and its environment.
- Infestation of *Ornithonyssus* and *Dermanyssus* spp. is eliminated by a combination of bathing and treating the host animal and environment as needed. In the case of wild animal sources, this may involve exterminating wild rats or not allowing wild pigeons onto a windowsill. Topical corticosteroid creams may be applied if needed.
- No additional treatment may be necessary for humans exposed to *Trixacarus*, *Sarcoptes*, and *Notoedres* spp. Topical lotions containing permethrin and oral ivermectin may be used to kill zoonotic *Sarcoptes scabiei*, but they are more necessary for the human variant. Resolution may be expedited by clipping fingernails, removing and cleaning jewelry, bathing regularly, and laundering clothing in hot water and drying on a hot dry cycle.
- Treatment of chiggers is aimed at relief of symptoms. Options include topical anesthetics, topical corticosteroids, intralesional corticosteroid injections, oral antihistamines, and application of ice to the lesion. Avoiding high-risk areas and using insect repellent will prevent further exposure.
- In all cases, affected individuals should seek the care of a physician and consult with a veterinarian.

RABBITS

- *Cheyletiella* spp. infestations can be treated using ectoparasitic shampoos and dips, permethrin, or topical amitraz formulations. Do not use fipronil because it can be fatal in rabbits. Clean the animal's environment by disinfecting its sleeping area, vacuuming exposed carpets, laundering exposed clothing, and disinfecting grooming supplies. Signs should resolve within 3 weeks of treatment.

FERRETS

- *Sarcoptes scabiei* infestation is treated using ivermectin at a dose of 0.2 to 0.4 mg/kg subcutaneously every 7 to 14 days for three doses. In-contact animals should also be treated. Lime sulfur or keratolytic shampoos are also used.

GUINEA PIGS

- *Trixacarus caviae* is also treated with ivermectin. Dosages vary from two 0.5-mg/kg subcutaneous doses 1 week apart to three doses of 0.2 to 0.4 mg/kg subcutaneously every 10 days. Oral ivermectin may not be as effective. Dusting with permethrin and carbamate powders may also be considered—use kitten doses. Treat all in-contact animals, and clean the house.

SMALL RODENTS

- *Dermanyssus* spp. and *Ornithonyssus* spp. infestations are best combated by removing wild animals and treating the environment. Parasitized pets may be bathed to remove mites. Symptomatic therapy is often the only therapy for rats; it consists of antihistamines and topical corticosteroids.
- *Notoedres* spp. have been treated with ivermectin (400 mcg/kg SC for a minimum of 8 weekly treatments; repeat until skin scrapings are negative in all infected animals), oral moxidectin (0.5% solution at 2.0 mg/kg), and topical moxidectin (0.5% solution at 0.5 mg/kg) or selamectin (6 to 12 mg/kg). Fox squirrels have responded to a single subcutaneous dose of ivermectin at 0.5 mg/kg.

BIRDS

- Hosts of *Ornithonyssus* and *Dermanyssus* spp. have been treated with topical acaricides such as gamma benzene hexachloride, pyrethroid, and organophosphate compounds. Removal of wild birds and infested nesting material from an area, as well as house cleaning and fumigation with pyrethroids, organophosphates, or carbamate-based acaricides, has been used to eliminate environmental sources. Treatment of *Dermanyssus* spp. may require only treatment of the host; treatment of *Ornithonyssus* spp. may require only environmental treatment.
- Treatment of chiggers focuses on prevention, by changing the animal's environment.

PREVENTION

- The most important method of prevention is minimizing exposure of humans and their pets to infested animals (wild or domestic).
- Pets should be kept away from wild animals, which may serve as reservoirs for mites.
- Pets should be kept in a clean environment that does not support the propagation of parasitic species.
- Prompt diagnosis of dermatologic disease in pets is necessary to decrease the risk of zoonotic exposure.
- If pets are known to be carriers of any type of acariasis, they should be treated as soon as possible. Gloves should be worn when suspect animals are handled.

REPORTING—NOTIFIABLE DISEASE

- Acariasis in humans and in animals is not reportable in the United States.
- Sarcoptic mange is reportable only in cattle.

PROGNOSIS

- In cases that are uncomplicated by secondary bacterial or rickettsial infection, zoonotic acariasis is normally self-limiting and carries a good prognosis for complete recovery in humans.
- In definitive host species, prognosis depends on the specific disease and the stage of progression, but if caught early enough, the prognosis for affected animals can be fairly good.

CONTROVERSY

Questions have arisen regarding whether certain mite species should actually be considered a zoonotic risk because of the lack of observed cases in the literature, as well as a large degree of host specificity. It is difficult to assess the frequency of these zoonoses in humans because they may be diagnosed inaccurately or overlooked at the time, but it seems reasonable to conclude that the potential does exist for interspecific spread of a variety of ectoparasites, both to and from humans.

PEARLS & CONSIDERATIONS

COMMENTS

- Although zoonotic acariasis may not itself pose a major public health threat, it is important not to overlook it when diagnosing and treating dermatologic conditions in humans.
  - Zoonotic mite infestations are often misdiagnosed because of lack of knowledge about their epidemiology; consequently, human and animal patients may not be receiving the most appropriate care.
  - Zoonotic acariasis should be considered on a differential list of human dermatides, especially when interaction with affected animals is noted in the history.
- Dermatologic conditions, often caused by ectoparasites, make up 25% of the cases in exotic pets presented for small animal consultations in general practice.

CLIENT EDUCATION

- Owners of exotic pets should be educated about the zoonotic potential of skin diseases that may develop in these animals.
- Many small mammals and birds can be carriers of various zoonotic acariases. Although spread to humans normally is self-limiting and even more infrequent than spread from dogs and cats, it is still possible.

SUGGESTED READINGS

Dobrosavljevic DD, et al: Systemic manifestations of Cheyletiella infestation in man, Int J Dermatol 46:397–399, 2007.

Engel PM, et al: Tropical rat mite dermatitis: case report and review, Clin Infect Dis 27:1465–1469, 1998.

Lucky AW, et al: Avian mite bites acquired from a new source—pet gerbils: report of 2 cases and review of the literature, Arch Dermatol 137:167–170, 2001.

McClain D, et al: Mite infestations, Dermatol Ther 22:327–346, 2009.

Menage J: An unusual zoonosis *(Trixacarus caviae)*, BMJ 331:1225, 2005.

Weese JS, et al: Parasitic diseases. In Weese JS, et al, editors: Companion animal zoonoses, Ames, IA, 2011, Wiley-Blackwell, pp 3–108.

CROSS-REFERENCES TO OTHER SECTIONS

Ectoparasites, Ferrets
Ectoparasites, Rabbits
Ectoparasites, Reptiles
Ectoparasitism, Birds
Skin Diseases, Guinea Pig
Skin Diseases, Hamster
Skin Diseases, Rats

AUTHOR: **MICHAEL V. CAMPAGNA**

EDITORS: **THOMAS M. DONNELLY AND SIMON R. STARKEY**

ZOONOSES

Animal Bites

BASIC INFORMATION

DEFINITION AND INFECTIOUS AGENT

In the United States, between 0.5 million and 2 million animal bites occur each year, but most are not reported. Animal bites account for 1% of emergency room visits. Although only 10% of animal bite wounds require professional medical attention, 1% to 2% requires hospitalization, and 10 to 20 human deaths occur each year. About 85% of animal bites harbor potential pathogens originating from the teeth and oral microorganisms (bacteria and viruses) of the biting animal or from the cutaneous bacteria of the victim. Fungi have rarely been reported.

EPIDEMIOLOGY

ANIMAL SPECIES—HOSTS AND/OR CARRIERS Dogs cause the majority of animal bites (80% to 90%), followed by cats (5% to 15%). Rodents, large mammals (e.g., bears), marine animals (e.g., seals), farm animals (e.g., horses, pigs), and reptiles inflict the remaining percentage (0 to 15%). Incidence surveys have not been reported for exotic small mammals; only individual case reports exist.

RISK FACTORS Children, especially between the ages of 2 and 10 years, are at highest risk for animal bite injuries. After dogs and cats, wild and pet rodents are the next most frequently biting group. These data emphasize the unpredictable nature of animals and the need for adult supervision when animals and children interact.

GEOGRAPHY AND SEASONALITY Most animal bites occur in warm weather (summer).

PATHOBIOLOGY

- Patients who present within 8 hours after injury usually present with crush injuries, disfiguring wounds, or the need for rabies or tetanus prophylaxis.
- Patients who present later than 8 hours after injury usually have established infection manifest as localized cellulitis, pain at the site of injury, and a purulent discharge. Fever, lymphangitis, and regional lymphadenopathy may occur. If dissemination of the microorganism occurs, sepsis, meningitis, and endocarditis may develop, although rarely.

CLINICAL PRESENTATION OF HUMANS

INCIDENCE IN HUMANS

Ferret bites

- Ferret teeth are slender but extremely sharp, easily penetrating skin. Ferret bites are not as severe as cat bites because of their smaller size; only one case of hand infection (due to recurrent *Mycobacterium bovis*) has been reported following a ferret bite in a 12-year-old boy. The true incidence of ferret bites is unknown. During an 11-month period in Arizona, the ratio of reported bites to the estimated pet population was 0.3% for ferrets compared with 0.4% for cats and 2.2% for dogs.
- In the 1980s and 1990s, ferrets were demonized, and numerous U.S. animal and veterinary organizations were opposed to keeping ferrets as pets because of their alleged unpredictable behavior and potential for rabies transmission. Since 2000, this has changed, and ferrets are considered "domesticated pets." However, California, Hawaii, New York City, and Washington, DC, still prohibit the sale or ownership of pet ferrets.
- The aspect of ferret behavior that concerned authorities was the unpredictability and unprovoked nature of many reported attacks. However, reports of severe injuries caused by ferrets are rare. In a 1986 review of 24 cases compiled by the California and Colorado state health departments, 10 were infants younger than 6 months old, many of whom were attacked while sleeping. In a few cases, attacks on infants, especially to the face, were severe, resulting in loss of ear and nose tissue. Attacks on sleeping infants are similar to those by wild rats and strongly suggest poor socioeconomic conditions of victims. Children who have recently finished feeding from a bottle have been bitten, suggesting that the smell of milk or formula may have prompted the attack.
- Concern about rabies is no longer a major issue because a vaccine (Imrab3, Merial) for ferrets has been available since 1990. The rabies concern was based on the tendency of ferrets to escape, approach rabies-infected wildlife, and develop rabies after returning home. The overall incidence of rabies in U.S. pet ferrets was 23 reported cases from 1960 to 2000 (0.6 cases per year). There has not been a case of rabies transmission from a ferret to a human.
- A 2007 study looking at laboratory ferrets being adopted as pets found a 91% success rate. Ferrets with limited socialization had less chance of making good pets, and behavioral issues (e.g., nipping, failure to litter train) were the most common reasons for not keeping the ferret.

Rabbit bites

- Bites from rabbits are rare, although rabbits of any age or gender (more frequent in intact rabbits) can show aggression to humans. Territorial issues motivate most rabbits to attack humans (e.g., rabbits confined to a small cage or hutch may attack when an owner tries to move the rabbit, clean the area, or replenish the feed). Rabbits usually attack a hand when it is placed into the cage, but in large areas where a rabbit has free range, the feet may be assailed. When danger is impending, the natural defense of rabbits is to run away (i.e., flight), but if a rabbit is confined and is unable to run away, it is more likely to defend itself (i.e., fight) by lunging at a person to bite or by standing up on its hind legs and attacking with its front limbs. Socialized house rabbits are known to nip at owners' feet and ankles when they are being ignored. This is not a form of aggression but may be misinterpreted as such by owners.
- Although *Pasteurella multocida* is a common infection of rabbits, only three reports have described isolation of *Pasteurella multocida* from patients after a rabbit bite (two cases involving finger and leg) or licking of a kerion celsi (an occipital or cranial dermatopathy secondary to tinea infection). In contrast, *Pasteurella canis* is the most common pathogen in infections from dog bites, and *Pasteurella multocida* is the most common isolate of cat bites. No other rabbit bite infections have been reported.

Guinea pig bites

- Bites from guinea pigs are exceedingly rare. Adult guinea pigs do not bite, and juveniles may nip.
- Two case reports of *Haemophilus influenzae* and *Pasteurella* species *(incertae sedis)* infections after guinea pig bites have been published.

Rat bites

- Bacteria grow in one-third of all rat bite wounds. Rats have a 14% carriage rate of *Pasteurella* spp. The risk of any type of infection after a rat bite is estimated as 1% to 10%.
- The biggest risk from rat bites is rat bite fever (RBF). Because rats have become popular as pets, children now account for more than 50% of RBF cases in the United States, followed by laboratory personnel and pet shop employees. The risk of RBF is unknown, as is the infectious dose of both *Streptobacillus moniliformis* and *Spirillum minus* for humans (see Rat Bite Fever).
- In recent years, transmission by pet rats of cowpox to other host species, including humans, has emerged in Europe. Cowpox is found primarily in Europe, where the natural hosts are thought to be small wild rodents, from which the virus occasionally spreads to domestic cats, cows, and humans.

Hamster bites

- Lymphocytic choriomeningitis (LCM) virus may be transmitted by Syrian hamster bites. However, the risk of hamsters transmitting LCM to the general population is overstated. Three of the largest outbreaks of LCM caused by hamsters in the United States were attributable to a single supplier in the late 1970s.
- The common house mouse, *Mus musculus*, is the natural host and principal reservoir of LCM virus. Pet rodents, including hamsters, become infected through contact with wild mice. Single cases of LCM have been epidemiologically linked to hamsters among transplant recipients (see Lymphocytic Choriomeningitis Virus).
- Two cases of *Pasteurella* peritonitis have been reported in peritoneal dialysis patients. These rare infections were the result of contamination of dialysis tubing by pet hamsters chewing the catheters.

Anaphylaxis after rabbit or rodent bite

- Severe anaphylaxis is a systemic reaction that affects two or more organs or systems and is caused by the release of active mediators from mast cells and basophils. A four-grade classification routinely places "severe" anaphylaxis in grades 3 and 4 (death could be graded as grade 5).
- The biggest risk to exotic pet owners is anaphylaxis after a bite, and to veterinarians and technicians, anaphylaxis after needlestick injury. Fifteen reports (more than all reports of pet rabbit and rodent bites) describe life-threatening anaphylaxis secondary to

rabbit, rat, Syrian and dwarf hamster, mouse, Mongolian gerbil, and prairie dog bites.

- Anaphylaxis following accidental needlestick injuries is described for rabbit, rat, and mouse tissue.
- Allergies consisting of rashes where animals are in contact with the skin, nasal congestion and sneezing, itchy eyes, and asthma are described for exposure to rabbits, rodents (including chinchillas and guinea pigs), and ferrets.

Bird bites

- Bird bites (e.g., rooster pecks, swan bites, bites resulting from owl attacks) have caused infection with *Streptococcus bovis, Clostridium tertium, Aspergillus niger, Pseudomonas aeruginosa,* and *Bacteroides* spp.
- Ocular injury, especially of children after rooster pecking, is frequently described.
- Cephalic tetanus and a brain abscess caused by rooster pecking the face have been reported.

Lizard bites

- Captive iguanas may react aggressively, and infection from iguana bites have been reported. *Serratia marcescens* and *Staphylococcus aureus* have been isolated from bite wounds.

Snake bites

- Each year, venomous snakes, mostly rattlesnakes and other vipers, bite about 8000 Americans. Extensive tissue necrosis predisposes the victim to infection from the snake's normal oral microbiota or from the fecal flora of its prey.
- The snake's oral microbiota and venom include predominantly anaerobes, such as *Bacteroides* spp. (especially *B. fragilis*), *Clostridium* spp., and *Propionibacterium acnes,* but also includes many species of aerobes, such as *Acinetobacter* spp., *Alcaligenes* spp., *Bacillus* spp., *Citrobacter* spp., *Corynebacterium* spp., *Enterobacter cloacae, Micrococcus* spp., *Proteus* spp., *Pseudomonas* spp., *Salmonella arizonae* and other salmonellae, *S. aureus,* coagulase-negative *Staphylococcus* spp., alpha-hemolytic streptococci, and *Streptococcus agalactiae.*

PHYSICAL FINDINGS IN INFECTED HUMANS

- Animal bites cause three types of wounds:
  - Lacerations (tears or evulsions)
  - Punctures
  - Crush injuries
- Most wounds in adults involve the arms, especially the hands. However, children aged from birth to 9 years of age are more likely to suffer wounds to the head and face.
- Wounds resulting from dog and large carnivore bites consist of lacerations and/or punctures. The "hole and tear" effect, whereby canine teeth anchor the person while other teeth bite, shear, and tear the tissues, results in stretch lacerations.
- In contrast, bites from domestic cats, ferrets, and rodents usually produce puncture wounds that can cause local abscesses. Although infection occurs in 3% to 18% of dog bites, 28% to 80% of cat bites result in infection.
- Bites from farm horses typically do not break the skin but cause severe crush injuries.

DIAGNOSIS

INITIAL DATABASE

Specimens for aerobic and anaerobic bacterial smears and cultures should be obtained from any infected bite wound.

ADVANCED OR CONFIRMATORY TESTING

A radiograph of the affected body part should be considered when a fracture is possible, or when bones or joints may have been penetrated.

TREATMENT

- Copious volumes of normal saline should be used for irrigation to reduce the bacterial load in the wound. Puncture wounds may be irrigated with a 20-mL syringe with an 18-gauge needle inserted into the wound in the direction of the puncture. Any foreign material should be removed.
- Infected wounds and those that are seen more than 24 hours after the bite should be left open.
- The usefulness of prophylactic antibiotics after animal bites continues to be debated. In a Cochrane review of eight randomized trials of mammalian bites comparing antibiotic prophylaxis with placebo or with no intervention, the authors concluded that prophylactic antibiotics did not appear to reduce the rate of infection after bites by cats or dogs. Wound type (puncture or laceration) also had no influence on the effectiveness of prophylaxis. However, the group did suggest that prophylactic antibiotics cause a statistically significant reduction in the rate of infection after bites on the hand or bites by humans.
- Empirical therapy for wound infection should consist of a combination of a [beta]-lactam antibiotic and a [beta]-lactamase inhibitor (usually amoxicillin/clavulanate). Empirical treatment for children who are allergic to [beta]-lactams consists of clindamycin plus trimethoprim/sulfamethoxazole. The second-generation cephalosporin, cefuroxime, is another option for monotherapy, but it should be used with caution in penicillin-allergic patients.
- Antimicrobial therapy should be given as a 3- to 5-day course of treatment to patients with moderate or severe wounds that are seen within 8 hours after the bite, with crush injury or edema, or for wounds that may involve bones or joints. This treatment is recommended for wounds to the hands; for punctures, particularly near a joint; and for wounds in patients with an underlying disease that may predispose to more serious infection.
- Patients with an overtly infected bite wound should be treated for 10 to 14 days. Purulent arthritis and osteomyelitis require even longer courses of treatment.
- Tetanus toxoid should be administered if a booster injection has not been given during the previous 5 years. Patients who have never been fully immunized may require a primary immunization series and simultaneous tetanus immunoglobulin administration.
- Rabies vaccination should be considered, especially in cases of wild animal bites. Rabies in rodents, including squirrels, hamsters, rats, and mice, is uncommon (see Rabies).
- Wild animals such as raccoons, skunks, bats, foxes, coyotes, bobcats, and other carnivores are often afflicted and should be considered rabid unless laboratory tests prove otherwise.
- The post-exposure rabies immunization schedule for unvaccinated persons includes the following:
  - Human rabies immunoglobulin, 20 μL/kg, which should be infiltrated around the wounds, with the remainder injected intragluteally; and
  - Human diploid cell vaccine, given on days 0, 3, 7, 14, and 28
- Elevation of the injured area is essential and should be continued for several days until edema has resolved. Hands with bite wounds should be immobilized with a splint for several days.

PREVENTION

- No direct evidence suggests that educational programs can reduce animal bite rates in children and adolescents. Educating children who are younger than 10 years of age in school settings could improve their knowledge, attitude, and behavior toward animals.
- Educating children and adolescents in settings other than schools should also be evaluated. High-quality studies that measure animal bite rates as an outcome are needed.

- To date, evidence does not suggest that educating children and adolescents is effective as a unique public health strategy to reduce animal bite injuries and their consequences.

REPORTING—NOTIFIABLE DISEASE

- Animal bites per se are not a federal notifiable disease.
- However, in all states and in many cities, doctors are required to report to state and local health department authorities any patient whom they see (in their office or in hospital) for an animal bite.

PROGNOSIS

Bites from exotic pets generally have a good prognosis if treated early. Risk of death is associated with rat bite fever, lymphocytic choriomeningitis virus, untreated anaphylactic shock, and envenomation from poisonous animals such as lizards, snakes, and fish.

PEARLS & CONSIDERATIONS

COMMENTS

- Approximately one-third of laboratory animal workers have occupational allergy to laboratory rodents and rabbits, and one-third of these have symptomatic asthma. Sensitization generally occurs within the first 3 years of employment; risk factors include atopic background, as well as the job description as it relates to the intensity of exposure. A symptomatic worker can reduce allergen exposure with personal protective devices.
- Specific immunoglobulin E to common aero-allergens and to domestic and laboratory animal allergens may be used to identify individuals who would benefit from further advice about managing their exposure.

CLIENT EDUCATION

- Children of all age groups are disproportionately represented in surveys of animal bites.
- The primary reason for mortality and morbidity in children in the Western world who are younger than 1 year of age is trauma (e.g., drowning in swimming pools, falls from stairs, burns); 41% of these incidents occur in the child's own home, again suggesting a role for oversight in risk mitigation.
- In contrast, dog bites in children represent only a small part of the burden of injury presenting to emergency departments (0.2% of emergency department visits).
- The unpredictable nature of animals requires adult supervision when animals and children interact.

SUGGESTED READINGS

Abrahamian FM, et al: Microbiology of animal bite wound infections, Clin Microbiol Rev 24:231–246, 2011.

Duperrex O, et al: Education of children and adolescents for the prevention of dog bite injuries, Cochrane Database Syst Rev (2): CD004726, 2009.

Jerrard D: Bites (mammalian), Clin Evid (Online) 914:1–8, 2006.

Medeiros IM, et al: Antibiotic prophylaxis for mammalian bites, Cochrane Database Syst Rev (1):CD001738, 2001.

CROSS-REFERENCES TO OTHER SECTIONS

Lymphocytic Choriomeningitis Virus
Pasteurella multocida
Rabies
Rat Bite Fever

AUTHOR: **THOMAS M. DONNELLY**

EDITOR: **SIMON R. STARKEY**

ZOONOSES

Chlamydiosis

BASIC INFORMATION

DEFINITION AND INFECTIOUS AGENT

- Psittacosis/ornithosis is a bacterial infection of humans caused by *Chlamydophila psittaci*. In birds, *C. psittaci* infection is referred to as *avian chlamydiosis*. *Psittacosis* refers to infection in humans transmitted by parrots; *ornithosis* refers to infection in humans transmitted by other birds. All *Chlamydophila* species are potential zoonotic pathogens, although *C. psittaci* is the most important and the best documented.
- The family Chlamydiaceae is divided into two genera:
  - Genus *Chlamydia* (*C. trachomatis*, *C. suis*, and *C. muridarium*)
  - Genus *Chlamydophila* (*C. abortus*, *C. caviae*, *C. felis*, *C. pecorum*, *C. pneumoniae*, and *C. psittaci*)
- Three new *Chlamydophila* species were derived from the previously classified *Chlamydia psittaci*: *Chlamydophila abortus*, *C. caviae*, and *C. felis*. This reclassification is controversial. Both old and new nomenclatures are used in the current literature; however, the latter recently has gained more widespread acceptance.
- Birds
  - *Chlamydophila* (formerly *Chlamydia*) *psittaci*
- Guinea pigs
  - *Chlamydophila caviae* (formerly known as the guinea pig inclusion conjunctivitis [GPIC] strain of *C. psittaci*)

SYNONYMS

In humans: psittacosis, ornithosis, chlamydiosis, parrot fever

In animals: avian chlamydiosis, mammalian chlamydiosis, chlamydial conjunctivitis

EPIDEMIOLOGY

ANIMAL SPECIES—HOSTS AND/OR CARRIERS

- *C. psittaci* has been identified in 460 avian species from 30 orders.
- Budgerigars and cockatiels appear overrepresented among pet birds. Poultry are also affected, and flock outbreaks can occur.
- *C. caviae* is specific for guinea pigs.

MODES OF TRANSMISSION

- Inhalation of elementary bodies (infectious, extracellular form of organism) in contaminated bedding, dust, and dander
- Ingestion of elementary bodies in feces and nasal or ocular secretions

CLINICAL PRESENTATION OF ANIMALS

- Ranges from acute and life threatening to subacute or chronic disease
- Acutely affected birds typically develop conjunctivitis and rhinitis with

naso-ocular discharge, variable dyspnea, ruffled feathers, lethargy, anorexia, and biliverdin-stained urates. Diarrhea may also be seen.
- Chronic disease may be associated with wasting and chronic naso-ocular discharge.
- Guinea pigs develop unilateral or bilateral conjunctivitis.

RISK FACTORS

- For birds
  - High stocking rates
  - Stressors such as inclement weather, transport, or other illness
  - Exposure to wild birds
- For guinea pigs
  - Unknown; however, stress and poor husbandry may play a role.

GEOGRAPHY AND SEASONALITY *C. psittaci* has a worldwide distribution. Prevalence of shedding may increase in summer months.

PATHOBIOLOGY

- Chlamydiae exist in two forms: an infectious but metabolically inactive elementary body that is relatively stable in the environment, and the metabolically active but noninfectious reticulate body.
- Infection is initiated when the elementary body attaches to susceptible cell membranes. The organism has a predilection for cells of the respiratory and gastrointestinal tracts, serous cavities, and reticuloendothelial system.
- Multiplication of the organism causes cell lysis; this, in conjunction with host immune response, causes the clinical signs and pathologic features of the disease.
- Common pathologic findings include air sacculitis, conjunctivitis, rhinitis, hepatosplenomegaly, perihepatitis, and military necrosis of the parenchymal organs.

CLINICAL PRESENTATION OF HUMANS

INCIDENCE IN HUMANS

- Typically fewer than 50 cases per year are reported in the United States. Many cases likely remain unreported.
- Prevalence is as high as 15% in caregivers at bird breeding facilities.
- Most cases occur after exposure to infected pet birds, usually cockatiels, parakeets, parrots, and macaws.

DISEASE FORMS/SUBTYPES

- Flulike syndrome
- Atypical pneumonia
- Septicemia

HISTORY, CHIEF COMPLAINT

C. psittaci

- Association with infected or high-risk animals
- Chief complaints of fever, malaise, headache, and hacking, typically nonproductive, cough

C. caviae

- Conjunctivitis

PHYSICAL FINDINGS IN INFECTED HUMANS

C. psittaci

- Typical: fever, malaise, myalgia, cough, pharyngeal edema, hepatomegaly, and a pink, blanching maculopapular rash
- Complicated: hepatitis, splenomegaly, hemolytic anemia, disseminated intravascular coagulation (DIC), endocarditis, myocarditis, pericarditis, and glomerulonephritis
- Neurologic complications such as hearing loss, cranial nerve palsy, cerebellar symptoms, and confusion can also occur.

C. caviae

- Conjunctivitis

INCUBATION PERIOD

5 to 15 days

DIAGNOSIS

DIFFERENTIAL DIAGNOSIS

C. PSITTACI

- Interstitial pneumonia due to:
  - *Mycoplasma pneumoniae*
  - *Coxiella burnetii*
  - *Legionella* spp.
  - Respiratory viruses

C. CAVIAE

- Inclusion conjunctivitis (*C. trachomatis*)
- Conjunctivitis due to allergy, bacteria, or virus

BIRDS

- Conjunctivitis/rhinitis: *Mycoplasma*, *Mycobacterium*, *Cryptosporidium* spp., primary bacterial, pigeon herpesvirus, foreign bodies
- Ruffled feathers and wasting: many infectious and noninfectious diseases

GUINEA PIGS

- Primary bacterial conjunctivitis, nasolacrimal duct obstruction, dacryocystitis

INITIAL DATABASE

HUMANS

- Serologic assay; greater than fourfold increase in complement-fixation (CF) titers
- Positive ELISA or microimmunofluorescence

BIRDS

- Complete blood count and plasma biochemistry panel: heterophilic leukocytosis often observed with or without a monocytosis; aspartate aminotransferase (AST) and bile acids may be elevated.
- Conjunctival cytologic examination may identify elementary bodies within epithelial or inflammatory cells.
- Radiographic imaging may demonstrate air sac thickening and/or hepatosplenomegaly.

GUINEA PIGS

- Conjunctival cytologic examination may identify elementary bodies within epithelial or inflammatory cells.

ADVANCED OR CONFIRMATORY TESTING

HUMANS

- Bacteriologic culture was the historic gold standard; currently used less because of the fastidious nature of the organism and specialized laboratory requirements and cost
- Antigen detection techniques use conjunctival swabs or blood polymerase chain reaction (PCR).

BIRDS

- Antigen detection techniques such as conjunctival, blood, choanal, or cloacal PCR or chlamydial cell wall antigen ELISA may also be used.
- Serologic assays such as immunofluorescence assay (IFA), enzyme immunoassay (EIA), or ELISA; sensitivity and specificity vary by species and laboratory
- Chronic or immunologic staining methods may be performed to identify intracytoplasmic inclusions of impression smears or histopathologic preparations of clinical or necropsy specimens.

TREATMENT

- Long-acting (5 to 7 days) doxycycline injections are the mainstay of animal treatment.
- Doxycycline or tetracycline has been used traditionally in humans with psittacosis. Azithromycin has been gaining popularity as treatment for psittacosis in humans.

PREVENTION

Protective measures include the following:

- When cleaning cages or handling infected birds, caretakers should wear protective clothing, which includes gloves, eyewear, a disposable surgical cap, and an appropriately fitted respirator with N-95 or higher rating.
- When necropsies are performed on potentially infected birds, wet the carcass with detergent and water to prevent aerosolization of infectious particles, and work under a biological safety cabinet or equivalent.
- Isolate newly acquired, ill, or exposed birds from other birds in the household and from noncaregiver humans.
- Avoid purchasing or selling sick birds.

REPORTING—NOTIFIABLE DISEASE

- Notification of U.S. federal health authorities is required.
- Notification of state health authorities varies by jurisdiction—contact local public health authorities and state department of agriculture.

PROGNOSIS

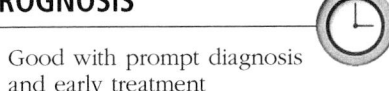

- Good with prompt diagnosis and early treatment
- Fair to guarded with delayed diagnosis or disseminated disease

CONTROVERSY

Veterinarians may be asked to declare a bird safe for residents of nursing homes or hospitals, or for persons with compromised immunity. Active client education is required, and the veterinarian should have knowledge of screening test sensitivity and specificity.

PEARLS & CONSIDERATIONS

COMMENTS

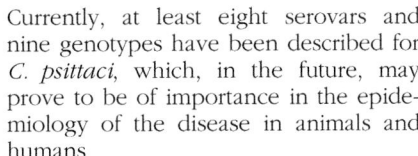

Currently, at least eight serovars and nine genotypes have been described for *C. psittaci*, which, in the future, may prove to be of importance in the epidemiology of the disease in animals and humans

CLIENT EDUCATION

- Avoid purchasing sick birds, especially those with signs characteristic of infection with *C. psittaci.*
- Use quarantine, maintain high levels of husbandry, and use personal protective equipment as indicated.
- Avoid purchasing guinea pigs with conjunctivitis:
  - Limit handling of affected guinea pigs.
  - Quarantine and wear gloves while handling infected animals.

SUGGESTED READINGS

Compendium of measures to control *Chlamydophila psittaci* infection among humans (psittacosis) and pet birds (avian chlamydiosis), St Paul, MN, 2010, National Association of State Public Health Veterinarians (NASPHV). http://www.nasphv.org/Documents/Psittacosis.pdf.

Kaleta EF, et al: Avian host range of *Chlamydophila* spp. based on isolation, antigen detection and serology, Avian Pathol 32: 435–461, 2003.

Lutz-Wohlgroth L, et al: Chlamydiales in guinea-pigs and their zoonotic potential, J Vet Med Assoc Physiol Pathol Clin Med 53:185–193, 2006.

CROSS-REFERENCES TO OTHER SECTIONS

Chlamydophila psittaci, Birds

AUTHOR: **SIMON R. STARKEY**

EDITOR: **THOMAS M. DONNELLY**

ZOONOSES

Cryptosporidiosis

BASIC INFORMATION

DEFINITION AND INFECTIOUS AGENT

- *Cryptosporidium* species are apicomplexan protozoan parasites. Members of this genus have been isolated from more than 150 mammalian species, as well as a broad range of birds, fish, and reptiles.
- *Cryptosporidium* preferentially infect enterocytes; however, other epithelial surfaces may become infected.
- Taxonomy among members of this genus is in constant flux; however, at the time of writing, 22 species are considered valid. Additionally, some 40 genotypes have been reported in the literature.

SYNONYMS

Disease

- In humans: None.
- In animals: None.

Organism

- The term *genotype* is synonymous with the term *cryptic species.* Historically, most genotypes were reported as *C. parvum* genotypes. For example, the cervine genotype was frequently recorded as *C. parvum* cervine genotype. Such genotypes are now reported as *Cryptosporidium* spp. cervine genotype.
- *C. cuniculus* is synonymous with *Cryptosporidium* rabbit genotype.
- *C. varanii* is synonymous with *C. saurophilum.*

EPIDEMIOLOGY

ANIMAL SPECIES—HOSTS AND/OR CARRIERS

Birds

- *Cryptosporidium* species have been isolated from more than 30 avian species. The predominant species affecting birds are *C. meleagridis* and *C. baileyi*, with the former demonstrating zoonotic potential, particularly among immune compromised individuals. *C. galli* was first reported in 1999 in chickens; the pathologic significance of this species is largely unknown in both birds and humans. This species has since been identified in a small number of psittacine and passerine birds.
- Several *Cryptosporidium* genotypes have been discovered among birds, particularly psittacines and passerines. The zoonotic potential of these genotypes is undetermined at this stage but is considered relatively low owing to the lack of confirmed human cases associated with these genotypes.
- *C. meleagridis* is most commonly observed among turkeys. The organism has also been isolated from chickens, game birds, and waterfowl. Recently, *C. meleagridis* has been reported in a small number of psittacine species.

Chinchillas

- Cryptosporidiosis has been identified in chinchillas for over 20 years. However, to the author's knowledge, no human cases of cryptosporidiosis have been attributed to chinchillas. Thus, the relative zoonotic risk posed by chinchillas to humans may be considered low.
- Molecular data are also lacking among cases of cryptosporidiosis in chinchillas. Such investigations would be useful in better characterizing the zoonotic risk posed by cryptosporidial infections in chinchillas.

Ferrets

- Reports of cryptosporidiosis among ferrets have appeared in the literature for over 20 years. However, as with chinchillas, no human cases of cryptosporidiosis have been attributed to ferrets, to the author's knowledge.

- Recent molecular investigations have demonstrated that the ferret has a unique genotype of *Cryptosporidium* that is conserved across wide geographic ranges. This genotype has not been identified in molecular epidemiologic studies of human cryptosporidiosis to date, further supporting the notion that *Cryptosporidium* ferret genotype is not zoonotic.

Gerbils

- Although immune competent and immune compromised gerbils *(Meriones unguiculatus)* are commonly used in the study of cryptosporidiosis, spontaneous infection with *Cryptosporidium* spp. has not been reported in this species, to the author's knowledge. Therefore, the zoonotic potential of gerbils with reference to *Cryptosporidium* is considered low.

Guinea pigs

- Reports of *Cryptosporidium* spp. among guinea pigs have appeared in the literature for over 40 years. The guinea pig was proposed to be the definitive host of *C. wrairi*, which received official species designation in 1971.
- Although it has been associated with clinical and subclinical infections in guinea pigs for over 40 years, *C. wrairi* is not known to cause disease in humans and is not considered a zoonotic species of *Cryptosporidium.*

Hamsters

- Infection with *Cryptosporidium* spp. has been reported in pet and laboratory hamsters (*Mesocricetus auratus, Phodopus sungorus,* and *Phodopus roborovskii*) for over 25 years. Molecular techniques have been applied to investigate the zoonotic potential of the cryptosporidial species and genotypes affecting hamsters.
- For example, in a recent Chinese study, zoonotic *C. parvum* was identified in 8 of 136 hamsters of various species obtained from a pet market in Zhengzhou. Other hamster isolates obtained in this study included *C. muris, C. andersoni,* and a newly defined hamster genotype. Therefore, hamsters should be considered as a potential source of human cryptosporidiosis.

Hedgehogs

- A few reports have described cryptosporidiosis in European hedgehogs *(Erinaceus europaeus).* Recently, *Cryptosporidium* spp. genotype belonging to the VIIa subtype family was identified in wild juvenile hedgehogs rescued and brought to rehabilitation centers in Europe. This genotype is closely related to *C. parvum* but is genetically distinct and is probably a hedgehog-specific *Cryptosporidium* spp. genotype with unknown zoonotic potential. One case of fatal cryptosporidiosis identified as *C. parvum* in an African hedgehog *(Atelerix albiventris)* from a U.S. zoo has been described. No human cases of cryptosporidiosis have been attributed to hedgehogs, to the author's knowledge.

Mice

- Pet, wild, and laboratory mice *(Mus domesticus)* are definitive hosts for *C. muris,* which has been isolated infrequently from humans and is considered to be of minor zoonotic concern.
- To the author's knowledge, genetically confirmed, zoonotic *C. parvum* has been reported in mice only once. In this report, five mice from Victoria, Australia, were shown to carry this organism. The mice might have obtained this organism from sheep with which they shared close proximity.
- Recent studies have demonstrated that mice also carry *Cryptosporidium* mouse genotypes I and II. To date, genotype I has been isolated from one human with clinical cryptosporidiosis in the Middle East. Genotype II has not been isolated from humans.
- The overall zoonotic risk of cryptosporidiosis posed to humans by mice is considered relatively small.

Rabbits

- *C. cuniculus* was first reported in 1979 in an asymptomatic adult female rabbit.
- *C. cuniculus* has subsequently been identified in laboratory, commercial, and wild rabbits.
- Prevalence among wild rabbits *(Oryctolagus cuniculus)* is approximately 7% based on studies conducted in Australia and the United Kingdom.
- The zoonotic potential of *C. cuniculus* was demonstrated in a 2008 waterborne outbreak in the United Kingdom.

Rats

- Pet and laboratory rats may be infected by a number of genotypes of *Cryptosporidium,* including rat genotypes I, II, and III and mouse genotype I. Based on current molecular epidemiologic studies, the three rat genotypes are not thought to be zoonotic. However, mouse genotype I may have zoonotic potential.

Reptiles

- *Cryptosporidium* infections have been reported in at least 57 species of reptiles. *Cryptosporidium serpentis* and *C. varanii* predominate in snakes and lizards, respectively.
- Occasionally *C. parvum* and *C. muris* are isolated from reptile feces. It is widely believed that these instances stem from passive transmission of *Cryptosporidium* spp. affecting rodent prey species, rather than true infections of the reptile hosts.
- To date, *C. serpentis* and *C. varanii* have yet to be identified from humans with cryptosporidiosis. Therefore, reptiles are not considered to pose a significant zoonotic risk to humans with reference to cryptosporidiosis.

MODES OF TRANSMISSION

- Fecal-oral transmission directly from the host or indirectly via multiple routes such as drinking of recreational water, food, or fomites.
- Oocysts have relatively thick walls and are environmentally resistant. This feature enhances the organism's ability to spread via indirect routes and its ability to cause large, often waterborne, outbreaks.

CLINICAL PRESENTATION OF ANIMALS

Birds

- *Cryptosporidium meleagridis* is most commonly observed among turkeys. The organism affects the epithelial cells of the small intestine and causes a severe diarrheal disease, particularly in poults. Additionally, birds may present with lethargy, anorexia, and huddling, and moderate flock mortality rates may be observed.
- *C. baileyi* causes bursitis and cloacal infection in chickens that may be detected histologically. However, this organism rarely leads to clinical disease.
- *C. baileyi* has, however, been reported to cause moderate to severe ocular and respiratory disease in more than 30 species of birds, including chickens, turkeys, and a number of caged, aviary, and pet bird species from multiple genera. Affected birds may present with oculonasal discharge, sneezing, and/or cough. Histopathologic evaluation of these birds may demonstrate sinusitis, air sacculitis, tracheitis, and/or pneumonia.
- Occasionally, *Cryptosporidium* species have been identified as a cause of nephritis and ureteritis in a variety of avian species. Clinical signs vary but may include anorexia, weight loss, and weakness characterized by pelvic limb paresis. Affected birds are typically immune suppressed by concurrent viral infections.

Chinchillas

- As with rabbits, cryptosporidiosis among chinchillas appears to be confined to younger animals. Despite relatively frequent anecdotal and unpublished reports of cryptosporidiosis among chinchillas, only a few publications can be found in the peer-reviewed literature.
- Affected animals develop anorexia, diarrhea, dehydration, and lethargy.

Death may occur, in spite of supportive care. Clinical cryptosporidiosis appears most common among stressed chinchillas such as those kept under poor conditions.

Ferrets

- Ferrets may be clinically or subclinically infected with *Cryptosporidium*. Clinical cryptosporidiosis appears to be more prevalent among juvenile ferrets and is characterized by anorexia, depression, and diarrhea. Death may occur in advanced cases.

Guinea pigs

- Despite the relatively high prevalence of *C. wrairi* in guinea pigs, clinical signs attributable to this organism are relatively rare. When clinical signs do occur, they are most common in juvenile guinea pigs, which present with failure to gain weight, weight loss, diarrhea, and death.

Hamsters

- Several peer-reviewed articles discuss both spontaneous and experimental cryptosporidiosis in hamsters. As with other animals, this condition tends to affect neonatal and juvenile hamsters to a greater degree than adults. Furthermore, cryptosporidiosis is more likely in immune suppressed adult hosts and/or those with concurrent disease.
- Clinically affected hamsters present with diarrhea and may develop hematochezia. Lethargy, listlessness, and death may occur, particularly among neonatal hamsters.

Mice

- Clinical cryptosporidiosis is rarely encountered in pet, laboratory, or wild mice. *C. muris* inhabits the gastric glands and appears to cause subclinical infection.

Rabbits

- *C. cuniculus* tends to cause subclinical infection in adult rabbits. *C. cuniculus* was first described in an asymptomatic adult female rabbit that had intestinal cryptosporidiosis. The rabbit demonstrated mild pathology of the ileum with blunted villi, a decrease in the villus-to-crypt ratio, and mild edema in the lamina propria. Later that year, two more rabbit cases were described in which intestinal pathology was similar to that in the first case.
- Several published reports describe severe and fatal cryptosporidiosis among juvenile and weanling rabbits. Affected rabbits typically are younger than 3 months of age and develop diarrhea, anorexia, lethargy, and occasionally death. Histopathologic examination has identified atrophy of the villi of the ileum.

Rats

- As with mice, clinical cryptosporidiosis is rarely reported in rats.

Reptiles

- *C. serpentis* is responsible for gastric infection in snakes. These animals typically develop anorexia, midbody swelling, lethargy, and weight loss. Infection with this organism may also occur in lizards; however, such infections are typically subclinical.
- *C. varanii* is typically an intestinal infection of lizards. Juveniles are affected more frequently than adults. This occurs with anorexia, weight loss, abdominal swelling, and death.

RISK FACTORS

Host

- The most important risk factor for the development of clinical cryptosporidiosis among humans and animals is immune suppression or an immature immune system.
- Immune suppression may be due to current infection such as Marek's disease in chickens or the human immunodeficiency virus (HIV) in people.
- Neonatal and juvenile/infant animals and humans are at greater risk of cryptosporidiosis owing to an immature immune system.

Environment

- Cryptosporidiosis occurs as the result of direct or indirect fecal-oral contamination. Personal and environmental hygiene and husbandry standards are important risk factors for the development of cryptosporidiosis in humans and animals.
- Outside of large waterborne outbreaks of human cryptosporidiosis, which often results from contamination or failure of water supply systems, most human cases stem from poor hand hygiene and contact with infected animals or humans (e.g., cryptosporidiosis is relatively common among veterinary students as the result of contact with infected calves).
- Among avian and exotic pets, an increased incidence of cryptosporidiosis appears to occur among animals kept in crowded conditions and those experiencing stress (e.g., cryptosporidiosis is observed more frequently among juvenile small mammals soon after transport from the breeder/wholesaler to pet stores).

GEOGRAPHY AND SEASONALITY

- *Cryptosporidium* species have a worldwide distribution, except for Antarctica.
- Statistically significant seasonality of infection among avian and exotic pets has not been reported to date.
- Seasonal infection has been reported among domestic and wild animals, as well as humans (e.g., a study of children in Spanish day care centers demonstrated a statistically significant increased prevalence of cryptosporidiosis during the winter months).
- In the United States, the number of cases reported to the national notifiable disease surveillance system shows a significant peak during the months of July, August, and September.
- California ground squirrels (*Spermophilus beecheyi*) were shown to have a significantly greater prevalence and rate of oocyst shedding during the summer.

PATHOBIOLOGY

- Cryptosporidia have a predilection for epithelial cells. Infection typically occurs in the small intestine, although other epithelial cells may be affected.
- The organism occupies a unique intracellular extracytoplasmic location. Intestinal epithelial cell infection causes malabsorptive and secretory diarrhea via functional and structural cellular changes such as altered sodium/water consumption, villous atrophy, and crypt hyperplasia.
- Oocysts are shed in an infectious, sporulated state. When ingested, oocysts excyst in the intestinal tract. The first phase of replication involves two phases of merogony. Meronts subsequently differentiate into male and female gamonts that form a zygote, ultimately developing into sporulated oocysts.
- Both thin- and thick-walled oocysts are produced. Thin-walled oocysts may infect other epithelial cells, perpetuating the infection and causing further epithelial damage and disruption. Thick-walled sporulated oocysts are infective when excreted. They are extremely infectious, with human ID_{50} (dose of an infectious organism required to produce infection in 50% of experimental subjects) of 10^2 oocysts in some studies.

CLINICAL PRESENTATION OF HUMANS

INCIDENCE IN HUMANS

- The prevalence of cryptosporidiosis is highest in developing nations, particularly those in which humans and cattle share close proximity.
- In developed nations, the prevalence of cryptosporidiosis is often highest among children attending day care and preschool facilities. In a Spanish study published in 1996, the period prevalence of cryptosporidiosis among children attending day care centers was 10% (17 of 170 children) over the 15-month study period.
- In 2008, the incidence of confirmed and probable cases of human cryptosporidiosis across the United States was 3.9 cases per 100,000 population. During this time, the incidence varied significantly by state, from 0.2 to 14

cases per 100,000 population in Hawaii and Wisconsin, respectively.

DISEASE FORMS/SUBTYPES

Intestinal cryptosporidiosis

- Is the most common form of human cryptosporidiosis. Among immune competent hosts, this condition presents as self-limiting watery diarrhea that may be associated with abdominal cramps, nausea, anorexia, and low-grade fever. In immune competent humans, diarrhea typically lasts 5 to 10 days but may persist for up to 4 weeks.
- Individuals with HIV infection and low CD4 cell counts may develop profuse, cholera-like diarrhea that may persist for many weeks. Infection in these individuals may be complicated by profound dehydration and malabsorption and may lead to death.

Biliary cryptosporidiosis

- This form of the disease often occurs as an extension of intestinal cryptosporidiosis among immune compromised individuals and may lead to severe cholecystitis, sclerosing cholangitis, and/or papillary stenosis.

Respiratory cryptosporidiosis

- As with biliary cryptosporidiosis, this form of the condition occurs as a rare extension of intestinal cryptosporidiosis, typically among immune compromised individuals. The organism may affect the epithelial cells lining the respiratory tract, causing sinusitis, tracheitis, and/or bronchopneumonia.

Disseminated microsporidiosis

- This advanced form of cryptosporidiosis is most often seen in patients with profound immune suppression in which the intestinal and biliary tracts, as well as the respiratory system, are affected. Prognosis is poor for patients with this form of the disease.

HISTORY, CHIEF COMPLAINT

History

- Persons affected by spontaneous cryptosporidiosis may recall exposure to animals with the potential for zoonotic transmission of the organism. Alternatively, they may report consumption of potentially contaminated water or foodstuffs such as fruits and vegetables.
- Small- and large-scale epidemics have been associated with pools and water parks and with contaminated municipal water supplies.

Chief complaint

- Diarrhea is the first and most common complaint among humans with most subtypes of cryptosporidiosis. Additional complaints such as abdominal pain, anorexia, nausea, and weight loss may occur with intestinal and/or biliary cryptosporidiosis. Cough, dyspnea, and increased respiratory secretions may be reported with the respiratory form of the disease.

PHYSICAL FINDINGS IN INFECTED HUMANS Watery diarrhea and dehydration are the most common physical findings among people with cryptosporidiosis. Upper right quadrant pain is reported among patients with biliary cryptosporidiosis. Dyspnea and increased respiratory secretions have been identified among patients with respiratory and disseminated cryptosporidiosis.

INCUBATION PERIOD The average incubation period for human intestinal cryptosporidiosis is 5 to 10 days, with a reported range of 2 to 28 days.

DIAGNOSIS

DIFFERENTIAL DIAGNOSIS

- Amebiasis
- Bacterial gastroenteritis
- Cyclosporiasis
- Giardiasis
- Isosporiasis
- Viral gastroenteritis

INITIAL DATABASE

- Fecal culture aids in ruling out other causes of infectious diarrhea and/or concurrent infection.
- Fecal ova and parasite screening employing concentration techniques with zinc sulfate or sugar solutions are often diagnostic.
- Modified acid-fast–stained fecal smears may be sufficient for the diagnosis of intestinal cryptosporidiosis.
- Stained sputum may be used to achieve a microscopic diagnosis in cases of respiratory cryptosporidiosis.

ADVANCED OR CONFIRMATORY TESTING

- Direct immunofluorescent antibody (IFA) techniques are available for use on clinical specimens. These techniques are sensitive and rapid; however, they require fluorescence microscopy, limiting their application to research and reference laboratories.
- Polymerase chain reaction (PCR) tests are being used with increasing frequency to diagnose cryptosporidiosis in humans and animals.
- DNA sequence analyses are used in outbreak settings to aid in determining the origin of the outbreak and to determine the likelihood of zoonotic versus anthroponotic transmission.

TREATMENT

- Many agents have been tried for the treatment of cryptosporidiosis in humans and in animals over the past 3 decades. Agents such as azithromycin, paromomycin, and hyperimmune bovine have been employed with variable success.
- In 2002, nitazoxanide oral suspension received FDA approval for use in children 1 to 11 years of age for the treatment of cryptosporidial diarrhea. This agent was approved for use in adolescents (aged 12+ years) and adults in 2005 based on a response rate of 96% in a double-blinded placebo-controlled clinical trial.
- In a gerbil model of biliary cryptosporidiosis published in 2006, nitazoxanide was found to be effective in reducing fecal oocyst shedding along with histopathologic evidence of ileal infection.
- Oral nitazoxanide at 150 mg/kg PO SID for 5 days yielded a greater than 95% reduction in oocyst shedding compared with untreated controls in a neonatal mouse model. In this same study, oral paromomycin at 50 mg/kg PO SID for 5 days yielded a greater than 98% reduction in oocyst shedding compared with controls.
- The author achieved laboratory-confirmed cure of clinical cryptosporidiosis in one ferret with a commercially available nitazoxanide oral suspension at 20 mg/kg PO twice daily for 5 days.

PREVENTION

HUMANS

- Thorough handwashing plays a pivotal part in the prevention of food-borne, animal-to-human and human-to-human cryptosporidiosis.
- Close supervision of children around potentially high-risk animals, such as hamsters and rabbits, is strongly advised.

ANIMALS

- Breeders, wholesalers, and distributors of avian and exotic pets should maintain the highest standards of husbandry possible and should reduce stress and overcrowding to the greatest degree possible.

REPORTING—NOTIFIABLE DISEASE

Cryptosporidiosis is reportable to federal and state authorities in the United States.

PROGNOSIS

The prognosis is excellent for immune competent humans and animals; however, juvenile or immune compromised individuals have a fair to guarded prognosis.

PEARLS & CONSIDERATIONS

COMMENTS

Cryptosporidiosis should be considered in all avian and exotic pets with acute or chronic diarrhea, particularly neonatal and juvenile members of those species mentioned in this chapter.

CLIENT EDUCATION

- Clients should be educated in the selection of healthy pets from high-quality breeders or retailers with impeccable husbandry and hygiene standards.
- Parents should be educated on the importance of hand hygiene in their children.
- Petting zoos and zoological gardens and sanctuaries should ensure that appropriate handwashing stations are provided in and around animal exhibits.
- Parents of children younger than 10 years of age and immune compromised persons are advised to consider the type of pet they acquire based on the relative risk of cryptosporidiosis and other zoonotic diseases.

SUGGESTED READINGS

Baishanbo A, et al: Efficacy of nitazoxanide and paromomycin in biliary tract cryptosporidiosis in an immunosuppressed gerbil model, J Antimicrob Chemother 57:353–355, 2006.
Chalmers RM, et al: *Cryptosporidium* sp. rabbit genotype, a newly identified human pathogen, Emerg Infect Dis 15:829–830, 2009.
Gibson SV, et al: Cryptosporidiosis in guinea pigs: a retrospective study, J Am Vet Med Assoc 189:1033–1034, 1986.
Molina-Lopez RA, et al: *Cryptosporidium baileyi* infection associated with an outbreak of ocular and respiratory disease in Otus owls *(Otus scops)* in a rehabilitation centre, Avian Pathol 39:171–176, 2010.
Sreter T, et al: Cryptosporidiosis in birds—a review, Vet Parasitol 89:313–319, 2000.

CROSS-REFERENCES TO OTHER SECTIONS

Birds
Cryptosporidiosis, Reptiles
Diarrhea, Birds
Endoparasites, Ferrets
Endoparasites, Rabbits
Ferrets
Hamsters
Intestinal Diseases, Hamsters
Intestinal Disorders, Rabbits
Rabbits
Reptiles

AUTHOR: **SIMON R. STARKEY**

EDITOR: **THOMAS M. DONNELLY**

ZOONOSES

Dermatophytosis

BASIC INFORMATION

DEFINITION AND INFECTIOUS AGENT

- Dermatophytosis is infection of the keratinized layer of the epidermis with fungi from the genera *Microsporum* and *Trichophyton* in humans and animals, and from the genus *Epidermophyton* in humans.
- Anthropophilic dermatophytes are found predominantly in humans and are rarely transmitted to animals.
- Geophilic dermatophytes are found predominantly in soil and are believed to survive by consuming decomposing fur, feathers, hooves, and other keratin sources.
- Zoophilic dermatophytes are found predominantly in animals, but can be transmitted to humans. Zoophilic dermatophytes tend to produce a pronounced inflammatory reaction in affected humans.
- The nomenclature of pathogenic dermatophytes is in flux. Molecular studies have indicated that the *Trichophyton mentagrophytes* complex consists of three or four separate species with five genotypes based on manganese-containing superoxide dismutase (MnSOD) gene sequence analysis. This complex contains both anthropophic and zoophilic isolates. The terminology used in this chapter represents the nomenclature currently used widely in clinical veterinary medicine and reported widely in clinical medical mycology articles. In the coming years, molecular epidemiology will become increasingly important in determining the origin of dermatophyte infection in humans and animals.

SYNONYMS

In humans: ringworm infection, dermatomycosis, tinea infection, trichophytosis, microphytosis

In animals: ringworm, keratinophilic mycosis

EPIDEMIOLOGY

ANIMAL SPECIES—HOSTS AND/OR CARRIERS

- Dermatophytosis has long been associated with rodents and rabbits. It is more common as a disease of rabbits and guinea pigs. It is uncommon in chinchillas, mice, and rats; rare in hamsters; and unreported in gerbils. The condition is rare in ferrets and African pygmy hedgehogs. Dermatophyte species most commonly identified in pet small mammals are listed below.

Rats, mice, and guinea pigs

- *Trichophyton mentagrophytes* var. *mentagrophytes*, *T. mentagrophytes* var. *quinckeanum*
- *Microsporum fulvum*, *M. gypseum*, *M. canis*

Rabbits

- *T. mentagrophytes* var. *mentagrophytes*
- *M. canis*

***European hedgehog* (Erinaceus europaeus) *and Central African (pygmy) hedgehog* (Atelerix albiventris)**

- *T. erinacei*

Chinchillas

- *T. mentagrophytes*
- *M. canis*
- *M. gypseum*

MODES OF TRANSMISSION

- Direct transmission
  - Contact with an infected or carrier animal can lead to establishment of zoophilic dermatophytosis in humans.
  - The young, the elderly, and immunocompromised individuals appear to be at greatest risk of developing dermatophytosis from their pets.
- Indirect transmission
  - Dermatophytes are environmentally stable, and humans and other animals can become infected via fomites.
- Person to person
  - It is rare for zoophilic dermatophytosis to spread from person to person.

CLINICAL PRESENTATION OF ANIMALS

Guinea pigs

- Dermatophytosis is common in guinea pigs; natural infection is always associated with *T. mentagrophytes* var. *mentagrophytes*.

- Lesions typically begin as broken hairs and circular, scaly alopecia initially occurring at the tip of the nose; these spread to the periocular, forehead, and pinnal areas. In severe cases, the dorsal sacrolumbar area is also affected, but the limbs and the ventrum are usually spared. Pruritus is usually minimal or absent.
- Some animals have more inflammatory lesions characterized by erythema, follicular papules, pustules, crusts, pruritus, and occasional scarring.

Rabbits

- Most cases in rabbits are caused by *T. mentagrophytes* var. *mentagrophytes.*
- Young rabbits are most prone to infection. Areas of patchy alopecia, broken hairs, erythema, and yellow crusting are typical. The lesions are pruritic, and secondary lesions occur on paws and toenail beds.
- *T. mentagrophytes* var. *mentagrophytes* can be isolated from the fur and skin of a significant minority of clinically normal rabbits.

Mice

- Clinical dermatophytosis is relatively rare in mice. When *T. mentagrophytes* var. *mentagrophytes* does induce lesions, they are most common on the face, the head, the neck, and the tail. These lesions have a scurfy appearance with irregular, patchy areas of alopecia, broken hairs, and scales, and variable degrees of erythema and crusting. Pruritus is usually minimal to absent.
- A more severe form of the disease occurs with *Trichophyton mentagrophytes* var. *quinckeanum.* The primary lesion is characterized by focal hair loss with the development of thick, yellow, saucer-shaped crusted lesions up to 1 centimeter in diameter called *scutula,* which consist of large quantities of dermatophyte mycelium and neutrophils.
- Asymptomatic mice represent a potentially large reservoir for zoonotic dermatophytosis. In one study, 12 of 20 pet store mice were found to be infected with *T. mentagrophytes* var. *mentagrophytes.* In 104 nonbreeder laboratory mice found to be infected with this organism, it was only observed clinically in 2 individuals.

Chinchillas

- Dermatophytosis is uncommon in chinchillas. Although *M. canis* and *M. gypseum* have been incriminated in outbreaks of spontaneously occurring dermatophytosis, *T. mentagrophytes* is the dermatophyte most commonly isolated.
- Small scaly patches of alopecia on the nose, behind the ears, or on the forefeet are seen in infected chinchillas. Lesions may appear on any part of the body, and in advanced cases, a large circumscribed area of inflammation with scab formation is not unusual. Although most mycologic studies of chinchillas are based on animals with clinical signs, *T. mentagrophytes* has been cultured in 5% of fur-ranched chinchillas with normal skins and in 30% of those with fur damage.

Rats

- Cutaneous lesions are most common on the neck and the back and, besides alopecia, have variable degrees of crusting and erythema. Pruritus is minimal to absent.
- *T. mentagrophytes* can be isolated from the hair coat of clinically normal rats and represents a potential zoonosis. However, because of its rarity in laboratory rats compared with mice and guinea pigs, it most likely poses a lesser potential zoonotic threat.

Ferrets

- Dermatophytosis is very rare in ferrets. One author described an outbreak of *M. canis* in his own ferret colony over a 3-year period. Lesions appeared as large circumscribed areas of alopecia and inflammation on all parts of the kit's body. Skin was thickened, red, and covered with scaling crusts. As kits became older, the lesions regressed, and clinical signs of ringworm were no longer apparent when the kits were fully grown.

RISK FACTORS Exposure to domestic or wild animals is a risk factor for zoophilic dermatophytosis in humans. Gardening and other activities involving contact with soil increase the risk for zoophilic and geophilic dermatophytosis in people.

GEOGRAPHY AND SEASONALITY

- Many dermatophytes have a worldwide distribution.
- Organisms grow best in warm, humid environments. Therefore, the prevalence of dermatophytosis is higher in tropical and subtropical areas.

PATHOBIOLOGY

- Dermatophytes grow in the nonliving keratin layer of the epidermis. However, inflammation, pain, and exudates occur secondarily to a local immune response within the dermis, and in subcutaneous tissues secondary to various dermatophyte antigens and products of metabolism.
- A degree of host adaptation occurs. Anthropophilic dermatophytes typically cause less pathology than zoophilic species.
  - Among the zoophilic dermatophytes, those species that likely had reduced co-evolution with humans appear to cause more severe disease in people. For example, zoonotic *T. erinacei* acquired from hedgehogs appears to induce a severely inflammatory and pruritic eruption in humans.

CLINICAL PRESENTATION OF HUMANS

INCIDENCE IN HUMANS The cumulative incidence of zoophilic dermatophytosis in the United States has been estimated at 2 million people per year.

DISEASE FORMS/SUBTYPES Dermatophytosis in humans is typically classified according to the location of the lesion(s).

- Tinea capitis is dermatophytosis of the scalp. Three subtypes have been identified:
  - Extothrix: with follicular destruction and arthoconidia formation on the outside of hair shafts. This form is often caused by zoophilic species such as *M. canis, M. gypseum, T. equinum,* and *T. vericosum.*
  - Endothrix: arthroconidia occur within the hair shaft. This form is caused by anthropophilic species.
  - Favus: crusting form of scalp dermatophytosis caused by anthropophilic strains
- Tinea corporis affects the glabrous skin of the body and may be caused by anthropophilic or zoophilic species.
- Tinea cruris affects the medial thighs, perineum, and buttocks. This is often caused by anthropophilic species.
- Tinea pedis and tinea unguium affect the feet and nails, respectively. These forms are most often caused by anthropophilic species.

HISTORY, CHIEF COMPLAINT

History

- Anthropophilic species: use of communal change rooms and showers, contact sports—particularly wrestling
- Zoophilic species: contact with animals, environments shared with animals, or fomites that have contacted infected animals

Chief complaint

- One or more erythematous, pruritic, and potentially exudative lesions
- Lesions may have failed to respond to treatment with steroids or antimicrobial therapy.

PHYSICAL FINDINGS IN INFECTED HUMANS

- Lesions often start as erythematous, scaly plaques. Lesions may progress to form extensive crusts, papules, vesicles, and potentially even bullae.
- Lesions vary in size, shape, and distribution; however, zoophilic dermatophytosis tends to affect areas that come into direct or indirect contact with animals, such as hands, arms, legs, face, scalp, or neck.
- Severe, pustular lesions known as *kerion* are most likely to occur in cases of zoophilic dermatophytosis.

INCUBATION PERIOD 1 to 3 weeks

DIAGNOSIS

DIFFERENTIAL DIAGNOSIS

- Atopic dermatitis
- Candidiasis
- Contact dermatitis
- Erythema multifome
- Parapsoriasis
- Psoriasis
- Pityriasis rosea
- Seborrheic dermatitis

INITIAL DATABASE

Microscopic examination of affected hairs, skin scales, or nail material digested with potassium hydroxide (KOH) can lead to diagnosis in many cases.

ADVANCED OR CONFIRMATORY TESTING

- Fungal culture is considered the gold standard in human and veterinary medicine.
- Molecular diagnostic techniques are being used more frequently in human medicine and in molecular epidemiologic studies.

TREATMENT

In humans
- Single, localized lesions many be treated with topical antifungals.
- Multiple, large, or severe lesions, as well as tinea unguium, are often treated with systemic antifungals such as terbinafine, or with an azole drug.

In small mammals
- Topical treatment may be effective for small, localized lesions; however, these products often mat the fur and may be ingested by the pet.
- The use of systemic antifungals such as terbinafine, or an azole drug (e.g., itraconazole).

PREVENTION

- Wash hands thoroughly after contacting any animal or potential fomite.
- Do not purchase small mammals with dermatoses or those from questionable facilities.
- Maintain high levels of hygiene and husbandry.
- Clean potential fomites, such as brushes, between use, or use specific items for animals housed individually or in groups.

REPORTING—NOTIFIABLE DISEASE

- Notification of federal U.S. health authorities is not required.
- Notification of state authorities varies by jurisdiction; contact local public health authorities and state department of agriculture.

PROGNOSIS

Good to excellent for humans and animals with appropriate therapy. Many cases resolve over weeks to months without intervention.

CONTROVERSY

Controversy surrounds the nomenclature of mycotic organisms of medical importance. Although resolution is important for academic and epidemiologic reasons, the implications for clinicians are limited at this time.

PEARLS & CONSIDERATIONS

COMMENTS

Up to 90% of infected cats are subclinical carriers of *M. canis.* Similar figures have not been established for small companion mammals; however, it must be anticipated that subclinical carriers do exist.

CLIENT EDUCATION

- Advise clients that children, the elderly, and immunocompromised individuals may be at greater risk of developing dermatophytosis by handling pets.
- Encourage good hygiene and personal protection.
- Educate clients to report skin lesions to their physician—whether or not their pet is clinically affected by dermatophytosis.
- Encourage owners to purchase outwardly healthy pets, free of obvious signs of disease or dermatoses, from reputable sources.

SUGGESTED READINGS

Burmester A, et al: Comparative and functional genomics provide insights into the pathogenicity of dermatophytic fungi, Genome Biol 12:R7, 2011.

Cafarchia C, et al: Molecular identification and phylogenesis of dermatophytes isolated from rabbit farms and rabbit farm workers, Vet Microbiol 154:395–402, 2012.

Chermette R, et al: Dermatophytoses in animals, Mycopathologia 166:385–405, 2008.

Donnelly TM, et al: Ringworm in small exotic pets, Sem Avian Exot Pet Med 9:82–93, 2000.

Fréalle E, et al: Phylogenetic analysis of *Trichophyton mentagrophytes* human and animal isolates based on MnSOD and ITS sequence comparison, Microbiology 153: 2466–2477, 2007.

Ghannoum MA, et al: Efficacy of terbinafine compared to lanoconazole and luliconazole in the topical treatment of dermatophytosis in a guinea pig model, Med Mycol 48:491–497, 2010.

AUTHOR: **SIMON R. STARKEY**

EDITOR: **THOMAS M. DONNELLY**

Encephalitozoonosis

BASIC INFORMATION

DEFINITION AND INFECTIOUS AGENT

- *Encephalitozoon* species are obligate intracellular eukaryotic microsporidian pathogens.
- Microsporidia are a diverse group of parasitic organisms, with more than 1200 recognized species in 143 genera. Recent phylogenetic evidence has indicated that these organisms are members of the fungal kingdom, or are closely related in a sister group.
- *Enterocytozoon bieneusi* and *Encephalitozoon intestinalis* have emerged over the past 25 years as common causes of chronic diarrhea in HIV-infected individuals. These pathogens also cause acute, self-limiting diarrhea in immunocompetent persons.
- Although less common, *E. cuniculi* and *E. hellem* have emerged as causes of localized infection (such as ocular lesions) or disseminated infection among immunocompromised persons.

SYNONYMS

Disease: In humans
- Often referred to as microsporidiosis. This term includes disease caused by

Enterocytozoon bieneusi and *Encephalitozoon* species, as well as several other microsporidial genera (e.g., *Pleistophora* spp., *Brachiola* spp.).

In animals

- Also known as microsporidiosis, particularly in canine and feline medicine

Organism

- *E. intestinalis* was initially known as *Septata intestinalis.*
- Three *E. cuniculi* strains have been defined on the basis of genetic variation. The term *strain* is used synonymously with the terms *genovar* and *genotype.*

EPIDEMIOLOGY

ANIMAL SPECIES—HOSTS AND/OR CARRIERS

Mammals

- *E. cuniculi,* the most common microsporidian infection in mammals, has been reported in rodents, foxes, monkeys, cats, dogs, sheep, goats, pigs, and llamas.
- Three strains of *E. cuniculi* have been defined based on the hosts from which the original isolates were characterized:
  - Strain I (rabbits)
  - Strain II (mouse)
  - Strain III (dogs)

Birds

- *E. hellem* has been associated with ocular and neurologic disease in various psittacines. Many of these birds have concurrent immune suppressive infections.
- Asymptomatic shedding of *E. hellem* appears to be particularly common among African lovebird parrots (*Agapornis* spp.) with concurrent psittacine beak and feather disease virus infection.
- A recent study from the Netherlands demonstrated *E. intestinalis, E. hellem, E. cuniculi,* and *Enterocytozoon bieneusi* in the feces of feral pigeons. Sequence analysis of the 18S SSU rRNA of these isolates demonstrated 99.6% to 100% homology with strains previously isolated from humans. It is unclear whether birds were actively shedding these organisms, or if sensitive molecular diagnostics detected organisms passing through the birds' intestinal tracts.

MODES OF TRANSMISSION

- Infection of most mammalian hosts with *E. cuniculi* occurs by ingestion or inhalation of spores from contaminated urine or feces that are shed by infected hosts. Infection by transplacental transmission and traumatic inoculation has been reported as well. Spores are moderately environmentally resistant and may survive 4 or more weeks under ideal conditions.
- Human-to-human transmission of *E. hellem* and *E. cuniculi* has been hypothesized but not proven.
- Definitive evidence of direct or indirect animal-to-human microsporidiosis has not been reported to date. However, substantial molecular epidemiologic and clinical data indicate that this is the most likely route of transmission. Several people infected with *E. cuniculi* strain I or III have reported ownership of, or recent contact with, rabbits or dogs, respectively. Additionally, a number of people with ocular *E. hellem* have reported bird ownership or contact.
- Additional evidence of the zoonotic potential of *E. cuniculi* has been demonstrated by successful experimental infection of rabbits with strains of human origin.

CLINICAL PRESENTATION OF ANIMALS

Rabbits

- Neurologic disease: ataxia, torticollis, head tilt, hind limb paresis, paralysis, seizures, collapse, nystagmus
- Urogenital disease: polyuria/polydipsia, weight loss, cystitis
- Ocular disease: cataract formation, uveitis—primary or phacoclastic

Psittacines

- Varies from asymptomatic shedding to keratoconjunctivitis. Acute death has been reported in lovebirds and budgerigars, particularly younger birds and/or those with concurrent immune suppressive infection.

RISK FACTORS

Rabbits

- A study in healthy pet rabbits in the United Kingdom failed to identify any of the following as potential risk factors for infection: husbandry, diet, breed, age, sex, body weight, vaccination status, health status, contact with *E. cuniculi*–positive rabbits, and preventive medicine routine.
- Presumptive risk factors include contact with infected urine, immune suppression, vertical transmission in utero, and an immature immune system.

Birds

- Immune suppression and concurrent infection are probable risk factors for serious disease associated with *E. hellem* infection. Studies performed to identify risk factors among asymptomatic shedders are lacking.

Humans

- Zoonotic transmission has not been proven for *E. cuniculi* or *E. hellem.* However, contact with infected or known host species or their urine or feces should be considered a risk factor, particularly among immune compromised individuals.
- Dogs may pose a zoonotic risk factor via ingestion of tissues from rabbits or mice infected with *E. cuniculi.* Ingestion of infected rabbit or mouse tissue could cause disease in humans as well.

GEOGRAPHY AND SEASONALITY

- Microsporidial infections in humans have a worldwide distribution, except for Antarctica. Infection with *E. cuniculi* has been diagnosed in rabbits in Europe, Africa, America, and Australia. The parasite was frequently encountered in laboratory rabbits, is rare in wild rabbits in the United Kingdom, and is common in commercial rabbitries in Europe and among wild rabbits in Australia. It is a newly emerging pathogen in pet rabbits. Incidence surveys in Europe suggest a 50% infection rate among pet rabbits.
- *E. hellem* has been identified among feral pigeons in Europe, in a wild, yellow-streaked Lory *(Chalopsitta scintillata)* in Indonesia, and among several species of captive psittacines in the United States.
- No seasonal variability has been detected among people with intestinal microsporidiosis in Brazil. Additionally, marked seasonal variability was not detected in a 1-year study of microsporidial loads in surface water in France.

PATHOBIOLOGY

- Parasite is ingested and carried in macrophages via blood to target organs—liver, kidney, intestines, central nervous system, lungs, and heart.
- Serum immunoglobulin (Ig)G antibody titers rise 3 to 4 weeks post infection and peak at 6 to 9 weeks.
- Spores are excreted in the urine from 1 month post infection until 3 months post infection, when shedding stops.
- Host cell is infected by injection of spore into cytoplasm using polar tube or phagocytosis.
- Spore multiplies, causing cell rupture and spore release to extracellular spaces.
- Spores infect surrounding cells and are passed via circulation to other organs.
- Chronic diffuse cellular infiltration and granuloma formation occur with mononuclear cell infiltration; clinical signs develop in relation to affected organs/tissues.

CLINICAL PRESENTATION OF HUMANS

INCIDENCE IN HUMANS

- A recent Japanese study demonstrated anti–*E. cuniculi* polar tube IgM antibodies among 36% of 380 apparently immune competent individuals. A previous study reported levels of 5% among pregnant French women and 8% among Dutch blood donors.

- These reports indicate that exposure to *E. cuniculi* appears to be relatively common, and that the disease is exceedingly rare among immune competent humans.
- Most clinical cases occur in HIV-positive individuals. Only six cases had been reported in the literature as of mid-2010 among persons immunocompromised for reasons other than HIV.
- *E. hellem* is more common among persons with HIV-induced immune suppression, although this organism appears to be an emerging cause of ocular infection among immunocompetent individuals.

DISEASE FORMS/SUBTYPES

Intestinal microsporidiosis

- This form is most common with anthroponotic *Enterocytozoon bieneusi* and *Encephalitozoon intestinalis.*
- Although more commonly associated with ocular, neurologic, or disseminated infection, *E. hellem* and *E. cuniculi* have been associated with intestinal microsporidiosis in humans.
- Clinical signs include chronic diarrhea, weight loss, nausea, vomiting, and abdominal pain.

Disseminated microsporidiosis

- May occur with *E. cuniculi, E. hellem,* and, less commonly, *E. intestinalis.*
- Organisms may replicate and cause cellular inflammation and death in one or more organ systems, leading to rhinitis/sinusitis, interstitial pneumonitis, nephritis, cystitis, cholecystitis, and cholangiohepatitis.

Central nervous system (CNS) microsporidiosis

- Encephalitis presenting as headaches and seizures may occur as a consequence of *E. cuniculi.*
- This may occur as the primary condition or as part of disseminated microsporidiosis.

Ocular microsporidiosis

- *E. cuniculi, E. hellem,* and *E. intestinalis* have been associated with ocular manifestations.
- Clinical signs include photophobia, epiphora, chemosis, and ocular pain.
- Deep stromal keratitides are more common in immune competent individuals, whereas a keratoconjunctivitis syndrome is more common among immune compromised individuals.
- As with CNS microsporidiosis, ocular manifestations may occur solely or in combination with disseminated disease.

HISTORY, CHIEF COMPLAINT

History

- A vast majority of cases of human microsporidiosis occur in immunocompromised persons, an overwhelming majority of whom are HIV-positive.
- Contact with animals known to harbor *Encephalitozoon* species is reported in a minority of cases of human microsporidiosis.

Chief complaint

- Fever is commonly observed in humans with most subtypes of microsporidiosis. Diarrhea is a common complaint among those with the intestinal form of the disease.

PHYSICAL FINDINGS IN INFECTED HUMANS Varies with disease subtype (see previous section)

INCUBATION PERIOD Incubation period varies with disease subtype; however, anti-*Encephalitozoon* IgM antibodies have been detected as soon as 10 days post infection in immunocompetent and immunodeficient Rhesus monkeys.

DIAGNOSIS

DIFFERENTIAL DIAGNOSIS

INTESTINAL MICROSPORIDIOSIS

- Giardiasis
- Cryptosporidiosis
- Bacterial gastroenteritis
- Viral gastroenteritis
- Inflammatory bowel disease

CNS MICROSPORIDIOSIS

- Toxoplasmosis
- Herpes simplex encephalitis
- Varicella-zoster virus encephalitis
- Cytomegalovirus encephalitis
- Arboviral encephalitides
- Lymphocytic choriomeningitis

OCULAR MICROSPORIDIOSIS

- Bacterial conjunctivitis
- Viral conjunctivitis
- Herpes simplex keratoconjunctivitis
- Trachoma *(Chlamydia trachomatis)*
- Ocular onchocerciasis *(Onchocerca volvulus)*

INITIAL DATABASE

- Fecal ova and parasite screening and fecal culture aid in ruling out other causes of intestinal microsporidiosis.
- Stained fecal smear is often sufficient for the diagnosis of intestinal microsporidiosis. Useful stains include Gram, trichrome, and Giemsa. Special stains, such as calcofluor, increase the sensitivity and specificity of microscopic techniques.
- Stained sputum, urine, and/or conjunctival scraping samples may be examined microscopically.

ADVANCED OR CONFIRMATORY TESTING

- Various immunologic tests have been developed over the past 20 years for clinical and research use; however, many have suffered from lack of specificity. Recent tests directed against the polar tube are considered much more specific.
- Direct immunofluorescence techniques are available and may be employed on a variety of samples such as sputum, urine, conjunctival scrapings, and feces.
- Immunohistochemical methods have been developed for biopsy and necropsy specimens.

TREATMENT

HUMANS

- Oral albendazole has traditionally been the treatment of choice for humans with disseminated or ocular microsporidiosis.
- Topical fumagillin has been advocated for use in cases of ocular microsporidiosis. This agent has been used to treat intestinal microsporidiosis via oral administration; however, it is seldom used because of the risk of drug-induced thrombocytopenia.

RABBITS

- Oral fenbendazole 20 mg/kg PO q 24 h × 28 d
- Covering broad-spectrum antibiosis, such as trimethoprim-sulfamethoxazole 30 mg/kg PO q 12 h or enrofloxacin at 10 mg/kg PO q 12 h × 10 d
- In acutely presenting cases, dexamethasone at 0.1-0.2 mg/kg SC q 48 h × 3 doses may also be given.
- Glucocorticoids should be used with care in rabbits because they may lower white cell counts and affect cell-mediated immune response thus limiting host defenses and increasing risk for other infections. Although one study showed 50% recovery rates in rabbits with neurologic signs treated with dexamethasone. A more recent study showed treatment with dexamethasone had no effect on neurologic score or on short- or long-term survival.
- Severe neurologic signs may require sedation of the rabbit with diazepam or midazolam at 0.5 mg/kg SC, IM, or IV.
- Prochlorpherazine 0.2-0.5 mg/kg PO q 8 h may be useful in rabbits with severe head tilt as it is used in humans with labyrinthitis.

PREVENTION

- Guidelines for the prevention of zoonotic microsporidiosis are not well defined because zoonotic transmission has not been definitively proven. However, immunocompromised individuals should be informed of the risks of owning pet rabbits and certain bird species.
- Because of fecal and urinary shedding of microsporidia, high-quality husbandry and hygiene should be emphasized.

REPORTING—NOTIFIABLE DISEASE

Microsporidiosis is not reportable to U.S. federal authorities. Reporting to local human and animal health authorities may be required.

PROGNOSIS

Prognosis is linked to early diagnosis, prompt treatment, and immune function of the infected person. People with CD4+ T cell counts lower than 100/microliter have a fair to poor prognosis in cases of disseminated or CNS microsporidiosis. Prognosis is good to excellent for immunocompetent individuals with intestinal microsporidiosis. Prognosis is also good for immunocompetent or immunocompromised individuals with ocular microsporidiosis.

CONTROVERSY

The relative zoonotic risk that pet rabbits and birds pose for causing microscopists in their owners is not well understood. Further molecular epidemiologic studies are required.

PEARLS & CONSIDERATIONS

COMMENTS

The host-parasite relationship has not been fully elucidated among rabbits and *E. cuniculi*. Even less is known about *E. hellem* among avian species. Clinicians are advised to educate clients on the potential risk and to consider microsporidiosis when asked to perform health screenings on animals entering nursing homes or facilities with immunocompromised populations, or on those owned by known immunocompromised individuals.

CLIENT EDUCATION

Owners of rabbits should be educated on the zoonotic potential of *E. cuniculi*. Owners of pet birds should be counseled despite greater lack of clarity on the true zoonotic potential that avian species pose.

SUGGESTED READINGS

Bart A, et al: Frequent occurrence of human-associated microsporidia in fecal droppings of urban pigeons in Amsterdam, the Netherlands, Appl Environ Microbiol 74:7056–7058, 2008.
Cama VA, et al: Transmission of Enterocytozoon bieneusi between a child and guinea pigs, J Clin Microbiol 45:2708–2710, 2007.
Didier ES: Microsporidiosis: an emerging and opportunistic infection in humans and animals, Acta Trop 94:61–76, 2005.
Mathis A, et al: Zoonotic potential of the microsporidia, Clin Microbiol Rev 18:423–445, 2005.
Sak B, et al: Unapparent microsporidial infection among immunocompetent humans in the Czech Republic, J Clin Microbiol 49:1064–1070, 2011.
Sulaiman IM, et al: Molecular characterization of microsporidiosis indicates that wild mammals harbor host-adapted *Enterocytozoon* spp. as well as human-pathogenic *Enterocytozoon bieneusi*, Appl Environ Microbiol 69:4495–4501, 2003.

CROSS-REFERENCES TO OTHER SECTIONS

Encephalitizoonosis, Rabbits

AUTHOR: **SIMON R. STARKEY**

EDITOR: **THOMAS M. DONNELLY**

ZOONOSES

Hantavirus

BASIC INFORMATION

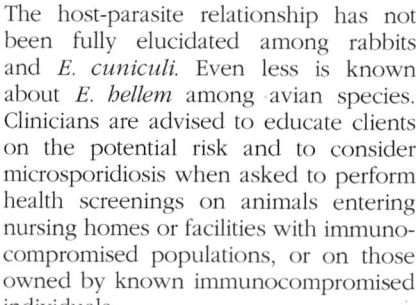

DEFINITION AND INFECTIOUS AGENT

Hantaviruses are members of the Bunyaviridae family, a group of negative-sense RNA viruses. Members of the genus *Hantavirus* are unusual among the Bunyaviridae insomuch as they are rodent-borne, whereas the other genera are arthropod-borne. The genus name is derived from the Hantaan River, from where the prototypic Hantaan virus was isolated in the mid-1970s as the cause of hemorrhagic fever with renal syndrome (HFRS), formerly known as Korean hemorrhagic fever. In 1993, the newly recognized Sin Nombre virus was isolated as the cause of Hantavirus (cardio-)pulmonary syndrome (HPS) in the United States. Other members of the genus have been associated with this syndrome throughout the Americas.

SYNONYMS

Organism

- The genus *Hanatvirus* contains more than 10 virus species (comprising Hantaan, Seoul, Puumala, Prospect Hill, Sin Nombre, El Moro Canyon, Bayou, Isla Vista, Black Creek Canal, Muleshoe, NY-1, and Andes) and 30 genotypes. Among these species, there is cause for confusion because several names are used synonymously.
- The prototypical cause of HPS, Sin Nombre virus, has also been called the Four Corners virus and the Muerto Canyon virus.
- Hantaan virus is also known as Korean hemorrhagic fever virus.

Disease

- In humans
  - HPS; Four Corners disease; in western Europe, nephropathia epidemica; in parts of eastern Europe and Asia, HFRS (Korean hemorrhagic fever); also many local names
- In animals
  - None

EPIDEMIOLOGY

ANIMAL SPECIES—HOSTS AND/OR CARRIERS

- In the Old World, Dobrava, Hantaan, Seoul, and Puumala viruses are known causative agents of HFRS and are associated with members of the subfamilies Arvicolinae (lemmings, muskrats, and voles) and Murinae (Old World rats and mice, including *Rattus rattus* and *R. norvegicus*).
- In the New World, Sin Nombre and related viruses and genotypes are considered causative agents of HPS and are associated with members of the subfamily Sigmodontinae (New World rats and mice).
- The principal reservoir for hantaviruses in the United States is the deer mouse *(Peromyscus maniculatus)*. Additional reservoir or spillover hosts include the cotton rat *(Sigmodon hispidus)*, the rice rat *(Oryzomys palustris)*, and the white-footed mouse *(Peromyscus leucopus)*.

- Various hantaviruses have been isolated from the house mouse *(Mus musculus)* in the United States, Latin America, and the Balkans. Isolation of a Puumala-like virus from *M. musculus* was associated with an outbreak of severe HFRS in humans in Serbia in 1988.
- To date, pet mice are not reported to be associated with human infection with any of the Hantaviruses. However, it is theoretically possible that horizontal transmission could occur to pet mice, subsequently leading to zoonotic disease in humans.
- Similarly, the principal reservoir of Seoul virus is the domestic rat *(R. norvegicus)*. Although detection in pet rats and subsequent zoonotic transmission to humans have not been reported, it is theoretically possible.
- Other common small mammal pet rodents and lagomorphs such as guinea pigs, hamsters, gerbils, and rabbits are not known to carry Hantaviruses.

MODES OF TRANSMISSION

- Direct transmission
  - Self-inoculation into oral or ocular mucous membranes after direct hand contact with rodent urine, droppings, or saliva is theoretically possible.
  - Bites inflicted by an infectious animal are considered a rare form of virus transmission to humans.
- Indirect transmission
  - The most common route of human infection is believed to be inhalation of infectious material. This commonly occurs during the process of cleaning dirt, dust, and debris contaminated with infectious rodent urine, droppings, or nesting material.
  - Ingestion of contaminated food is theorized to cause human infection with Hantaviruses.
- Person to person
  - Considered extremely rare, it has been reported in a single outbreak of Andes virus in Argentina in 1996.

CLINICAL PRESENTATION OF ANIMALS

Hantaviruses appear to have co-evolved with their rodent hosts, and overt disease and pathology are minimal to nonexistent.

RISK FACTORS

- Close proximity to reservoir species through infestation of dwellings, camping in rodent-infested areas, and cleaning of sheds and other areas likely frequented by rodents.
- Occupational hazard: farmers, pest exterminators, military personnel in endemic areas

GEOGRAPHY AND SEASONALITY

- Members of the genus *Hantavirus* have a worldwide distribution; however, viral species and genotypes appear to have regional distributions based in part on reservoir host range.
- Infection with Dobrava, Hantaan, Seoul, and Puumala viruses and subsequent HFRS or nephropathia endemica are most common in Korea, China, Russia, the Balkan states, and Scandinavia.
- Infection with Sin Nombre and related viruses with subsequent HPS is most common in Brazil, Chile, Argentina, and Paraguay. Within the United States, HPS is most common in southwestern states.
- HFRS incidence increases in spring and summer and is believed to relate to increased exposure of humans to reservoir species and their excreta and secretions in the environment.
- Paradoxically, in the United States, HPS incidence increases in autumn, as a consequence of increased movement of rodents indoors.

PATHOBIOLOGY

- Pathogenesis is not completely understood.
- Likely due to many factors causing immune-mediated damage to infected endothelial cells, leading to an increase in cell permeability
- Activation of classical and alternative complement pathways is believed to play a role in HFRS pathobiology. Highest levels of complement activity coincide with the peak of clinical signs.
- Cytotoxic T cells are important in virus clearance; however, these cells damage and destroy infected endothelial cells and cause inflammation and organ damage.

CLINICAL PRESENTATION OF HUMANS

INCIDENCE IN HUMANS

- In the United States, a total of 560 cases of HPS were reported to the Centers for Disease Control and Prevention (CDC) between 1993 and mid-December 2010.
- Among members of the South Korean military from 1995 to 1998, between 40 and 64 cases per 100,000 occurred each year.
- Estimated incidence of nephropathia endemica in Sweden is 20 cases per 100,000 each year.

DISEASE FORMS/SUBTYPES

HFRS

- Most commonly associated with Hantaan virus in Asia and Dobrava virus in the Balkans. Fatality rates vary between 5% and 15% for these viruses. Seoul virus tends to cause a milder form of HFRS in Asia and is associated with a case fatality rate of less than 5%.
- The average patient with this syndrome is moderately to severely afflicted and develops characteristic renal pathology.
- Five stages are well recognized in most cases of HFRS. Chronologically, they include the following:
  - Febrile: 3- to 5-day duration of fever, headache, chills, and photophobia. Patients may develop erythema of the face, neck, and thorax.
  - Hypotensive: This phase may be as short as a few hours or may last up to 2 days. It is characterized by nausea, vomiting, and thrombocytopenia. Blood pressure falls, and severe and potentially fatal shock ensues.
  - Oliguric: This phase lasts several days to 2 weeks and is characterized by oliguria and production of isosthenuric urine. CNS signs such as depression or coma may ensue. Hemorrhagic complication may develop during this phase.
  - Polyuric: This phase occurs as renal function improves, but it leads to the production of large volumes of hyposthenuric urine.
  - Convalescent: Renal function continues to improve, but fluid and electrolyte imbalances remain for several weeks.

Nephropathia endemica

- Considered a less severe form of HFRS in which renal dysfunction may be moderate or severe, but the hemorrhagic manifestations of HFRS are typically absent.
- Symptoms include fever, headache, and myalgia with vomiting and diarrhea.
- Occurs in Scandinavia and western Russia and is associated with Puumala virus. The reservoir host in this region is the Bank Vole *(Myodes glareolus)*.

HPS

- Initial clinical signs are nonspecific and include fever, chills, myalgia, headache, cough, and abdominal pain.
- Characteristic respiratory signs develop a few days later. These range from mild hypoxemia to progressive respiratory failure and shock. Complications may include disseminated intravascular coagulation, myocardial dysfunction, and cardiac arrhythmias. The case fatality rate may reach 40%.
- HPS is associated with Sin Nombre virus in the southwestern United States. Other proposed causative agents in the United States include Bayou, Black Creek Canal, and New York viruses.

HISTORY, CHIEF COMPLAINT

History

- Exposure to wild rodents and/or their excreta and secretions through occupational, recreational, or domestic exposure

Chief complaint

- Fever, headache, and chills are prominent early signs. Additional signs may develop as previously described, depending on the infecting virus and disease syndrome.

PHYSICAL FINDINGS IN INFECTED HUMANS Varies with disease subtype (see previous section)

INCUBATION PERIOD

- HFRS and nephropathia endemica: 1 to 6 weeks after exposure
- HPS: 1 to 4 weeks

DIAGNOSIS

DIFFERENTIAL DIAGNOSIS

HFRS

- Hemolytic-uremic syndrome
- Leptospirosis
- Rickettsial disease
- Lyme disease
- Pyelonephritis
- Streptococcal disease (and poststreptococcal glomerulonephritis)
- Malaria

HPS

- Acute respiratory distress syndrome
- Pneumonic plague
- Q fever
- Tularemia
- Influenza

INITIAL DATABASE

- History of exposure to rodent in the preceding 1 to 6 weeks will increase index of suspicion.
- Altered coagulation profile
- Elevated blood urea nitrogen (BUN), creatinine, and liver enzymes
- Urinalysis reveals hematuria and proteinuria.

ADVANCED OR CONFIRMATORY TESTING

- ELISA may be used to detect anti-hantaviral immunoglobulin (Ig)M in the acute phase of illness.
- Immunohistochemical methods may be used to detect hantaviruses in biopsy (often renal) or necropsy specimens.
- Reverse transcriptase polymerase chain reaction (RT-PCR) may be performed on whole blood to aid in the diagnosis of hantaviral infection.

TREATMENT

- In humans, treatment revolves around supportive care, with emphasis on fluid management and, where appropriate, dialysis for HFRS.
- Advanced cardiovascular and respiratory support is indicated for cases of HPS.
- Use of the antiviral ribavirin leads to reduced mortality if it is used in the first few days of onset of either syndrome.

PREVENTION

- Reduce risk of exposure to rodent excreta and secretions
  - Workers professionally dealing with rats should wear personal protective working clothes and ideally a properly fitted N100 respirator.
  - Those cleaning dusty areas likely frequented by rodents should first wet the area with dilute chlorine solution to minimize aerosolization of the virus.
  - Dwellings should be adequately sealed to prevent rodent entry.
  - Food and trash should be secured to prevent attracting rodents.

REPORTING—NOTIFIABLE DISEASE

Notification of U.S. federal health authorities is required.

PROGNOSIS

Varies with disease subtype, rate of diagnosis, and sophistication of treatment. The antiviral, ribavirin, may improve prognosis if given early in the course of treatment.

PEARLS & CONSIDERATIONS

COMMENTS

To date, pet rodents and lagomorphs have not been demonstrated to pose significant risk to humans. However, clinicians should remain cognizant of the possibility that hantaviruses may infect zoological collections, breeding facilities, and individual pet rodents.

CLIENT EDUCATION

Clients should minimize the entry of wild rodents into their dwellings and should prevent direct or indirect contact between pet rodents and wild rodents.

SUGGESTED READINGS

Antoniasis A: Direct genetic detection of Dobrava virus in Greek and Albanian patients with hemorrhagic fever with renal syndrome, J Infect Dis 174:407–410, 1996.

Diglisic G, et al: Isolation of a Puumala-like virus from *Mus musculus* captured in Yugoslavia and its association with severe hemorrhagic fever with renal syndrome, J Infect Dis 169:204–207, 1994.

Klein SL, et al: Emergence and persistence of hantaviruses, Curr Top Microbiol Immunol 315:217–252, 2007.

Olsson GE, et al: Hantaviruses and their hosts in Europe: reservoirs here and there, but not everywhere? Vector Borne Zoonotic Dis 10:549–561, 2010.

Settergren B: Clinical aspects of nephropathia epidemica (Puumala virus infection) in Europe: a review, Scand J Infect Dis 32:125–132, 2000.

Vaheri A, et al: How to diagnose hantavirus infections and detect them in rodents and insectivores, Rev Med Virol 18:277–288, 2008.

AUTHOR: **SIMON R. STARKEY**

EDITOR: **THOMAS M. DONNELLY**

ZOONOSES

Leptospirosis

BASIC INFORMATION

DEFINITION AND INFECTIOUS AGENT

- Leptospirosis is a systemic bacterial infection in animals or humans caused by any of the pathogenic *Leptospira* species.
- Leptospires are spirochetes.
- Nomenclature is in flux; however, it is widely accepted that approximately 20 species and more than 200 serovars exist. Pathogenicity varies by species and by serovar.
- Small mammal–associated leptospirosis has been linked to various serovars of *L. interrogans, L. kirschneri,* and *L. borgpetersenii.*

SYNONYMS

The large number of synonyms given to leptospirosis throughout the years and in many parts of the world demonstrates the diagnostic difficulty that clinical signs and sources of infection have presented to physicians and veterinarians.

- In humans
  - Mud fever, rice field fever, swamp fever, swineherd disease, Weil's disease, seven-day fever, cane cutter's disease, Japanese autumnal fever, Fort Bragg fever, hay makers disease, mouse fever, swineherd's disease, canicola fever
- In animals
  - Canicola disease in dogs, moon blindness (ophthalmia periodica) in horses, Stuttgart disease

EPIDEMIOLOGY

ANIMAL SPECIES—HOSTS AND/OR CARRIERS

- Rodents are the only major group of animals that can carry leptospires in kidneys and shed them throughout their lifespan without clinical manifestations.
- In addition to rodents, a subclinical carrier state is seen in some wildlife species (e.g., raccoons, opossums, European hedgehogs).
- Clinical disease has been identified in horses, cattle, sheep, swine, and dogs.
- A few cases of human leptospirosis have been directly linked to pet and laboratory rats and mice, and to pet guinea pigs. Rabbits *(Oryctolagus cuniculus)* have been implicated in occasional cases in Europe; however, it is not clear whether the rabbits were domestic or wild.
- In 2005, human leptospirosis was transmitted to two men in Japan by southern flying squirrels imported from the United States.

MODES OF TRANSMISSION

- The disease is usually transmitted via direct or indirect contact between mucous membranes and/or compromised skin and urine, secretions, or contaminated water from infected animals.
  - Leptospires do not survive well in acid urine but remain viable in alkaline urine. Consequently, herbivores and animals whose diet produces alkaline urine are relatively more important as shedders than are producers of acid urine.
- Occasionally, the disease may be transmitted between animals, or between animals and humans, via ingestion of infected animals.
- Rarely, the disease is directly transmitted through the bite of an infected animal.

CLINICAL PRESENTATION OF ANIMALS

Rats and mice

- These rodents are subclinical carriers, and clinical signs rarely develop.

Guinea pigs

- Vasculitis, disseminated intravascular coagulation, and death have been induced experimentally with pathogenic strains of *L. interrogans* var. *icterohaemorrhagiae.*
- Sudden death occurred in 20 of 50 guinea pigs owned by a German man shortly before he was hospitalized with leptospirosis caused by *L. interrogans* var. *bratislava.* Three surviving guinea pigs were positive for this serovar.
- This condition may be underreported in domestic guinea pigs.

RISK FACTORS

- Exposure to wildlife
- Poor husbandry/sanitation
- Active shedding of leptospires by rodents can go unrecognized until persons handling the animals become infected.

GEOGRAPHY AND SEASONALITY

- Worldwide distribution
- Most prevalent in tropics and areas with alkaline soils. Most U.S. cases originate in Hawaii.

PATHOBIOLOGY

- Current understanding is that all serovars are potential pathogens to humans and animals.
  - Previously, specific serovars were ascribed to specific species of animals.
- Humans are considered a dead end host for leptospiral transmission.
- Leptospiral infections in humans (and animals) are highly variable in clinical signs:
  - Clinical literature on human leptospirosis contains numerous combinations of symptoms that often end in a "surprising" final diagnosis of leptospirosis after positive serologic and isolation tests.
- Pathologic findings are as confusing as symptoms and depend on the affected organ system.
  - Human leptospirosis does not produce any gross or microscopic pathognomonic lesions.

CLINICAL PRESENTATION OF HUMANS

INCIDENCE IN HUMANS

- Incidence in United States (1974-1999) was 0.05 per 100,000 people; in Germany (1998-2003), 0.06 per 100,000 people.
- Fewer than 200 cases per year in the United States

DISEASE FORMS/SUBTYPES

- In humans, leptospirosis varies from a mild syndrome to a severe and potentially life-threatening condition that even with supportive therapy has 10% mortality.
- Anicteric form
  - Most cases (90%) involve mild, self-limiting disease in two stages:
    - Septicemic stage lasts about 1 week.
    - Immune stage may occur a few days after first stage. Hallmark is aseptic meningitis.
- Icteric form (Weil's disease)
  - Severe form of leptospirosis characterized by renal failure, hepatic dysfunction, thrombocytopenia, and hemorrhagic complications
  - Biphasic course with persistence of fever, jaundice, and azotemia
- Hemorrhagic pulmonary leptospirosis, an emerging leptospiral syndrome, may occur.

HISTORY, CHIEF COMPLAINT Abrupt onset of fever, headache, and myalgia

PHYSICAL FINDINGS IN INFECTED HUMANS

- Anicteric form
  - Fever, conjunctival suffusion, severe myalgia, skin rash, lymphadenopathy, hepatomegaly, splenomegaly, and meningitis

- Icteric form (Weil's disease)
  - Jaundice, persistence of fever, azotemia, uveitis, hemorrhage, vascular collapse

INCUBATION PERIOD Approximately 10 days (range of 3 to 20 days, depending on route of infection, dosage and virulence of organism)

DIAGNOSIS

DIFFERENTIAL DIAGNOSIS

- Brucellosis
- Rat bite fever (see Rat Bite Fever)
- Rocky Mountain spotted fever (*Rickettsia rickettsii*)
- Lyme disease
- Hantavirus (see Hantavirus)
- Tularemia (see Tularemia)
- Cat-scratch disease
- Chlamydiosis (see Chlamydiosis)

INITIAL DATABASE

- In humans
  - Elevated white blood cell count, elevated liver enzymes, albuminuria, and increased urine sediment
  - Culture of blood/CSF in first 10 days of illness; culture of urine after first 7 days and for up to 30 days after onset of illness
- In small mammals
  - Clinicopathologic changes may not be encountered in subclinical carriers.

ADVANCED OR CONFIRMATORY TESTING

- Serologic testing is imperative owing to variability in clinical signs.
  - Immunoglobulin (Ig)M ELISA and microscopic agglutination test (MAT) for IgG and IgM are widely employed to detect single high or paired rising titers against various serogroups of leptospires.
- PCR assays performed on whole blood, serum, CSF, or biopsy specimens are gaining favor for the rapid diagnosis of leptospirosis in humans. However, most PCR assays cannot identify infecting serovar, which has epidemiologic and public health significance.
- Serologic or PCR testing may be performed on small mammals. Commercially available tests are limited. Contact local commercial and university laboratories for information.

TREATMENT

Penicillin, doxycycline, ceftriaxone, and streptomycin have all been used in humans and animals with leptospirosis.

PREVENTION

- Prevent exposure of pet rodents and small mammals to wild rodents.
- Infection most frequently results from handling of infected pet rodents (contaminating hands with urine) or from aerosol exposure during cage cleaning:
  - Maintain high levels of husbandry in pets' cages.
  - Wash hands thoroughly after handling pets.
  - Avoid contacting pets or their enclosures if breaks in the skin exist.

REPORTING—NOTIFIABLE DISEASE

- Notification of U.S. federal health authorities is not required.
- Notification of state authorities varies by jurisdiction—contact local public health authorities and state department of agriculture.

PROGNOSIS

- Good in most human cases
- Guarded to poor for cases of Weil's disease and pulmonary hemorrhagic leptospirosis
- Good to excellent for most small mammals owing to subclinical carrier state. Exception may be guinea pigs in which acute death has been epidemiologically linked to leptospirosis.

CONTROVERSY

- Veterinarians may be asked to declare small mammals safe for residents of nursing homes, hospitals, or schools, or for persons with compromised immunity. Active client education about zoonoses is critical. Routine testing of pet mammals for leptospirosis is not commonly performed, but this may change in the future.
- The prevalence of leptospiral shedding in the pet small mammal population is largely unknown. Significant scope is available for research in this area.

PEARLS & CONSIDERATIONS

COMMENTS

- Although human leptospirosis is considered rare in developed countries, low but persistent rates of illness and death have been reported.
- Because of its nonspecific clinical features, lack of awareness among physicians, and difficulties in isolating the organism and performing serologic testing, the incidence of leptospirosis is likely underestimated.
- Wild rats are a well-documented source of human infection with *Leptospira*. However, pet rats are reported rarely as a source of infection.
- Carrier rates for laboratory-bred and -maintained rodents in the United States are unknown but probably low. Leptospirosis in persons handling laboratory animals has been primarily associated with mice.
- Leptospirosis has been reported in a wide variety of mammalian and nonmammalian species. Increased vigilance is suggested for this reemerging zoonosis.

CLIENT EDUCATION

- Clients should be encouraged to seek outwardly healthy pets from reliable sources.
- High standards of husbandry and personal hygiene should be encouraged among owners of small mammals.
- The practice of adopting feral rats should be actively discouraged.
- Clients reporting fever of unknown origin or unusual flulike symptoms should be directed to their physician and advised to mention the potential of zoonotic disease from their pets.

SUGGESTED READINGS

Adler B, et al: Leptospira and leptospirosis, Vet Microbiol 140:287–296, 2010.

Gaudie CM, et al: Human *Leptospira interrogans* serogroup *icterohaemorrhagiae* infection (Weil's disease) acquired from pet rats, Vet Rec 163:599–600, 2008.

Pischke S, et al: Of guinea pigs and men—an unusual case of jaundice, Z Gastroenterol 48:33–37, 2010.

Strugnell BW, et al: Weil's disease associated with the adoption of a feral rat, Vet Rec 164:186, 2009.

CROSS-REFERENCES TO OTHER SECTIONS

Chlamydiosis
Hantavirus
Rat Bite Fever
Tularemia

AUTHOR: **SIMON R. STARKEY**

EDITOR: **THOMAS M. DONNELLY**

ZOONOSES

Lymphocytic Choriomeningitis Virus

BASIC INFORMATION

DEFINITION AND INFECTIOUS AGENT

Lymphocytic choriomeningitis virus (LCMV) is a rodent-borne virus. It is the prototypic virus of the Arenaviridae family and can cause substantial neurologic disease known as lymphocytic choriomeningitis—particularly among prenatal and immune compromised humans. The common house mouse, *Mus musculus*, is the natural host and principal reservoir of LCMV. However, wild, pet, and laboratory rodents (rats, guinea pigs, hamsters) can also be infected. Humans are typically infected through close proximity to wild mice and their droppings, or to infected pet rodents. The immune system plays a major role in the outcome of this viral infection, ranging from predominantly inapparent infection in healthy individuals to severe neurologic disease among immunocompromised individuals.

EPIDEMIOLOGY

ANIMAL SPECIES—HOSTS AND/OR CARRIERS

- LCMV is found on all continents where the common house mouse has been introduced. Mice are often clinically unaffected and may shed the virus throughout their lives.
- Pet rodents such as guinea pigs, rats, and hamsters represent an additional source of human infection. These species are not thought to be natural reservoirs; rather they become infected through contact with wild mice.
- Infection has been reported among other wild rodents, including the yellow-necked field mouse *(Apodemus flavicollis)*, the wood mouse *(A. sylvaticus)*, and the bank vole *(Myodes glareolus)*.
- Rats are naturally resistant to the virus.

MODES OF TRANSMISSION

- LCMV is excreted in urine, feces, and saliva of infected rodents. Rodent blood is also infectious.
- Direct transmission
  - Scratches or bites inflicted by infectious animals may transmit the virus directly.
  - Handling of infectious animals or their tissues or infectious excreta may lead to infection through existing cuts or self-inoculation of the oral mucosa.
- Indirect transmission
  - Inhalation of dust contaminated with infectious material
  - Ingestion of food contaminated with rodent urine or feces
  - Contact with fomites, such as rodent bedding, poses significant risk.
- Person to person
  - Occurs vertically between an infected woman and her fetus
  - Known to occur horizontally after organ transplant from an infected donor

CLINICAL PRESENTATION OF ANIMALS

***House mouse* (Mus musculus)**

- Clinical signs are usually absent among house mice infected with LCMV in utero or in the neonatal period. These animals typically shed the virus for life. Some animals may develop clinical signs such as growth retardation, unkempt fur, hunched posture, ascites, and, rarely, death.
- Mice infected later in life are more likely to develop the aforementioned clinical signs, or to die acutely from the virus.

***Golden hamster* (Mesocricetus auratus)**

- Hamsters are likely infected via contact with wild house mouse populations in breeder facilities, pet stores, or owners' residences.
- Although not considered a host species, a significant proportion of golden hamsters may remain clinically unaffected by LCMV. Hamsters can transmit the virus for at least 8 months.
- Clinical signs have been reported in hamsters and are often protracted. The disease is characterized by a wasting disease. Early signs include decreased activity and appetite, and unkempt coat. Later signs include weight loss, hunched posture, blepharitis, convulsions, and eventually death.

***Guinea pig* (Cavia porcellus)**

- Tend to be clinically affected with greater frequency than hamsters. Clinical signs are similar to those seen in hamsters, although hind limb paresis/paralysis is a common clinical sign in guinea pigs.

RISK FACTORS

- Direct or indirect exposure to house mice and their excrement
- Occupational exposure: veterinarians, laboratory animal technicians, pet store employees, farmers, pest control personnel
- Residents with house mouse infestations in their homes or apartments

GEOGRAPHY AND SEASONALITY

- There is a worldwide distribution of LCMV.
- Incidence increases among humans in autumn and winter as wild rodent populations move indoors.

PATHOBIOLOGY

- The study of LCMV biology and pathobiology has added significantly to the understanding of the fields of immunology and virology.
- LCMV acts in a paradoxical manner on the immune system with reference to the role that cellular immunity—particularly T cells—plays in its pathobiology and natural history.
  - CNS signs observed in humans and rodents affected later in life are attributable to cytotoxic T cells and natural killer cells attacking virus-infected cells within the meninges, causing a localized inflammatory response.
  - Conversely, T cell downregulation is critical for the development of persistent shedders among house mice infected in utero or in the early neonatal period.
  - This apparent paradox was critical in the discovery and definition of the concept of major histocompatibility complex (MHC) restriction.
- Although they are adapted hosts, house mice do suffer pathologic consequences of being lifelong shedders. The main consequence is the development of anti-LCMV antibodies by B cells and subsequent antigen-antibody complex deposition and immune-mediated glomerulonephritis.

CLINICAL PRESENTATION OF HUMANS

INCIDENCE IN HUMANS Human seroprevalence in the United States is reported to range between 2% and 5%.

DISEASE FORMS/SUBTYPES

- May remain completely subclinical in many humans; however when apparent, the disease tends to be biphasic
- First phase
  - Fever, lethargy, myalgia, headache, and vomiting. Less common symptoms include pharyngitis, orchitis, myocarditis, and/or alopecia.
- Second phase
  - Can be mild or may go unnoticed in immune competent individuals
  - Occurs after a 2- to 4-day respite from initial symptoms
  - Includes aforementioned symptoms, as well as neurologic signs ranging

from increasing lethargy to encephalitic signs and nuchal rigidity
- Hemorrhagic fever syndrome
  - Occurs during the second phase in immune compromised individuals
  - Leads to reduced respiratory function, worsening neurologic function, leukopenia and thrombocytopenia, coagulopathy, hepatic and renal dysfunction, and petechiae and ecchymoses in multiple organs
- Transplacental infection
  - Occurs in the fetus of women who develop viremia during the first and second trimesters
  - The virus acts as a neuroteratogen, causing chorioretinopathy, hydrocephalus, microcephalus, lissencephaly, and potentially fetal death.

HISTORY, CHIEF COMPLAINT

History
- Workplace exposure to wild, domestic, or laboratory rodents
- Domestic exposure to wild rodents, particularly household infestations with *M. musculus*
- Keeping of pet rodents as pets
- Transplant recipient

Chief complaint
- Fever, headache, lethargy, and sore neck typically noted 1 to 3 weeks after exposure to rodents

PHYSICAL FINDINGS IN INFECTED HUMANS Vary with immune competence of the host, but typically nuchal rigidity

INCUBATION PERIOD Typically varies from 1 to 3 weeks

DIAGNOSIS

DIFFERENTIAL DIAGNOSIS
- Enterovirus meningitis
- Togaviruses
- Herpes simplex virus encephalitis
- Influenza virus
- Cat-scratch disease
- Dengue fever
- Leptospirosis
- Typhoid

INITIAL DATABASE
- Leukopenia and thrombocytopenia may be observed.
- Cerebrospinal fluid may demonstrate low glucose levels and elevated white cell counts. Fluid will be bacterial culture negative.

ADVANCED OR CONFIRMATORY TESTING
- Virus isolation performed using Vero cells (in specialized BSL-4 laboratory).
- Single elevated or rising antibody titers detected with immunoglobulin (Ig)G and IgM ELISA, IFA, or complement fixation techniques.
- Real-time reverse transcriptase polymerase chain reaction (RT-PCR) is used in research and epidemiologic settings and is gaining acceptance in clinical settings for use on sera, CSF, and biopsy and necropsy specimens.
- Immunohistochemistry performed on liver biopsy specimens or necropsy specimens

TREATMENT

- In humans, treatment is mainly supportive; however, immunoglobulins and the antiviral ribavirin sometimes are used experimentally in immunocompromised patients.
- Treatment generally is not attempted in animals.

PREVENTION
- Humans should minimize contact with wild rodents and their excreta by ensuring high levels of sanitation within their dwellings, by sealing buildings to prevent rodent entry, and by using pest control services where necessary.
- Occupationally exposed individuals should wear gloves when handling rodents and should take additional precautions, such as use of an N95 respirator, when working with or near high-risk animals such as house mice.
- Keep small exotic mammals indoors, and prevent exposure to wildlife and wild rodents.

REPORTING—NOTIFIABLE DISEASE
- Notification of U.S. federal health authorities is not required.
- LCMV-related disease is reportable in only three U.S. states (Wisconsin, Massachusetts, Arizona) and in one city (New York City).

PROGNOSIS

Prognosis in humans is generally excellent with a case fatality rate of less than 1% reported. Prognosis is dramatically worse for humans infected in utero, with risk of fetal death or severe neurologic sequelae exceeding 80%.

CONTROVERSY
- The risk of hamsters transmitting LCMV to the general population may be overstated. Three of the largest outbreaks of LCMV attributable to hamsters in the United States were attributable to a single supplier in the late 1970s. Single cases have subsequently been epidemiologically linked to hamsters among transplant recipients.
- Recent infection among organ transplant recipients has been associated with pet hamsters. The relative risk posed by these animals should be considered among recipients and in review of the donor history. Additionally, persons immunocompromised by any cause may best be advised against keeping pet rodents.

PEARLS & CONSIDERATIONS

COMMENTS
- Although very uncommon among exotic companion mammals, veterinarians are advised to remain cognizant of the possibility of LCMV as a diagnosis among these species, particularly in endemic areas.
- The name lymphocytic choriomeningitis does not describe the naturally occurring disease in rodents, since choriomeningitis is rare in such animals and naturally infected mice usually show no clinical signs. The name applies mainly to the results of intracerebral inoculation of mice and the meningitic complication of the human disease.

CLIENT EDUCATION
- Advise clients of the risks of this organism, with particular reference to children and immunocompromised persons.
- Maintain pets indoors; control wild rodent populations and their access to pet rodents.

SUGGESTED READINGS

Amman BR, et al: Pet rodents and fatal lymphoplasmacytic choriomeningitis in transplant patients, Emerg Infect Dis 13:719–725, 2007.

Bowen GS, et al: Laboratory studies of a lymphocytic choriomeningitis virus outbreak in man and laboratory animals, Am J Epidemiol 102:233–240, 1975.

Gregg MB: Recent outbreaks of lymphocytic choriomeningitis in the United States of America, Bull World Health Organ 52: 549–553,1975.

Jay MT, et al: The arenaviruses, J Am Vet Assoc 227:904–915, 2005.

AUTHOR: **SIMON R. STARKEY**

EDITOR: **THOMAS M. DONNELLY**

Mycobacterium marinum Granuloma

BASIC INFORMATION

DEFINITION AND INFECTIOUS AGENT

- Aquarium-borne *Mycobacterium marinum* granuloma is a superficial skin infection characterized by papular and/or ulcerating subcutaneous single or often multiple nodules limited to cooler areas of the body (e.g., hands, feet). Some infections consist of chains of granulomatous, inflamed, pustular lesions extending along the hand and arm. *M. marinum* granuloma is the most frequent "atypical" cutaneous mycobacteriosis.
- *M. marinum* (formerly known as *M. balnei*) is a slowly growing ubiquitous waterborne organism that grows optimally at temperatures around 30°C (86°F). It belongs to Runyon group I (the photochromogens) atypical mycobacteria, which produce a yellow carotene pigment when exposed to a strong light. Together with *M. fortuitum* and *M. chelonae*, the bacterium is one of the agents of fish mycobacteriosis (piscine tuberculosis), a chronic progressive disease that results in disseminated infection, emaciation, and death for more than 150 fish species.

SYNONYMS

Fish tank granuloma, fish fancier's finger, swimming pool granuloma

EPIDEMIOLOGY

ANIMAL SPECIES—HOSTS AND/OR CARRIERS

- *M. marinum* is a pathogen of fresh and saltwater fish. It naturally infects at least 150 fish and frog species, as well as freshwater eels and oysters.
- Dolphins, manatees (dugongs), and other aquatic mammals can also be infected.
- *M. marinum* infections have been observed in African toads and in a ball python.

MODES OF TRANSMISSION

- Transmission of fish mycobacteriosis is not well established. The disease is thought to be spread among fish by:
  - Ingestion of infective material
  - Transovarian transmission in viviparous fish
  - Direct transmission from water contact
  - Entrance through dermal wounds
  - Vector organisms (e.g., aquatic insects) as intermediate hosts
- It is likely that several modes of transmission exist, and that they are case, host, and mycobacterial species specific.

CLINICAL PRESENTATION OF ANIMALS

- Affected fish may be cachectic and frequently show skin changes consisting of pigment changes, loss of scales, blood spots with eventual formation of ulcers, and fin and tail rot.
- Microscopically, miliary tubercles may be found in virtually every organ system.

RISK FACTORS Stress caused by overcrowding, poor water quality, or contaminated food sources

GEOGRAPHY AND SEASONALITY

- *M. marinum* is widely distributed.
- Fish mycobacteriosis is reported commonly in aquaculture and ornamental fish.

PATHOBIOLOGY

- The temperature of human skin is advantageous for the establishment of superficial infection.
- The organism usually is acquired through abrasions, lacerations, or punctures sustained in an aquatic environment (e.g., aquarium, swimming pool).

CLINICAL PRESENTATION OF HUMANS

INCIDENCE IN HUMANS

- *M. marinum* infection in humans is comparatively rare.
- Annual incidence in the United States is 0.27 confirmed cases per 100,000 inhabitants.
- Approximately 50% of infections with known exposures are aquarium related; remaining cases are related to fish or shellfish injury, or to injury associated with saltwater or brackish water.

DISEASE FORMS/SUBTYPES

- Superficial infection
  - Lesions typically occur on:
    - Hands and fingers in aquarium owners
    - Elbows, knees, and feet in swimming pool–related cases
    - A common feature is the spread of lesions in a proximal fashion along the line of the lymphatics (sporotrichoid spread), although this does not usually cause axillary pain or lymphadenopathy.
- Deep tissue infection
  - Usually involves the hand (and sometimes the wrist) and develops as a result of misdiagnosis, administration of systemic corticosteroids to diminish inflammatory reactions (25% of all cases), and delayed treatment
    - Tenosynovitis (most common)
    - Osteomyelitis
    - Septic arthritis
    - Sclerokeratitis
  - In 50% of deep tissue infections involving the hand and wrist, carpal tunnel syndrome occurs.
- Disseminated systemic illness
  - Immune suppressed patients on corticosteroid therapy are affected most frequently and may develop cutaneous, pulmonary, or visceral infection.

HISTORY, CHIEF COMPLAINT

- Development of single or multiple asymptomatic granulomas on hands of aquarium owners.
- Placing unprotected hands into fish tank.
- More than 75% of reported cases involve the hand, usually the dominant right hand.

PHYSICAL FINDINGS IN INFECTED HUMANS

- Superficial lesions
  - One to six lesions appear as chronic erythematous plaques, verrucous papules (1.0 to 2.5 cm), or nodules
  - Lesions may ulcerate and drain purulent material.
  - Most lesions are asymptomatic.
  - Symptoms, if present, include slight tenderness and discharge.
  - Lymphadenopathy occurs rarely.
  - Occasionally, spread in a sporotrichoid fashion occurs.
- Deep tissue infections
  - Superficial lesions may invade deeper tissues through attempted self-excision, by intralesional cortisone injection, or by incomplete surgical excision that is not combined with appropriate antibiotics.
  - These infections are more destructive and are more resistant to treatment than are superficial lesions.
  - Diffuse edema at the site of infection
  - Slight fullness may be palpated at the site of affected tendon sheath.
  - Unlike in pyogenic infections, the dorsum of the hand does not swell, and a throbbing pain does not occur.
  - Joint limitation may occur with subsequent development of draining sinus tracts.
  - Systemic complaints, fever, and lymphadenopathy are usually absent.

- The erythrocyte sedimentation rate is usually normal, and radiographic findings are nonspecific.

INCUBATION PERIOD The incubation period ranges from 2 weeks to 2 months.

DIAGNOSIS

DIFFERENTIAL DIAGNOSIS

- Bacterial infection
  - Nocardia, syphilis, yaws, tularemia
- Fungal infection
  - Sporotrichosis, coccidioidomycosis, blastomycosis, histoplasmosis
- Neoplasia
  - Common warts, benign or malignant tumors
- Miscellaneous
  - Sarcoidosis, cutaneous leishmaniasis, gout, rheumatoid arthritis, iodine or bromine granuloma

INITIAL DATABASE

- Culture of secretions from skin lesions may lead to diagnosis of *M. marinum*, but culture from tissue biopsies is more sensitive.
- Concomitant histopathologic examination of tissue biopsy specimens
- Diagnosis relies primarily on isolation of the organism by staining or culture.

ADVANCED OR CONFIRMATORY TESTING PCR is not available.

TREATMENT

- Superficial lesions—antibiotics
  - Minocycline has long been considered the drug of choice.
  - Clarithromycin and doxycycline have been equally efficacious; however, resistance to doxycycline is described.
  - Ciprofloxacin has good in vitro activity.
  - Treatment should be continued for 6 to 12 weeks.
- Deep tissue infection
  - Deeper tissue involvement requires surgical intervention (e.g., excision, tenosynovectomy, synovectomy, arthrodesis, incision and drainage of infected bones or joints).
- Treatment time
  - Overall median treatment time in 63 reported superficial lesion cases was 3.5 months; in deep tissue infection, 11 months.

PREVENTION

- Education
  - Among 40 tropical fish salesmen, only 6 (15%) knew this disease well; 30 (75%) ignored it.
- Personal protection
  - Wear gloves when immersing hands in a fish tank.
- Elimination and disinfection
  - Destroy all fish from a contaminated aquarium. Disinfect aquarium with 5% calcium hypochlorite solution before adding other fish.

REPORTING—NOTIFIABLE DISEASE

Notification of U.S. federal health authorities is not required.

PROGNOSIS

- The time lag between appearance of lesion and correct diagnosis ranges from a few weeks to a few years.
- Left untreated, 80% of lesions resolve completely in about 14 months.
- Factors associated with a poor prognosis for deep tissue infection include persistent pain, presence of a draining sinus tract, and previous local injection of corticosteroids.

PEARLS & CONSIDERATIONS

COMMENTS

- The tuberculin skin test is often positive in *M. marinum* infection but has low predictive value because cross-reacting antigens are present in various mycobacteria.
- Efforts to control mycobacteriosis in aquaculture through culture practices or feed supplements have met with mixed success. Currently, no drugs have been approved by the Food and Drug Administration (FDA) for the treatment of mycobacteriosis in fish, leaving depopulation and facility disinfection as the only options.

CLIENT EDUCATION

- Establish a quarantine area or tanks that are separate from existing populations, in which new fish can be held to prevent zoonotic pathogens and other disease agents (i.e., viral, bacterial, parasitic, and fungal) from entering clients' fish populations.
- Hold new fish in quarantine for 30 to 45 days to allow development of any clinical signs. However, chronic infection with *Mycobacterium* spp. may not be evident.
- Have clients seek veterinary guidance before purchasing fish, and have them arrange prepurchase examinations by a veterinarian when expensive or large numbers of fish are involved. However, it can be difficult to impossible to determine whether a fish is persistently infected with *Mycobacterium* spp. Inspection of facilities and assessment of the health status of existing fish populations can provide indications of zoonotic risk.
- Advise clients to deal with fish and feed suppliers that have a reputable history and that provide veterinary certificates of health for purchased fish.
- Advise clients to have regularly scheduled appointments for fish examinations or site visits.

SUGGESTED READINGS

Lowry T, et al: Aquatic zoonoses associated with food, bait, ornamental and tropical fish, J Am Vet Med Assoc 231:876–880, 2007.
Petrini B: *Mycobacterium marinum*: ubiquitous agent of waterborne granulomatous skin infections, Eur J Clin Microbiol Infect Dis 25:609–613, 2006.

CROSS-REFERENCES TO OTHER SECTIONS

Bacterial Disease, Fish

AUTHOR: **THOMAS M. DONNELLY**

EDITOR: **SIMON R. STARKEY**

ZOONOSES

Pasteurella multocida

BASIC INFORMATION

DEFINITION AND INFECTIOUS AGENT

Pasteurellacea are small, nonmotile Gram-negative bacilli to coccobacilli that make up part of the normal flora of the nasopharynx and the proximal gastrointestinal tract of many animal species, including common livestock, as well as many pet species. The taxonomy of Pasteurellaceae is in flux; however, at the time of writing, the species of greatest zoonotic concern is *Pasteurella multocida*, followed by *P. dagmatis* and *P. pneumotropica*. Biochemical differentiation of *P. multocida* from *P. dagmatis* is technically challenging and is not possible with many commercial kits. Therefore, it is believed that these organisms have been and continue to be misreported in the literature with some frequency.

SYNONYMS

In humans: pasteurellosis
In animals: pasteurellosis, snuffles (respiratory pasteurellosis in rabbits)

EPIDEMIOLOGY

ANIMAL SPECIES—HOSTS AND/OR CARRIERS

P. multocida

- Among exotic companion animals, infection and asymptomatic colonization are most commonly seen in rabbits.
- Organism is isolated less frequently from rats and mice.
- *P. multocida* has also been isolated from a number of diseased marsupials, including Virginia opossums, mouse opossums, kangaroos, wallabies, and potoroos.

P. pneumotropica

- Among exotic companion animals, this organism has been isolated from rats, mice, hamsters, and gerbils.
- Some prevalence studies have shown that up to 95% of outwardly healthy laboratory mice carry *P. pneumotropica*.

P. dagmatis

- Has been isolated predominantly from the oral cavity of dogs and cats, and less frequently from rats.
- Given the inability of many commercial biochemical systems to differentiate *P. dagmatis* from *P. multocida*, it is likely that the prevalence of *P. dagmatis* has been underestimated to date.

MODES OF TRANSMISSION

- Direct transmission
    - Humans
        - A vast majority of *Pasteurella* spp. infections in humans are directly attributable to *P. multocida* or to *P. canis* associated with dog or cat bite and/or scratch wounds.
        - *P. multocida* infection occasionally has been reported in humans after exposure to cats or dogs in the absence of bites or scratches. Infection in these cases has been theorized to occur secondary to direct contact with infectious secretions, as may occur when an animal licks a human.
        - Over the past 70 years, fewer than 10 published human cases of *Pasteurella* spp. infections have been directly attributed to rabbit-, rodent-, or marsupial-inflicted wounds. Infections in humans have not been directly attributed to any avian species.
        - Transmission via inhalation of infectious secretions has been theorized but is not yet proven, as is the case with vector-borne transmission.
    - Animals
        - Transmission may occur via direct contact with infectious secretions or excretions or through inhalation of aerosols.
- Indirect transmission
    - Humans
        - As with direct transmission, indirect routes of infection have been theorized to play a role in *Pasteurella* species infection in humans after animal exposure in the absence of bites or scratches. These cases are believed to occur secondary to indirect contact with infectious secretions or excretions.
        - Two cases of *Pasteurella* spp. peritonitis have been attributed to contamination of dialysis tubing by hamsters biting the tubes in patients undergoing peritoneal dialysis.
    - Animals
        - Transmission may occur via indirect contact with infectious secretions or excretions, particularly by fomites.

CLINICAL PRESENTATION OF ANIMALS

P. multocida

- Rabbits
    - Rhinitis with mucopurulent nasal discharge and sneezing
    - Ocular discharge associated with dacryocystitis/conjunctivitis
    - Head tilt associated with otitis interna/media
    - Cutaneous swellings associated with abscesses
    - Dyspnea associated with upper airway disease, pneumonia, and/or thoracic abscessation
    - Systemic illness, malaise, and abdominal masses associated with abdominal abscessation and/or pyometra
    - Mastitis
    - Orchitis
- Marsupials
    - Anorexia, lethargy, and mucopurulent nasal discharge
    - Sudden death without premonitory signs of illness
    - Regional lymphadenopathy and lymph node abscessation
    - Orchitis
- Rodents
    - Clinical disease attributable to *P. multocida* is considered relatively rare in rodents. The organism has been associated with natural infection causing head tilt and otitis media/interna in mice.

P. pneumotropica

- Rodents
    - Dyspnea associated with pneumonia occurring as spontaneous single cases or rarely as large outbreaks have been reported among laboratory mice. Dyspnea may also occur secondary to pleural abscesses.
    - Conjunctivitis among weanling laboratory mice
    - Abdominal masses associated with organ and/or peritoneal abscesses
    - Dermatitis and subcutaneous abscesses
    - Reproductive disorders such as infertility and metritis

P. dagmatis

- Rodents
    - This organism is considered to be a commensal in rats and has yet to be associated with clinical disease.

RISK FACTORS

Animals

- In most instances, *Pasteurella* species are commensal organisms.
- Stress has long been associated with induction of clinical disease among several species of animals, including rabbits, rodents, and marsupials.
    - Stressors may include overcrowding, transport stress, introduction of

new animals/altered hierarchy, concurrent disease, and heat stress.
- Glucocorticoid therapy–induced immune suppression increases the risk of opportunistic *Pasteurella* infection.

Humans
- Bite or scratch wounds inflicted by cats or dogs represent the greatest risk factor among humans.
- Close contact with dogs and cats, especially with exposure to saliva, may pose a risk for infection in the absence of bite/scratch wounds. Risk is increased among people with preexisting skin lesions.
- Immune suppression and preexisting disease increase the risk of *Pasteurella* infection and systemic manifestations in humans.
- *Pasteurella* species infections secondary to wounds inflicted by exotic companion animals are extremely rare, with only several reports in the literature over the past century:
  - A 1969 report documented localized *P. multocida* infection secondary to a bite inflicted by an opossum *(Didelphis virginiana)* under laboratory conditions.
  - One report from 1995 involved severe *Pasteurella* "SP" group infection from a guinea pig bite to the finger of a healthy 31-year-old woman.
  - Two reports of *P. multocida* from rabbit bites can be found in the literature. One involved an immune suppressed individual.
  - Human cases of *Pasteurella* infection have not been associated with pet or aviary birds.

GEOGRAPHY AND SEASONALITY
- *Pasteurella* species have a worldwide distribution. Retrospective studies have failed to demonstrate any seasonality with human infections secondary to bites.
- *Pasteurella* infection among exotic companion mammals does not appear to demonstrate seasonality.

PATHOBIOLOGY
- The presence of a capsule among many strains of *P. multocida* increases pathogenicity by preventing effective phagocytosis of the organisms.
- Lipopolysaccharides are an important target of humoral immunity and are required for pathogen replication and clinical disease in vivo.
- Most *P. multocida* strains produce sialidases, which aid in providing the organism with a carbon source and in defeating host cell defenses such as mucin.

CLINICAL PRESENTATION OF HUMANS
- Most patients have a history of dog- or cat-inflicted wounds. Local infections are well established as soon as 3 hours after a bite wound, and clinical signs such as localized pain, swelling, and redness occur within 12 to 24 hours.
- Additional presentations may occur (see Disease Forms/Subtypes, below) for additional information.

INCIDENCE IN HUMANS Although the incidence of *Pasteurella* species infection is not readily calculable, it has been estimated that more than 5 million dog and cat bites occur in the United States each year. Of these, an estimated 800,000 wounds necessitate medical care. It has been estimated that between 3% and 18% of dog bites and between 28% and 80% of cat bites become infected. *Pasteurella* species are commonly cultured from dog and cat bite wounds; thus a conservative estimate of the annual incidence of wound-associated *Pasteurella* species infections in the United States would be 30,000 to 40,000 cases.

DISEASE FORMS/SUBTYPES
- Local infection
  - The most common type of infection stems from local infection of a dog- or cat-inflicted wound. As noted previously, this form of infection has occurred occasionally secondary to exotic companion mammal bites.
  - Within 24 hours, infected wounds become erythematous and painful, and a purulent discharge is often noted. A trivial bacteremia/septicemia with mild fever may ensue.
  - Common complications include local abscess formation and tenosynovitis.
  - Less frequent, but not uncommon, complications include cellulitis, edema, lymphangitis, osteomyelitis, and septic arthritis.
- Respiratory infection
  - *P. multocida* occurs as a commensal in the upper airway of humans, along with severe respiratory disease such as pneumonia and pleural abscessation.
  - Clinical disease is typically associated with trauma, infection, or immune compromise. It is most commonly seen in patients with chronic underlying respiratory disease.
  - Patients may have a history of atraumatic contact with farm animals, cats, or dogs.
- Systemic infection
  - A variety of systemic manifestations may occur, including brain abscessation, bacterial peritonitis, septicemia, and abdominal abscessation.
  - About half of all patients with systemic manifestations have a history of animal exposure.
  - Patients typically have concurrent disease causing immunosuppression.

HISTORY, CHIEF COMPLAINT Most human cases of *Pasteurella* infection are associated with dog- or cat-inflicted wounds. Patients typically present for treatment of the wounds themselves and/or of wound infections often manifesting as pain, swelling, and erythema.

PHYSICAL FINDINGS IN INFECTED HUMANS See Disease Forms/Subtypes, above.

INCUBATION PERIOD Among *Pasteurella* species, infections associated with bite wounds and signs of infection typically manifest within 12 to 24 hours (range, 3 hours to 3 days).

DIAGNOSIS

DIFFERENTIAL DIAGNOSIS
Infections associated with:
- *Actinobacter* species
- *Actinomyces* species
- *Clostridium* species
- *Haemophilus* species
- *Neisseria* species
- *Proteus* species
- *Staphylococcus* species
- *Streptococcus* species

INITIAL DATABASE
- History of animal-inflicted wounds or exposure to livestock, dogs, or cats
- Gram stain of wound exudates, blood, and/or CSF fluid may yield a high index of suspicion.
- Culture of abscess material, wound exudates, CSF fluids, or blood is typically part of the initial database and often allows the diagnosis to be achieved.

ADVANCED OR CONFIRMATORY TESTING
- Biochemical tests are typically employed to identify *Pasteurella* species in clinical laboratories.
- PCR testing of abscess material, wound exudates, CSF fluids, or blood is used with increased frequency in clinical and research settings for the diagnosis and differentiation of species of *Pasteurella.*

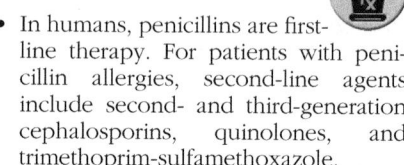

TREATMENT
- In humans, penicillins are first-line therapy. For patients with penicillin allergies, second-line agents include second- and third-generation cephalosporins, quinolones, and trimethoprim-sulfamethoxazole.
- Penicillins and quinolones are commonly employed in the treatment of exotic companion mammals, particularly rabbits, with *Pasteurella multocida* infection.

PREVENTION

- Reduce risk of exposure to rabbit/rodent bites.
  - Workers professionally dealing with rodents should wear personal protective working clothes and gloves.
  - In laboratories, use purpose-bred rodents that are free of *Pasteurella* species.
  - Children who are around pets should always be supervised by adults.
- Educate workers and pet owners to report pet bites and serious scratches.
  - Meticulous wound treatment is necessary.
  - After an animal bite (see Animal Bites) or scratch, the wound should be cleaned thoroughly and reported to a physician.

REPORTING—NOTIFIABLE DISEASE

Notification of U.S. federal health authorities is not required.

PROGNOSIS

- Generally good to excellent for local and regional infections. Chances of complete return to function are reduced in cases of osteomyelitis and septic arthritis.
- Prognosis is good for patients with meningitis given prompt diagnosis and effective treatment.

CONTROVERSY

The relative frequency of *P. dagmatis* infection may be underestimated given the inability of many commercial systems to differentiate this organism from *P. multocida*. Increased molecular studies and/or advanced biochemical testing of *Pasteurella* isolates will shed light on this facet of the disease in the coming years.

PEARLS & CONSIDERATIONS

CLIENT EDUCATION

Although exotic companion mammals appear to pose little risk with regard to *Pasteurella* species infection, the following advice should be given to clients:

- Children, the elderly, and immunocompromised individuals who are handling pet rabbits and/or rodents may constitute a special risk group.
- Encourage good hygiene and personal protection.
- Educate clients to report pet bites to their physician.
- Any bite or scratch wound should be cleaned thoroughly.

SUGGESTED READINGS

Boisvert PL: Human infection with *Pasteurella leptiseptica* following a rabbit bite, J Am Med Assoc 17:1902–1903, 1941.

Campos A, et al: Hamster bite peritonitis: *Pasteurella pneumotropica* peritonitis in a dialysis patient, Pediatr Nephrol 15:31–32, 2000.

Donnio PY, et al: Characterization of *Pasteurella* spp. strains isolated from human infections, J Comp Pathol 130:137–142, 2004.

Freeman AF, et al: *Pasteurella aerogenes* hamster bite peritonitis, Pediatr Infect Dis J 23:368–370, 2004.

Harper M, et al: *Pasteurella multocida* pathogenesis: 125 years after Pasteur, FEMS Microbiol Lett 265:1–10, 2006.

Hubbert WT, et al: *Pasteurella multocida* infections. I. *Pasteurella multocida* infection due to animal bite, Am J Public Health Nations Health 60:1103–1108, 1970.

Lion C, et al: *Pasteurella* "SP" group infection after a guinea pig bite, Lancet 346:901–902, 1995.

Silberfein EJ, et al: Aortic endograft infection due to *Pasteurella multocida* following a rabbit bite, J Vasc Surg 43:393–395, 2006.

CROSS-REFERENCES TO OTHER SECTIONS

Animal Bites
Pasteurellosis, Rabbits (Section I)
Rat Bite Fever

AUTHOR: **SIMON R. STARKEY**

EDITOR: **THOMAS M. DONNELLY**

ZOONOSES

Plague

BASIC INFORMATION

DEFINITION AND INFECTIOUS AGENT

Plague is caused by the Gram-negative, bipolar staining, nonmotile bacillus *Yersinia pestis*. This organism has been responsible for some of the largest epidemics in human history and is currently responsible for several thousand deaths each year around the world. Plague causes an acute, febrile condition that is often fatal if left untreated, or if treatment is delayed.

SYNONYMS

In humans: bubonic plague, pneumonic plague, septicemic plague, black death

In animals: feline plague, rodent plague, sylvatic plague

EPIDEMIOLOGY

ANIMAL SPECIES—HOSTS AND/OR CARRIERS

- Commensal (human-associated) rats (*Rattus rattus* and *R. norvegicus*) are an important worldwide reservoir of *Y. pestis*.
- In the United States, wild rodents such as ground squirrels, rock squirrels, and prairie dogs serve as important reservoirs.
- Domestic cats have been responsible for a number of human cases in the United States since the mid-1970s.

MODES OF TRANSMISSION

- Direct transmission
  - Scratches or bites inflicted by infectious animals
  - Handling of infectious animal tissues, such as butchering wild rodents and small game
- Indirect transmission
  - May occur among cat owners and veterinarians treating cats with respiratory symptoms secondary to the plague
  - May also affect wildlife rehabilitators, veterinarians, and good Samaritans caring for infected reservoir species
  - Is a relatively common form of human-to-human infection
- Vector-borne transmission
  - Fleas are the principal vectors of plague. Approximately 30 flea species are believed to be plague vectors.
  - Once infected, certain flea species may remain infectious for up to 1 year.

  - Urban plague has been linked to *Xenopsylla cheopis*, a common flea of the *Rattus* species.
  - In North America, *Oropsylla montana* is considered to be the predominant vector in sylvatic plague.
  - Cat fleas *(Ctenocephalides felis)* are considered relatively poor vectors for plague.
  - The human flea *(Pulex irritans)* has been known to transmit the plague under crowded conditions.
- Person to person
  - Occurs secondary to inhalation of droplets from the cough of a person with pneumonic plague

CLINICAL PRESENTATION OF ANIMALS

***Prairie dogs* (Cynomys *species*)**

- Plague is an acutely fatal disease of prairie dogs. Epizootics have been responsible for the complete extinction of entire colonies of black-tailed prairie dogs *(Cynomys ludovicianus)*.
- Concern regarding plague in prairie dogs stems from their role as the main food source for the endangered black-footed ferret.

Mustela species

- The black-footed ferret *(Mustela nigripes)* was first thought to be resistant to *Y. pestis* owing to the relative resistance seen in carnivores (other than domestic cats). A 1991 study appeared to support this theory because eight domestic ferrets *(Mustela putorius furo)* and two Siberian polecats *(M. eversmannii dauricus)* survived infection via subcutaneous inoculation without developing clinical signs.
- However, a case report in 1994 described a case of fatal plague in a captive black-footed ferret likely exposed to infected prairie dogs (*Cynomys* species) after escaping its enclosure.
- In November of 1997, 27 of 30 black-footed ferrets accidentally exposed to plague-infected food either died or were missing and presumed dead within 48 hours of ingestion of the contaminated prairie dog meat at the U.S. Army's Pueblo Chemical Depot.
- The most common clinical signs observed in these ferrets were lethargy and hematochezia. Necropsy findings include peripheral lymphadenopathy, pulmonary consolidation and edema, foamy blood in the nares, cervical lymphadenopathy, and gastrointestinal and mesenteric lymph node hemorrhage.
- A subsequent experimental infection study in Siberian polecats demonstrated a high fatality rate, with death occurring at or before day 12 post infection in 29 of 33 animals—a case fatality rate similar to that seen in the black-footed ferret accidentally exposed at the Pueblo Chemical Depot. Clinical signs in experimentally infected polecats included lethargy, decreased fecal production, green-colored diarrhea, wheezing, coughing, dyspnea, hematochezia, and ataxia.

Squirrels

- Squirrels, particularly ground squirrels, serve reservoir species of *Y. pestis*. The California ground squirrel *(Otospermophilus beecheyi)* appears to be partially resistant to the plague. An experimental infection study demonstrated that 28% of squirrels inoculated with 6070 organisms or fewer died acutely, 19% survived and seroconverted, and 53% survived without seroconversion.
- This resistance may have implications for the study of the ability of *Y. pestis* to persist between epizootics.

RISK FACTORS

- Hunting reservoir species in endemic areas
- Exposure to arthropod vectors in endemic areas
- Caring for wildlife or domestic pets potentially infected with plague
- Keeping of guinea pigs indoors and their use as food in Andean countries have been associated with plague in humans.
- Contact with infected humans, particularly those with pneumonic plague

GEOGRAPHY AND SEASONALITY

- *Yersina pestis* has a worldwide distribution.
- Prevalence of plague is greatest in developing nations.
- In the United States, most human cases originate in Arizona, Colorado, California, New Mexico, and Texas.
- Typically, prevalence peaks among wildlife and humans in spring and summer, associated with increased arthropod vector activity. However, a second peak is seen in late autumn and winter months and is associated with small game hunting.

PATHOBIOLOGY

- The genetic basis of *Y. pestis* pathogenesis is a subject of much research because the organism diverged from the enteric pathogen *Y. pseudotuberculosis*, allowing comparative genomics to determine virulence factors.
- One key facet of the pathogenicity of the plague within mammalian hosts revolves around its ability to reside in phagocytes and to resist phagocytosis. A lipopolysaccharide plays a key role in this process, as do coagulase and fibrinolysin, which are encoded by the gene, *pla*. These latter enzymes likely contribute to the often fatal disseminated intravascular coagulation seen as a consequence of septicemic plague.
- A plasmid-acquired phospholipase D is considered an evolutionarily recent addition to virulent strains of *Y. pestis*; it appears to allow the pathogen to survive within the flea midgut, thus allowing for arthropod-borne transmission of the plague.

CLINICAL PRESENTATION OF HUMANS

INCIDENCE IN HUMANS On average, 10 to 15 cases are reported each year in the United States.

DISEASE FORMS/SUBTYPES

Bubonic plague

- The most common clinical presentation of the plague among humans
- Sudden-onset fever, chills, and headache occur after a 1- to 8-day incubation period. Patients may also experience myalgia, weakness, diarrhea, and/or abdominal pain. Painful lymphadenopathy occurs typically in the groin, but may also occur in the axillae or neck. These lesions are referred to as *buboes*.
- Without appropriate treatment, this form of the condition may lead to secondary pneumonic plague and/or disseminated sepsis.

Pharyngeal plague

- This form occurs from ingestion of infectious secretions, excretions, or meat.
- Symptoms include fever, pharyngitis, and painful cervical lymphadenopathy.

Pneumonic plague

- This form is highly infectious and may occur via inhalation of infectious aerosol droplets from the cough of an infected human or from respiratory secretions of infected animals.
- Laboratory workers may also be exposed to infection via this route in the course of their work.
- Patients with bubonic or septicemic plague may develop pneumonic plague from hematogenous spread of the organism to the lungs.
- Patients with this form of the disease may or may not have peripheral lymphadenopathy.
- Patients present with sudden-onset fever, chills, productive cough, dyspnea, and/or hemoptysis.

Septicemic plague

- This form is most common among elderly or immunocompromised humans. Symptoms occur rapidly and include abdominal pain, nausea, vomiting, and diarrhea.
- Endotoxic shock rapidly ensues, and patients quickly become moribund and die. Case fatality rate approaches

100% without appropriate and prompt antimicrobial administration.
- Peripheral lymphadenopathy is uncommon in this form of the disease, increasing the degree of difficulty in diagnosing the condition.

Meningeal plague
- Clinical signs include fever, headache, and nuchal rigidity. Lymphadenopathy is common, and axillary buboes are associated with a greater incidence of the meningeal form.

HISTORY, CHIEF COMPLAINT

History
- Exposure to wild animals or vectors through high-risk activities, including hunting of small game, camping, and contact with wildlife, especially in endemic areas.
- Contact with sick cats in endemic areas, especially outdoor cats known to hunt reservoir species

Chief complaint
- Varies with route of infection and disease subtype but typically includes sudden-onset fever, headache, and lethargy

PHYSICAL FINDINGS IN INFECTED HUMANS Vary with disease subtype (see previous section)

INCUBATION PERIOD Varies with disease form but is typically 1 to 8 days

DIAGNOSIS

DIFFERENTIAL DIAGNOSIS
- Anthrax
- Brucellosis
- Bacterial pneumonia
- Cat-scratch disease
- Dengue fever
- Leptospirosis
- Malaria
- Reye's syndrome
- Rocky Mountain spotted fever (*Rickettsia rickettsii*)—early stages
- Septic shock
- Tonsillitis
- Tularemia
- Typhus

INITIAL DATABASE
- Several complete blood count parameters, including neutrophilic leukocytosis and thrombocytopenia, may be altered in patients with plague.
- Peripheral blood smears may demonstrate the organism.
- Gram stain of cerebrospinal fluid, sputum, or lymph node may demonstrate small Gram-negative coccobacilli.
- Blood culture may yield a diagnosis of plague in a variable percentage of cases.
- Chest radiographs may demonstrate variable infiltrates through lung lobe consolidation.

ADVANCED OR CONFIRMATORY TESTING
- Rising antibody titers to the F-1 antigen of *Y. pestis* are considered diagnostic.
- Direct immunofluorescence tests are available and may be employed on culture samples to speed diagnosis.
- An immunohistochemical detection method is available for use on paraffin-embedded tissues.

TREATMENT
- In humans, treatment with streptomycin, gentamicin, chloramphenicol, doxycycline, or ciprofloxacin
- Treatment generally is not attempted in animals.

PREVENTION
- Humans should minimize contact with arthropod vectors by using insect repellents and by wearing long-sleeved shirts and pants, especially in areas with known vectors and/or endemic plague.
- Wear cut-resistant gloves while processing wild game, and cook game meat thoroughly.
- Keep small exotic mammals indoors, and prevent exposure to wildlife and wild rodents.
- Take preventive measures when treating or caring for wildlife, especially reservoir species, in endemic areas.

REPORTING—NOTIFIABLE DISEASE
Notification of U.S. federal health authorities is required.

PROGNOSIS
Varies with disease subtype and rate of diagnosis and treatment. Prognosis is generally poor to grave with pneumonic and septicemic forms of the disease.

CONTROVERSY
Risk posed by exotic companion mammal pets is considered relatively small, with the exclusion of prairie dogs. However, the relative risk is not well quantified, especially among those pets kept in endemic areas, where exposure to reservoir species and/or arthropod vectors may occur.

PEARLS & CONSIDERATIONS

COMMENTS
Although very uncommon in exotic companion mammals, veterinarians are advised to remain cognizant of the possibility of plague as a diagnosis among these species, particularly in endemic areas.

CLIENT EDUCATION
- Advise clients of the risks associated with this organism.
- Maintain pets indoors, and control arthropod vectors in endemic areas.

SUGGESTED READINGS

Bizanov G, et al: Experimental infection of ground squirrels *(Citellus pygmaeus Pallas)* with *Yersinia pestis* during hibernation, J Infect Dis 54:198–203, 2007.

Castle KT, et al: Susceptibility of the Siberian polecat to subcutaneous and oral *Yersinia pestis* exposure, J Wildl Dis 37:746–754, 2001.

Gabastou JM, et al: An outbreak of plague including cases with pneumonic infection, Ecuador, 1998, Trans R Soc Trop Med Hyg 94:387–391, 2000.

Hinnebusch BJ: Role of *Yersinia* murine toxin in survival of *Yersinia pestis* in the midgut of the flea vector, Science 296:733–735, 2002.

Lowell JL: Identifying sources of human exposure to plague, J Clin Microbiol 43:650–656, 2005.

Matchett MR, et al: Enzootic plague reduces black-footed ferret *(Mustela nigripes)* survival in Montana, Vector Borne Zoonotic Dis 10:27–35, 2010.

Pauli JN, et al: A plague epizootic in the black-tailed prairie dog *(Cynomys ludovicianus)*, J Wildl Dis 42:74–80, 2006.

Williams ES, et al: Experimental infection of domestic ferrets *(Mustela putorius furo)* and Siberian polecats *(Mustela eversmanni)* with *Yersinia pestis*, J Wildl Dis 27:441–445, 1991.

Williams ES, et al: Plague in a black-footed ferret *(Mustella nigripes)*, J Wildl Dis 30: 581–585, 1994.

AUTHOR: **SIMON R. STARKEY**

EDITOR: **THOMAS M. DONNELLY**

ZOONOSES

Rabies

BASIC INFORMATION

DEFINITION AND INFECTIOUS AGENT

- Rabies is caused by a number of related rhabdoviruses belonging to the genus *Lyssavirus.* Members of this genus are unique among rhabdoviruses in their ability to replicate in mammalian central nervous system (CNS) tissue. Different strains of rabies virus are adapted to particular animal species that serve as reservoir hosts. Rabies is perhaps the most feared zoonosis because it is almost always fatal in the absence of appropriate postexposure prophylaxis (PEP).
- From Latin *rabere* = to rave

SYNONYMS

In humans: lyssa, hydrophobia
In animals: "La rage" [French], mad dog

EPIDEMIOLOGY

ANIMAL SPECIES—HOSTS AND/OR CARRIERS

- Rabies viruses can affect any mammal; however, they typically are maintained in a geographic region or ecologic niche via adapted strains circulating in reservoir hosts:
  - Bat rabies is widespread throughout the United States, and rabid bats have been encountered in all 48 continental states.
  - Raccoon rabies is endemic along most of the Eastern seaboard and represents a significant amount of the animal rabies reported in the United States.
  - Red fox rabies variant is maintained in a small area in northern Vermont and New Hampshire and far western Maine. It is the major variant in Western and Central Europe.
  - Gray foxes maintain a second fox variant that occurs in Texas and Arizona.
  - Skunks represent a major reservoir both geographically and in terms of the number of cases identified nationwide each year. One reservoir covers much of the central part of the United States from Montana to Texas and from Wyoming to Ohio. The other reservoir covers much of California.

MODES OF TRANSMISSION

- Direct transmission
  - Saliva of animals infected with rabies is infectious several days to weeks before clinical signs are apparent, until the animals dies.
  - The virus typically enters the body via a bite, through an open wound such as a scratch, or by contact with mucous membranes. Other secretions or excretions are not considered infectious.
- Indirect transmission
  - Infection by inhalation has occurred infrequently in people entering caves frequented by bats and in laboratory settings.
- Person to person
  - Person-to-person transmission has occurred very rarely in cases of corneal or organ transplantation.

CLINICAL PRESENTATION OF ANIMALS

- After an incubation period typically lasting weeks to months, animals will manifest furious or dumb forms of the disease. One form will predominate at a given point in time; however, both forms can occur during the course of infection in a single animal.
- Furious
  - Animals may appear irritable, aggressive, and hypersexual and may experience hyperptyalism. They may bite or scratch humans or other animals without provocation; they may roam and attack inanimate objects. Abnormal vocalizations may develop, and convulsions are often noted.
- Dumb
  - Animals experience marked lethargy and paralysis that originates at the head and neck, and progresses in a descending manner before culminating in death.
- Small mammals
  - The overall incidence of rabies in U.S. pet ferrets was 23 reported cases from 1960 to 2000 (0.6 cases per year).
  - Rabies is relatively rare in small synanthropic (live near humans) and feral rabbits and rodents. The reasons are unclear but probably are more behavioral than biological.
  - Of 87,700 cases of animal rabies reported in the United States from 1992 to 2002, only 621 occurred in rodents or lagomorphs. Most (559) occurred in groundhogs *(Marmota monax)* and were most likely a result of den contact with infected skunks or raccoons.
  - Despite its rarity, rabies has been reported in pet rabbits, guinea pigs, and ferrets.
    - Both dumb and furious rabies are described after natural infection and experimental inoculation in these species.
  - Unilateral pelvic limb paresis or paralysis has been reported as an early clinical sign in domestic rabbits. Other signs in rabbits include anorexia, mild hyperptyalism, biting at inanimate objects, and nonspecific neurologic signs.
  - Postexposure prophylaxis was required for a resident of New York State who was bitten by a pet guinea pig that had been infected with raccoon rabies. The animal was in thin body condition and had epiphora and poor coat condition 7 days after biting the owner, at the time of euthanasia. Neurologic signs were not detected in this animal.
  - Rabies has been reported in wild rodents sometimes kept as pets, such as chipmunks and squirrels.

RISK FACTORS

- Exposure to wild animals, particularly known rabies vectors
- Greatest risk is from pets housed outdoors in endemic areas.

GEOGRAPHY AND SEASONALITY

- Rabies has a worldwide distribution with the exception of a small number of Pacific and Caribbean islands, including Hawaii.
- Rabies may have a higher prevalence in spring and summer, although this may be confounded by increased ease of identification and capture of rabid animals in warmer seasons of the year.

PATHOBIOLOGY

- *Lyssavirus* enters the body at the site of a bite or other break in the skin, or via the mucous membranes.
- Virus replicates locally and then slowly travels through sensory and motor nerves to the CNS, where it causes encephalitis.
- Virus then spreads to salivary glands and other organs via peripheral nerves. Once the organism replicates within salivary glands, the host becomes capable of infecting other animals or humans.

CLINICAL PRESENTATION OF HUMANS

INCIDENCE IN HUMANS

- Incidence varies greatly between developed and developing nations. The greatest disease burden occurs in Asia, with approximately 31,000 cases per year. Africa has the second

greatest incidence, with 24,000 cases per year.
- Fifteen cases were reported in humans in the United States from 2003 to 2008.

DISEASE FORMS/SUBTYPES
- Classic encephalitic rabies (furious rabies)
  - Characterized by hyperexcitability and hydrophobia
- Paralytic (dumb) rabies
  - Characterized by flaccid muscle weakness
- Nonclassical atypical
  - Neuropathic pain, focal brainstem signs, monoclonus, and other neurologic signs

HISTORY, CHIEF COMPLAINT

History
- Association with wildlife, particularly reservoir species
- Contact between pet and reservoir species
- Close proximity to bats, in a dwelling or recreationally

Chief complaint
- Bite, scratch, or contact with saliva of wild or domestic animal may be reported.
- Anxiety, fever, malaise, and headache
- Pain, irritation, or altered sensation at the site of the bite
- Sensitivity to light
- Hydrophobia

PHYSICAL FINDINGS IN INFECTED HUMANS
- Wound(s) may be observed or reported in infected people.
- Mydriasis and hyperptyalism may be observed.
- Variable neurologic signs (e.g., paresis/paralysis, inability to swallow, altered mentation, hydrophobia, seizures, delirium) may occur.

INCUBATION PERIOD
- In humans, typically 20 to 90 days (although incubation of several years has been reported)
- In other mammals, variable incubation period extending typically from weeks to months

DIAGNOSIS

DIFFERENTIAL DIAGNOSIS

For fever, malaise, and headache:
- Brucellosis
- Leptospirosis
- Rocky Mountain spotted fever (*Rickettsia rickettsii*)
- Lyme disease
- Tularemia
- Cat-scratch disease
- Streptococcal disease

For encephalitic signs:
- Viral encephalitis
- Bacterial meningitis

INITIAL DATABASE
- Thorough medical history often provides the greatest evidence early in the course of the disease in humans.
- CSF fluid analysis may indicate increased white blood cell (WBC) count, elevated lactate, and/or elevated protein level.
- Hydrophobia is considered pathognomonic for furious rabies in humans.
- Evidence or knowledge of exposure to wildlife will increase the index of suspicion for domestic and pet animals.

ADVANCED OR CONFIRMATORY TESTING

HUMANS
- Antemortem
  - Direct fluorescent antibody test (DFA) or reverse transcriptase polymerase chain reaction (RT-PCR) on punch biopsy of skin from the nuchal region
  - DFA on corneal impressions
  - In vitro virus isolation from saliva
  - Virus neutralization assay on serum (for evidence of rabies antibody)
  - Virus neutralization assay on cerebrospinal fluid (for evidence of rabies antibody)
  - RT-PCR performed on saliva
  - RT-PCR or DFA on antemortem brain biopsy
  - Molecular techniques are gaining favor for the antemortem diagnosis of rabies in humans.

ANIMALS
- Typically, postmortem immunohistochemistry of the hippocampus, cerebellum, and brainstem

TREATMENT

HUMANS
- Until recently, the disease was considered almost uniformly fatal once established. Supportive and palliative care was provided.
- To date, survival after rabies encephalitis has been well documented for six patients.
- Physicians are advised to consider using the Milwaukee protocol for rabies treatment. This protocol has saved the life of one person, who developed rabies without being given preexposure or postexposure prophylaxis. The protocol subsequently failed in several other human cases.

ANIMALS
- No treatment is available for animals.
- Euthanasia and appropriate postmortem testing are recommended for suspect animal cases after government-mandated quarantine period is observed.

PREVENTION
- Ferrets should be vaccinated with an approved vaccine on an appropriate schedule. No vaccines have been approved for other small mammal pets.
- If pets must be housed outside, they should be protected from predators and potentially rabid animals. The use of two layers of caging material separated by a space may enhance protection afforded to outdoor pets.
- Any person whose pet is bitten or exposed to potential rabies vectors should contact his or her veterinarian and local public health officials.

REPORTING—NOTIFIABLE DISEASE
- Notification of U.S. federal health authorities is required.
- Notification of local and state health and agriculture authorities is required.

PROGNOSIS

In humans and animals, the prognosis is grave.

CONTROVERSY
- Because bites from pet small mammals are frequent events, veterinarians must be concerned with rabies.
  - However, no case of human rabies has ever been reported as resulting from bites by pet rodents or rabbits.
  - The risk of humans acquiring rabies from other pet small mammals (excluding rodents and rabbits) appears negligible but is not well quantified. Consequently, each incident must be considered on a case-by-case basis.

PEARLS & CONSIDERATIONS

COMMENTS
- Dogs are infectious for up to 13 days before clinical signs appear and then continue to shed virus in saliva until death.
- The total period of infectivity likely varies among species and is not known in most small mammals. Thus, quarantine guidelines for these species are difficult to determine. Protocols established for carnivores will likely serve as guidelines until these data become available.
- Wounds from bats often go undetected among people and domestic animals. Hence, postexposure prophylaxis (PEP) is recommended in many states for people in close proximity to bats.

CLIENT EDUCATION

- Advise clients that no rabies vaccine is available for small mammals except ferrets, so prevention is essential.
  - Discourage owners from keeping small mammals outside or from allowing them outside without constant, close supervision.
- Advise ferret owners to vaccinate their pets in accordance with local and/or state laws.
- Encourage owners:
  - To consult their veterinarian if their pet is exposed to a potentially rabid animal.
  - To consult local health department officials if exposed to potentially rabid wildlife or if their pets may have been exposed.

SUGGESTED READINGS

Dowda H, et al: Naturally acquired rabies in an eastern chipmunk *(Tamias striatus)*, J Clin Microbiol 19:281–282, 1984.

Eidson M, et al: Rabies virus infection in a pet guinea pig and seven pet rabbits, J Am Vet Med Assoc 227:932–935, 2005.

Hu WT, et al: Long-term follow-up after treatment of rabies by induction of coma, N Engl J Med 357:945–946, 2007.

Karp BE, et al: Rabies in two privately owned domestic rabbits, J Am Vet Med Assoc 215: 1824–1927, 1999.

AUTHOR: **SIMON R. STARKEY**

EDITOR: **THOMAS M. DONNELLY**

ZOONOSES

Rat Bite Fever

BASIC INFORMATION

DEFINITION AND INFECTIOUS AGENT

Rat bite fever (RBF) consists of three bacterial diseases in humans that are clinically similar yet distinctive syndromes. Illness may result from infection by *Streptobacillus moniliformis* after a rat bite or from ingestion of contaminated food. RBF due to *Spirillum minus* is a separate disease.

SYNONYMS

Disease

- RBF, streptobacillary RBF, streptobacillary fever, or streptobacillosis
  - Infection after a rat bite or animal bite from which *S. moniliformis* is isolated
- Haverhill fever or erythema arthriticum epidemicum
  - Disease transmitted via consumption of *S. moniliformis*–infected water or by milk or food contaminated with rat excreta
- Sodoku, spirillary RBF, spirillary fever, or spirillosis
  - RBF caused by infection with *S. minus*
  - "Sodoku" is Japanese word meaning "rat" (so) "poison" (doku).
  - Until 1942, all cases of RBF had been considered to be sodoku.

Organism

- *Spirillum minus* was named in 1924. However, the organism is not on the Approved List of Bacterial Names because no type or reference strain for this taxon has been identified. It is considered a species *incertae sedis* (Latin for "species sits uncertain") that does not belong to the genus *Spirillum*.

EPIDEMIOLOGY

ANIMAL SPECIES—HOSTS AND/OR CARRIERS

- *S. moniliformis*
  - Rats are natural hosts and asymptomatic carriers. The organism is a commensal flora of the nasopharynx in rats.
  - It has been reported in other rodents (mouse, spinifex hopping mouse, gerbil, guinea pig) and in carnivores (cat, dog) and other animals (calf, turkey, koala, monkey).
  - RBF has occurred after bites of mice (rare) and of dogs.
  - No confirmatory evidence suggests that other animals from which *S. moniliformis* has been isolated act as transmitters of RBF.
- *S. minus*
  - Rats are natural hosts and asymptomatic carriers.
  - It is assumed that *S. minus* does not occur in rat saliva but rather in the blood. Only if lesions are present in the oral mucosa is *S. minus* transferred to the animal's saliva.
  - It has been reported in mice and guinea pigs.
  - Carrier rates among rats vary widely in different geographic regions.

MODES OF TRANSMISSION

- Direct transmission
  - *S. moniliformis* and *S. minus* can be transmitted by bite from rats.
  - *S. moniliformis* is infrequently transmitted by bite from carrier animals (mouse and dog).
- Indirect transmission (only with *S. moniliformis*; not with *S. minus*)
  - Bites from rat-eating carnivores (dogs)
  - Rat feces–contaminated food, milk, and water
  - Animal contact (rats and mice) and/or contaminated environment
    - 30% of patients report no known rat bite.
    - In some human streptobacillary infections, close contact with the oral flora of pet rats through kissing and sharing of food may have been the route of transmission.
- Person to person
  - Never reported for *S. moniliformis* or *S. minus*

CLINICAL PRESENTATION OF ANIMALS

- *S. moniliformis*
  - Rats
    - Generally resistant—no disease is seen
  - Other species
    - Purulent lesions
    - Cutaneous abscesses (dogs, guinea pigs)
    - Pneumonia (calves, koalas, guinea pigs, mice)
    - Polyarthritis (mice, turkeys)
    - Cervical lymphadenitis (mice, guinea pigs)
    - Fatal septicemia (mice, spinifex hopping mice)
- *S. minus*
  - The microorganism does not appear to be pathogenic in animals.

GEOGRAPHY AND SEASONALITY

- Streptobacillary RBF has been reported worldwide.
- RBF by *S. minus* was first described in Japan and occurs predominantly in Asia.
  - Infection has also been diagnosed in Europe and the United States.

PATHOBIOLOGY

- *S. moniliformis*
  - Pathogenesis is not well established because of rarity of disease and low mortality.
  - Bacteremia and septicemia always occur.
  - Immunologic mechanisms may contribute to polyarthritis.
  - Susceptibility of mammalian species to infection by many microorganisms is genetically based. These observations extend to humans.
    - In one report of two persons bitten by the same rat, only one developed RBF.
    - A brother and sister in contact with (but not bitten by) the same pet rat both contracted RBF.
- *S. minus*
  - Pathogenesis is not well established because of rarity of disease and low mortality.

CLINICAL PRESENTATION OF HUMANS

INCIDENCE IN HUMANS

- Because rats have become popular as pets, children now account for more than 50% of cases in the United States, followed by laboratory personnel and pet shop employees.
  - Bacteria grow in one-third of all rat bite wounds. The risk of any type of infection following a rat bite is estimated at 1% to 10%. The risk of RBF is unknown, as is the infectious dose of both *S. moniliformis* and *S. minus* for humans.
  - Surveys of *S. moniliformis* human clinical isolates show the following:
    - An equal incidence between males and females
    - 50% of isolates are from patients 9 years old or younger
    - 83% of suspected RBF cases with positive diagnosis involved a known rat bite or exposure to rodents.
    - 70% of exposures occurred from a wild rat, 21% were from a laboratory rat, and 9% were from a pet shop rat.

DISEASE FORMS/SUBTYPES

- *S. moniliformis*
  - Bacteremia and septicemia
    - Abrupt onset of high fever
    - Headache, chills, vomiting, and rash
    - Petechial rash develops over the extremities, in particular, the palms and the soles, but sometimes is present all over the body.
    - In 20% of cases, the rash desquamates.
    - Infants and children may experience severe diarrhea resulting in loss of weight.
    - Mortality in 7% to 13% of untreated patients
  - Post bacteremia
    - Polyarthritis develops in 50% to 70% patients.
      - Joints commonly affected are knees, ankles, wrists, elbows, and shoulders.
      - Arthritis may be suppurative or nonsuppurative.
      - Joint fluid usually is highly inflammatory with predominance of polymorphonuclear leukocytes.
    - Endocarditis develops in approximately 50% of patients with previously damaged heart valves, usually as the result of rheumatic fever.
      - Endocarditis mortality is approximately 55%.
- *S. minus*
  - Clinical features overlap with *S. moniliformis.*
  - Reaction often occurs at bite wound after healing.
  - Lymphadenitis is more common.
  - Mortality is lower.

HISTORY, CHIEF COMPLAINT

- Rat bite followed by fever, chills, myalgias, arthralgias, headache, and vomiting
- Many patients report symptoms suggestive of an upper respiratory tract infection.
- If a bite has occurred, it typically heals quickly.
- Significant regional lymphadenopathy is not seen.

PHYSICAL FINDINGS IN INFECTED HUMANS

- The initial presentation of RBF is nonspecific.
- 75% of patients develop a rash that may appear maculopapular, petechial, or purpuric.
- Appearance of this rash, especially of hemorrhagic vesicles, in the setting of an otherwise nonspecific set of disease signs and symptoms should strongly suggest the diagnosis of RBF.

INCUBATION PERIOD

- *S. moniliformis*
  - 3 to 10 days (usually 1 to 3 days, with average of 5 days)
  - Ingested *Streptobacillus* is approximately 1 to 3 days, with longest reported period of 16 days.
- *S. minus*
  - 7 to 21 days (may be as short as 2 days or may extend to several weeks)

DIAGNOSIS

DIFFERENTIAL DIAGNOSIS

RBF has a nonspecific presentation with a broad differential diagnosis:

- Brucellosis
- Leptospirosis (see Leptospirosis)
- Rocky Mountain spotted fever (*Rickettsia rickettsii*)
- Lyme disease
- Tularemia (see Tularemia)
- Cat-scratch disease
- Viral exanthems (Coxsackie virus B, Epstein-Barr virus)
- Disseminated sexually transmitted diseases (secondary syphilis, gonococcal arthritis)
- Streptococcal disease
- Drug reactions
- Systemic lupus erythematosus

INITIAL DATABASE

- Isolation of *S. moniliformis* from blood culture, abscess, synovial fluid, or wound. However, this is difficult and sometimes unsuccessful because of fastidious growth of the organism and the need for special growth media.
- *S. minus* cannot be grown in bacterial culture. Initial diagnosis relies on direct visualization of characteristic spirochetes with Giemsa stain, Wright stain, or darkfield microscopy.

ADVANCED OR CONFIRMATORY TESTING

- *S. moniliformis*
  - For humans, currently no validated serologic tests are available, but such assays are in use in monitoring of laboratory animals for *S. moniliformis.*
  - PCRs have been used for purposes of screening (in animals) and diagnosis (in humans).
- *S. minus*
  - Serologic tests or PCR are not available for diagnostic efforts.
  - In cases of suspected infection, blood or wound aspirates are injected intraperitoneally into guinea pigs or mice for diagnostic purposes. After successful infection, spirochetes may be detected after 5 to 15 days in the blood using darkfield microscopy.

TREATMENT

- No treatment in rats
- In humans, treatment for both *S. moniliformis* and *S. minus* infections is primarily with penicillin

PREVENTION

- Reduce risk of exposure to rat bites.
  - Workers dealing professionally with rats should wear personal protective working clothes and gloves.
  - In laboratories, use commercially reared specific pathogen–free (SPF) rats that are free of *S. moniliformis*.
- Owners buying pet rats from pet stores are at greater risk than laboratory animal care staff:
  - Children handling pet rats may be a special risk group.
  - 14% of RBF cases in children involved exposure to a rat at school.
- Owners rescuing wild rats are at greatest risk.
- If bitten by a rat, promptly clean and disinfect the wound.

REPORTING—NOTIFIABLE DISEASE

Notification of U.S. federal health authorities is not required.

PROGNOSIS

- *S. moniliformis*
  - Good with early reporting, meticulous wound care, and parenteral penicillin therapy
  - Death in approximately 10% of untreated cases (usually associated with late reporting)
- *S. minus*
  - Lower mortality in untreated cases

CONTROVERSY

- Efficacy of antimicrobial prophylaxis is unknown.
- Possible explanations for rare diagnosis of RBF include the following:
  - True incidence is low despite common exposure.
  - Low index of suspicion exists among physicians.
  - Streptobacillosis and spirillosis mimic other systemic and atypical infections.
  - Difficulty has been associated with culturing *S. moniliformis* in the past (rapid PCR tests now exist).

PEARLS & CONSIDERATIONS

COMMENTS

- The nonspecific initial presentation combined with difficulties in culturing the causative organism produces significant risk of delay or failure in diagnosis.
- Inbred mice show different strain susceptibility to *S. moniliformis*. In outbred pet mice, infection may not cause clinical signs. Therefore, there is a low risk that the bite of a pet mouse housed with or near pet rats may transmit RBF.
- Publications do not always distinguish between the high prevalence of *S. moniliformis* in wild rats compared with laboratory rats.
  - Infection of laboratory rats and mice with *S. moniliformis* is very rare.
  - Over a 2-year period, Charles River Laboratories cultured 1500 laboratory rats and 7200 laboratory mice for *S. moniliformis*, and all were negative. The organism was not found in submitted samples from research animal facilities or from research-bred animals.

CLIENT EDUCATION

- Encourage good hygiene and personal protection.
  - Practice regular handwashing and avoid hand-to-mouth contact when handling rats or cleaning rat cages.
- Advise clients that children handling pet rats may be a special risk group.
  - Adults should closely supervise children younger than 5 years of age, to prevent bites and hand-to-mouth contact.
- If bitten by a rat, the wound should be cleaned thoroughly and reported to a physician.

SUGGESTED READINGS

Elliott SP: Rat bite fever and *Streptobacillus moniliformis*, Clin Microbiol Rev 20:13–22, 2007.

Gaastra WR, et al: Rat bite fever, Vet Microbiol 133:211–228, 2009.

CROSS-REFERENCES TO OTHER SECTIONS

Leptospirosis
Tularemia

AUTHOR: **THOMAS M. DONNELLY**

EDITOR: **SIMON STARKEY**

ZOONOSES

Salmonellosis

BASIC INFORMATION

DEFINITION AND INFECTIOUS AGENT

- *Salmonella* are Gram-negative, facultative anaerobic rod-shaped bacteria belonging to the family Enterobacteriaceae. There are more than 2500 distinct serovars (serotypes), which are defined by the lipopolysaccharide (O), flagellar protein (H), and capsular (Vi) antigens. Many serovars are adapted to particular animal species.
- In humans, the most common agents are *S. enterica* subspecies *enterica* serovar Typhimurium and *S. enterica* subspecies *enterica* serovar Enteritidis. *S. enterica* subspecies *enterica* serovar Typhi, the causative agent of typhoid fever, and *S. enterica* subspecies *enterica* serovar Paratyphi are found only in humans. Most *Salmonella* serovars have animal reservoirs and are potentially zoonotic.
- β-Lactamase–mediated antimicrobial resistance is common. Antibiotic resistance in *Salmonella* species has been linked to the use of antibiotics in animal agriculture.

SYNONYMS

Disease

- In humans
  - Nontyphoid salmonellosis
- In animals
  - Songbird fever, fowl typhoid, Pullorum disease

Organism

- There is considerable room for confusion in the nomenclature of *Salmonella* species. Initially, species were named according to host species and nature of disease. Later, non–host-specific serovars were named according to the location in which they were isolated. However, an official ruling from the Judicial Commission of the International Committee on the Systematics of Prokaryotes (Opinion 80) in 2005 declared that there are only two species of

Salmonella: *S. enterica* and *S. bongori*. Six subspecies of *S. enterica* are officially recognized: *enterica*, *arizonae*, *diarizonae*, *houtenae*, *indica*, and *salmae*. Later that year, a third species, *S. subterranean*, was also recognized.
- Interested readers are directed to review Volume 55 of the *International Journal of Systematic and Evolutionary Microbiology* (2005) for further discussion of this ruling and the taxonomic implications, as well as a list of synonyms.
- Clinicians, bacteriologists, and pathologists, particularly in human medicine, still use the older terminology with some frequency. Therefore, *S. enterica* subspecies *enterica* serovar Typhi is often written simply as *S. typhi*.

EPIDEMIOLOGY

ANIMAL SPECIES—HOSTS AND/OR CARRIERS

Birds

- Poultry
  - Poultry are considered one of the principal reservoirs of *Salmonella*. Hundreds of serovars have been isolated from poultry, many without causing discernible disease in these birds. Poultry are considered a significant reservoir of zoonotic *Salmonella*, acquired through foodborne disease or fecal-oral contamination after handling pet poultry (often chicks and ducklings).
- Psittacines
  - Parrots are very rarely associated with salmonellosis in humans. Reports in the literature describing human salmonellosis associated with pet, aviary, and wild psittacines are sparse.
- Wild birds
  - Several outbreaks of human salmonellosis have been epidemiologically linked to wild songbirds in the United Kingdom, New Zealand, and Scandinavia. The role of wild birds in human salmonellosis may be underestimated.

Hedgehogs

- Both African pygmy and European hedgehogs have been associated with human salmonellosis in North America and Europe. The asymptomatic rate of carriage is relatively high and has been reported to be as 25% and 28% in European and African pygmy hedgehogs, respectively.

Rabbits

- An outbreak of salmonellosis among 29 Italians in 1997 was linked to the consumption of roasted rabbit. However, given that the rabbit was considered well cooked, the infection was likely a result of poor sanitary conditions in the restaurant.

Rodents

- A recent multi-state cluster of rodent-borne outbreaks of human salmonellosis in the United States was associated with pet hamsters, rats, and mice. Rodents may serve as definitive hosts for certain *Salmonella* and as incidental hosts for others.
- In the summer of 2010, a total of 34 people in 17 states were found to be infected with a matching serovar of *S. enterica* subspecies *enterica*. A case-controlled epidemiologic investigation linked the outbreak to handling of frozen rodents used as reptile feed.
- In 1967, an outbreak occurred in a Canadian family. The human cases were attributed to the family's guinea pig breeding operation.

Reptiles and amphibians

- Human salmonellosis has been associated with a large number of reptiles and amphibian species. Reptiles may have subclinical infection rates as high as 90%. *Salmonella* has been identified in all reptiles examined to date.
- Turtles with a shell length less than 4 inches have been banned from sale in the United States under Federal Regulations since 1975. This ban was imposed as small children were considered at risk because they are likely to place small turtles in their mouths.

Ferrets

- To the author's knowledge, no published reports have described human salmonellosis attributable to ferrets.

MODES OF TRANSMISSION

- *Salmonella* is primarily considered a foodborne disease of animal origin. A susceptible human host ingests food or water that is contaminated with feces from an infected animal.
- Person-to-person transmission can occur by the fecal-oral route or by food handlers who are shedding organisms and contaminated food items as the result of substandard handwashing practices.
- Direct animal-to-human transmission can also occur via fecal-oral contamination. This form often occurs among young children with poor hand hygiene standards.
- Water from contaminated tropical fish aquaria: *Salmonella* organisms are believed to originate not directly from fish but from "carrier water" in which tropical fish are transported, or from water containing infected amphibians and reptiles reared in tanks nearby.
- Infection can occur sporadically or in large outbreaks involving thousands of individuals with a common exposure. Contaminated peanut butter and peanut paste were the sources of a multistate outbreak of *S. enterica* subspecies *enterica* serovar Typhimurium infection for people and pets through contamination of processed foods and pet treats.
- Vertical (transovarial) transmission may occur in birds and in reptile species.

CLINICAL PRESENTATION OF ANIMALS

Poultry

- *Salmonella enterica* subspecies *enterica* serovar Pullorum is the causative agent of Pullorum disease, which can cause high mortality rates among young chickens and turkeys. Morbidity and mortality vary among adult birds depending on strain pathogenicity and host susceptibility. Affected birds demonstrate anorexia and weakness and heat-seeking behavior and often die in a matter of days. Most mortality occurs in birds younger than 3 weeks of age. Survivors often become lifelong carriers, with the organism localizing to the ovary.
- *S. enterica* subspecies *enterica* serovar Gallinarum is the causative agent of fowl typhoid. The epidemiologic and clinical picture is similar to that of Pullorum disease; however, fowl typhoid affects older birds to a greater degree than Pullorum disease.

Psittacines

- Salmonellosis is considered a rare clinical entity in psittacines. Affected birds are often immune suppressed as the result of concurrent disease and/or stress. Affected birds may present with diarrhea, anorexia, and maldigestion/malabsorption. Septicemia may ensue, and birds may develop hepatitis, nephritis, and/or endocarditis. Sudden death may also occur.
- In a 2001 outbreak among Lories and Lorikeets in a U.S. zoological collection, birds developed sudden-onset lethargy and dyspnea. The fatality rate was 22% among the 45 birds in the exhibit. Histopathologic examination revealed hepatitis, splenitis, bacterial emboli in multiple organs, and enteritis.

Wild songbirds

- Outbreaks of salmonellosis and sudden death have been reported in various songbird species over the past four decades. Recent, well-publicized outbreaks have occurred in Scotland and northern England. Birds are often found dead with no premonitory signs. Outbreaks have been epidemiologically linked to wild bird feeders.

Ferrets

- Ferrets are rarely affected by *Salmonella* species. When infection occurs, it is often attributed to infected food. Afflicted ferrets demonstrate fever, lethargy, and diarrhea that may be bloody.

Hedgehogs

- Asymptomatic carrier rates among African pygmy hedgehogs are reportedly as high as 28%. Clinical disease may ensue in some carrier animals and often presents as anorexia, diarrhea, weight loss, and lethargy.
- African pygmy hedgehogs have been associated with at least 10 human cases of salmonellosis in Canada and with 1 case in the United States. *S. enterica* subspecies *enterica* serovar Tilene was isolated from infected individuals and a number of hedgehogs associated with the outbreaks.

Rabbits

- Salmonellosis is not considered a common condition among rabbits. However, clinical disease has been reported and is associated with sepsis and acute death seen with or without diarrhea, depression, and pyrexia. The most common *Salmonella* isolated from affected rabbits is *S. enterica* subsp. *enterica* serovar Typhimurium.

Rodents

- Rats and mice appear to be asymptomatic carriers of *Salmonella.* Hamsters and guinea pigs may develop diarrhea, septicemia, and death.

Reptiles

- Disease or death attributed to salmonellosis is rarely reported in reptiles, despite their high rates of *Salmonella* carriage.

Fish

- *Salmonella* has not been regarded as a fish pathogen, and few reports have described the isolation of *Salmonella* from fish. Individual case reports of zoo- or aquaria-maintained fish suggest that *Salmonella* is transmitted to affected fish by "carrier water" from infected amphibians and reptiles reared in different tanks nearby, or that affected fish are fed contaminated feed (fish feed meal or live fish). One-third of shipments of aquarium snails and aquarium frogs have been found contaminated with *Salmonella.*

RISK FACTORS

- Poor hand and food hygiene is considered a key risk factor for the development of salmonellosis among humans.
- Decreased immune competence due to young or advanced age, or to concurrent illness, is considered a risk factor among humans and animals for the development of clinical salmonellosis.
- Crowding, stress, and poor husbandry have been associated with increased risk of clinical salmonellosis among a variety of animal species.

GEOGRAPHY AND SEASONALITY

- Incidence among humans appears to increase in spring and summer months.
- Incidence is higher in developing nations, particularly those in the tropics.

PATHOBIOLOGY

- Stomach acidity plays a major protective role in the prevention of salmonellosis among hosts ingesting this organism.
- Once in the small intestine, salmonellae attach to epithelial cells within Peyer's patches via fimbriae. The organisms are then transported to the lamina propria.
- Virulence factors are an active area of research. These factors are carried on transmissible plasmids and on chromosomes of the organism, and they mediate uptake into epithelial cells and survival within phagosomes among other processes.
- Host factors contribute to the degree of pathology observed in humans and animals. Concomitant and often immunosuppressive illnesses such as HIV have been associated with more severe systemic or nonintestinal salmonellosis.

CLINICAL PRESENTATION OF HUMANS

INCIDENCE IN HUMANS An estimated 1.4 million persons develop salmonellosis in the United States each year. This leads to approximately 14,800 hospitalizations and more than 400 deaths. In addition to individual cases or small clusters, outbreaks may occur nationally, or at the local or regional level. In 2008, an epidemic affecting more than 1400 people was linked to contaminated peppers.

DISEASE FORMS/SUBTYPES

Gastroenteritis/enterocolitis

- This is the most common form of nontyphoid salmonellosis. Patients develop an acute onset of profuse diarrhea, sometimes with frank blood. Patients also experience fever, abdominal pain, cramps, nausea, and vomiting.

Focal disease

- When the organism crosses the intestinal lamina propria and enters the systemic circulation, focal disease may occur in any organ of the body. Typically, organs with preexisting pathologies are affected.

HISTORY, CHIEF COMPLAINT

History

- Recent contact with symptomatic or asymptomatic pets or zoological specimens, particularly ducklings, chicks, reptiles, and rodents
- Foodborne disease may be associated with the consumption of almost any foodstuff; however, recent consumption of beef, poultry, or eggs may be associated with increased risk of salmonellosis.

Chief complaint

- Voluminous, watery, and occasionally bloody diarrhea is a common presenting sign.
- Fever, abdominal pain, and cramps are also commonly observed with nontyphoidal salmonellosis.

PHYSICAL FINDINGS IN INFECTED HUMANS

- Diffuse abdominal pain/tenderness and dehydration are the most common physical findings in humans.
- Low-grade fever (38°C to 39°C [100.4°F to 102.2°F]) is common in the acute phase.
- Rectal examination or visualization of stool may indicate blood.

INCUBATION PERIOD In humans, the incubation period for gastrointestinal salmonellosis varies between 6 and 73 hours. Symptoms typically last 1 to 12 days, with fever often abating within 48 hours.

DIAGNOSIS

DIFFERENTIAL DIAGNOSIS

- Campylobacteriosis
- Cryptosporidiosis
- Cyclosporiasis
- Colibacillosis *(Escherichia coli)*
- Listeriosis
- Shigellosis
- Intestinal yersiniosis
- Viral enteritis

INITIAL DATABASE

- Fecal ova and parasite screening aids in ruling out other causes of diarrhea.
- Fecal culture is commonly employed in the diagnosis of salmonellosis.
- Complete blood count and biochemistry are of little diagnostic value in most cases of nontyphoid salmonellosis.

ADVANCED OR CONFIRMATORY TESTING

- Serologic tests are considered to lack sensitivity and specificity in humans.
- Blood and/or bone marrow cultures may be required in cases of bacteremia or septicemia. Sensitivity is greatest early in the disease course. Bone marrow may be required if previous antibiotherapy has been employed.
- PCR tests are being developed for clinical use; however, concerns over sensitivity have been raised.

TREATMENT

- Treatment in humans may take the form of supportive care alone or may involve provision of antibiotherapy with agents such as ampicillin, amoxicillin, chloramphenicol,

fluoroquinolones, gentamicin, and trimethoprim/sulfamethoxazole.
- Treatment of asymptomatic carriers is not advised because of concerns about the development of multidrug-resistant serovars of *Salmonella*.
- Clinically affected animals may be treated with supportive care and, if deemed necessary, an appropriate antimicrobial for the species being treated.

PREVENTION

- Thorough handwashing plays a pivotal part in the prevention of foodborne, animal-to-human, and human-to-human salmonellosis.
- Close supervision of children around high-risk animals such as reptiles, rodents, and poultry, particularly chicks and ducklings, is strongly advised.
- Prevent children from placing hands in ornamental fish aquaria, and avoid high-risk behaviors, such as cleaning aquaria in sinks. In one outbreak of salmonellosis linked to aquaria, 70% of cases were seen in children younger than 10 years of age.
- Breeders, wholesalers, and distributors of pets and commercial animals are advised against the prophylactic use of antimicrobial agents.
- The Centers for Disease Control and Prevention has advised that reptiles and amphibians should not be kept in households with children younger than 5 years old.
- Multidrug-resistant *Salmonella* infections in employees and clients of small animal veterinary clinics and animal shelters have been reported and were the result of direct and indirect contact with infected animals.
  - Veterinarians and animal technicians should wash their hands after handling pets, especially after handling feces.
  - Reduce exposure to feces by wearing rubber or disposable gloves, and by removing gloves and washing hands immediately after finishing a task that involves contact with animal feces.
  - Take measures to reduce splashes of feces to the mouth when hosing or cleaning animal areas.
  - Clean and disinfect all surfaces contaminated with feces.
  - No eating should be allowed in animal treatment and holding areas.

REPORTING—NOTIFIABLE DISEASE

Salmonellosis is reportable to U.S. federal health authorities.

PROGNOSIS

- Prognosis is excellent for immunocompetent individuals infected with intestinal salmonellosis. The mortality rate associated with nontyphoid *Salmonella* outbreaks in the United States between 1985 and 1991 was less than 0.5%. Mortality rates increase among the very young and the elderly, as well as in the immunocompromised.
- A chronic carrier state may occur in less than 1% of nontyphoid *Salmonella* cases.

PEARLS & CONSIDERATIONS

COMMENTS

- Salmonellosis should be considered in all avian and exotic pets with acute diarrheal illness or acute death with necropsy findings consistent with sepsis, particularly those species mentioned in this topic.
- Given the high prevalence of asymptomatic shedding among reptiles, it is prudent to consider all reptiles as carriers and to take appropriate precautions.
- Although isolation of *Salmonella* from ornamental fish tanks is reportedly low (0.4% to 8.0%), 60% of adults with salmonellosis have reported that fish in their aquarium had been sick or died during the week before their illness.

CLIENT EDUCATION

- Clients should be educated in the selection of healthy pets from high-quality breeders or retailers with impeccable husbandry and hygiene standards.
- Parents should be educated on the importance of hand hygiene in their children.
- Petting zoos and zoological gardens and sanctuaries should ensure that appropriate handwashing stations are provided in and around animal exhibits.
- Parents of children younger than 10 years and immunocompromised persons are advised to consider the type of pet they acquire based on the relative risk of salmonellosis and other zoonotic diseases.
- Reptiles and amphibians should not be kept in households that include pregnant women or children younger than 5 years of age.
- Brochures and guidelines for clients have been prepared by several professional organizations (e.g., American Veterinary Medical Association, Association of Reptilian and Amphibian Veterinarians).

SUGGESTED READINGS

Centers for Disease Control and Prevention: Salmonellosis associated with chicks and ducklings—Michigan and Missouri, Spring 1999, Morb Mortal Wkly Rep 49:297–299, 2000.

Craig C, et al: African pygmy hedgehog–associated *Salmonella tilene* in Canada, Can Commun Dis Rep 23:129–131, 1997.

Fish NA, et al: Family outbreak of salmonellosis due to contact with guinea pigs, Can Med Assoc J 99:418–420, 1968.

Kaye DK, et al: The parakeet as a source of salmonellosis in man: report of a case, N Engl J Med 264:868–869, 1961.

Mermin J, et al: Reptiles, amphibians, and human salmonella infection: a population-based, case-control study, Clin Infect Dis 38(Suppl 3):S253–S261, 2004.

Swanson SJ, et al: Multidrug-resistant *Salmonella enterica* serotype *Typhimurium* associated with pet rodents, N Engl J Med 356:21–28, 2007.

Woodward DL, et al: Human salmonellosis associated with exotic pets, J Clin Microbiol 35:2786–2790, 1997.

CROSS-REFERENCES TO OTHER SECTIONS

Bacterial Diseases, Fish
Salmonella, Reptiles

AUTHOR: **SIMON R. STARKEY**

EDITOR: **THOMAS M. DONNELLY**

Tularemia

BASIC INFORMATION

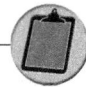

DEFINITION AND INFECTIOUS AGENT

Tularemia is an acute febrile and often granulomatous illness of humans and a variety of mammals caused by the small intracellular Gram-negative coccobacillus *Francisella tularensis*. Two major subspecies exist with varying pathogenicity. *Francisella tularensis tularensis* (Jellison type A) is considered the more pathogenic of the two subspecies. Human case fatality rates without treatment can be as high as 15% with this organism. This subtype is also highly infectious, with rabbit LD50 (dose that kills half of tested group) reported to be as low as 14 organisms in rhesus macaques *(Macaca mulatta)*. The second major subspecies, *Francisella tularensis holarctica* (Jellison type B), is considerably less pathogenic, and human fatalities are rare with this subspecies.

SYNONYMS

In humans: rabbit fever, Francis disease, deer-fly fever, O'Hara's disease, market men's disease
In animals: rabbit fever, deer-fly fever

EPIDEMIOLOGY

ANIMAL SPECIES—HOSTS AND/OR CARRIERS

- *F. tularensis* has been identified in more than 200 wild and domestic mammals, as well as birds, amphibians, fish, and arthropods. Host species and vectors vary by geographic region.
- In the United States, cottontail rabbits (*Sylvilagus* spp.), jackrabbits (*Lepus* spp.), beavers, moles, squirrels, muskrats, meadow voles, and sheep are prone to the disease, which is often fatal.
- Domestic rabbits *(Oryctolagus cuniculus)* are not considered a significant source of infection among humans, perhaps because of the increased tendency to keep rabbits indoors and away from arthropod vectors.
- Arthropod vectors in the United States include the wood tick *(Dermacentor andersoni)*, the dog tick *(D. variabilis)*, the lone star tick *(Amblystoma americanum)*, and the deer fly *(Chrysops discalis)*.
- *F. tularensis* is stable in certain environments and may remain viable for months in water and sediment.

MODES OF TRANSMISSION

- Vector-borne transmission
  - Most human cases in the United States are arthropod borne, leading to the ulceroglandular form of the disease.
- Direct transmission
  - Exudates from skin lesions, blood, and respiratory secretions may be infectious.
  - Contact with an infected animal carcass (typically wild rabbits) can lead to the ulceroglandular form of the disease. Although the organism may penetrate intact skin, it is likely that minor skin lesions in the host facilitate penetration of the organism.
  - Contact of infectious secretions with host mucous membranes may also induce the ulceroglandular form of the disease.
  - Ingestion of contaminated meat or water may lead to an oropharyngeal or typhoidal tularemia.
  - One report describes a child developing ulceroglandular tularemia secondary to a bite wound inflicted by a pet hamster shortly before it died. Another report discusses a child who acquired the disease after being bitten by a pet squirrel.
- Indirect transmission
  - Tularemia may be acquired after inhalation of aerosolized infectious material.
  - During an outbreak in Martha's Vineyard, Massachusetts, a primary pneumonic tularemia was epidemiologically linked to the use of lawnmowers/brush cutters. Thus, aerosolization of infected rabbits or other infected wildlife was proposed as the route of transmission.
  - It is likely that this route of transmission contributes to tularemia, which is the second most frequent laboratory-acquired infection in the United States, according to a 1976 report.
- Person to person
  - Never reported for *F. tularensis*

CLINICAL PRESENTATION OF ANIMALS

Most small rodents and rabbits affected by this organism die rapidly from the disease.

Hamsters

- The common hamster *(Cricetus cricetus)* is believed to be a reservoir of tularemia in eastern Europe. Hamster hunting appears to be a significant risk factor for the development of ulceroglandular tularemia. Experimental infection of two common hamsters led to death on the 8th and 9th days after infection. Both hamsters experienced apathy soon after inoculation, and necropsy findings were consistent with septicemia.
- A pet hamster (species not reported) was associated with a case of ulceroglandular tularemia in a 3-year-old boy in Colorado in 2004. The hamster died shortly after biting the child. Five other hamsters purchased by the family also died. The main clinical sign observed in the hamsters was diarrhea. The pet store reported unexpectedly high mortality among other hamsters in the store. Fifteen of 18 clients were traced, and 8 reported that hamsters died within 2 weeks of purchase. Only one live hamster was available for testing, and this pet was negative for *F. tularensis* by serologic analysis and culture. It was hypothesized that wild rodents entering the pet store infected the hamsters.

***Black-tailed prairie dogs* (Cynomys ludovicianus)**

- In 2002, approximately 250 of 3600 wild-caught prairie dogs that passed through a Texas commercial facility died.
- Clinically affected animals were lethargic, dehydrated, and emaciated. All dead or dying animals confirmed to have *F. tularensis* also demonstrated submandibular lymphadenopathy and were believed to have the oropharyngeal form of the disease, likely secondary to cannibalism.
- A proportion of surviving animals were seropositive and continued to shed *F. tularensis*, suggesting that prairie dogs may act as chronic carriers of this organism.

Cottontail rabbits* (Sylvilagus *species) and jackrabbit/hare* (Lepus *species)

- Considered a common reservoir species in Europe and North America. Necropsy findings are consistent with septicemia and often include acute focal necrosis of the liver, spleen, and/or bone marrow.
- Hemorrhagic enteritis, typhlitis, and intestinal lymphadenitis have been documented among hares in Sweden.

Squirrels

- Ground squirrels, particularly the California ground squirrel *(Otospermophilus beecheyi)*, are known reservoir hosts of *F. tularensis*. McCoy and Chapin, who investigated plague in *O. beecheyi* in 1911 and 1912 described the organism. The disease produced a

clinical syndrome similar to plague, in which squirrels would die acutely of a septicemic condition.
- A child developed ulceroglandular tularemia after being bitten by a 6-month-old squirrel that had been kept as a pet. The animal died shortly after biting the child.

Guinea pigs and domestic rabbits
- Because of the lack of literature on the natural occurrence of tularemia in these species, it has been speculated that they may be partially resistant to the disease, or may not be exposed with sufficient frequency for natural cases to occur.

RISK FACTORS

Humans
- Exposure to arthropod vectors through outdoor activities
- Contact with potentially infected small mammals through hunting, by eating undercooked game meat, through wildlife rehabilitation, or providing veterinary services.
- Laboratory personnel, particularly those in microbiology, clinical pathology, and necropsy/autopsy departments

Companion mammals
- Exposure to arthropod vectors
- Exposure to infected rodents and other wildlife

GEOGRAPHY AND SEASONALITY
- In the United States, incidence is highest in western and south central states.
- Increased incidence has recently been seen in spring/summer and is likely associated with increased exposures to arthropod vectors.
- Historically, an increased incidence was seen in late fall and winter and was associated with small game hunting season and increased exposure to infected animals.

PATHOBIOLOGY Investigation into the virulence factors of *F. tularensis* is ongoing and appears to involve outer wall proteins that enable the bacterium to survive within macrophages. This ability contributes to the granulomatous nature of this disease when it affects epithelial surfaces and regional lymph nodes.

CLINICAL PRESENTATION OF HUMANS

INCIDENCE IN HUMANS Annual incidence in the United States is estimated to be approximately 200 cases per year. This condition is likely underreported.

DISEASE FORMS/SUBTYPES

Ulceroglandular tularemia
- Most common form of the disease. Typically results from vector inoculation or penetration of skin by organism. Leads to onset of fever, myalgia, headache, and often recumbency several days after exposure. A papule forms at the site of inoculation and often develops into a granulomatous lesion that may ulcerate. Regional lymphadenopathy often ensues.

Oculoglandular tularemia
- Conjunctival inoculation leads to an often severe and typically unilateral purulent conjunctivitis with concomitant periorbital edema and cervical lymphadenopathy. Often severe secondary ophthalmic conditions may ensue, such as corneal ulceration and even globe rupture.

Oropharyngeal tularemia
- Oral inoculation with infectious material may occur after ingestion of undercooked, infected meat or via contaminated water. This leads to stomatitis/pharyngitis with regional lymphadenopathy. This form may affect the entire gastrointestinal (GI) tract with mesenteric lymphadenopathy, vomiting, diarrhea, and GI hemorrhage. The case fatality rate may exceed 50% with this form of the disease.

Pneumonic tularemia
- This form can occur after inhalation of infectious material and is a common route by which tularemia is acquired in the laboratory.
- At least one case of pneumonic tularemia was associated with inhalation of infectious material after wild rabbits were aerosolized by a lawn mower.
- This form may also occur secondary to hematogenous spread to the lungs in cases initially presenting as other subtypes of the disease.
- Patients often present with dry cough, variable dyspnea, and pleuritic pain. Radiographic changes vary from patchy pulmonary infiltrates to lobar pneumonia and/or severe hemorrhagic pleural effusion.

Typhoidal tularemia
- This form occurs secondary to *F. tularensis* bacteremia. Clinical signs and symptoms include fever, chills, headache, myalgia, and malaise. Pneumonia is common with this form. Skin lesions and lymphadenopathy are often absent, making diagnosis more difficult.

HISTORY, CHIEF COMPLAINT

History
- Exposure to wild animals or vectors, especially through high-risk activities such as hunting small game, camping, and landscaping/gardening in endemic areas

Chief complaint
- Varies by disease syndrome but often includes fever, chills, headache, myalgia, and malaise, with or without skin lesions, lymphadenopathy, ocular lesions, respiratory symptoms

PHYSICAL FINDINGS IN INFECTED HUMANS Vary by disease form (see Disease Forms/Subtypes, above)

INCUBATION PERIOD Varies with disease form but often is as short as 3 to 5 days

DIAGNOSIS

DIFFERENTIAL DIAGNOSIS
- Anthrax
- Brucellosis
- Leptospirosis (see Leptospirosis)
- Rocky Mountain spotted fever (*Rickettsia rickettsii*)
- Lyme disease
- Cat-scratch disease
- Rat bite fever
- Streptococcal disease
- Plague (see Plague)
- Chlamydiosis/Psittacosis
- Q fever

INITIAL DATABASE
- Baseline blood tests offer little diagnostic value in identification of tularemia, apart from aiding in the exclusion of other diseases.
- 20% to 30% of patients will have sterile pyuria.
- Routine blood culture is often negative.

ADVANCED OR CONFIRMATORY TESTING

HUMANS
- Tube agglutination testing is the most common serodiagnostic used in human medicine. Cross-reaction may occur with pathogens such as *Salmonella*, *Yersinia*, and *Legionella* species.
- Culture of infectious exudates or blood may be performed at reference laboratories. Specific cysteine culture media are required.
- PCR tests are being developed for rapid, sensitive, and specific diagnosis of the condition. These tests are being developed for wound material and for other potentially infectious exudates such as ocular discharge and sputum.

ANIMALS
- Necropsy specimens are used most often in the diagnosis of tularemia in animals. Direct antibody and immunofluorescence assay (IFA) tests may be used on various exudates and tissue samples to facilitate rapid and accurate diagnosis. An immunohistochemical technique has been described for paraffin-embedded tissue sections.
- Researchers and public health authorities focusing on diagnosis and typing of *F. tularensis* among animals are also using molecular techniques.

TREATMENT

- In humans, the treatment of choice is streptomycin. Gentamicin and amikacin have also been used.
- In animals, because of the rapidly fatal nature of the infection and its zoonotic potential, treatment is rarely attempted.

PREVENTION

- Humans should minimize contact with arthropod vectors by using insect repellents and by wearing long-sleeved shirts and pants, especially in areas with known vectors and/or endemic tularemia.
- Wear cut-resistant gloves while processing wild game, and cook game meat thoroughly.
- Keep small exotic mammals indoors, and prevent exposure to wildlife and wild rodents.
- Thoroughly wash bite wounds inflicted by any animal, and report to physician.

REPORTING—NOTIFIABLE DISEASE

Notification of U.S. federal health authorities is required.

PROGNOSIS

Varies with form of the disease

CONTROVERSY

The relative risk posed by nontraditional pets, especially wild-caught animals, is not well quantified.

PEARLS & CONSIDERATIONS

COMMENTS

Tularemia is extremely rare in common exotic pets such as guinea pigs and domestic rabbits. However, clinicians are advised to consider this condition, especially in endemic areas and among pets with increased risk of disease, such as those living outdoors.

CLIENT EDUCATION

- Advise clients of the risks associated with this organism.
- Maintain pets indoors, and control arthropod vectors in endemic areas.
- Thoroughly wash all wounds, and report to physician.

SUGGESTED READINGS

Avashia SB, et al: First reported prairie dog-to-human tularemia transmission, Texas, 2002, Emerg Infect Dis 10:483–486, 2004.

Donnelly TM, et al: Laboratory-acquired lymphadenopathy in a veterinary pathologist, Lab Anim (NY) 29:23–25, 2000.

Feldman KA, et al: An outbreak of primary pneumonic tularemia on Martha's Vineyard, N Engl J Med 345:1601–1606, 2001.

Gyuranecz M, et al: Susceptibility of the common hamster *(Cricetus cricetus)* to *Francisella tularensis* and its effect on the epizootiology of tularemia in an area where both are endemic, J Wildl Dis 46:1316–1320, 2010.

Magee JS, et al: Tularemia transmitted by a squirrel bite, Pediatr Infect Dis J 8:123–125, 1989.

Petersen JM, et al: Tularemia: emergence/re-emergence, Vet Res 36:455–467, 2005.

CROSS-REFERENCES TO OTHER SECTIONS

Leptospirosis

Plague

AUTHOR: **SIMON R. STARKEY**

EDITOR: **THOMAS M. DONNELLY**

A

Abdomen pain, in small mammals, 682
Abdominal breathing tube, in birds, 537
Abdominal distention
  in hamsters, 285-287, 296
  in rabbits, 384
"Abdominal" fluid, in birds, 153-154
Abdominal ultrasound, in ferrets, 431
Abdominocentesis, 538
  in birds, 154
  in hamsters, 286
Abducent nerve deficit, 581
Abnormal molt, 7-8
Abrasion, in birds, 232-234
Abscesses
  in birds, 147-149, 148f
  in guinea pigs, 278-280
  in hamsters, 297
  in invertebrates, 2-3
  periapical
    in degus, 321
    in guinea pigs, 256
    in hamsters, 290
    in rabbits, 355-360
  preputial, 314
  in rabbits, 331-332, 332f
  in reptiles, 71-74, 520-521
Acariasis, 690-694
  in birds, 690-691
  in ferrets, 691
  in guinea pigs, 278-280, 691
  in hedgehogs, 326
  in rabbits, 690-694
  in reptiles, 98-99
  in rodents, 691
Acaricides, 12
Acetaminophen toxicity, in ferrets, 464-465
Acetylcholinesterase, 212
Acquired dental disease, in rabbits, 355-360
Acrodont teeth
  in lizards, 143, 145
  in reptiles, 132
Acroeimeria spp., 87-89
Acroporid corals, infectious diseases of, 9-10
Activated charcoal, in birds, 227
Acute hepatitis, 115
Acute liver disease, in reptiles, 104
Acute myxomatosis, 399
Acute phase proteins, 618
Acute renal disease, in ferrets, 491-494
Acute renal failure
  in ferrets, 491-494
  in rabbits, 412-413
Acute respiratory distress syndrome, 572
Acyclovir, herpesvirus infection in reptiles treated with, 106
Adenovirus infection
  diarrhea in reptiles caused by, 94
  enteritis caused by, 182
  in guinea pigs, 277
  in reptiles, 74-75, 94
Adiposity, in rabbits, 401-402
Adrenal disease, in ferrets, 430-432
Adrenal gland disease, in ferrets, 430-432

Page numbers followed by "f" indicate figures, and "t" indicate tables.

Adrenal neoplasia, in ferrets, 430-432
Adrenal panel, in ferrets, 598-599
Adrenal tumors, in ferrets, 430-432
Adrenocortical disease, in ferrets, 430-432
"Aeromonas" disease, 40-41
Aeromonas salmonicida, 17
African bullfrogs
  gastrointestinal overload in, 56
  hypovitaminosis A in, 57
African grey parrots
  amylase in, 602-603
  Aspergillus spp. in, 155, 156f
  cardiac disease in, 157
  Chlamydophila psittaci in, 163
  circumscribed abscess in, 148f
  enteritis in, 182
  feather picking in, 184-185
  fungal granulomas in, 156f
  mycoses in, 204
  papillomas in, 215
  proventricular dilatation disease in, 222-225
  submandibular abscess in, 148f
African hedgehogs
  cardiomyopathy in, 323-324
  wobbly hedgehog syndrome in, 327
Agema, 130-131
Aggression
  differential diagnosis of, 590
  in rabbits, 337-338
  in reptiles, 75-77
Air sac carcinoma, in birds, 236
Air sac tube placement, in birds, 537
Alanine aminotransferase, 599-600
Albendazole, 121
  encephalitozoonosis treated with, 429
  neurocysticercosis treated with, 376
Albumin, 600
Aleutian disease, 433-434, 453, 492
Alk phos, 601
Alkaline phosphate, 601
Alkalinity, water, 45
Allergic dermatitis, in hamsters, 297
Allopurinol, 102
  in birds, 192, 229
  hyperuricemia treated with, 192
Allylamines, mycoses in birds treated with, 205
Alofia spp., 130
Alopecia
  in degus, 318
  differential diagnosis of, 572
  in ferrets, 432f
  in guinea pigs, 278-280
  in invertebrates, 3-4
  in rabbits, 360-364
  in small mammals, 669
Alpha-amylase, 602-603
Aluminum hydroxide, 188, 247
AM, 602-603
Amantadine, in birds, 224
Amazon parrots
  amylase in, 602-603
  cardiac disease in, 157
  central nervous system signs in, 209f
  cloacal papillomas in, 215
  feather picking in, 184-185
  lead toxicity in, 193f
  round cell sarcoma in, 237f
American foulbrood, 4-5
Amikacin, 136-137
  in birds, 218, 231
  lower respiratory tract disease treated with, 142
  in reptiles, 521
Aminophylline, in birds, 218
Ammonia, 44, 45t-46t, 601-602
Ammonia poisoning, 47-48
Ammonia toxicosis, 47-48
Ammonium, 601-602
Amoebiasis, in amphibians, 48-49
Amoebic colitis, in reptiles, 100-101
Amoebic enteritis
  in amphibians, 48-49
  in reptiles, 100-101
Amoebic nephritis, 48-49
Amoxicillin
  bacterial enteritis in birds treated with, 182
  in ferrets, 460
Amoxicillin/clavulanic acid
  in ferrets, 476
  in hedgehogs, 326
  in rats, 246
  respiratory tract disease in rats treated with, 248
Amphibian(s)
  ammonia toxicosis in, 47-48
  amoebiasis in, 48-49
  anemia in, 646
  azurophil count in, 604
  basophil count, 606
  cholesterol in, 613
  chromomycosis in, 49-50
  cloacal prolapse in, 51-52
  coccidiosis in, 52-53
  corneal lipidosis in, 53-54
  dangerous antibiotics in, 582
  dehydration in, 70
  emergency care in, 519
  erythrocytes in, 644-645
  flagellate enterocolitis in, 55-56
  gastrointestinal foreign body in, 56-59
  gastrointestinal overload in, 56-59
  general emergency care in, 519
  granulomas in, 61
  handling of, 520
  heteropenia in, 632
  heterophilia in, 632
  hypovitaminosis A in, 57-59, 58f
  mycobacteriosis in, 59-60, 59f
  nematodiasis in, 60-62
  neutrophilia in, 631
  nutritional secondary hyperparathyroidism in, 62-64
  restraint of, 520
  salmonellosis in, 727
  saprolegniasis in, 64-65
  septicemia in, 65-67, 66f
  sudden death in, 654
  thermal tolerance of, 70
  trauma in, 67-68
  vomiting in, 68-69
  weight loss in, 70-71, 655
  wound management in, 67-68
  xanthomatosis in, 53-54
Amphibian Ringer's solution, 53, 65-66

Amphibian tuberculosis, 59-60
Amphotericin B
  aspergillosis in birds treated with, 156
  in birds, 218, 231
  chromomycosis treated with, 50
  in ferrets, 440
  mycoses in birds treated with, 205
Amprolium hydrochloride, 88, 449
AMS7, 602-603
Amylase, 602-603
Amylodinium, 34
Amyloidosis
  in birds, 201
  in hamsters, 295-297
  in rabbits, 413
Anabolic steroids, in birds, 196
Anal fold dermatitis, in guinea pigs, 271-272
Anaphylaxis, in ferrets, 500-501
Anchor worm, 21-22
Androstenedione, 598-599
Anemia
  in birds, 149-151
  of chronic renal failure, 414, 493
  differential diagnosis of, 573
  in ferrets, 462-463
  laboratory tests for, 643-646
  nonregenerative, 644
  red blood cell count, 643-646
  regenerative, 644
Anesthesia
  in ferrets, 552
  in fish, 513-514
  hypothermia prevention during, 566-567
  in invertebrates, 504
  MS 222, 513-514
  in rabbits, 547-549, 552
  in rats, 547-549
  vomiting caused by, 68
Angiocardiography, in birds, 158
Angiotensin-converting enzyme inhibitors
  in ferrets, 459
  in rabbits, 342
Animal bites, 694-697
Anisognathism, 356
Anorexia
  in birds, 151-153
  in chinchillas, 309
  differential diagnosis of, 573
  in guinea pigs, 253-254
  in rabbits, 333-334, 334f, 384
  in small mammals, 670
Anseriformes
  ascites in, 153
  viral diseases in, 240
Anterior uveitis, in rabbits, 426-428
Anterior vena cava, for blood collection in small mammals, 550
Antibiotic responsive enteritis, 465
Antibiotic-associated enterocolitis, 291-293
Antibiotics. *See also* Antimicrobials
  cloacal prolapse in birds treated with, 166
  periodontal disease treated with, 133
  Salmonella spp. treated with, 144-145
  in sugar gliders, 328
Antidiuretic hormone, 647
Antiemetics, in birds, 227
Antifungals, in ferrets, 440
Antihelmintics, 121
Antimicrobials. *See also* Antibiotics
  bacterial diseases in fish treated with, 18-19
  periodontal disease treated with, 133
  proliferative spinal osteopathy treated with, 136
  Salmonella spp. treated with, 144-145
  septicemia in amphibians treated with, 66
  ulcer disease in koi treated with, 41
AP, 601
Aphanomyces spp., 24-26
Apical abscessation, in rabbits, 355-360
Aplastic anemia, in ferrets, 462-463
Apocrine adenoma, in rabbits, 351
Aqui-S, 514
Arachnids
  fungal infections in, 8-9
  septicemia in, 4
Arctic fox rabies, 722
Argulus spp., 21-22
Armillifer spp., 130
Arterial blood pressure, 549
Arteriolar nephrosclerosis, in hamsters, 285-286, 295-296
Arteriosclerosis, in rabbits, 341-342
Arthritis, in rabbits, 334-336
Arthropods
  dysecdysis in, 7-8
  ectoparasites in, 12-13, 505-506
  fluid administration in, 508
  fungal infections in, 8-9
Arthroscopy, in rabbits, 336
Articular gout
  in birds, 191-192
  in reptiles, 101-103
Ascaro L15, 650-651
Ascites
  in birds, 153-154, 196, 203
  differential diagnosis of, 574
  in fish, 20-21
  in hamsters, 285-286
Asian water dragons
  abscesses in, 71
  dysecdysis in, 95
  periodontal disease in, 132
  rostral damage in, 143
Aspartate aminotransferase, 195, 603-604
Aspergillosis, in birds, 155-157, 205-206
Aspergillus spp., 91, 202
Aspiration pneumonia, in birds, 208
Assisted shedding, in reptiles, 522-523
AST, 603-604
Ataxia
  in birds, 159-161, 207
  description of, 595
Atherosclerosis
  description of, 612
  in rabbits, 341-342
Atrioventricular block, in ferrets, 456-458
Atropine sulfate
  in birds, 160, 213
  organophosphate toxicity treated with, 213
  in rabbits, 427
Atypical myxomatosis, 399
Atypical water mold, 24
Aural abscesses, in reptiles, 72-73, 72f, 521
Autoimmune hepatitis, in rabbits, 384
Avascular necrosis of the plantar aspect of the feet, 407-409
Avian bornaviruses, 222
Avian chlamydiosis, 161-163
Avistraint, 543
Azithromycin
  in chinchillas, 304
  Chlamydophila psittaci treated with, 163
  chronic respiratory disease in rats treated with, 250
  in rabbits, 359
Azoles, 205-206
Azotemia
  differential diagnosis of, 574
  in ferrets, 491-494
  in rabbits, 412-415
  in rats, 247
Azurophil count, 604
Azurophilic monocyte, 604

B

B cells, 625-627
Bacillus piliformis, 202
Bacillus thuringiensis, 4
Bacterial dermatitis
  in guinea pigs, 279
  in rats, 252
  in reptiles, 77-79
Bacterial diseases
  in fish, 17-20
  in invertebrates, 4-5
Bacterial mastitis, 397
Bacterial skin infection, in reptiles, 77-79
Bacterial stomatitis, in reptiles, 132-134, 145-147
Baculovirus, 16
Bad molt, 505-506
Balanoposthitis, 313-315
Baldness. *See also* Alopecia
  in invertebrates, 3-4
"Balloon disease", 51-52
Basal cell carcinoma, in birds, 234
Basal cell tumors, in birds, 234
Basal metabolic rate, 539
Basilic vein, 546
Basilisks
  abscesses in, 71
  rostral abrasions in, 78
Basophil count, 604-606
Bat rabies, 722
Bath antibiotics, 19
Baycox. *See* Toltrazuril
Baytril, 136
Beak and feather disease, psittacine, 239-240, 241f
Beaks, overgrown, 213-214, 215f
Bearded dragons
  adenovirus infection in, 74-75
  calicivirus infection in, 79
  hepatic lipidosis in, 103-105
Becaplermin, 30
Behavioral disorders
  in degus, 318-319
  in rabbits, 337-338
  in sugar gliders, 328-329
Bell's horned frogs, calicivirus infection in, 79
Benazepril, 342
Bendrofluazide, in rabbits, 394
Benedensia spp., 23
Benzimidazoles, 121, 370
Benzocaine, 514
Besmottia spp., 87-89
Bicalutamide, 490
Bile acids, 104, 195, 606-607, 607t
Bili, 608
Biliary cryptosporidiosis, 702
Biliary cystadenoma, 385f
Bilirubin, 608
Biliverdin, 117, 608
Biopsy
  in birds, 169, 217
  fine-needle, in rabbits, 359
  skin, in birds, 178
Birds. *See also* African grey parrots; Amazon parrots; Cockatiels; Cockatoos; Macaw(s); Parrot(s); Psittacines
  abdominocentesis in, 154
  abscesses in, 147-149
  acariasis in, 690-691
  air sac tube placement in, 537
  alkaline phosphate in, 603
  amylase in, 602-603
  anemia in, 149-151, 646
  anion gap in, 635
  anorexia in, 151-153

Birds *(Continued)*
ascites in, 153-154
aspergillosis in, 155-157
aspiration pneumonia in, 208
basophil count, 605-606
beaks
overgrown, 213-214, 215f
trimming of, 214, 215f
bile acids in, 606, 607t
bites by, 696
blood collection in, 546-547, 547f
blood transfusion in, 151
bumblefoot in, 147-149, 219-221, 220f
calcium fluid deficit in, 172
calcium in, 197-198, 610-612
cardiac disease in, 157-158
cataracts in, 211, 212f
central nervous system signs in, 159-161, 209f
chlamydiosis in, 211, 697-699
Chlamydophila psittaci in, 159, 161-163, 230
chloride in, 612
chorioretinitis in, 211
chronic egg laying in, 164-165, 196
chronic sinusitis in, 230-231
claws, overgrown, 213-214, 215f
cloacal prolapse in, 165-166, 215
coelomocentesis in, 538
conjunctivitis in, 167-168, 211
constipation in, 168-170
corneal ulceration in, 211
creatinine in, 615
crop infusion in, 538-539, 539f
crop stasis in, 170-171, 226
crop thermal burn in, 152f
cryptosporidiosis in, 181, 204, 699-701
dangerous antibiotics in, 582
dehydration in, 171-172
diarrhea in, 173-175, 173f, 222
duodenostomy in, 539-540
dystocia in, 175-177
E-collars in, 540
ectoparasitism in, 177-178
emaciation in, 180-181
encephalitozoonosis in, 706
endoscopy in, 169, 186, 217, 223, 537f
enteritis in, 181-183
eosinophil count in, 616-617
erythrocytes in, 644-645
esophagostomy in, 540-541
feather picking in, 184-185
fluid therapy in, 541-542
follicular stasis in, 185-186
force-feeding of, 152f
foreign bodies in, 186-189
fractures in, 189-191, 233
gastrointestinal foreign bodies in, 186-189
globulins in, 618-619
glucose levels in, 619-622
gout in, 191-192
handling of, 543-544
heavy metal toxicity in, 192-194
heme oxygenase produced by, 608
hepatic lipidosis in, 194-197
heteropenia in, 632-633
heterophilia in, 632-633
hypercholesterolemia in, 195f
hyperglycemia in, 619-622
hyperkalemia in, 640
hypocalcemia in, 197-198
hypokalemia in, 641
hypoproteinemia in, 541
hypotensive shock in, 541
hypovitaminosis A in, 199-201
ileus in, 168-170, 222

Birds *(Continued)*
intraosseous administration of fluids in, 542, 543f
intravenous administration of fluids in, 542, 542f
lipase levels in, 624-625
lithium heparin for, 625
liver disease in, 201-203
lung wash in, 545, 546f
lymphocytosis in, 626
lymphopenia in, 626-627
megabacteriosis in, 203-204
mites in, 177-178
monocytosis in, 628
mycoses in, 204-206
nail trimming in, 214, 215f
nasal flush in, 544, 544f-545f
neurologic disease in, 159-161, 207-209
neutrophilia in, 630-631
ocular lesions in, 209-212
ocular trauma in, 211
organophosphate toxicity in, 212-213
overgrown beaks and claws in, 213-214
pain management in, 233
papillomas in, 215-216, 235
peritoneal fluid accumulation in, 538
phlebotomy in, 546-547
plasma globulins in, 618
pneumonia in, 217-218
pododermatitis in, 219-221, 220f
polytetrafluoroethylene toxicity in, 217, 221
proventricular dilatation disease in, 169, 222-225, 223f
pulmonary edema in, 218
regurgitation in, 225-227
renal disease in, 228-229
restraint of, 543-544, 543f
reticulocyte count in, 643
salmonellosis in, 727-728
seizures in, 207-209
sinusitis in, 230-231
soft tissue edema in, 179-180
stress hyperglycemia in, 622
thrombocytes in, 638
thrombocytopenia in, 639
total protein in, 642
tracheal foreign bodies in, 186-188
tracheal wash in, 545, 546f
trauma in, 232-234
tuberculosis transmission to, 180
tumors in, 234-236
uric acid in, 649-650
uveitis in, 211
venipuncture in, 546-547, 547f
viral diseases in, 239-242
vomiting in, 196, 225-227
zinc toxicity in, 192-194, 650
Bismuth subsalicylate, in birds, 174
Bite wounds, 536, 536f
Bites, animal, 337-338, 694-697
Black band disease, 9-10
Black death, 719-721
"Black patch necrosis", 17
"Black robber" syndrome, 16
Bladder atony, in rabbits, 392-394
Bladder overdistention, in rabbits, 392-394
Bladder stones, in guinea pigs, 282-283
Bleeding disorder, 575
Blepharedema, 111
Blepharitis, in birds, 210
Blister disease, in reptiles, 77-79
Bloat
in chinchillas, 308-311
in guinea pigs, 258-259
in rabbits, 378-381, 380f
"Bloated abdomen" syndrome, 16

β-Blockers
in ferrets, 459
in rabbits, 340
Blood collection. *See also* Venipuncture
in birds, 546-547, 547f
in ferrets, 550, 645
in fish, 518-519, 519f
in rabbits, 550
in reptiles, 533-534
in small mammals, 549-550
Blood gases, 549
Blood insulin, 107
Blood pressure
in chelonians, 523
in green iguanas, 523
in guinea pigs, 549
in hamsters, 549
in iguanas, 523
in mice, 549
in rabbits, 549
in rats, 549
in reptiles, 523-524
in snakes, 523
Blood transfusion
anemia in birds treated with, 151
in small mammals, 551-552
Blood urea nitrogen, 608-609, 609t
Blue powder, 650-651
Blue-tongued skinks
adenovirus infection in, 74-75
dysecdysis in, 95
entamoebiasis in, 100
Boa constrictors, 143
Body surface area conversions using the Meeh coefficients, 610
Boil, 147-149
Bone marrow aspiration and core biopsy, 552-553
Bone marrow hypoplasia, in ferrets, 462-463
Booklungs, 11
Bordetella bronchiseptica, 276-278
Bothriocephalus acheilognathi, 27-28
Botulism, 377
Box turtles
aural abscess in, 72f
dysecdysis in, 95
vitamin A therapy in, 111-112
Bradycardia, 590
Branchiomyces spp., 24
Branchiomycosis, 24-26
Brittle bones, 62-64
Broken bones, in birds, 189-191
Bronchial disease, 575
Bronchoalveolar lavage, 553-555
Bronchodilators
in rabbits, 368
in rats, 250
Bronchoscopy, in small mammals, 553-555
Brookynella, 33-34
"Bubble disease", 51-52
Bubonic plague, 719-721
Budgerigars
amylase in, 602-603
ascites in, 153
cloacal prolapse in, 165-166
Knemidokoptes spp. in, 177
neoplasia in, 237f
ocular lesions in, 209
Bumblefoot
in birds, 147-149, 219-221
in guinea pigs, 273-275, 274f
in rabbits, 407-409
BUN, 608-609, 609t
Buoyancy disorder, 36-37, 37f
Buphthalmia, in rabbits, 338-341, 340f
Buphthalmos, in hamsters, 294

Buprenorphine
in chinchillas, 304
in degus, 320
in ferrets, 553, 562
in guinea pigs, 253, 267, 269, 283, 568
in hamsters, 286, 289, 568
in hedgehogs, 325
in mice, 567
in rabbits, 380, 553, 562, 567
in rats, 567
in sugar gliders, 328
Burmese pythons, 143
Buserelin, 484
Butorphanol, 190
in ferrets, 553, 562
in guinea pigs, 568
in hamsters, 568
in hedgehogs, 325
in mice, 567
in rabbits, 553, 562, 567
in sugar gliders, 328

C

Cabergoline, in rats, 244
Cachexia
in birds, 180-181
in guinea pigs, 253-254
Calcium
deficiency of. *See* Hypocalcemia
laboratory tests, 610-612
Calcium carbonate, 45
Calcium channel blockers, in ferrets, 459
Calcium disodiumversenate, in birds, 160, 169, 193
Calcium glubionate, 83, 123-124, 330
Calcium gluconate
in birds, 160, 176, 198, 200
in sugar gliders, 330
Calcium glycerophosphate, in birds, 160
Calcium lactate, in birds, 160
Calciuria, in rabbits, 392
Calicivirus infection
in rabbits, 381-383
in reptiles, 79-80
California desert tortoises, 118
Campylobacter spp., 434-435
Campylobacteriosis, 434-435
Canaries
amylase in, 602-603
coccidiosis in, 181
Cancer
in hedgehogs, 324-325
ovarian, in ferrets, 482-484
skin, in ferrets, 495-496
testicular, in rabbits, 419
Candidiasis, in birds, 205-206
Cane cutter's disease, 711
Canicola disease, 711
Canicola fever, 711
Canine distemper virus, 444-445
CANV, 80-82, 90-92
Capillaria spp., 27, 182
Capnography, 548
Capsalids, 22-24
Carapacial infection, 77-79
Carbimazole, in guinea pigs, 261
Carbonic anhydrase inhibitors, 339-340
Carbuncle, in birds, 147-149
Cardiac disease
in birds, 157-158
in chinchillas, 301-302
in ferrets, 456-460
in hamsters, 287-288
in reptiles, 82-84
Cardiac ultrasound, 557
Cardiocentesis, 533
Cardiomyopathy
in chinchillas, 301-302
in ferrets, 458
in hedgehogs, 323-324
Cardiopathy, in chinchillas, 301-302
Cardiopulmonary-cerebral resuscitation, in reptiles, 524-525
Cardiovascular disease
in rabbits, 341-342
in reptiles, 82-84
Caries
in chinchillas, 302-305
in degus, 320-321
Carnitine supplementation, 104
Carp, spring viremia of, 35
Carp pox, 43-44
Carprofen
in ferrets, 553, 562
in guinea pigs, 568
in rabbits, 553, 562, 567
in rats, 567
Caryospora spp., 87-89
Castration, in small mammals, 555-557
Cataplexy, 594t
Cataracts
in birds, 211, 212f
in Chinese hamsters, 293
in ferrets, 435-437
in guinea pigs, 268-269
in rabbits, 342-344, 374f
in sugar gliders, 329
Catfish, enteric septicemia of, 17
Caudal vertebral chordoma, 437-438
Cecotrophal soiling of perineum, 387
Cefotaxime
in birds, 218
pain management uses of, 190
Ceftazidime, 18, 136-137
in chinchillas, 313
pain management uses of, 190
in reptiles, 521
Celecoxib, in birds, 169, 175, 227
Celiotomy, in fish, 516-517
ß-Cell tumor, 469-471
Cellulitis
in rabbits, 362
in reptiles, 71-74
Central nervous system disorders, 575-576
Central nervous system microsporidiosis, 707
Central nervous system signs
in birds, 159-161, 209f
in chelonia, 657
differential diagnosis of, 576
in lizards, 658
in reptiles, 657-659
in small mammals, 671
in snakes, 659
Cephalexin, in hedgehogs, 326
Cephalic vein, 550
Cephalobaena spp., 130
Cervical vertebral chordoma, 437-438
Cestodaria spp., 27
Cestodes
in fish, 27-28
in guinea pigs, 264
praziquantel for, 27-28, 183
in rabbits, 374-376
Chameleons
adenovirus infection in, 74-75
bacterial stomatitis in, 143
periodontal disease in, 134
pseudogout in, 103
vitamin A therapy for, 112
Cheek pouch disorder, in hamsters, 288-290
Cheek pouch eversion, 288-290, 289f
Cheek pouch impaction, 288-290
Cheek pouch prolapse, 288-290
Cheek teeth
in chinchillas, 303
in guinea pigs, 256
in hamsters, 290-291
in rabbits, 356-357
Cheek teeth disorders
in chinchillas, 303
in guinea pigs, 255-258
in hamsters, 290-291
Cheilitis, in guinea pigs, 254-255
Chelation therapy, in rabbits, 377
Chelonians. *See also* Tortoises; Turtles
bacterial dermatitis in, 78
bacterial stomatitis in, 145-147
blood pressure in, 523
blood urea nitrogen in, 609t
central nervous system signs in, 657
dysecdysis in, 95-97
dystocia in, 528
fracture repair in, 126
gallbladder in, 116
hepatic lipidosis in, 103-105
hypervitaminosis A in, 78, 108
hypovitaminosis A in, 96, 110
injections in, 532-533
Mycoplasma spp. in, 143
pain management in, 109
paraphimosis in, 128
phlebotomy in, 534
proliferative spinal osteopathy in, 136
shell fractures in, 126
stomatitis in, 145-147
Chemical vapor deposition, 428-430
Chemotherapy
in birds, 236, 239
in ferrets, 470, 472, 473t-474t, 474-475
lymphoma treated with, 472, 473t-474t, 474-475
in rabbits, 395-396
Cherry eye, in rabbits, 344-345, 346f
Cheyletiella parasitovorax, 366-367, 691
Chickens
central nervous system signs in, 161f
coccidiosis in, 181
cryptosporidiosis in, 181
enteritis in, 182
heavy metal toxicity in, 188f
thyroid hormones in, 649t
Chiggers, 692
Chilodonella, 33-34
Chinchillas
anorexia in, 309
blood urea nitrogen in, 609t
cardiac disease in, 301-302
castration in, 556
cryptosporidiosis in, 699-701
dental disease in, 302-305
dermatophytosis in, 306, 704
echocardiography in, 558t
fur disorders in, 305-308, 307f
gastrointestinal disorders in, 308-311, 311f
heart murmurs in, 301
lead levels in, 624
lymphocyte count variations in, 627
ocular disorders in, 311-313
ovariohysterectomy in, 565-566
penile disorders in, 313-315, 316f
teeth in, 302-305
Chinese hamsters
cardiac disease in, 287-288
cataracts in, 293
Chitin inhibitors, 21-22
Chlamydia
in reptiles, 141, 143
treatment of, 143

Chlamydiosis, 697-699
in birds, 211, 697-699
in reptiles, 84-85
Chlamydophila abortus, 84
Chlamydophila caviae, 268-269, 698
Chlamydophila felis, 84
Chlamydophila pneumoniae, 84
Chlamydophila psittaci, 159, 161-163, 182, 184, 230, 697-699
Chlamydophilosis, in reptiles, 84-85
Chloramphenicol
in birds, 160, 211
in chinchillas, 304, 315
in ferrets, 476
in guinea pigs, 254, 265, 267, 279, 281, 284
in hamsters, 289-290
in rabbits, 370
respiratory tract disease in rats treated with, 248
Chloride, 612-613
Chlorine toxicity, 45t-46t
Choanal papilloma, 216f
Cholangiocarcinoma, in birds, 235
Choleoeimeria spp., 87-89
Cholestasis, in birds, 203
Cholesterol, 613-614
Choline supplementation, 104
Chondroma, in birds, 235
Chondrosarcoma, in birds, 235
Chordoma, in ferrets, 437-438, 438f
Chorioretinal scarring, 210
Chorioretinitis
in birds, 211
in rabbits, 426-428
Choroiditis, in rabbits, 426-428
Chromoblastomycosis, 49-50
Chromodacryorrhea, in rats, 242-243
Chromomycosis, 49-50
Chronic bee paralysis, 16
Chronic blepharitis, 111
Chronic egg laying, in birds, 164-165, 196
Chronic interstitial nephritis, 492
Chronic progressive nephrosis, 246
Chronic renal failure
in ferrets, 491-494
in hamsters, 295-297
in rabbits, 412-415
in rats, 245-247
Chronic respiratory disease, in rats, 249-250
Chronic sinusitis, in birds, 230-231
Chrysosporium anamorph of *Nannizziopsis viesii*, 80-82, 90-92
Cimetidine
in birds, 174, 227
in ferrets, 438, 452
Ciprofloxacin
anaerobes treated with, 227
in birds, 231
in guinea pigs, 269
lower respiratory tract disease treated with, 142
in reptiles, 521
Circling, 159-161, 590
Circovirus, 181, 202
Cisapride
in birds, 227
in guinea pigs, 254
in rabbits, 380, 388
Cisplatin, in birds, 236
CK, 614
"Clagging", 387
Clarithromycin, in ferrets, 460
Clawed frogs, mycobacteriosis in, 59
Claws, overgrown, 213-214, 215f
Clindamycin, in rabbits, 376
Clinical crown, 302
Cloacal papillomas, in birds, 215
Cloacal prolapse
in amphibians, 51-52
in birds, 165-166, 215
in reptiles, 85-87
Cloacopexy, 166
Cloacoplasty, 166
Cloacoscopy, 527
Clomipramine, cloacal prolapse in birds treated with, 166
Closantel, 23
Clostridial enteritis, in rabbits, 385-390
Clostridial enterotoxemia, in rabbits, 385-390
Clostridium difficile, 291-293
Clotrimazole, aspergillosis in birds treated with, 156
Clove oil, 514
Cnemidocoptes mites, in birds, 210
Coagulopathies, in birds, 149, 203
Coccidiosis
in amphibians, 52-53
in birds, 173, 181-182
in ferrets, 448-450
in rabbits, 346-348, 348f, 383, 385-390
in reptiles, 87-89
Cochlear nerve deficit, 581
Cockatiels
amylase in, 602-603
Chlamydophila psittaci in, 167
cloacal prolapse in, 165-166
conjunctivitis in, 167-168
egg binding in, 176f
feather picking in, 184-185
hepatic lipidosis in, 195f
zinc concentrations in pancreas of, 160, 193
Cockatoos
amylase in, 602-603
cardiac disease in, 157
cloacal prolapse in, 165-166, 166f
feather picking in, 184-185
oviduct prolapse in, 166f
proventricular dilatation disease in, 169, 222-225
Coeliotomy, prefemoral, 528
Coelom, distended, 584
Coelomic cavity fluid aspirate, in fish, 510
Coelomic fluid, in birds, 153-154
Coelomocentesis, 538
Colchicine, 203
in birds, 192, 229
hyperuricemia treated with, 192
"Cold", 230-231
Coliform enteritis, 387
Colitis, in chinchillas, 308-311
Collagenous hamartoma, in rabbits, 351-352
Colloids, 560-561
Colonic prolapse, in reptiles, 86-87
Colonoscopy, 467
Colubrids, metronidazole dosing in, 137-138
Columbiformes, viral diseases in, 240
Complete AV block, in ferrets, 456-458
Congenital hip dislocation, in rabbits, 416-417
Congenital limb adduction, in rabbits, 416-417
Congestive cardiomyopathy, 323-324
Congestive heart failure
in ferrets, 458
in rabbits, 341-342
Conjunctivitis
in birds, 167-168, 211
in chinchillas, 311-313
cryptosporidial, in birds, 167
differential diagnosis of, 577
in guinea pigs, 268-269
in hamsters, 294
Conjunctivitis *(Continued)*
hemorrhagic, in birds
in rabbits, 349-351, 353, 423-424
Constipation
in birds, 168-170
in chinchillas, 308-311
differential diagnosis of, 577
in reptiles, 660
Constipative mucoid enteropathy, 364-365
Constrictive toe syndrome, 179-180, 180f
Contrast radiography, in birds, 169
Contusion, in birds, 232-234
Conures
amylase in, 602-603
proventricular dilatation disease in, 169, 222-225
Conversion factors, 578
Convulsions, in birds, 159-161
Copepods, 21-22
Copper
ectoparasites treated with, 34
monogeneans treated with, 23-24
Copulatory organ prolapse, in reptiles, 86
Corals, acroporid, 9-10
Corneal edema, in rabbits, 426
Corneal lipidosis, in amphibians, 53-54
Corneal ulcers
in birds, 211
in chinchillas, 311-313
differential diagnosis of, 580
in guinea pigs, 268-269
Coronaviral disease, in ferrets, 452-454
Coronavirus, 387
Corticosteroids
in birds, 233, 236
in ferrets, 438, 443, 450, 453, 470
in prairie dogs, 317
in rabbits, 396, 430
Corynebacterium kutscheri, 248-249
Cotton fur syndrome, in chinchillas, 305-308
Cotton skin, 64-65
"Cotton wool disease", 17
COX-2 inhibitors, in birds, 224
Coxal apodeme fractures, 15
CPCR, 524-525
CPK, 614
Cranial nerve deficits, 581
Creat, 615
Creatine kinase, 614
Creatine phosphokinase, 614
Creatinine, 494, 615
Crohn's disease, 465-467
Crop burns, 227
Crop fistulas, 227
Crop impaction, in birds, 170-171
Crop infusion, in birds, 538-539, 539f
Crop stasis, in birds, 170-171, 226
Crop thermal burn, in birds, 152f
Crotalid calicivirus, 79-80
Crustaceans
ectoparasites in, 21-22
septicemia in, 4
Cryptobia, 28-29
Cryptococcal infection, in ferrets, 439-441
Cryptococcosis, in ferrets, 439-441
Cryptococcus gatti, 439-441
Cryptococcus neoformans, 205, 439-441
Cryptosporidial conjunctivitis, in birds, 167
Cryptosporidiosis, 699-703
in birds, 181, 204, 699-701
in chinchillas, 699-701
in ferrets, 699-701
in gerbils, 700
in guinea pigs, 700-701
in hamsters, 700-701
in hedgehogs, 700
in mice, 700-701

Cryptosporidiosis *(Continued)*
in rabbits, 387, 700-701
in rats, 700-701
in reptiles, 89-90, 137, 700-701
Cryptosporidium baileyi, 700
Cryptosporidium cunulus, 700
Cryptosporidium meleagridis, 700
Cryptosporidium saurophilum, 89-90
Cryptosporidium serpentis, 89-90
Cryptosporidium wrariri, 264
Crystalloid fluids, 560-561
Cuban tree frogs, 53
Cubirea spp., 130
Cutaneous abscesses, in reptiles, 72
Cutaneous lymphoma
in ferrets, 496
in rabbits, 420f
Cutaneous masses, in rabbits, 351-352
Cutaneous papilloma, in birds, 235
Cuticle
retention of, 7-8
shedding of, 7
Cyanobacteria, in invertebrates, 4
Cyclitis, in rabbits, 426-428
Cyniclomyces guttulatus, 264, 309
Cyprinids, 24
Cystadenocarcinoma, in birds, 235
Cystadenoma, in birds, 235
Cystic mastitis, 397
Cystic ovarian disease, in birds, 185-186
Cystic ovaries
in gerbils, 299-300
in guinea pigs, 269-271
Cysticercosis, 374-376
Cystitis, in ferrets, 498-500
Cystoliths, 394
Cystoscopic stone removal, in guinea pigs, 283
Cytoplasmic polyhedrosis viruses, 16

D

Dacryocystitis, in rabbits, 352-354, 355f
Dacryocystorhinography, 353-354
Dacryosolenitis, in rabbits, 352-354
Dactylogyrus spp., 22-23
Decoquinate, 449
Deer-fly fever, 730-732
Deferoxamine, 203
Degenerative joint disease, in rabbits, 334-336
Degenerative myelopathy, 327-328
Degus
behavioral disorders in, 318-319
castration in, 556
dental disease in, 319-322
diabetes mellitus in, 322-323
dysecdysis in, 95
ovariohysterectomy in, 565-566
Dehydration
in amphibians, 70
in birds, 171-172
in invertebrates, 5-6
weight loss caused by, 70
Demodectic mange, 298
Demodectic mites, 251, 297-298
Demodicosis
in ferrets, 447
in guinea pigs, 279
Dental abscess, in rabbits, 355-360
Dental disease
in chinchillas, 302-305
in degus, 319-322
in ferrets, 441-442
in guinea pigs, 255-258
in hamsters, 290-291
in rabbits, 355-360
Dental infection, in rabbits, 359
Dental malocclusion
in chinchillas, 302-305
in degus, 319-322
in rabbits, 355-360
Dental spurs, in rabbits, 357
Dermal fibrosis, in rabbits, 362
Dermanyssus spp., 177-178, 690-694
Dermatitis
bacterial
in guinea pigs, 279
in rats, 252
in reptiles, 77-79
in guinea pigs, 278-280
necrotizing mycotic, 91
pododermatitis
in birds, 219-221, 220f
in guinea pigs, 273-275, 274f, 278-280
in hamsters, 298
in rabbits, 407-409, 408f
in rabbits, 361
in rats, 251-252
Dermatomycosis, in reptiles, 90-92
Dermatophilosis, in reptiles, 92-93
Dermatophilus chelonae, 92-93
Dermatophilus congolensis, 92-93
Dermatophytes, 703
in birds, 205
in rabbits, 360
Dermatophytosis, 703-705
in chinchillas, 306, 704
in ferrets, 704
in guinea pigs, 278-280, 703-704
in hamsters, 298
in hedgehogs, 326
in mice, 704
in rabbits, 360-364, 704
in rats, 251-252, 704
Dermatosepticemia, 65-67, 66f
Dermatosis, 582
Dermocystidium koi, 24-25
Dermopathies, in rabbits, 360-364
Dermoplasty, 394
Desiccation, 5-6
Deslorelin, in rats, 244
Dexamethasone
in prairie dogs, 317
in rabbits, 373
Dexamethasone sodium phosphate, in birds, 160
Dextran 70, 561
Dextrose, in birds, 160
Diabetes mellitus
in degus, 322-323
differential diagnosis of, 583
in ferrets, 620
in rabbits, 620
in reptiles, 107-108
Diagnostic sampling
in fish, 510-511
in invertebrates, 504-505
in reptiles, 525-526
in snails, 504-505
Diarrhea
in birds, 173-175, 173f, 222
in chinchillas, 308-311
differential diagnosis of, 583
in guinea pigs, 263-266
in rabbits, 384
in reptiles, 93-95, 104, 661
in small mammals, 672
Diazepam
in birds, 160
in rabbits, 373
seizures in birds treated with, 193, 208, 224
in sugar gliders, 330
Diazoxide, 470
Diclofenac, 313
Diesingia spp., 130
Difluorbenzuron, 22
Digoxin
in birds, 158
in ferrets, 459
in hamsters, 288
in rabbits, 342
1,25-Dihydroxycholecalciferol, 123
Dilatative cardiomyopathy, 157
Dilated cardiomyopathy
in ferrets, 458
in hedgehogs, 323-324
Dimercaptosuccinic acid, in birds, 160, 169, 193
Dimetridazole, 29
Dinoflagellates, 33-34
Diphenhydramine, in rats, 252
Diplococcal infection, in rats, 248-249
Dirofilaria immitis, 443-444
Dirofilariasis, 443-444
Disinterest in food, in birds, 151-153
Disseminated collagenous hamartomas, in rabbits, 360-364
Disseminated idiopathic myositis, 478-479
Disseminated intravascular coagulation, in hamsters, 287
Disseminated microsporidiosis, 702, 707
Dissolved oxygen, 44, 45t-46t
Distemper, in ferrets, 444-445, 500
Distended coelom, 584
Diuretics, in rabbits, 342
DMSO, 133
Doxorubicin, 396, 470
Doxycycline
bacterial enteritis in birds treated with, 182
in birds, 196
Chlamydophila psittaci treated with, 163, 167
chronic respiratory disease in rats treated with, 250
in hamsters, 289-290
Lawsonia intracellularis treated with, 293
in rabbits, 376
respiratory tract disease in rats treated with, 248
D-penicillamine, in birds, 160-161
Drooling, 590
Dropsy, in fish, 20-21
Duck virus enteritis, 182
Ducklings, ascites in, 153
Duodenostomy, in birds, 539-540
Dwarf hamsters, skin diseases in, 297-299
Dwarf rabbits, encephalitis in, 369
Dysautonomia, in rabbits, 364-365, 387
Dysbacteriosis
in chinchillas, 308-311, 315
definition of, 309
in guinea pigs, 264
Dysecdysis
in chelonians, 95-97
in invertebrates, 7-8, 505-506
in lizards, 95-97
in reptiles, 95-97
in snakes, 78, 95-97
Dysorexia, in guinea pigs, 253-254
Dysphagia, 590
Dysplasia, in rabbits, 397-398
Dyspnea, 585, 674
Dystocia
in birds, 175-177
differential diagnosis of, 585
in guinea pigs, 275-276
in reptiles, 526-528
Dysuria, in rabbits, 392-394

E

Ear canker, 403-405
Ear mange, 403-405
Ear mites, in ferrets, 445-446
Eastern equine encephalitis, 182
ECG, 558-559
Echinococcus granulosus cyst, 384
Echocardiography
in birds, 158
in rabbits, 342
in small mammals, 557, 558t
Eclampsia, in ferrets, 486-487
Eclectus, proventricular dilatation disease in, 222-225
E-collars
in birds, 540
in small mammals, 558
Ectoparasites, 98. *See also* Parasites
in arthropods, 505-506
in birds, 177-178
ciliated, 33-34
in crustaceans, 21-22
dysecdysis caused by, 96
in ferrets, 447
in fish, 20-22, 33-34
flagellated, 33-34
in guinea pigs, 278-280
in invertebrates, 12-13, 505-506
in rabbits, 361, 363, 366-367, 367f
in rats, 251-252
in reptiles, 98-99
Ecydsis, 7-8
Edema
in birds, 179-180
in fish, 20-21
soft tissue, in birds, 179-180
Edwardsiella tarda, 17
Egg binding
in birds, 175-177
in reptiles, 526-528
Egg laying, chronic, 164-165, 196
Ehlers-Danlos–like syndrome, 362
Eimera spp.
in amphibians, 52-53
E. chinchillae, 308-309
E. stiedai, 346
in reptiles, 87-89
EKG, 558-559
Electrocardiography
anesthesia monitoring using, 548
in birds, 158
in ferrets, 457
in rabbits, 342
in small mammals, 558-559, 559t
Electrocution, 368-369, 369f
Electrolytes, in rabbits, 377
Electromyography, in birds, 208
Elenia spp., 130
Elizabethan collars
in birds, 540
in small mammals, 558
Elodontoma, 316-322
Emaciation
in birds, 180-181
differential diagnosis of, 586
Embryonal nephromas, in rabbits, 413
Emergency care
in amphibians, 519
in fish, 512
Emesis
in amphibians, 68-69
in reptiles, 136-138
Enalapril
in birds, 158
in hamsters, 288
in hedgehogs, 324
Encephalitis, in rabbits, 369-371
Encephalitozoon cuniculi, 339, 342-344, 369, 371, 374f, 375, 413, 426-430, 705-708
Encephalitozoonosis, 705-708
in birds, 706
in psittacines, 706
in rabbits, 371-374, 429, 706-707
in small mammals, 706
Encephalomeningitis, 369-371
Endocardiosis, 458
Endocarditis, in reptiles, 83
Endocrine neoplasias, in birds, 235
Endometrial adenocarcinoma, in rabbits, 426f
Endometriosis, in rabbits, 425
Endometritis, in guinea pigs, 284
Endoparasites. *See also* Parasites
in ferrets, 448-450, 449f
in rabbits, 374-376
Endoscopy, in birds, 169, 186, 217, 223, 537f
Endotracheal tube, 548, 562
End-tidal CO_2, 548
Enilconazole
in birds, 218
in guinea pigs, 269
Enrofloxacin, 18, 39, 137
bacterial enteritis treated with, 182
in birds, 160, 182, 218, 231
in chinchillas, 304, 313
chronic respiratory disease in rats treated with, 250
in degus, 321
in ferrets, 476
in guinea pigs, 253, 265, 269, 281, 284
in hamsters, 289-290
in hedgehogs, 326
Lawsonia intracellularis treated with, 293
lower respiratory tract disease treated with, 142
in prairie dogs, 317
in rabbits, 394
in rats, 247
in reptiles, 521
in sugar gliders, 328
Entamoeba invadens, 100-101
Entamoebiasis, in reptiles, 100-101
Enteric septicemia of catfish, 17
Enteritis
in birds, 181-183
in chinchillas, 308-311
in ferrets, 451-452
in guinea pigs, 263-266
in rabbits, 385-390
Enterocolitis, 728
flagellate, 55-56
Enterotomy, 189, 455
Enterotoxicosis, in rabbits, 385-390
Entomopathogenic systemic mycoses, 8-9
Eosinophil count, 616-617
Eosinophilic enteritis, 465
Eosinophilic gastroenteritis, 465
in ferrets, 450, 453
Epidermal necrosis, 91
Epiphora
in chinchillas, 303, 311-313
in guinea pigs, 268-269
in rabbits, 352-354
Episodic weakness, 594t
Epitheliotropic T-cell lymphoma, 471-475
Epizootic catarrhal enteritis, 451-452, 465
Epizootic ulcerative syndrome, 24
Ergasilus spp., 21
"Eroded mouth syndrome", 17
Erythrocytic virus, 114-115
Erythrodermatitis, in koi, 40-41
Erythromycin
bacterial enteritis in birds treated with, 182
Chlamydophila psittaci treated with, 168
Escherichia coli, 309, 475-477
Esophageal achalasia, 477-478
Esophageal foreign bodies, in ferrets, 454
Esophageal probe, 548
Esophagostomy, in birds, 540-541
Estivation, 5-6
Estradiol, 598-599
Estrogen toxicosis, in ferrets, 462-463
Estrogen-induced bone marrow depression, in ferrets, 462-463
Estrus-associated anemia, in ferrets, 462-463
Eugenol, 51, 514
European brown hare syndrome virus, 383
European foulbrood, 4-5
Euthanasia, in invertebrates, 506
Exophthalmia, 235, 290
Exophthalmos
in guinea pigs, 268-269
in hamsters, 294
Exoskeleton repair, in invertebrates, 507-508
Eye discharge, in guinea pigs, 268-269
Eye lesions, in birds, 209-212
Eyelid diseases, in birds, 210-211

F

Facial nerve deficit, 581
Falconiformes, viral diseases in, 240
False pregnancy, 411-412
Famotidine, 247
Fatty eye, in guinea pigs, 268-269
Fatty infiltration of the liver, in birds, 194-197
Fatty liver disease, in reptiles, 103-105
Fatty liver syndrome, in birds, 194-197, 201
Feather digest, 178
Feather lice, 177-178
Feather picking, in birds, 184-185
Feather plucking, 184-185
Feather trauma, 184-185
Fecal examination, in reptiles, 529
Fecal sample collection, in reptiles, 525-526
Fecal wet mount, in fish, 510-511
Feeding tube placement
in birds, 539-541
in rabbits, 559-560
in rodents, 559-560
Feline plague, 719-721
Femoral neck anteversion, in rabbits, 416-417
Fenbendazole, 121
Capillaria spp. treated with, 182
in chinchillas, 310
Chlamydophila psittaci treated with, 168
encephalitozoonosis treated with, 429
in ferrets, 449
giardiasis treated with, 449
in guinea pigs, 265, 267
nematodes treated with, 28, 137, 293
in rabbits, 373
spirochid trematodes treated with, 83
Fenthion, 21
Ferret(s)
acariasis in, 691
acetaminophen toxicity in, 464-465
adrenal disease in, 430-432
adrenal panel in, 598-599
alanine aminotransferase in, 599-600
Aleutian disease in, 433-434, 453, 492
alopecia in, 432f
anemia in, 646
anesthesia in, 552
atrioventricular block in, 456-458
bile acids in, 607t
bites by, 695
blood collection in, 550, 645
blood transfusion in, 551-552

Ferret(s) *(Continued)*
blood urea nitrogen in, 609t
Campylobacter spp. disease in, 434-435
cardiac disease in, 456-458
castration in, 556
cataracts in, 435-437
chemotherapy in, 470, 472, 473t-474t, 474-475
chordoma in, 437-438, 438f
coccidiosis in, 448-450
creatinine in, 494, 615
cryptococcosis in, 439-441
cryptosporidiosis in, 699-701
dental disease in, 441-442
dermatophytosis in, 704
diabetes mellitus in, 620
dirofilariasis in, 443-444
distemper in, 444-445, 500
ear mites in, 445-446
ectoparasites in, 447
endoparasites in, 448-450, 449f
enteritis in, 451-452
eosinophilic gastroenteritis in, 450, 453
epizootic catarrhal enteritis in, 451-452, 465
erythrocytes in, 645
gastritis in, 460-461
gastrointestinal foreign bodies in, 454-456, 456f
giardiasis in, 448-450
glucose levels in, 619-622
granulomatous inflammatory syndrome of, 452-454
heart disease in
atrioventricular block, 456-458
structural, 458-460
Helicobacter mustelae-associated gastritis and ulcers in, 460-461
hepatobiliary disease in, 461-462
hyperestrogenism anemia in, 462-463
hyperglycemia in, 619-622
ibuprofen toxicity in, 464-465
inflammatory bowel disease in, 465-467
influenza in, 468-469
insulinoma in, 469-471
lymphoma in, 471-475
mast cell tumors in, 496f
mastitis in, 475-477
megaesophagus in, 477-478, 478f
mites in, 445-446
myofascitis in, 478-479
neonatal disease in, 479-481
osteoma in, 481-482, 482f
ovarian neoplasia in, 482-484
ovarian remnant syndrome in, 484-485
ovariohysterectomy in, 564-566
parasites in, 447-450, 449f
periodontal disease in, 441-442
plague in, 720
platelets in, 639
pregnancy toxemia in, 486-487
proliferative bowel disease in, 487-488
prostatic disease in, 488-491
rabies in, 722
renal cysts in, 495f
renal disorders in, 491-494, 495f
respiratory tract disorders in, 440
salmonellosis in, 727
seizures in, 470
skin tumors in, 495-496
splenomegaly in, 497-498
systemic coronaviral disease in, 452-454
thrombocytopenia in, 639
thyroid hormones in, 649t
toxoplasmosis in, 448-450
trichobezoars in, 454, 456f
ulcers in, 460-461

Ferret(s) *(Continued)*
upper respiratory disease in, 469f
urethral catheterization of, 570
urethral compression in, 488-490
urethral obstruction in, 488-490, 499
urolithiasis in, 498-500
vaccine reactions in, 500-501
Ferret enteric coronavirus infection, 451-452
Fibrinous pleuritis, 392f
Fibroma, in birds, 234
Fibropapillomatosis, 105-106
Fibrosarcoma
in birds, 234
in rabbits, 351
Filarial nematodes, in reptiles, 121
Filarid worms
in amphibians, 61
in reptiles, 83
Fin clip, in fish, 510-511
Finasteride, 490
Finches
coccidiosis in, 181
conjunctivitis in, 167-168
cryptosporidiosis in, 181
Fine-needle aspiration or biopsy, in rabbits, 359
Finquel, 513-514
FIP-like disease of ferrets, 452-454
Fipronil, 11
in hedgehogs, 326
lice treated with, 178
ticks treated with, 178
First-degree AV block, in ferrets, 456-458
Fish
acid-base regulation in, 635-636
anesthesia in, 513-514
ascites in, 20-21
azurophil count in, 604
bacterial diseases in, 17-20
basophil count, 606
blood urea nitrogen in, 609t
calcium in, 611-612
cestodes in, 27-28
diagnostic sampling in, 510-511
dropsy in, 20-21
ectoparasites in, 20
ciliated, 33-34
crustacean, 21-22
flagellated, 33-34
edema in, 20-21
emergency care in, 512
eosinophil count in, 616-617
flukes in, 22-24
fungal diseases in, 24-26
gastrointestinal nematode and cestode parasites in, 27-28
gastrointestinal protozoal parasites in, 28-29
head and lateral line erosion in, 30-31
heteropenia in, 632
hyperkalemia in, 640
hypokalemia in, 641
intracoelomic injections in, 512-513, 513f
intramuscular injections in, 512-513, 513f
lymphocystis in, 32-33
lymphocytosis in, 626
lymphopenia in, 626-627
monocytosis in, 628
MS 222 anesthesia in, 513-514
nematodes in, 27-28
neutrophilia in, 631
oral medications in, 514-515
protozoal parasites in
ectoparasites, 33-34
gastrointestinal, 28-29
salmonellosis in, 728
spring viremia of carp, 35

Fish *(Continued)*
surgical principles in, 516-517
swim bladder disease in, 36-37, 37f
tank pond therapy in, 517-518
total protein in, 642
trauma in, 38-40
venipuncture in, 518-519, 519f
viral diseases in, 42-43
viral epidermal hyperplasia in, 43-44
water quality for, 44-46
wound management in, 38-40
Fish fancier's finger, 715-716
Fish louse, 21-22
Fish tank granuloma, 715-716
Flaccid paresis, in rabbits, 376-378
Flagellate enterocolitis, 55-56
Flavobacterium columnare, 17, 19
Flexibacter maritimus, 17
Flies, in birds, 177-178
Floppy rabbit syndrome, 376-378, 378f
Florida gopher tortoises, 118
Flu, 230-231, 468-469
Fluconazole
aspergillosis in birds treated with, 156
complications of, 156
Flucytosine, 440-441
Fluid therapy
in birds, 541-542
in invertebrates, 508
in rabbits, 560-561
in rodents, 560-561
Flukes, in fish, 22-24
Flunixin meglumine, in ferrets, 476
Fluoropyrimidines, mycoses in birds treated with, 205-206
Fluoxetine, 328
Flurbiprofen, 313
Flutamide, 490
Flystrike, 367f
Follicle-stimulating hormone, 430
Follicular cysts, in guinea pigs, 269-271
Follicular stasis, in birds, 185-186
Food aggression, in rabbits, 337-338
Food allergy, 465
Force feeding, in fish, 514-515
Foreign body obstruction, in rabbits, 379
Formalin
ectoparasites treated with, 34
ich treated with, 34
monogeneans treated with, 23
saprolegniasis treated with, 25
Fort Bragg fever, 711
Fowl typhoid, 726-729
Fractures
in birds, 189-191, 233
greenstick, 190
incomplete, 190
open, 190
pathologic, 190
in reptiles, 125-127
Francis disease, 730-732
Francisella tularensis, 730-732
Fregate Island giant tenebrionid beetles, 8
Freshwater head and lateral line erosion, 30-31
Frogs, 79
Fungal diseases
in birds, 204-206
in reptiles, 80-82
Fungal infections
in fish, 24-26
in invertebrates, 8-9
of skin, in reptiles, 90-92
superficial, 8-9
systemic, 8-9
Fungal pathogens, abscesses/granulomas caused by, 2

Fungal pneumonia, in birds, 155-157
Fur changes, in small mammals, 684
Fur disorders
in chinchillas, 305-308, 307f
in degus, 318-319
Fur mites, in guinea pigs, 279
Fur ring, 313-315
Fur-chewing, in chinchillas, 305-308
Furosemide
ascites treated with, 154, 179
in birds, 158, 221
in chinchillas, 301
in ferrets, 459
in hamsters, 288
in hedgehogs, 324
in rabbits, 342
Fur-slip, in chinchillas, 305-308
Furuncle, in birds, 147-149
Furunculosis, in koi, 40-41
Fusariomycosis, 90-92
Fusus coli, 386

G

Galliformes, 240
Gallinaceous birds, ascites in, 153
Gammaglutamyl transferase, 617-618
Gangrenous mastitis, in ferrets, 475-477
Gas bubble disease, 45t-46t
Gastric decompression, in guinea pigs, 259
Gastric dilatation and volvulus
in guinea pigs, 258-259
in rabbits, 379-381
Gastric disorders, in rabbits, 378-381, 380f
Gastric hypomotility/stasis, in rabbits, 378-381
Gastric stasis
differential diagnosis of, 586
in rabbits, 385-390
Gastric torsion, in guinea pigs, 258-259
Gastric tubing, in fish, 514-515
Gastric tympany
in guinea pigs, 258-259
in rabbits, 378-381
Gastric ulceration, in rabbits, 379
Gastritis, 137
in ferrets, 460-461
in rabbits, 378-381
Gastroenteritis, 728
Gastroesophageal sphincter incompetence, 137
Gastrointestinal disorders
in chinchillas, 308-311, 311f
in rabbits, 378-381
Gastrointestinal foreign bodies
in amphibians, 56-59
in ferrets, 454-456, 456f
Gastrointestinal hypomotility/stasis, in rabbits, 385-390
Gastrointestinal obstruction, in rabbits, 386
Gastrointestinal overload, in amphibians, 56-59
Gastrokinetic drugs, in birds, 224, 227
Gavage
in birds, 538-539, 539f
in fish, 514-515
Geckos, dysecdysis in, 95
Generalized muscular weakness, in rabbits, 376-378
Gentamicin
in birds, 231
in guinea pigs, 269
Gerbils
blood urea nitrogen in, 609t
chromodacryorrhea in, 242-243
cryptosporidiosis in, 700
ovarian disease in, 299-300
Gerrhosaurid herpesvirus 1, 105-106
Gerrhosaurid herpesvirus 2, 105-106
Gerrhosaurid herpesvirus 3, 105-106
GI foreign body, in ferrets, 454-456, 456f
Giardia duodenalis, 308-309
Giardiasis
in amphibians, 55-56
in ferrets, 448-450
Gigliolella spp., 130
Gill maggots, 21-22
Gill snip/scrape, in fish, 510-511, 511f
Glaucoma
in hamsters, 294
in rabbits, 338-341
Glob, 618-619
Globulins, 618-619
Glomerular filtration rate study, 529
Glomerulonephritis, 612
Glossopharyngeal nerve deficit, 581
Glucocorticoids, in rabbits, 373
Gluconeogenesis, 619
Glucose, 619-622
Glucosuria, 107, 322-323
Glutamate dehydrogenase, in birds, 195
α-Glutaryltransferase, 617-618
Gluten hypersensitivity, 465
Glycogenolysis, 619
Going light, in birds, 180-181, 203-204
Golden eagles, *Aspergillus* spp. in, 155
Goldfish, swim bladder disease in, 36-37, 37f
Gonadal tumors, in ferrets, 482-484
Gonadotropin-releasing hormone agonists
in ferrets, 463, 484
in guinea pigs, 270
in rats, 244
Goshawks, *Aspergillus* spp. in, 155
Goussia spp., 87-89
Gout
in birds, 191-192
in reptiles, 101-103
Grand mal seizures, 594t
Granulomas
in amphibians, 61
in birds, 153
in invertebrates, 2-3
Mycobacterium marinum, 715-716
Granulomatous inflammatory syndrome of ferrets, 452-454
Granulosa cell tumors, in gerbils, 300
Grass sickness, 364-365
Gray patch disease, 105-106
Green diarrhea, in ferrets, 451-452
Green iguanas
blood pressure in, 523
blood urea nitrogen in, 609t
dysecdysis in, 95
entamoebiasis in, 100
proliferative spinal osteopathy in, 135-136
Green sea turtles, entamoebiasis in, 100
Green slime, in ferrets, 451-452
Green tree pythons, 85, 143
Greenies, in ferrets, 451-452
Greenstick fracture, 190
"Ground glass" appearance, 154
Gryodactylus spp., 22-23
Guinea pigs
acariasis in, 691
anorexia in, 253-254
bile acids in, 607t
bites by, 695
blood pressure in, 549
blood urea nitrogen in, 609t
castration in, 556
cheek teeth disorders in, 255-258
cheilitis in, 254-255
cryptosporidiosis in, 700-701
dangerous antibiotics in, 582
Guinea pigs *(Continued)*
dental disease in, 255-258
dermatophytosis in, 278-280, 703-704
diabetes mellitus in, 621
echocardiography in, 558t
electrocardiography in, 559t
gastric dilatation and volvulus in, 258-259
hyperthyroidism in, 260-261, 261f
hypovitaminosis C in, 262-263, 267
incisor teeth disorders in, 256
intestinal disorders in, 263-266
intubation technique in, 562-563
intussusception in, 568
Kurloff cell in, 627
leptospirosis in, 711
lymphocytic choriomeningitis virus in, 713
neurologic disorders in, 266-267
neuro-otitis in, 267f
ocular disorders in, 268-269
ovarian cysts in, 269-271, 271f, 284
ovariohysterectomy in, 564-566
periapical abscesses in, 256
perineal sac impaction in, 271-272
pneumonia in, 276-278
pododermatitis in, 273-275, 274f, 278-280
pregnancy and parturient disorders in, 275-276
rectal impaction in, 271-272
rectal prolapse in, 568
respiratory tract disease in, 276-278
seizures in, 266-267
skin diseases in, 278-280
skull of, 257f
strept zooepidemicus in, 280-282
teeth in, 255-258
thyroid hormones in, 649t
tularemia in, 731
urolithiasis in, 282-283, 283f
uterine disorders in, 284-285, 285f
vaginal disorders in, 284-285
"Guppy killer disease", 33-34
Gut stasis
in birds, 170-171
in rabbits, 385-390
Gyakuten disease, 36-37, 37f
Gyrfalcons, *Aspergillus* spp. in, 155

H

Hair loss. *See also* Alopecia
in invertebrates, 3-4
Hairballs, in rabbits, 378-381
Haloperidol, 328
Hamartomas
in prairie dogs, 316
in rabbits, 351-352, 360
Hamster(s)
abdominal distention in, 285-287, 296
abscesses in, 297
amyloidosis in, 295-297
bites by, 695
blood pressure in, 549
blood urea nitrogen in, 609t
cardiac disease in, 287-288
castration in, 556
cheek pouch disorder in, 288-290
conjunctivitis in, 294
cryptosporidiosis in, 700-701
dangerous antibiotics in, 582
dental disease in, 290-291
glaucoma in, 294
intestinal disorders in, 291-293, 292f
intussusception in, 568
lymphocytic choriomeningitis virus in, 713
ocular disorders in, 293-295, 295f
ovariohysterectomy in, 564-566
pododermatitis in, 298

Hamster(s) *(Continued)*
proptosis in, 294
rectal prolapse in, 568
renal disease in, 295-297
skin diseases in, 297-299, 299f
thyroid hormones in, 649t
tularemia in, 730
Hamster enteritis, 291-293
Hamster polyomavirus, 286, 297
Handling
of amphibians, 520
of birds, 543-544
of invertebrates, 509-510, 509f
of rabbits, 568-569
of reptiles, 530-531
of rodents, 568-569
Hantaan virus, 708
Hantavirus, 708-710
Hantavirus pulmonary syndrome, 709-710
Hantavirus spp., 708-710
Hard pad disease, 444-445
Harderian gland
prolapse of, 344-345, 346f
secretions from, 353
Hardness, water, 45
Hay makers disease, 711
HCT, 622-623
Head and lateral line erosion, 30-31
Head tilt
in birds, 159-161, 208
differential diagnosis of, 590
in rabbits, 428-430
Heart disease
in chinchillas, 301-302
in ferrets, 456-460
in reptiles, 82-84
Heart murmurs, in chinchillas, 301
Heartworm disease, in ferrets, 443-444
Heavy metal toxicity, in birds, 150, 152, 160, 192-194
Hedgehogs
amylase in, 602-603
blood urea nitrogen in, 609t
cardiomyopathy in, 323-324
cryptosporidiosis in, 700
neoplasia in, 324-325
salmonellosis in, 727-728
skin diseases in, 325-326, 326f
wobbly hedgehog syndrome, 327-328
Helicobacter mustelae-associated gastritis and ulcers, 460-461
Helicobacter-associated gastric disease, 460-461
Helminthiasis, in amphibians, 60-62
Helminths, in rabbits, 374-376
Hemagglutination inhibition assay, in birds, 241
Hemangiolipoma, in birds, 235
Hemangioma, in birds, 234
Hemangiosarcoma
in birds, 234
in ferrets, 497
in rabbits, 351
Hematocrit, 622-623
Hematophagous parasite, 149
Hematuria
differential diagnosis of, 587
in rabbits, 393, 414
Heme oxygenase, 608
Hemipenal abscesses, in reptiles, 72-73, 521
Hemipenile prolapse, in reptiles, 85-87, 128-130
Hemipenis amputation, 129, 130f
Hemochromatosis, 201
Hemolymph, 504
Hemoparasites, in birds, 149
Hemorrhagic disease, in rabbits, 381-383
Hemorrhagic fever with renal syndrome, 709-710, 714
Henderson-Hasselbalch equation, 633-634
Henophidia, 113
Hepatic coccidiosis, 383-385
Hepatic disease, 115-117
Hepatic disorders, in rabbits, 383-385
Hepatic encephalopathy, in birds, 159, 196, 203
Hepatic failure, 587
Hepatic lipidosis
in birds, 194-197
in ferrets, 454
in rabbits, 384
in reptiles, 103-105
Hepatic steatosis, in birds, 194-197
Hepatitis, 115-117
Hepatobiliary disease, in ferrets, 461-462
Hepatocellular damage, 116
Hepatomegaly, 186
Hepatopathy, in rabbits, 383-385
Hepatosis, 115-117
Herbivores
dietary recommendations for, 124
high-protein diets in, 139
Herpesvirus infections
in birds, 182
in koi, 31-32
in reptiles, 105-106
Heteropenia, 629-633
Heterophils, 629-633
Hexamita
in amphibians, 55-56
in fish, 28-29
Hip dysplasia, in rabbits, 416-417
Histiocytic enteritis, in rabbits, 385-390
Histomoniasis, 181-182
"Hitra" disease, 17
HLLE, 30-31
"Hole in the head", 30-31
Honey bees
American foulbrood in, 4-5
chronic bee paralysis in, 16
European foulbrood in, 4-5
mites in, 13f
Hookworms, in amphibians, 60-62
Horned frogs
gastrointestinal overload in, 56
hypovitaminosis A in, 57
Human chorionic gonadotropin
in ferrets, 484
follicular stasis treated with, 186
in guinea pigs, 270
Human herpesvirus type 1, 312
Human recombinant erythropoietin, 415
Humans
acariasis in, 690-694
cryptosporidiosis in, 701-702
hantavirus in, 708-710
leptospirosis in, 711-712
microsporidiosis in, 705-708
Mycobacterium marinum granuloma in, 715-716
Pasteurella multocida in, 717-719
plague in, 719-721
rat bite fever in, 724-726
salmonellosis in, 726-729
Hyalohyphomycosis, 90-92
Hydrochlorothiazide, in rabbits, 394
Hydrocoelom, 61
Hydrogen peroxide, for *Aphanomyces* spp., 25
Hydrogen sulfide toxicity, 45t-46t
Hydrometra, in rabbits, 425
Hydronephrosis, 492
Hydrophobia, 722-724
Hydrophthalmia, 338-341
Hydrophthalmos, 338-341
Hydroxyzine, in rats, 252
Hyperadrenocorticism, 298, 430-432
Hypercalcemia, 588, 610
Hypercalciuria, 282
Hypercholesterolemia, 613
in amphibians, 53-54
in birds, 195f
Hyperesthesia, 590
Hyperestrogenism anemia, in ferrets, 462-463
Hyperglycemia, 107-108, 322-323, 619-620
Hyperinsulinism, 469-471
Hyperkalemia, 588, 640
Hyperlipidemia, 195, 588
Hyperlipidosis, in amphibians, 53-54
Hypernatremia, 647
Hyperparathyroidism, nutritional secondary
in amphibians, 62-64
in reptiles, 121-125, 128
in sugar gliders, 329-330
Hyperphosphatemia, 247, 493
Hypersplenism, 497
Hyperthyroidism, 96, 260-261, 261f, 649
Hypertonic saline, 561
Hypertrophic cardiomyopathy, in ferrets, 458
Hyperuricemia, in birds, 191
Hypervitaminosis A
in chelonians, 78
in reptiles, 108-109
Hypervitaminosis D, 636
Hypervitaminosis E, 200
Hypoadrenocorticism, 626
Hypoalbuminemia, ascites caused by, 153
Hypocalcemia
in birds, 197-198
persistent
in reptiles, 121
signs of, 123
in sugar gliders, 329-330
Hypoglossal nerve deficit, 581
Hypoglycemia
in birds, 195
in ferrets, 469
in sugar gliders, 329
Hypokalemia, in birds, 195
Hypoparathyroidism, 636
Hypoproteinemia, 541
Hypotensive shock, 541
Hypothermia prevention, during anesthesia, 566-567
Hypoventilation, 548
Hypovitaminosis A, 57-59
in birds, 199-201
in chelonians, 96
in lizards, 96
in reptiles, 110-112
Hypovitaminosis C, in guinea pigs, 262-263, 267
Hypovitaminosis D, 637

I

Iatrogenic hypervitaminosis, in reptiles, 108-109
IBD, 113-114
Ibuprofen
in ferrets, 562
in guinea pigs, 568
in mice, 567
in rabbits, 553, 562
in rats, 567
toxicity, in ferrets, 464-465
"Ich", 33-34
Ichthyophoniasis, 24, 26
Ichthyophonus hoferi, 24-26
Ichthyophonus multifiliis, 33-34

Ichthyosporidiosis, 24
Icosahedral virus, 16
Idiopathic primary myocardial failure, 323-324
Iguanas
bile acids in, 116
blood pressure in, 523
blood urea nitrogen in, 609t
cloaca palpation in, 139f
dysecdysis in, 95
entamoebiasis in, 100
glomerular filtration rate in, 140
Iguanid herpesvirus 1, 105-106
Iguanid herpesvirus 2, 105-106
Ileus
in birds, 168-170, 222
in ferrets, 455
in hamsters, 285-286
in rabbits, 385-390
Imidacloprid, 367
Immunofluorescent assay, in birds, 241
Inappetence, 151-153, 333-334
Incisor teeth disorders
in guinea pigs, 255-258
in hamsters, 290-291
Inclusion body disease of snakes, 113-114, 113f
Incomplete fracture, 190
Incontinence, urinary
differential diagnosis of, 588
in rabbits, 392
Infectious diseases of acroporid corals, 9-10
Infectious pododermatitis, in birds, 219-221, 220f
Infectious stomatitis, in reptiles, 132-134, 145-147
Inflammatory bowel disease, 387, 465-467, 589
Influenza, in ferrets, 468-469
Infraorbital sinus abscesses, in birds, 148
Ingluviotomy, 227
Injections
in fish, 512-513, 513f
in reptiles, 531-533
Injury
in birds, 232-234
in invertebrates, 15-16
Insectivores, dietary recommendations for, 124
Insects
dehydration in, 5-6
fungal infections in, 8-9
septicemia in, 4
Insulinoma, in ferrets, 469-471
Insulin-secreting tumors, 469-471
Interferon, in birds, 224
Internal abscesses, in reptiles, 72
Interstitial cell tumors, in rabbits, 419
Intestinal cestodes, in fish, 27-28
Intestinal coccidiosis
in amphibians, 52
in rabbits, 346-348, 348f
Intestinal cryptosporidiosis, 702
Intestinal disorders
in guinea pigs, 263-266
in hamsters, 291-293, 292f
in rabbits, 385-390
Intestinal feeding tube placement, in birds, 539-540
Intestinal microsporidiosis, 707
Intestinal nematodes, in fish, 27-28
Intestinal parasites, diarrhea caused by, 173
Intestinal stasis, in rabbits, 385-390
Intoxication, in invertebrates, 11-12
Intracoelomic injections
in fish, 512-513, 513f
in reptiles, 531-533
Intramuscular injections, in fish, 512-513, 513f
Intranuclear coccidiosis, 87-89
Intraosseous administration of fluids, in birds, 542, 543f
Intraosseous catheters, in small mammals, 561-562
Intravenous administration of fluids, in birds, 542, 542f
Intubation technique, in small mammals, 562-563
Intussusception
in birds, 165
in chinchillas, 308-311
in guinea pigs, 568
in hamsters, 568
in mice, 568
Invertebrates
abscesses in, 2-3
alopecia in, 3-4
anesthesia in, 504
bacterial diseases in, 4-5
dehydration in, 5-6
diagnostic sampling in, 504-505
dysecdysis in, 505-506
dysecdysis in, 7-8
ectoparasites in, 12-13, 505-506
euthanasia in, 506
exoskeleton repair in, 507-508
fluid administration in, 508
fungal infections, 8-9
granulomas in, 2-3
handling of, 509-510, 509f
intoxication in, 11-12
mites in, 12-13
mycoses in, 8-9
panagrolaimidae oral nematodes in, 13-14
pesticide exposure in, 11-12
poisoning in, 11-12
restraint of, 509-510, 509f
trauma in, 15-16
viral diseases in, 16-17
wounds in, 15-16
Iodine-131, in guinea pigs, 261
Ipronidazole, *Histomonas* spp. treated with, 182
Iridocyclitis, in rabbits, 426-428
Iridovirus infection, in reptiles, 114-115
Iron dextran, 150
Islet cell adenocarcinoma, 469-471
Islet cell tumor, 469-471
Isoflurane, in amphibians, 51
Isopods, 13, 21-22
Isospora
in amphibians, 52-53
in reptiles, 87-89
Isoxsuprine, 179
Itraconazole
aspergillosis in birds treated with, 156
chromomycosis treated with, 50
dermatomycosis in reptiles treated with, 91-92
in guinea pigs, 269, 280
in hedgehogs, 326
Ivermectin
ascariasis treated with, 326
Capillaria spp. treated with, 182
Cheyletiella parasitovorax treated with, 367
Chlamydophila psittaci treated with, 168
in ferrets, 443, 446
mites treated with
in birds, 178
in ferrets, 446
in guinea pigs, 279
in invertebrates, 12
Ivermectin *(Continued)*
in lizards, 99
in rats, 252
in snakes, 99
pentastomes treated with, 131
Psoroptes cuniculi treated with, 366-367

J

Japanese autumnal fever, 711
Jasad, 650-651
Jaundice, in rabbits, 384
Jills, 462-463
Jugular vein, 546

K

K^+, 640-642
Kaolin/pectin, in birds, 174
Keratitis
in chinchillas, 311-313
in hamsters, 294
Ketoprofen, in rabbits, 398
Ketosis, in rabbits, 409-410
KHV, 31-32
Kidney disease
in ferrets, 491-494
in hamsters, 295-297
in rats, 245-247
Kidney failure
in birds, 228-229
in ferrets, 491-494
in hamsters, 295-297
in rats, 245-247
Kidney stones, in guinea pigs, 282-283
Kingsnakes, adenovirus infection in, 74-75
Kiricephalus spp., 130
Kits, 479-481
Klossiella spp., 87-89
Knemidokoptes spp., 177, 214
Koi
fungal infection of, 26f
herpes virus infection in, 31-32
monogeneans in, 23
surgery in, 517f
ulcer disease in, 40-41
viral epidermal hyperplasia in, 43-44
Komodo dragon, entamoebiasis in, 100
Kurloff cells, 627

L

Laboratory tests
adrenal panel in ferrets, 598-599
alanine aminotransferase, 599-600
albumin, 600
alkaline phosphate, 601
ammonia, 601-602
amylase, 602-603
aspartate aminotransferase, 603-604
azurophil count, 604
basophil count, 604-606
bile acids, 606-607, 607t
bilirubin, 608
blood urea nitrogen, 608-609, 609t
body surface area conversions using the Meeh coefficients, 610
calcium, 610-612
chloride, 612-613
cholesterol, 613-614
creatine kinase, 614
creatinine, 615
eosinophil count, 616-617
gammaglutamyl transferase, 617-618
globulins, 618-619
glucose, 619-622

Laboratory tests *(Continued)*
hematocrit, 622-623
lead, 623-624
lipase, 624-625
lymphocyte count, 625-627
monocyte count, 628-629
neutrophil-heterophil count, 629-633
pH, 633-636
phosphorus, 636-637
platelet count, 637-639
potassium, 640-642
protein, 642-643
red blood cell count, 643-646
reticulocyte count, 646-647
sodium, 647-648
thyroid hormones, 648-649
total protein, 642-643
uric acid, 649-650
zinc, 650-651
Labryinthomyxa marina, 8
Labyrinthitis, 403-405, 428-430
Lactated Ringer's solution, 560
Lagomorphs, myxomatosis in, 398-401
Lagovirus, 383
Lameness, 589, 677
Laser cyclophotocoagulation, 340
Lateral saphenous vein, 550
Latex cryptococcal antigen test, 440
Lawsonia intracellularis, 291-293, 387, 487-488
Lawsonia-associated diarrhea, 487-488
L-Carnitine, 196
Lead
laboratory tests for, 623-624
toxicity, in birds, 192-194
Leiomyosarcoma
in birds, 235
in rabbits, 351
Leiperia spp., 130
Leopard tortoises, 94
Lepidopterans
cytoplasmic polyhedrosis viruses in, 16
nuclear polyhedrosis viruses, 16
Leptospirosis, 711-712
Lernaea spp., 21
Leuprolide acetate, 166, 186
in ferrets, 490
in rats, 244
Levamisole
ascarids treated with, 183
nematodes treated with, 28
Leydig cell tumors, in rabbits, 419
L-Gulonolactone oxidase, 262-263
Lice
in birds, 177-178
in guinea pigs, 279
Limb amputation, in invertebrates, 15
Lingual squamous metaplasia, 57-59
Lip sores, in guinea pigs, 254-255
Lipase, 624-625
Lipemic serum, in birds, 195, 195f
Lipid keratopathy, in amphibians, 53-54
Lipid storage disorders, in amphibians, 53-54
Lipofuscinosis, in birds, 201
Lipoma, in birds, 234
Liposarcoma
in birds, 234
in rabbits, 351
Lithium heparin, 625
Liver disease
ascites associated with, 153
in birds, 201-203
in rabbits, 383-385
in reptiles, 115-117
Liver failure, 589
Liver fluke, 384
Lizards
acrodont dentition in, 143, 145
bites by, 696
blood urea nitrogen in, 609t
central nervous system signs in, 658
Chrysosporium anamorph of *Nannizziopsis viesii* in, 80-82
dysecdysis in, 95-97
dystocia in, 527-528
entamoebiasis in, 100
gallbladder in, 116
handling of, 530-531
hemipenal plugs in, 129
hepatic lipidosis in, 103-105
hypovitaminosis A in, 96
injections in, 532
mites in, 99
nutritional secondary hyperparathyroidism in, 122
pain management in, 109
paraphimosis in, 128
periodontal disease in, 132-134
phlebotomy in, 534
pneumonia in, 141-143
reovirus infections in, 140-141
respiratory tract disease in, 141-143
restraint of, 530-531
stomatitis in, 145-147
vitamin A therapy in, 111
Loggerhead genital-respiratory herpesvirus, 105-106
Loggerhead musk turtles, entamoebiasis in, 100
Loggerhead orocutaneous herpesvirus, 105-106
Loose stool, in reptiles, 93-95
Lop-eared rabbits, encephalitis in, 369
Loperamide, 188
Lories, coccidiosis in, 181
Lower motor neuron bladder, in rabbits, 392-394
Lower respiratory disease, in birds, 217-218
Lower respiratory tract disorders, in rabbits, 390-392
Lower urinary tract disorders, in rabbits, 392-394
Lower urinary tract infection, in ferrets, 498-500
Lufenuron, 22
Lung, eye, and trachea disease, 105-106
Lung carcinoma, in birds, 236
Lung wash
in birds, 545, 546f
in reptiles, 535
Lungworms, 60-62
Luteinizing hormone, 430
Lymphoblastic lymphoma, in ferrets, 471-475
Lymphocystis, in fish, 32-33
Lymphocyte count, 625-627
Lymphocytic choriomeningitis virus, 713-714
Lymphocytosis, 626
Lymphoma
chemotherapy for, 472, 473t-474t, 474-475
in ferrets, 453, 471-475
splenomegaly caused by, 497
Lymphopenia, 626-627
Lymphoplasmacytic encephalomyelitis, 222-225
Lymphoplasmacytic enteritis, 465
Lymphoplasmacytic gastritis, 203
Lymphosarcoma
in birds, 235
in ferrets, 471-475
in rabbits, 395-396, 413
Lymphs, 625-627
Lyssa, 722-724
Lyssavirus, 722-724

M

Macaw(s)
amylase in, 602-603
blood collection in, 547f
cloacal papillomas in, 215
erythrocytes in, 644
feather picking in, 184-185
foreign bodies in, 189f
oral papillomas in, 215
proventricular dilatation disease in, 169, 222-225, 224f
venipuncture in, 547f
zinc levels in, 651t
Macaw wasting syndrome, 222-225
Macrorhabdus ornithogaster, 203
Mad dog, 722-724
Malachite green
Aphanomyces spp. treated with, 25
saprolegniasis treated with, 25
Malassezia dermatitis, 362
Malignancy, in hedgehogs, 324-325
Malignant lymphoma, 351
in ferrets, 471-475
in rabbits, 395-396
Malignant melanoma
in birds, 235
in rabbits, 351
Malignant peripheral nerve sheath tumors, in rabbits, 351-352
Malocclusion, in rabbits, 355-360
Mammary gland disorders, in rabbits, 397-398
Mammary mass, in small mammals, 680
Mammary tumors, in rats, 243-245, 245f
Mange
demodectic, 298
ear, 403-405
in ferrets, 447
notoedric, 326
psoroptic, 403-405
in rabbits, 403-405
sarcoptic, 279, 447
Mannitol
head trauma in birds treated with, 208
in rabbits, 339-340
Marine equivalent *Cryptocaryon irritans*, 33-34
Marine equivalent *Uronema*, 33-34
Marine head and lateral line erosion, 30-31
Marine ich, 33-34
Market men's disease, 730-732
Maropitant, 188
Mast cell tumors, 496f
Mastitis
in ferrets, 475-477
in rabbits, 397-398
Mean corpuscular hemoglobin concentration, in birds, 150
Mean corpuscular value, in birds, 150
Mebendazole, 23
Medial metatarsal vein, 546
Medicated foods, in fish, 514-515
Meeh coefficients, for body surface area conversions, 610
Megabacteriosis, in birds, 203-204
Megacolon syndrome, 387
Megaesophagus, in ferrets, 477-478, 478f
Melarsomine, in ferrets, 443
Melatonin
in ferrets, 432, 490
in rats, 244
Melena, 203
Melissococcus pluton, 4
Meloxicam, 109
in amphibians, 51, 68
in birds, 166, 169
in chinchillas, 304

Meloxicam *(Continued)*
cloacal prolapse treated with, 51, 166
constipation in birds treated with, 169
in degus, 320
in ferrets, 476
in guinea pigs, 253, 267, 269, 283
in hamsters, 286, 289
in hedgehogs, 325
in mice, 567
in prairie dogs, 317
in rabbits, 398, 408, 553, 562, 567
in rats, 567
in sugar gliders, 328
Meningeal plague, 721
Merrillite, 650-651
Metabizium anisopliae, 8
Metabolic acidosis, 634
Metabolic alkalosis, 634
Metabolic bone disease
in amphibians, 62-64
in sugar gliders, 329-330
Metabolic neuropathies, in birds, 159
Methimazole, in guinea pigs, 261
Methionine, 104
Methylprednisolone sodium succinate, in ferrets, 438
Metoclopramide
in birds, 224, 227
in guinea pigs, 254
in rabbits, 389
Metomidate, 514
Metopimazine, 188
Metronidazole
amoebiasis treated with, 49
anaerobes treated with, 227
antibiotic-associated enterocolitis treated with, 293
in chinchillas, 304, 310
cryptosporidiosis treated with, 137
entamoebiasis treated with, 101
in ferrets, 449
flagellate enterocolitis treated with, 55
giardiasis treated with, 449
in guinea pigs, 254, 265, 269
in hamsters, 290
Hexamita treated with, 29-30
Lawsonia intracellularis treated with, 293
Spironucleus treated with, 29-30
Mice
amylase in, 603
blood pressure in, 549
blood urea nitrogen in, 609t
chromodacryorrhea in, 242-243
cryptosporidiosis in, 700-701
dermatophytosis in, 704
intussusception in, 568
leptospirosis in, 711
lymphocytic choriomeningitis virus in, 713
rectal prolapse in, 568
thyroid hormones in, 649t
Microhematocrit method, 645
Microhepatica, 201
Microsporidiosis, 705-708
Milk thistle, 203, 384
Mites
in birds, 177-178
demodectic, 251, 297-298
ear, 445-446
in ferrets, 445-446
fur, 279
in invertebrates, 12-13
in lizards, 99
ophioptid, 98
parasitic, 12-13
predatory, 13
in rats, 251
Mites *(Continued)*
in reptiles, 98-99
saprophytic, 12-13
sarcoptic
in hamsters, 297-298
in rats, 251
in snakes, 98-99
in tortoises, 99
trombiculid, 98
in turtles, 99
Mollusks
ectoparasites in, 12-13
fluid administration in, 508
Monitor lizards, entamoebiasis in, 100
Monocyte count, 628-629
Monocytic leukemia, 628
Monocytosis, 628-629
Monogenean parasites, 22-24
Moon blindness, 711
Morphine
in ferrets, 553, 562
in mice, 567
in rabbits, 553, 562, 567
in rats, 567
Mosquitoes, in birds, 177-178
Motile aeromonad infection, 17-18
Mouse fever, 711
Mouth rot, in reptiles, 132-134, 145-147
Moxidectin, in ferrets, 443-444
MRM, 249-250
MS 222 anesthesia, 513-514
Mucoid enteropathy, 347, 387, 390f, 621
Mucometra, 425
Mucor ramosissimus, 91
Mucosa-associated lymphoid tissue lymphoma, 471-475
Mud fever, 711
Murine respiratory mycoplasmosis, 249-250
Mustela putorius furo, 461
Mycobacteriosis
in amphibians, 59-60, 59f
in fish, 17-19
in reptiles, 117-118
Mycobacterium spp.
in birds, 202
in fish, 17
granulomas, 153
lower respiratory tract disease caused by, 141
M. marinum granuloma, 715-716
M. tuberculosis, 117-118
Mycoplasma spp.
M. pulmonis, 249-250
in reptiles, 118-120, 141-143
Mycoses
in birds, 204-206
in invertebrates, 8-9
Mycosis fungoides, in ferrets, 471-475
Mycotic granulomatosis, 24
Mycotic infection, in birds, 155-157
Myelography, in birds, 208
Myelolipoma, in birds, 234-235
Myelosuppression, 472
Myenteric ganglioneuritis, 222-225
Mynahs
ascites in, 153
coccidiosis in, 181
Myocardial disease, in rabbits, 341-342
Myocarditis, 157
Myofascitis, 478-479
Myxomatosis, 398-401
Myxosarcoma, 351

N

Na, 647-648
Na^+, 647-648
N-Acetylcysteine, 196, 269, 317
Nail trimming, in birds, 214, 215f
Narcolepsy, 594t
Nasal discharge, 589
Nasal flush, in birds, 544, 544f-545f
Nasal irrigation, in birds, 544, 544f-545f
Nasolacrimal cannulation, of rabbits, 563-564
Nasolacrimal duct inflammation, in rabbits, 352-354
Natt-Herrick method, 637-638
Nausea, in birds, 225-227
Navigator. *See* Nitazoxanide
Nebulization
in birds, 218, 231
in rats, 250
Necrobacillosis, in rabbits, 360-364
Necrotizing acute disease, in Texas tortoises, 91
Necrotizing mycotic dermatitis, 91
Necrotizing typhlitis, 182
Nematodes
in fish, 27-28
in hamsters, 293
panagrolaimidae oral, in tarantulas, 13-14
in rabbits, 374-376
in reptiles, 137
Nematodiasis
in amphibians, 60-62
in rabbits, 375, 387, 389
in reptiles, 120-121
Neobenedenia spp., 23
Neonatal disease, in ferrets, 479-481
Neoplasia
in birds, 159
in hedgehogs, 324-325
Nephrocalcinosis, 246
Nephropathia endemica, 709
Nephropathy
in ferrets, 491-494
in hamsters, 295-297
in rats, 245-247
Nephrotic syndrome, in hamsters, 295
Neurofibrosarcoma, in rabbits, 351-352
Neuroglycopenia, 469
Neurologic deficits, in birds, 207-209
Neurologic diseases and disorders
in birds, 159-161, 207-209
in guinea pigs, 266-267
Neurologic signs, 590
Neuro-otitis, in guinea pigs, 267f
Neuropathic gastric dilatation, 222-225
Neutropenia, 472
Neutrophil-heterophil count, 629-633
Neutrophilia, 629-633
Neutrophil-polymorphonuclear cells, 629-633
New tank syndrome, 47-48
Newcastle disease, 182
NH^{4+}, 601-602
Nitazoxanide
coccidiosis treated with, 88
cryptosporidiosis treated with, 90, 137, 702
Nitrate, 45, 45t-46t
Nonsteroidal anti-inflammatory drugs
in birds, 169, 224, 229, 236
constipation treated with, 169
in ferrets, 453
in rabbits, 336, 358, 380, 393, 398, 406, 408, 427
Nontyphoid salmonellosis, 726-729
Normosol, 560-561
Notoedres muris, 691
Notoedric mange, 326
Nuclear polyhedrosis viruses, 16
Nursery web spider, baculovirus in, 16
Nutritional disorders, in sugar gliders, 329-330

Nutritional neuropathies, in birds, 159
Nutritional osteodystrophy, 329-330
Nutritional secondary hyperparathyroidism
in amphibians, 62-64
in reptiles, 121-125, 128
in sugar gliders, 329-330
Nutritional support
in birds, 227, 233
in guinea pigs, 265, 275-276
Nystagmus, in birds, 159-161
Nystatin
in birds, 205-206, 227
in guinea pigs, 265

O

Obesity, in rabbits, 401-402
Obstipation, in birds, 168-170
Ocular disorders
in chinchillas, 311-313
in guinea pigs, 268-269
in hamsters, 293-295, 295f
in small mammals, 681
Ocular hypertension, 338-341
Ocular lesions
in birds, 209-212
in rabbits, 372
Ocular microsporidiosis, 707
Ocular trauma, in birds, 211
Oculoglandular tularemia, 731
Oculomotor nerve deficit, 581
Odontoma, in prairie dogs, 316-318
Odontoprisis, 590
17-OH progesterone, 598-599
O'Hara's disease, 730-732
Oil gland, 237-239
Olfactory nerve deficit, 581
Omega-3 fatty acids
hyperuricemia in birds treated with, 192
in rabbits, 415
Omeprazole
in birds, 227
in ferrets, 452
Oomycetosis, 64-65
Open fracture, 190
Ophioptid mites, 98
Ophthalmia periodica, 711
Ophthalmic neonatorum, 479-481
Ophthalmic surgery, in fish, 516
Ophthalmologic lesions, in birds, 209-212
Opioids
in guinea pigs, 259
in rabbits, 394, 398, 408
Opisthotonos, 590
OPMV, 127-128
Optic nerve deficit, 581
Oral cavity abscesses, in reptiles, 72
Oral medications, in fish, 514-515
Oral nematodes, panagrolaimidae, in tarantulas, 13-14
Oral papillomas, in birds, 215
Orbital abscess, in birds, 148
Orchiectomy, 555-557
Organ prolapse, in reptiles, 85-87
Organophosphates
acetylcholinesterase binding by, 212
ectoparasites treated with, 21-22
monogeneans treated with, 23
toxicity, in birds, 212-213
Ornithonyssus spp., 177-178, 251, 690-694
Ornithosis, 161-163, 697-699
Oropharyngeal tularemia, 731
Orthomyxoviridae, 468-469
Orthopedics, in reptiles, 125-127
Oryctolagus cuniculus, 381
Osteoarthritis, in rabbits, 334-336
Osteoarthrosis, in rabbits, 334-336
Osteoma
in birds, 235
in ferrets, 481-482, 482f
Osteomyelitis, 133-134, 521, 536
Osteosarcoma
in birds, 235
in rabbits, 351
Otitis, in rabbits, 403-405, 429
Otitis externa, 403-405, 429
Otitis interna, 403-405
Otitis labyrinthitis, 403-405
Otitis media, 403-405, 429
Otoacariasis, 403-405
Otodectes cynotis, 445-446
Ovarian cancer, in ferrets, 482-484
Ovarian cysts
in gerbils, 299-300
in guinea pigs, 269-271, 271f, 284
Ovarian disease, in gerbils, 299-300
Ovarian neoplasia
in ferrets, 482-484
in gerbils, 299-300
Ovarian neoplasms, in birds, 235
Ovarian remnant syndrome, in ferrets, 484-485
Ovarian tumors
in ferrets, 482-484
in gerbils, 299-300
Ovariectomy, 564-566
Ovariohysterectomy, 284, 406, 463, 564-566
Ovariohysterovaginectomy, 564-566
Overgrown beaks and claws, in birds, 213-214, 215f
Overweight, in rabbits, 401-402
Oviductal neoplasms, in birds, 235
Oviductal prolapse
in amphibians, 51-52
in birds, 166f
in reptiles, 86
Ovocentesis, 527
Oxycentesis, 176
Oxygen therapy
in birds, 218, 221
in prairie dogs, 317
Oxymorphone, in rabbits, 567
Oxytetracycline, *Chlamydophila psittaci* treated with, 163, 167
Oxytocin, in birds, 176

P

Pacheco's disease, 182
Packed cell volume, 150, 622-623
Packed red cells, 622-623
Paecilomycosis, 90-92
Paenibacillus larvae, 4
Pain
in birds, 233
in rabbits, 567
in rodents, 567
Painful abdomen, in small mammals, 682
Panagrolaimidae oral nematodes, in tarantulas, 13-14
Pancreatectomy, 470
Pancreatic tumors, in birds, 235
Panuveitis, in rabbits, 426-428
Papillomas, in birds, 215-216, 235
Papillomatosis, 165, 215-216
Papillosum cyprinid, 43-44
Paracetamol, 464
Parakeets, 229f
Paralysis, in birds, 159-161, 207, 212-213
Paramyxovirus infection, in reptiles, 127-128
Paraphimosis
in chinchillas, 313-315
in reptiles, 128-130
Parasambonia spp., 130
Parasites. *See also* Ectoparasites; Endoparasites; Lice; Mites
diarrhea in reptiles caused by, 94
in ferrets, 447-450, 449f
monogenean, 22-24
in rabbits, 361, 363, 366-367, 367f, 374-376
in rats, 251-252
in reptiles, 98-99, 662
Parasitic mites, in invertebrates, 12-13
Paraspidodera uncinata, 264
Parathyroid hormone, 123
Paresis
in birds, 159-161, 207
in rabbits, 335
in small mammals, 683
Parovarian cyst, in guinea pigs, 269-271
Parrot(s)
amylase in, 602-603
Aspergillus spp. in, 155
cardiac disease in, 157
coelomic cavity of, fungal plaque in, 156f
feather picking in, 184-185
restraint of, 543-544, 543f
vitamin A deficiency in, 199-201, 199f
Parrot fever, 161-163
Partial seizures, 594t
Parturient disorders, in guinea pigs, 275-276
Parvovirus, 94
Passeriformes, 240
Passerines, 209
Pasteurella dagmatis, 717
Pasteurella multocida, 369, 405-407, 425, 428-430, 717-719
Pasteurella pneumotropica, 717
Pasteurellosis, 405-407, 717-719
Pathologic fractures, 190
Pb, 623-624
Pelonia spp., 130
Pelvic limb fractures, 126
Penguins, *Aspergillus* spp. in, 155
Penicillamine, in birds, 169, 193, 227
Penicillin, in rabbits, 422
Penile disorders, in chinchillas, 313-315, 316f
Penis prolapse, in reptiles, 128-130
Pentastomiasis, 130-131
Periapical abscesses
in degus, 321
in guinea pigs, 256
in hamsters, 290
in rabbits, 355-360
Periarticular fibrosis, 335
Pericarditis, 392f
Perineal dermatitis, in rabbits, 361-362
Perineal sac impaction, in guinea pigs, 271-272
Periodontal disease
in chinchillas, 302-305
in degus, 319-322
in ferrets, 441-442
in lizards, 132-134
in reptiles, 132-134, 145-147
Periorbital abscess, in birds, 148
Periprostatic cysts, in ferrets, 488-491
Peritonitis, 538
Periurethral cysts, in ferrets, 488-491
Persistent estrus, 484-485
Persistent hyperglycemia, in reptiles, 107-108
Persistent hypocalcemia, in reptiles, 121
Pesticide exposure, in invertebrates, 11-12
pH, 44, 633-636
Phacoemulsification, 436
Phaeohyphomycosis, 90-92
Phantom pregnancy, 411-412
Pharyngeal plague, 720
Pheasants, cryptosporidiosis in, 181
Phenobarbital sodium, in birds, 160, 208
Phenoxybenzamine, in ferrets, 490

Phimosis, in chinchillas, 313-315
Phlebotomy
in birds, 546-547
in reptiles, 533-534
Phosphate, 636-637
Phosphorus, 636-637
Physaliferous cells, 438
Physical vapor deposition, 428-430
Pica, 187, 454
Pigeons
coccidiosis in, 181
enteritis in, 181
Piloerection, 501f
Pimobendan, 342
in ferrets, 459
in hamsters, 288
Pimple, in birds, 147-149
"Pine-cone" disease, 20-21
Pink belly disease, 65-67
Pinworms, in rabbits, 374-376
Pionus parrots
Aspergillus spp. in, 155
mycoses in, 204
Piperacillin, 137
lower respiratory tract disease treated with, 142
Pirhemocyton spp., 114-115
Piscinoodinium, 34
Pituitary tumors
in birds, 235
in rats, 243-245, 245f
Plague, 719-721
Plasmalyte, 561
Plastral infection, 77-79
Platelet count, 637-639
Plumbism, 192-194, 623-624
Pneumococcal infection, in rats, 248-249
Pneumonia
in birds, 217-218
in guinea pigs, 276-278
in reptiles, 141-143
Pneumonic plague, 719-721
Pneumonic tularemia, 731
Pododermatitis
in birds, 219-221, 220f
in guinea pigs, 273-275, 274f, 278-280
in hamsters, 298
in rabbits, 407-409, 408f
Poisoning, in invertebrates, 11-12
Pollakiuria, 413
Polposipus herculaenus, 8
Polychromatophilic erythrocyte, 646-647
Polycystic kidney disease, in hamsters, 286, 295-297
Polycythemia, 622, 643
Polydipsia, 392-393, 591-592
Polyhedrosis viruses, 16
Polymer fume fever, 221
Polymethyl methacrylate, antibiotic-impregnated
for pododermatitis
in birds, 220
in rabbits, 408-409
for septic arthritis in rabbits, 336
Polymyositis, 478-479
Polyostotic hyperostosis, 186
Polyphagia, 591
Polytetrafluoroethylene toxicity, 217, 221
Polyuria, 392-393, 591-592
Pond turtles, bacterial dermatitis in, 78
Poor body condition, in birds, 180-181
Porocephalus spp., 130
Positive-pressure ventilation, 368
Posterior uveitis, in rabbits, 426-428
Post-estrus anemia, in ferrets, 462-463
Potassium, 640-642
Potassium bromide, in birds, 160
Povidone-iodine, fungal infections treated with, 9
Prairie dogs
blood urea nitrogen in, 609t
odontoma in, 316-318
plague in, 720
tularemia in, 730
Pralidoxime chloride, organophosphate toxicity treated with, 213
Praziquantel
cestodes treated with, 27-28, 183, 265, 293
in chinchillas, 310
monogeneans treated with, 23
spirochid trematodes treated with, 83
trematodes treated with, 168, 183
Prazosin, in ferrets, 490
Prednisolone
in birds, 160
in ferrets, 470
in guinea pigs, 269
in rabbits, 395
Prednisolone sodium succinate, in birds, 160
Prednisone
in ferrets, 450, 453, 470, 473t
in prairie dogs, 317
Preen gland, 237-239
Prefemoral coeliotomy, 528
Pregnancy disorders, in guinea pigs, 275-276
Pregnancy toxemia
in ferrets, 486-487
in guinea pigs, 275-276
in rabbits, 409-410
Preovulatory egg binding, in birds, 185-186
Preputial abscess, 314
Pressure sores, in rabbits, 407-409
Primary hyperparathyroidism, 637
Prochlorperazine, in rabbits, 370
Progesterone, 598-599
Progressive syndrome of acquired dental disease, in rabbits, 355-360
Prokinetics, in rabbits, 388
Prolapse, in reptiles, 663
Proliferating pool, 629
Proliferative bowel disease, 453, 465, 487-488
Proliferative colitis, 465, 487-488
Proliferative enteritis, in rabbits, 385-390
Proliferative ileitis, 291-293
Proliferative spinal osteoarthropathy, in reptiles, 135-136
Proliferative spinal osteopathy, in reptiles, 135-136
Proligestone, 484
Prolonged immersion treatment, in fish, 517-518
Propentofylline, wing tip edema treated with, 179
Proptosis, 294
Prostaglandin E2, in birds, 176
Prostaglandin $F_{2\alpha}$, 412
Prostatic abscess, in ferrets, 488-491
Prostatic cysts, in ferrets, 488-491
Prostatic disease, in ferrets, 488-491
Prostatitis, in ferrets, 488-491
Prostatomegaly, in ferrets, 488-491
Protein overload nephropathy, 296
Protozoal parasites. *See also* Cestodes; Nematodes
in birds, 201
in fish, 28-29
in rabbits, 374-376, 387
in reptiles, 100-101
Proventricular adenocarcinoma, in birds, 235
Proventriculotomy, 188-189, 227
Proventricular dilatation disease, in birds, 169, 222-225, 223f
Proventricular dilatation syndrome, 222-225
Pruritus, in rabbits, 360-364
Pseudocapillaroides xenopi, 61
Pseudochylous ascites, 153
Pseudocyesis, 411-412
Pseudogout, 103
Pseudomonas spp., 142
P. aeruginosa, 312-313
Pseudopregnancy, in rabbits, 411-412
Pseudopterygium, in rabbits, 349-351
Pseudotuberculosis, 248-249
Psittaciformes, 239-240
Psittacines
basal metabolic rate of, 539
beak and feather disease, 239-240, 241f
blood collection in, 546
cardiac disease in, 157
cloaca of, 216
crop stasis in, 226
cryptosporidiosis in, 181
encephalitozoonosis in, 706
proventricular dilatation disease in, 222-225
salmonellosis in, 727
Psittacosis, 161-163, 167, 697-699
Psoroptes cuniculi, 366-367, 404
Psoroptic mange, 403-405
Psoroptic scabies, 403-405
Pullorum disease, 726-729
Pulmonary edema
in birds, 218
in rabbits, 368
Pulse oximetry, 549
Pustule, in birds, 147-149
Putting to sleep, 506
Pyelonephritis
in ferrets, 492
in rabbits, 412-415
Pyoderma
in guinea pigs, 278-280
in hamsters, 298
in rats, 251-252
Pyometra, 286, 425
Pyometra endometritis, in guinea pigs, 284
Pyrantel pamoate, ascarids treated with, 183
Pyrethins, 447
Pyrethrin
lice treated with, 178
ticks treated with, 178
Pyrimethamine, in rabbits, 376
Pythonella spp., 87-89

Q

Quail
cryptosporidiosis in, 181
ulcerative enteritis, 182
Quaker parrots, feather picking in, 184-185

R

Rabbit(s)
abdominal distention in, 384
abscesses in, 331-332, 332f
acariasis in, 690-694
alkaline phosphate in, 603
amylase in, 602-603
anesthesia in, 547-549, 552
anorexia in, 333-334, 334f, 384
arthritis in, 334-336
behavioral disorders in, 337-338
biliary cystadenoma in, 385f
biliverdin in, 608
bites by, 695-696
blood pressure in, 549
blood transfusion in, 551-552
blood urea nitrogen in, 609t
buphthalmia in, 338-341, 340f

Rabbit(s) *(Continued)*
calcium in, 610-612
cardiovascular disease in, 341-342
castration in, 556
cataracts in, 342-344, 374f
cherry eye in, 344-345, 346f
cholesterol in, 613
coccidiosis in, 346-348, 348f, 387, 389
conjunctival disorders in, 349-351, 353
conjunctivitis in, 423-424
cryptosporidiosis in, 700-701
cutaneous lymphoma in, 420f
cutaneous masses in, 351-352
dacryocystitis in, 352-354, 355f
dangerous antibiotics in, 582
dental disease in, 355-360
dermatophytosis in, 360-364, 704
dermopathies in, 360-364
diabetes mellitus in, 620
diarrhea in, 384
dysautonomia in, 364-365, 387
echocardiography in, 558t
ectoparasites in, 361, 363, 366-367, 367f
electrocardiography in, 559t
electrocution in, 368-369, 369f
encephalitis in, 369-371
encephalitozoonosis in, 371-374, 706-707
endoparasites in, 374-376
epiphora in, 352-354
erythrocytes in, 645
feeding tube placement in, 559-560
fibrinous pleuritis in, 392f
floppy rabbit syndrome in, 376-378, 378f
fluid therapy in, 560-561
gastric disorders in, 378-381, 380f
glaucoma in, 338-341
glucose levels in, 619-622
grass sickness in, 364-365
handling of, 568-569
hemorrhagic disease in, 381-383
hepatic disorders in, 383-385
hepatic lipidosis in, 384
hyperglycemia in, 619-622
hypervitaminosis D in, 413-414
intestinal disorders in, 385-390
intubation technique in, 562-563
lead
blood levels of, 624
toxicity caused by, 389, 624
lower respiratory tract disorders in, 390-392
lower urinary tract disorders in, 392-394
lymphosarcoma in, 395-396, 413
mammary gland disorders in, 397-398
myxomatosis in, 398-401
nasolacrimal cannulation of, 563-564
nematodiasis in, 375, 387, 389
obesity in, 401-402
otitis in, 403-405
ovariohysterectomy in, 564-566
pain management in, 368, 562
pain recognition in, 567
pasteurellosis in, 405-407
pericarditis in, 392f
platelet count in, 639
pododermatitis in, 407-409, 408f
pregnancy toxemia in, 409-410
pseudopregnancy in, 411-412
pseudopterygium in, 349-351
renal disorders in, 412-415
restraint of, 568-569
salmonellosis in, 727-728
splayleg in, 416-417
staphylococcosis in, 417-419
testicular tumors in, 419
third eyelid protrusion in, 344-345
thrombocytopenia in, 639

Rabbit(s) *(Continued)*
thymoma in, 420-421
torticollis in, 371f
treponematosis in, 421-422
tularemia in, 730-731
upper respiratory tract disorders in, 423-424
uterine disorders in, 424-426
uveitis in, 426-428
vestibular disease in, 428-430
Rabbit calicivirus disease, 381-383
Rabbit fever, 730-732
Rabbit gastrointestinal syndrome, 378-381, 385-390
Rabbit syphilis, 421-422
Rabies, 722-724
Raccoon rabies, 722
Radiographs
in birds
for ascites, 154
for proventricular dilatation disease, 223
for regurgitation/vomiting evaluations, 226
for renal disease evaluations, 228
in guinea pigs, 259
Radiotherapy, in birds, 236
Raillietiella spp., 130
Rain rot, 92-93
Rainbow boas, 95
Ranavirus disease, 114-115
Ranitidine, 247
in ferrets, 452
in guinea pigs, 254
in rabbits, 388
Rapid tissue degeneration, 10
Rat(s)
alkaline phosphate in, 603
amylase in, 603
anesthesia monitoring in, 547-549
bile acids in, 607t
bites by, 695
blood pressure in, 549
castration in, 556
chromodacryorrhea in, 242-243
cryptosporidiosis in, 700-701
dermatophytosis in, 251-252, 704
intubation technique in, 563
leptospirosis in, 711
mammary tumors in, 243-245, 245f
ovariohysterectomy in, 564-566
pituitary tumors in, 243-245, 245f
renal disease in, 245-247
respiratory tract disease in
acute, 248-249
chronic, 249-250
skin diseases in, 251-252
Streptobacillus moniliformis in, 724
thyroid hormones in, 649t
Rat bite fever, 724-726
Rat fur mite, 251
Rattlesnakes
calicivirus infection in, 79
metronidazole dosing in, 137-138
Recombinant tissue-plasminogen activator, 211
Rectal impaction, in guinea pigs, 271-272
Rectal prolapse
in amphibians, 51-52
in chinchillas, 308-311
in guinea pigs, 568
in hamsters, 568
in mice, 568
Red blood cell count, 643-646
Red cell distribution width, in birds, 150
Red fox rabies, 722
Red leg disease, 65-67, 66f
Red spot disease, 24

Red tears, in rats, 242-243
Red-footed tortoises, 100
Red-tailed hawks, 155
Regranex, 30
Regurgitation
in birds, 225-227
differential diagnosis of, 592
in reptiles, 136-138, 664
Renal azotemia
in rabbits, 412-415
in rats, 247
Renal coccidiosis, in amphibians, 52
Renal compromise, in birds, 228-229
Renal cystic disease, 492
Renal disease
in birds, 228-229
in hamsters, 295-297
in rats, 245-247
in reptiles, 138-140
Renal disorders
in ferrets, 491-494, 495f
in rabbits, 412-415
Renal failure
in birds, 228-229
differential diagnosis of, 593
in ferrets, 491-494
phosphorus levels affected by, 636
in rabbits, 412-415
Renal fibrosis, in rabbits, 413
Renal insufficiency
in ferrets, 491-494
in rabbits, 412-415
in rats, 247
Renal reserve, 412, 491
Renal tumors, in birds, 236
Renin-angiotensin-aldosterone system, 647
Reovirus infections
in birds, 202
in reptiles, 140-141
Reproductive tract abscess, in birds, 148
Reptiles. *See also specific reptile*
abscesses in, 71-74, 520-521
acariasis in, 690
adenovirus infection in, 74-75
aggression in, 75-77
alkaline phosphate in, 603
assisted shedding in, 522-523
azurophil count in, 604
bacterial dermatitis in, 77-79
basophil count, 605-606
bite wounds in, 536, 536f
bites by, 696
blood collection in, 533-534
blood pH in, 635-636
blood pressure in, 523-524
blood urea nitrogen in, 609t
calcium in, 610-612
calcium-to-phosphorus ratio in, 637
calicivirus infection in, 79-80
cardiac disease in, 82-84
cardiopulmonary-cerebral resuscitation in, 524-525
central nervous system signs in, 657-659
chlamydophilosis in, 84-85
chloride in, 612
cloacal prolapse in, 85-87
coccidiosis in, 87-89
constipation in, 660
creatinine in, 615
cryptosporidiosis in, 89-90, 137, 700-701
dangerous antibiotics in, 582
defensive behavior in, 76
dermatomycosis in, 90-92
dermatophilosis in, 92-93
diarrhea in, 93-95, 104, 661
dysecdysis in, 95-97
dystocia in, 526-528

Reptiles *(Continued)*
ectoparasites in, 98-99
entamoebiasis in, 100-101
eosinophil count in, 616-617
erythrocytes in, 645-646
fecal examination in, 529
fecal sample collection in, 525-526
fracture repair in, 125-127
fungal disease in, 80-82
glomerular filtration rate study in, 529
glucose levels in, 619-622
gout in, 101-103
handling of, 530-531
hepatic lipidosis in, 103-105
herpesvirus infections in, 105-106
heteropenia in, 632-633
heterophilia in, 632-633
hyperglycemia in, 107-108
hyperkalemia in, 640
hypervitaminosis A in, 108-109
hypokalemia in, 641
hypovitaminosis A in, 110-112
inclusion body disease of snakes, 113-114, 113f
injections in, 531-533
intracardiac injections in, 531
intracoelomic injections in, 531-533
iridovirus infection in, 114-115
kidneys of, 140
lead placement in, 524t
liver disease in, 115-117
lung wash in, 535
lymphocytosis in, 626
lymphopenia in, 626-627
medication administration in, 531-533
mites in, 98-99
monocytosis in, 628
mycobacteriosis in, 117-118
Mycoplasma spp., 118-120
nematodes in, 137
nematodiasis in, 120-121
neutrophilia in, 630-631
nutritional secondary hyperparathyroidism in, 121-125
orthopedics in, 125-127
paramyxovirus infection in, 127-128
paraphimosis in, 128-130
parasites in, 662
pentastomes in, 130-131
periodontal disease in, 132-134, 145-147
phlebotomy in, 533-534
pneumonia in, 141-143
prolapse in, 663
proliferative spinal osteoarthropathy in, 135-136
rain rot in, 92-93
regurgitation in, 136-138, 664
renal disease in, 138-140
reovirus infections in, 140-141
reproductive behavior in, 76
respiratory tract disease in, 141-143
restraint of, 530-531
salmonella in, 143-145
salmonellosis in, 141, 143-145, 727-728
sampling collection in, 525-526
swellings in, 665
territorial behavior in, 76
thermal burns in, 536
thrombocytes in, 639
thrombocytopenia in, 639
total protein in, 642
tracheal wash in, 535
transtracheal sample collection in, 525-526
unspecific problem/not doing well algorithm for, 666
uric acid in, 649-650
urinalysis in, 525-526

Reptiles *(Continued)*
vomiting in, 136-138, 667
weight loss in, 668
wound care in, 535-536
Reserve crown, 302
Respiratory acidosis, 634-635
Respiratory alkalosis, 634
Respiratory cryptosporidiosis, 702
Respiratory rate, 548
Respiratory tract disease and disorders
in ferrets, 440
in guinea pigs, 276-278
in rabbits, 390-392, 423-424
in rats
acute, 248-249
chronic, 249-250
in reptiles, 141-143
Restraint
of amphibians, 520
of birds, 543-544, 543f
of invertebrates, 509-510, 509f
of rabbits, 568-569
of reptiles, 530-531
Restrictive cardiomyopathy, in ferrets, 458
Retained molt, 7-8
Retained shed
in invertebrates, 7-8
in reptiles, 95-97
Reticulated boas, 143
Reticulated pythons, 71
Reticulocyte count, 646-647
Retinochoroiditis, in rabbits, 426-428
Retrobulbar abscess, in hamsters, 294
Retrobulbar fat prolapse, 345
Rhabdias infection, 60-62
Rhabdomyoma, in birds, 235
Rhabdomyosarcoma, in rabbits, 351
RHD virus, 383
Rheumatoid arthritis, 335
Rhinitis, in rabbits, 423-424
Ribavirin, in birds, 224
Rice field fever, 711
Ringtail, 251
Ringworm
in guinea pigs, 278-280
in rats, 251-252
Rodent(s). *See also* Mice; Rat(s)
acariasis in, 691
anesthesia monitoring in, 547-549
bites by, 695-696
blood transfusion in, 552
castration in, 556
feeding tube placement in, 559-560
fluid therapy in, 560-561
glucose levels in, 619-622
handling of, 568-569
intubation technique in, 562-563
pain recognition in, 567
restraint of, 568-569
salmonellosis in, 727-728
Rodent plague, 719-721
Rodentolepis nana, 309
Romet-30, 18-19
Rose-breasted cockatoos, 157
Rostral abrasions, 536
Rotavirus, 182, 387
Rough-legged hawks, 155
Round cell sarcoma, 237f
Roundworms
in amphibians, 60-62
in fish, 27-28
Rubber jaw, 62-64
Runny nose, in birds, 230-231
Runny stool, in birds, 173-175
Russian hamsters
cataracts in, 293
cheek pouch disorder in, 288

S

"Saddleback", 17
S-adenosyl-methionine, 196
Salamander
hypovitaminosis A in, 58f
mycobacteriosis in, 59f
Salinity, 45
Salmonella, in reptiles, 143-145
Salmonella spp., 143-145, 264, 726-729
Salmonellosis, 726-729
in rabbits, 387
in reptiles, 141, 143-145
Salpingohysterectomy, 166
"Salt-water furunculosis", 17
Sambonia spp., 130
Sampling collection, in reptiles, 525-526
San Miguel sea lion virus, 79-80
SAP, 601
Saprolegnia spp., 24
Saprolegniasis
in amphibians, 64-65
in fish, 24-26
Saprophytic mites, 12-13
Sarcocystis, 201
Sarcocystis spp., 87-89
Sarcoptes scabiei, 690-691, 693
Sarcoptic mange, 279, 447
Sarcoptic mites
in hamsters, 297-298
in rats, 251
Scabies
in ferrets, 447
in guinea pigs, 278-280
Scaly leg mite, 177
Scent gland abscesses, in reptiles, 72-73, 521
Schellackia spp., 87-89
Schmorl's disease, 360-364
Scintigraphy imaging, in birds, 208
Scurvy, in guinea pigs, 262-263
Sebaceous adenitis, in rabbits, 362
Sebaceous gland carcinoma, in rabbits, 351
Sebekia spp., 130
Second-degree AV block, in ferrets, 456-458
Seizures
in birds, 159-161, 207-209
differential diagnosis of, 590, 593-594, 594t
in ferrets, 470
grand mal, 594t
in guinea pigs, 266-267
partial, 594t
Selamectin, 252, 279, 326, 367, 446
Selfia spp., 130
Self-mutilation, in rabbits, 360-364
Seminomas
in birds, 235
in rabbits, 419
Septic arthritis, in rabbits, 334-336
Septicemia
in amphibians, 65-67, 66f
in arachnids, 4
enteric, of catfish, 17
Septicemic cutaneous ulcerative disease, 78
Septicemic plague, 719-721
Serous cysts, in guinea pigs, 269-271
Serpulina pilosicoli, 182
Sertoli cell tumors
in birds, 235
in rabbits, 419
Serum glutamic-pyruvic transaminase, 599-600
Serum protein, 642-643
Seven-day fever, 711
Shedding disorder, in reptiles, 95-97
Shell fractures, in chelonians, 126
Shell rot, 90-92
Shell trauma, in invertebrates, 507-508
Short-tongue syndrome, 57-59

Silkworms, 8
Simethicone
 in birds, 224
 in guinea pigs, 254
Sin Nombre virus, 708
Sinusitis, in birds, 230-231
Skin abscesses
 in hamsters, 298
 in rats, 252
Skin biopsy, in birds, 178
Skin cancer, in ferrets, 495-496
Skin diseases
 in guinea pigs, 278-280
 in hamsters, 297-299, 299f
 in hedgehogs, 325-326, 326f
 in rats, 251-252
Skin neoplasia, in ferrets, 495-496
Skin scrape
 in birds, 178
 in fish, 510
Skin tumors, in ferrets, 495-496
Skunks, 722
Sludgy urine, in rabbits, 392-394
Sludgy urine syndrome, in rabbits, 392-394
Small mammals. *See also* Chinchillas; Ferret(s); Gerbils; Guinea pigs; Hedgehogs; Mice; Rabbit(s); Rat(s)
 abdomen pain in, 682
 alopecia in, 669
 anesthesia in
  hypothermia prevention during, 566-567
  monitoring of, 547-549
 anorexia in, 670
 blood collection in, 549-550
 blood transfusion in, 551-552
 bone marrow aspiration and core biopsy in, 552-553
 bronchoscopy in, 553-555
 bumps in, 678
 castration in, 555-557
 central nervous system signs in, 671
 dangerous antibiotics in, 582
 diarrhea in, 672
 dyspnea in, 674
 echocardiography in, 557, 558t
 E-collars in, 558
 electrocardiography in, 558-559, 559t
 eosinophil count in, 616-617
 fur changes in, 684
 hyperkalemia in, 640
 hypokalemia in, 641
 intraosseous catheters in, 561-562
 intubation technique in, 562-563
 lameness in, 677
 lumps in, 678
 lymphopenia in, 626
 mammary mass in, 680
 monocytosis in, 628
 neutropenia in, 631-632
 neutrophilia in, 630-631
 ocular changes in, 681
 ovariohysterectomy in, 564-566
 painful abdomen, 682
 paresis in, 683
 reticulocyte count in, 643
 skin changes in, 684
 urinary changes in, 687
 vaginal discharge in, 685
 weight loss in, 686
Snails
 dehydration in, 5-6
 diagnostic sampling in, 504-505
 estivation in, 5-6
 intoxication in, 11
Snakes
 bites by, 696
 blood collection in, 533-534
Snakes *(Continued)*
 blood pressure in, 523
 blood urea nitrogen in, 609t
 central nervous system signs in, 659
 Chrysosporium anamorph of *Nannizziopsis viesii* in, 80-82
 Cryptosporidium in, 90
 dysecdysis in, 78, 95-97
 dystocia in, 526-528
 gallbladder in, 116
 handling of, 530-531
 hemipenal trauma in, 129
 inclusion body disease of, 113-114, 113f
 injections in, 532
 mites in, 98-99
 Mycoplasma spp. in, 143
 necrotizing mycotic dermatitis in, 91
 paraphimosis in, 128
 phlebotomy in, 533-534
 pneumonia in, 141-143
 proliferative spinal osteopathy in, 135-136
 reovirus infections in, 140-141
 respiratory tract disease in, 141-143
 restraint of, 530-531
 rostral abrasions in, 78
 stargazing by, 113f
 stomatitis in, 134f, 145-147
 vomiting in, 136-138
Snapping turtles, 78
Snowy owls, 155
Snuffles, 405-407, 423-424, 717-719
Sodium, 647-648
Soft tissue edema, in birds, 179-180
Soft tissue swelling, in birds, 179-180
Softshell turtles, bacterial dermatitis in, 78
Songbird fever, 726-729
Sore hocks, in rabbits, 407-409
Sour crop, in birds, 170-171
Spay, 564-566
Spider(s). *See also* Tarantulas
 ectoparasites in, 505-506
 fungal infections in, 8-9
 restraint of, 509-510, 509f
Spider tortoises, entamoebiasis in, 100
Spinal accessory nerve deficit, 581
Spinal osteoarthropathy, in reptiles, 135-136
Spinal osteopathy, in reptiles, 135-136
Spinal reflexes, in birds, 159
Spiracles, 11
Spirillum minus, 724-726
Spirochetosis, 182
Spirochid trematodes, in reptiles, 83
Spironucleus, 28-29
Splayleg, 416-417
Splenectomy, in ferrets, 498f
Splenomegaly
 in birds, 163f
 in ferrets, 497-498
Spongiform leukoencephalopathy, 327-328
Spring viremia of carp, 35
Squamous cell carcinoma
 in birds, 235
 in rabbits, 351
Squamous metaplasia, 57-59, 111
Squirrels, 720
Staphylococcosis, in rabbits, 417-419
Staphylococcus aureus, 273, 407, 417-419
Stargazing, 113f
Status epilepticus, in birds, 160
"Step-mouth", 356
Stick insect, 7f
Stomach worms, 375, 379
Stomatitis
 in lizards, 145-147
 in reptiles, 132-134, 145-147
 in snakes, 145-147
Strept zooepidemicus, 280-282
Streptobacillus moniliformis, 724-726
Streptococcal bacteria, 17
Streptococcal lymphadenitis, 280
Streptococcus iniae, 17, 19
Streptococcus pneumoniae, 248-249, 276-278
Streptococcus zooepidemicus, 280-282
Streptomycin, bacterial enteritis in birds treated with, 182
Strigiformes, viral diseases in, 240
Strongyloides infection, in amphibians, 60-62
Stuck-in cast, 7-8
Subluxation of hip, in rabbits, 416-417
Submandibular abscess, in birds, 148, 148f
Subspectacular abscesses, in reptiles, 72-73, 144, 521
Subtriquetra spp., 130
Sucralfate, 174, 188, 227
Sudden death, in amphibians, 654
Sugar gliders
 behavioral disorders in, 328-329
 nutritional disorders in, 329-330
Sulfadiazine
 in ferrets, 449
 in rabbits, 376, 449
Sulfadimethoxine
 coccidiosis treated with, 88
 in rabbits, 384
Sulfamethoxine, coccidiosis treated with, 182
Sulfonamides, in rabbits, 347
Suppurative nephritis
 in hamsters, 295-297
 in rabbits, 412-415
 in rats, 245-247
Suppurative pododermatitis, in rabbits, 407-409
Suppurative pyelonephritis
 in hamsters, 295-297
 in rats, 245-247
Surgery, in fish, 516-517
SVCV, 35
Swamp fever, 711
Swans, 155
Swellings, in reptiles, 665
Swim bladder disease, 36-37, 37f
Swimming pool granuloma, 715-716
Swineherd disease, 711
Sylvatic plague, 719-721
Syncope, 594t
Synovial cell carcinoma, in birds, 235
Syrian hamsters
 cardiac disease in, 287-288
 cheek pouch disorder in, 288-290
 echocardiographic parameters in, 287
 skin diseases in, 297-299
Systemic coronavirus-associated disease, 452-454

T

T_3, 648-649
T_4, 648-649
T cells, 625-627
Taenia pisiformis, 374
Tail chordoma, in ferrets, 438f
Tail vein, for blood collection in small mammals, 550
Tamoxifen
 follicular stasis treated with, 186
 in rats, 244
Tank pond therapy, 517-518
Tapeworms
 in fish, 27-28
 in rabbits, 362, 374-376
Tarantulas
 alopecia in, 3-4
 dehydration in, 5-6, 6f
 fluid administration in, 508

Tarantulas *(Continued)*
intoxication in, 11
limb amputation in, 15
panagrolaimidae oral nematodes in, 13-14
restraint of, 509-510, 509f
trauma in, 15
worms in, 13-14
Teflon toxicity, 221
Tenpuku disease, 36-37, 37f
Teratoma, in rabbits, 419
Terbinafine
aspergillosis in birds treated with, 156
dermatomycosis in reptiles treated with, 91-92
in guinea pigs, 269, 280
in hedgehogs, 326
Terramycin, 18-19
Testicular cancer, in rabbits, 419
Testicular tumors
in birds, 235
in rabbits, 419
Tetracyclines, in birds, 196
Tetrahymena, 33-34
Texas tortoises, necrotizing acute disease in, 91
Thermal burns, 536
Thiabendazoles, 446
Thiacetarsamide sodium, 443
Thiazide diuretics, in rabbits, 394
Third eyelid protrusion, 344-345
Third-degree AV block, in ferrets, 456-458
Thoracentesis, in ferrets, 443
Thoracic limb fractures, 126
Thoracic vertebral chordoma, 437-438
Thrombocytopenia, 639
Thrombocytosis, 638
Thymoma
in birds, 235
in rabbits, 420-421
Thyroid hormones, 648-649
Thyroidectomy, in guinea pigs, 261
Thyrotoxicosis, in guinea pigs, 260-261
Thyroxine, 260, 648-649
Ticarcillin/clavulanic acid
in birds, 169, 231
constipation treated with, 169
Ticks
in birds, 177-178
in reptiles, 98-99
Tilapia, 24
Tissue adhesives, 15
Tissue prolapse, in reptiles, 85-87
TMS, 513-514
Tobramycin, in guinea pigs, 269
Toddia spp., 114-115
Toltrazuril
coccidiosis treated with, 88
in guinea pigs, 265
in rabbits, 347
Tongue worms, 130-131
Tooth fracture, in ferrets, 441-442
Tooth overgrowth
in chinchillas, 302-305
in degus, 319-322
Tooth root abscess, in rabbits, 355-360
Torticollis
in birds, 159-161
in rabbits, 371f, 428-430
Tortoise herpesvirus 1, 105-106
Tortoise herpesvirus 2, 105-106
Tortoises. *See also* Chelonians; Turtles
blood urea nitrogen in, 609t
entamoebiasis in, 100
handling of, 531
mites in, 99
necrotizing acute disease in, 91
reovirus infections in, 140-141
Tortoises *(Continued)*
restraint of, 531
upper respiratory tract disease in, 118-120
Total ammonia nitrogen, 47
Total protein, 642-643
Toucans
ascites in, 153
coccidiosis in, 181
Toxic nephropathy, 492
Toxic neuropathies, in birds, 159
Toxicity, in invertebrates, 11-12
Toxoplasma spp., 375, 448-450
Toxoplasmosis
in ferrets, 448-450
in rabbits, 376, 429
TP, 642-643
TPP, 642-643
Tracheal aspiration, in birds, 545, 546f
Tracheal irrigation, in birds, 545, 546f
Tracheal wash
in birds, 545, 546f
in reptiles, 535
Tracheobronchial tree, 555f
Tracheostomy, 317
Transmissible ileal hyperplasia, 291-293
Transtracheal lavage, in birds, 218
Transtracheal sample collection, in reptiles, 525-526
Trauma
in amphibians, 67-68
ascites caused by, 153
in birds, 232-234
in fish, 38-40
in invertebrates, 15-16
in tarantulas, 15
Traumatic neuropathies, in birds, 159
Tree boas, 143
Trematodes
in birds, 201
in reptiles, 83
Tremors, 159-161, 590
Treponema paraluiscuniculi, 421-422
Treponematosis, in rabbits, 362, 421-422
Treponemiasis, 421-422
Tricaine methanesulfonate, 51, 513-514
Tricaine-S, 513-514
Trichlorfon
ectoparasites in fish treated with, 21
monogeneans treated with, 23
Trichobezoars
in ferrets, 454, 456f
in rabbits, 378-381
Trichoblastoma, in rabbits, 351-352
Trichodina, 33-34
Trichoepithelioma, in rabbits, 351
Trichofolliculoma, 279
Trichomonas, 201
Trichomoniasis, in amphibians, 55-56
Trichophyton spp., 82
Trichostrongylid nematode worm, in rabbits, 374-376
Trigeminal nerve deficit, 581
Trimebutine, in guinea pigs, 254
Trimethoprim/sulfamethoxazole
antibiotic-associated enterocolitis treated with, 293
bacterial enteritis treated with, 182
in birds, 182, 231
in chinchillas, 304, 310, 315
coccidiosis treated with, 52-53, 88
in degus, 321
in guinea pigs, 254, 265, 279, 284
in hamsters, 290
in hedgehogs, 326
in rabbits, 347, 373, 384
in rats, 246
in sugar gliders, 328
Trixacarus caviae, 278-280, 691, 693
Trochlear nerve deficit, 581
Trombiculid mites, 98
Tropical rat mite, 251
Tube feeding, in fish, 514-515
Tularemia, 730-732
Tumors
in birds, 234-236
in hedgehogs, 324-325
in rats, 243-245, 245f
uropygial gland, 238f
Turkeys
cryptosporidiosis in, 181
enteritis in, 182
histomoniasis in, 181
Turtles. *See also* Chelonians; Tortoises
bacterial dermatitis in, 78
blood pH in, 635
blood urea nitrogen in, 609t
entamoebiasis in, 100
handling of, 531
hypervitaminosis A in, 110f
mites in, 99
restraint of, 531
Salmonella spp. in, 144
vitamin A therapy in, 111-112
Tylenol, 464
Tylosin
Chlamydophila psittaci treated with, 167
chronic respiratory disease in rats treated with, 250
Tympany
in chinchillas, 308-311
in guinea pigs, 264-265
Type I hypersensitivity reaction, in ferrets, 500-501
Typhlitis
in chinchillas, 308-311
in rabbits, 385-390
Typhoidal tularemia, 731
Tyzzer's disease, 291-293, 384, 387

U

Ulcer disease, in koi, 40-41
Ulcerative colitis, 465-467
Ulcerative dermatitis
in guinea pigs, 279
in koi, 40-41
in rats, 251-252
Ulcerative enteritis, in quail, 182
Ulcerative keratitis, in chinchillas, 311-313
Ulcerative mycosis, 24
Ulcerative pododermatitis, in rabbits, 407-409
Ulcerative skin disease, in koi, 40-41
Ulceroglandular tularemia, 731
Ultrasound
ascites in birds, 154
in birds, 154, 169, 202
Umbilical-placental entanglement, in ferrets, 479-481
Underweight, in guinea pigs, 253-254
Undigested food in droppings, 595
Upper respiratory disease
in ferrets, 469f
in rabbits, 423-424
in tortoises, 118-120
Upper respiratory tract disorders, in rabbits, 423-424
Urate coloration, 595
Urate oxidase, 229
Urea nitrogen, 608-609, 609t
Uremia
in ferrets, 491-494
in rabbits, 412-415
in rats, 247
Ureteral stone obstruction, in rabbits, 413

Urethral catheterization, of ferrets, 570
Urethral compression, in ferrets, 488-490
Urethral obstruction
  in ferrets, 488-490, 499
  in guinea pigs, 283
Urethritis, in rabbits, 392
Uric acid, 102, 595, 649-650
Urinalysis, in reptiles, 525-526
Urinary bladder prolapse, in reptiles, 86
Urinary calculi
  in ferrets, 498-500
  in guinea pigs, 282-283
Urinary incontinence
  differential diagnosis of, 588
  in rabbits, 392
Urinary sludge syndrome, in rabbits, 392-394
Urinary tract disorders, lower, in rabbits, 392-394
Urolithiasis, 393
  in ferrets, 498-500
  in guinea pigs, 282-283, 283f
  in rabbits, 392-394
Uronema, 33-34
Uropygial gland
  anatomy of, 237-238, 238f
  diseases of
    abscesses, 148
    in birds, 148, 237-239
  tumor of, 238f
Uropygial gland tumors, 235
Ursodeoxycholic acid, 196, 203
Uterine adenocarcinoma, in rabbits, 425
Uterine disorders
  in guinea pigs, 284-285, 285f
  in rabbits, 424-426
Uterine prolapse
  in birds, 165-166
  in guinea pigs, 284, 285f
Uterine torsion, in guinea pigs, 284
Uveitis
  in birds, 211
  in guinea pigs, 268-269
  in rabbits, 426-428

V

Vaccine reactions, in ferrets, 500-501
Vaginal discharge, in small mammals, 685
Vaginal disorders, in guinea pigs, 284-285
Vaginal prolapse, in guinea pigs, 284
Vaginitis, in guinea pigs, 284
Vagus nerve deficit, 581
Valvular heart disease, in ferrets, 458
Vasodilators, in rabbits, 342
Veiled chameleons, pseudogout in, 103
Venereal spirochetosis, 421-422
Venipuncture. *See also* Blood collection
  in birds, 546-547, 547f
  in fish, 518-519, 519f
Venous transfusion, 551-552
Vent disease, 421-422
Ventricular adenocarcinoma, in birds, 235
Vesicular exanthem of swine, 79-80
Vestibular disease, in rabbits, 428-430
Vestibulocochlear nerve deficit, 581
Vibramycin, *Chlamydophila psittaci* treated with, 167
Vibravenös, 163
Vibrio spp., 17
Vibriosis, 17
Viral diseases
  in birds, 239-242
  in fish, 42-43
  in invertebrates, 16-17
Viral epidermal hyperplasia, 43-44
Viral hemorrhagic disease, 381-384
Visceral gout
  in birds, 191-192, 201
  in reptiles, 101-103
Visceral larval migrans, 429
Vitamin A
  deficiency of, 111, 199-201
  dietary sources of, for reptiles, 110-111
  hyperuricemia in birds treated with, 192
  intoxication, in reptiles, 108-109
  therapeutic applications of, 111-112
  water-soluble forms of, 111
Vitamin B_1, in birds, 160
Vitamin C, in guinea pigs, 254, 262-263, 265, 280
Vitamin D_3, 62-64, 124
  in birds, 176
Vitamin D deficiency, in birds, 199-201
Vitamin E
  in birds, 160, 199-201
  deficiency of, 199-201
Vomiting
  in amphibians, 68-69
  in birds, 196, 225-227
  differential diagnosis of, 592
  in reptiles, 136-138, 667
Voriconazole, 91-92

W

Waddycephalus spp., 130
Warble fly infestation, in rabbits, 362-363
Wasting syndrome, in amphibians, 70-71
Water chemistry, 44-46
Water deprivation test, in birds, 228-229
Water dragons
  dysecdysis in, 95
  rostral abrasions in, 78
  wound management in, 77f
Water quality, for fish, 44-46
Waterfowl, cryptosporidiosis in, 181
Watermold infection, 64-65
"Wave-mouth", 356
Weakness, 595
Weight loss
  in amphibians, 70-71, 655
  differential diagnosis of, 596
  in guinea pigs, 253-254
  in reptiles, 668
  in small mammals, 686
Weil's disease, 711
Wet eye, in chinchillas, 311-313
Wet tail, 291-293
White band disease, 9-10
White muscle disease, in birds, 199-201
White pox, 9-10
White's tree frogs, 53
"White-spot disease", 33-34
Wing tip swelling, 179-180
"Winter kill", 24
Wobbly hedgehog syndrome, 327-328
Wood turtles, 100
Worms. *See also* Roundworms; Tapeworms
  anchor, 21-22
  hookworms, 60-62
  lungworms, 60-62
  pinworms, 374-376
  stomach, 375, 379
  in tarantulas, 13-14
  tongue, 130-131
Wound(s)
  in amphibians, 67-68
  in birds, 232-234
  in fish, 38-40
  in invertebrates, 15-16
  in reptiles, 535-536
Wound dressings, for guinea pigs, 274
Wrongful shed, in reptiles, 522-523
Wryneck, 428-430

X

Xanthoma
  in amphibians, 53-54
  in birds, 235
Xanthomatosis, in amphibians, 53-54

Y

Yellow fungus disease, 80-82, 90-92
Yellow-pigmented bacteria, 17-20
Yersinia pestis, 719-721
Yersinia pseudotuberculosis, 182

Z

Zinc
  laboratory tests for, 650-651
  toxicity, in birds, 192-194, 650
Zoonoses
  animal bites, 694-697
  chlamydiosis, 697-699
  cryptosporidiosis, 699-703
  dermatophytosis, 703-705
  encephalitozoonosis, 705-708
  hantavirus, 708-710
  leptospirosis, 711-712
  lymphocytic choriomeningitis virus, 713-714
  Mycobacterium marinum granuloma, 715-716
  Pasteurella multocida, 717-719
  plague, 719-721
  rabies, 722-724
  rat bite fever, 724-726
  salmonellosis, 726-729
  tularemia, 730-732
Zoospores, 92